The Transformation of Pediatrics

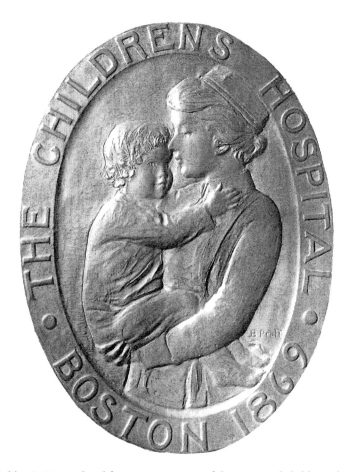

The Children's Hospital seal featuring an image of the nurse and child was designed in March 1916 by Bostonian and noted American sculptor Bela Lyon Pratt (1867–1917). It was the vision of Dr. Harold C. Ernst, a hospital bacteriologist, and friend of Bela Pratt. It was first used for Children's Hospital School of Nursing diplomas in 1916. It hung in the main hall of Children's Hospital on Huntington Avenue in the early 20th century and currently resides in the lobby of the Wolbach Building.

The
Transformation
of
Pediatrics

*How a Pediatric Department and Its Residency
Influenced American Pediatrics*

*A 125-Year History
(1882–2007)*

Frederick H. Lovejoy, Jr., MD

Science History Publications/USA
division
Watson Publishing International LLC
Sagamore Beach
2015

First published in the United States of America
by Science History Publications/USA
a division of Watson Publishing international LLC
Post Office Box 1240, Sagamore Beach, MA 02562-1240, USA
www.shpusa.com

Library of Congress Cataloging-in-Publication Data
Lovejoy, Frederick H., Jr., author.
    The transformation of pediatrics: how a pediatric department and its residency influenced
American pediatrics: a 125-year history (1882–2007) / Frederick H. Lovejoy, Jr.
       p.;   cm.
    Includes bibliographical references and index.
    ISBN 978-0-88135-499-7—ISBN 0-88135-499-6
    I. Title. [DNLM: 1.   Boston Children's Hospital.   2.   Hospitals, Pediatric—
history—Boston.   3.   Internship and Residency—history—Boston.   4.   History, 19th
Century—Boston.   5.   History, 20th Century—Boston.   6.   History, 21st Century—
Boston.   7.   Pediatrics—education—Boston.   8.   Pediatrics—history—Boston.   WS 28
AM4]
    RJ102.5.B66
    362.198920009744'61--dc23
                                                                                          2015035717

Designed and typeset by Publishers' Design and Production Services, Inc.

Second printing, April, 2021
Manufactured in the USA.

To Jill, my loving wife, our children, Phoebe, Ted, and Charlie and their spouses, and our grandchildren, all always supportive on this glorious journey.

Foreword

DAVID G. NATHAN, MD

FREDERICK LOVEJOY has been the right arm of no less than five chairs of the Department of Medicine at the Boston Children's Hospital where he had been a resident and then a staff member since the late 1960s. During his long tenure on the quarter deck of that remarkable department and the Department of Pediatrics at Harvard Medical School, he has kept his eyes wide open and his pen at the ready. Like the late Clement Smith, an inveterate notetaker and diary keeper and a man with an elephantine memory, Lovejoy offers, in this labor of love, his account of the history of the Department of Medicine at Children's and the training of its housestaff over 125 years as well as the major national and world events that shaped the department's development.

Why such a book at this time about Boston Children's Hospital; why that particular hospital and that department? Children's hospitals have a short appearance on stage in the relatively brief history of American medicine. Boston Children's, arguably the most prestigious of them, did not exist until 1869, when a group of dissident child-oriented physicians bolted from the Massachusetts General Hospital because they believed that children were being ignored in that setting. A decade or two later they were joined by the Sisters of St. Margaret, a group of Episcopal nuns determined to help them to establish a hospital for "the sick and maimed poor children of Boston." Their aim was to focus their attention on those children, and the early leaders did so by emphasizing nutrition, clinical descriptions in the Oslerian tradition, and careful explorations of surgical corrections (there being little that medicine had to offer other than love).

Science as we know it today did not become emphasized at Boston Children's until the post–World War II era of James Gamble, Sidney Farber, and John Enders. It was in this period that Charles A. Janeway began his 28-year leadership of the department and developed subspecialty pediatrics and first-class clinical research. Lovejoy joined Janeway as his clinical right arm along with William Berenberg, a fine general pediatrician. Lovejoy eventually became the Berenberg Distinguished Professor of Pediatrics at Harvard and remains today completely devoted to the excellence of Janeway's beloved department. The four chairs who followed Janeway built on his precepts, and Lovejoy carefully documents that subsequent history as a faithful description of the modern history of pediatrics.

So this book offers much more than a review of the 10 chairs of pediatrics, their departments, and the evolution of housestaff training that have occurred over the past 125 years. It is actually an account of the growth and development of national academic pediatrics in the United States. Today, there are several fine children's hospitals, many of them fortified by Boston Children's graduates, and there are excellent pediatric research programs from coast to coast. They are all modeled on the approaches that Charles A. Janeway adopted in those post–war years, and they are enormously successful. Though Lovejoy has confined his account to the events that transpired at Boston Children's, they have been replicated in one way or another in a number of great children's hospitals throughout the country. Those who care about the health of children in the future would do well to study this book. We are now facing conditions that threaten the very foundations of academic medicine. Lovejoy reminds us of what can be accomplished for children if we have the will.

David Nathan, MD, was physician-in-chief of the Children's Hospital from 1985 to 1995 and president of the Dana-Farber Cancer Institute from 1995 to 2000.

Foreword

JOSEPH B. MARTIN, MD, PHD

O N SEPTEMBER 23, 1906, a large gathering on the front steps of a new
campus led by the distinguished Harvard University President Charles
W. Eliot heralded the beginning of a new century for Harvard Medical School.

Five majestic Beaux-Arts buildings constituted with Vermont marble transformed a cow pasture, the Ebenezer Francis estate, into a new vision. This was
the new Harvard Medical School on Longwood Avenue, relocated from a site
on Boylston Avenue in downtown Boston.

The Harvard Medical School complex grew over the next 10 years with the
addition of the Peter Bent Brigham Hospital in 1913 and in 1914, the Children's
Hospital. Today, the Longwood Medical Area is one of the largest concentrations
of clinical care, education, and biomedical research in the world.

In this wonderful volume, my friend Fred Lovejoy begins even earlier, with
the formation of the Children's Hospital in South Boston in 1869, shortly after
the Civil War. It traces the story of the evolution over the decades that led to the
international reputation of the Children's Hospital as one of the preeminent leaders in education, research, and clinical care for children, both locally and abroad.

Lovejoy traces the remarkable story of the largest department of the
Children's Hospital—the Department of Medicine—through generations of
leadership.

The complexity of the relationships within the Harvard Medical community
with its independent hospitals and the relationships of this whole complex to a
major university are important issues to consider in this 21st century. Dr. Lovejoy
repeatedly demonstrates the critical relationships that exist between a medical

school and a teaching hospital and outlines not only the positives but also some of the challenges that are faced.

As dean of the Faculty of Medicine from 1997 to 2007, I had the opportunity to work closely with Fred Lovejoy and other leaders of the Boston Children's Hospital. I am honored to be included among those who are grateful to Fred for his outstanding leadership in the Harvard community. During my deanship, Fred was always available, always present when issues arose to build and create the connections of our two communities. I will be forever grateful to him for his leadership and for the effort put forward in this volume telling the details of this wonderful example of academic and medical history.

Joseph B. Martin, MD, PhD, was dean of the Faculty of Medicine at Harvard Medical School from 1997 to 2007.

Introduction

The *Transformation of Pediatrics* is my effort to record and describe how a pediatric department and its residency influenced American pediatrics over a 125 year period of time. The book focuses on residents and the impact of national influences as well as the Children's Hospital, the medical department and its faculty on the training of young physicians. Why a book predominantly focused on house officer training? To serve the sick as a physician is a great privilege. Accomplishing this important task requires both excellent training and the development of superior personal attributes. Little has been written exploring in depth these pivotal years in a physician's life. This book examines and records the training program at the Children's Hospital over a 125-year period, beginning with the first house officer in 1882 and ending in 2007, when I relinquished my role as program director of the residency. In some places, however, I have mentioned events that occurred after 2007 but before the book was submitted for publication.

One of the great joys in my life was having the opportunity to come to the Children's Hospital as a resident in my mid-20s. Little did I know I would still be here nearly 50 years later and that I would spend 27 years directing the hospital's residency program. Over the decades, I have served and observed a rich tapestry of people and remarkable work accomplished in the vineyard of service to sick children.

During my four years as chief resident, I was fortunate to have a very close personal mentor in Dr. Charles Janeway, physician-in-chief at the Children's Hospital from 1946 to 1974, who shared with me the history of those who went before. And as associate physician-in-chief, I was also privileged to work closely with the four subsequent physicians-in-chief, enabling me to witness the history of the Department of Medicine as it was being made. This department, the hospital, and national influences have had—and continue to have—a significant impact on the training program at the Children's Hospital.

In writing this book, I made the decision early on to explore the history of our training program as objectively and accurately as possible for a medical audience. Thus, the book is targeted toward faculty, residents, and fellows who are currently training, or who have trained or worked, at the Children's Hospital over the past 40 to 50 years; academic physicians throughout the U.S. concerned with the training of physicians and the development of departments and programs in support of that mission; medical educators associated with medical schools and their affiliated hospitals; and medical libraries, academic hospitals, and organizations that support physician training.

Specifically, the book focuses on the training of pediatric medical residents rather than training in other disciplines, such as surgery, psychiatry, anesthesiology, etc. Children's Hospital department chairs and their faculty as well as the institution itself, its buildings, and its many programs are discussed, as they impact and influence the training of medical residents. The history is organized by eras of departmental leadership, which provides both a convenient and familiar way to present information. However, the history of the very distinguished surgical departments is unfortunately omitted due to space constraints. The last chapter is written with the purpose of discussing some of the lessons learned from my nearly three decades as residency program director.

This book may be read from cover to cover, delved into through specific times and chapters that relate to one's time at Children's Hospital, or studied in an effort to acquire perspective on the education and training of young physicians over the decades. It is also hoped that it will be of use to future historians who wish to study a remarkable training program.

Through my association with Dr. Janeway and other mentors, as well as my own personal experience, I have been able to accumulate a rich history of the Children's Hospital and its training of pediatricians. This book, *The Transformation of Pediatrics*, is a humble effort to faithfully record this period of history and the preceding decades back to 1882.

Acknowledgements

FOR THIS BOOK, I have depended predominately on primary references written by major players in the history of the Department of Medicine and the hospital. Annual reports as well as *Physician-in-Chief* newsletters, which were written in close proximity to the various years under consideration, provided an accurate record of events. The majority of the annual reports are the work of the 10 physicians-in-chief and have served as an important substrate of departmental activities, upon which the training program was superimposed. The hospital's *Year in Review* and Harvard Medical School's *Dean's Review*, while compiled by institutional writers, are similarly timely and thus offer an accurate recording of events and institutional change. Other primary reference sources included original articles published in professional journals as well as books.

I have also depended upon a large number of departmental committee reports and summaries, including especially the minutes of the Residency Program Training Committee, Residency Strategic Planning Committee reports, and the Harvard Medical School Pediatric Executive Committee minutes for academic promotions. I have also drawn from a number of materials personally saved from the date of my arrival as a resident at the hospital, including senior resident dinner speeches, graduation exercise brochures, and house officer show playbills, all of which have offered a rich tapestry of the culture of the residency. I am very grateful to Alison Clapp, hospital librarian, and Sheila Spalding and Alina Morris, hospital archivists, for access to invaluable hospital letters, reports, and materials, as well as a treasure trove of pictures of housestaff and faculty over a 125-year period. Finally, I am deeply grateful to Susan Brooks, not only for sharing her photographs of the housestaff but also for her extensive knowledge compiled over many years with the training program and its house officers.

The book undoubtedly benefited from information gathered during interviews carried out with a number of house officers, and I am indebted to them. They have offered important perspectives of how house officer life was both the same and very different in each of the eras in which they trained. Their honest appraisals and perspectives have been faithfully recorded and add much to the description of the evolving life of the housestaff. Much of the unpublished background information came from both short and long conversations with the faculty. Most important were frequent conversations with Charles Janeway, Mary Ellen Avery, David Nathan, Philip Pizzo, and Gary Fleisher, facilitated by the positions I held under each. Additionally, I am grateful to William Berenberg, Robert Haggerty, Joel Alpert, and Bob Masland, who as senior mentors and close friends, shared with me important vignettes of hospital lore. I also thank my younger colleagues, including Jonathan Finkelstein, Robert Vinci, Ted Sectish, and Vincent Chiang, who directed the residency during the modern era and offered invaluable insights for my benefit.

I wish to thank David Nathan, Joseph Martin, Georges Peter, and Mary Beth Gordon, who read the whole text from cover to cover, making invaluable suggestions. David Nathan and Joseph Martin offered their thoughts from the perspective of local senior physicians highly knowledgeable about academic medicine, residency training, and the institutions involved. Georges Peter, as a senior academic pediatrician at Brown Medical School and longtime friend, offered his detailed and careful critique to the great benefit of the manuscript. Mary Beth Gordon, who served as a resident and chief resident at the Children's Hospital, offered her invaluable perspective as a recent house officer. I also thank Mark Rockoff, Bob Vinci, and Jean Emans, senior leaders at the Children's Hospital and Boston Medical Center, who read selected chapters with a critical eye.

The book went through innumerable drafts to achieve the final product. This would never have occurred without the dedication, expertise, and persistence of Barbara Roach, Cindy Chow, Lauren Codd, and Rose-Marie Bussey in the Department of Medicine. I am deeply grateful to all four. I also wish to thank Alan Lightman, Russell Robb, Thomas Piper, John Graef, Richard Bachur, Mary Beth Son, Anne Stack, Jeffery Burns, Elizabeth Woods and Scott Podolsky, whose editorial suggestions did so much to improve the manuscript. Finally, I am especially grateful to my current chief, Gary Fleisher, and the hospital's presidents, James Mandell and Sandra Fenwick, whose constant support throughout this project allowed it to come to fruition.

I am very grateful to David Nathan and Joseph Martin for writing forewords to this book. Both have carried out with great dedication and distinction major leadership roles at the Children's Hospital and Harvard Medical School, as described in chapters 6 and 7. Further, for me, they have been extremely close colleagues and friends over many years. We all share a deep appreciation and affection for the institutions we have served and thus, their contribution to this book is particularly meaningful.

Finally, I wish to express my most profound appreciation to my publisher, Neale Watson, and his colleague, Mark Bergeron, for the tremendous expertise, wisdom and guidance that they have brought to this effort. This book has been the grafeful beneficiary of their years of experience and for this I am deeply grateful.

I am also grateful to Pat Cleary, whose editorial experience and capability as well as her remarkable attention to content and factual detail greatly enriched the final version of the text. We worked closely and happily together over a year to record a history that is accurate and a manuscript that is hopefully enjoyable for the reader, informative for the historian, and a pleasurable journey for faculty and housestaff alike who have labored in the vineyards of healing at the Children's Hospital.

Contents

Commonly Used Abbreviations

AAMC	Association of American Medical Colleges
AAP	American Academy of Pediatrics
ABP	American Board of Pediatrics
ACGME	Accreditation Council for Graduate Medical Education
AMSPDC	Association of Medical School Pediatric Department Chairmen
APPD	Association of Pediatric Program Directors
APS	American Pediatric Society
ARP	Accelerated Research Pathway of the American Board of Pediatrics
BCRP	Boston Combined Residency Program
BMC	Boston Medical Center
BWH	Brigham and Women's Hospital
CAAP	Committee on Academic Appointments and Promotions (at the Children's Hospital)
CCHP	Comprehensive Child Health Program (at the Children's Hospital)
CDC	Center for Diseases Control
CHB/BCH	Children's Hospital Boston/Boston Children's Hospital
CHMC	Children's Hospital Medical Center
CIR	Committee on Interns and Residents in New York City
CPC	Clinical Pathological Conference

GME	Graduate Medical Education
IRP	Integrated Research Pathway of the American Board of Pediatrics
JAMA	Journal of the American Medical Association
JAR	Junior Assistant Resident
JPN	Joint Program in Neonatology (at the Children's Hospital)
MECL	Medical Emergency Clinic (at the Children's Hospital)
MGH	Massachusetts General Pediatrics
MOPD	Medical Outpatient Pediatric Department (at the Children's Hospital)
NCI	National Cancer Institute
NEJM	New England Journal of Medicine
NICHD	National Institute of Child Health and Human Development
NICU	Neonatal Intensive Care Unit
NIH	National Institutes of Health
PEC	Pediatric Executive Committee (at Harvard Medical School)
PGA	Pediatric Group Associates (at the Children's Hospital)
PGY-I, II, III	Post Graduate Year I, II, III
PICU	Pediatric Intensive Care Unit
PL-I, II, III	Pediatric Level I, II, III
RDS	Respiratory Distress Syndrome
RPTC	Residency Program Training Committee
RRC	Residency Review Committee (of ACGME)
SAP	Special Alternative Pathway of the American Board of Pediatrics
SPR	Society for Pediatric Research
Sub-I	Sub-Internship at Harvard Medical School
USMLE	United States Medical Licensing Examination

CHAPTER I

The Medical House Officer

A Resident's Life in 1905, 1966, and 2005

INTERNSHIP AND RESIDENCY is a pivotal time in the training of physicians. It follows four years of formal education in medical school and precedes either the practice of medicine or further training as a fellow in a subspecialty area. Residency is perhaps the most intense and most formative phase in a young physician's life. This training is unique among the professions, a similar period of practical training in one's chosen calling not existing in business, law, or education. And it is unique in its wedding of education with service. Years later, physicians recall their residency with remarkable clarity and nostalgia. Stories and events are remembered as if they occurred yesterday. Personal friendships endure over a lifetime. The core elements of a physician—knowledge, skills, and attitudes—are firmly cemented during this critical period. It is, in fact, during this time that the mind and soul of a physician are formed.

The residency of today is very different from the residency of a century ago. It has changed slowly, but when viewed over 125 years, its evolution is dramatic. To capture a sense of this remarkable change, the life of a house officer in 1905, 1966, and 2005 is offered in three letters composed by the author and written to their families, reflecting the thoughts and life of three fictional house officers at the Children's Hospital during each of these times. (See Figures 1 through 3 for images that represent each of these eras.) The subsequent seven chapters will examine in greater detail the rationale and nature of this change.

Medical House Officer Reflections[1]

June 14, 1905

Dear Mother and Father,

I thought I would tell you about my life as an interne now that I have been here for three months. The hospital is located on Huntington Avenue, next to Symphony Hall and across the street from the park where the Boston Red Stockings play. It is a three-story building that opens out to an avenue (so-called Avenue of the Arts) and the trolleys that pass by. The patients are located on 20-bed wards with high ceilings, large ceiling-to-floor windows, sun balconies, and an open fireplace. Current practice emphasizes the benefits of fresh air and sunlight for the treatment of rickets and tuberculosis. We have been at this location since 1882. Plans are underway to move to the Francis Farm at the border of Brookline.

Our patients are mainly from Boston. Generally poor and often of Irish descent, they are all two years or older. Those less than two years are admitted to the West End Nursery on Blossom Street near the Massachusetts General Hospital. We remain very concerned about infectious diseases and outbreaks of infections in the hospital, so parents are able to visit only a few hours each week. We screen and do not admit to the hospital patients with measles, diphtheria, scarlet fever, whooping cough, and chickenpox. Of 1,500 admitted inpatients last year, there were more orthopedic patients being treated for tuberculosis of the bones and rickets than medical patients. The outpatient clinics saw 5,500 medical and surgical patients last year. The older physicians tell me our diagnoses are more precise than in the past, with the most common diagnoses on the medical wards being pneumonia, rheumatic fever, typhoid fever, and tuberculosis. In the outpatient department, we see a lot of bronchitis, diarrhea, eczema, and cases of improper feeding. The length of stay of our hospitalized patients is about two and one-half weeks. This is much shorter than before because of new treatments and because we can now transfer patients with chronic illnesses to a convalescent home in Wellesley. We try hard to obtain autopsy permission from parents of children who die. We feel we can benefit from the findings at autopsy because it assists us in diagnosing disease more accurately in the future.

The housestaff and nurses are the permanent staff on the floors. As part of the housestaff, I am called a junior house physician. There is a lot resting on my shoulders since the attendings, as we call the attending physicians who form the more senior hospital staff, are here only sporadically. We are small in number and

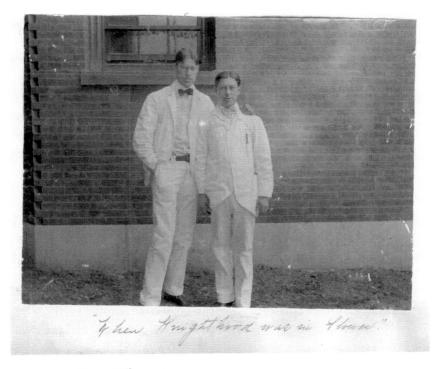

"When Knighthood was in flower."

FIGURE 1   House Officers, circa 1902

House officers at the turn of the century were male, formally dressed with high-collared shirt and tie, white pants, short white jackets, and dark shoes. The hair was often parted down the middle. (From the scrapbook of Edith Pollard Ralston, a Children's Hospital Nursing School graduate in 1901)

all men as medical house officers this year. We will all have a training period of 15 months, so we should get to know each other very well. Only five years ago, an interne served for just six months, lived and ate at the hospital, and cared for patients only on the wards. They were assisted by externes who cared exclusively for outpatients and did not live or eat at the hospital. We now care for patients on both the inpatient and outpatient services, and while we receive no salary, we do receive room and board. We are required to return to the wards at night only in the case of emergencies. Fifteen months without a vacation seems awfully long. This coupled with having to obtain permission from the superintendent to be absent overnight makes for a pretty monastic life. We are also required to get permission from the superintendent to invite a friend in for a meal at the hospital.

We report for administrative matters to the superintendent and for medical matters to the attending physician for the month. The six or seven attending physicians are from well-known Boston Brahmin families. They have private practices in the city but assume responsibility for the patients in the hospital three to four months at a time each year. They are present on the wards only infrequently, however, and for a relatively short period of time. On occasion, we see the consulting senior staff. These men are famous names in pediatrics who once served as attending physicians. Medical students also come to the hospital to learn pediatrics, fourth-year students in the outpatient department, third-year students two mornings each week on the wards. They all want to end up at a Harvard hospital for their training, so they work hard. Our nurses are Children's Hospital trained at the School of Nursing and are excellent.

All in all, life is busy, but I am learning a great deal from my colleagues and the attending staff. I feel like I have joined a second family.

Sincerely,

Elijah

Medical House Officer Reflections[2]

December 9, 1966

Dear Mom and Dad,

I thought I would catch you up on my life after six months as a junior assistant resident (JAR) in medicine at The Children's (we shorten Children's Hospital to "The Children's," but our competitors think we are a bit too full of ourselves). Life is so busy but also so exciting. I am learning a great deal every day, and I feel extremely fortunate to be taught by the medical giants in pediatrics. Boston is different than New York, Children's is different than Bellevue, and my junior year is different from my intern year. The patients are sicker and more specialized here, but there is more help from faculty and nursing and social work staff. I still miss the independence of Bellevue. We believed we ran the show there, less so here, but we learn more here. More about this later.

The faculty are really impressive—big names who have written the books. Dr. Janeway, our chief, is a fantastic teacher, incredibly knowledgeable about all of pediatrics. We admire him greatly. Dr. Berenberg is his right-hand man, has a lot of private patients, and has been here since 1942, when Richard Smith served as physician-in-chief. He delivers both the good and the bad news for Dr. Janeway.

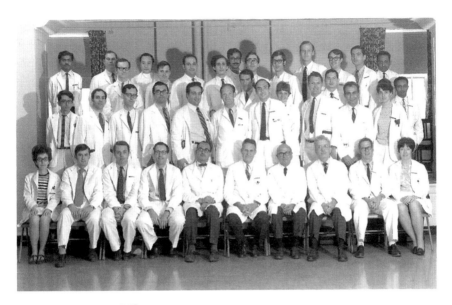

FIGURE 2   House Officers, circa 1968

House officers in the late 1960s were still formally dressed, with collared white shirt and tie or dentist-type high-collared shirts, white pants, white short jacket, and white or dark shoes. The women wore blouses, skirts, and short white jackets.

He orders a lot of tests to make a diagnosis. We call them Berenberg-a-grams. The big giants are Dr. Nadas in cardiology, Dr. Diamond in hematology, Dr. Farber in tumor therapy, Dr. Shwachman in cystic fibrosis, Dr. Neuhauser in radiology, and Dr. Clement Smith in neonatology. It is a bit more formal here, and we have to make appointments to see the division chiefs. They are always very welcoming, but we are still a little nervous in their presence. The younger doctors, like David Nathan in hematology, Fred Rosen in immunology, Sam Katz in infectious disease, and Frank Fellers in kidney disease are really good. They come onto the wards at all hours and are great teachers.

Sherwin Kevy is an older, really seasoned chief resident. His title is assistant to the physician-in-chief, and his responsibility is us. His knowledge is really encyclopedic. We meet with him every morning in the blood bank. If we don't get our white counts, tuberculin tests, and urinalysis results into the chart quickly, he can really ream us out. When we can't diagnose a patient, we go to Dr. Kevy; he always can! The senior residents look out for us and tell us how to stay out of trouble.

I have gotten into trouble twice so far. Dr. Gross (he is the most famous surgeon here) had a patient with a bleeding ulcer who he was going to operate on. I thought this six-year-old boy was bleeding from his nose and swallowing his blood. The surgical resident agreed with me. Dr. Gross wasn't happy, but we were right. The second episode was a yellow baby in the nursery. Dr. Diamond ordered phenobarbital for the infant (it removes bilirubin more rapidly from the body). He was a private patient, so I asked his private pediatrician if it was okay. Boy, did I get into trouble. It's a new treatment, and Dr. Diamond wants to publish a paper about it, but he is afraid that he will be beaten out by a neonatologist in California. He wasn't happy; said he would speak to Dr. Janeway about me. I thought I would be on the next bus home, even though I was right to do what I did. I saw Dr. Janeway yesterday; he said it was handled, not to worry about it. I am still here!

My fellow house officers are great. They have welcomed me in. There are 36 of us, 14 interns, 14 juniors, and eight seniors. I admire the five women housestaff greatly. They work remarkably hard and carry their load as well if not better than the guys. The senior residents (SARS, as we call them) tend to be more seasoned because many have spent several years doing research at the National Institutes of Health (NIH), while others have been in the Berry Plan (that's the government's plan that defers our military service of two years until we are trained as specialists). They tend to be older and more experienced as leaders and as researchers and thus are a great resource for us. The residents in the NIH group have already decided on a subspecialty direction and consequently tend to be more focused and more knowledgeable about diseases in their chosen specialty.

The first two years of the residency cover most specialties in either the inpatient or outpatient setting. The senior year is the year for being a supervisor. There is not much autonomy in the junior year, something we wish we had more of. There is a bit of a hierarchy both in the residency as a whole and between the three different medical residency classes. The residents who work in the MOPD (Medical Outpatient Pediatric Department) and those who work in the affiliated residency program spend the majority of their time in the hospital's outpatient clinics and in the affiliated hospitals (Beverly and North Shore Hospitals). If they perform very well, they often move into our residency. It's a bit of a first-class, second-class system, but many residents are from foreign countries, and thus learning the American medical system before moving into the more intense traditional residency makes sense.

I have made some good friends from outside the U.S.: Charlie Phornphutkul from Thailand, David Lobo from Venezuela, and Francisco Tome from Honduras. We also have an exchange with a hospital in London (I think it is called St. Mary's Hospital). We send a senior to them and they similarly send one to us. They do less laboratory testing in England and depend more on the history and physical examination. I think their influence helps to make us better doctors. Dr. Janeway is very much committed to international pediatrics. This is why we have so many physicians from foreign countries here. He feels that when they go back to their countries, they will have an important influence on health care.

The nurses are all pediatric trained, are really good with kids, and are a tremendous help. We even have play therapy ladies here and play therapy rooms for the kids. For the kids with rheumatic fever, psychiatric diseases, and other chronic diseases, they have public school teachers who come in each day so the kids will not fall too far behind in their work. I think all of these are advantages of a children's hospital oriented to kids and, I believe, seen less in pediatric units in a general hospital.

I am in a pretty consistent pattern of rotations now. I change every 30 days. Most rotations in the first year are on the general inpatient services, while in the second year, many rotations are in the subspecialties—tumor therapy, psychiatry, neurology, cardiology, and neonatology. In addition to being on duty 12 out of 14 days over a two-week period, I am on every other night and every other weekend, which comes out to Monday, Wednesday, Saturday, and Sunday nights in the first week, and Tuesday, Thursday, and Friday nights in the second week. I generally sleep four to five hours when on duty but especially in the winter months, I hear I will get less sleep. Each day on the inpatient services is quite similar: in the morning, we have work rounds followed by X-ray rounds, then teaching rounds; a formal conference over lunch; workup of patients in the afternoon; a teaching conference around 5 p.m.; and then sign out in the early evening. If I'm off for the night, I leave around 7 p.m., and if on, I am generally up until midnight or after. We often have teaching rounds at 10 p.m. led by the senior or junior for the interns and, on occasion, students. I enjoy these greatly because they are low-key and we learn a lot.

The outpatient rotations are a bit easier. We follow our continuity patients in the Family Health Care Program the same afternoon each week. I am caring for a girl with burned-out myocarditis (a viral infection of the heart muscle), who is in and out of heart failure. She is from South Boston. I have become close to her and her family, and I hope she will get better. I feel it is a privilege to be a resident at Children's, and I am proud to be here. My first week of vacation (two weeks in total for the year) starts after Christmas. I look forward to going skiing and sleeping.

I miss you!

Ted

Medical House Officer Reflections[3]

April 23, 2005

Dear Grandma,

I'm writing this note to you with just three months to go until I complete my residency and move on to Emergency Medicine. It has been a wonderful three years of incredibly hard work, successes in the care of my patients, and some very sad losses. I have tended to bond most with my fellow women housestaff (can you believe we outnumber the men two to one?) and especially those who have spouses (nearly half of our class is married, and many have kids). The unmarried women housestaff complain there are not enough men (for dates) and they will never get married! The number of pregnancies in our class has grown over the three years to one-fourth of the class. A big class helps with maternity leave. I am very close to my interns, who I supervise frequently this year. They are really smart. I have a very close relationship with my fellow senior residents. They are my best friends. We have lived through an intense and personally challenging period together. We are a big class, but it feels like we are really a big and very close family.

We are divided into categorical residents (people like me who are pursuing fellowships), primary care residents (who have a strong interest in general pediatrics, prevention of disease, and inner city and underserved patients), and medicine-pediatric residents who spend two years in pediatrics and two years in internal medicine at the Brigham and Women's Hospital. The medicine/pediatric residents add a body of knowledge that is very enriching for those of us training in pediatrics.

The three years have passed very rapidly, slowly at first but rapidly now. The learning curve in the first year was steep. We had lots of general pediatrics,

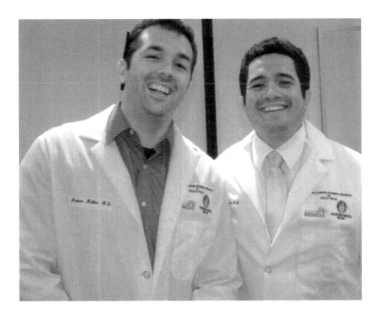

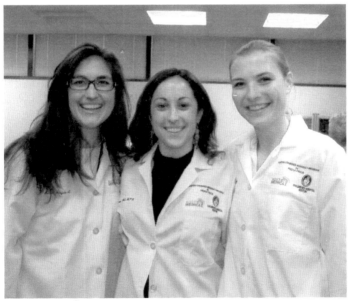

FIGURE 3   House Officers, circa 2005

Housestaff in the new millennium are less formally dressed. Dress includes
shirts, pants, blouses, and skirts as well as hospital scrubs or laboratory coats.
Beards and mustaches are typically absent. All are neatly groomed.

neonatology, and emergency room rotations with some subspecialty exposure in cardiology and adolescent medicine. The second year involved a lot of subspecialty rotations and, as a result, was a bit isolating. This third year has been the plum; we run the wards, supervise the interns and call the shots (of course with our attendings, to whom we are responsible). We have a three-month rotation when we learn about research and academic medicine and work on research projects. My project on Kawasaki disease went really well. It affects the major arteries in the body, and no one really knows what causes it. Although it can be frightening, the good news is that most patients make a good recovery. I received departmental funding and presented my work at the major pediatric meeting in Denver in April. It was a blast, and people said I did a good job. My fellow residents presented as well and did a great job. I am so proud of them and our hospital.

Being able to spend time at the Children's Hospital and Boston Medical Center is what makes this residency great. At Children's we get lots of training, see very sick patients, and see many unusual diseases that only come to a hospital with a stellar reputation like Children's. At Boston Medical Center, we see the bread-and-butter cases. We have less supervision from above, so we have real autonomy in our decision-making. This is great because we have less independence at Children's. The Children's doctors are typically specialists with great knowledge of specific diseases; the Boston Medical Center doctors are superb generalists. The combination has made me a better doctor. Children's has become a complex network with not just community physicians sending in patients, but now surrounding hospitals doing the same. We seem to compete with other pediatric hospitals in Massachusetts for patients.

There are over 700 faculty in the Department of Medicine at Children's, and some we see a great deal. They tend to be our department chairs and program directors. We have a very comfortable relationship with our attendings. It is more informal than in the past, and we can freely ask them questions. We learn a great deal as a result. We have gone to Red Sox games with them. It is a collegial relationship. They tend to come out of our housestaff and are often young.

We generally get along well with the nurses and have a good relationship with them. The nurses can make your life a great deal easier, allowing you to get some sleep and not interrupting you when you are in a teaching conference. They are a bit tougher on us women than on the men. I am not sure why. There are also lots of support staff here, IV teams, pediatric nurse practitioners, social workers, and play therapists who are great for the patients and help us out immensely as well. There are even clowns who are wonderful for the patients . . . and us! Ours is very much a team approach to the care of the patients.

The diseases we see vary from the common (asthma, diabetes, pneumonia, diarrhea, urinary tract infections) to the complex and very serious (such as acute chest syndrome in sickle cell disease or acute respiratory failure). We frequently consult with doctors who specialize in various areas of medicine. Many attendings tell me it is different today than in the past when there were a lot of acute illnesses (meningitis, epiglottitis, acute rheumatic fever, Reye syndrome). Now there is acute illness on top of chronic disease (for example, children with genetic or metabolic diseases with acute infections). There are many patients with G-tubes (for feeding), lines for giving antibiotics, and tracheotomy tubes. The hospitalizations are often very short (two to three days) or alternatively quite long with chronic illnesses. They push us hard to get the patients out as quickly as possible. The parents are great. They are more knowledgeable today than in the past. They ask a lot of questions and know a lot about the disease their child has as a result of information available on the Internet. They expect us to know the answers. I think they perhaps respect us less than in the past.

There is a lot of paperwork because we need to document carefully what we do. We spend too much time in front of the computer, and our class has been pushing our interns to go to the bedside more. We do fewer procedures than in the past because the fellows want to do them as well. I guess this is okay, but my technical skills in starting IVs, inserting lines, doing lumbar punctures, and suturing are perhaps not as strong as they should be. Fortunately, we do more procedures at Boston Medical Center, so this is helpful.

Residency has been an incredible experience. It clearly has its extreme highs and its extreme lows. The Children's Hospital is a very academic, Type A environment. The standards are extremely high. A great deal is asked and expected of us, and there is pressure on us to deliver. I went to the memorial service for parents whose children we had not been able to save. It was so sad; I cried all the way home in the car. People have no idea how tough residency is. At times, especially in the first two years, I have been both physically and mentally exhausted—burnt out. The senior year is easier in this regard.

Residency is part of the training of a doctor, I guess, but it is tough. Now there is an 80-hour work week limit to prevent burnout and errors, but that is not perfect either. I have to leave at a specified hour irrespective of the condition of my patients and turn them over to another resident. I don't like that. The attendings and nurses become the continuity, not me, and I also don't like that. I worry that with shortened hours there is not enough time for me to learn all the new information. It is interesting that as an intern, I worried that I didn't belong here; as a junior, I worried about making a mistake; and as a senior, I worry I will not have learned enough and will not be good enough. I wonder whether there should be a fourth year of residency. Still, all in all, it's been a great year.

Jim sends his best. He is incredibly busy but happy working at the bank. He is doing very well, and I am proud of him. I'll sign off now and go to bed. I miss you and can't wait to see you.

Love,

Lucy

CHAPTER II

The Rotch/Morse/Schloss Era

Residency as an Apprenticeship
1882–1923

"In contrast to now-a-days, there were only two medical house
officers. The Junior looked after the outpatients in the morning
and assisted the Senior on the wards in the afternoon . . ."

—James L. Gamble in 1954, reflecting on
being a house officer in 1912,

THE CHILDREN'S HOSPITAL opened its doors in 1869. Its birth was highly
influenced by the development of medicine in Boston, New York, and Philadelphia, both before and after the Civil War. Before we turn to the Children's
Hospital's early years, and the training of its housestaff, it is useful to examine
the medical profession and its early approach to medical education from the
national perspective.

The National Perspective[1]

In the post–Revolutionary War period in the United States, medicine was
thought by many to be an inferior profession, often populated by the middle
and lower classes of society. The highly talented went into law and the ministry
rather than medicine. Few entering the field had graduated with honors. Medicine actually occupied a limited segment of a physician's time, as he carried out
multiple important roles for his community and society, such as sitting on the
boards of charitable organizations. By the first half of the 19th century, however,

medicine had become more demanding, leaving less time to take on community-oriented roles. Thus the status of physicians rose, while their involvement in socially oriented projects declined.

Prior to the Civil War, education for a medical career did not follow a fixed pattern. Whether a physician went to medical school or not and for how long was highly variable. Medical education was carried out in proprietary schools (medical schools owned by the professors and operated for profit). Educational requirements in these schools were very loose. Even young men without a high school degree could enter medicine. Generally two years in length, the coursework followed no regular progression, with students choosing the sequence for the classes they took. There was no laboratory work, and the didactic lecture

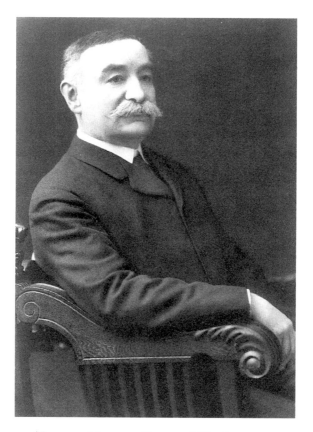

THOMAS MORGAN ROTCH, MD, 1893–1914

Dr. Rotch trained 134 housestaff using the apprenticeship model during his 21 years as chair of the Department of Medicine before his death in 1914.

was the means of instruction. The practice of medicine was learned through apprenticeships carried out in the preceptor's office or patients' homes.

Apprenticeships had no standard content. Few training positions existed in hospitals, and those that did were not awarded competitively but rather based on social connection. Once trained, a physician had to set out on his own to acquire patients. As a result, a successful practice was often uncertain since it was dependent upon the acquisition of prominent patients and appointment to a medical college or hospital. The professional elite with hospital appointments did not identify with practitioners, who were often less well trained and less socially connected.

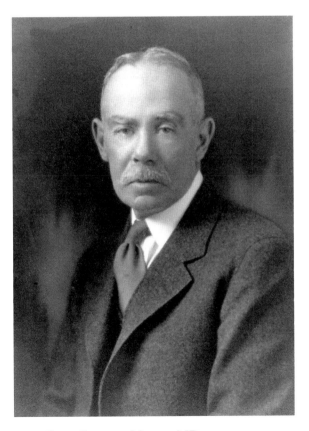

JOHN LOVETT MORSE, MD, 1914–1921

Dr. Morse trained 69 housestaff using the apprenticeship model during his eight years as chair of the Department of Medicine, with World War I being waged during much of his tenure.

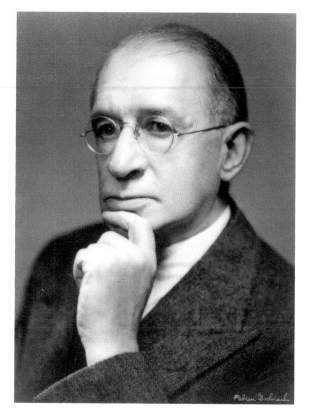

OSCAR MENDERSON SCHLOSS, MD, 1921–1923

Dr. Schloss trained 23 housestaff during his brief
chairmanship of the Department of Medicine before returning
to New York. He introduced the scientific method and the
residency system into the training of housestaff during his two
years in Boston.

Reform Brings Structure

In the 1870s, Charles William Eliot, president of Harvard College, and Daniel
Coit Gilman, president of Johns Hopkins University, began to champion and
lead reform in the profession. But change occurred very gradually. Medical school
was extended from four months to two years, then to three years and, ultimately,
four. Physiology, chemistry, pathology, anatomy, and the laboratory were added
to the curriculum. All courses had to be passed to graduate. The quality of the
students slowly improved while the number applying decreased. Medical education as a field of graduate study became grounded in basic science, the focus

of the first two years, with the last two devoted to clinical care in the hospital. Clinical research also assumed greater importance.

Most teaching hospitals were built in proximity to medical schools, thereby fostering an emphasis on research and education. Internships were started and later residency was introduced at the Johns Hopkins University School of Medicine for specialized training after internship. Hospital house officers now had a shared professional identity. By 1923, a sufficient number of internship positions existed nationwide to accommodate all graduates. At Harvard, professors began to receive small salaries for their hospital work rather than being paid by dividing up patient fees. These reforms ultimately resulted in the melding of education and research with hospital practice.

The effect of these reforms in the 1870s and after was to narrow the portals of entry into medical school, with less recruitment from the lower and middle classes. Fewer applied to the proprietary schools, resulting in less income generated by these schools and hastening their closure. Similarly, the few medical schools solely for women began to close as Johns Hopkins University School of Medicine and others accepted women. But as the number of positions became limited, women had increasing difficulty obtaining admission to medical school. Many schools restricted the number of women to 5% of a given medical school class, a quota system that would not change until the 1950s and 1960s. The training of "elite" physicians also resulted in fewer physicians electing to work in rural and depressed areas of the country. Policies of discrimination limited admission of Jews and blacks to medical schools. And discrimination also extended to immigrant physicians who came to the U.S. looking for a position in a hospital. They often had to find jobs in "ethnic" hospitals that cared for Jewish, Catholic, or German patients.

By the turn of the 20th century, the American Medical Association (AMA), the Carnegie Foundation, and Abraham Flexner, who would gain recognition as a critic of medical education, began to focus on the quality of medical schools. The Flexner Report of 1910 severely criticized American medical schools for their commercialism and low standards. The medical reform galvanized by the Flexner Report was necessary largely due to the failure of the proprietary schools and apprenticeship systems to translate the growing body of scientific knowledge into clinical practice.

Second-rate schools that didn't measure up to the higher standards championed by Eliot, Gilman, and Flexner and increasingly expected of all medical schools by the profession were either closed or merged with stronger schools. The assimilation of medical education into the university gradually increased the separation between academic medicine and private practice. Unsalaried part-time "visits" (physicians in private practice who "visited" to see their patients or who served as ward or clinic attendings) had been beneficial to hospitals and had helped to lower hospital costs. Affiliation with a hospital was also beneficial to a practitioner for the prestige that it garnered. But the Flexner Report now argued for full-time clinical professors similar to full-time basic science professors. The medical schools at Johns Hopkins, Yale University, the University of Chicago, the University of Rochester, Vanderbilt University, and Washington University constructed their clinical departments in the early 1900s to be full time. Others, notably Harvard, continued to depend on part-time visits who supported themselves through their practices.

Evolution of Hospitals and Care

By the time the Children's Hospital opened in 1869, the mandate of hospitals in general had already changed more than once. They evolved from institutions that served religious purposes in the Middle Ages to the almshouses of the colonial period in America. These almshouses became a substitute household for people who were poor or sick and without a home. Their residents became a family. Almshouses and the early American hospitals transitioned from "familial" homes to "bureaucratic" institutions. They became paternalistic, with patients entering because of the generosity of their benefactors. These institutions served a general welfare function, housing the aged, the orphaned, the ill, and the debilitated—only incidentally caring for the sick.[2] Unkempt and overcrowded, the almshouse was often a place of indignity and neglect. They separated the sick from their homes and families and were often seen as a place to die. They did, however, serve an important medical and social function by giving young physicians experience under supervision working with the poor and thereby making a valuable contribution to the community.

Their successor was the public charity hospital. The trustees and superintendents were powerful, deciding on admissions to free beds, which were often privately endowed. This system gave legitimacy to many citizens' philanthropic intentions as well as social prominence through service on hospital boards. As donations failed to cover costs, hospitals gradually turned to their patients. These private patients were generally treated alongside the "ward" patients, although some private rooms were eventually created.

Following the Civil War, surgery began to flourish with the birth of anesthesia and antisepsis. Surgeons could now operate not just on the extremities but on the body's internal organs. Increases in surgical volume allowed for both growth and profit for hospitals. With antisepsis, hospitals became safer places, thereby allowing their evolution from the sustenance of chronic invalids to the care of potentially curable patients. Length of stay dropped from a month or more, to weeks in the mid-1880s, to 18 days at Boston City Hospital in 1900.

Medical Education

The birth of education reform had its genesis in theories of experimental medicine, conceptualized in France and Germany in the mid-1800s, later championed by Eliot and Gilman in the United States in the 1870s, and brought to national attention by the Flexner Report in 1910. The focus of the major reform was on medical school education, and prior to the release of Flexner's report, the pedagogy of medical learning had already been revised. Rote memorization, the lecture, and the apprenticeship in the office or home were replaced by problem solving, critical thinking, evaluation of information, and learning in laboratories and on the wards.

Further change came from within the medical profession, its medical schools, and its hospitals. The core concepts of education reform included laboratory work on scientific subjects; house officer training with patient care responsibility; refinement of the physical examination; the centrality of the hospital for patient care and teaching anatomical location of disease in organs; understanding and application of the germ theory; the birth of therapeutics (aspirin and chloral hydrate); experimental and statistical methods in research as applied to disease; and the realization that knowledge is not static but evolves, leading to an emphasis on scientific publication and a proliferation of journals.

By the early 20th century, clinical bacteriology, hormones and vitamins, antitoxin therapy for infectious diseases, thyroid extract for myxedema, vaccines for rabies and typhoid fever, and new diagnostic techniques (the stethoscope, EKG, X-ray, hematologic and serologic tests) had significantly changed the face of clinical care. As noted by Paul Starr, growing medical knowledge, the attractiveness of medical careers, and achievements of medical research resulted in a rising "professional authority" and an increased prestige for medicine.[3]

Universities, Medical Schools, and Hospitals

The efforts of President Eliot in Boston led to a wedding of the university and the medical school and influenced changes in the rest of the country. His presence as the chair at Harvard Medical School faculty meetings in the latter part of the 1800s resulted in the creation of a truly academic graduate school with educational rigor. And the close affiliation of the university and medical school led to demanding entrance requirements and a science-based curriculum. A perhaps unintended result, however, was the separation of academic medicine from medical practice as academic physicians became more like university professors with greater research and teaching responsibilities.

While medical schools wished to affiliate with hospitals to gain access to the patients needed for third- and fourth-year student teaching, hospitals were less enamored of affiliating with the university and medical school. Progressive medical education emphasized the thorough and active study of a limited number of patients, with the hospital and dispensary becoming the clinical laboratory of study for students. Hospital trustees, however, carefully protected their autonomy and stewardship over their hospitals. They permitted student education reluctantly and only as long as it was carefully supervised.

Johns Hopkins University School of Medicine and the medical schools at the University of Michigan and the University of Pennsylvania owned their hospitals and appointed the teaching faculty. Here, student teaching thrived more easily. Student education in hospitals and medical schools with separate boards of trustees proceeded with greater difficulty. Hospitals, however, gradually came to realize that education and research improved care through the more careful study of diseases. The intellectual climate of the teaching hospital, in turn, attracted the best young physicians and, as noted by the greatly admired Harvard Professor of Medicine Francis Peabody, "The teaching hospital became synonymous with a good hospital."[4] Gradually, the benefits were to be seen as mutual for school and hospital alike, and by 1923, both became convinced that they were indispensable to each other's welfare, though for different reasons.

The House Officer—Early Origins and Pre- and Post-Civil War Periods

The first American hospitals were established successively in Philadelphia, New York, and Boston. The faculty in these hospitals had initially been trained in Edinburgh and London and later in Paris, Vienna, and Berlin and thus were heavily influenced by the European model of training. The first system of training in London in 1617 involved apothecaries. Immersed in an apprenticeship-type model, they followed their teachers on rounds, observing and assisting in treatment. This system evolved in the mid-1660s in the hospitals of London (St.

Bartholomew's, Guy's, St. Thomas', and St. George's) into a system of students and apprentices (called pupils or dressers), who observed, practiced dissection, treated accident cases, and paid tuition for the privilege. They continued to be called resident apothecaries until the mid-1800s when they were designated resident medical officers.

This apprenticeship system was thus transferred to the colonies and in 1751 to the Pennsylvania Hospital. In 1773, the apprentices began living at the hospital in order to learn the art of medicine because there was no medical college in the country at the time.[5] The first such house physician was Jacob Ehrenzeller, who was appointed in 1773 and served for five years. At the Philadelphia General Hospital, "house pupils" in 1789 were required to pay $100 a year for their in-house exposure. By 1813, entrance requirements for hospital service included working for a recognized practitioner for one to two years and attending a course of medical lectures.

In New York by 1809, hospital appointment required one year of preceptorship, a formal course of lectures, and a third year as a non-resident hospital assistant. Formal teaching by the hospital faculty was notably absent in this pre–Civil War period. By 1870, candidates for hospital employment in New York were required to have three years of medical study (which included the preceptorship). Called junior walkers, or senior walkers, they received orders, dressed wounds, took histories, and ate their meals at the hospital but lived at home. The most senior house officer, the house physician or house surgeon, supervised the walkers in the care of the patients. The house physician or house surgeon lived in the hospital and was accountable to the attending physician.[6]

The earliest house officers in Boston were appointed at the Massachusetts General Hospital (MGH). In 1830, nine years after the admission of the first patient, the hospital trustees appointed their first house officer, an apothecary who had completed one year of training as a medical student. He and other early house officers lived in-house, were required to have studied medicine for a year, and were paid an annual salary of $50. By 1846, their numbers had doubled, and in 1849, they acquired a new medical nomenclature, house pupil, "a title that they bore with honor for generations."[7,8]

The terms pupil, dresser, walker, house physician, and house surgeon were used in the 1700s and well into the late 1800s. The term interne was used in France but was not used in the U.S. until the late 1800s. In France, the position of interne was very senior, representing the final stage of training for the elite who had considerable specialized clinical and pathological experience. The term intern in the United States (or interne with an e) was saved for the position between medical school and residency.[9] In 1872, among 178 U.S. hospitals with medical house officers, only nine were connected with a medical college, and only 36 hospitals provided teaching and instruction.[10]

The house officer in the pre–Civil War period had to compete for an internship position, often taking an outpatient appointment first as an externe, or working as a clinical research assistant for an older physician. Alternatively, he could serve as a stand-in in a practice or fill in for a physician during the summer.[11] He—only men were chosen—had to be ambitious, well connected, have a patron, and be approved by the trustees and/or the medical board of the hospital. In short, getting a house officer position was a "courting ritual" that necessitated the applicant calling on his patron and trustees or the hospital manager. Being successful required academic accomplishment, social status, a tenacity of purpose, and often a prior short-term appointment as a student in the hospital or clinic. This process of admission resulted in a less uniform career path and length of appointment. It also led to inconsistencies in nomenclature. The first-year house officer was referred to as either a house pupil or interne. The amount of training varied, but typically he had little prior experience, lived and slept in the hospital, provided the bulk of daily care, was unpaid, and generally served for less than one year. These men were the eyes and ears of the attending physician. They and the nurses were the continuity of care for the patients.

Following the Civil War, the house officer system further evolved. With the need for more house officers, levels of training became graded (externe, interne, and resident physician). The increasing complexity of medicine resulted in longer training, differing titles, the creation of different specialties by the early 20th century (surgery, medicine, orthopedics, pediatrics, radiology, gynecology, ophthalmology, and otolaryngology), and graded levels of training among the housestaff. Internship became a prerequisite for residency. House officers were often unpaid but received room and board (as they lived in the hospital) as well as uniforms. Training gradually became more formal and standardized. Clinical opportunities and credentials were important for the next rung on the training ladder (for house officers) and for patient referrals (for attending physicians). Further reform in the early 1900s created the formal hospital appointment process. Hospital appointments were coordinated to occur following medical school graduation. Successful completion of final examinations determined graduation from medical school and admission to internship. By 1920, the house officer system of today was fully in place.

The Visit and the Administration

Between 1840 and 1900, the hospital became integral to medical careers and well-defined roles emerged. The attending or visiting physician was often a graduate of the hospital's housestaff training program. Attending physicians, or attendings, were reappointed each year. They served in the hospital for three to four months of the year, with eight to nine months spent in their practices, thus their influence was limited. Although unpaid, the prestige of the hospital appointment enhanced their ability to attract patients. These doctors were the upper crust of society, while their patients were generally poor and, in Boston, often Irish, creating an economic and social distance between patient and physician. At retirement, they became consulting physicians, an honorific title.

The superintendent (manager) of the hospital served the trustees, hired and fired, and was a sort of business partner to the trustees. This person, who had no medical background, oversaw all administrative matters, while the visit was responsible for all medical matters.

By the turn of the century, the hospital was made up of a community of students, internes, externes, resident physicians, junior and senior visits, consulting physicians, nurses, and the superintendent. All were highly dependent on the hospital. Patients were the clinical material for learning, teaching, and research. Wealth, social position, being white and male, and socially respected were the tickets to success in the hospital setting.

The Children's Hospital—The Early Years[12]

The modest new Children's Hospital situated in Boston's South End was heavily influenced by the social and cultural norms of the day. It was rooted in the medical progress being made following the Civil War and influenced in particular by advances in Boston. We will examine the rapid growth and development of the hospital in the early years from the perspective of the institution's mission as well as the development of its clinical, education, and research programs. We will also see how the concept of post-graduate medical education (internship and residency) evolved and gained momentum from the late 1880s to the early 1900s, from what was initially an apprenticeship system to a formal medical training program.

Throughout this book, the hospital, for purposes of brevity, will be referred to as (the) Children's Hospital. In fact, it was Children's Hospital from 1869 until 1922, when the name was changed to the Children's and Infants' Hospital. Then, in 1948, it became the Children's Medical Center and kept that name until 1959, when the word Hospital was added: Children's Hospital Medical Center. Jump ahead to 2000, when it garnered a new name, Children's Hospital Boston, which would remain in effect until 2012. Since then, this storied institution has been known as Boston Children's Hospital.

Rutland Street, 1869–1870 and Washington and Rutland Streets, 1870–1882

The Children's Hospital opened on July 19, 1869, as a 20-bed facility in a brick townhouse at 9 Rutland Street in Boston's South End. This opening followed a prior failed attempt at the establishment of a similar facility for children, the Children's Infirmary, which opened in 1847 on Washington Street and closed 18 months later. That institution was believed to have failed because of "the deep rooted and commendable feeling which prompts the mother to cling to her sick and suffering child, rather than entrust it to those whose motives she has never learned to fathom."[13] The first annual report of the Children's Hospital, published in 1870 (six months after the hospital's opening), in its bylaws states its objectives to be: 1) The medical and surgical treatment of sick children; 2) Instruction in the diseases of children; and 3) Instruction of young women in the duties of nurses and nursery maids. The hospital saw its central mission to be the care of the poor and the "little waifs who crowd our poor streets."[2,14]

As noted in its third annual report, the hospital was thus initially created for both moral and physical benefit, stressing a spiritual role, including a degree of medical fatalism along with social activism, and stressing the need for those dying to spend their last days "in a home of equality, comfort and peace." The hospital served "as an alternative home for the poor, offering order, purity and kindness, a salubrious haven where they would be nursed, fed, kept clean and safe," and where the children would receive "positively Christian nurture." To protect the children from deleterious influences and to enhance physical and spiritual care, visiting hours in stark contrast to today were restricted to one hour per day, only on weekdays, and to one relative at a time. The hospital's first patient was a seven-year-old girl diagnosed with a fracture of the radius. She was discharged entirely well after a stay of one month.[13] In the hospital's first five months, 30 patients were admitted. Many had suffered fractures but many others had serious medical diseases.[13] Remarkably, there were no deaths.

In 1870, within a year of its opening, the hospital was relocated to a second site, in a larger building on the corner of Washington and Rutland Streets

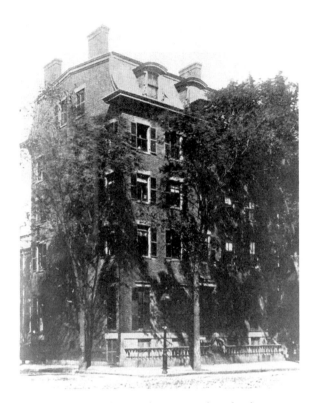

FIGURE I   Children's Hospital at Washington and Rutland Street, circa 1870

Located in Boston's South End from 1870 to 1882 and containing 27 beds, this hospital would antedate the Children's Hospital's first internes and externes in 1882.

(Figure 1) and remained at this location for 12 years. This hospital contained 27 beds (Figure 2). During this time, the hospital evolved gradually from its earlier social and moral orientation to a more medical approach. In the outpatient setting in particular, the child's illness was cared for. Moral improvement gradually disappeared as a goal of hospital care. Additionally, the hospital became less of a charity hospital for the poor as patient revenue began to supplement donations and medical care became the central mission.

It is important to note that the opening of the Children's Hospital was not met with universal enthusiasm.[14] The MGH in 1869 had approximately 160 hospitalized children and infants among its 1,200 annual admissions. In addition, the MGH had secured the philanthropic support of the dominant families in Massachusetts; the creation of the Children's Hospital served as an impediment to financial support from these ancestor-oriented donors.[15] The MGH

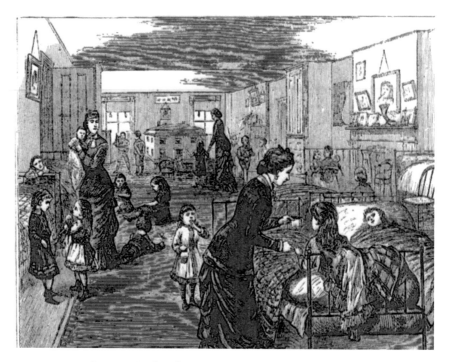

FIGURE 2   A Patient Ward in the Hospital on Washington and Rutland Streets, circa 1881

Wards were large and crowded with metal cribs and children in beds and playing on the floor. (From *Leslie's Illustrated Newspaper*, December 10, 1881)

actively tried to convince the public that the proposed Children's Hospital was not needed and that they were fully able to care for the city's sick children. The competition became more intense as the MGH in its annual reports stressed its fine ability to care for children as well as the many advantages of mingling children and adults on the same ward, and finally, the "inspiration and good cheer spread by the stoicism of the children."[16] The Children's Hospital countered by noting "the gloomy and forbidding appearance of the ward of a general hospital."[17] Over time the intensity of this rivalry lessened, however present-day academic pediatricians may find similarities in some of the attitudes of today and yesteryear among the two Harvard teaching hospitals that care for children.

Huntington Avenue, 1882–1914

A growing patient population in the early 1880s begged for an increased number of beds as well as a medical and surgical housestaff to care for them. The 27

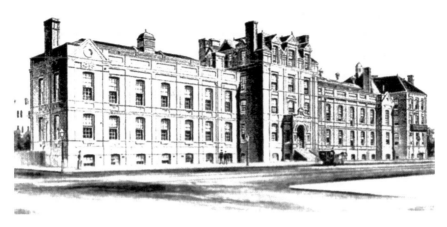

FIGURE 3   Children's Hospital on Huntington Avenue, circa 1882

This hospital, constructed with the $95,000 raised by the first Children's Hospital capital campaign, contained 60 beds, with another 36 added in 1890. It would be the site of training for Dr. Thomas Morgan Rotch's housestaff from 1882–1914.

beds in the Washington and Rutland Street facility were simply inadequate. So in December 1882, the hospital again moved, this time to the north side of Huntington Avenue next to the site where Boston's Symphony Hall would be constructed 20 years later (Figure 3).

Built to house patients from ages 2 to 12, it contained two 20-bed wards, five private rooms, and three rooms for "special cases" (Figure 4). Notably, children less than 2 years old were not cared for at this facility because of fears of the spread of infection. The building had high ceilings, many windows, and sun balconies for sunlight and fresh air. Its average census was 37 at a daily cost of $1.22 for each patient. A house physician's room was located close to the wards and next to the dining room and scullery (the part of the pantry used for prepping food and washing dishes).

In 1888, six years after the move to Huntington Avenue, a location was acquired on Washington Street for a separate outpatient building. Medical patients were seen on the second floor of this new facility by the visiting physicians and externes. One year later, a new east wing for the Huntington Avenue Hospital was constructed, with the first floor accommodating two wards of eight to 10 beds and the second floor containing three smaller wards with a total of 14 beds and four single rooms. Sleeping and relaxing space for the housestaff was located on the third floor. The addition of the east wing allowed for an increase

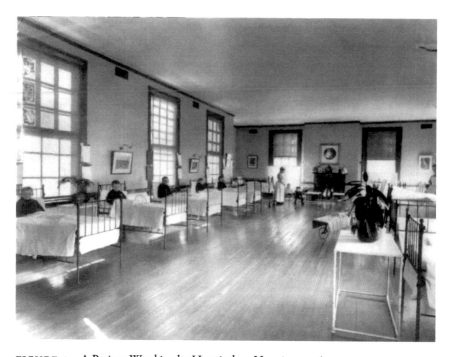

FIGURE 4   A Patient Ward in the Hospital on Huntington Avenue

The patient wards in the hospital on Huntington Avenue were large, with high ceilings and generous windows to provide light, fresh air, and ventilation. The wards had fireplaces for heat and often a balcony.

in the daily census to 73. The patients in the new inpatient wing were cared for by the visiting physician and medical interne.

From the time of the hospital's founding in 1869 until 1882, medical admissions (884) equaled surgical admissions (870). But the move to the Huntington Avenue location and its subsequent expansion, coupled with the improved patient safety achieved thanks to antisepsis, asepsis, and surgical anesthesia, resulted in surgical admissions (6,390) increasing to be double medical admissions (3,536) for the period 1883 to 1900.[18]

The number of admitted patients, often now with more complex disease and longer hospitalization due to the subacute and chronic nature of their disease, required a facility more suited for prolonged care. The Wellesley Convalescent Home and the Heart Hospital in Brookline only partially addressed this problem. Still, conditions were over-crowded and additional facilities that were clearly necessary would come on line at a later time. By 1912, the inpatient wards were handling 1,729 patients (565 medical and 1,104 surgical).

Treatment of orthopedic diseases, deformities of infantile paralysis, rickets, osteomyelitis, bowlegs, and knocked knees established the Children's Hospital as a modern hospital and thereby purged from the hospital's mission "removing threatening urchins from the streets and transforming them into cultured and disciplined children."[19] The successful treatment of orthopedic disease also led to the admission of not only the poor but now the middle class and even wealthy patients. Medical advances also resulted in a broader range of medical admissions. The hospital had clearly moved from social activism directed at the poor to medical activism focused on serving the children of the whole community. It had also become a general hospital for the care of children afflicted with medical and surgical diseases, thereby becoming an attractive site for the training of young physicians.

The medical staff at the Children's Hospital evolved as hospital privileges became increasingly important. The "consulting" staff consisted of older and distinguished physicians and the "visiting" (attending) staff of younger more active physicians who supervised the internes. A visiting physician, or just the "visit," a term mentioned earlier, was often from a Brahmin family, served for three to four months each year, came in infrequently, and was not paid. Hospital appointments were limited, creating an elite professional group, and sowing the early seeds of future challenges in town–gown relationships. The elite physician, in turn, resented the authority of the trustees and superintendent who tried to obtain as much work from each physician as possible with only a hospital appointment in return. Very gradually, the influence of the trustees diminished and physician control increased. The trustees no longer entered into the details of admission and management as they had during the first 13 years of the hospital's existence on Rutland Street and Washington and Rutland Street. The superintendent of the hospital now took on that role.

Longwood Avenue, 1914–1923

By the early 1900s, it was again clear that insufficient space had become a pressing problem. As cogently stated in the annual report for the year 1905, "a number of beds should be waiting for the children, and not that the children should wait for the beds." With an average daily inpatient census of 75, children with pneumonia, gastroenteritis, and other acute infections often had to be turned away. The annual report for 1908 recorded an outpatient census of 27,197 patients (7,391 medical patients) and an inpatient census of 1,729 (661 medical patients) with many complaints of overcrowding.

The first architectural rendering of the new Hunnewell Building with a steeple (rather than a dome, which was ultimately installed) appeared in the annual report for 1910, accompanied by a request for financial support (Figure 5). The building was named for Francis Welles Hunnewell, a generous contributor to the hospital and its president from 1901 until his death in 1918. In fact, there were three major donors to the construction of the Hunnewell Building. Francis Hunnewell's gift supported construction of the west wing, while the estate of Anne White Vose funded construction of the east wing, and the central administration wing was made possible by the estate of Helen Angier Ames. In April 1914, the new facility on Longwood Avenue was opened with great fanfare by James M. Curley, mayor of Boston, A. Lawrence Lowell, president of Harvard University, and Charles Coolidge, the building's architect. Constructed on farmland that had been owned by Ebenezer Francis, it was located next to Harvard Medical School, which had relocated from the Back Bay in Boston to the area in 1906. This new building—and its address (300 Longwood Avenue)—would become a well-known, signature landmark and a nostalgic remembrance for innumerable medical and surgical trainees in years to come. Equally recognizable is the iconic picture of special cows, which provided tuberculosis-free milk, grazing peacefully opposite the entrance to the Hunnewell Building (Figure 6).

This new facility was much larger and better organized, allowing for increased efficiency in serving and caring for its patients. The new Hunnewell Building served a number of purposes, housing not only patients but house

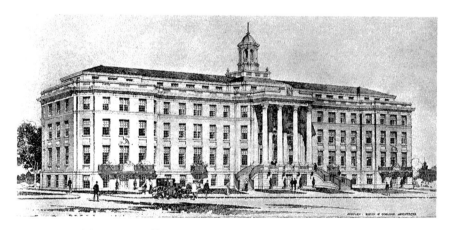

FIGURE 5   The Hunnewell Building, circa 1910

This architectural rendering, with a steeple rather than a dome, was used to raise financial support for the new hospital to be built on the Francis Farm on Longwood Avenue, next to the newly constructed Harvard Medical School.

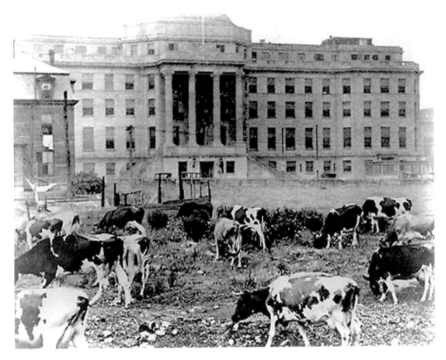

FIGURE 6   Specially bred cows grazing in 1919
Kept in a field across from the Hunnewell Building, these cows provided tuberculosis-free milk for patients at the Children's Hospital.

officers, nurses, and members of a religious order of nuns trained as nurses. The first floor of the main wing had room for physician examining rooms, staff rooms, and a library. The house officers' quarters and a chapel were on the second floor, while the Ladies Aid Association was located on the third floor along with rooms for maids; beds for private patients were found on the fourth floor. The west wing was largely devoted to outpatient care but also had laboratories, rooms for lectures, a gymnasium, a hospital dispensary, and a ward for private patients and for those children who needed to be isolated. The east wing, known as Vose House, accommodated 70 nurses and the nuns from the Episcopal Sisterhood of St. Margaret.

In a perfect example of form following function, the central dome of the Hunnewell Building was made of quartz glass that allowed ultraviolet light to enter, thereby enhancing vitamin D stores in the children. In addition, behind the Hunnewell Building, there were five pavilion buildings (two, each with two stories for medicine and orthopedics, and two, each with a single story for surgery) as well as one building just for surgical operating rooms. These separate buildings were constructed with two goals in mind, to prevent the spread of highly contagious infections and to afford ample sunlight and ventilation. Medical patients were housed in the pavilion building known as Ward 1 (Figure 7). (The terms pavilion building and ward building were used interchangeably.) All pavilion buildings were connected by unheated connectors—the lowest level for pipes and heating and the other connectors for transport of food and supplies by motorized carts as well as passage of patients, parents, physicians, and nurses. A central, open courtyard contained one small shack for airing mattresses between admissions. This courtyard also served as a recreation area for doctors, nurses, patients, and other hospital staff.

Ward 1 contained two wings of 10 beds each and an isolation room, with the head nurse's station placed between the two wings. The pavilion buildings were built for ventilation, exposure to fresh air and sun, and control of spread of infection. The piazzas and balconies were constructed to enjoy maximum sunlight, and each ward had a solarium.

Three additions occurred on the Longwood campus prior to 1923. On November 14, 1921, a 46-bed private-patient floor (16 patients in double bedrooms and 30 patients in single bedrooms) was opened in the Vose House, located in the east wing of the Hunnewell Building (provision had been made for the nurses with the purchase of a hotel on the corner of Longwood and Huntington

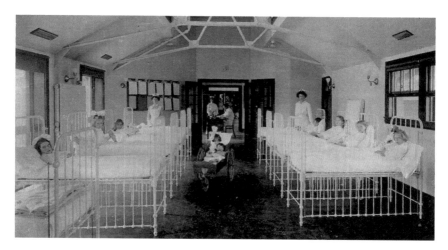

FIGURE 7   Patients in a Pavilion Building

The patient wards in the pavilion buildings were divided by specialty—medical, surgical, and orthopedic—and connected by unheated connectors.

Avenues). Long championed by the staff physicians for their patients, this addition was well received.

In 1923, a pavilion for the Infants' Hospital was opened on the Children's Hospital campus (behind the current Wolbach Building) with babies and children less than 2 years old now admitted and cared for by Children's Hospital nurses and housestaff. This new pavilion presented the opportunity for housestaff to see and treat diseases in newborns and young infants. Prior to this time, children younger than 2 had been cared for in the Thomas Morgan Rotch Jr. Memorial Building (the current Wolbach Building) on Shattuck Street. That building had proven to be ill-suited for the care of infants, lacking isolation facilities and being inefficient for hospital use. It was sold to Harvard University and became the home of the Harvard School of Public Health. The Children's Hospital eventually repurchased the building.

Finally, in September of 1922, a laboratory building was completed with James Gamble as its director. Located behind the Hunnewell Building's west wing, it enhanced the hospital's clinical laboratory capacity and served as the location for hematology, immunology, bacteriology and infectious disease clinical analyses and research. This building also served as the site for Gamble's investigation of disorders of metabolism as well as some of the most important research work of the hospital over the next 25 years. It was a significant sign to the housestaff of the importance of research, both in their training and for their future academic careers.[20]

Between 1914 and 1923, the hospital and medical service grew rapidly in both patient volume and complexity as well as in the number of faculty attendings and housestaff. This growth would slow briefly in 1917 and 1918 due to World War I, only to accelerate in the early 1920s with new buildings, an enlarged faculty and housestaff, and a new scientific orientation on the medical service with the arrival of Drs. Oscar Schloss and James Gamble.

Departmental Leadership, 1893–1923

First Chair of the Department of Medicine

The leadership of the Department of Medicine was formally conferred upon Dr. Thomas Morgan Rotch (photo, front of chapter) in 1893, 24 years following the hospital's founding in 1869 and 11 years after the appointment of the first medical housestaff in 1882.[21] He served in that capacity until 1914, training 134 house officers during his tenure. Rotch was born in Philadelphia in 1849, his forbearers associated with whaling and shipping in New Bedford, Massachusetts. He graduated from Harvard Medical School in 1874, spent two years studying abroad in Germany, and served both the Children's Hospital and the Infants' Hospital from 1884 to 1914. His academic contributions included the percentage system of the contents of milk for infant feeding and his 1,100-page pediatric textbook, *The Hygiene and Medical Treatment of Children*, which was the classic text of the time. Upon his death in 1914 and after serving 21 years as physician-in-chief, he was succeeded by John Lovett Morse, his loyal associate physician for five years.

Second Chair of the Department of Medicine

Dr. John Lovett Morse lived from 1869 to 1940 (photo, front of chapter).[22] Born in Taunton, Massachusetts, he received his medical training at Harvard Medical School. Morse had a most successful and "fashionable" private practice, was a lucid and clear teacher, and capably oversaw hospital arrangements and teaching matters as physician-in-chief from 1914 to 1921. He served as president of the American Academy of Pediatrics, the American Pediatric Society, and the pediatric section of the American Medical Association. He trained 69 house officers between 1914 and 1921.

Third Chair of the Department of Medicine

When looking for a successor to Dr. Morse, the highly influential Harvard Medical School Dean David Linn Edsall initiated the first national search for a new, fulltime, pediatric chief—this time with investigative as well as clinical capabilities. The search identified Dr. Oscar Menderson Schloss (photo, front of chapter).[23] Schloss was born in Cincinnati, graduated from Johns Hopkins University School of Medicine in 1905, and received his house officer training in New York. He was appointed professor of pediatrics at Cornell University Medical College in 1919, at the age of 37, based upon his highly productive scholarly work, which was often presented at American Pediatric Society meetings. He served as physician-in-chief in Boston for a period of less than two years, from 1921 to 1923, training 23 house officers.

He returned to Cornell due to a number of misunderstandings involving his personal laboratory space, financial commitments made to him and his faculty, and issues involving the leadership of the Children's Hospital and the Infants' Hospital. His loyal resident Arthur F. Anderson, looking back over Schloss' two years of stewardship, noted a number of significant accomplishments, including "the fusion of investigative and clinical aspects of pediatric teaching and practice,

the establishment of the residency system, the erection of the Pediatric Laboratory Building . . . the appointment of Dr. James L. Gamble . . . to the Staff, and
the establishment of clinical medicine upon a university basis."[14]

These three pediatric leaders, Rotch, Morse, and Schloss, trained 226 house
officers at the Children's Hospital over a 30-year period. They launched the
careers of such iconic future national leaders and prior house officers at the Children's Hospital as James Gamble, Bronson Crothers, Lewis Webb Hill, Richard
Smith, Fritz Talbot, and Samuel Levine and formulated the structure and rules
of operation of house officer training, much of which stands as their legacy today.

The Faculty, 1882–1923

The medical staff was small in number from the time of the opening of the hospital in 1869 until the arrival of the first housestaff in 1882. The physicians in
those years included A.M. Sumner, F.G. Morrill, and J.P. Oliver as physicians;
H.C. Haven and T.M. Rotch as assistant physicians; and F.H. Brown, one of
the hospital's founders, as consulting physician. Establishing an early important
linkage with Harvard Medical School, several of the hospital's physicians and
surgeons were also appointed as instructors at Harvard Medical School. By the
time Thomas Morgan Rotch was appointed head of the medical service, the staff
had increased in size at all three levels of appointment. Drs. Rotch and Herbert
Leslie Burrell, a hospital surgeon, published a 367-page *Medical and Surgical
Report* in 1895 both for internal staff use as well as use external to the hospital.
In 1905, Dr. Rotch, as evidence of his growing power and influence, published the
first medical department report in the hospital's annual report. Prior to that time,
all departmental reports were issued as part of the board of manager's report.

With medical education an integral part of the job description of the faculty,
the staff now actively taught the housestaff and students and were productive
in scholarship. Over a five-year period, Dr. Rotch published two books and 27
manuscripts, and Dr. Morse published one book and 31 manuscripts, setting a
clear example for the housestaff of an expectation of scholarly work and output,
a requirement even for—or especially for—the department chiefs.

At the time of the announcement of John Lovett Morse's chairmanship in
1914, the number of medical students (four to six in the outpatient department
and six to 10 on the inpatient service), the large number of graduate house physicians coming from afar, and an ever-increasing number of housestaff necessitated
a larger faculty, with Drs. P.H. Sylvester and E.T. Wyman joining the staff as
junior assistant physicians. The departure of some faculty served to compound

the staffing shortage. Maynard Ladd left to head the Department of the Diseases of Children at the Boston Dispensary as did three outpatient physicians (one to the Infants' Hospital, one to the fledgling Boston Floating Hospital, and one to North Carolina). To this was added the attrition of the war years, with as many as four departing for military service in 1917, their roles filled by a "corps of young women," community physicians, and alumni. By 1918, an additional seven staff departed to the war effort and a similar depletion was also seen in the housestaff. The number of visiting graduate physicians decreased as well. Medical students were most helpful in filling in, both in the inpatient and outpatient settings.

Stability returned after the war. Distinguished visiting scientists were now appointed to the staff, adding a rich diversity of scientific expertise for the faculty and housestaff alike, and included: Drs. H.C. Ernst (bacteriologist), O.K. Folin (chemist), W.B. Cannon (physiologist), S.B. Wolbach (pathologist) and R. Hunt (pharmacologist). Bronson Crothers was appointed neurologist in 1920. With the arrival of Oscar Schloss as chair of the Department of Medicine in 1921, the staff included a number of revered clinicians and teachers, including James Gamble and Richard Smith as associate physicians; Philip Sylvester and Edwin Wyman as assistant physicians; Harold Stuart and Louis Webb Hill as junior assistant physicians; and Maurice Briggs, long-serving secretary of the Children's Hospital Medical Alumni Association, and Mary Putnam, a private practice pediatrician in Lexington who was one of the few early female practitioners in eastern Massachusetts, as clinical assistant physicians. The majority of these attendings had served as house officers during the tenures of Drs. Rotch and Morse, setting a precedent for hiring from within—a pattern still in existence today, some 98 years later.

The Children's Hospital—Housestaff and Medical Education, 1882–1923[24]

The Housestaff

There were no housestaff from 1869 to 1882, during the period of time that the hospital was located first on Rutland Street and then on Washington and Rutland Streets. The first three appointments occurred in 1882, 13 years after the opening of the hospital and were necessitated by a growing number of admissions. The two internes were Henry S. Otis and George Haven, and the single externe was F.W. Knowles, Jr. (In the early years as noted previously in this chapter, interne and externe ended with an "e.")

The appointment of these three men occurred roughly 100 years after the first house physician appointment in Philadelphia in 1773, and 50 years after the first house officer appointment in Boston at the MGH in 1830. While little is known about them, all three were most likely of Brahmin heritage, consistent with the nature of appointments at that time. The internes lived in the hospital and were primarily responsible for the inpatients. The medical externe lived and took his meals outside the hospital and was responsible for outpatients. In fact, the Children's Hospital Rules of 1894 indicated that it was forbidden for the externe to "live in the hospital or take any meals therein, except when acting in the absence of, or assisting, the interne."[25] The higher level of responsibility for the interne when contrasted with the externe, reflects the perceived increased complexity of inpatient care when compared with outpatient care. When an interne or externe was absent, his position was often filled by a medical student.

The nomenclature for housestaff has changed over the years. During the Rotch/Morse/Schloss era, medical externe, medical interne, house physician, and resident physician were used. Starting in the 1920s and continuing for roughly the next two decades, the terms house physician, medical house officer, and resident physician were used. Commencing in 1945 and for the next 50 years, the terms for these trainees were intern, resident, and ambulatory (or outpatient) resident, and since 1995, the terms categorical or primary care (PL-1, -2, or -3) residents have been used. When speaking generally of all trainees, from the opening of the hospital until about 1945, the term house officer was often used. From that point until the present, trainees have been called residents or housestaff (with interns subsumed under both terms). In this book, the terms house officer and housestaff will be used interchangeably, the only exception being in the Blackfan/Smith era when house officer referred to junior trainees and resident physician to senior trainees.

When the first *Rules and Regulations for House Officers* was published in 1894, it illustrated the hospital's carefully laid out expectations of its housestaff in training. The interne and externe served for a period of six months but with different patient responsibilities, suggesting a hierarchy: the interne superior to the externe. In the early 1900s, the term senior and junior house physician was substituted for interne and externe, respectively; with the senior house physician caring for inpatients and the junior house physician responsible for outpatients. Their duration of service was now 15 months. Simultaneously, the hospital and its staff were training a large number of practicing pediatricians from different parts of the country (called graduate physicians). In the early 1900s, the number of housestaff increased to meet a growing clinical demand. (Figures 8–11)

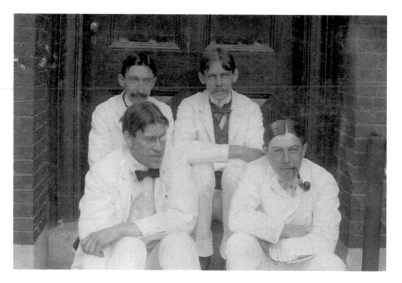

FIGURE 8   House Officers, circa 1901

Four house officers, "The Big Four," at the turn of the 20th century, neatly dressed in whites outside the hospital on Huntington Avenue. (From the scrapbook of Edith Pollard Ralston, a Children's Hospital Nursing School graduate in 1901)

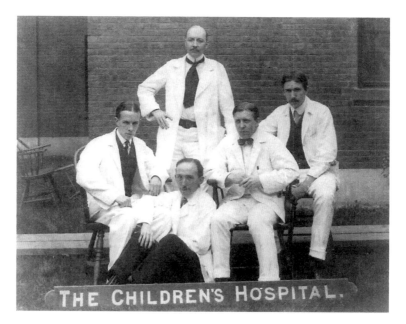

FIGURE 9   Housestaff, circa 1902

The house officers at the turn of the century posing formally for their yearly photograph.

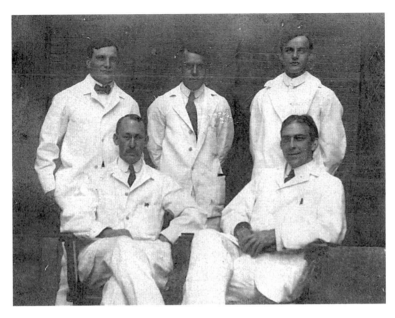

FIGURE 10   Housestaff, circa 1905

Five house officers in 1905, including Dr. Fritz Talbot in the front row on the right,
who later became chief of the Children's Service at the Massachusetts General
Hospital. (From the scrapbook of Edith Pollard Ralston, a Children's Hospital
Nursing School graduate in 1901)

The year 1909 was notable for the training of Richard Smith (future chief of
medicine at the Children's Hospital); 1912 for the training of Bronson Crothers, James Gamble, and Edwin Wyman (all three stalwarts of the Department
of Medicine); 1914 for the training of Frank Ober (future chief of orthopedics
at the Children's Hospital); 1917 for the training of Alton Goldbloom (future
chief of pediatrics at Montreal Children's Hospital); and 1922 for the training of
Samuel Levine (future chief of pediatrics at Cornell University Medical College).
The annual report for the year 1913 used the term resident for the first time, in
reference to the appointment of Henry J. Fitz-Simmons. This use of the term
resident reflected a higher level of responsibility and authority.

In 1914, the housestaff consisted of seven men: one resident, three house
physicians, and three graduate house physicians. Further drawing upon the reliable use of the hospital for teaching of Harvard Medical School students, this
group of housestaff was joined by a cadre of fourth-year students working in the
outpatient setting one afternoon each week, third-year students working on the
wards two mornings each week, and second-year students who also spent time

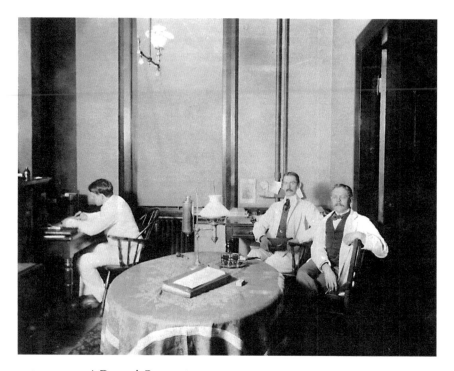

FIGURE 11   A Doctor's Room, circa 1910

Staff physicians and a medical student in a doctor's conference room, where teaching and charting took place.

in the hospital setting. This medical student involvement was most helpful in 1917 and 1918 when the war effort depleted the number of housestaff and the medical students were called in as invaluable replacements.

By the first year of Oscar Schloss' tenure as Department of Medicine chair, in 1921, the housestaff had grown to 13, with one resident, three house physicians, and 9 to 10 graduate house physicians. The resident training system Dr. Schloss introduced was based on his experience in training at Johns Hopkins Hospital in Baltimore; the system had been conceptualized there by Drs. William Osler and William Halsted in the mid-1890s. It offered the advantage of service by a housestaff with greater experience and training, who then were able to assume increased responsibility in running and leading the service. It is further interesting to note that the leadership of both the nursing service and the resident staff were listed together in the annual reports, perhaps reflecting the continuous nature of their service to their patients, as contrasted with the attending staff, whose service was more sporadic.

TABLE I　Medical Housestaff Statistics

	Average Number/Year (by decade)				
	1880s	1890s	1900s	1910s	1920s
TOTAL	2	3	6	8	13
Male/Female	2/0	3/0	6/0	8/0	13/0
Chief Residents	0	0	0	0	0

From the first appointment of housestaff in 1882 until Dr. Schloss left in 1923, 226 house officers were trained at the Children's Hospital. The average number of house officers trained per year by decade is shown in Table 1.

Education of Nurses

The bylaws of the newly opened hospital at 9 Rutland Street on March 22, 1869, stated as its third objective, "Instruction of young women in the duties of nurses and nursery maids."[26] When the hospital opened, there were no trained nurses in the United States. Florence Nightingale had established the first training school for nurses at London's St Thomas' Hospital only a few years earlier. In fact, the Episcopal Sisterhood of St Margaret, founded in England as a nursing order trained in the tradition of Florence Nightingale, came to the U.S. in 1873 to take charge of the small new hospital for children in Boston.

In the first annual report, the managers of the hospital indicated that they wished "to initiate a system hitherto untried in Boston of instruction to young women in the middle and lower classes in the duties of nurses."[27] Twenty years after this expressed intent in the bylaws, on May 5, 1891, the first graduating nursing class received diplomas (Figure 12).[28] Though no formal vote was taken to establish a nursing school, the date of 1889 has been accepted as the date of organization of the school. Thus within seven years of each other, instruction of medical house officers (1882) and instruction of student nurses (1889) had begun at the Children's Hospital, thereby establishing a tradition of commitment to education alongside the care of patients.

Bylaws and Rules

The *By-laws of the Corporation* (March 22, 1869, article 13) had provided for a future housestaff: "When deemed necessary for the good of the Hospital, one or more Medical House Officers should be selected by the Medical Staff,

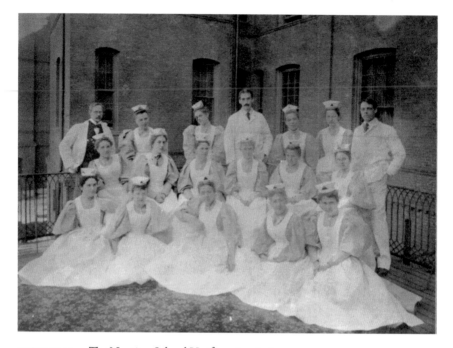

FIGURE 12   The Nursing School Uniform in 1896

Nursing students from the sixth graduating class. The nurses "strawberry box" caps had narrow bands that reflected the number of years of education, with a wider band replacing the narrow bands upon graduation.

after examination, subject to the approval of the Board of Managers. They shall have the immediate medical care of the patients, subject to the direction of the Medical Staff; shall, if required, perform the duties of pharmacist, and keep the medical and surgical record."[29] The bylaws thus set the stage for selection of housestaff based on demonstrated capacity, careful selection by the medical staff, and ultimate approval by the lay board of managers. They also assured housestaff supervision by the medical staff, with responsibility for matters of clinical care and maintenance of the medical chart.

The Hospital Rules of 1894 tell us much about the nature of clinical care in the hospital:[30]

a. Rules, page 2: "Members of the Medical Staff shall not continue patients in the Hospital for periods longer than three months."

b. Rules, page 2: "Patients shall not be admitted under the age of two years or over the age of twelve, unless in cases of emergency."

　c.　Rules, page 10: "No case which is suspected to be one of diphtheria, measles, variola, varicella, scarlet fever, erysipelas, or whooping cough shall be admitted to the Hospital unless it has first been examined and found to be free from these diseases."

　d.　Rules, page 11: "Every patient must receive a disinfecting bath from head to foot before returning to the general ward."

These rules created a setting in which hospitalization was carefully regulated. The strict attention to the dangers of contagion and spread of viral exanthems and bacterial infections was recognized as critical for the safety of all patients. This reflected a concerted effort to reverse the prior held belief that hospitals were dangerous and primarily a place to die. As mentioned earlier, the basis for housing children under 2 in a separate location was concern about spreading infections from the older children to the youngest patients. This dictate changed gradually, with the Infants' Hospital being moved to a separate building on the Children's Hospital campus in 1923 and its eventual incorporation into the main hospital in 1959.

Rules and Regulations for 1905

A slightly enlarged housestaff operated under an extensive set of rules established in the *Children's Hospital By-laws for Housestaff* in 1905.[31] They tell us much about the hospital life of a house officer. The housestaff (house physicians) were seen as the "representatives of the visiting staff, during their absence, in all medical matters." They were "answerable in matters of administration to the Superintendent." They were to carry out "the directions of the visiting staff implicitly; directing under their guidance the treatment and care of all patients . . . and shall attend promptly to any duties assigned by the Superintendent." As an early indication of a hierarchy among house officers, "they [senior house physicians] are to consider that the junior house officers on the medical side . . . are under their direction, and all junior assistants are expected to perform such duties as may be delegated to them by the senior house physician . . ." The house physician was able to leave his assistant in charge when absent, but both could not be absent simultaneously. House physicians were expected to refer all hospital administrative matters regarding "patients and attendants requiring reprimand or discipline to the Superintendent."

　The medical house officer's work was "devoted to the medical wards." They were required to "keep such records of patients as the visiting staff directed"; enter in a book "the name and treatment of all cases of accident"; and "not publish any report or other communication in regard to any case in the hospital, except with the approval and in the name of the physician in whose service the case has been treated." Finally, "all orders given by the house officer . . . must be written in the order book," and "no medicine shall be given or treatment changed except by written order of a member of the visiting staff or a house officer."

Clearly, the house officer of that day was required to follow strict regulations. Housestaff guidelines of today, while more flexible, have their roots, lexicon, and rules of operation in the past. The house officer was required to report a contagious case requiring isolation as well as a child who was dangerously ill to the physician-in-charge and the superintendent. All orders for the comfort of the patients had to be "issued not later than seven p.m., except for emergency cases," and "it was not expected that the house officer will visit the wards after eight p.m., except in emergencies, or upon call." The house officer's absence from the wards after 8 p.m. stands in stark contrast to the long hours overnight carried out by today's housestaff.

Finally, even the rules of house officer daily living were clearly laid out, "house officers are not allowed vacations during their time of service, but leave of absence may be granted in case of necessity, by application to the Superintendent." The house officer may "not be absent over night without permission from the Superintendent," and finally, "house officers shall notify the office before inviting friends to meals." Clearly, the rules of employment were strict and carefully enforced with the expectation that they be honored and met.

Reflections

James Gamble, when reflecting in 1954 on his internship in 1912 noted, "Also, in contrast to now-a-days, there were only two medical house officers. The Junior looked after the outpatients in the morning and assisted the Senior on the ward in the afternoon. My companions were Bronson Crothers, who was my senior, and then Ed Wyman became my junior. The house officers' rooms were in the basement . . . their windows looked up at the sidewalk and I remember that they received large quantities of dust from Huntington Avenue. The uppermost windows in the central part of the building served an important purpose. They provided an excellent view of proceedings in the Red Sox [Boston Red Stockings] ballpark across the way. [The original park was situated where the buildings of Northeastern University currently reside.] The wards were . . . much more spacious than our modern wards. There was an open fireplace. It was a most pleasant and gracious room. In the medical ward three or four of the beds were usually occupied by patients with typhoid fever and an occasional polio patient was admitted to the open ward without qualm."[32]

Richard Smith, subsequently physician-in-chief from 1942 to 1946, recalled that in his house officer days of 1909 "the junior member of that group was sent to a newsstand across Huntington Avenue every Thursday noon for the new *Saturday Evening Post* . . . after the Thursday lunch, the senior house officer always read aloud to his little flock of underlings the new installment of whatever continued story the *Post* was then running . . ."[33]

Inpatient and Outpatient Diseases

A review of the census data for the hospital from 1884 to 1922 allows for an understanding of the clinical environment as well as the nature of the diseases cared for by the housestaff. Taken from five annual reports over a 38-year period, in Table 2, one can see that surgical admissions outnumbered medical inpatient admissions generally by a 2:1 to 3:1 ratio, and that medical outpatient visits equaled surgical visits by the early 1920s.

The medical housestaff cared for 50 to 110 admissions per year, with the larger number after the turn of the century most likely explained by a shortening of the length of stay (hospitalization) and facilitated by the creation of Children's Hospital–affiliated chronic-care facilities (Wellesley Convalescent Home, Sharon Sanitorium). Examination of outpatient visits reveals that here, too, surgical visits exceeded medical visits initially, but by the turn of the century medical visits equaled surgical visits as therapeutic interventions became more available for medical illnesses.

The nature of diagnoses initially were quite general and inexact (debility, gastrointestinal diseases, improper feeding, intestinal indigestion) but became more precise over time. On the inpatient services, infectious diseases predominated (pneumonia, typhoid fever, diphtheria, tuberculosis, scarlet fever, and measles), with pneumonia and typhoid fever the most prevalent. Diseases of the heart (mitral valve stenosis and regurgitation, chronic valvular disease), kidney disease (nephritis), lymphoid system diseases (chronic hypertrophy of the tonsils and adenoids) followed. Infant mortality was so great in 1882 from diarrhea that the West End Nursery and Infants' Hospital and other institutions caring for babies had to close during the summer months. However, a diagnosis of diarrhea is absent from the hospital's inpatient admissions records.[34] This is explained by the fact that children under 2 were in the Infants' Hospital on Blossom Street in

TABLE 2   Hospital Inpatients and Outpatients 1884–1922

Annual Report Number	Year Data Collected	Total Hospital Inpatients	Medical Inpatients/ Surgical Inpatients	Number of Medical Inpatients/ Number of Medical Housestaff	Total Hospital Outpatients	Medical Outpatients/ Surgical Outpatients	Inpatient Diagnoses (by prevalence)	Outpatient Diagnoses (by prevalence)
16	1884	304	98/170	98/2 = 49	601	266/344	1. Debility 2. Typhoid Fever 3. Heart Disease 4. Pneumonia 5. Gastrointestinal Diseases	N/A
26	1894	675	190/449	190/3 = 63	2,360	1,094/1,266	1. Pneumonia 2. Diphtheria 3. Typhoid Fever 4. Tuberculosis 5. Scarlet Fever	1. Improper Feeding 2. Diarrhea 3. Eczema 4. Bronchitis 5. Pertussis
34	1902	1,519	548/971	548/5 = 110	5,536	2,711*/1,825**	1. Pneumonia 2. Rheumatic Fever 3. Typhoid Fever 4. Measles 5. Tuberculosis	1. Improper Feeding 2. Bronchitis 3. Diarrhea 4. Eczema 5. Improper Diet

44	1912	565*/1,104**	565/8 = 71	5,569	2,306*/3,263**	1. Pneumonia 2. Intestinal Indigestion 3. Tuberculosis 4. Rheumatic Fever 5. Typhoid Fever	1. Regulation of Feeding 2. Intestinal Indigestion 3. Malnutrition 4. Duodenal Indigestion 5. Hypertrophy of Tonsils
54	1922	573*/4,416**	573/12 = 48	11,510	5,446*/5,894**	1. Pneumonia 2. Rheumatic Fever 3. Nephritis 4. Tuberculosis 5. Chronic Hypertrophy of Tonsils & Adenoids	1. Regulation of Feeding 2. Nasopharyngitis 3. Vaccination 4. Bronchitis 5. Otitis Media

N/A: Not available

*Includes Medicine and Neurology

**Includes Surgery, Orthopedics, Throat, and Gynecology as surgery began its differentiation (sub-specialization) after the turn of the century the West End neighborhood of Boston and were not seen by Children's Hospital physicians until the Infants' Hospital moved to the Children's campus in 1923.

On the outpatient side, problems of feeding were the primary reason for bringing a child to be seen, followed by gastrointestinal disease (diarrhea, intestinal indigestion, malnutrition), and finally less serious problems (eczema, bronchitis, otitis media, and nasopharyngitis). In general, infectious diseases predominated in the inpatient setting, while that distinction belonged to gastrointestinal ailments in the outpatient setting.

A chronologic review of those diseases requiring the attention of the medical staff offers an understanding of the daily work of the housestaff. Initially, the diagnoses tended to be less specific in the 1870s and early 1880s. Debility (weakness) made up 78% of 124 admissions in 1881. The prevalence of diphtheria and typhoid fever and the perceived importance of the germ theory led to the hiring of a hospital bacteriologist in 1895 and the creation of the first clinical laboratory.

The research and written scholarship of the faculty in the early 1900s illustrates the areas of clinical care of the day and thus the focus of housestaff care: John Lovett Morse—polio, meningitis, jaundice, nephritis, fever, scurvy, intussusception with purpura; Charles Dunn—rheumatic fever, tuberculosis, pneumonia, diarrhea; William Palmer Lucas—vaccination for dysentery, anaphylaxis to antitoxin, cerebrospinal fluid in meningitis; and Thomas Morgan Rotch—the use of X-ray, volvulus, pyloric stenosis, milk feeding.

By 1915, children with prolonged hospitalization for such prevalent chronic diseases as tuberculosis, diabetes, nephritis, rheumatism, chorea, and carditis were transferred to the Heart Hospital in Brookline, the Wellesley Convalescent Home, and the Sharon Sanitorium. With the polio epidemic of 1916, the opening of a polio clinic three mornings each week became necessary as well as the hiring of a resident pathologist and a second bacteriologist to help with diagnosis and care. Polio was becoming an increasing focus of housestaff care, reaching its peak in the 1950s. Many cases of diphtheria were admitted to the throat service. The increasing research focus of the staff on the etiology and treatment of chorea and nephritis and the role of protein sensitization in eczema and asthma led to calls for a research laboratory (to be built in 1922 with the arrival of James Gamble).

The 50th annual report, for the year 1918, took note of an increasingly active clinical laboratory with analyses of throat, sputum, spinal fluid, blood, and pleural fluid specimens. Commonly identified organisms included pneumococcus, streptococcus, staphylococcus, diphtheria, gonococcus, and mycobacteria. The annual report for 1919 drew attention to the specialized clinics set up to care for specific diseases seen with some frequency, including a nutrition clinic; an anaphylaxis, syphilis and tuberculosis clinic; and a heart clinic. It further noted research on gas bacillus and indigestion, stool input and output studies, and mechanisms of fever. All of these studies required that additional chemists and bacteriologists be added to the staff. In the annual report for the year 1922, Oscar Schloss wrote about Frederick Banting's groundbreaking research work with "the active principle of the internal secretion of the pancreas" and the hope that this held for children cared for with diabetes.

Departmental Education

From its inception, the Children's Hospital had medical education as one of its core values. Initially focused on the education of house officers and nurses, after the turn of the 20th century its focus broadened to include the education of medical students and graduate physicians. The annual report for 1906 noted, "The increasing importance of the hospital as an educational center should also be emphasized, not only in the opportunity for study on the wards given to physicians and medical students, but in the increased amount of instruction given to the nurses . . ." The annual report for 1912 stated that there were four to six students at all times in the outpatient department and that visits were made regularly to the wards by the staff with groups of students. Reflecting the hospital's national prominence and influence, the same report also noted more than 50 graduate physicians from all parts of the U.S., Canada, and beyond taking courses on diseases of children with the staff and studying both in the outpatient department and on the wards. The report further reflected on "how widely the influence of the hospital extends and how much good it does . . ." The annual report for 1916 paid a compliment to the graduate physicians: "These students serve as a source of inspiration to everyone connected with the hospital to do their very best." That same report noted that all but the youngest members of the staff were faculty members of the pediatric department at Harvard Medical School. The annual report for 1917 referenced a decrease in graduate physicians due to World War I, while the annual report for 1918 said that "the war has taught at least one lesson, namely that no one was working hard enough before the war, and that if five or six can carry the work of the Department, more can carry the work better and undertake much original investigation."

Career Achievements

In the Rotch/Morse/Schloss era, many housestaff graduates emulated their teachers in terms of their future careers. They pursued careers heavily focused on the care of the pediatric patient, generally based out of an office practice. Some also worked in hospitals, in dispensaries, or as consultants. Most taught students and residents in the context of their hospital responsibilities. In that sense, they emulated their chiefs, Rotch and Morse. Very few, until the 1910s and 1920s, pursued a more traditional academic career with a significant focus on research, thus pursuing a career similar to Schloss and the model espoused by William Welch, Halsted, and Franklin Mall at Johns Hopkins. Many achieved remarkable success, with six from the Rotch years, one from the Morse years, and one trained during the Schloss years deserving particular mention.

Charles Hunter Dunn was a 1900 graduate of Harvard Medical School and served as an interne at the Children's Hospital in 1902 under Thomas Morgan Rotch. Dunn subsequently served as an attending at the Children's Hospital and was in charge of anti-meningococcal serum produced by the Rockefeller Laboratories for distribution and use in New England. He published a two-volume text entitled *Pediatrics* and many monographs. Dunn was a member of the American Pediatric Society and its treasurer from 1910 to 1921. He served as the chief of service at the Infants' Hospital, resigning from this post in 1922 over conflicts with Harvard Medical School and Dean David Edsall.[35]

Fritz Bradley Talbot received his AB and MD degrees from Harvard University and was an interne at the Children's Hospital in 1905. A serious scholar and researcher, his focus was on intake and output studies of protein, carbohydrate, and fat; skin testing for anaphylaxis; and determination that certain types of asthma are due to egg white. His interest in the physiology of digestion led to an enhanced understanding of a number of gastrointestinal diseases. Talbot was an active member of the American Pediatric Society and served on its council and as its president in 1935–1936. He was also secretary of the New England Pediatric Society. He rose to become chief of the children's service at the MGH and professor of pediatrics at Harvard Medical School.[36]

Richard Mason Smith received his AB degree from Williams College and his MD from Harvard Medical School in 1907. He served as a house officer under Thomas Morgan Rotch in 1909 and was a close colleague of John Lovett Morse. Throughout his career, he was a highly successful practitioner, with one of the largest practices in Boston. He organized and ran a course on child hygiene at Harvard Medical School. Smith was a founding member of the American Pediatric Society and the Massachusetts Public Health Council, as well as a trustee of his alma mater, Williams College. He served as the fifth physician-in-chief of the Children's Hospital, from 1942 to 1946.[37]

Bronson Crothers received his AB and MD degrees from Harvard University and interned at the Children's Hospital under Thomas Morgan Rotch in 1912. He was a major in the U.S. Army. Crothers' special focus was on neurologic conditions in children, and he carefully studied the effects of birth injury on the central nervous system. He served as a faculty member at Harvard Medical School and developed and led pediatric neurology at both the Infants' Hospital and the Children's Hospital. He was an active member and president of the American Academy of Pediatrics and president of the American Pediatric Society in 1950–1951.[38]

James Lawder Gamble received his AB degree from Stanford University and his MD in 1910 from Harvard Medical School. He interned under Thomas Morgan Rotch at the Children's Hospital in 1912 and did further study in Vienna and Germany. He was brought back to the Children's Hospital by Oscar Schloss to run the newly constructed research laboratory in 1922. His outstanding research focused on fluid and electrolyte balance and the physiology and pathology of extracellular fluid. Gamble was appointed professor of pediatrics at Harvard Medical School. He served as the interim physician-in-chief at the time of the death of Department of Medicine Chair Kenneth Blackfan in 1941. He was a member of the Association of American Physicians, the American Society for Clinical Investigation, and the American Academy of Pediatrics, and was the first president of the Society for Pediatric Research, from 1929 through 1931, and also served as president of the American Pediatric Society in 1943–1944.[39]

Edwin Theodore Wyman graduated from Tufts College Medical School and completed his internship under Thomas Morgan Rotch in 1912. He was a major in the Indian Regiment of the British Army and was awarded the British Military Cross. He was a highly successful pediatric practitioner and a consultant to the Norwood, Fitchburg, and Burbank Hospitals, all in Massachusetts. The focus of Wyman's writings was on heliotherapy, milk, and rickets and he co-authored the textbook *The Infant and the Young Child* with John Lovett Morse and Lewis Webb Hill. In 1930, he was president of the New England Pediatric Society.[40]

Lewis Webb Hill received his AB and MD degrees from Harvard University and was an interne under John Lovett Morse in 1915. As an instructor at Harvard Medical School, the focus of his publications was on nephritis, infant nutrition, and eczema. Hill was a member of the American Academy of Pediatrics, American Medical Association, the American Pediatric Society, and the Aesculapian Club at Harvard Medical School. He was president of the New England Pediatric

Society. He co-authored a book entitled *Classics of the American Shooting Field*, a compilation of shooting stories.[41]

Samuel Zachary Levine received his AB degree from the College of the City of New York and his MD from Cornell University Medical College in 1920. He served as a house officer under Oscar Schloss in 1923. His research focused on metabolism, ketosis, respiratory exchange, and elimination of water through the skin. Levine rose to professor of pediatrics at Cornell University Medical College and physician-in-chief at New York Hospital. He was a member of the Harvey Society, the American Pediatric Society, and in 1937 served as president of the Society for Pediatric Research and president of the pediatric section of the New York Academy of Medicine. He also served as president of the American Pediatric Society in 1959–1960.[42]

The Howland Award is the highest honor bestowed on an academic pediatrician each year by the American Pediatric Society. Three of the eight would be Howland Award winners: Gamble in 1955, Bronson Crothers in 1960, and Samuel Levine in 1964.

Summation

The leadership of Rotch, Morse, and Schloss did not focus on the curriculum or the content of medical education for the housestaff. These eras would nonetheless produce a remarkable number of talented housestaff who would become the early leaders in American pediatrics.

CHAPTER III

The Blackfan/Smith Era

Formalized Training and an Educational Curriculum

1923–1946

*"During my residency, there were only 10 to 12
on the medical housestaff but what we lacked
in numbers, we made up in hours . . ."*

—R. Cannon Eley, reflecting on his time as a house officer in 1929

T HE CHILDREN'S HOSPITAL became a truly academic institution during the Blackfan/Smith era. The movement in this direction had in fact begun during the Schloss era, but that period was so brief that the evidence of academic accomplishments was less clear. The focus of the Rotch/Morse era was clinical, centered on patient care, but it gave birth to a faculty who would become the academic engine of the Blackfan/Smith era. The Blackfan era in turn would produce renowned department leaders from the housestaff, including Drs. Randolph Byers, R. Cannon Eley, Charles McKhann, Louis K. Diamond, Charles May, and Clement Smith. And it was during the constrained time of the war years in the Smith era that a plethora of additional future academic leaders would emerge from the housestaff, including Drs. Harry Shwachman, Alexander Nadas, and William Berenberg. The Blackfan/Smith era of house officer education was built within a national context of growth and maturation in internship and residency training.

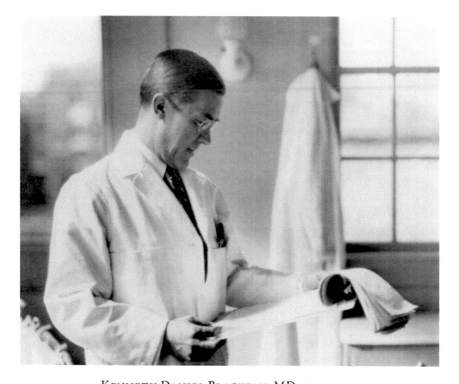

KENNETH DANIEL BLACKFAN, MD, 1923–1941

Dr. Blackfan trained a stellar group of housestaff during his 18 years as chair of the Department of Medicine. It was the "heroic era," not only for the department but also for the training of the future leaders in pediatrics.

The Children's Hospital and the Department of Medicine[1]

By the time of Kenneth Blackfan's ascendency to the chairmanship in 1923, the hospital (the Hunnewell Building, five pavilion buildings, and the Infants' Hospital) had been on the Longwood campus for nearly 10 years (Figures 1–3); the Infants' Hospital would be moved from what is now the Wolbach Building on Shattuck Street and integrated into the Children's Hospital campus in 1923. The time was ripe for a burst of expansion funded by modest hospital philanthropy and community support. The first change, in 1925, involved the purchase, renovation, and furnishing of several small townhouses on Longwood Avenue (at the current site of the Enders Building) for additional housestaff living quarters to supplement the existing space in the Hunnewell Building (Figure 2).

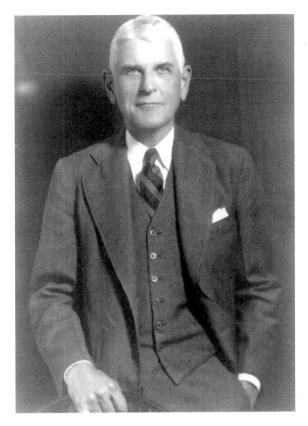

RICHARD MASON SMITH, MD, 1942–1946

Dr. Smith trained a highly capable group of housestaff during
his four short years as chair of the Department of Medicine,
this accomplished with a severely depleted staff as a result of
World War II.

In 1927, a second floor was added to the Laboratory Building, located behind
the west wing of the Hunnewell Building (Figure 2). The second floor included
a beautiful 22-by-31–foot pine-paneled room called the "Lab Study," plus four
additional laboratory rooms for the study of nutrition, blood, and infectious
diseases (Figures 4 and 5). Housestaff and faculty spent many productive hours
of study in this room, an important gathering spot for collegial interaction. The
"Lab Study" also served as a conference room for the teaching of housestaff on
the weekends and was long remembered by residents as the location of Sydney
Gellis' probing exploration of housestaff knowledge during the Charles Janeway
era. Given anonymously "in memory of Anne 1918–1926," the "Lab Study" was

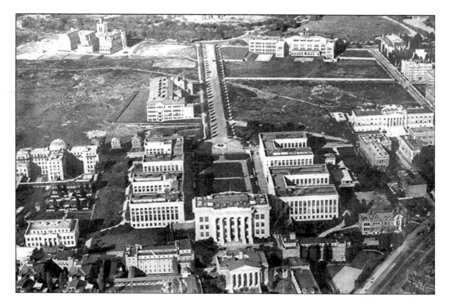

FIGURE 1   The Harvard Medical Area, circa 1921

On the left is the domed Hunnewell Building, the pavilion buildings, and the Infants'
Hospital (in the current Wolbach Building), and in the center are the buildings of Harvard
Medical School.

torn down in 1965 and reconstructed in a similar style in the 1990s in the current
hospital library as the "Gamble Reading Room."

In 1928, three floors of the east wing of the Hunnewell Building were
vacated by nursing, with the nurses temporarily housed in the Hotel Harvard
at the corner of Longwood Avenue and Huntington Avenue until moving to
their spacious new quarters in the Gardner House in 1930. An underground
tunnel between the Hunnewell Building and the Gardner House provided the
nurses with rapid and safe access to the hospital. This relocation made room
for the private wards on the first, second, and third floors, where the housestaff
ultimately worked in the late 1930s and 1940s (Figure 2). The private physician
offices of Drs. Diamond, Eley, and later Nadas were on the fourth floor.

The Bader Building was opened for neurology and psychiatry in 1930 on
the corner of Vila (now Blackfan) and Van Dyke (now Shattuck) Streets (Figure
2). This building became an important site for the education of house officers in
neurologic disease and "disturbances of mental life." The first floor contained a
gym and pool, the second floor a muscle training facility and waiting room, the
fourth and fifth floors were home to the neuropsychiatric ward service. Heliotherapy and ultraviolet light therapy were on the sixth floor.

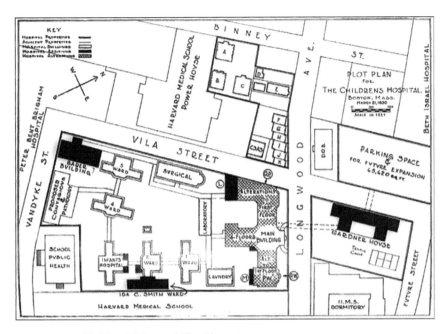

FIGURE 2   Children's Hospital Plot Plan, circa 1930

The Hunnewell Building, the pavilion buildings (Wards 1, 2, 4, and 5), and the Surgical Building were opened in 1914. The Laboratory Building opened in 1922, and the Infants' Hospital (opened in 1914) moved to a pavilion building on the campus in 1923. The Gardner House, Ida C. Smith Ward (also known as the Ida C. Smith Building), and Bader Building all opened in 1930. A–K houses purchased by Children's Hospital were used for house officer quarters. Van Dyke Street is now Shattuck Street and Vila Street is Blackfan Street.

Construction in the 1930s

Hunnewell West saw small improvements in the late 1930s and early 1940s in the record room on the first floor and the medical clinics on the second floor, as well the construction of a new otolaryngology unit on the third floor and a new X-ray department on the fourth floor (Figure 2). In addition, Ward I Lower (the Prouty Ward) was refurbished with a new porch and awnings, a new tile floor, new paintings, and tables and chairs. Ward I Upper was on the second floor. Three floors on the backside of the central wing of the Hunnewell Building were remodeled for the housestaff. The second floor contained a living room, a housestaff dining room, billiard room, and hospital library, while the third floor and two mezzanine floors provided well-furnished single rooms for the housestaff, in close proximity to the patients in the Hunnewell Building as well as the pavilion buildings.

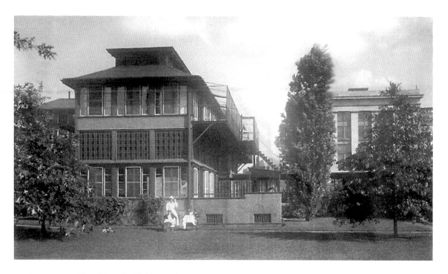

FIGURE 3   Pavilion building, circa 1930

The pavilion buildings differed only in height. One building was for medical patients, while another was home to orthopedic patients. The other three were devoted to general surgery and surgical patients.

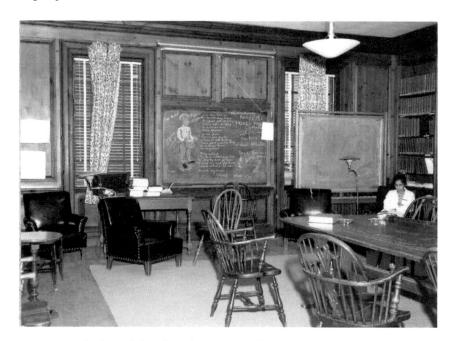

FIGURE 4   "Lab Study" in the Laboratory Building

The pine-paneled library on the second floor of the Laboratory Building was used and loved by housestaff and faculty alike.

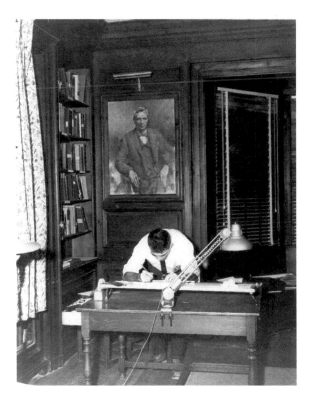

FIGURE 5   "Lab Study" in the Laboratory Building

A staff member hard at work in the library, with the portrait of James L. Gamble painted by Alexander James in the background.

As reflected upon in 1992 by Donald Fyler, a member of the medical housestaff in 1945 under Dr. Richard Smith, the Hunnewell Building was "The Hospital." The physicians' dining room on the ground floor served steaks every Friday and was "a gold mine of medical banter, stories, jokes and gossip." The telephone operator's booth was next to the dining room. "There were no beepers, only overhead paging. If you didn't answer the page, cigarette smoking, tough, long-standing employee, Josie Daly, got your attention with some-off color remark, repeated if you didn't promptly answer." The manually operated elevator was on the first floor. "As you got in the elevator you were treated to the latest joke. The operator, who had been around for years, assumed the responsibility to have a new joke every day." On the third floor was the ear, nose and throat department, where Drs. Carlyle Flake and Charles Ferguson held forth: "Flake serene, reserved and refined and Fergie ebullient, smiling, breathlessly stuttering, collected an impressive display of foreign objects retrieved from the bronchi of choking children."[2]

The final moves in the early 1930s included the opening of the Isolation and Pathology Building in 1931 and in 1934, the creation of semiprivate wards on the first floor and the fourth floor (Ward VII) in the east wing of the Hunnewell Building for private polio cases (Figure 2). Pathology, located in the Isolation and Pathology Building, was assigned to the basement, while an infectious diseases research laboratory (for Dr. McKhann in the 1930s and for Dr. Janeway in the 1940s) was located on the first floor. Two house officer rooms were located on the second floor, and isolation rooms as well as classrooms were found on the third and fourth floors. Built 62 years after the hospital's opening, the isolation rooms importantly now allowed the Children's Hospital to take care of its young patients with contagious diseases rather than sending them to Boston City Hospital as they had done in the past. Initially, the isolation unit was open five to six months each year (opening year round in the early 1940s) and focused its attention on protecting against cross infection through the use of separate rooms and by the aggregation of the more contagious patients (measles and chickenpox) on the upper floor and less contagious patients on the lower floor. There were no wards or cubicles. Ultimately at peak polio season, as many as 10 Drinker artificial respirators were in use at one time. Specially trained nurses delivered care to the patients on these units. The housestaff began their work on an isolation unit rotation in this building led by Drs. McKhann, Eley, and John Davies in the mid-1930s, and by Drs. Janeway and Davies in the 1940s.

Construction in the 1940s

A quiet period in hospital construction and renovation of close to 10 years then ensued, until the war years necessitated some modifications for efficiency and to keep costs down in 1942. This included closing the housestaff dining room and repurposing that space, combining the private and public admitting offices in one area in the Hunnewell Building, and establishing a blood and plasma bank. Although these changes were originally intended to be temporary, they remained in effect after the war. The following year, the building committee of the board of trustees began, with the assistance of the architectural firm Coolidge Shepley Bulfinch and Abbott and the construction firm Stone and Webster, to conceptualize a new inpatient facility to replace the pavilion buildings (ultimately the

Farley Building). Built in 1914, the pavilion buildings had become too expensive to heat, and the transportation of food and laundry was too slow and labor intensive.

Finally, in 1945 at the end of World War II, the hospital purchased the nearby Carnegie Building from the Carnegie Foundation. Connected by a bridge to the Bader Building and contiguous to the soon to-be-constructed Jimmy Fund Building, this building housed infectious disease laboratories for Drs. J.F. Enders, F.C. Robbins, and T.H. Weller, who would share a Nobel Prize in 1954, as well as one of the first seizure units in the U.S. for William Lennox. Additional changes in 1945 included a new hematology research laboratory for Louis K. Diamond, new examining rooms in the Hunnewell Building, and the construction of an additional floor for the Isolation and Pathology Buildings.

While the 1920s, 1930s, and 1940s saw much physical growth in the hospital footprint, beneficial for both patient care and housestaff education, larger changes were on the horizon following World War II, with the construction of facilities necessary to support the newly conceptualized Children's Medical Center.

Medical Diseases[3]

An understanding of the diseases cared for in the 1920s, 1930s, and the first half of the 1940s can offer an understanding of the patients cared for by the housestaff on the inpatient and outpatient services. As is shown in Table 1, hospital inpatient and outpatient statistics remained relatively stable between 1924 and 1945; the number of medical inpatients, however, more than doubled while medical outpatient visits decreased.

TABLE 1   Inpatient and Outpatient Statistics

	1924	1932	1940	1945
Hospital				
Inpatient Admissions	5,004	5,842	5,808	5,878
Outpatient Visits	57,693	67,466	63,374	54,750
Medicine				
Inpatient Admissions	733	1,030	1,813	1,907
Outpatient Visits	23,478	24,215	25,473	20,356

1920s

The most common medical diseases cared for in 1923 included pneumonia, encephalitis, chorea, tuberculosis, rheumatic fever, and nephritis (the majority caused by viral or bacterial pathogens). By system, the most common on the medical inpatient service (in descending order of frequency) were: pulmonary, central nervous system, otolaryngology, gastrointestinal, and circulatory diseases. In the outpatient department, the corresponding list read as follows: gastrointestinal, otolaryngology, skin, and pulmonary diseases. The number of hospital inpatient beds gradually increased to meet the rising demand, with 150 hospital beds in 1914, 211 by 1926, and 265 by 1931. The number of medical clinics grew as well to include heart, luetic (syphilis), diabetes, celiac, skin, anaphylaxis, nutrition, eczema, Schick (diphtheria), premature, breast feeding, well-baby, neurology, hematology, and Infants' Hospital discharge clinics.

Dr. Harold Stuart was appointed director of the Medical Outpatient Pediatric Department (MOPD) in 1927 to lead and administrate the growth in outpatient visits and to organize a teaching program for the housestaff (who would now rotate into the specialty clinics). On the inpatient side, the incidence of polio grew in frequency throughout the 1920s as did the incidence of rheumatic fever, bacterial meningitis, viral encephalitis, and their sequelae. A metabolic ward was opened in 1923 to care for patients with diabetes, nephritis, and epilepsy, and by 1930, Medical Ward I was filled with children with seizures, celiac, diabetes, and kidney diseases. The role of prevention of disease was evident with the establishment of a well-baby clinic, a vaccination clinic for smallpox, and a diphtheria antitoxin clinic.

The relocation of the Infants' Hospital in 1923, followed by the Bader Building and the isolation unit in 1930, and in 1931 respectively, clearly made the Children's Hospital a "general" hospital able to care for children of all ages and with all diseases. The volume of private patients grew in the 1920s but never exceeded the number of ward (non-private) patients. New facilities to support clinical care also came online and included a new X-ray department, a new record room, and a new bacteriology department, all in 1926. In addition, a new hospital physician call system and new respiratory support machines for polio cases were added in 1928 and 1929.

Finally, research by the faculty began to be focused on the most prevalent and problematic clinical diseases. The Drinker artificial respirator used in the treatment of polio (James Wilson and Charles McKhann); treatment of lead poisoning (Bronson Crothers and Randolph Byers); and the study of water metabolism (James Gamble) were all major clinical research efforts focused on common diseases. Because all had clinical implications for patients cared for on the hospital wards, the housestaff had frequent contact with superb role models who were deeply invested in clinical research.

1930s

Respiratory support and care of the polio patient and the treatment of bacterial disease with antibiotics defined the era of the 1930s and thus became both a focus of house officer care and the development of ancillary systems with accompanying departments to bolster that care.

Chronic disease and its care was also a new challenge. Congenital heart disease patients because of new diagnostic abilities were increasing in number. They joined children with rheumatic fever as a focus for inpatient and outpatient care, with the chronic sequelae of both requiring long-term care at the Wellesley Convalescent Home. Further, chronic sequelae associated with polio, diabetes, and nephritis fostered development of follow-up facilities to enhance the long-term care of these diseases. A child guidance clinic was also established in 1921, a first indication of a new focus on maintenance of health. In the new isolation unit, the epidemiology of disease was becoming more clearly defined. Scarlet fever and whooping cough made up one-third of all admissions, followed by chicken pox, diphtheria, measles, mumps, and tuberculous meningitis. By 1938–1939, the isolation unit was seeing 168 admissions each year during the six months it was open. This was especially significant in light of the fact that typhoid fever and smallpox had become a thing of the past, and ultraviolet light was becoming more effective as a barrier to cross-infection for the highly contagious measles and chickenpox.

By the 1930s, of 348 inpatient hospital beds, the medical service occupied 104, with 44 for children, 50 for infants, and 10 for premature infants. The early 1930s also saw continued growth in the number of private inpatients and the establishment of a semiprivate ward in the Hunnewell Building. An occupational therapy department was created in 1933, followed by a photography department in 1934, and the social service department grew as it became increasingly indispensable for the effective placement of patients following hospitalization. In the annual reports for 1938 and 1939, Dr. Kenneth Blackfan praised the work of the social service department, noting its essential role in care. Finally, to assist with more efficient patient care, a centralized record room was established in 1936.

Again, the research of the faculty offers an indication of the important clinical diseases of the time and those illnesses with which house officers became most familiar. The annual report in 1933 takes note of research on rickets, epilepsy, scarlet fever, dehydration, abnormal kidney physiology in Bright's disease (post-streptococcal glomerulonephritis), and antisera treatment of *Haemophilus influenzae* disease. The bacteriology laboratory, led by LeRoy Fothergill and with assistance from John Davies and Warren Wheeler, was particularly active in studies focused on *Haemophilus influenzae* meningitis, antisera treatment of bacterial disease, the immunology of pertussis, and the permeability of the cerebrospinal fluid membrane to antibiotics. In the clinic, allergic diseases and milk sensitivity, recurrences of rheumatic fever, and the early treatment of neonatal syphilis were a particular focus. Studies were also being carried out on leukemia; inadequate iron intake as a cause of anemia; hypocalcemia in rickets and its association with seizures; sodium, potassium, and CO_2 abnormalities in dehydration; and finally, immunity in *Haemophilus influenzae* disease. Interestingly, in collaborative research efforts, Harvard Medical School, Rockefeller University, the Commonwealth of Massachusetts laboratories, and the bacteriology laboratory at the Children's Hospital all collaborated to carry out important research on 30 cases of Eastern equine encephalitis. This demonstrated the broader impact of the research efforts of the department and its growing focus and emphasis on research.

The summer of 1938 saw a major summer outbreak of polio; 20% of all cases of polio in Massachusetts were cared for at the Children's Hospital. A room-size respirator able to care for up to four patients at one time was created in the basement of the Infants' Hospital. Seventeen polio cases were cared for over 16 months. Patient overflow from the isolation unit necessitated expansion into the basement of the Infants' Hospital. Admissions to the isolation unit continued to increase throughout the mid-1930s, especially in children less than 2 years of age.

In 1937, sulfa drugs (Prontylin, sulfanilamide, and sulfapyridine) were introduced into clinical care. This effective antimicrobial therapy significantly changed the work of the housestaff and created a revolutionary change in the treatment of meningitis, pneumonia, sepsis, and pyelonephritis caused by the streptococcus, pneumococcus, *Haemophilus influenzae*, and colon bacillus. Repeated lumbar punctures for the administration of antisera now became a thing of the past. Dilantin was also first used in 1938, affording the opportunity to treat childhood convulsive disorders. Simultaneously, to support optimal antibiotic therapy, the use of the bacteriology laboratory grew (to accurately determine the infecting organism) as did the chemistry laboratory (to determine optimal drug levels) and the hematology laboratory (to assess adverse effects caused by the antibiotics). As an illustration of the growth in the use of these laboratories, the bacteriology laboratory in 1928 handled 10,240 specimens; by 1938, that number and grown to 14,584 specimens and by 1939, 21,174 specimens. Chemistry and clinical pathology saw a similar growth in activity.

The annual report of 1939 also noted a further administrative reorganization of the medical clinics with general medicine, neurology, cardiac, eczema, thyroid, and endocrine clinics open in the morning, and the luetic, celiac, diabetes, allergy, rheumatic fever, and child health and development clinics in the afternoon, indicating a further differentiation and subspecialization in the outpatient department.

1940s

The first half of the 1940s, as mentioned before, saw the medical service adjusting to the impact of World War II. Faculty and housestaff numbers were depleted, new construction was put on hold, and research was focused on studies that would enhance the war effort. It was a period of extremely hard work that nonetheless engendered great satisfaction among those left behind working at the Children's Hospital. They came to feel that they were doing important work both for the children they served as well as for the country at war.

Volume on the medical service remained robust in 1940 and only thereafter did outpatient visits decrease while inpatient admissions continued to rise. In fact, private admissions in 1940 were up 18% and ward admissions were up 51%, when contrasted with 1939. Infections caused by streptococcus and meningococcus were now routinely treated with sulfa drugs, while both sulfa drugs and antisera were used to treat pneumococcus and *Haemophilus influenzae*. There remained no satisfactory treatment for tuberculosis. In the outpatient setting syphilis became less and less frequent, while rheumatic fever grew in prevalence. The Wellesley Convalescent Home and the Sharon Sanitorium were increasingly used for long-term care.

To assist with fewer available faculty, interns in 1941 began to assume rotations in the outpatient department and by 1941 the annual report noted the increased efficiency of operations of that department as a result of the interns' hard work. By 1942, the isolation unit stayed open all 12 months of the year, just in time for major polio outbreaks in 1943 and 1945. In fact, in 1945, of 534 cases in the Commonwealth of Massachusetts, 164 were cared for at the Children's Hospital. In 1943, penicillin first became available for use, carefully rationed for distribution by C.A. Janeway and J.A. Davies. In fact, so precious and limited in availability was penicillin that the urine of treated patients was collected so that the penicillin could be captured and made available for reuse. Psychologically based diseases were seen with increased frequency in the medical outpatient department, including psychogenic pain, obesity, and behavioral problems. By 1945, faculty began to return from the war to assume their leadership positions, L.W. Hill of the allergy clinic, R.C. Eley of postgraduate education, and C.D. May as director of the MOPD.

Research performed by the faculty continued unabated and perhaps with an increased intensity during the war. Nonmilitary research was also active and often groundbreaking. Its outcomes frequently involved and impacted care administered by the housestaff. Bronson Crothers and Randolph Byers continued their important studies of the sequelae of cerebral palsy, brain injury, and lead poisoning; James Gamble and Alfred Shohl intensified their work on fluid, electrolyte, and amino acid parenteral nutrition; Charles Janeway pursued his important studies on albumin and gamma globulin and their clinical use in immunodeficiency and infectious diseases; Louis K. Diamond intensified his work on blood grouping, RH and ABO incompatibility, and their role in the pathogenesis of erythroblastosis; Alan Butler and Nathan Talbot pursued their study of synthetic hormones for use in endocrine diseases of childhood, and Charles May and Harry Shwachman began their pursuit of intestinal enzyme deficiency in celiac disease and cystic fibrosis. Finally, Clement Smith, on returning from Michigan, began his studies of the physiology of the newborn and premature infant.

Departmental Leadership

The leadership of Kenneth Blackfan and Richard Smith spanned 22 years, from 1923 to 1946. Kenneth Blackfan served as chief of the Department of Medicine in what Clement Smith called "A Heroic Era," from 1923 to 1941[4] and Richard Smith served four years, from 1942 through 1945.

Blackfan's long tenure of chairmanship and remarkable leadership skills stabilized and developed the Department of Medicine as well as a remarkable number of junior faculty, many of whom passed through residency and went on to important national leadership positions. He was ably assisted by the senior faculty he had inherited from Drs. Rotch, Morse, and Schloss, including Bronson Crothers, Harold Stuart, Richard Smith, and Lewis Webb Hill. Emulating what he had observed under John Howland, his renowned chief at Johns Hopkins, he gathered around him in the first half of his tenure, Richard Smith, James Gamble, and Charles McKhann and in the second half, James Wilson, Louis

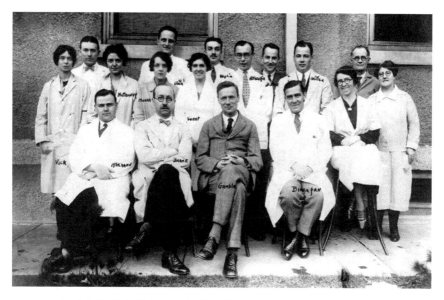

FIGURE 6   Medical Staff, Kenneth Blackfan Era, circa 1928

In front row from left to right are Drs. McKhann, Drake, Gamble, and Blackfan. In the
second row, Dr. Fothergill is fifth from the left, while in the third row, Dr. Butler (wearing a
suit) is fourth from the left.

K. Diamond, Charles May, Alan Butler, R. Cannon Eley, Randolph Byers, and
Clement Smith (Figures 6 and 7). Nearly all of these faculty, who were superb clinicians and teachers and thus powerful role models for the housestaff, remained
at the Children's Hospital and Harvard Medical School for their entire careers.
James Wilson left in 1937 to join the faculty of Wayne State University School
of Medicine; Charles McKhann went to the University of Michigan Medical
School in 1940 and then later to the Case Western Reserve University School
of Medicine; Alan Butler and Nathan Talbot joined the Children's Service at
the Massachusetts General Hospital in 1941; and Clement Smith left in 1943 to
join the Children's Hospital of Detroit as medical director (gratefully to return
in 1945).

Fourth Chair of the Department of Medicine

Kenneth Daniel Blackfan (photo, in front of chapter) was born in Cambridge,
New York, on September 8, 1883. His father, Henry S. Blackfan, practiced medi-
cine in Cambridge for many years. Kenneth Blackfan entered Albany Medical
College in 1901 and graduated at the top of his class in 1905. The year following

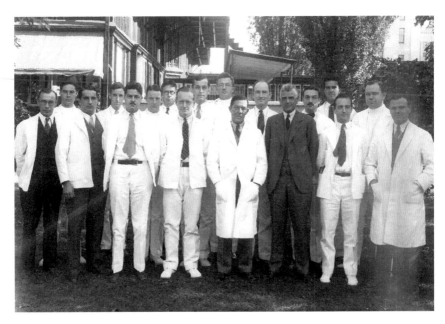

FIGURE 7   Medical Staff, Blackfan Era, circa 1931

A later picture of the Blackfan staff. In the front row from left to right: Drs. Fothergill (far left in short coat) and Diamond (second from left); Drs. Blackfan (in center with long white coat), and Richard Smith (in dark suit next to Blackfan).

his graduation was spent in pathology and bacteriology at the Albany Hospital. He then entered practice with his father. In 1908, he decided on a pediatric career and set out for Philadelphia in 1909 with a letter of introduction from Dr. Richard Pierce, a pathologist and mentor to Dr. Blackfan at the Albany Hospital. He was received by Drs. Sam Hamill and David Edsall, later to become dean of Harvard Medical School, who found a position for him as resident-in-charge at St. Vincent's Foundling Hospital in Philadelphia.

A short year later in 1911 he joined Dr. John Howland as an assistant in pediatrics at Washington University School of Medicine and a resident at St. Louis Children's Hospital. When Dr. Howland relocated to Baltimore the following year, Blackfan followed him, becoming a resident physician on the pediatric service at the Harriet Lane Home and remaining in that role until 1917. During this time, he went from instructor in pediatrics at Johns Hopkins University School of Medicine to assistant professor, and then in 1919 to associate professor. Blackfan became a full professor of pediatrics in 1920 as part of his brief sojourn to the University of Cincinnati College of Medicine.

That same year, he married Lulie A. Bridges of Louisville, Kentucky, and gained a stepson from his wife's first marriage. "Her son became as much of a son to Kenneth Blackfan, as any child could be . . . "[5] In 1923 at the age of 40, he was recruited to Boston as chair of pediatrics at Harvard Medical School; at the same time, he was appointed chief of medicine at the Children's Hospital and director of the Infants' Hospital. Ironically, as reported by Edwards (Ned) A. Park, "Dr. Howland never thought he [Dr. Blackfan] was university material . . . ." but, in Dr. Park's words, "Harvard never made a better choice."[6] Like Blackfan, Park had served under John Howland. Park, a mentor of great importance to Charles Janeway, had been head of the dispensary while Blackfan was in charge of the wards at Johns Hopkins Hospital. They remained close friends throughout their lifetimes.

In his early years at Johns Hopkins, Blackfan's research focused on hydrocephalus. Later, it turned to dehydration in diarrhea. He showed that fluid depletion was more dangerous than acidosis and undertook the treatment of dehydration by the injection of saline solution into the peritoneal cavity. In Boston, his research interests shifted to blood dyscrasias and hematologic disorders. This work culminated in his textbook *Atlas of the Blood in Childhood*, co-authored with Louis K. Diamond and published in 1944 after Blackfan's death.[7] While all of his own research was clinical in nature, he carefully followed the biochemistry, nutrition, and hematology research of his faculty with great interest.

Kenneth Blackfan was deeply interested in clinical medicine, clinical investigation, and teaching. According to his longtime chief resident and colleague James Wilson, his order of priorities were: a) the department, b) the patient, c) the student, and d) the resident.[8] He was loved and respected by his students, who called him "The Little Giant" (Figure 8).[9,10] His "devoted attitude to teaching of medical students was so apparent that sometimes his residents felt treated unfairly."[11] He was not a skillful lecturer, but his teaching of housestaff and students on the wards was close to perfection.[12] He often said a lazy or "a poor student first suggested to him a poor instructor."[13] As described by Wilson, he believed that one became a good doctor by "doing pediatrics," that one didn't become a well-rounded physician without "a real interest in progress of medical knowledge and some participation in research," and that a physician "must place the wellbeing of each individual patient before all else, including the demands of teaching and research."[14]

Blackfan believed the most effective learning came through "responsible contact with a patient," and that the most effective teaching was at the bedside or in

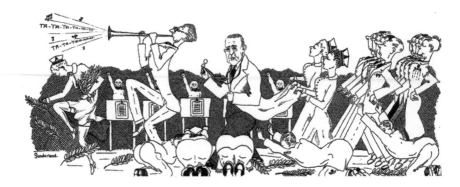

FIGURE 8   Kenneth Blackfan on Rounds: "The Processional"

A famous cartoon by Douglas A. Sunderland, MD, published in the *Journal of Pediatrics* shows Chief Resident James Wilson leading the procession followed by Dr. Blackfan, nurses, and housestaff.

the clinic. His ward rounds were relatively formal, focused around the analysis of a clinical problem (Figure 9). He believed strongly as a part of residency training in the integration of clinical and laboratory work and thus of having his residents spend a year in the biochemical or bacteriology laboratories before they started their clinical work (the origins of starting an internship in the laboratory before beginning as a house officer at the Children's Hospital). Relative to the modeling of patient care, "no child's interest was expected to be sacrificed to the demands of teaching and research, or to hospital routines, rules and customs."[15] Further, "He disliked discharging children against advice," and "he always objected to the use of the word case in reference to a patient . . . ."[16] Years later, faculty who trained as housestaff under Blackfan would with great reverence and respect recount with perfect memory to their students the principles of medical care and teaching espoused by Blackfan and transmitted both by example and through the spoken word. The Housestaff Rules of 1935 clearly articulate the high standards set by Kenneth Blackfan. The resident's absolute dedication to the assiduous care of the sick child with sensitive and regular communication with the child's parents is evident throughout these rules.

As one of the very few educated in the early 1900s who did not have a part of his training in European clinics,[17] he was an expert clinician, quite unassuming, thorough, determined, completely reasonable, and very kind with a capacity for real sympathy. Many felt his greatest contributions included the development of teachers, encouraging the research of his staff, and fostering the growth of the department. He was a member of the Society for Pediatric Research, the

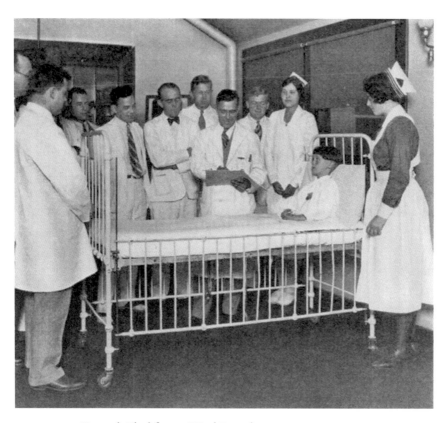

FIGURE 9   Kenneth Blackfan on Ward Rounds, circa 1929

Kenneth Blackfan reviewing notes at the bedside with his assistant Charles McKhann (at the end of the bed) and Cannon Eley (next to Dr. Blackfan on his right).

American Academy of Pediatrics, the Association of American Physicians, and the American Society for Clinical Investigation. He served on the Council of the American Pediatric Society from 1926 to 1933 and as its president in 1938. He was appointed to the first editorial board of the *Journal of Pediatrics* in 1932 when the journal was founded. When Edsall resigned as dean of Harvard Medical School in 1934, Blackfan was asked to consider the job. He declined the offer because the deanship was not a full-time job. In addition, he did not want to give up pediatrics.[18]

He loved his home in Brookline, which he and his wife planned in considerable detail. He also loved his cottage on the lake in Cambridge, New York, and its surrounding cottages for visiting guests. He suffered throughout his chairmanship from the pain of tic douloureux and residual effects of an anesthetic face, tongue, and eye on one side following surgery. The final years of his life were complicated by neoplastic disease.[19] Kenneth Blackfan, at age 58 after serving as physician-in-chief for 18 years, died on November 29, 1941, a week before the attack on Pearl Harbor. He died in Louisville, Kentucky, while taking a sabbatical year from his teaching and administrative duties due to his illness.[20]

During the difficult, roughly six-month period after Blackfan's death and prior to the appointment of a new chairman, James Gamble shouldered the challenges of departmental leadership. Then in June 1942, Richard Mason Smith was appointed chairman of the Department of Medicine. Both men were ably assisted by both senior and junior men, to whom extra burden had been added by the departure of other valued faculty to the war effort. The Department of Medicine faculty throughout the mid- and late 1930s included between 38 to 40 physicians and even increased to 47 physicians during the war years (Figures 10 and 11). This was due to an influx of younger associate and assistant physicians joining the staff. A large number of experienced faculty, such as R.C. Eley, C.D. May, H.N. Pratt, F.C. Robbins, H. Shwachman, and H.C. Stuart left the hospital to join the war effort.

The junior ranks were filled by women (Drs. L. Francis (later McMackin), G. Hutchins (later Moll), D. Moore, and A. Nauen), many of whom graduated from housestaff training at the Children's Hospital (Figure 10). This group of

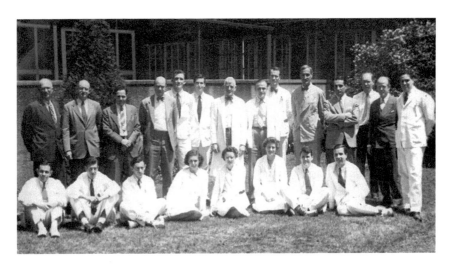

FIGURE 10   Medical Staff, Richard Smith Era in the Prouty Garden, circa 1944

Dr. Richard Smith's staff and housestaff during the war years, showing women house officers in the front row. In the second row, Dr. Richard Smith is in the middle and to his left Drs. Berenberg, Ferris, Stuart, Diamond, Pratt, Davies, and an unidentified house officer.

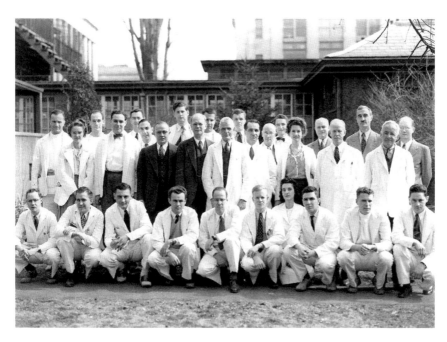

FIGURE 11   Medical Staff, Richard Smith Era, circa 1946

Dr. Richard Smith's staff in 1946, with future Nobel Prize winner Tom Weller in the front row (fifth from right). In the second row, Dr. Smith in the middle in long white coat, with Randolph Byers on his right and William Berenberg next to Dr. Byers. Dr. Diamond is on Dr. Smith's left, and to his left, Drs. Hubbard and Hutchins, the first female resident at the Children's Hospital.

dedicated physicians would assure that the clinical and teaching services continued to function effectively, while others maintained ongoing research efforts, much of it focused on studies to assist in the war effort.

Fifth Chair of the Department of Medicine

Dr. Richard Smith (photo, in front of chapter) served as physician-in-chief at the Children's Hospital and as the Thomas Morgan Rotch professor of pediatrics at Harvard from 1942 to 1946.[21] His was a fortuitous appointment. A superb clinician with excellent diagnostic acumen and a very skilled administrator, he steered the department through the challenging war years. He grew up in Northfield, Massachusetts, and graduated from the Mount Hermon School, Williams College, and Harvard Medical School. A resident in 1909 under Rotch, he served with James Gamble as the senior visiting physician throughout Kenneth Blackfan's tenure. He was a revered pediatrician, making house calls on the children of Beacon and Marlboro Streets, and applying his considerable diagnostic skills to complex pediatric problems at the Children's Hospital.

He was described as energetic and optimistic, with a certain elegance of style. A medical statesman, he founded and headed the Department of Child Health at the Harvard School of Public Health and served as president of the American Academy of Pediatrics. He was an author of more than 40 original articles, many focused on anomalies and infections of the urinary tract. Smith also authored two books, *The Baby's First Two Years* and *From Infancy to Childhood*, and served as chair of the committee on publications of the Massachusetts Medical Society. His leadership was the ideal transition for the Department of Medicine between the Blackfan and Janeway years.

The war years were difficult for the hospital, the faculty, and the housestaff. Physical plant renovations necessary for clinical care were postponed, and faculty, at the mercy of the Procurement and Assignment Division (the medical recruitment office for the government), were in increasing numbers sent overseas. Housestaff similarly were recruited, placing additional stress on the faculty remaining at the hospital. The need for encouragement for the hospital's staff, housestaff, and nurses is captured in George Von L. Meyer's (the hospital manager's) closing summary in the annual report for the year 1941, "Glory and praise will be to him who fulfills his job cheerfully, unselfishly and without thought of reward, till the battle is won."

There were other adjustments. Faculty investigation was diverted to research necessary for the war effort, including: Butler, Wilson, and Smith—the effects of low atmospheric pressure; Janeway—studies of human serum albumin used in the treatment of shock; Diamond—studies of blood grouping and blood banking; and Gamble—studies of water requirements and the effect of water deprivation on castaways. Fritz Talbot came out of retirement and his emeritus status and helped to strengthen medical student teaching in the fourth year, both at the Massachusetts General Hospital and the Children's Hospital. Students now carried out their clinical rotations year round instead of nine months each year.

On the clinical side, Charles Janeway became head of the isolation unit in 1942; Eliot Hubbard ran the outpatient department; Nathan Talbot, the endocrine clinic; William Lennox, who had joined the staff in 1944, the new seizure unit; James Gamble, assisted by Alfred Shohl, the metabolism unit and chemistry laboratory; and Louis Diamond, the blood grouping laboratory. Because these research and clinical faculty worked long hours in the hospital, they had considerable contact with the housestaff, this serving to enhance their roles as teachers, mentors, and role models. The outpatient department, into which the interns and residents now rotated, changed greatly. Diagnostic workups were now done on an outpatient rather than inpatient basis, assisted by new capabilities that had become available: X-ray, chemistry, EKG, electroencephalography, and psychometric testing. All supported outpatient evaluations as well as inpatient care.

In early 1945, faculty began to return from the war. Housestaff, older and more experienced as a result of their involvement in the war sought residency positions in large numbers. The department prepared itself for expanding clinical and research responsibilities as part of the newly envisioned Children's Medical Center.

The National Perspective

Development of Internships

Internship was created because of the ever-increasing body of information to be learned.[22,23] It was viewed as a way to round out the learning experience for medical students. Some Midwestern schools saw it as a fifth year of medical school. However, most educators favored a hospital-based, practical experience. Before World War I, the majority of internships were one to two years in length. They existed as a service to the hospital but with little accompanying educational experience. Initially, because few positions were available to medical school graduates, internship was reserved for the elite. Landing one was highly competitive as they were "the ticket" for future jobs in hospitals or prestigious practices. Hospitals, in turn, increasingly came to view the internship as an effective way to meet both patient care and manpower needs. Medical schools happily saw internships as a way to fulfill the school's educational responsibilities to its students without directly assuming control of that experience. Medical schools contributed educational content to the programs but did so without authority. Gradually, internship came to be viewed as the final and necessary experience for general practice.

While service predominated and education was sporadic and variable from hospital to hospital, a number of forces combined to direct greater attention toward the intern's education. Interns began to select the programs where education by the faculty was excellent and resident responsibility for patient care was valued. In 1914, the first listing of available internships in U.S. hospitals was published. At that time, only one-half of graduates in the United States could obtain internships. By 1932, sufficient openings existed in hospitals to supply 95% of graduates with internships.[24] As the number of jobs grew, the elite status of internship gave way to the view that internship was a necessary component of training for all physicians.

The Council on Medical Education of the American Medical Association began examining hospitals to approve internships and in 1919 published its *Essentials for Approved Internship*, thereby converting internship from "on the job training" to an educational process. Failure to comply with the educational standards of the Council on Medical Education resulted in disapproval as a site for training. Internships assured education though conferences, lectures, rounds, and other formal and informal instruction; added a teaching component as a result of instruction of medical students; offered the opportunity to participate in clinical research; and through limitation on the number of patients cared for, afforded the opportunity for reading and study of patients' diseases.[25] By 1939, only 344 unfilled positions existed among internships in the United States, but by 1945, the number of internships was increasing faster than the production of graduates by medical schools.[26] Two-year internships disappeared by World War II, and the growth in the number of residencies continued at a robust pace.

As the number of unfilled slots in academic hospitals and especially community hospitals increased even further, foreign medical graduates began to fill these positions. These unfilled slots, in turn, placed increasing pressure on hospitals to successfully recruit interns, a feat that was accomplished through an increased emphasis on excellent education, improved salaries and living conditions, and increased intern responsibility for patients under their care. City hospitals, academic hospitals, and hospitals with large ward services thrived. Aging community hospitals, hospitals with large numbers of private patients, and less prestigious hospitals did not fare as well in filling open slots. The Hill–Burton Act (passed in 1946 by Congress to build new hospitals and renovate and expand older hospitals following World War II) helped to correct this deficiency in house officer manpower by enhancing the attractiveness of hospitals to perspective intern and resident applicants.

Finally, internships, which initially were "rotating" (rotation among all clinical areas), "straight" (a focus on medicine or surgery), or "mixed" (a cross between "rotating" and "straight"), began to be seen as the first year in the training of a resident in medicine, surgery, pediatrics, gynecology, neurology, and psychiatry. As the residency movement began to flourish, internships were increasingly incorporated into these various specialties.

Development of Residencies

The modern residency had its origins at Johns Hopkins Hospital in the 1890s, modeled after the German university clinic "house assistant."[27,28] Developed by medical giants William Osler, chief of medicine, and William Halsted, chief of surgery at Johns Hopkins Hospital, the residency appointment was to follow internship and was seen as an intensive educational experience so as to become proficient in a field of practice. The selected resident was among the chosen; in William Osler's words, "a superior man who wishes to do scientific hospital work."[29] The resident was trained to become a future academic leader in medicine, with the capacity to do important research and to develop new knowledge and scholarship. However, two other models were created that challenged this hospital-based model; one combined clinical work with a formal degree such as an MS or ScD (instituted after World War I at Harvard, Columbia, and New York University), and the other consisted of short fee-driven, six-week courses with a resultant certificate of achievement. The number of residencies and residents were relatively few prior to and immediately after World War I. Most were created by Johns Hopkins' disciples such as Harvey Cushing at the Peter Bent Brigham Hospital in Boston, Kenneth Blackfan at the University of Cincinnati College of Medicine and then at Harvard Medical School, and George Heuver, a surgical protégé of Halsted, at Cornell University Medical College. These residencies were small in size, reserved for the elite, generally three years in length, and relatively few in number.

Following World War I, the number of residencies grew dramatically. Published in 1925, the first list of residencies contained 29 programs.[30] In 1928, *The Essentials of Residency* was published, giving guidance on the nature of "an approved" residency program. By 1929, the number of residencies had increased to 1,909 and existed in the majority of disciplines.[31] As the hospital-based model achieved wider and wider acceptance, the graduate school degree model and the six-week course model began losing their popularity and were phased out by the late 1930s. The current residency model developed rapidly in the 1930s. The number of slots was pyramidal in nature and the levels of responsibility and authority increased from "assistant resident," to "senior assistant resident," to the pinnacle "resident" (or in some cases, chief resident). The "resident" (chief resident) often served for a number of years as an assistant to the department chairman—Kenneth Blackfan serving as John Howland's chief resident for six years at Johns Hopkins and Charles McKhann and James Wilson serving for similarly extended periods of time for Kenneth Blackfan in Boston. In addition, the resident's rotations often involved sicker and more complex patients than those cared for by the interns, and the degree of responsibility assumed by the resident increased with each subsequent year.

By the 1930s, while the residency was no longer just for the elite and had become the accepted model of training, all was not well. There were problems in lack of uniformity of training, low standards, and, as noted, until the late 1930s residual commercial courses and degree programs.

National Oversight Boards

The first specialty board (ophthalmology) was established in 1917, the pediatric board in 1933, and by 1937, 14 boards had been established under the auspices of the Advisory Board of Medical Specialties (ABMS).[32] ABMS served, however, in an advisory capacity. The hospital maintained local control, with only minimal input from the medical school. While each board had its own rules and regulations, certification as a specialist in a given discipline generally required completion of an approved residency, followed by several years of practice and successful completion of an examination. All these initiatives served to enhance and upgrade the quality of the residency. By the mid-1940s there were more residencies than internships, and there was no body limiting the growth in the number of residencies that were proving so beneficial to hospitals. As a result, during World War II there were as many as 1,500 residency vacancies. In fact, residency had become less elite. As the body of specialized knowledge increased, the time was ripe for the beginning of the fellowship movement, which developed and flourished following World War II.

The university had never wanted responsibility for the residency, and by the 1940s, control of the residency had been fully transferred by default to the hospital and to the profession. As the boards became the protectors of the quality of the *resident graduates*, the Residency Review Committee of the Accreditation Council on Graduate Medical Education (ACGME) became the protector of the quality of the *residency program*. This took on particular importance as the hospital assumed increasing responsibility (and authority through the department chairman) of the residency. Stringent rules and regulations, long work hours, low or absent salaries, and excessive service demands with less attention to resident education became evident. These negative factors were ameliorated by the innate professionalism of the resident (unions that existed in other lines of work in the 1930s and 1940s had not found traction in medicine), the ability of the resident to pick the hospital of his or her choice for residency that offered the best teaching and independence in care, and the small "family" nature of the faculty/resident relationship that created a comfortable and supportive environment. An area of confusion and even conflict surrounded the role and status of the house officer as a trainee versus employee; this would become an increasing challenge in future years.

Educational Mission and Rules and Regulations[33]

The annual reports during the Rotch/Morse/Schloss era and early Blackfan era were relatively silent on the goals and the philosophy of the training of house officers.[34] This clearly changed in the Blackfan/Smith era when the hospital superintendent, Ida C. Smith, and later the manager, George Von L. Meyer, and the physician-in-chief, Kenneth Blackfan, regularly commented on the training curriculum, the goals and mission of the training program, and the impact of external forces on the program.[35] (The hospital superintendent and later manager are akin in responsibility to the current combined roles of the hospital chief executive officer and chief operating officer.)

The teaching function of the hospital was clearly articulated in the annual report for the year 1923: "It is now generally recognized that medical teaching and research act as a stimulus to the best kind of medical and surgical care of patients. The entire hospital and Outpatient Department of the Children's Hospital are used for the training of medical students and the teaching of graduates in medicine. The teaching is done, under close supervision, with careful regard for the patients, by instructors chosen from the faculty of the Harvard Medical School. The visiting medical and surgical staff of the Hospital is composed of these teachers." This statement also emphasized the central teaching role of the hospital for medical student education and the interdependence of the two institutions.

Medical education, however, was not solely for students and housestaff. Mirroring what was occurring at a national level, it was also for postgraduate education, thereby fulfilling an additional central educational mission of the hospital, to serve as a source of continuing education for practicing physicians. These graduate physicians, through their exposure to clinical care and research as "fellows in research," acquired new information and knowledge and then carried their experiences back to their practices and throughout the United States, enhancing the influence of the hospital and contributing to the welfare of sick children. This endeavor achieved its most profound impact following World War II in the postgraduate courses of R. Cannon Eley and in the international training programs of Charles A. Janeway. In the 65th annual report in the mid-1930s, Kenneth Blackfan emphasized the central role of the educational mission of the hospital and department, noting, "Students are the best spur and whip I know." And in an annual report published immediately prior to World War II, the hospital expressed particular satisfaction in the achievements of its medical and surgical departments in furthering the quality of medicine through its graduates and "in the work that they are doing to raise the standards of medicine in all parts of the United States and in many foreign lands."

Training Requirements

The influence of the American Board of Pediatrics can first be seen in 1934 when it instituted board certification and promulgated new house officer training requirements, specifically 16½ months of house officer training (a level comparable to interns and junior residents today) and 12 months or more of resident training (a level comparable to senior residents today). This influence would extend in time to training requirements for clinical fellows. Training requirements for housestaff and fellowship *programs* would ultimately be assumed by the ACGME's residency review committees with oversight over postgraduate training in all specialties and subspecialties. The Board of Pediatrics would maintain its role of certification of competency of *residents* and *fellows*.

Throughout the 1930s, the curriculum of the housestaff at the Children's Hospital was widened in keeping with board recommendations and included exposure to general and subspecialty clinics, the Boston Lying-In (the site for education in the care of the newborn infant), the isolation and the neurological units, the admitting department, the private ward services, and the Convalescent Home in Wellesley, Massachusetts and the Sharon Sanitorium in Sharon, Massachusetts. In annual reports during this period, Kenneth Blackfan emphasized the importance of housestaff coming from "Class A" medical schools, thereby helping to assure the highest quality interns and residents for the training program. In addition, he strongly emphasized the great importance of housestaff clinical exposure during residency for their future careers in medicine.

The World War II years moved the emphasis from an enriched curriculum and longer duration of training to one that was focused on a shorter educational experience and reduced breadth of clinical exposure, often with less supervision. An important educational change occurred as interns now increasingly began to work in the MOPD to cover for faculty involved in the war effort. There also were fewer graduate physicians available to help out. Residents moved rapidly to faculty staff positions following residency. All housestaff and faculty worked harder. Yet all knew that this situation was temporary and soon the housestaff ranks began to fill with returning physicians, who in Richard Smith's words in the annual report for 1945, "were well experienced, well-seasoned and capable of excellent judgment."

House Officer Rules and Regulations

Much can be learned about the life of a house officer in the Blackfan era through the Rules for House Officers published by the hospital in 1928. These rules clearly indicate that the superintendent was the head of, and had overall responsibility for, the hospital under the board of managers: "the Visiting Staff has charge of the patients under the Superintendent," and the "Senior House officer is in charge of his service under the Visiting Staff and the Superintendent." The reporting structure of the visiting staff to the superintendent, in contrast to the chief of service today, is clearly evident in these regulations. The hierarchy of house officer reporting structure is also evident. The junior house officer was responsible to the senior house officer, and was "to obey his orders, except that orders from the Visiting Staff or Superintendent annul those of the Senior House Officer." Consults could not be called by a house officer without the permission of the visiting physician staff; the junior house officer could serve as the admitting physician but was "not at liberty to refuse on his own responsibility any patient recommended by a member of the Staff" and, if he suspected a contagious disease, this matter required referral to the superintendent. Pathologic, bacteriologic, and serologic slips were "to be filled out with extreme care" (as were death certificates) and "no record of any case shall be taken, copied or published . . . without the consent or direction of the Superintendent." Communication with parents was clearly a priority and an important responsibility; house officers were expected to see all parents during visiting hours from 2 to 4 p.m. on Saturday before leaving the hospital.

The rules were equally stringent relative to house officer behavior: "smoking is forbidden in the hospital, except in the house officer's quarters . . ., no music or noise will be allowed . . . after 10:30 p.m., no books or magazines are to be taken from the Library, and no house officer may be away all day or overnight, or leave the hospital for a vacation, without the permission of the administration," again emphasizing the supervisory role of the superintendent over housestaff activities and the strict rules under which the house officer lived. Because the hospital lacked isolation facilities until 1931, rules for the handling of cases suspected or known to be contagious in nature were also carefully laid out in great detail in the 1928 rules.

The Housestaff Rules of 1935 contained a marked change in emphasis and tone.[36] The chief of the Department of Medicine now clearly ran the medical service. Medical education, house officer clinical rotations, and teaching rounds and conferences were laid out in great detail. The schedule of the day and expectations in the area of patient care on each rotation were clearly enunciated. Medical students were responsible to house officers and house officers to senior or junior residents. All housestaff were responsible to the visiting physician and their "appointed" associate visiting physician, the latter "who acts as advisor to the residents and house officers." House officer rules had now been liberalized but continued to be written down in great detail so that the responsibilities of a house officer were clear. This is in contrast to today where the rules are embedded in the housestaff culture ("a hidden curriculum") and passed down each year largely by word of mouth.

Each house officer enjoyed a two-week vacation once "all discharge records are finished and a substitute has been secured acceptable to the Chief of Service." Each house officer and resident had every other night and every other weekend off duty, "provided his work is up-to-date and his patients are in condition to be left under another's supervision." A strong sense of responsibility for one's patient at all times whether on or off duty was seen as an essential characteristic of the good doctor. The call schedule of every other night and every other weekend off would last for 30 years until the mid-1960s. Currently, considerable reflection and discussion is occurring over the meaning of *responsible* patient care, especially with regard to trainee work schedules and the impact of those schedules on patient safety.

A typical schedule for week one included overnight duty on Monday, Wednesday, and Saturday and Sunday nights and for week two, on Tuesday, Thursday, and Friday nights. "Married men can be accepted as house officers or residents only with a clear understanding that their time on duty will be the same as for others." They were required to remain in the hospital at all times when on duty and to live in their assigned rooms while on call. These restrictive rules made marriage quite infrequent in the period between the two world wars. House officers could function as "acting resident" in the absence of their resident. "Residents and house officers should change their posts at different times so that an entirely new staff shall not take charge of a group of patients at any time," this in contrast to today when change of shifts occur at the same time to allow for coordinated planning among multiple services and caregivers. They "should take care to be in touch with the telephone operator at all times and should not go out of hearing of the call bell without notifying the operator. The operator should also be notified when each man leaves the hospital." The importance of immediate availability on a service is evident in these orders. Senior medical students or "clinical clerks" (medical students) were told that "much interesting and instructive experience can be gained at night, Sundays and holidays" and clinical clerks were instructed to supply themselves with a microscope, hemocytometer, otoscope, ophthalmoscope, stethoscope, tape measure, and percussion hammer. The value of student learning through observation and being present on the service as much as possible is evident in these instructions.

Additional Rules and Regulations

Relative to laboratory data, "laboratory methods must not be used to the exclusion of the important information which may be gained from a careful and thoughtful consideration of the facts obtained from the history and physical examination." Relative to the admission of patients, this "important administrative function that often requires tact and judgment, should not take over the detailed diagnostic and therapeutic duties of the resident and house officer in charge of the patient." Financial matters as well as admission to the private ward were to be decided upon by the admitting department and the parents. Again contagion was to be ruled out, notes brief, admissions not detailed, the ward personnel notified about a patient by the admitting resident, and the parent interviewed by the inpatient staff before leaving the hospital. The function of the admitting department was one of triage and efficient transfer of the patient to the ward service and its staff for care. Admissions would continue in this manner until the mid-1980s when emergency department physicians began to fully work up the patient in the emergency room before transferring the child to the floor.

The medical record of the house officer on the floor was to emphasize why the patient was admitted and a full history, physical examination, and provisional diagnosis was to be completed and placed in the chart promptly. The discharge summary, done within a week of discharge (a more liberal policy than today), was to be "concise, informative and as interesting as possible" and suitable to be sent to the referring physician. The completeness of the record was reviewed at "history meeting" each week with the associate visiting physician ("resident advisor") for accuracy, completeness, correct grammar, and correct classification of disease. The resident advisor's responsibility was quite similar to the hospitalist of today, though with a greater administrative role and less of a clinical role than occurs currently. "Interesting cases" were selected for discussion with Dr. Blackfan at Friday's chief's conference.

A high standard for communication with parents was emphasized both in its nature and its timing. It was to be done in a "sympathetic, simple and consistent" manner and be "honest and understandable to avoid destroying the parent's confidence in the care their child was receiving." It was to occur on admission, daily by phone between 6:30 p.m. and 7:30 p.m., on Saturdays between 2 p.m. and 4 p.m., and on discharge.

The most difficult communication for a house officer involved the death of a child. In addition to reporting and explaining the death to the best of their ability, house officers were also expected to obtain permission for an autopsy whenever possible. Autopsies often provided a cause of death and were thus valuable for clinical, educational, and research purposes. Occasionally, they served a legal purpose in a medical legal case. If the medical examiner refused the case, the house officer was instructed to obtain an autopsy. House officers needed to obtain written permission from both parents for an autopsy and have the death certificate witnessed upon its completion.

In the case of medical emergencies, a clear order of individuals to be called was laid out for the housestaff (in descending order of priority); during the day, resident advisors; visiting staff; Drs. Kenneth Blackfan, Charles McKhann, and James Wilson; and at night, resident advisors; James Wilson and Charles McKhann; visiting staff; and Kenneth Blackfan. This list clearly shows the faculty Blackfan most depended upon for the clinical service and for supervision of the housestaff.

Finally, all active residents had to have a temporary medical license and "strikers" (unpaid substitutes for house officers) could only be used with the approval of the director of the hospital.

The Housestaff

Housestaff training matured remarkably during the tenure of Kenneth Blackfan. While men of significant stature were trained in the Rotch/Morse/Schloss years, housestaff training during that early era was essentially an apprenticeship with little emphasis on house staff education. House officers were relatively few in number. The length of training was brief, and there was little progression of authority and responsibility based on length of training (with the only change being in nomenclature from junior to senior house officer). Rotations through different services experienced by all house officers were just beginning.

In 1923, two different types of postgraduate training existed: housestaff (house physicians and resident physicians) and graduate physicians. The latter were men who had received prior residency training and came to the Children's Hospital for a refresher course (today called continuing medical education [CME] courses). They attended clinics, teaching and staff conferences, and participated in investigation. Some were volunteers and some were paid by Harvard Medical School. All carried their experiences with them, spreading what they had learned throughout the U.S. The housestaff nomenclature in descending order of seniority included resident physician and assistant resident physician (comparable to a PL-3 today), house officer or house physician (comparable to a PL-2 today), and intern (comparable to a PL-1 today). This system of titles existed until World War II, when the laboratory-based internship year was eliminated, and the length of training of a house officer and resident was reduced in length. As the war years ended, greater differentiation among the residency years was reinstated, and the commencement of clinical fellowships in hematology and general pediatrics began.

During the Blackfan and Smith eras, as shown in Table 2, there were on average 13 house officers in the 1920s, 17 in the 1930s, and 12 to17 in the first half of the 1940s.

A group of remarkable men were trained in the 1920s and 1930s, and they were joined by women who entered the training program in the 1940s. The first women housestaff were appointed in 1942, specifically Gretchen Hutchins as resident on July 1, 1942, and Lillian Francis as house officer on July 13, 1942. In the annual report for 1941, Acting Physician-in-Chief James Gamble had this to say about the executive committee's decision to accept women as interns and residents: "This does not imply a disadvantage to the intern service. On the contrary, the quality of our service is better sustained by taking well trained physicians [women] than accepting men applicants whose qualifications are below our established standards." Writing in the following year's annual report, Richard Smith noted, "It is hoped that it [accepting women as house officers] may become a permanent policy." (Figures 10 and 11)

These and subsequent appointments of women had been necessitated by the depleted number of male housestaff. Dr. Clifford S. Grulee, Jr., a house officer under Dr. Blackfan, reported that the first aborted attempt at a female house

TABLE 2   Medical Housestaff Statistics

Average Number/Year (by decade)							
	1880s	1890s	1900s	1910s	1920s	1930s	1940–1945
Total	2	3	6	8	13	17	12–17
Male/Female	2/0	3/0	6/0	8/0	13/0	17/0	15/1–2
Chief Residents	0	0	0	0	0	0	0

officer appointment occurred in the late 1930s. He recalled the following in a letter: "Prior to the late thirties the idea of a female house officer was unthinkable. Imagine Dr. Blackfan's surprise when a petite, attractive and very intelligent Filipino lady arrived to start her residency training. It apparently had not occurred to anyone that . . . Children's Hospital only appointed males to its housestaff. Her room and meals were finally arranged for in the nursing residence, and she was put to work as a research fellow."[37]

The first clinical fellows were appointed in 1944 in hematology under Louis K. Diamond, specifically Drs. R. Denton, S. Israels, and F.L. Plachte. In 1945, four fellows, three in hematology, Drs. D.H. Clement, A.L. Luhby, and E.A. Gregory and one in general pediatrics, Dr. I. Dogramaci, later to become Secretary General of the International Pediatric Association, were appointed.

A large number of distinguished future leaders were trained during the Blackfan era. The first two appointments by Dr. Blackfan in 1923 were such, Charles McKhann as a resident and Dr. Randolph Byers as a house officer. They would be joined in the 1920s, 1930s, and 1940s by a large number of remarkable housestaff as is shown in Table 3.

Curriculum and Rotations[38]

The resident curriculum saw gradual but constant changes in the organization and structure of rotations throughout the Blackfan/Smith era.[39] When Kenneth Blackfan assumed leadership of the department, the typical length of training for a house officer was 15 months.

The first extension in the length of training took place in 1930, when it was expanded to 21 months. For a given house officer, 12 of the 21 months were spent in rotations on the general medical wards of the Children's Hospital as well as the Infants' Hospital; three months on the surgical, orthopedic, and otolaryngology services; three months in the isolation unit; and three months in the MOPD and in the well-baby and "newly born" clinic (Figures 12–14). The most senior of the group served as director of the MOPD. This 21-month period was always preceded by a year of training in a general hospital or research exposure in a specialty department (bacteriology or pathology).

In 1933, the 21 months of training was further divided, 15 months for a house officer and six months for a resident. House officers were appointed at three-month intervals, in contrast to today when all begin in mid- to late June of a given year. The house officer spent six months on the general medical wards, six months on the wards of the Infants' Hospital, and three months on

TABLE 3   Selected Medical Housestaff During the Blackfan and Smith Eras

1920s			
R.K. Byers	(1923)	R. Ganz	(1926)
S.H. Clifford	(1929)	C.G. McKhann	(1925)
R.C. Eley	(1929)	A.H. Washburn	(1924)
G.M. Guest	(1925)	J.L. Wilson	(1929)
H.E. Gallup	(1928)		
1930s			
J.M. Baty	(1939)	C.D. May	(1939)
D.H. Clement	(1939)	A.S. Ross	(1932)
J.A. Davies	(1934)	C.A. Smith	(1931)
L.K. Diamond	(1931)	L. Snedeker	(1933)
E.C. Curnen, Jr.	(1939)	W.J. Turtle	(1935)
L. Fothergill	(1930)	P.V. Woolley, Jr.	(1937)
1940s			
F.H. Allen	(1942)	F.C. Moll	(1946)
W. Berenberg	(1944)	A.S. Nadas	(1943)
M. Birdsong	(1941)	R.S. Paine	(1944)
J.H. Dingle	(1940)	W. Pfeffer, Jr	(1946)
I.A. Dogramaci	(1946)	E.L. Pratt	(1944)
E.C. Dyer	(1941 and 1946)	D.G. Prugh	(1944)
B.G. Ferris	(1948) *	F.C. Robbins	(1941)
L. Francis	(1944)	L. Schwab	(1944)
G. Haydock	(1946)	H. Shwachman	(1940)
J.P. Hubbell, Jr.	(1947) *	N. Talbot	(1940)
G. Hutchins	(1946)	W.M. Wallace	(1942)
C. Lowe	(1946)	T.H. Weller	(1942 and 1946)

(*Last year of house officer training)

the otolaryngology and neurology services, while the resident served for three months as director of the MOPD and three months on the isolation unit.

In 1934, the American Board of Pediatrics requirements changed from 21 months to 28½ months, in which 16½ months was spent as a house officer and 12 months as a resident. In response to the board's directives, the schedule of

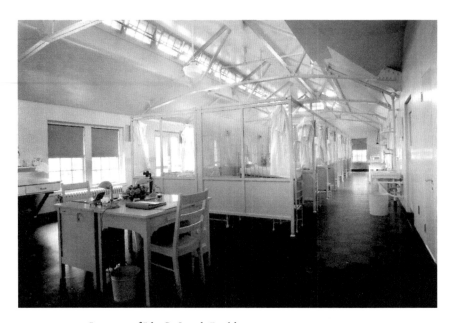

FIGURE 12   Interior of Ida C. Smith Building, circa 1930s

This photo shows a nursing station and cubicles, with hand washing sinks on the right.

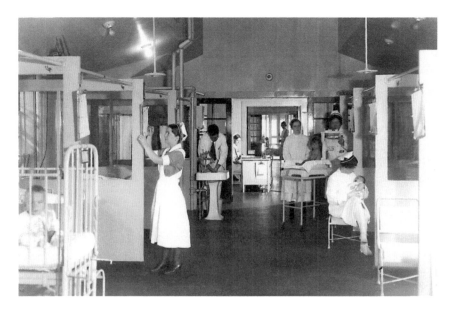

FIGURE 13   Ward in the Infants' Hospital

This photo shows a ward in the Infants' Hospital, with a nursing student wearing the traditional cap, staff nurses, and a house officer at the sink.

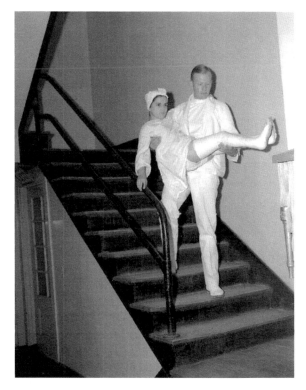

FIGURE 14   House Officer and Patient in the 1920s
Taken before elevators, this photo shows a house officer
carrying a patient down the stairs.

rotations was further differentiated for a house officer into eight two-month
rotations plus two weeks for vacation, for a total of 16½ months. For a resident,
rotations were divided into three four-month blocks (Table 4) for a total of 12
months. As before, this 28½-month training was preceded by a year in a general
hospital or in a specialty department. As is shown in Table 4, the rotations
included general ward services, specialty services (neuropsychiatric, isolation,
newborn, admitting), and the outpatient department.

By 1937, the resident's duration of training was extended from 12 months to
16½ months, for a total duration of training of 32 months plus one month for
vacation. This, coupled with the intern year of 12 months training, resulted in
a total length of training of 45 months—nine months longer than today! The
resident's 16½ months of training consisted of: four months on the Children's
Upper and Lower, four months on the Infants' Upper and Lower, four months

TABLE 4   Housestaff Rotations in 1934

House Officer Rotations (Two months on each service)	Resident Rotations (Four months on each service)
Service 1 Children's Lower	Service 1 Children's Upper and Lower
Service 2 Neuropsychiatric Ward	Service 2 Infants' Upper and Lower
Service 3 Infants' Upper	Service 3 Isolation Unit or the MOPD
Service 4 Children's Upper	
Service 5 Infants' Lower	
Service 6 Boston-Lying In, MOPD, Specialty Clinics	
Service 7 Admitting, MOPD	
Service 8 Isolation Unit, MOPD	

MOPD: Medical Outpatient Pediatric Department

on Admitting and on the Infants' Ward, four months on the isolation unit or in the MOPD, and two weeks for vacation. The resident's 16½ months was further differentiated into time as an assistant resident and time as a resident.

Two pathways were available to those interested in taking the certifying examination of the American Board of Pediatrics. Option one was a practice pathway that included 12 months of internship, 16½ months of house officer training, and 24 months of practice, for a total of 52½ months. The second option was an academic pathway that included 12 months of internship, 16½ months of house officership, and 16½ months of residency, for a total of 45 months of training.

As the war began, the length of house officer training was dramatically shortened. By 1942, the internship year was eliminated, house officership was reduced from 16 ½ months to 12 months, and the residency was also shortened. A year later, house officer training was further reduced in length to nine months and, while the residency years still existed, the number of both house officers (now called interns) and residents was significantly reduced. In 1943, the housestaff at Children's Hospital consisted of nine interns, three assistant residents, and one resident, placing a heightened workload on the housestaff as well as the junior faculty. Thus both the residents and the faculty, sacrificed during the war years. By 1945, as World War II ended, the residency at Children's Hospital experienced an influx of older and more experienced men wishing to complete their residency. In fact by 1945, the resident positions were filled until January of

1947. The residency was now poised to begin a period of growth and expansion in the number of young men and women to be trained during the Janeway years.

Reflections

The tone of the Blackfan and Smith era for housestaff is captured by reflections of the faculty, often offered many years after they served as residents.

The hours of work and the nature of that work as well as the hospital environment in which the housestaff labored was very different from today as captured in comments by R. Cannon Eley, a house officer and devoted faculty member, concerning his training during this period. "During my internship and residency there were only 10 to 12 on the medical housestaff, but what we lacked in numbers, we made up in hours."[40] And reflecting on the nature of hospital work, Louis K. Diamond wrote, "I was assigned to Dr. Charles F. McKhann (Dr. Blackfan's right hand man) and saw Dr. Blackfan often. Charles F. McKhann worked my tail off but did he teach me pediatrics."[41] Further commenting on salary, living quarters, and board, Diamond went on to say, "I lived in Vanderbilt Hall in a room for $4/week and managed to eat but not to get fat on about $15/week . . . and even saved a few dollars."

The housestaff as we have seen were all men until the war years. The hospital culture did not encourage marriage during training as noted by Randolph K. Byer's reflections, "When I arrived for internship in September in 1921, the hospital [Massachusetts General Hospital's emergency department] was dumbfounded and didn't know what to do. No one had ever had the temerity to be married after being appointed to one of their internships."[42]

The war years were the needed impetus for admission of women with the supportive backing of Drs. Gamble and Richard Smith. Yet not all accepted the change easily. When the first female intern, Lillian Francis, commenced her first day of work, a senior doctor announced, "It has come to this!"[43]

Finally, issues of adequate salary and living quarters were not a high priority. The privilege of working at the institution was felt to be more than sufficient compensation, as noted again by this reflection of Louis K. Diamond, "Dr. Blackfan offered me a pediatric appointment for October 1928 if I'd study hematology and start a blood laboratory under him, instead of going to New York Hospital. Accepted. No question of any pay or living quarters . . . . In due time we'd see what could be found."

Clearly a culture of professional behavior was a well understood guiding principle of Dr. Blackfan's: "a sense of responsibility for his patients at all times whether he is off duty or not is an essential characteristic of the good doctor."[44] R. Cannon Eley's reflections add emphasis to this culture, "Interns had two nights off every alternate weekend. If a patient was admitted when an intern was going off duty, the intern could not leave the Hospital and turn the case over to his relief, but had to follow the patient to the conclusion of the case, no matter how much time it took out of his night off."[45]

Career Achievements

Among the limited number of housestaff in the Blackfan/Smith era, a remarkable number went on to make important contributions to American pediatrics (Table 5). The Society for Pediatric Research and the American Pediatric Society were relatively young organizations, making the number of presidents from the Children's Hospital quite remarkable.

In the arena of honors, Louis K. Diamond and Alexander Nadas were invited to give the Blackfan lecture; Charles D. May, Louis K. Diamond, Nathan B. Talbot, and Harry Shwachman received the E. Mead Johnson Award for outstanding research achievements; and Louis K. Diamond and Clement Smith received the highly prestigious Howland Award from the American Pediatric Society.

TABLE 5   Career Achievements

Department Chairs	
James Baty	Tufts University School of Medicine
Mac Lemore Birdsong	University of Virginia School of Medicine
Edward Curnen	Columbia University College of Physicians and Surgeons
R. Cannon Eley	Brown University Medical School
Edward Pratt	University of Cincinnati School of Medicine
Frederick Robbins	Case Western Reserve University School of Medicine
Alan Ross	McGill University School of Medicine
Nathan Talbot	Harvard Medical School
James Wilson	University of Michigan Medical School
Warren Wheeler	University of Kentucky College of Medicine
Paul Woolley	Wayne State University School of Medicine

TABLE 5   Career Achievements *(Cont.)*

Presidents of Pediatric Organizations		
American Academy of Pediatrics	Richard Smith	1940
	Stuart Clifford	1957
American Pediatric Society	Alfred Washburn	1960
	James Wilson	1963
	Clement Smith	1965
	Alan Ross	1967
	Louis K. Diamond	1968
	Warren Wheeler	1972
	Edward Pratt	1975
	Alexander Nadas	1982
Society for Pediatric Research	Charles McKhann	1936
	William Wallace	1957
	Edward Pratt	1958
Editors of *Pediatrics*	Charles May	
	Clement Smith	

Summation

Clement Smith, in his carefully chronicled early history of the hospital, *The Children's Hospital of Boston, Built Better than They Knew*, has called the Blackfan era "a heroic era" and indeed it was. Great strides were made in the treatment of diseases, the faculty grew and assumed leadership roles in Boston and beyond, and formalized training and an educational curriculum instituted by both Blackfan and Smith allowed residency training to enter the modern age. This period of time prepared the hospital and the department well for the remarkable growth in graduate medical education that would ensue following World War II.

CHAPTER IV

The Janeway Era

Residency with a National and
International Impact
1946–1974

"When you are surrounded by giants, their presence
made you reach to a higher level . . ."

~ Fred Mandell, reflecting on his time as a house officer in 1969

IN 1946, DR. CHARLES A. JANEWAY was appointed chairman of the Department of Medicine. He served for 28 years, until 1974, as the Thomas Morgan Rotch professor of pediatrics at Harvard Medical School and physician-in-chief at the Children's Hospital. This period was a time of expansion and optimism for academic medicine, with the creation of new medical schools, the initiation and rapid growth of the National Institutes of Health (NIH), the infusion of new federal research dollars, and remarkable acceleration in subspecialty medicine. The Children's Hospital in Boston would see the formation of the Children's Medical Center in 1948 and the Children's Hospital Medical Center in 1959, new physical facilities added to its campus (the Farley, Fegan, and Enders Buildings), and stable and capable administrative and departmental leadership. The Department of Medicine, in turn, would witness significant growth in its faculty as well as maturation in its three core missions of care, research, and education. While Charles Janeway's tenure is widely recognized for the development of the department's medical divisions and his contributions to international pediatrics, great progress in research, the training of academic leaders, and his innovations

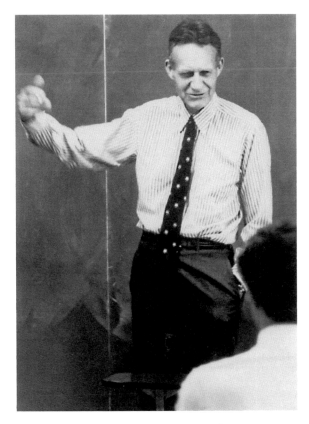

CHARLES ALDERSON JANEWAY, MD, 1946–1974

Dr. Janeway trained over 1,000 housestaff during his 28 years
as chair of the Department of Medicine. He introduced
significant innovations in the curriculum and educated a cadre
of leaders who have had a national and international impact.

in residency and fellowship training—both in the U.S. and abroad—also stand
out among his most significant accomplishments.

The Children's Hospital and the Department of Medicine

Extraordinary medical progress is evident in the post–World War II years when
contrasted with the 1930s and '40s. This was especially true in the areas of biochemistry, microbiology, and pharmacology. The development of sulfonamides
in the late 1930s and penicillin in the early 1940s led to a marked reduction in

the life-threatening nature of ear and mastoid infections, pneumonia, osteomyelitis, scarlet fever, and meningitis. New drugs were being developed to control the growth of malignant cells, and the introduction of ACTH and cortisone heralded a new era of hormonal therapy. Synthetic diets were being constructed to bypass biochemical blocks found in metabolic diseases that often resulted in mental retardation, an example being the avoidance of phenylalanine in patients with phenylketonuria. Finally, improved tissue culture techniques enabled the discovery and ultimately the production of vaccines to control measles, rubella, and polio. The chemist and biologist "had placed the equivalent of a sharp scalpel in the hands of the physician."[1] This evolution in patient care as a result of effective new therapies deeply altered the natural history of the diseases that housestaff treated on the wards and in the clinics.

Driven by these advances, the pattern of hospitalization changed markedly. A growing appreciation of the advantages of caring for a child at home and the significant cost associated with prolonged care in the hospital also had an impact on which children were hospitalized and for how long. Numerous changes were taking place in outpatient care as well. Total medical outpatient visits increased in part due to remarkable increases in the number of visits to the emergency room, and the development of subspecialties further fueled outpatient growth.[2]

A transition was also underway in childhood morbidity and mortality. Infectious disease, the major cause of mortality in the pre–World War II era, was replaced by prematurity, congenital malformations, accidents, malignancy, and chronic diseases. Morbidity from acute illness, which occupied much of the house officer's time, continued to increase as the hospital served a larger number of Boston's inner-city children. In addition, pediatricians and the community hospitals were referring more complex patients for evaluation and treatment to the Children's Hospital. These statistics were augmented by the "new morbidities," children with behavioral problems, learning disabilities, and variations in development.

All of these changes resulted in significant pressures on the Department of Medicine. They included the need to train more physicians with general pediatric skills (general hospital-based physicians, pediatric housestaff, and community physicians) as well as academic consultants with subspecialty pediatric skills. The resultant increase in staff, in turn, generated increased demand for more modern inpatient and outpatient facilities and greater use of the hospital's resources. At the same time, burgeoning research activity led to a heightened demand for new research space.

As shown in Tables 1 and 2, for the period between 1946 and 1970, a significantly changed inpatient and outpatient picture for the Department of Medicine emerged. When considering short-term admissions for the period between 1946 and 1970, annual admissions increased by approximately 56%, length of stay decreased from 15 days to 9.5 days, and hospital days (the number of days in which a patient stays overnight) had stabilized around 34,000 per year. Long-term admissions fell markedly, reaching a nadir in 1966 and then rising gradually until reaching 346 admissions in 1970; length of stay had decreased progressively, from 70 days to 16 days, resulting in hospital days falling precipitously, from 32,692 to 5,580. In the aggregate, total medical admissions increased from 2,725 in 1946 to 3,880 in 1970 and represented one-third of all hospital admissions.[3] This growth in the volume of inpatients as well as more rapid turnover of patients placed heightened emphasis on inpatient care for the housestaff and led to more intense and longer hours of work when on duty.

In the ambulatory department, the number of medical visits more than tripled between 1946 and 1970, rising to 87,523 in 1970 and making up 47% of

TABLE 1   Medical In-patient Services Admissions

	1946–47	1956–57	1966–67	1968–69	1969–70*
Short-Term Admissions					
Admissions	2,261	2,917	3,527	3,545	3,534
Hospital Days	33,926	26,484	35,315	34,389	33,608
Average Stay per Admission (Days)	15	8.4	10	9.7	9.5
Long-Term Admissions					
Admissions	464	253	146	282	346
Hospital Days	32,692	20,757	6,801	5,905	5,580
Average length of Stay per Admission (Days)	70	82	47	21	16
Total Medical Admissions†	2,725	3,007	3,673	3,827	3,880
Total Admissions, All Services	—	—	12,133	12,153	12,379
Percent Admissions, Medical Service	—	—	—	31.5%	31.3%

* Figures include Cardiology, which became a separate department in 1970.

† Statistics for Medical patients on all Nursing Divisions

TABLE 2　Medical Ambulatory Service

Visits to Clinics	1946–47	1956–57	1966–67	1968–69	1969–70
Family Health Care Unit	—	2,839	4,308	3,148	4,639
Outpatient Department	13,470	7,701	5,677	10,847	9,296
Adolescent Unit	—	4,807	7,801	5,509	4,980
Medical Subspecialty Clinics	10,890	10,057	15,285	16,753	17,307
Emergency Clinic	—	5,506	41,631	43,936	51,301
TOTAL VISITS (Medical)	24,360	30,910	74,702	80,193	87,523
TOTAL VISITS (All Services)	—	—	154,697	172,350	185,204
PERCENT MEDICAL VISITS	—	—	48.5%	46%	47%

all hospital outpatient visits (Table 2). This increase was explained primarily by a 10-fold increase in emergency room visits between 1956 and 1970 reflecting the increasing importance of the emergency room for the delivery of care and the education of the house staff. Medical subspecialty and family health care unit clinic visits also showed increases in volume, while Medical Outpatient Pediatric Department (MOPD) visits decreased and adolescent unit visits varied over the same time period.[4] A pattern was now established with the emergency clinic (in the later Janeway years called emergency department) and the general medical clinics being largely the domain of the housestaff and the specialty clinics the domain of a growing cadre of clinical fellows. The rapid growth in the volume of emergency department visits was a reflection of the increased use of this 24-hour service by inner city children and their families at the Children's Hospital and throughout the U.S.

Changes in the Nature of Disease

The face of pediatric disease was undergoing noticeable change. Poliomyelitis, which occupied so much time and effort in the Blackfan era, was one such example. The last big epidemic occurred at the Children's Hospital in the summer of 1955 and following that difficult year, the number of cases of polio began to drop due to the increasing availability and use of the Salk vaccine and later the Sabin vaccine.

The Isolation Building, so important in the Blackfan era, was enlarged by three additional floors in 1949 to care for patients who required strict isolation. In the 1950s, however, the need for isolation slowly decreased. Isolation of patients infected with resistant bacteria was achieved by individual isolation rooms in the Farley Building. By 1963, no polio cases were admitted to the hospital.

What we had come to expect when confronted with rheumatic fever was also changing. Hospitalization for the disease in the 1940s and 1950s frequently resulted in stays of up to four—or even 12—months and many patients were re-hospitalized for recurrences. By the 1960s, the duration of the initial attack was shortened, recurrences were eliminated by penicillin prophylaxis, and the number of hospitalized days plummeted. The House of the Good Samaritan on Binney Street was converted from a facility solely for the care of rheumatic fever to the care of chronic medical diseases such as rheumatoid arthritis and hemophilia. Torn down in the early 1980s to make room for construction of the Brigham and Women's Hospital, the House of the Good Samaritan had been established in 1860 for patients with tuberculosis. In the late 1860s, it took on an orthopedic focus for children with rickets, and as that disease disappeared, by the early 1920s, it was used predominantly for children with rheumatic fever convalescing from rheumatic heart disease. Housestaff began to rotate through the Good Samaritan in the early 1950s.[5]

Further impacting the ongoing changes in pediatric medicine were the advent of vaccines, gamma globulin, and antimicrobial therapy, which reduced the risk of infection to the point that generous hours for parental visiting, play therapy, and in-hospital schooling were instituted to better meet the child's psychological needs. All of these changes in the nature of medical diseases seen in the hospital setting as well as enhanced interdisciplinary care made it more difficult for attendings to oversee minute-to-minute changes in care, thereby enhancing the role of the housestaff as the primary custodians of patient care.

In 1970, 224 deaths were recorded on the medical service, accounting for 5.8% of the 3,880 admissions that year. The major causes of death had changed, with their percentage distribution as follows: neoplastic disease (38%), congenital malformations (15%), diseases of the newborn (15%), heart disease (13%), and unknown causes (8%). Infection made up only 6% of all deaths.[6] These figures stand in stark contrast to the Rotch, Morse, Schloss, Blackfan, and Smith eras when infections, including diarrhea, typhoid, tuberculosis, pneumonia, polio, and common viral exanthems, were in aggregate by far the most common causes of death at the Children's Hospital.

Subspecialty Medicine

The 1960s and 1970s saw a remarkable maturation of the divisions in the Department of Medicine. This significantly impacted the nature of the diseases cared for in the inpatient and outpatient settings, thereby altering the focus of resident education. Separate wards devoted to specialized care (cardiology, tumor therapy, psychiatry, and neurology) resulted in month-long rotation exposures for the housestaff to subspecialty disease. New subspecialty clinics sprang up as diseases were aggregated for care in the outpatient department. The emergency room with its vast volume of common diseases became an excellent educational site for residents, and community hospital rotations (North Shore Children's Hospital and Beverly Hospital) presented an opportunity to learn community-based pediatrics. The growth in the subspecialty divisions and the care that they carried out served to differentiate the pre–World War II experience from the post–World War II experience for the housestaff.

Inpatient Setting

By the early 1960s, with the hospital's newly instituted open-door admission policy (admitting all patients regardless of their ability to pay), inpatient services were very busy with more complex patients. The beds were now full; the patients were sicker.

During the 1950s when the patient volume was decreasing, the courtesy staff (community physicians who were given privileges to admit patients to the hospital) were invited to care for their patients in the hospital. This resulted in more physicians with whom the housestaff had to interact, risking a diminished sense of personal responsibility by house officers for the care of these private patients. Technology and testing were proliferating. The nature of disease was leading to interdepartmental integration of care (for example, medical and surgical treatment of heart disease), and interdisciplinary care now involved social workers, psychologists, education specialists, play therapists, and pharmacists. The hospital setting was indeed a more complex and busier environment for the house officer.

Outpatient Setting

As previously noted, the needs of urban Boston children with acute illness had swelled the emergency room volume. The Children's Hospital had become a community hospital for Boston. Referrals also increased from community pediatricians and from community hospitals to the emergency department for subsequent triage to the MOPD, diagnostic or subspecialty clinics, or the inpatient service. Emergency room care was imperfect because of its episodic nature, but it was a rich educational experience for the housestaff.

The general medical and subspecialty clinics meanwhile grew in complexity. The MOPD cared for difficult chronic illnesses too complex and too time consuming for the busy practicing physician, specifically functional disorders, behavioral problems, learning disabilities, developmental delay, enuresis, and encopresis. These conditions would become an important part of the complete training of a house officer, especially those entering practice. The growth of the divisions in the Department of Medicine led to increased subspecialty clinic volume, a number of new clinics, and the need to offer both general care as well as care of specific diseases. The aggregation of rare diseases in a single specialty clinic offered advantages for improved patient care and disease-specific support groups for parents, as well as opportunities for clinical research and for teaching residents and fellows. Congenital heart disease, diabetes, cystic fibrosis, hematology, and endocrine clinics were now joined by newly established genetic, arthritis, phenylketonuria, hemophilia, infectious disease, and pulmonary clinics.

For the resident, the very busy hospital in the 1960s and 1970s was a wonderful educational environment as long as the tasks associated with patient care were carefully balanced with education and learning. Janeway, as a Johns Hopkins graduate, was most likely mindful of the interdependency of patients and medical education and of the memorable quote of William Osler, "He who studies medicine without books sails on uncharted seas, but he who studies medicine without patients does not go to sea at all."[7] The balance between education and service would become an increasing challenge during the Mary Ellen Avery and David Nathan eras still to come.

Program Development and Building Construction

The Children's Hospital Center was conceptualized during the war years. Initially, it was an organizational integration of existing institutions and later involved a sizable construction effort encompassing the Farley, Fegan, and Enders Buildings. The integration of institutions within the Children's Hospital had, in fact, begun when the Infants' Hospital moved to the Longwood campus (Figure 1). By 1923, the care of children less than two years of age by faculty and housestaff in the Infants' Hospital had become fully integrated with the care of children in the Children's Hospital. As reported in a 1951 publication, the Sharon Sanitarium, the House of the Good Samaritan, and the Children's Cancer Research Foundation administratively and organizationally joined the Children's Hospital, thereby forming the Children's Medical Center.[8,9] By the 1960s and 1970s, with long hospitalizations for rheumatic diseases becoming

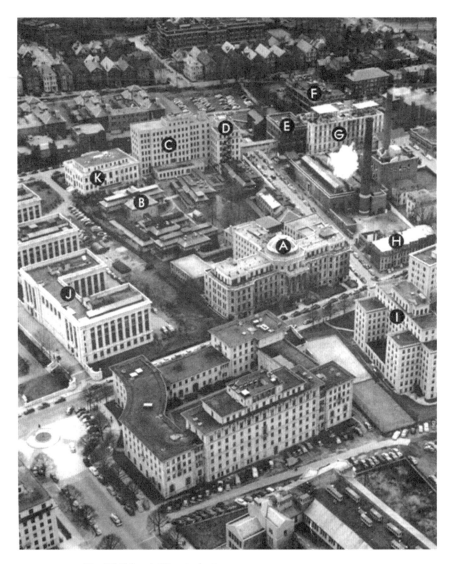

FIGURE 1   The Children's Hospital, circa 1950

This photo shows the Children's Hospital in 1950, including the Hunnewell Building (A), the cottages and the Infants' Hospital (B), the Pathology and Isolation Building (C), the Bader Building (D), the Carnegie Building (E), the House of the Good Samaritan (F), the Jimmy Fund Building (G), House officer quarters (H), the Gardner House (I) Harvard Medical School (J), the old Harvard School of Public Health, now the hospital's Administration Building (K).

less common, the wards of the House of the Good Samaritan became filled with chronic diseases, including diabetes, osteomyelitis, endocarditis, and hemophilia. This institution was also home to cutting-edge clinical research in the endocrine division, led by John Crigler, division chief and author of one of the most influential papers in endocrinology ever published in *Pediatrics*, specifically describing the first use of glucocorticosteroid treatment of congenital adrenal hyperplasia. It also housed the group led by Benedict Massell, renowned for his clinical work and research efforts related to rheumatic fever. Medical house officers during the Janeway years cared for all of these patients as a part of their inpatient rotation assignments.

The Sharon Sanitarium was founded in 1891 for the care of tuberculosis and later it, too, turned its attention to rheumatic fever and polio. In 1946 it was incorporated into the Children's Hospital, specifically as an inpatient floor (the Sharon Cardiovascular Unit) in the Farley Building, with medical house officers regularly rotating through. Here they witnessed firsthand the medical benefits of close collaboration of medical and surgical expertise in the care of cardiac disease. Finally, the Children's Cancer Research Foundation, dedicated to the treatment of children with cancer, garnered broad financial support and a new physical home, the Jimmy Fund Building on Binney Street (across the street from the current Smith and Dana-Farber Cancer Institute Buildings).[10,11] The National Cancer Institute of the U.S. Public Health Service, the Variety Clubs of New England, the Boston Braves, and the film industry all provided funding. Children with cancer were admitted for their inpatient care to the tumor therapy floor on the eighth floor of the Farley Building. The medical housestaff supervised by the oncology faculty actively cared for these patients during their tumor therapy rotation.

The Farley Building, first conceptualized during the war and named for the hospital's president John Wells Farley (1944–1959), was completed in 1956 (Figure 2). All of the pavilions were razed to make room for the Farley Building except the Ida C. Smith Building (which housed Park Gerald's genetic research efforts and the adolescent unit during the Janeway and Avery eras and today houses the Massachusetts and Rhode Island Regional Center for Poison Control and Prevention) and the Laboratory Building. The Farley Building contained the medical and surgical inpatient units as well as the radiology department and clinical laboratories. It was also the site of the cardiology, the tumor therapy, the newborn, and neurology services and thus was the major site of training of housestaff throughout the Janeway and Avery eras. Its beds would be moved to a new clinical building in 1986, later named the Berthiaume Family Building, but

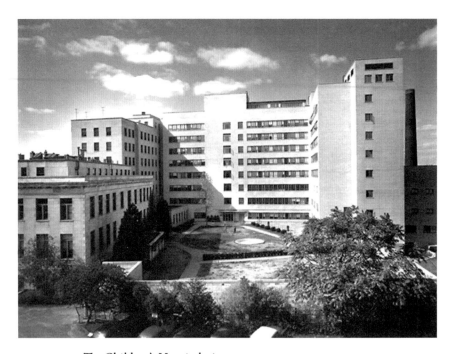

FIGURE 2 The Children's Hospital, circa 1955

This photo shows the Administration Building (now the Wolbach Building) on the left, the new Farley Building in the center and on the right, and the Prouty Garden in the center.

it still stands today, housing clinical laboratories, ambulatory procedure units, administrative support offices, and the hospital's cafeteria.

The Fegan Building was completed in 1967, replacing the crowded ambulatory clinics located in the Hunnewell Building. The Fegan Building was named in honor of its benefactor, a Brookline resident and an heiress to her grandfather's fortune from the clipper ship trade. Eleven stories high and located behind the Hunnewell Building (center and east wings), it housed a vast array of medical and surgical clinics and became a major site for general and subspecialty work carried out by the housestaff, fellows, and faculty. The space located between the Farley Building, the Ida C. Smith Building, and the Fegan Building was to be a parking lot. The Prouty family, which had supported the refurnishing of one of the pavilion buildings, Medical Ward I, thoughtfully decided that it should instead be a garden for the enjoyment of staff and patients alike, and wisely specified that it could never be infringed upon by new building construction. Its gardens and space, designed by the firm of Frederick Law Olmstead, remain today a respite from the surrounding concrete and intensity of the hospital's work and a joy for all who visit (Figures 2 and 3).[12] As space becomes increasingly constrained in the current era on the Longwood campus, remaining faithful to the Prouty family's initial wish and intention has become increasingly difficult and is a cause of considerable consternation even today.

The last large building to be completed during the Janeway era was the new Research Building (in 1976 named the Research Laboratories in honor of John Franklin Enders, Children's Hospital faculty member and 1954 Nobel Prize recipient for his work with the poliovirus). It replaced the laboratories that existed in the Laboratory Building. The research work of James Gamble, Allan Butler, William Wallace, Jack Metcoff, and Robert Schwartz, which focused on the regulation of body fluids and their composition, took place in this building, so too Louis K. Diamond's research in hematology, David Gitlin's work in immunology, and Charles D. Cook's work on respiratory mechanics. In 1964, this revered building was taken down to make room for construction of the hospital entrance to the Farley Building on Blackfan Street and the later-to-be-constructed Fegan Building. Temporary research quarters were created (above the hyperbaric chamber and under the current hospital library) for basic research, which included genetics under Park Gerald, hematology under David Nathan,

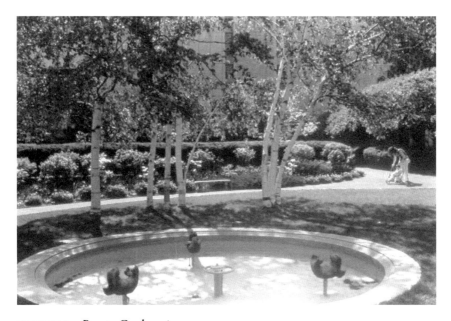

FIGURE 3   Prouty Garden, circa 1970s

Thanks to the Prouty family's generosity, this garden at Children's Hospital serves as a cherished gift to patients, families, and visitors who enjoy its open space, beauty, and serenity.

immunology under Fred Rosen, and nephrology under Francis Fellers. This juxtaposition of disciplines allowed for intellectual collaboration as well as the sharing of costly equipment. Clinical investigation was simultaneously pushed forward by the creation of the Clinical Research Center, capably led by John Crigler and located on Division 20, one of the wards in the Farley Building. "Divisions" replaced the nomenclature of wards from the Blackfan era. The floors were divided into divisions based on the type of care needed and consisted of one-, two-, and four-bed rooms.

Thirteen stories tall, the Enders Building had floors for patients with mental retardation, medical and surgical research, animal laboratories, and the Enders Auditorium (to be renamed in 2010 in honor of deeply admired and brilliant Children's Hospital surgeon Judah Folkman). It was physically enlarged by about 40% in the 1980s under the leadership of David Nathan when junior and senior Howard Hughes Medical Institute investigators were appointed. While the housestaff spent relatively little time in this building, it reflected the hospital's active pursuit of new knowledge in the conquest of disease. The housestaff, through the example set by both the physical structures as well as the individuals who labored in these buildings, came to fully appreciate the importance of excellent research in confronting medical disease. In turn, this culture became an important example and compass for their future careers.

With the demolition of the Laboratory Building, the housestaff lost a lovely library for reading and reflection. As temporizing solutions, the medical and surgical services built their own departmental libraries in the Hunnewell, Farley, Bader, and Fegan buildings, and the hospital built a small library on the first floor of the Hunnewell Building. An anonymous donor gave a small medical library (housed in a prior patient room) for use by the medical housestaff while on call on the seventh floor of the Farley Building. All existed until the construction of the new hospital library (and the reconstruction of the old "Lab Study" room of a prior era as the Gamble Reading Room, although not with the original wood) in the 1990s.[13]

The care of the newborn in the Blackfan/Smith era occurred in the Infants' Hospital. In the early 1930s, a new ward was added to the Boston Lying-In Hospital, providing an air-conditioned nursery for infants born prematurely. The Lying-In Hospital was located at the junction of Longwood and Louis Pasteur Avenues. In 1933, Stuart Clifford was made pediatrician-in-chief responsible for the care of the premature and newborn at the Children's Hospital, the Infants' Hospital, and the Boston Lying-In Hospital. The housestaff rotated to all three institutions for care of the newborn and premature infant until the arrival of

Dr. Avery in 1974. From that time forward, neonatal care would be carried out at the Children's Hospital, the Brigham and Women's Hospital, and the Beth Israel Hospital.[14]

None of the pavilion buildings remain from the original 1914 hospital plan, but the Ida C. Smith building, built in 1930, still stands. In 1974, it became the home of Roswell Gallagher and Robert Masland's adolescent unit. This unit became an important site for the education of Harvard medical students and medical housestaff.

Departmental Leadership

Sixth Chair of the Department of Medicine

Charles A. Janeway (photo, front of chapter) assumed chairmanship of the Department of Medicine at the Children's Hospital in 1946. In 1942, when a 20-bed isolation unit opened at the Children's Hospital, Janeway moved from his infectious disease position at the Peter Bent Brigham Hospital to assume a similar role at the Children's Hospital. He was, in fact, being "groomed" by four years of "on the job" training at the Children's Hospital for his subsequent responsibilities as physician-in-chief.[15]

Janeway came from an illustrious medical family. Grandson of Dr. Edward Janeway, professor of pathology, dean of Bellevue Medical College, and responsible for the description of the (Janeway) lesions in bacterial endocarditis, Charles Janeway was born in New York City in 1909. His father, Dr. Theodore Janeway, was the first full-time professor of medicine and physician-in-chief at Johns Hopkins Hospital. He attended the Calvert School in Baltimore, Milton Academy in Massachusetts, and Yale College in New Haven, graduating in 1930. His first two years of medical school were spent at Cornell, his last two at Johns Hopkins. These years included the happy occasion in July 1931 of his marriage to Betty Bradley, a Vassar College graduate and social work student at Simmons College.

Medical school was followed by two years of medical residency on Harvard's fourth medical service at Boston City Hospital under Soma Weiss. (Harvard Medical School, Boston University School of Medicine, and Tufts University School of Medicine all had responsibility for medical and surgical services at the Boston City Hospital.) He spent the next year as an assistant resident in medicine at Johns Hopkins Hospital. He then returned to Boston for two years of fellowship training, from 1937 to 1939, in bacteriology and immunology under Professor Hans Zinsser at Harvard Medical School. This training would germinate his lifelong interest in infection and immunity. In 1939, he moved to the Peter Bent Brigham Hospital under his old chief Soma Weiss, with responsibility for the infectious disease service. The following year, Soma Weiss introduced Janeway to Edwin Cohn, who was leading a wartime effort at Harvard Medical School studying the products of plasma fractionation, the use of albumin as a plasma expander in the treatment of shock, and the use of gamma globulin to prevent hepatitis. Janeway participated actively in clinical trials with the Cohn group while continuing his own studies of beta hemolytic streptococcus, the mode of action of sulfa drugs, and immunotransfusion for the treatment of sepsis. Janeway's move to the Children's Hospital was precipitated by several changes in the early 1940s. Kenneth Blackfan's death in 1941 opened the position of physician-in-chief at the Children's Hospital. This was followed by Soma Weiss' death in 1942 and the selection of George Thorn as physician-in-chief of the Peter Bent Brigham Hospital. Janeway remained at the Children's Hospital until his death in 1981.

Charles A. Janeway's impact would be far reaching at the Children's Hospital and Harvard Medical School as well as nationally and internationally.[16] He saw health and disease as a "seamless whole" from biology to behavior.[17] He developed 19 subspecialty divisions, ranging from somatic disciplines such as hematology, immunology, infectious disease, and cardiology to psychiatry, adolescent medicine, and family health care. These divisions became an extraordinary resource for the education of students, house officers, and subspecialty fellows. He, in fact, built the largest academic pediatric service in the United States.

Remarkably, Janeway continued his research until the mid-1960s while administering the large and burgeoning Department of Medicine. His research group accomplished major advances in immunology and an enhanced understanding of immune deficiency diseases (along with Ogden Bruton at Walter Reed Hospital and Fred Rosen, Sherwin Kevy, and David Gitlin at the Children's Hospital), describing the first four cases of X-linked agammaglobulinemia during an address given at a Society for Pediatric Research meeting.[18] He also initiated the clinical use of gamma globulin in the treatment of agammaglobulinemia and forged a better understanding of the thymus gland, lymphocyte, and complement complexities. With Gitlin and Rosen, he studied plasma proteins in the nephrotic syndrome and showed that foreign proteins could produce nephritis in rabbits. Additionally, he demonstrated that serum complement was involved in nephritis. In the late 1950s and 1960s, he focused on the metabolism of albumin and serum globulins, furthered an understanding of the pathogenesis and complications of agammaglobulinemia, and described new immunodeficiency diseases.

In the 28 years of his stewardship, Janeway attracted over 1,000 young trainees to his housestaff, training them as generalists, subspecialists, and academic leaders. He was an active participant on a weekly basis at all teaching conferences involving the housestaff. He felt strongly that education must have a scientific basis. Janeway also believed that the psychosocial aspects of medical care were essential to the complete training of a pediatrician. He thought that clinical medicine was optimally taught at the bedside and emphasized the importance of an in-depth history and physical examination linking the pathophysiology of the disease with the psychosocial elements of the illness.

A proponent of the Socratic method of teaching over didactic lectures, he held that medicine is not a "spectator sport," but that the resident learns best by "doing" under careful supervision.[19] He laid out four principles of effective residency education. First, "teaching above all must be by example" carried out in "a training program in which service is an integral part." Janeway fervently believed that "service is the hallmark of our profession." Second, he emphasized that increasing responsibility over the years of training was critical, but always under the watchful eye of diligent supervisors to assure optimal care. Third, he believed that effective education occurred through problem solving rather than rote learning. Finally, he reasoned that "teaching must be as relevant as possible to the demands of society, both in the present and in the future."[20,21] Charles Janeway believed internship and residency were the last vestiges of the apprentice system, in which one learns under the supervision of a master.[22,23] He emphasized the importance of graded responsibility and warned against over-emphasis of service at the expense of education.

While less in evidence to the residents and fellows, Janeway's contribution to international pediatrics was monumental. During his sabbaticals and overseas trips for the International Pediatric Association, Louis K. Diamond, chief of hematology/oncology, and William Berenberg, a superior generalist pediatrician trained under Richard Smith, assumed Janeway's role, serving as interim chief. His greatest contributions were made through his involvement with the Iran Foundation in developing the medical school in Shiraz between 1955 and 1971 (serving as the foundation's president from 1958 to 1965); through his work with the International Pediatric Association from 1956 to 1971 (serving as chair of its executive committee from 1962 to 1968 and as its president from 1968 to 1971); and through the development of a new medical school in the Cameroons between 1973 and 1978.

Awards and recognitions were many and included serving as president of the Society for Pediatric Research in 1954 and of the American Pediatric Society in

1971; the naming of the Child Health Center in his honor in St. Johns, New-foundland, in 1966; and the most prestigious award in academic pediatrics, the Howland Medal, on April 26, 1978.

A revered chief with the highest personal integrity, human compassion, patience, objectivity, and unpretentiousness of manner, he was a man of few words but very deep thoughts and a "humanist first and foremost."[24] He stepped down from his leadership of the department in 1974, turning over the reins to the first woman to lead the department at the Children's Hospital, Dr. Mary Ellen Avery.

Medical Divisions and Faculty

The faculty of the Department of Medicine was relatively small immediately prior to and during World War II. However, it grew rapidly following the war due to increased federal funding for research, an economy stimulated by the war, and growth in the number of young physicians training in medical schools throughout the United States. While the clinical faculty grew in concert with new physical plant facilities (the Farley and Fegan Buildings), research space remained limited until the opening of the Enders Building in 1970. Growth in the faculty came about both through expansion in the limited number of prior existing divisions and the establishment of new divisions. Younger men and women trained as fellows in these divisions and then filled the ranks of the faculty.

Early in the Janeway years, house officers had frequent contact with senior faculty attendings; in the later years as the department grew, that contact was less frequent, replaced by more extensive interactions with junior attendings. For the reader of this book, a review of the divisions and their faculty is useful to understand the nature of the diseases studied and cared for. These diseases, in turn, had a major impact on the educational content experienced by the housestaff. In addition, both junior and senior faculty in the divisions served as powerful role models, attracting talented housestaff into their specialties. Examples of that influence are illustrated within each division.

Inpatient Divisons

The hematology division throughout the majority of the Janeway era was led by Louis K. Diamond. Revered by the fellows and faculty, he was considered by many to be the "father of American pediatric hematology."[25] His establishment of the blood grouping laboratory led to a new focus on chromosomal abnormalities, thereby spawning the Division of Genetics.

Research in the hematology division was carried out in the Laboratory Study Building and later in space under the current library. In 1932, Diamond and James Baty, both Children's Hospital house officers, with their chief Blackfan, were the first to unite three separate neonatal syndromes, anemia, jaundice, and hydrops as clinical manifestation of erythroblastosis fetalis.[26] Louis K. Diamond and Fred Allen's subsequent work on the Rh factor as the cause of erythroblastosis fetalis led to the development of exchange transfusion and the subsequent prevention of brain damage from bilirubin buildup (kernicterus).

Diamond and Sherwin Kevy led an extremely active blood banking service, which worked in close collaboration with cardiac surgery. Herbert Strauss oversaw the coagulation laboratory and targeted clinical coagulation disorders and hemophilia. This work and subsequent important scholarship by others, which focused on iron deficiency anemia, aplastic anemia, hereditary blood diseases, and coagulation disturbances, led to a rich educational experience in hematology for the medical housestaff.[27,28] With ambulatory pediatrics, it was the first division to accept clinical fellows during the war, and over the subsequent years, it attracted the most outstanding of fellows as trainees. Children's Hospital house officers and subsequently highly distinguished academic physicians, Park Gerald, Sam Lux, Herbert Abelson, and Harvey Cohen, were trained as fellows in this division.

During the last five years of Janeway's leadership, the hematology division was led by David G. Nathan. Trained in internal medicine, David Nathan's broad knowledge of hematology and biochemistry resulted in many important studies of the red cell membrane and accompanying diseases such as hereditary spherocytosis, sickle cell disease, thalassemia, and newly described hemolytic anemias.

The Division of Infectious Diseases had its genesis in the Blackfan era with the active involvement of Charles McKhann, R. Cannon Eley, and John Davies. It developed its scientific underpinnings with the movement of John Enders from Edwin Cohn's wartime efforts in protein chemistry in the quadrangle at Harvard Medical School to the Carnegie Building and the Children's Hospital, culminating in the development of the ability to grow viruses in tissue culture. It was this achievement that led to a 1954 Nobel Prize for Enders, Fred Robbins, and Tom Weller.

The greatly admired John Enders focused his research on vaccinia, coxsackie, polio, and cytomegalovirus (CMV). The author, along with other young house officers in the late 1960s, observed Dr. Enders with respectful awe. "We saw him walking the halls, shoulders stooped, pipe in his mouth. We heard the stories of his brown-bag lunches, his simple tastes, his frugality, his modesty, and his great integrity. His magnificent life ended at age 88 in September 1985 at his summer home in Connecticut, while reading T.S. Eliot aloud to his wife and daughter."

Tom Weller (later professor at the Harvard School of Public Health) focused his research on polio and rubella; George Miller (later John Enders Professor at Yale University School of Medicine) on Epstein-Barr virus (EBV); Sam Katz (later chair of the Department of Pediatrics at Duke University School of Medicine) and Anna Mietus on measles; and Fred Robbins (later dean at Case Western University School of Medicine) on poliovirus.

The 1960s and 1970s brought a new focus on bacterial infection, with an understanding of bacterial genetics and metabolism and bacterial resistance to antimicrobials, led by David Smith, an ex-chief resident at the Children's Hospital, who trained in the Department of Bacteriology and Immunology at Harvard. He was joined by Pierce Gardner and Arnold Smith, both favorites of the housestaff in the 1960s and 1970s. David Smith's iconic work (along with his colleague Porter Anderson) focused on *Haemophilus influenzae* type b and ultimately led to the development of the vaccine and the elimination of *Haemophilus influenzae* type b invasive disease, the highly prestigious Lasker Award in 1968, and the E. Mead Johnson Award in 1975. As vaccination against polio, measles, rubella, diphtheria, and tetanus became widespread, the common contagious diseases of the past became less prevalent and were replaced by *Haemophilus influenzae* type b, pneumococcus, meningococcus, and gram-negative bacterial disease as well as bacterial and fungal diseases occurring in the compromised host.

John Enders initially, followed by Samuel Katz and then David Smith, led the Division of Infectious Diseases during the Janeway era. Children's Hospital house officers David Carver, Samuel Katz, Sidney Kibrick, John Modlin, Richard Moxon, and Georges Peter were all trained in this important division. Prestigious honors came to Children's Hospital housestaff who pursued careers in infectious disease and included the presidency of the American Pediatric Society (Sam Katz); E. Mead Johnson Award (Tom Weller, Fred Robbins, David Smith); Distinguished Pediatric Infectious Disease Society awardees (Sam Katz and Georges Peter); president of the Infectious Disease Society of America (Catherine Wilfert); and Nobel Prize recipients (Tom Weller, Fred Robbins, and Carleton Gajdusek).

The immunology division was initially directed by Charles Janeway and then by Fred Rosen, who was just beginning his distinguished and lifelong association with the hospital and the department. The laboratory for protein studies was supervised by David Gitlin. Both Gitlin and Rosen had been Children's Hospital house officers and trainees of Charles Janeway, and both went on to make major contributions to the discipline of immunology.

Research in the division focused on a number of immunologic diseases as well as disorders of the complement system, including hereditary angioneurotic edema and deficiency of the third component of complement, seen in renal and collagen vascular disease. Among a group of patients with nephrosis, this research team described progressive glomerulonephritis; among children with recurrent bacterial infections they identified agammaglobulinemia. In the clinic, they studied hereditary disorders of copper metabolism (Wilson's disease); disorders affecting serum proteins (nephrosis); and rheumatologic disorders such as rheumatoid arthritis and lupus erythematosis.

Drs. Janeway, Rosen, Harvey Colten, and Martin Klemperer were active teachers of the housestaff, both on the inpatient service and in the clinic, and attracted to their fellowship very capable medical housestaff, including, among others, Richard Johnston, Raif Geha, Irwin Gelfand, Robertson Parkman, and Richard Insel. Richard Johnston, David Gitlin, Fred Rosen, Erwin Gelfand, and Raif Geha went on to win the E. Mead Johnson Award for their pioneering work in immunology. David Gitlin and his son Jonathan Gitlin, a house officer in the Avery era, would become the only father–son recipients from Children's Hospital of this prestigious award. In 1996, Johnston served as president of the American Pediatric Society and in 2008 was a Howland Award recipient.

The cardiology division thrived under Hungarian born Alexander Nadas, becoming a free-standing, separate department at the end of the Janeway era. Nadas had served as a volunteer outpatient resident at the Children's Hospital in 1942, exhibiting outstanding clinical skills. After moving to Michigan and receiving another MD degree in 1945, he returned to Massachusetts, where he practiced general pediatrics in Greenfield. In 1949, Janeway invited Nadas to develop a pediatric cardiology program. Stimulated by advances in the surgical correction of congenital malformations of the heart and great vessels by Robert Gross in Boston and Drs. Alfred Blalock and Helen Taussig at Johns Hopkins Hospital in the late 1930s and 1940s, Nadas gathered a fine group of physiologists, pathologists, and cardiologists. He developed a top-flight fellowship training program and a large clinical volume on both the inpatient Sharon cardiovascular unit and in the outpatient clinic.[5]

Nadas was ably assisted by: Donald Fyler, who directed the catheterization laboratory, the New England Regional Infant Cardiac Program, and ultimately the cardiac registry; Richard Van Praagh, who as cardiac pathologist studied the embryologic origin of congenital heart disease and correlated disease with morphologic changes; Greer Monroe, who studied factors affecting the performance of heart muscle; Walter Gamble, who developed fiber-optic systems to record hemodynamic changes; Warren Gold, who studied regulation of the pulmonary circulation; Grant LaFarge, who worked in the artificial heart program; Paul Hugenholtz, who studied electric forces produced by the heart; and Bill Plauth, who focused on the natural history of heart disease.

Children's Hospital house officers Welton Gersony, Amnon Rosenthal, Robert Freedom, and Tom Graham trained in cardiology during the Janeway era and went on to distinguished careers in cardiology beyond Children's Hospital, all serving as chairs of divisions of cardiology, respectively, at Columbia University College of Physicians and Surgeons, the University of Michigan Medical School, the University of Toronto School of Medicine, and the Medical University of South Carolina. Amnon Rosenthal received the prestigious Founders Award in 2003 from the cardiology section of the American Academy of Pediatrics (Alexander Nadas being its first recipient in 1988).

The study of rheumatic fever, which took place in the House of the Good Samaritan, was ably led by Benedict Massell.[29] The disease by now was clearly shown to be caused by group A beta hemolytic streptococcus. Increasingly, the focus turned to its prevention through the use of penicillin, both to shorten hospitalization and prevent recurrences. The large number of inpatients with rheumatic fever on the seventh floor of the Farley Building (Division 37) began to decrease in the late 1950s as a result of these efforts. The effect of this change as perceived by the housestaff was dramatic. The intricacies of the diagnosis and treatment of rheumatic fever became a thing of the past in the early 1970s, only to recur briefly but with increased virulence in the mid-1990s.

The Division of Genetics, which became part of the Department of Medicine in 1966, grew out of the hematology division and was led by Park Gerald, who had been trained both as a house officer and hematology fellow at the Children's Hospital. A clinical genetic laboratory was established in the 1960s in the Ida C. Smith Building to study the biochemical manifestations of genetically induced diseases. Park Gerald focused his studies on disturbances of hemoglobin synthesis, Mary Louise Efron on disorders of amino acid metabolism, and Joseph Kennedy on phenylketonuria (PKU). The division consulted at the Boston Lying-In Hospital, the Beth Israel Hospital, and the Brigham and Women's Hospital; taught the housestaff on the hospital's inpatient service; and ran the genetics and PKU clinics. By the 1970s, a cytogenetics laboratory was added to the biochemical genetics laboratory. However, the prominent position that genetics would ultimately hold in pediatric medicine was yet to arrive on the wards and in the clinics. It would assume great importance in the Nathan, Philip Pizzo, and Gary Fleisher eras.

The metabolism division was led by James Gamble until 1951, then by William Wallace until 1952, followed by Jack Metcoff until 1955, and finally by Robert Schwartz until 1958. Children's Hospital house officers Malcolm Holliday, Jack Metcoff, Robert Schwartz, and Sumner Yaffe all trained as fellows in this remarkable division. Metcoff was nationally recognized for his studies of the pathogenesis and treatment of nephrosis and for the use of hemodialysis in children, Holliday for his studies of growth and nutrition in uremic children, and William Wallace for his studies of the composition of urine. James Gamble, as a result of his investigation of fluid and electrolytes, studies of extracellular fluids, and "Gamblegrams" accrued many recognitions and honors, including presidency of the Society for Pediatric Research and the American Pediatric Society as well as the highly prestigious Howland Award. The metabolism division was eventually subsumed by the renal and endocrine divisions, led respectively by Francis Fellers and John Crigler.

The renal division mirrored its parent division, with a focus on metabolic diseases such as cystinuria and its treatment with penicillamine, vitamin D metabolism and bone disease, studies of the feasibility of repeated dialysis with John Merrill at the Peter Bent Brigham Hospital, long-term management of the nephrotic syndrome, and classification of a plethora of evolving renal diseases. The division's future chief Bill Harmon trained as a resident during the Janeway era and later as a fellow in nephrology in the early to mid-1970s.

The endocrine division, led by John Crigler, with its laboratory efforts located in the House of the Good Samaritan and supervised by Norman Gold, focused its attention on the regulation of growth and the many metabolic processes regulated by the hypothalamus. The clinical wing of the Division of Endocrinology, which provided multiple consultations and special laboratory studies, targeted diseases of carbohydrate and lipid metabolism, uses for growth hormone, regulation of calcium metabolism, clinical manifestations of hypoglycemia, the management of diabetes, and the effects of neurosurgical ablation of craniopharyngioma. Crigler, initially trained by Lawson Wilkins at Johns Hopkins Hospital and further trained at the Massachusetts Institute of Technology, and Gold were assisted by Joseph Fisher, an adult endocrinologist from the Brigham and Women's Hospital. Endocrinology would further grow in size and academic stature under the outstanding leadership of Joseph Majzoub and would become a popular and highly sought after career destination for some of the best Children's Hospital house officers.

Rapid development of neonatology occurred following World War II. The clinical service was led by Stewart Clifford until the mid-1960s and neonatal research by Clement Smith until the early 1970s. Clifford focused his attention on clinical studies of the premature infant, the syndrome of post maturity, and prenatal factors responsible for cerebral palsy; Clement Smith studied alterations of respiration and circulation on extra-uterine life in the newborn as well as the broader physiology of the newborn. The housestaff rotated at the Boston Lying-In Hospital for their instruction in the care of the newborn. In addition, a neonatology unit was opened on the fifth and then seventh floor of the Farley Building, initially on Division 25 and then in 1964 on Division 37. It cared for newborns with neonatal disease requiring the hospital's subspecialty services (congenital heart disease, erythroblastosis, sepsis, and neurologic disorders). The housestaff from the Children's Hospital and the Massachusetts General Hospital rotated through this unit, where over 100 exchange transfusions were assiduously performed yearly by the housestaff. James Drorbaugh led an important study on the follow-up of infants at the Boston Lying-In, although the housestaff were only peripherally involved in this activity. Nicholas Nelson, future chief of pediatrics at Pennsylvania State University School of Medicine, Peter Auld, neonatologist at Cornell University Medical College, and William Cochran, future chair of neonatology at the Beth Israel Hospital, would go on from their training in pediatrics and neonatology at the Children's Hospital to distinguished careers in neonatology.

Although not freestanding divisions, significant work occurred in the allergy, nutrition, and pulmonary clinics. Each of these predominately outpatient disciplines were designated as divisions by the end of the Janeway era and the beginning of the Avery years. The leadership of the allergy clinic, run for so many years by Lewis Webb Hill until his retirement, was assumed by Harry Mueller in the mid-1950s. Mueller was assisted by Irving Bailet. Harry Mueller, a clinical allergist, focused his interests on insect bites, Irving Bailet on the treatment of asthma. The high prevalence of allergic disease resulted in an extremely active clinical inpatient and outpatient service.

The nutrition clinic cared for children with cystic fibrosis, celiac disease, and disorders of nutrition and was led by Harry Shwachman, chief of the Division of Laboratories of Clinical Pathology. The Children's Hospital, as a result of Shwachman's extensive experience and great dedication to patients with cystic fibrosis, became a renowned center for the treatment of this condition. Dr. Shwachman's work gradually lengthened survival and improved quality of life for these children. He also focused his attention on disaccharide enzyme deficiency diseases involving the small bowel, celiac disease, and with Louis Kopito, the measurement of lead levels in plumbism and copper in blood and urine in Wilson's disease. This important work ultimately resulted in the formation of the Division of Gastroenterology and Nutrition, led by Richard Grand, a prior resident in the mid-1960s at the Children's Hospital, and later by Allan Walker, a division chief appointee in the Avery era. The Harry Shwachman Award was established in Shwachman's honor in 1984 by the North American Society for Pediatric Gastroenterology and Nutrition. Richard Grand, a revered Children's Hospital clinician and investigator of gastrointestinal disease, received the award in 1993.

The pulmonary clinic was established to support the laboratory work on respiratory physiology established under Charles D. Cook. Mary Ellen Wohl, who carried out her research at the Harvard School of Public Health, soon joined the clinic and began her many contributions to pulmonary medicine. The respiratory therapy service, which collaborated closely with the housestaff on the inpatient services, also worked closely with Drs. Cook and Wohl. All three of these disciplines—allergy, nutrition, and pulmonary—would morph into full-fledged powerful divisions in the Avery era and would become extremely important sites for housestaff education.

Outpatient Divisions

Ambulatory pediatrics became a relatively new and critical area for housestaff education. In fact, Dr. Janeway was well ahead of others in championing it as an essential part of a pediatric resident's training. It included the MOPD, the emergency department, the medical consultation service, the adolescent medicine clinic, and the family health care unit. It was led briefly by Charles D. May and Sydney Gellis in the late 1940s, followed by John Tuthill (1950–1954), Charles D. Cook (1954–1964), Thomas Cone (1964–1973), and Melvin Levine from 1974 onward. John Graef became the first full-time leader of the emergency department.

The work of ambulatory pediatrics was supplemented by the adolescent medicine unit and the family health care unit. J. Roswell Gallagher, initially a school physician at Phillips Andover Academy and recruited to Children's Hospital by Janeway, established the first adolescent medicine clinic in the United

States at the Children's Hospital in 1951 as well as the first academic training program in this discipline in the United States. Considered the "father of adolescent medicine" in the United States, he published his classic textbook on medical care of the adolescent in 1960, 1966, and 1976.[30,31]

Adolescent medicine was predominately an outpatient specialty and handled a heavy clinic volume of both old and new patients. Special cardiac and endocrine clinics, precepted respectively by Somers Sturgis and John Crigler, were developed for adolescent patients, and division staff supervised the inpatient care of adolescent patients on the seventh floor, Division 37, in the Farley building. Roswell Gallagher's and then Robert Masland's model of care of the adolescent patient was copied by adolescent units throughout the United States. The division's future chief Jean Emans trained as a resident in pediatrics and then in adolescent medicine as a fellow in the early 1970s. Encouraged by Dr. Janeway, she set up the first pediatric and adolescent gynecology service with Donald Goldstein and also authored the text *Pediatric and Adolescent Gynecology*, now in its sixth edition, with him. She would ultimately hold the Mary Ellen Avery Professorship in Pediatrics at the Harvard Medical School.

The child health division initially led by Harold Stuart evolved into the Family Health Care Program in 1955, led first by Robert Haggerty, then by Joel Alpert, and finally by Richard Finebloom (both Haggerty and Alpert were Janeway's chief residents). They were assisted by John Kosa and Leon Robertson for research and Margaret Heagarty for clinical care. Janeway and Dane Prugh had received a Commonwealth Fund Grant to "develop a program that would care for children in their homes and provide an educational opportunity for medical students and pediatric residents to learn about the social and psychological influences on the health of children."[32] The Family Health Care Program was so named because it cared for the whole family, emphasized health through prevention, and cared for the sick as well as providing preventative services. Haggerty and Alpert further developed the program by creating a robust training site for students, residents, and fellows and by building a strong research unit that demonstrated the beneficial effects of care for families over time. This clinical service served as an excellent site for resident continuity clinic training and was thus important in enhancing Janeway's view of the optimal training of a resident. The Family Health Care Program was discontinued early in the Avery era.

Neurology, capably led for so long by Bronson Crothers and then Randolph Byers, was a critical discipline in the education of housestaff. It focused on a number of diseases, including lead poisoning, infections of the central nervous system, the neurologic sequellae of birth injury, cerebral palsy, and psychiatric disease. Along with Frank Ford from Johns Hopkins and Bernard Sacks from New York, Bronson Crothers received the recognition of "father of child neurology."[33] With the arrival of L. Lahut Uzman as the first Bronson Crothers professor of neurology in 1962, neurology became its own department. Similar to the creation of cardiology as its own department, Janeway felt that when a division had achieved sufficient size and success it deserved independent status as a hospital department. However, this did have the adverse effect of neurology being seen less as a core part of Department of Medicine activities and therefore not central to the training of the medical housestaff. In the ensuing years, neurology rotations existed for the housestaff but never with the centrality experienced prior to 1960. Uzman's untimely death a short time after joining the Children's Hospital led to the appointment of Charles Barlow as neurologist-in-chief. During Barlow's subsequent 27-year tenure, a Mental Retardation and Developmental Disabilities Research Center sponsored by the National Institutes of Health (NIH) was established as well as the Longwood Neurology Residency Program.

The work in neurology was capably carried out by the neurology staff, by William Berenberg (for handicapped children), and by Allen Crocker (in the developmental unit). The first seizure unit in the United States dedicated to the study of childhood epilepsy was started by William Lennox (an early recipient of the Lasker Award, in 1951) in the early 1940s during the Smith era. It was then led by Cesare Lombroso and brought into the newly formed neurology department. Similarly, psychiatry, which had started in the Department of Medicine under Dane Prugh in 1947, was established as an independent department in 1955 under George Gardner (1953–1970) and later Julius Richmond (1971–1977). Its inpatient division (Division 72 in the Judge Baker Guidance Center and subsequently named the Richmond service) became an important site for housestaff education.

The National Perspective

Internship and Residency

Prior to World War II, interns outnumbered residents. Internships were often two years in length and were "rotating" (involving rotations through medicine, surgery, pediatrics, and obstetrics and gynecology). The programs were pyramidal in nature, and the attending staff was actively involved with the housestaff in patient care. This would change following the war as the number of residents grew, exceeding by several fold the number of interns and thereby creating a residency structure with equal numbers of housestaff in each year. As the amount of knowledge to be learned in a given specialty expanded, there was too much to master; with the encouragement of subspecialty boards, gradually straight medicine, surgery, and pediatric internships began to replace rotating internships (these internships becoming part of the internal medicine, surgery, and pediatric residency structure of training).

As the housestaff grew in number and expertise, the faculty depended increasingly on them for chores ("scut work"), for performing procedures, for making clinical care decisions and for teaching medical students (the housestaff often holding a concomitant medical school title for this purpose). The house officer's workload grew, the patients were sicker, and the turnover rate was more rapid due to a progressive shortening of length of stay. The faculty and the hospitals depended more and more on the housestaff. Competition among the best national training programs became intense in an effort to attract the best and the brightest. Community hospitals, also depending on housestaff for manpower, began to compete for the best trainees by offering better salaries and medical school affiliation.

Housestaff compensation, which in 1955 included room and board and a small stipend ($25 a month for interns), grew rapidly after the introduction of Medicare and Medicaid, with interns by 1970 earning $7,000 a year.[34] By the mid-1950s the number of national training slots exceeded the number of available U.S.-trained medical students, and hospitals—particularly community hospitals—turned to foreign medical graduates. Higher salaries were now used by hospitals to enhance recruitment. Importantly, this allowed aspiring future physicians, who before could not afford it, to enter medicine, enhancing diversity of backgrounds in the resident staff. Nonetheless, income remained modest and residents also turned to moonlighting at other hospitals during their off hours to earn extra money to pay back medical school loans and support growing families. This practice was strongly supported by residents, while it was frowned on by the hospital's administration. This difference in opinion was accentuated when work hour regulations to prevent house officer fatigue became an important issue in the late 1990s.

Internship and residency were now required for all housestaff. But gradually, residency was no longer a sufficient credential for an academic career. No longer did it offer a trainee the necessary knowledge and skills to be "cutting edge" in specialty care. In short, one had to sub-specialize in a fellowship to gain mastery over a field of medicine and to pursue an academic career.

Fellowship Training

With so much emphasis on specialization, fellowships began to proliferate. Subspecialty training became the means for mastering a clinical subspecialty and developing the research skills necessary for an academic career. Many of the best fellowships emphasized research training over clinical training. In contrast to residents who were paid by clinical dollars, fellows were paid by grants from the NIH, medical schools, or the university. By the 1960s, fellowship numbers nationally exceeded residency numbers in large academic teaching centers. Residents took on the primary role of care provider for inpatients, the fellows the role of consultant, often creating friction among trainees ("turf wars"). By 1970, many fellows were entering the private practice of their specialty and caring for their patients in community hospitals, where they began to demand the necessary technology to carry out this specialized care. This led to competition for patients with the academic centers that had trained them.

Resident Life

Prior to World War II, house officer training involved long hours and hard work but was compensated by a sharp learning curve, housestaff collegiality, and the honor of training in a prestigious academic center. The family atmosphere and the total immersion in house officer training and life, however, gradually began to disappear following the war.

As the house officer numbers grew, there were too many residents to live in hospital quarters. More began to live at home on their nights off. Frequency of night call had decreased, such that by the mid-1970s, many training programs were every third night on call. There was an increased desire for leisure time and personal enjoyment. Marriage and children became more common. All of this resulted in a loss of the family atmosphere of house officer training. The paternalistic rules of the 1930s and 1940s were no longer accepted. Dress in the hospital became less regimented and hair became longer. Often house officers were less responsive to the practicing volunteer faculty than the academic faculty. They frequently felt that the practicing faculty made care decisions without consulting them and with insufficient evidence-based information. The practicing faculty, in turn, felt that residents were uppity, made decisions without consulting *them* and often appropriated their patients for the ward services. These attitudinal changes were accompanied by opposition to the Vietnam War and the growing rebellion of youth throughout the U.S.

There was more and more to do (sicker patients, more scut work, ever constant pagers) and moonlighting had crept in, all of which resulted in sleep deprivation, negative mood swings, and increased stress. Managing large housestaffs and maintaining a happy training environment was becoming an increasing challenge. Finally, all of these changes fueled the debate over residency as an educational versus service experience. House officer rights found a voice in the proliferation of housestaff associations in the late 1960s and early 1970s (to negotiate with "the administration" over living conditions, salary, and benefits) and in limited cases, to unionized housestaff in Boston, New York, and Chicago.[35] Clearly, with the increasing importance of residents and fellows in the care of hospitalized patients had come greater complexities regarding their organization and management.

Residency Training

The medical residency grew remarkably during Charles Janeway's tenure as chairman. Between 1946 and 1974, over 1,000 house officers were trained, 587 in the traditional residency and 155 in the Medical Outpatient Pediatric Department (MOPD) residency, and many others in the affiliated, coordinated, and part-time residencies. The traditional residency grew rapidly following World War II, with young doctors returning from Europe and the Pacific anxious to get on with their medical training. As shown in Table 3, by 1951 the traditional residency had reached 30, by the late 1950s 30 to 40; by 1974, it had reached 50 to 60 residents. Representative pictures of faculty and housestaff during the Janeway era are shown in Figures 4–6.

TABLE 3   Medical Housestaff Statistics

	1880s	1890s	1900s	1910s	1920s	1930s	1940–1945	1945–1959	1960s	1970s
Total	2	3	6	8	13	17	12–17	25–30	30–40	50–60
Male/Female	2/0	3/0	6/0	8/0	13/0	17/0	15/1–2	5%*	10%*	25%*
Chief Residents	0	0	0	0	0	0	0	1–4	2–4	2

*Percentage of women on the housestaff

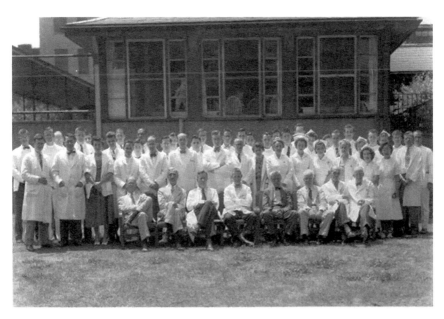

FIGURE 4   The Early Janeway Era, 1949–1950

In the front row from left to right: Randolph Byers, Harold Stuart, Clement Smith, Charles Janeway, James Gamble, Bronson Crothers, Cannon Eley, and John Davies.

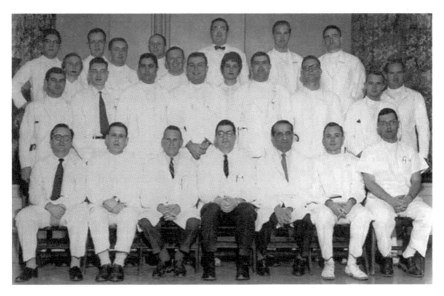

FIGURE 5   The Mid-Janeway Era, 1960–1961

The Janeway Housestaff in the early 1960s showing (in the front room) Charles Janeway (third from left), and to his left, Chief Resident David Carver and Louis K. Diamond.

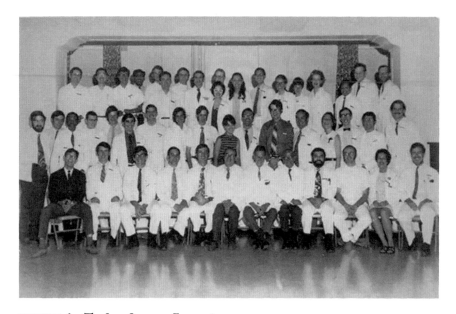

FIGURE 6   The Late Janeway Era, 1969–1970

The Janeway Housestaff near the end of his chairmanship, showing in the middle of the first row (sixth from left) Sherwin Kevy, and to his left, Charles Janeway and William Berenberg.

In the Blackfan/Smith era, house officers' titles were relatively simple, with the senior men called "residents" and the junior men "medical house officers." Women first entered the housestaff in 1942 during the middle of World War II and the first house officer of color in the early 1950s. A new nomenclature was adopted by the hospital following World War II and included the following designations: intern, junior assistant resident (JAR), senior assistant resident (SAR), senior resident (also called SAR), and chief resident. Intern equated with PGYI (post graduate year 1) in our current nomenclature, JAR with PGYII (post graduate year 2), and SAR with PGYIII (post graduate year 3). In the 1950s, there were fewer interns than junior and senior residents because entry into the residency often followed an internship in internal medicine, a pediatric internship elsewhere, or a pathology internship. In 1951, the housestaff included four interns, 13 junior residents, and eight senior residents, but by 1968, there were 14 interns, 14 junior residents, and eight senior residents (as fewer supervisory experiences existed, a smaller number of SARs were needed). In the early Janeway years, the residency generally lasted for two years, but by the mid-1960s, the residency was generally three years in duration.

Dr. Janeway created six different residency tracks during his 28 years of leadership. The differences in make-up and content reflected his foresight and belief in the value of flexibility in residency structure and curriculum. They consisted of the Traditional Residency, the Medical Outpatient Pediatric Department Residency, the Affiliated Residency, the Coordinated Residency, the Part-Time Residency, and the St. Mary's Exchange Residency. Four of these tracks began early in the Janeway era, the Traditional Residency in 1946, continuing the program established so effectively in the Blackfan/Smith era, the Medical Outpatient Pediatric Department (MOPD) Residency in 1947, the Affiliated Residency in 1951, and the St. Mary's Exchange Residency in 1951. Two began relatively late in the Janeway era, the Part-time Residency in the mid-1960s and the Coordinated Residency in 1969.

Traditional Medical Residency

This residency track, the largest of the six, was based on several educational foundations, including exposure of residents to the core content of pediatric training in the first year (general inpatient, outpatient, general surgery, and emergency department pediatrics) and subspecialty pediatrics (cardiology, neonatology, tumor therapy, hematology, and neurology) in the second year. At the conclusion of these two years, the resident would have had an intensive experience with the diagnosis and treatment of a broad array of diseases in children. In addition, through rotations in the outpatient department, in the family health care unit, and in community hospitals, the resident gained exposure to community-based care and comprehensive pediatric care.

During the third year of training, education was further developed on the principle of choice so as to best equip residents with the skills needed for their future careers. These choices consisted of the traditional senior year, which included supervising on the three general ward services, the emergency department, an admitting department rotation, a community hospital rotation, a teaching resident rotation (with responsibility for the medical students) and two elective months; or direct entry after the second year into subspecialty fellowship training in a wide variety of clinical and investigative specialties (such as cardiology, hematology, endocrinology, and infectious diseases) or more general fields such as adolescent medicine and family health care. Residents pursuing these options often were headed to careers in academic medicine. Alternatively, senior residents might pursue a year in the ambulatory department, where they would have considerable exposure to general medical and subspecialty behavioral and developmental clinics as well as the emergency service. These residents often proceeded into practice careers in pediatrics.

A critical part of the training of all residents throughout the 1960s and 1970s and championed by Robert Haggerty and Joel Alpert (future department chairs at the University of Rochester and Boston University medical schools, respectively) was involvement with continuity of care (care of the pediatric patient over time). This was accomplished through the following of a pregnant woman and the care of her child following delivery in the family health care unit or the care of the pediatric patient (often initially cared for on the hospital wards or emergency department) in a hospital-based residency continuity clinic into which the resident rotated one-half day each week.

Years later, residents of the program remember vividly their early rotations at the Children's Hospital. As reflected upon by Richard Johnston, "During the 1960s and for years thereafter the Boston Lying-In Hospital was located across Longwood Avenue from the Children's Hospital. I moved from an air-conditioned medical school in the South and began my residency at the Lying-In in the summer of 1963. The lasting memories of that rotation include the gentlemanly, kind, and laconic personality of Clement Smith, director of the newborn service, and the nursery itself. To my amazement and horror, the normal newborns were housed in a single large room ventilated by very large open windows with a view toward downtown Boston. Thus, along with the breeze blowing over the babies was the soot and airborne efflux of the city."[36]

Medical Outpatient Pediatric Department (MOPD) Residency

This residency was introduced in 1947. MOPD residents served for one to two years in the outpatient clinics and community hospitals. Many pursuing this track were physicians returning from the military service and ultimately headed for community practice. One such resident was Sterling MacDonald, the first to enter this program in 1947, who subsequently entered and ultimately led a fine pediatric practice on the North Shore of Massachusetts, where he remained his entire career. This program was led by a number of distinguished faculty, including John Tuthill in the 1950s, Charles Cook in the 1960s, and Thomas Cone in the 1960s and 1970s. Cone was ably assisted in the 1970s in the MOPD by Melvin Levine, who ultimately succeeded him as chief of the Division of General Pediatrics (the new name for the Medical Outpatient Department) under Dr. Avery and John Graef, who was chief resident from 1970 to 1972 and then director of the emergency department. A number of distinguished physicians were trained in the MOPD program, including Roger Ashley, Joel Bass, Diane Kittredge, Jeffery Maisels, Paul McCarthy, Victoria Meguid, Elias Milgram, Heather Palmer, Keith Reisinger, and Margaret Sharfstein.

Affiliated Residency

The Affiliated Residency was established in 1951, and its curriculum lasted for one to two years. This residency was structured to allow residents to rotate into the Children's Hospital from other training programs, including the Roger Williams Program and the Rhode Island Hospital Program, both in Providence; the Massachusetts General Hospital Program; the Springfield Hospital Program, and others. These residents rotated in the outpatient department and clinics, the emergency department, several inpatient services, and community hospitals, including North Shore Hospital, Beverly Hospital, the Beth Israel Hospital, Mount Auburn Hospital, the Springfield Hospital, and the U.S. Naval Hospital in Chelsea. These residents often moved into positions in the Traditional Residency. Most ultimately proceeded into pediatric practice.

The Coordinated Residency

Formally instituted in 1969, this residency was run by Barry Adels and lasted for three years. It was created for the large number of residents coming from other countries to the Children's Hospital, a practice so very typical of the Janeway years. Prior to 1969, these foreign-born residents had been incorporated into the MOPD program and the Affiliated program. The residents in the Coordinated Residency Program rotated into the outpatient clinics and community hospitals. Their curriculum, similar to the Affiliated and MOPD residencies, lasted for one to two years. Some particularly capable residents moved from this program into the Traditional Residency Program. This formal program for foreign residents was not fully successful because of feelings of inferior citizenship by those involved and a lack of enthusiastic support for the program among some of the senior faculty. Charles Janeway, however, continued to bring pediatricians from other countries for a variety of educational experiences both before and after this program ended.

Part-time Residency

Dr. Janeway's belief in flexibility in the residency and its curriculum was strongly held. This was particularly so for the education of foreign physicians. It was also very true for married women who shouldered family obligations. As he noted in the hospital's annual report in 1964, "An interesting phenomenon of recent years has been the growing group of young women whose medical careers have been interrupted by marriage and the raising of young children, returning to complete their pediatric hospital training by working on a part-time basis."

In the late 1960s, Janeway successfully sought permission from the Board of Pediatrics to create a curriculum for a shared residency (two house officers assuming one residency slot). This track was used most successfully during the last five years of his chairmanship.[37] Directed by the outpatient chief resident, John Graef, six house officers (five women and one man) took advantage of this program between 1969 and 1974.[38] Today as they look back on their experience, they are adamant that it made all the difference in allowing them to complete their residency. Five of six who were eligible and wished board certification were successful in that pursuit and subsequently pursued academic careers; one established a highly successful practice in Massachusetts. To this day, they are grateful to the program and to Charles Janeway for an opportunity that was unique at that time and unavailable elsewhere in the country. Janeway would say, "We are pleased that it has been possible to introduce sufficient flexibility into our educational program to meet the needs of an able group of future physicians, whose obligations to their families must be met simultaneously."[39] This was 20 to 40 years before the interest in part-time residencies of today.

St. Mary's Exchange

The St. Mary's Exchange was a highly innovative curricular program introduced in 1952. Planned by Charles Janeway and Reginald Lightwood from England, it involved an exchange of senior residents from the Children's Hospital and registrars (equivalent to clinical fellows in training in a subspecialty or the general area of pediatrics in the U.S.) from St. Mary's Hospital in London (Figure 7). The exchange lasted for each registrar or senior resident from six months to a full year. The program, which ran for 25 years until 1977, involved 35 residents from the Children's Hospital and 26 registrars from St. Mary's Hospital. The Children's Hospital residents are listed in Table 4.

Children's Hospital residents rotated in a number of settings during their London stay, including Paddington Green Children's Hospital (one of the first hospitals in London devoted solely to children), St. Mary's and St. Charles Hospitals, and at differing times to Princess Louise Hospital and the neonatal unit at Harron Road.[40] The London registrars assumed all the rotations of the

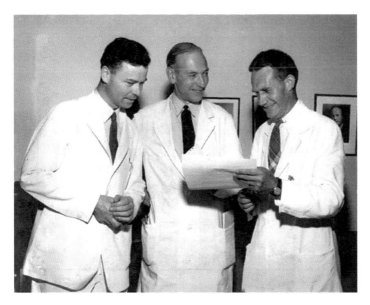

FIGURE 7   The First Blackfan Lecture, circa 1952

Dr. Janeway is shown on the right, Dr. Reginald Lightwood from St.
Mary's Hospital in the center as the first Blackfan lecturer and Henry Giles
exchange resident from St. Mary's Hospital in London on the left.

TABLE 4   Participants in the Exchange Residency with St. Mary's Hospital,
London, (1952–1977)

Children's Hospital Residents

Barry Adels	William B. Gurfield	John F. Modlin
Joel J. Alpert	Allen J. Hinkle	Murray E. Pendleton
W. Bruce Anderson	Mackenzie W.G. Hume	Patricia A. Rompf
Walter R. Anyan	Peter Humphreys	David Rush
Robert B. Berg	Richard A. Insel	John A. Spargo
Abraham B. Bergman	Samuel L. Katz	Victor C. Strasburger
Irma D. Brown	Howard E. Kulin	John W. G. Tuthill
Paul H. Dworkin	William Maniscalco	Larry J. Wasser
Lowell E. Fox	Larry Martel	Christopher Wilson
Stephen E. Gellis	Sanford J. Mathews	Sumner Yaffe
Ronald Gold	William C. Mentzer	Peter M. Zawadsky
Robert A. Goodell	Denis R. Miller	

traditional medical residency as a senior supervising resident at the Children's Hospital. The first residents in 1952 to participate were John Tuthill and Murray Pendleton from Boston and the first registrars included John Reinhold and John Davis from London.

Among the Children's Hospital residents who participated, many familiar names appear. The same is true among the registrars; these include John Davis, Henry Giles, Tom Oppe, Andrew Riggs, Donald Barltrop, John Lloyd-Still, Kim Oates, and Tom Lissauer. Among the senior residents on the list, six became department chairs (Drs. Alpert, Bergman, Dworkin, Katz, Modlin, and Wilson) and among the registrars a similar number became professors and chairs of renown at various medical schools (including Tom Oppe at St. Mary's Hospital Medical School, John Davis at Cambridge University, Donald Barltrop at Westminster, and Kim Oates at the University of Sydney).

The lessons learned by U.S. residents were invaluable. As noted by Joel Alpert at the 50th anniversary celebration in 2002: "For the Americans, there was the introduction to the National Health Service and the knowledge that no patient in the U.K. faced a financial barrier to needed health care . . . The Americans found an enhanced emphasis on history taking and physical examination skills. The importance of clinical skills remained with almost every American in the Exchange as did the genuine admiration for the U.K.'s social commitment to removing the financial barrier to medical care in time of need."[41] And as Tom Lissauer from St. Mary's Hospital noted: "Those of us who went to the U.S. were introduced to the exciting possibilities of high-tech medicine and the requirement that our opinions be backed by evidence."[42]

These experiences were remembered many years after. Abraham Bergman recalled, "On my first day on the ward on Paddington Green, I wrote feeding orders on an infant. Sister Webster said, 'Dr. Bergman, don't you think I know how to feed a baby?' She sure did. It never happened again."[43] And Murray Pendleton recalled, "My first day of rounds with Dr. Lightwood—my being admonished for ordering an X-ray to confirm a case of pneumonia since the physical findings were sufficient for the diagnosis."[44]

Samuel Katz had been a St. Mary's Exchange resident in 1956, and when he assumed the chairmanship of the Department of Pediatrics at Duke University School of Medicine, he contacted infectious disease colleague and friend (and Children's Hospital house officer and infectious disease fellow in the early 1970s) Richard Moxon, chair of pediatrics at Oxford University and John Davis, chair of pediatrics at Cambridge University, to develop a similar exchange between Duke, Oxford, and Cambridge. When conceived in 1986, the Cambridge program was too small to be able to supply a house officer on alternate years, but the Duke/ Oxford program flourished. At a 2002 gathering marking the 15th anniversary of the Duke/Oxford Exchange (1986–2001), Katz noted that while the enthusiasm for the exchange remained high, its cost—$35,000 annually—and the requirements placed on the respective residents and registrars to meet medical licensure qualifications made the exchange more difficult.[45] This residency exchange program was ahead of its time. Today, it is commonly duplicated in rotations involving U.S. residents in developing countries throughout the world (an example being the current rotation of Boston Combined Residency Program residents in Lesotho, Africa). It is perhaps fitting that the final event at the reunion in 2002 of this remarkable program should end with a celebratory dinner at the houses of Parliament and in the Winston Churchill Dining Room.[46]

Foreign Medical Graduates

Clearly one of Charles Janeway's unique contributions to residency was his desire to train individuals from foreign countries and then send them back to their own countries to assume leadership roles. This formed the basis for the Coordinated Residency Program, previously mentioned. Importantly, he did this not to fill unfilled residency positions for the purpose of providing service, but rather from a deep desire to positively impact world health by training the brightest and best, who would then return to their home countries carrying forth what they had learned at the Children's Hospital. Many, in fact, did exactly that and outstanding contributions to world health were made as a result of Janeway's view of pediatrics from a more global perspective. He pursued this approach despite some rather significant concerns and even objections from his own faculty, who thought that this endeavor might dilute the high quality of the traditional training program.

In the 1964 annual report, Dr. Janeway stated, ". . . we have a very real obligation to assist in the training of the best among the multitude of foreign physicians who are flocking to this country for medical training."[47] He utilized three types of experiences for foreign physicians: a) post-graduate courses organized by the Harvard Medical School for students from foreign countries to study the scientific basis of modern pediatrics in preparation for their subsequent entry into American residencies; b) formal residency training for those sufficiently proficient in the English language; and c) advanced clinical and research fellowship training in a specialized field for established pediatric teachers and faculty. In the same report, he noted with some pride that when he traveled, he frequently met former Children's Hospital resident trainees in airports throughout the world, including "Frankfort, Paris, Rome, Athens, Cairo, Beirut, Ankara, Teheran, Karachi, Bombay, New Delhi, Madras, Colombo, Djakarta, Surabaya, Hong Kong, Singapore, Manila, Taipei, and Honolulu."[48]

In the 1966 annual report, Janeway discussed the advantages and successes as well as disadvantages and, on occasion, failures of the foreign medical graduate program at the Children's Hospital.[49] He reflected on the reasons why these residents came to be trained in the U.S., including a "youthful desire to see the world, genuine desire for better medical training, desire for prestige and the hope of a better job at home, and pay as a house officer which far exceeds a professor's full-time salary in their own country."[49] He further noted that health manpower needs in the U.S. were being "aided handsomely by those countries which can least afford it." If these physicians returned to their countries, Janeway felt all was for the best. However, he wrote, ". . . unfortunately, a fair number do not return permanently, many are not properly trained to meet the real needs of their countries, and often they are not optimally utilized upon their return, but may find themselves relegated to inferior positions by their elders who are less well trained but jealous of their own prestige."[49] Ending on an optimistic note and remembering the countries he visited during his sabbatical years (Korea, Japan, Taiwan, Hong Kong, the Philippines, Thailand, India, Iran, and Egypt), he noted the fine reputation the Children's Hospital enjoyed around the world but concluded that, as a result, "the flood beats upon our doorstep more than most."[49]

Writing in the 1970 annual report, after the Coordinated Residency Program had been discontinued, Janeway reflected somewhat sadly that although the program had been greatly improved by Dr. Adels, "its participants felt like second class citizens, even though they were often more experienced than our regular residents." As a result, he noted there was now a single large housestaff in which "we neither discriminate against women nor against foreign citizens."[50]

Many graduates of foreign medical schools who did post-graduate training under Dr. Janeway later ascended to highly important positions in their own countries. One was Dr. Francisco Tome, who went on to head the Hospital of Honduras as well as the Central American District of the American Academy of Pediatrics. He had started as an observer at the Children's Hospital, then a student at the Harvard School of Public Health, and finally a fully integrated member of the residency.[51] A second was Dr. David Lobo from Caracas, Venezuela, who served as a resident in the Traditional Residency Program prior to returning to his country to lead the Children's Hospital in Caracas. Other important examples include Charlie Phornphutkul, who went on to become dean of Thailand Medical School, and Nabil Kronfol, future president of the Lebanese Health Care Management Association in Beirut. Jon Rohde, a Janeway trainee, became chair of the James P. Grant School of Public Health in Daka, Bangladesh, in recognition of his important contributions to international health. Dr. Janeway's willingness to make adjustments needed by newly arrived foreign medical graduates as they became proficient in the English language and comfortable in the U.S. medical culture was essential to their success. Many years later, they would attribute their training in the U.S. and Dr. Janeway's personal interest in them as major contributors to their subsequent professional success.

Chief Residency

The earliest reference to the chief resident and his role is found in the late 19th century on the surgical service of William Halsted at Johns Hopkins Hospital, specifically in a reference to a senior resident who had demonstrated sufficient competence in his craft to be allowed to manage and operate on patients with minimal supervision.[52] In the early 20th century, the surgical model was extended to medical, pediatric, and psychiatric services and included the responsibility for helping to train young interns and residents. By 1940, the Commission on Graduate Medical Education suggested that the chief resident "should have the responsibility for developing programs for at least a portion of the conferences, seminars and meetings."[53] This responsibility was also perceived to be helpful once the chief resident became a staff member.

In the Blackfan era, the most senior of the resident staff was considered to be the chief resident, if not formally so designated. There is reference in 1931 to Louis K. Diamond serving as the chief resident; others of similar renown followed in that role, including Clement Smith, Warren Wheeler, Clifford Grulee Jr., and Edward Pratt. Also, as noted before, Kenneth Blackfan had served as chief resident (in role if not in title) for John Howland at Johns Hopkins Hospital for a number of years, and he in turn created a similar role for James Wilson—future chair of pediatrics at the University of Michigan—at the Children's Hospital as the perennial assistant to the chief in the 1930s.

Dr. Janeway formally institutionalized a similar role and nomenclature for the chief resident, who after several years became assistant to the physician-in-chief.[54] In the mid-'60s, he appointed Sherwin Kevy to the position, a post that he would hold for seven years, two years as chief resident and five as assistant to the physician-in-chief (Figure 8). Kevy would become an icon to innumerable classes of house officers, known for his extensive knowledge of pediatrics, his excellent teaching ability, and his fine clinical acumen. [The author would be similarly appointed in 1970 for four years, two years as chief resident and two years as assistant to the physician-in-chief.] The assistant to the physician-in-chief was a faculty member (and no longer a resident) and served for a number of years offering continuity in care and teaching of the resident staff, a role that a chief resident appointed for six months to a year was unable to fulfill. The assistant to the physician-in-chief led the housestaff program, worked daily with the residents, and was the stand-in for the chief on matters clinical and educational. This role and title were discontinued in the Avery and Nathan years, with more seasoned faculty needed to organize and run the clinical services and with the chief residents appointed for a 12-month period.

The chief residents in the Janeway era served for six months to two years, with most serving for one year. A total of 48 chief residents, as shown in Table 5, were appointed by Charles Janeway.

All were male, save Lisbeth Hillman and Juanita (Judy) Lamar, although Gretchen Hutchins had served in that role during World War II under Dr. Richard Smith. The chief resident's area of responsibility was assignment to either the inpatient or the outpatient service, with two or more chief residents cross covering each other at night. Fred Robbins, although appointed by Richard Smith, was

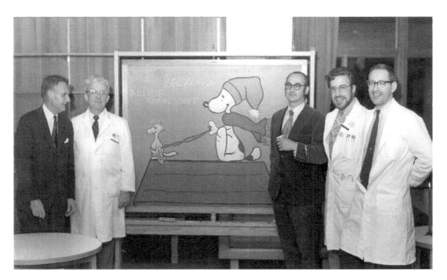

FIGURE 8   Holiday Greetings, 1972

Dr. Janeway and Tom Cone are shown on the left with Sherwin Kevy (third from left), John Graef, and Fred Lovejoy (Dr. Janeway's chief residents) in the chief's office at the time of the holiday season.

TABLE 5   Charles A. Janeway's Chief Residents

1947	Frederick C. Robbins, Jr.	1960–1961	David H. Carver
1948	Robert J. McKay, Jr.		A.A. Douglas Moore*
1949–1950	Charles D. Cook	1961–1962	Robert A. Goodell
1951	John D. Kennell		Joel J. Alpert*
1952	Leonard Apt	1962–1963	Thomas Adams
	Edward A. Mortimer, Jr.*		David H. Smith
	Harrie R. Chamberlin*	1963–1964	John L. Green
1953	John R. Hartmann		James R. Hughes
	Alexander Blum*	1964–1965	M. David Atkin
1954	Maurice M. Osborne, Jr.		Myron Johnson
	Charles V. Pryles*	1965–1966	Sherwin V. Kevy**
1955	Robert J. Haggerty	1966–1967	Sherwin V. Kevy**
	Willard B. Fernald*		Michael J. Maisels*
1955–1956	Mohsen Ziai	1967–1968	Sherwin V. Kevy**
	Samuel Katz		Robert Rosenberg*
	Lewis B. Anderson*	1968–1969	Sherwin V. Kevy**
	Philip Adler*	1969–1970	Sherwin V. Kevy**
1956–1957	Peter A. Auld		Robert Reece*
	John Whitcomb*	1970–1971	Frederick H. Lovejoy, Jr.
	Seymour Zoger*		John W. Graef*
	Lisbeth Hillman*	1971–1972	Frederick H. Lovejoy, Jr.
1957–1958	Charles Andrew Rigg		John W. Graef*
	Michael Braudo*		Roger Ashley*
	Richard L. Lester, Jr.*	1972–1973	Frederick H. Lovejoy, Jr.**
	William London*	1973–1974	Frederick H. Lovejoy, Jr.**
1958–1959	Sherwin V. Kevy		Elias Milgram*
	James N. Montgomery*	1974–1975	John A. Phillips
1959–1960	Sherwin V. Kevy		Juanita Lamar*
	John P. Eckert*		
	Walter S. James*		

*(MOPD) Medical Outpatient Pediatric Department Chief Resident
**Assistant to the Physician-in-Chief

Dr. Janeway's first chief resident, while Jim McKay was the first chief resident chosen by Dr. Janeway. Steeped in hospital lore is the story of Robbins, who was departing his position as chief resident and asked the incoming chief resident, Jim McKay, to relieve him earlier than planned so that he might return to his laboratory work. Reluctantly McKay, who was a resident at Babies Hospital in

New York City, agreed. It was December 1947, the laboratory (the Enders Laboratory) grew the poliovirus in tissue culture shortly thereafter, and the Nobel Prize followed in 1954 for a remarkably young Fred Robbins.[55] From that day forward, Dr. Janeway never had any difficulty filling his chief residency positions!

A number of chief residents went on to lead medical school pediatric departments, Fred Robbins at Case Western Reserve, Jim McKay in Vermont, Charles Cook at Yale, Edward Mortimer at the University of New Mexico, Bob Haggerty in Rochester, Sam Katz at Duke, David Carver in Toronto, Joel Alpert at Boston University, and David Smith in Rochester. Drs. Robbins, Cook, Haggerty, Katz, Kevy, Alpert, Smith, Lovejoy and Graef went on from their chief resident positions to serve on the faculty at the Children's Hospital. One reason why so many chiefs pursued academic careers was Dr. Janeway's way of involving them in curriculum planning, the overall educational process, and hospital policy. They also participated actively in the teaching of Harvard Medical School students (Figure 9). The joy of being a generalist for one or more years augmenting one's medical knowledge and skills, coupled with the prestige of the position (with potential subsequent appointment to the faculty), made for a highly coveted position among the housestaff. When Mary Ellen Avery assumed the chairmanship in 1974, she appointed two chief residents each year thereafter, now with the sharing of administrative, clinical, and teaching responsibilities.

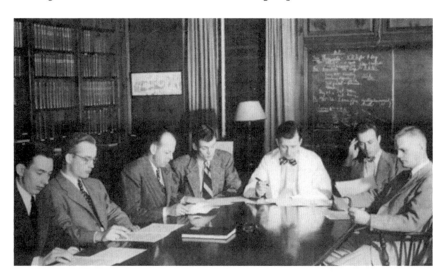

FIGURE 9   Instruction of Harvard Medical School students, circa 1950
The photo shows instruction of fourth-year Harvard Medical School students in the "Lab Study."

Medical Teaching

Housestaff education was led in the 1940s and 1950s by Louis K. Diamond, Edward Pratt, and Sydney Gellis and in the 1960s and 1970s, by William Berenberg and Sherwin Kevy for the inpatient service and by Tom Cone and Joel Alpert for the outpatient service. In fact, Bill Berenberg and Tom Cone served as the primary senior leaders for inpatient and outpatient education of the housestaff and deserve great credit for the quality of training of house officers in the program. A rich offering of teaching conferences was constantly created for the residents and students, thereby maintaining an active focus on medical education.[56] These conferences were well attended by the housestaff, which was smaller than today and thus one's absence was more easily noticed. Dr. Janeway also set the expectation that his faculty be present, especially for grand rounds and chief rounds. In addition, while some teaching sessions were enjoyed more than others by the housestaff, their overall quality and the culture of inquiry and learning was exceedingly strong.

Senior rounds occurred daily from 10 to 11 a.m and were reserved for the senior residents only. This tradition was carefully guarded by the seniors until the early 2000s, when these rounds were opened to the junior residents. Drs. Janeway, Berenberg, and Kevy were the primary faculty in attendance. Additional faculty members were not included as they are today, with the best teachers being selected to participate by the current senior residents. Several presentations by the seniors on the ward services were given. The presentations were of recently admitted patients, thus the cases were relatively "fresh" and not fully "worked up." The discussions were oriented around a differential diagnosis and the diagnosis as well as the treatment plan. There was also the opportunity for the chiefs to communicate policy directives concerning the hospital, residency issues, communication with community physicians, etc. In addition, senior rounds provided the chance for follow-up and closure on a past difficult or complex case, often with added encouragement from Dr. Janeway to a senior resident to write up the case for publication. Attendance by the residents was always excellent, and the conference was remembered years later as being highly influential and formative in the residency experience.

Chief's rounds occurred each Thursday afternoon in the Division 34 classroom (located on the surgical floor of the Farley Building). The room held approximately 80 people comfortably; however, generally 90 or more students, residents, faculty, and nurses were in attendance. Consequently, the residents often sat (uncomfortably) on the ascending staircase. Each year, the residents would lobby (unsuccessfully) for a larger room, with Janeway firmly explaining a fully filled smaller room was better than a half filled larger room—the former enhancing collegiality and more active discussions. Charles Janeway and the division chiefs sat in the front row with junior faculty and senior and junior housestaff behind them. Nurses were encouraged to attend and did.

The chief resident facilitated the session. The case was presented by the housestaff; the X-rays reviewed by the radiologist; the patient and parent present with Dr. Janeway (or Drs. Diamond or Berenberg in Dr. Janeway's absence) pointing out the pertinent physical findings; and the case was then discussed in a relatively free-flowing manner by the "front row." Dr. Janeway would call on his faculty to comment. The case to be discussed was generally known ahead of time so the faculty could prepare (so not to be caught flat footed). Occasionally, the housestaff would complain that the discussion was too anecdotal and inadequately informed by the literature. Long presentations by the faculty were not encouraged; the opportunity to observe how the faculty reasoned and thought through a problem was encouraged. Housestaff and student opinions were actively solicited. Despite occasional criticism, this conference was highly popular and extremely well attended.

Grand rounds and clinical pathological conference (CPC) were held on Wednesdays, initially for two hours and later for one hour (with grand rounds three times each month and CPC once a month). They were held in the Jimmy Fund Auditorium (located between the Carnegie Building and the current Smith and Dana-Farber Buildings). Both were for the hospital community—faculty, fellows, housestaff, students, nurses, and community physicians. Generally, 125 to 150 individuals attended. They were more formal than chief's rounds. A topic was covered. The case was presented, the patient (or parent) was interviewed with pertinent findings demonstrated (in contrast to today's practice), and presentations were made by several faculty (and on occasion housestaff). Considerable discussion of the case then followed. Topics were often selected by the chief resident; controversial diagnostic or management issues with opposing positions presented were particularly popular. These were hospital grand rounds with surgical and other medical departments (psychiatry, neurology, cardiology, etc.) often attending.

CPCs were modeled after the very popular case reports in *The New England Journal of Medicine*, edited for more than two decades by Dr. Benjamin Castleman, a pathologist at the Massachusetts General Hospital. The case was presented and carefully discussed by a faculty member with a "clinical diagnosis" made. This was followed by the student diagnosis and then a presentation, "anatomical diagnosis," and discussion orchestrated by the pathologist. Drs. Sidney Farber, Benjamin Landing, John Craig, and Gordon Vawter led this conference over the years, with selected CPCs from the Children's Hospital (edited by Drs. Farber and Vawter) published in the *Journal of Pediatrics*. Mike Liberman and John Graef presented the first CPC given by the housestaff, a precursor to subsequent resident participation at grand rounds and CPCs. As new technology allowed for more accurate diagnosis and post-mortem examinations became less common and relevant, the CPC began to lose its essential role. This conference became less frequent in the 1970s. A second **resident pathology conference** was held on Mondays from 4:30 to 5:30 p.m. in the pathology department. Attended and led by Drs. Farber and Janeway, the purpose of this pathology conference was to review the gross and microscopic findings of a recent death on the medical service. As autopsies became less frequent, it, too, began to lose its essential nature and was gradually phased out during Dr. Avery's tenure as chief.

Dr. Janeway's ward rounds occurred from 4 to 5 PM once a week alternating between Division 27 (for children from 1 month to 4 to 5 years) and Division 37 (for children from ages 4 to 5 up through adolescence). The rounds were attended by the housestaff, students, and nurses. The senior resident for the floor selected the case in consultation with the chief resident, and the rounds were always held at the bedside. The case (which was not made known to the chief before the rounds) was presented by the student or junior resident. Then the chief (or his substitute) would carefully question the parent and when possible the child. The setting in which the child grew up was always carefully explored. Then following careful hand washing (as an example to the housestaff), the child was meticulously examined, physical findings demonstrated, and the housestaff encouraged to feel the enlarged spleen, ballot the ascites, examine the tender swollen knee, or describe the observed rash. This would take the first half hour. The chief would then discuss the case and engage in a Socratic dialogue with those students and housestaff present. Teaching was as much by example as by spoken word. Laboratory results were carefully interpreted but not over emphasized (in contrast to the history and the physical examination). The rounds ended with a discussion of the treatment plan and the expected rate of improvement. The rounds ended promptly at 5 p.m. A very similar approach was used on Mondays at noon with the medical students. Considered in retrospect, a minimum of four hour-long sessions each week with the chief (chief's rounds, senior rounds, ward rounds and grand rounds) was a remarkable commitment of the department chair's time, a phenomenon less seen today because of the current administrative burdens of the job.

Life as a House Officer

For a house officer, this was an era of giants. Janeway, Diamond, Nadas, Farber, Robert Gross, and Edward Neuhauser were seen as innovative pioneers whose discoveries were thought to be long lasting, even permanent. As noted by Fred Mandell (a house officer in 1969) years later, "When you were surrounded by giants, their presence made you reach to a higher level. You felt it was an honor to be among them and to be part of the Children's Hospital. You felt an over-whelming commitment to teach well and to give the best care to your patients."[57] Implied in this reflection is the view of the housestaff of the 1960s, who saw themselves as the major caregivers on the inpatient services, with the faculty playing less of a minute-to-minute oversight role. This deep focus on patient care by the housestaff and the somewhat peripheral involvement of the faculty disrupted the prior family-oriented culture among the faculty and the residents. A close collegiality between the two was now less evident. The paternalistic role of the faculty was also less accepted by the housestaff, especially in the late 1960s and early 1970s.

The hospital was a relatively formal place in the early 1950s. Interns were taught to call their senior teachers "Doctor," and the use of first names did not occur until one's senior resident year. All but student nurses were called "Miss" by the housestaff. This was especially true for nurse supervisors, who were seen as very powerful. All male housestaff wore clean regulation whites, including white dentist-style shirts, short white coats and white pants (all changed almost daily due to concerns with infection), and white shoes. Feelings of inadequacy and worries about lack of knowledge were frequent. Similarly, fears of misman-agement of a patient or making an error were also commonplace, with feelings of "sick with anxiety" occurring in even the most competent resident.[58] These feelings persist today and are one of the reasons why residents work so hard to avoid making an error. The hospital limited visiting hours in the early 1950s. The medical service allowed only one hour for visiting each evening and the surgical service two hours each week, only on Sundays. The rationale offered was "too much disruption, too many tears." Parents were excluded from the treatment room when a procedure or test was to be carried out.[58]

The night call in the 1940s, 1950s, and early 1960s was every other night and every other weekend (Monday, Wednesday, Saturday, Sunday, Tuesday, Thursday, and Friday over a two-week period). By the 1970s, it had been liberalized to every third night and every third weekend. Vacation was initially for one week each year, then two weeks in the 1950s and 1960s, and finally three weeks each year in the 1970s. Patient volume and thus the work of a house officer was often dictated by the prevalence of infectious diseases. Winter and spring tended to be busier than the summer and fall. Today's house officer may be busier due to the large number of laboratory tests, the need for rigorous documentation, and the large number of admissions each night and turnover each day (due to a length of stay today of 4 to 5 days, in contrast to 8 to 10 days in the 1950s, 1960s, and 1970s). Yet the house officers in the Janeway era did their own CBCs (complete blood count tests), urine analyses, spinal fluid analyses, and tuberculin tests, and then transported these fluids to the laboratory and started their own intravenous lines and performed their own cutdowns (surgical placement of a catheter into a vein) on the floors. The emergency room was the location for diagnosis and decisions on admission (or return to home), the wards the location for the work-up.

Resident learning came less from formal conferences and more from work on the wards. As reflected upon by Fred Mandell, later an astute and greatly admired practicing pediatrician, "You learned pediatrics by listening, watching, and through the example of your teachers. Your most significant learning came from the hour-to-hour care of your patients. Being available and being responsible was the credo of the day. We depended on each other and that defined our camaraderie. We considered it an honor to be among our fellow residents."[57]

And as noted by Dr. Suzanne Boulter, a resident in the late 1960s and later a school physician at St. Paul's School and practicing pediatrician in Concord, New Hampshire, "We were paid $3,600/year as an intern and $6,000/year as a junior resident, the increase due to a 'heal-in' at Boston City Hospital. We didn't have time to spend our money so the amount mattered little. We were on every other night and every other weekend and with generally 2 to 3 hours of sleep. It was the hardest experience of my life. It changed me as a person. It made me feel I could cope with anything, no matter how tough in the future. My principles and ethics were developed here. They were clarified and encoded in me." And reflecting further, Boulter said, "There wasn't a good balance in my life but I learned the meaning of total commitment. We were told we were lucky to be here and we were."[58]

The senior residents in the 1960s and 1970s tended to be older, and some were married with children. This was because many had served in the military as part of the draft and Berry Plan (a national initiative to train physicians as specialists before being called into the armed services as officers) or had acquired research experience at the National Institutes of Health. Other residents had often served at a public city hospital prior to coming to the Children's Hospital, where they were given more latitude in independent decision-making. This allowed them to serve as "junior executives" in their supervisory role as senior residents.[59] Norman Spack, himself a senior resident in the late 1960s and a future faculty member in endocrinology, had this observation about senior residents: "They avidly protected the prerogative of their junior house officers to write orders and to make their own decisions on their patients. They invited nurses to attend their work rounds and respected the wisdom and experience of the senior nurses. Finally, senior rounds were very active and even contentious, with seniors strongly advocating for their decisions and attendings often serving as arbitrators around hotly debated issues."[59]

The house officer in the Janeway era was indeed very busy, and on many nights would get only one or two hours of sleep. The call rooms were not on the floors of the hospital but rather in the small, white houses lining Longwood Avenue or in the Hunnewell Building. Haircuts tended to be relatively short until the late 1960s, when the hair became longer. When suggested that this looked somewhat unprofessional, the house officer's plaintive retort was, "It's what's inside my head that is important, not what is on top of it!" In the 1940s and 1950s, meals for the housestaff when on call were taken in the faculty dining room. Visitors could be invited but had to be paid for. Tables in the faculty dining room were covered with linen tablecloths and fine silver was used. The faculty dining room was discontinued in the late 1950s, replaced by a hospital-wide dining room for all hospital personnel and families of patients. Although strongly advocated for by some senior faculty because of its collegial atmosphere, the faculty dining room was never recreated in the hospital.

As reflected upon by Richard Johnston, a resident in the early 1960s, "residents in the Department of Pediatrics were paid about $145 a month after taxes. Rent for my wife, infant son, and me in a safe building across from the Isabella Stewart Gardner Museum was $115 a month. (This was the time of the Boston Strangler.) There were other benefits; however, food in the hospital cafeteria was free to house staff. We could eat all meals in the cafeteria, the post-call day ending about suppertime. The hospital provided a special bonus: three yellow certificates a month that would allow the resident's family to eat, theoretically, three free meals. In our case, my wife wheeled our son to the cafeteria nightly and submitted one yellow certificate. Now, the cashiers who received the certificates were ladies who looked and behaved like grandmothers. When they had recorded the use of the certificate instead of cash, they simply handed back the certificate, which we used again and again. In this way my family and I were well fed and I wore clean clothes on $30 a month."[60]

Life as a woman was not easy. As remembered by Suzanne Boulter years later, "We felt there were no female role models. We were the pioneers. We had to be as good as or better than the men. We never wanted to show our weak side. We never cried. We felt it was important for us to succeed so as to open the path for the women who followed. My second night on call I was exhausted at 4 a.m., went to the on-call rooms, but there was no place for women to sleep so I went back to the nursery and slept there. I spoke to David Weiner [the future hospital director] the next day and he fixed it. Still it was difficult because as a woman I did not want to rock the boat. Dating was the hardest. There was no time, you were too tired. If you told a date you were a resident they didn't understand the life and they were frankly intimidated. It wasn't a plus as today; it was a turnoff. I began to tell them I was an X-ray technician. That was more normal."[58]

Dr. Janeway was a strong advocate, as noted in the minutes of the hospital's executive committee, for fair and adequate housestaff salaries: "interns and residents are not only students of medicine, but are productive members of society, providing the bulk of medical care for patients with serious illness. They ought to receive adequate compensation, comparable to that earned by other young professionals such as teachers and lawyers, at the start of their careers."[56] When this became a hospital issue in the early 1960s, he chaired a committee that contrasted the Children's Hospital house officer salaries with those throughout the country. House officer salaries prior to that time had been based on the view that, "hard work itself and the educational experience of working in an outstanding hospital" was sufficient reward.[61] The resultant increase in salaries led to very few applicants turning down an offer of a residency position at the Children's Hospital.

The House Officer Association, started in the mid- to late 1960s and led by Alan Rozycki, a superb former Dartmouth football player and later faculty member in Hanover, became an effective body for progress in medical education and living conditions. The housestaff went to considerable lengths to plead to the administration for increased salary, as reflected here: "I remember one house officer pleading poverty and applying for state unemployment, only to be told by an unamused Dr. Janeway it was Children's or unemployment; he chose Children's!"[57] In the early 1970s, Jan Breslow, a future distinguished physician-scientist and president of the American Heart Association, advocated for an increase in house officer salaries. As president of the Housestaff Association, he, Phil Landrigan, a future department chair in New York City, and John Graef, lobbied successfully, obtaining Dr. Janeway's full support, with a resultant 30%

increase in a resident's salary. The Housestaff Association also became a strong participant in advocating for a robust educational system for the housestaff.

Dinners in faculty homes were a common practice. Following a month of ward attending, the faculty would invite the three to four housestaff plus students for a relaxing and much appreciated dinner in their home. Holiday parties were common over the Christmas holidays. A limited numbers of days off to enjoy the holidays at home (with cross coverage) occurred over Christmas and New Year's. The housestaff show had its genesis in the early 1960s when the housestaff would go to the Gamble's farm in Taunton, Massachusetts (and later the Eley's farm in New Hampshire) and put on a play.[62] While lacking in the musical and dancing talent of today's shows, the shows, especially in the late 1960s and early 1970s, were an opportunity for merriment and a few digs at the faculty. To be the chief with long dancing eyebrows for the evening [Dr. Janeway] was the most sought-after role.

Internship selection became a more formal process as the housestaff grew in size over the 1950s, 1960s, and 1970s. Applicants were interviewed by the senior faculty throughout the preceding weeks. The senior faculty would then meet for a single evening prior to submission of the match list to review the applicants and submit the final list. Dr. Janeway would run the meeting; the chief resident would keep the list at the blackboard; the considered opinion of the senior faculty was carefully solicited.[62] By 1970, 15 interns were matching to a program of 58 house officers. That year, 20% graduated from Harvard Medical School and 28% were women.[63]

And with some nostalgia one house officer of that era, William Cochran, a house officer in the 1950s and later a greatly respected neonatologist at the Beth Israel Hospital, reflected, "I remember playing tennis on the Gardner House tennis courts, the yearly house officer show in the Jimmy Fund Auditorium, the parties at the visits'[ward attendings] homes, senior rounds in Sherwin Kevy's tiny blood bank office with its smell of pipe tobacco, and the bedrooms in the small white houses on the current site of the Enders Building with their white sheets, white pillow cases, thin white blankets, and telephones."[64]

Dr. Janeway's personal and professional impact on the life of his trainees during residency would last for a lifetime. Dan Cohen, a senior resident in the early 1970s, recently related to the author the following illustrative story of Dr. Janeway's remarkably impactful teaching style: "One day I asked Dr. Janeway to come over to Division 27 to see a two-year-old child with classical Still's disease. As Dr. Janeway entered the room, he took off his starched white coat and washed his hands before sitting down to talk with the child's young mother. After talking with her, he got up, washed his hands a second time and then examined the child. After examining the child he shared his thoughts, asked the mother if she had any questions and promised to return to see her child again the next day. He then got up and washed his hands a third time before leaving the room.

As we all congregated to discuss the case, one of the students asked Dr. Janeway why he washed his hands three times. Dr. Janeway looked down at his hands, paused momentarily, and said the following: 'I washed my hands when I entered the room because I did not want to bring any bacteria in or out of this child's environment. I washed my hands the second time, before examining the child, because I sensed the mother needed additional reassurance. Washing my hands the second time was intended to send a message to the mother that I really cared about her child and wanted the child to be absolutely safe.' Hand washing for Dr. Janeway was both about preventing the spread of infection and about demonstrating caring and concern for this mother's child. This lesson was carefully noted by each of us."[65]

Career Achievements

Among the 1,000-plus housestaff trained during the nearly 30-year tenure of Charles Janeway, an amazing number of academic and leadership accomplishments were achieved by the remarkable graduates of his training program. It is impossible to completely record the extensive list of division chiefs or to highlight the research accomplishments of the group, and these lists do not include innumerable notable fellowship trainees in the Janeway era (who were not housestaff). Particular accomplishments in the world of academic pediatrics are, however, worth noting.

Thirty-two department chairs came from the era commencing in 1946 and 1947. They include Fred Robbins, chair at Case Western Reserve School of Medicine, and James McKay, long-time chair at the University of Vermont School of Medicine, extending to John Modlin, past chair of the Department of Pediatrics at Dartmouth Medical School, and Paul Dworkin, currently chair of pediatrics at the University of Connecticut Medical School. The remarkably large list of chairs from the Janeway era in the United States and Canada is shown below (Table 6). This list does not include chairs in foreign countries. A partial list of those individuals includes Richard Moxon at Oxford University, Thomas Oppe at St. Mary's Medical School, John Davis at Cambridge University, Nabutako Matsuo in Tokyo, Moshen Ziai in Iran, and Kim Oates at the University of Sydney in Australia. Of significance, this list does not include any women, although Betty

TABLE 6   Department Chairs

Herbert T. Abelson	University of Chicago School of Medicine; University of Washington School of Medicine
Joel J. Alpert	Boston University School of Medicine
Lewis A. Barness	University of South Florida School of Medicine
Spencer Borden	Harvard Medical School; University of Pennsylvania School of Medicine
George W. Brumley	Emory University School of Medicine
David H. Carver	University of Toronto School of Medicine; New Jersey Medical School
Harvey J. Cohen	Stanford University School of Medicine
Charles D. Cook	Yale University School of Medicine; SUNY Downstate College of Medicine
C. William Daeschner, Jr.	University of Texas Medical Branch, Galveston
Paul H. Dworkin	University of Connecticut School of Medicine
Lewis E. Gibson	Loyola University Chicago School of Medicine
Eli Gold	University of California at Davis School of Medicine
Richard B. Goldbloom	Dalousie University School of Medicine
Robert J. Haggerty	University of Rochester School of Medicine and Dentistry
Richard B. Johnston, Jr.	University of Pennsylvania School of Medicine
Samuel L. Katz	Duke University School of Medicine
Philip J. Landrigan	Mount Sinai School of Medicine, New York
Nobutake Matsuo	Keio University School of Medicine, Tokyo
R. James McKay	University of Vermont College of Medicine
Stanley A. Mendosa	University of California at San Diego Medical School
Jack Metcoff	University of Chicago School of Medicine
John F. Modlin	Dartmouth Medical School
Edward A. Mortimer, Jr.	University of New Mexico School of Medicine
E. Richard Moxon	University of Oxford, England
George A. Nankervis	Northeastern Ohio Universities College of Medicine
Nicholas M. Nelson	Pennsylvania State University School of Medicine
Philip A. Pizzo	Harvard Medical School
Frederick C. Robbins, Jr.	Case Western Reserve University School of Medicine
Jimmy Simon	Bowman Gray School of Medicine
David H. Smith	University of Rochester School of Medicine and Dentistry
Jon B. Tingelstad	East Carolina University School of Medicine
William M. Wallace	Case Western Reserve University School of Medicine

Lowe and Mildred Stahlman were pioneers in leadership roles in the Academy of Pediatrics and the American Pediatric Society, respectively (Tables 7 and 9).

Achievements in leadership of the American Academy of Pediatrics (AAP) (5), the Society for Pediatric Research (SPR) (4), the American Pediatric Society (APS) (6), the American Board of Pediatrics (ABP) (4), ABP sub-boards of pediatrics (4), and Editors of *Pediatrics* (2) are shown in Tables 7–12.

TABLE 7   Presidents of the American Academy of Pediatrics

R. James McKay	1970–1971
Robert J. Haggerty	19841–985
Betty A. Lowe	1993–1994
Joel J. Alpert	1998–1999
Thomas McInerny	2012–2013

TABLE 8   Presidents of the Society for Pediatric Research

Frederick C. Robbins, Jr.	1962
Charles R. Scriver	1976
Richard B. Johnston, Jr.	1981
Harvey J. Cohen	1989

TABLE 9   Presidents of the American Pediatric Society

Frederick C. Robbins, Jr.	1973
Mildred T. Stahlman	1984
Lewis A. Barness	1985
Samuel L. Katz	1986
Charles Scriver	1994
Richard B. Johnston, Jr.	1996

TABLE 10   American Board of Pediatrics

Presidents	Herbert T. Abelson	1997
	Jon B. Tingelstad	1998
Secretary-Treasurer	C. W. Daeschner, Jr.	1974–1982
	Herbert T. Abelson	1995

TABLE 11   American Board of Pediatrics Subspecialty Boards

Chair of the Sub-Board of Pediatric Cardiology	Amnon Rosenthal	1987–1988
Chair of the Sub-Board of Pediatric Hematology/ Oncology	William Mentzer	2002–2003
Chairs of the Sub-Board of Neonatology	Nicholas Nelson	1983–1984
	M. Jeffery Maisels	1987–1988

TABLE 12   Editors of the Journal *Pediatrics*

Robert J. Haggerty, Co-Editor	1974
James McKay, Associate Editor	1974

Finally achievements of Janeway housestaff graduates are recognized through multiple awards and honors, including selection to give the annual Blackfan Lecture (7), Harvard Medical School Teaching Awards (4), the E. Mead Johnson Award (13), the prestigious Howland Award (7) and the Nobel Prize (3) (Tables 13–17). The remarkable number of E. Mead Johnson Award winners bears witness to the great importance placed by the Children's Hospital

TABLE 13   Blackfan Lecturers

Charles Scriver	1975
D. Carleton Gajdusek	1981
Robert J. Haggerty	1987
Samuel L. Katz	1992
E. Richard Moxon	1994
Mildred Stahlman	1997
Fred S. Rosen	2006

TABLE 14   Harvard Medical School Teaching Awards

William Cochran	1981, 1992
Shah Khoshbin	1984, 2000, 2003
Frederick H. Lovejoy, Jr.	1979, 1981, 1986
Samuel E. Lux, IV	1982, 1983, 1984

TABLE 15   E. Mead Johnson Award

Frederick C. Robbins	1953
Thomas H. Weller	1953
David Gitlin	1956
Park S. Gerald	1962
C. Carleton Gajdusek	1963
Charles R. Scriver	1968
Fred S. Rosen	1971
David H. Smith	1975
Erwin W. Gelfand	1981
Samuel E. Lux	1983
Jan L. Breslow	1984
John Phillips	1984
Raif S. Geha	1986

TABLE 16   American Pediatric Society Howland Award

Lewis A. Barness	1993
Mildred T. Stahlman	1996
Robert J. Haggerty	1998
Samuel L. Katz	2000
Richard B. Johnston, Jr.	2008
Charles R. Scriver	2010
Philip A. Pizzo	2012

TABLE 17   Nobel Prizes

Frederick C. Robbins, Jr.	1954
Thomas H. Weller	1954
D. Carleton Gajdusek	1976

and Harvard Medical School on research. The number of Howland Award winners, given for outstanding lifetime contributions to academic pediatrics, is also particularly noteworthy.

These numbers fail to recognize other prestigious positions, such as deans of medical schools, which include Frederick C. Robbins, Jr., at Case Western

Reserve Medical School, Steven Spielberg at Dartmouth Medical School, Philip Pizzo at Stanford Medical School, and Jonathan E. Fielding at the UCLA School of Public Health; leaders of the divisions of the National Institutes of Health, such as Sumner Yaffe; commissioners of public health, such as Jonathan Fielding (in Massachusetts and Los Angeles County); hospital presidents, such as Jonathan Bates; vice chancellors of health systems, such as Mark C. Rogers at Duke University Medical Center; and members of the National Academy of Sciences and/or the Institute of Medicine, including among others Jan L. Breslow, Jonathan E. Fielding, Philip J. Landrigan, Philip A. Pizzo, and Mark C. Rogers. These lists do, however, show the tremendous impact of Janeway's housestaff graduates and their great influence on American pediatric medicine in the second half of the 20th century.

Summation

Greatly revered, deeply respected and universally extolled for many years to come, Dr. Janeway's 28 years as chairman created a halcyon era for the Department of Medicine. He firmly established the department's divisional structure and helped both old and new divisions to mature such that many were recognized for their clinical and research accomplishments being among the best throughout the United States. Secondly, his long tenure of leadership allowed him to train in the department's residency and fellowship programs outstanding academic physician leaders who then went on to populate and lead departments and divisions throughout the U.S. His impact through his trainees would be witnessed by American pediatrics for many years after his passing. Thirdly, he committed time and immense effort to the needs of the world's children, traveling the globe and offering his wisdom and advice for the betterment of health care throughout the world. Finally, his personal characteristics: high intelligence, fine bedside teaching skills, great modesty, remarkable wisdom and perspective, and a deep commitment to the needy and the underserved earned him great affection and deep respect.

Janeway in his usual reserved, thoughtful, and understated way was deeply committed to the professional and personal development of housestaff, fellows, and junior faculty. He saw in them the future of pediatrics. In his waning years, as if to offer one last bit of advice while there was still time, he reflected quietly on the beach in Annisquam to his great friend Bob Haggerty, "Bob, bet on youth."

CHAPTER V

The Avery Era

Program Development and Maturation
1974–1984

*"You meet lots of senior clinician-scientists, and you learn from these
people as to what success looks like and what pitfalls look like . . ."*

—Norman Rosenblum, reflecting on his
time as a house officer in 1985

T HE SELECTION OF DR. MARY ELLEN AVERY as the seventh physician-in-
chief of the Children's Hospital and the Thomas Morgan Rotch professor
of pediatrics at Harvard Medical School was a seminal event. Her appointment
was announced by Robert H. Ebert, MD, dean of the Faculty of Medicine at
Harvard Medical School and by Leonard W. Cronkhite, Jr., MD, president of
the Children's Hospital. The selection of a woman to one of the most prestigious
academic positions in the country was notable. In fact, her appointment in 1974
signaled several firsts, the first woman to be the physician-in-chief at the Children's Hospital and the first woman to chair a clinical department at Harvard
Medical School.[1]

Her opportunities—and challenges—were great. The opportunities included
the chance to build a strong neonatology program, recruit new talented divisional
leadership, and further develop a robust residency program. A top-flight scientist,
Dr. Avery was an early pioneer in pediatrics. Her work on surfactant deficiency
was groundbreaking, and as a role model, she recruited many women at every
level into pediatrics.

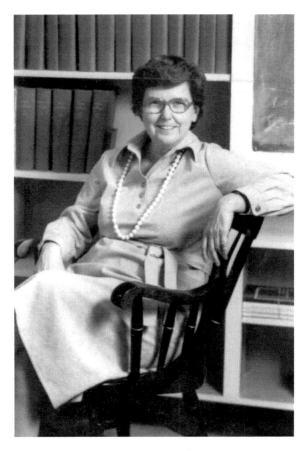

MARY ELLEN AVERY, MD, 1974–1984

Dr. Avery trained 250 housestaff during her tenure as Chair
of the Department of Medicine. She emphasized scientific
training in the curriculum and was a role model and strong
advocate for women in pediatrics.

Counted among her challenges was the need to establish a state-of-the-art
practice plan with a sound billing system. This was made more difficult by the
fact that the two large moneymakers for the department, cardiology and oncology, were no longer part of the Department of Medicine. Cardiology was now a
separate department, and oncology had been incorporated into the Dana-Farber
Cancer Institute. Further, Dr. Avery followed one of the most revered and loved
figures in American pediatrics, Charles Janeway. Although Dr. Janeway was
one of her most ardent supporters during her tenure, some of the senior faculty
in the Department of Medicine who had trained or served under Dr. Janeway

were still very loyal to him and the programs that he had established, making it challenging for Dr. Avery to institute needed policy changes.

Mary Ellen (or Mel, as she was known to colleagues and friends) Avery assumed the helm of the department with confidence, energy, and a new direction and purpose. Her prior training and experience had prepared her well for this new role.

The Children's Hospital and The Department of Medicine

Significant Hospital Events[2]

Major events in the 1970s included the resignation of Leonard Cronkhite as president of the Hospital in 1977 after 15 years of leadership to become the president of the Medical College of Wisconsin, and the appointment of his successor, David Weiner, a young and very talented University of Michigan School of Public Health graduate. The year 1977 also saw the appointment of the hospital's psychiatrist-in-chief, Julius Richmond, as surgeon general of the United States. As a result of a major snowstorm in February 1978, that year became known as the "Year of the Blizzard," with over three feet of snow closing down Boston and eastern Massachusetts. It strained the hospital's resources but cemented a spirit of teamwork throughout the hospital. Later that year, the Massachusetts Poison Control System opened at the Children's Hospital; this regionalized emergency information service served all citizens of the Commonwealth of Massachusetts. An innovative model of emergency information and care for the poisoned patient, it grew out of the Boston Poison Information Center, which had been started by Bob Haggerty and later run by Joel Alpert, both house officers in the Janeway era and future pediatric department chairmen.[3] The decade ended with the hospital celebrating its 110th anniversary in 1979.

The early 1980s ushered in the 10th anniversary of the renal transplant program, the deaths of Drs. Janeway, John Davies, Harry Mueller, and Richard Smith, all hospital giants, and the retirement of Drs. Alexander Nadas and Thomas Cone, both Department of Medicine stalwarts. That period also saw the return of the remarkable general surgeon Hardy Hendren as chief of surgery, the appointment of Bernardo Nadal-Ginard as chief of the Department of Cardiology, and the honoring by the hospital of Nobel Prize Laureate John Enders. The year 1983 witnessed the retirement of longtime, devoted Board of Trustees' President William Wolbach (the hospital's administrative building, the Wolbach Building, was later named in his honor) and the installation of a new board chair, David Kosowsky; the 20th anniversary of the Clinical Research Center; the 100th anniversary of James Gamble's birth; the 15th anniversary of the Developmental Evaluation Clinic; and the 10th anniversary of the Joint Program in Neonatology. In 1984, the first liver transplantation at the Children's Hospital was performed on a 15-month-old boy, and the hospital received its DoN (Determination of Need) designation for the construction of a new inpatient facility.

Patient Care[4]

During Leonard Cronkhite's tenure, in the 1960s and '70s, the Children's Hospital had been moving inexorably away from being a hospital for children with common pediatric diseases to a highly specialized hospital, where difficult cases in the region and beyond could be referred. "Regionalized" pediatric care, in which local hospitals managed less complex problems with more complex cases referred to specially oriented hospitals such as the Children's Hospital, was the accepted model of care in the late 1960s and early 1970s. The regional infant cardiac program initiated by Alexander Nadas and his longtime associate Donald Fyler to treat congenital cardiac problems was one example; the national—and even international—referrals to the orthopedic service for correction of scoliosis, led by Department of Orthopedic Surgery Chair John Hall, was another. The renal dialysis program exemplified a similar accomplishment in regionalization.

Remarkable medical advances were generating a need for new operating rooms, expanded recovery rooms, and enlarged radiology facilities. By the mid-1970s, advances in medical technology had made it possible to perform open-heart surgery, transplant organs, and implant artificial devices such as pacemakers. New medicines and drugs were reducing the burden of disease and shortening the length of hospital stay. These initiatives in the aggregate synergized the development of the specialty divisions in the Department of Medicine and assured that the Children's Hospital residency and fellowships were the place to train if one envisioned an academic pediatric career.

When David Weiner assumed the hospital presidency in 1977, controlling spiraling costs while simultaneously continuing to deliver the highest quality of care, had become the hospital's paramount challenge. This task was made more difficult by the ever-increasing severity and complexity of care, which necessitated more intensive care facilities and more highly trained personnel. By the early 1980s, a new concept for the containment of costs had entered the market place, "price competition." The idea was that competition among hospitals would ultimately reduce cost. Opponents argued that a competitive (rather than region-alized) approach would compromise quality of care, harm the existing system, and deny access to many groups of patients. A tertiary care teaching hospital was particularly vulnerable in such a system because of its higher costs related to medical education, development of research technology, higher intensity of care, and treatment of the medically indigent.

Forces in the Commonwealth of Massachusetts began to exert a major influence during the first half of the 1980s. Legislation and regulatory efforts to reduce reimbursement for health care represented a formidable challenge. The state's hospital cost control legislation, also known as Chapter 372, sought to limit rising health care costs while simultaneously maintaining services. Blue Cross/Blue Shield instituted a new system of prospective reimbursement for hospitals, whereby the hospital was paid a set amount for services rendered. The federal government initiated cutbacks in entitlements for those unable to pay for health care and curtailed funds for research. The housestaff and the training program were protected from these new realities of hospital economics mainly because the residency was seen as being within the purview of the medical and surgical departments.

Both the climate of cost constraint and the increasing complexity of patient care necessitated new approaches. The hospital adjusted, ratcheting up its phil-anthropic efforts, reducing its operating expenses, altering its efforts focused on the critically ill and the tertiary and even quaternary care patient, positioning itself to increasingly care for HMO and inner-city patients, and continuing to strengthen its referral relationships with private practitioners.

Hospital Construction[5]

The building of the hospital as we know it today had occurred over the previous two decades, with the opening of the Farley Building in 1956, the Fegan Building in 1967, and the Enders Research Building in 1970. Upon this sturdy foundation, smaller, but no less significant, internal construction occurred.

In 1976, a new neonatal intensive care unit was built and a new recreation room was added to Division 37 as an adjunctive form of therapy for the hospital's adolescent patients. Two years later, a Comprehensive Child Health Program (CCHP) was opened, along with a diagnostic test center, made possible by a gift from the Children's Hospital League. In 1980, the new 36-bed medical–surgical intensive care unit opened on the fifth and sixth floors of the hospital, with the fifth floor constructed to serve cardiovascular and general surgical patients and dedicated to Robert Gross, surgeon-in-chief from 1947 to 1967, and the sixth floor designed to serve neurosurgical, orthopedic, and medical patients and dedicated to Robert Smith, who served as anesthesiologist-in-chief from 1946 to 1980. Also in 1979, the Ronald McDonald House, a much-needed home-away-from-home for pediatric cancer patients and their families opened in a renovated Victorian house at 229 Kent Street in nearby Brookline.

The year 1980 saw the dedication of the new Cystic Fibrosis Research Center, made possible by the cooperative efforts of the Children's Hospital and the Massachusetts chapter of the Cystic Fibrosis Foundation, as well as the construction of an all-important bridge over Blackfan Street connecting the Enders and Hunnewell Buildings, thereby joining research with clinical care efforts. In addition, four new beds were added to the neonatal intensive care unit in 1980. In 1981, the emergency room waiting room was renovated and a new house officer lounge was constructed on the first floor of the Surgical and Radiology Pavilion Building, which connected the Farley and Hunnewell Buildings. This was made possible thanks to a gift from Geraldine Nelson, a volunteer in the blood bank during World War II, a generous donor, and a great friend of the trustees and staff at the hospital. In the same year, patient activity rooms on Division 35 (for the cardiology service) and Division 26 (for the orthopedic service) received a facelift.

On June 28, 1981, the old power plant on Blackfan Street was demolished to make room for the new inpatient hospital, ultimately to be renamed the Berthiaume Family Building. In 1982, the Surgical and Radiology Pavilion was completed. Finally in 1983, a new enlarged and modern neonatal medical intensive care unit opened. The majority of these improvements occurred in the arena of patient care and as such, positively impacted housestaff life both in clinical care and in medical education.

Departmental Leadership

Seventh Chair of the Department of Medicine

Mary Ellen Avery (photo, front of chapter) was a native of Camden, New Jersey. Her father owned a manufacturing company; her mother was vice principal of a high school. She attended Wheaton College, a fine liberal arts college in Norton, Massachusetts, majoring in chemistry and graduating in 1948 summa cum laude. Wheaton, where she later served as a trustee from 1965 to 1985, was an ideal site for her education and personal maturation. She reflected upon her time there, "I was a big fish in a small pond. I was recognized as a serious student and I had a ball."[6]

Johns Hopkins University School of Medicine was well known for its willingness to accept women as medical students, and Mary Ellen Avery was one of four women in a class of 90 (along with Betty Hay, subsequently a basic science department chair at Harvard Medical School) to be admitted in the fall of 1948. Following a very successful four years, she accepted a highly coveted position as a house officer at Johns Hopkins Hospital. However, her training was interrupted in the fall of 1952 when she was diagnosed with pulmonary tuberculosis. She was admitted to the Trudeau Sanatorium in Saranac, New York, in the Adirondacks for rest and treatment. She returned to her residency a year later, completing her senior year in 1957 and then moving to Boston for a neonatology fellowship at the Harvard School of Public Health and the Children's Hospital with Clement Smith.

While working with Jere Mead, a highly creative professor of physiology at the Harvard School of Public Health and comparing the lungs of premature infants who died of respiratory distress syndrome (RDS) with those of healthy animals, she noted a higher than normal lung surface tension and the absence of a foam-like substance (surfactant) in the lungs of the infants with RDS (also known as hyaline membrane disease). This suggested that RDS was characterized by a deficiency of surfactant, which normally serves to prevent atelectasis of the lung. This observation explained the clinical findings noted in these very sick premature infants. This seminal work was published in 1959 with Mead as a landmark publication in the *American Journal of Diseases of Children*, "Surface Properties in Relation to Atelectasis and Hyaline Membrane Disease."[7,8]

As subsequent studies confirmed this discovery, Dr. Avery's reputation soared. Her scholarship between 1959 and 1965 included classic papers on neonatal physiology in *The New England Journal of Medicine*, *Science*, and *Nature*. Later, working with Mont Liggins in New Zealand, Dr. Avery noted that steroids accelerated lung development in fetal lambs and when given to pregnant women before delivery, reduced the risk of RDS in the treated versus untreated premature infants. Finally, later in her career, Avery and her colleagues were able to observe that the administration of commercially available surfactant into the lungs of premature infants with RDS markedly reduced both disease severity and mortality. In 1964, Avery published her textbook *The Lung and Its Disorders in the Newborn Infant*. From the initial work and imagination of a young neonatology fellow and with the help of generous mentors, the face of a dreaded and lethal disease had been significantly altered.

Following four years as Eudowood associate professor of pulmonary diseases of children at Johns Hopkins University School of Medicine and pediatrician-in-charge of newborn nurseries, Dr. Avery was recruited to become professor and chair of pediatrics at McGill University School of Medicine. At McGill, she initiated new programs in developmental pharmacology and neonatal circulatory physiology and developed robust training programs in pediatrics and neonatology.

Five years later in 1974, she moved to the Children's Hospital and Harvard Medical School. Interestingly, Harvard had twice before tried to woo her to Boston unsuccessfully. In 1971, Dr. Janeway had attempted to entice Avery and pediatric geneticist Charles Scriver to come to the Children's Hospital. The following year, Dr. Herbert Abrams, chair of the Harvard Medical School search committee, sought to interest her in the position of director of perinatal medicine at the Children's Hospital, the Boston Hospital for Women, and the Beth Israel Hospital. Simultaneously, her mentor and friend Helen Taussig was making her aware of Johns Hopkins' desire to bring her back to Baltimore.[9] Ultimately it was when the Children's Hospital needed a new departmental leader that Harvard succeeded. Avery had the same excellent academic background

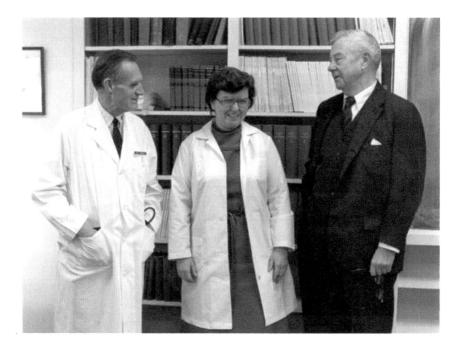

FIGURE 1   The New Physician-in-Chief, circa 1974

Mary Ellen Avery appearing in the first year of her tenure with the prior chief, Charles Janeway, on her right and her longtime mentor and colleague Clement Smith on her left.

as Kenneth Blackfan, James Gamble, and Charles Janeway (Johns Hopkins University School of Medicine) and Alton Goldbloom and Alan Ross (McGill University School of Medicine), all of whom had served as residents or faculty at the Children's Hospital. Janeway, in fact, became one of her strongest supporters throughout her tenure of leadership (Figure 1). Additional strong senior faculty supporters included Drs. Enders, Clement Smith, Nadas, and John Crigler (Figure 2). Clement Smith became her most important mentor and supporter over the years. After the death of his first wife, he married Mary Bunting Smith, president emerita of Radcliff College, and together they became close social friends and valued professional advisors to Dr. Avery.

Dr. Avery chaired the Department of Medicine for 10 years, from 1974 to 1984, and oversaw a steady growth in its academic productivity. She supported well-established programs in the Divisions of Hematology/Oncology, Cardiology, Immunology, Adolescent Medicine, and Infectious Diseases and fostered rapid growth in the Divisions of Neonatology, General Pediatrics, Pulmonary

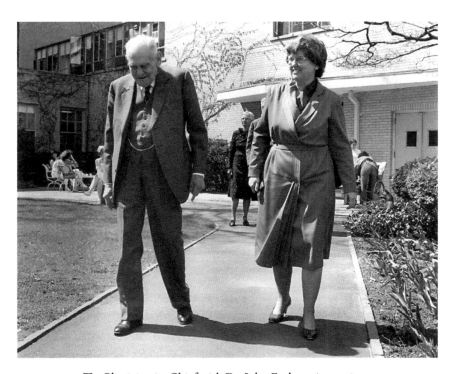

FIGURE 2   The Physician-in-Chief with Dr. John Enders, circa 1981

Drs. John Enders and Mary Ellen Avery during a stroll through the Prouty Garden at the Children's Hospital, followed by Mary Bunting Smith.

Medicine, and Genetics. She championed an academic orientation in the residency program and encouraged women wishing to pursue careers in pediatrics and research. Between 1975 and 1985, revenues from research increased from $4 million to $13 million dollars, departmental publications increased from 150 a year to over 250, and a significant rise occurred in the number of books published by the faculty.[10]

Dr. Avery garnered many academic honors.[11] While in Montreal, she was elected a fellow of the American Academy of Arts and Science, received the prestigious E. Mead Johnson Award with her McGill colleague Charles Scriver, and served as president of the Society for Pediatric Research. During her chairmanship at Harvard, she was elected to the Institute of Medicine and was honored with the Henry D. Chadwick Medal from the Massachusetts Thoracic Society and the Edward Livingston Trudeau Medal from the American Lung Association, all in recognition of her contributions to the reduction in neonatal mortality as a result of her scientific investigation and discoveries in respiratory distress syndrome.

Honors following her chairmanship included presidency of the American Pediatric Society, election to the National Academy of Science, the Virginia Apgar Award, and in 2005, the Howland Award, given by the American Pediatric Society. She was elected president of the American Association for the Advancement of Science in 2004, the first pediatrician to be so honored. In addition, she was the first recipient of the Philipson Prize in Pediatric Medicine from the Nobel Committee in 1998 for her "outstanding scientific achievement in neonatology, pulmonology and for her leadership during a critical phase of development of neonatology, and for her successful endeavor to maintain the bonds in neonatology and pediatrics."[12] At the time of her receipt of the National Medal of Science from President Bush in 1991, she was cited as one of the founders of neonatal intensive care and "a major advocate for improving access to care of all premature and sick infants."[11] When she received an honorary doctorate of science from her alma mater, Wheaton College, the citation read, "Mary Ellen Avery, physician, scientist, teacher, administrator and trustee, you have honored your profession and your college by your unique achievements in a field of extraordinary importance to unborn generations."[13]

She exemplified through her practice of medicine her commitment to the highest quality of pediatric care. In a "Conversation with Mary Ellen Avery, physician" in the *Harvard Magazine* in 1977 she stated, "My style is to be the total physician . . . I undress them [the children] myself because I learn a lot while I'm doing it . . . I usually weigh the child myself . . . I send all my own X-rays."[14] Her commitment to training ran deep, "I brought eight people with me from McGill and set up neonatology here, people who had been in that training program [at McGill University School of Medicine] in which I was engaged in prenatal medicine and research."[14]

And finally in *Pediatrics: the Practice of Preventive Medicine* at a Rockefeller Archive Center Conference in May 1982, she laid out some of her views on education and care.

> "For the house officer, the issues of newborn screening, genetic counseling, care of a child with chronic illness, provision of emotional support to a family, mobilization of community resources, identification of a pioneering approach to treatment have provided a memorable experience. In my view, that experience is a model of the best way to educate a young physician. The science is essential. Commitment to a patient over a period of time is all too unusual but equally essential if we are to teach responsibility for an individual for whom we are to provide the best possible care."[15]

Dr. Avery stepped down from her departmental leadership in 1984. She had successfully pulled the hospitals in Boston together, first around collaborative efforts in neonatology (the Joint Program in Neonatology involving the Children's Hospital, the Brigham and Women's Hospital, and the Beth Israel Hospital). She spearheaded a similar effort in gastroenterology (the Children's Hospital and the Children's Service at the Massachusetts General Hospital), but this did not sit well with the senior faculty in her department. The complex competitive history in pediatrics between the Massachusetts General Hospital and the Children's Hospital lay just below the surface, and reappeared as a result of her efforts to unite the two divisions of gastroenterology. At the Children's Hospital, the result was a serious splitting of the departmental faculty, with a number of the senior faculty opposing the plan. This disagreement, along with issues surrounding academic appointments, led to Dr. Avery's decision to step down as chair.

Following her chairmanship, she was in great demand nationally and internationally as a visiting professor.[16] She continued to receive honorary degrees and prestigious awards. Additionally, she made major contributions in mentoring young pediatricians throughout the country, advising physicians and hospitals in the underdeveloped world, and leading renowned national organizations.

In 2014, Harvard Medical School, the institution she had served so faithfully, established the Mary Ellen Avery Professorship in Pediatrics in the field of newborn medicine. Bestowed upon Terrie E. Inder, MD, PhD, MBChB, as the nominated incumbent, this was a fitting tribute to the first woman to chair a clinical department at Harvard Medical School.

A true pioneer in pediatrics, Mary Ellen Avery's achievements were highly important for pediatrics and the care of premature infants. Her life was one of firsts: the first woman to hold the Thomas Morgan Rotch professorship in pediatrics, the first woman to be president of the Society for Pediatric Research, and the first pediatrician to lead the American Association for the Advancement of Science. Her work on surfactant deficiency in hyaline membrane disease established her as a world-renowned investigator. In addition, she was a greatly respected role model for women physicians and strived successfully to help them break their own glass ceilings.

Faculty Leadership

Departmental faculty leadership on the Children's Hospital's senior appointments committee for full professor promotions included Drs. Avery, Fred Rosen, and Nadas and on the medical staff executive committee, Drs. Avery, Rosen, Nadal-Ginard, and a medical chief resident.[10,17] During the Avery era, the Harvard Medical School Pediatric Executive Committee, responsible for academic appointments and promotions, included for the Children's Hospital, Drs. Avery, David Nathan, Fred Rosen, Park Gerald, Harvey Colten, Nadal-Ginard, Samuel Latt, and Kenneth McIntosh, and for the Massachusetts General Hospital, Drs. Nathan Talbot, Donald Medearis, Jack Crawford, and Allan Walker.[18] The internship selection committee was chaired by William Berenberg, the fellowship oversight committee by David Nathan, and medical student education by the author. The author served as Dr. Avery's associate physician-in-chief and chair of the residency training committee commencing in 1980 through the end of her chairmanship, with responsibility for the educational curriculum of the housestaff.

The staff of the Department of Medicine showed steady growth during Dr. Avery's tenure. Full-time staff increased to nearly 200 by 1984, with a part-time staff of over 100. The number of clinical fellows ranged between 120 and 125 each year. The housestaff numbered 68, with approximately 22 to 24 interns entering the program every year.

Divisional Leadership[19]

The divisional leadership that Avery inherited from Janeway was notable for its seniority and strength and included Drs. Nadas, Robert Masland, Crigler,

Nathan, Rosen, David Smith, Gerald, Berenberg, Allen Crocker, and T. Berry Brazelton. Many would remain in their leadership positions throughout Dr. Avery's chairmanship, while others were replaced by highly competent inside or outside leaders, including Drs. Harvey Colten, Raif Geha, Melvin Levine, Peter Goldman, Jan Breslow, Richard Grand, McIntosh, Alice Huang, Latt, Warren Grupe, Arthur Rhodes, Denise Streider, Mary Ellen Wohl, William Taeusch, and Barry Smith. Many division chiefs were prior Children's Hospital residents, including Drs. Nadas, Berenberg, Brazelton, Crocker, Geha, Levine, Grand, Rosen, David Smith, and Gerald. Remarkably, while senior in responsibility and extremely busy running their divisional and laboratory enterprises, all were clinically available and thus well known to the housestaff.

Cardiology became a separate department at the Children's Hospital in the Janeway era but remained part of the Department of Pediatrics at Harvard Medical School for purposes of academic appointments and promotions. The division and then the department were most capably led by the charismatic and much-admired pediatric cardiologist Alexander Nadas from 1950 until 1982, a period of 33 years. Nadas saw the importance of cardiac catheterization in delineating abnormalities in pulmonary and cardiovascular physiology associated with congenital cardiac malformations. His textbook, initially authored alone and then with Donald Fyler, *Pediatric Cardiology*, became the classic in the field. When Nadas stepped down in 1982, the helm of leadership was assumed by Bernardo Nadal-Ginard. Nadal brought new concepts in molecular biology to explore cardiac development.

Throughout his career, Alexander Nadas was a stalwart and loyal lieutenant to both Drs. Janeway and Avery. If Helen Taussig was called the "mother of pediatric cardiology," Alexander Nadas could most certainly be considered the "father of pediatric cardiology."[20] Important future leaders in cardiology at the Children's Hospital who were house officers in the Avery era and who were trained by Drs. Nadas and Nadal included Jane Newburger, future associate cardiologist-in-chief; Roger Breitbart, who would receive the Society for Pediatric Research Young Investigator Award; and Steven Goldstein, a recipient of the E. Mead Johnson Award. Other distinguished housestaff alumni were Phil Saul, an electrophysiologist and chief of pediatric cardiology at the Medical University of South Carolina, and John Cheatham, a cardiac catheterization interventionist at Ohio State University School of Medicine.

Robert Masland led the Division of Adolescent Medicine throughout Avery's tenure. His devoted leadership from 1967 to 1992, a period of 25 years, resulted in steady growth in the referral of adolescent patients cared for in the outpatient adolescent clinic as well as on the inpatient medical service (Division 37). The adolescent division also became a magnet for Harvard medical students, and their subsequent exposure to the hospital served as an important opportunity for recruitment to the pediatric residency in the Department of Medicine. Bob Masland also had a superb eye for talent, and in the Nathan era he would serve as a highly effective chairman of the intern selection committee. The division trained from the housestaff such future leaders in adolescent medicine as Victor Strasburger at the University of New Mexico School of Medicine, Janice Key at the Medical University of South Carolina, and Elizabeth Woods and Norman Spack at the Children's Hospital in Boston.

The recruitment of the highly capable immunologist Harvey Colten had occurred under Janeway.[21] Colten assumed the leadership of Harry Mueller's allergy division early in Avery's tenure. In the late 1970s, he was asked to lead the new cystic fibrosis division (later called Cell Biology) with the leadership of the allergy division passing to a young and highly talented Raif Geha, a house officer in the early 1970s and a Fred Rosen trainee during the Janeway years. Colten went on to become a distinguished pediatric department chair at Washington University School of Medicine in St Louis. Important trainees in allergy from the housestaff in the Avery era and trained by Raif Geha included Donald Leung, a recipient of the E. Mead Johnson Award, Dale Umetsu, who had a distinguished career at Stanford University School of Medicine prior to returning to the Children's Hospital in 2005, during the Gary Fleisher era, and Michael Young, a practicing allergist with special expertise in peanut allergy.

Melvin Levine, a Rhodes scholar and Children's Hospital house officer in the late 1960s, was selected and trained to assume the leadership of the Division of General Pediatrics, the position long held by his mentor Thomas Cone. He served in that capacity throughout Dr. Avery's tenure and made major contributions to the diagnosis, treatment, and education of children with attention deficit, reading and learning disorders, and children with special needs challenges. These difficult and complex medical problems became a part of the core general pediatrics ambulatory curriculum and thus a most important part of residency training. On his departure to the University of North Carolina to run a major program, Judy Palfrey was appointed from within as the new division chief. Important trainees of Melvin Levine's who were prior Children's Hospital housestaff included Leonard Rappaport, who went on to become division chief of behavioral and developmental medicine under Gary Fleisher, and Paul Dworkin, who later became a distinguished chair of pediatrics at the University of Connecticut School of Medicine. In addition, Lynn Haynie and William Barbaresi held important faculty and leadership positions in the Divisions of

General Pediatrics and Behavioral and Developmental Medicine during the Philip Pizzo and Fleisher eras.

Clinical pharmacology was established as a Harvard Medical School program in the Avery era and was located at the Children's Hospital, the Beth Israel Hospital, and the Brigham and Women's Hospital. Its leadership at the Children's Hospital was assumed by Peter Goldman upon his recruitment from the National Institutes of Health, a position he held for the majority of Avery's time as departmental leader. The highly successful development of the statewide poison control system as well as the adverse drug surveillance program, led by Allen Mitchell, occurred under his watch.

John Crigler led endocrinology with great distinction from 1966 to 1988, which spanned the Janeway, Avery, and Nathan tenures. The division incorporated within it the Division of Metabolism when its chief, Jan Breslow, a brilliant former Harvard medical student and Children's Hospital resident, left for Rockefeller University in 1984. Crigler also led the hospital's Clinical Research Center for a considerable period of time. Crigler established a pediatric endocrine fellowship training program, one of 11 such programs started by trainees of Lawson Wilkins, chief of endocrinology at Johns Hopkins University School of Medicine.[22]

Richard Grand, a Janeway trainee in the mid-1960s, led gastroenterology from 1972 until 1983, when it was combined as a joint division under Allan Walker and housed at both the Children's Hospital and the Massachusetts General Hospital. Grand, after a distinguished career at the Floating Hospital and Tufts Medical School, returned to the gastroenterology division at Children's Hospital in the Pizzo era and focused his efforts on developing the Inflammatory Bowel Disease Center and offering his knowledge and wisdom to innumerable young trainees. The division focused its research on gastrointestinal host defense and its clinical efforts on gastrointestinal, nutritional, and hepatic disorders. Drs. Grand and Walker attracted many highly talented Avery house officers to gastroenterology, including Dr. Steve Altschuler, later president of the Children's Hospital of Philadelphia; David Piccoli, later chief of the Division of Gastroenterology at the Children's Hospital of Philadelphia; Dr. Alan Leichtner, later clinical chief of the Division of Gastroenterology at the Children's Hospital and vice chair for clinical affairs in the Department of Medicine under Gary Fleisher; and Colin Rudolph, later chief of gastroenterology at the Medical College of Wisconsin. Maureen Jonas and Jeffrey Hyams, Avery trainees, also went on to hold important positions, respectively, in the development of hepatology at the Children's Hospital and as chief of gastroenterology at the University of Connecticut School of Medicine.

The hematology/oncology division was developed and led most ably by David Nathan for 16 years, from 1968 to 1984. Appointed by Janeway and following in the long and distinguished footsteps of Louis K. Diamond, Nathan developed the pediatric hematology and oncology program at the Dana-Farber Cancer Institute and the Children's Hospital into the premier program in the country. Many of the top leaders in hematology and oncology in the country from the 1950s to today were trained in its stellar fellowship program, led successively by Diamond, Nathan, and Samuel Lux from the mid-1940s to the mid-2000s. A number of housestaff in the Avery era, attracted to this highly popular training program during David Nathan's tenure as division chief, went on to receive prestigious awards: the Society for Pediatric Research Young Investigator Award (Alan Schwartz, Edward Prochownik), the E. Mead Johnson Award (Stuart Orkin, Alan Schwartz, Jonathan Gitlin) and membership in the National Academy of Science and the Institute of Medicine (Stuart Orkin, Alan Schwartz). Over a nearly 60-year period of time, this division would attract the most talented housestaff, not only from the Children's Hospital but from hospitals throughout the U.S., training them superbly such that they would be pivotal in advancing knowledge and understanding of life-threatening diseases in both disciplines.

Fred Rosen, the first Gamble professor of pediatrics at Harvard Medical School, inherited the Division of Immunology leadership from his mentor and chief Charles Janeway in 1968. He led the division in a distinguished manner throughout the Avery era until 1985, a period of 17 years, before becoming the president of the Center for Blood Research in the Nathan era. Building on Janeway's work on the role of gammaglobulin in immune deficiency disorders, Rosen's work focused on abnormalities in host defense, the hyper IGM syndrome, hereditary angioneurotic edema, C_2 and C_3 deficiency, and factor 1 deficiency in the alternative pathway. Important Rosen trainees from the Children's Hospital housestaff during the Janeway and Avery eras included Richard Johnston, Raif Geha, Erwin Gelfand, and Robertson Parkman. This division incorporated within it the clinical disciplines of allergy, dermatology, and rheumatology, adding an important basic science underpinning for a more complete understanding of these diseases.

Additional Divisions

David Smith led the Division of Infectious Disease until 1975. A chief resident of Janeway's in the early 1960s, a scientist trained in bacterial pathogenesis at

Harvard Medical School, and a greatly admired academic physician, he left to assume leadership of pediatrics at Strong Memorial Hospital in Rochester, following in the footsteps of Robert Haggerty, who was also a chief resident and faculty member in the Janeway era. Smith's pioneering studies, with his indispensable colleague Porter Anderson, who carried out the chemistry of the work that resulted in the development of the *Haemophilus influenzae* vaccine, led to his receiving wide recognition for his work. Dr. Avery then recruited Alice Huang as director of laboratories and Kenneth McIntosh, an internist and outstanding virologist from the University of Colorado School of Medicine, as clinical chief. Together, they turned the division's focus from bacterial disease to viral disease, returning to its rich heritage under Enders, Thomas Weller, Frederick Robbins, and Samuel Katz. McIntosh continued to most capably lead the division throughout the Avery and Nathan eras for a period of 20 years. This division trained from the housestaff such distinguished future chairs of pediatrics as Margaret Hostetter at Yale University School of Medicine, John Schreiber at Tufts University School of Medicine, and John Modlin at Dartmouth Medical School. Long seen as a core component of pediatrics, the division's faculty, including Drs. McIntosh, Donald Goldmann, Edward O'Rourke, Richard Malley, and Sandra Burchett, were viewed over the years as among the best teachers on the faculty.

The renal division was led throughout the Avery era by Warren Grupe, a fine clinical nephrologist and medical educator, who developed a national reputation for his studies on the use of alkylating agents in the treatment of steroid-resistant nephrosis. He left near the end of Dr. Avery's chairmanship to become chief of pediatrics at Rainbow Babies and Children's Hospital in Cleveland. William Harmon, a house officer in the Janeway era and at the beginning of the Avery era, pursued investigation of the use of hemodialysis in young children, and Julie Inglefinger, a future associate editor of *The New England Journal of Medicine*, carried out studies on hypertension in children. The division recruited from the housestaff important trainees, including Alan Krensky, future recipient of the Society for Pediatric Research Young Investigator Award; Lisa Guay Woodford, future president of the Society for Pediatric Research; Norman Rosenblum, future vice chair for research at Toronto Sick Children's Hospital; and Ellis Avner, future chair of pediatrics at Case Western Reserve University School of Medicine in Cleveland.

The Division of Clinical Genetics was founded in 1965, and Park Gerald, a close protégé of Louis K. Diamond, was appointed as its chief. Gerald developed both the clinical and laboratory wings of the division until 1983, when Samuel

Latt, who studied and advanced techniques for chromosomal identification and the molecular basis of many genetic syndromes, assumed the division's leadership. Louis Kunkel, a talented member of the division, extended this work by exploring genes related to specific diseases, and in particular muscular dystrophy. Stuart Orkin similarly bridged hematology and genetics through his molecular studies of thalassemia. Both would achieve wide recognition for their pioneering and highly innovative work. Particularly distinguished geneticists and house officers from the Avery era included Bruce Dowton, future medical school dean in New South Wales in Australia and Alan Guttmacher, future director of the National Institute of Child Health and Human Development.

Denise Streider was recruited by Janeway to run the first pulmonary function laboratory at the Children's Hospital and was appointed by Avery to lead the pulmonary division. Streider was succeeded by Mary Ellen Wohl in 1980, when she departed to join the Children's Service at the Massachusetts General Hospital to carry out a similar role. This division underwent great development and maturation under Wohl's leadership during the Nathan era.

Dr. Avery brought William Taeusch plus a large number of neonatology fellows from Montreal to the newly formed Joint Program in Neonatology. The program was created by a memorandum of understanding between the three involved hospitals and, as mentioned earlier, was located at the Children's Hospital, the Brigham and Women's Hospital, and the Beth Israel Hospital. With Mary Ellen Avery's assistance, Bill Taeusch developed the Division of Neonatology into a highly successful and very large clinical operation. Barry Smith assumed brief leadership of the division in 1984 when Taeusch took over responsibility for the infant follow-up program. Michael Epstein then led the division before becoming the vice president of the Children's Hospital.

Important, future distinguished neonatologists attracted into neonatology by the division and house officers during the Avery era included Diana Bianchi at Tufts University School of Medicine, who in 2013 was inducted into the Institute of Medicine in recognition of her work on prenatal genomics and DNA diagnosis; Sessions Cole at Washington University School of Medicine in St. Louis; and Charles Simmons at Cedars Sinai Medical Center in California. DeWayne Pursley became pediatrician-in-chief at the Beth Israel Hospital in Boston; Devn Cornish, chief of pediatrics at Emory University School of Medicine; and Gary Silverman, chief of the Division of Neonatology, first at the Children's Hospital and subsequently at the Children's Hospital of Pittsburgh.

Clinical Services

Three senior clinicians and former Richard Smith and Charles Janeway trainees held important departmental and divisional roles under Avery. They were William Berenberg, a highly revered practicing academic pediatrician and valued mentor to innumerable housestaff and chief of the Services to Handicapped Children; Allen Crocker, chief of Mental Retardation and Developmental Disabilities; and T. Berry Brazelton, the nationally recognized chief of the Division of Child Development. Dr. Berenberg became a national leader in the treatment of cerebral palsy, Crocker led the developmental center for evaluation of children with mental retardation and developmental disabilities with great dedication, and T. Berry Brazelton became widely recognized for his clinical observations of maternal–infant interaction and the development of the Brazelton Neonatal Behavioral Assessment Scale. He would go on to receive the Presidential Citizens Medal, the nation's second highest civilian honor for exemplary deeds of service, from President Obama. All three were major influences on the life and careers of Harvard medical students and the Children's Hospital housestaff.

Finally, while not part of the Department of Medicine, the Department of Neurology, under the superior leadership of Charles Barlow and later Joseph Volpe, recruited outstanding house officers from the Avery era into neurology, including Nina Schor, future chair of pediatrics at the University of Rochester School of Medicine and Dentistry; Scott Pomeroy, future chair of neurology at the Children's Hospital; Edwin Zalneraitis, future pediatric program director at the University of Connecticut School of Medicine; and Bruce Korf, future chair of genetics at the University of Alabama School of Medicine at Birmingham.

All of these Department of Medicine division chiefs thus recruited a large number of clinical fellows from the residency training program at the Children's Hospital, with many becoming junior faculty members. They and their staffs were powerful teachers and role models on a daily basis for the housestaff.

The Department of Medicine

Patient Care

Inpatient admissions to the medical service, including the general ward services (Medical Team A for patients ages 2 months to 6 years on Division 27, Medical Team B for adolescent and young adult patients on Division 37, and Medical Team C for ages 6 to 12 on Division 39) as well as the subspecialty services (cardiology, neonatal intensive care unit, psychosomatic unit, Clinical Research Center, neurology, and oncology) ranged from a low of approximately 7,800 in 1977 to nearly 8,800 by 1984. Total patient days ranged from approximately 43,500 in 1977 to 47,000 by 1984 (representing over 55% of the hospital's inpatient volume), with the mean length of stay in 1984 being seven days.[23] The clinics in the outpatient department, which included the specialty clinics, the Comprehensive Child Health Program (CCHP), the medical diagnostic clinic (MDC), and the Martha Eliot Health Center, ranged from approximately 45,000 visits in 1975 to 67,000 visits in 1984.[10, 17] Finally, volume in the medical emergency room rose only modestly over the 10-year period, increasing from 37,000 to 43,000 visits.[10,17] All in all, a steady growth in clinical volume reflected a growing emphasis on clinical care as a dependable source of income for the hospital and the department and a rich substrate for housestaff education.

During the 10 years of Dr. Avery's leadership, the volume, complexity, and severity of illness in all hospital settings also increased. The most dramatic increases in volume were seen in the number of teenagers and young adults cared for in both the inpatient and outpatient settings, in the complexity of patients seen in the emergency department, and in the increase in outpatients presenting with school difficulties and behavioral disorders. Asthma, cystic fibrosis, diabetes, heart disease, cancer, and premature infants occupied a significant proportion of the resident's time. Complex, time-consuming, and costly therapies, including bone marrow transplantation (for aplastic anemia, leukemia, Wiscott Aldrich syndrome), renal dialysis and kidney transplantation, plasmapheresis, and intensive care support for premature infants, constituted particularly intensive work that led to important clinical advances during the Avery era. Regionalized care and referral for cardiac and neoplastic disease as well as childhood injuries (drug and household product poisoning, lead poisoning, child abuse) would also undergo considerable growth.

Preventive pediatrics and early intervention in delayed development, school dysfunction, and behavioral issues became a major focus in the Comprehensive Child Health Program and subspecialty clinics. Neonatal mortality fell while morbidity simultaneously rose. Genetic prenatal testing impacted care and preventive approaches for thalassemia, sickle cell disease, and other hereditary disorders. The *Haemophilus influenzae* vaccine dramatically altered housestaff exposure to patients with the prior common and generally severe "H flu" diseases, including epiglottitis, septic arthritis, meningitis, and pneumonia, leading to their elimination from the hospital wards. Penicillin and factor replacement essentially ended, respectively, rheumatic fever and hemophilia on the inpatient services.

Basic and Clinical Research

Research dollars awarded to the faculty of the Department of Medicine showed a progressive increase, reaching $13 million in 1984 at the end of the Avery era.[10] The divisions of hematology/oncology followed by neonatology and general pediatrics were the most successful in acquiring these funds. Research dollars emanated from federal sources (National Institutes of Health and the Centers for Disease Control and Prevention), private foundations (Robert Wood Johnson, March of Dimes, American Cancer Society, American Heart Association, and the Hood and Cystic Fibrosis Foundations), and the Massachusetts Department of Public Health. Two-thirds of the dollars funded research carried out in the John F. Enders Pediatric Research Laboratories, the other one-third in the clinical setting. These dollars funded two-thirds of faculty salaries. This figure remained remarkably high, though falling to approximately 50% of faculty salaries in the aggregate in subsequent eras. These figures reflect the department's emphasis on research—a fact well evident to the housestaff.

A few examples of basic research efforts included the prenatal diagnosis of hemoglobinopathies and immune deficiency syndromes, regulation of surfactant production in fetal life, new techniques for chromosome identification, basic T and B cell as well as complement studies, molecular studies of viral disease, and development of monoclonal antibodies. Examples of clinical investigation include therapeutic trials for asthma, chelation therapy for removal of iron in thalassemia, indomethacin for patent ductus closure, vaccine trials for *Haemophilus influenzae*, new chemotherapies for cancer, use of hemoglobin A_{1C} to monitor the control of blood sugar in diabetes, studies of growth retardation in renal disease, and evaluation of performance in the preschool population. The housestaff had considerable exposure to the implementation of the research carried out in the clinical setting, although they had little involvement as a participant in or author of the research itself.

The National Perspective

The 1970s ushered in a period of housestaff militancy that interrupted the tranquil nature of residency present in the preceding two decades. Issues in training that had been just below the surface emerged with great intensity. The place of women and minorities in the medical profession as well as a focus on the social needs of the poor and the underserved became celebrated causes for housestaff protests. The baton of the Janeway era of 27 years had been passed to a scientifically trained faculty, who thanks to numerous advances, were now faced with diseases and patient care of a more complex and intense nature. The correct balance of education and service became a central theme over the ensuing decades.

Housestaff Activism

The medical student and housestaff tended to be deferential in the 1950s and 1960s. Only the yearly student and housestaff shows afforded the rare opportunity to be less so and even then, only mildly critical of faculty and teachers. Activism, however, surfaced in the mid- to late 1960s in the form of protests against racism and the Vietnam War, coupled with efforts to support the needs of the community and the poor. Students made important inroads and gained a place at the decision-making tables in colleges and medical schools. By the mid-1970s, these students, now house officers, carried their passion for social change into the arena of graduate medical education.

Housestaff became concerned with issues involving their training, pay, hours of work, and working conditions. They, in fact, had a right to be concerned. Their salaries were modest, their hours long, and the support staff to assist with routine patient care–related tasks few.[24] In addition, personal and family time, marriage and children, maternity leave, and more liberal vacations were only just becoming part of the culture of the day. These changes were enhanced as more women entered the housestaff. Finally, a resident's status as hospital employee versus student was yet to be clarified.

The first Committee on Interns and Residents (CIR) was formed in New York City in the late 1950s.[25] Its predecessors, the Interne Council of Greater New York, organized in 1934, and the Interne Council of America (ICA), organized in 1936, had been relatively ineffective during the late 1940s and 1950s. By the mid-1960s the CIR was negotiating successfully with the city for better salaries and benefits. By 1972, the group represented all housestaff in 18 municipal hospitals in New York City. In fact, by 1972, 80% of all hospitals in the U.S. had organized housestaff associations.[25] These associations also advocated for universal health insurance, programs for the treatment of substance abuse, and elimination of discrimination of any kind. They were against war and championed socially responsible positions and corrective actions by their hospitals.

They saw themselves as hospital employees who should be paid a salary; their hospitals saw them as students and paid them a student stipend. In 1975, the CIR undertook a strike in New York City against the 100-hour workweek and 50 hours of continuous work without rest. The strike ended with the signing of a two-year contract and, among other concessions, the stipulation that no housestaff "shall be required to perform on-call duty more frequently than one night in three . . ."[25] Housestaff associations viewed hospital administrators as outdated, out of touch, and behind the times. Hospital administrators saw hard work as a part of housestaff training and their actions as unprofessional. Hospital concerns were inflamed by the housestaff's use of their free time for moonlighting. In fact, by 1977, 78% of third-year residents and 41% of second-year residents were moonlighting.[26] These tensions only heightened housestaff activism in the 1970s and sharpened their focus on a better and higher standard of living.

Housestaff associations developed methods that resulted in formidable leverage. By focusing on the inadequacy of their working conditions, they were able to negatively or positively influence those applicants applying to their program. This leverage became important to their success in achieving some of their demands (better salaries, benefits, and the right to moonlight). In 1976, the National Labor Relations Board, however, ruled that housestaff were, in fact, students, not employees, and as a consequence, their housestaff associations were not permitted to bargain as unions.[25] In 1980, when the Supreme Court upheld this decision, the strength of the housestaff associations began to wane, and many of the associations dissolved or continued to exist only as social organizations. Happily, at that point, faculty–housestaff relationships, which had been severely strained, began to improve. Despite the Supreme Court decision, the basic issue of whether graduate medical education was a service or education had not been resolved. This issue would assume great importance over the next 30 years, first in the Libby Zion case in New York City in the 1980s and subsequently in work hour regulations of the 1990s and 2000s. It would not be resolved until the early 2000s when a court decision ruled that housestaff were employees (*Mayo Foundation v. U.S.*).

Women and Minorities

The place of women and minorities in medicine also assumed center stage in the 1970s and 1980s, with inroads first made in medical schools and only later in the hospital setting. In the 1960s, only 6% to 7% of doctors in the U.S. were women, far less than the percentage of women in medicine in Europe.[27] Empowered by the feminist movement in the U.S. and Title IX of the Higher Education Amendment of 1972 (which banned sex discrimination in education programs receiving federal aid), admission of women to medical schools soared to 28% in 1979 and 42% by 1994.[28] These gains resulted in a growing number of women entering residency and especially residencies such as pediatrics, medicine, psychiatry, family practice, and obstetrics and gynecology.

Similarly underrepresented minority medical school enrollment, including African Americans, Mexican Americans, American Indians, and mainland Puerto Ricans, grew from 3% in 1968 to 10% in 1974, and plateaued at 10% in 1984. Black enrollment rose from 2.7% in 1968 to 7.5% in 1974.[28,29] Mexican American enrollment rose 11-fold, and Native American and Puerto Rican enrollment rose 20-fold over the same period.[28,29] These gains were achieved because of significant funding emanating from the Commonwealth, Sloan, Macy, and Robert Wood Johnson Foundations as well as a supportive climate created by the civil rights gains made in the 1960s. Significant pushback, however, came about as a result of the Bakke case in 1978 in which the Supreme Court ruled against the use of quotas as a benchmark in medical school admission policy.[28] In addition, admission of minorities to residency lagged significantly behind medical school admissions and by 1994, even more concerning was the fact that only 2.4% of faculty members in U.S. medical schools were black.[30] Recognizing that the efforts of the past had been inadequate, "Project 3,000 by 2000" was introduced by the Association of American Medical Colleges (AAMC), with a goal of enrolling 3,000 students from underrepresented minority groups in U.S. medical schools by the year 2000.[31] This laudable undertaking was unfortunately unsuccessful and the ambitious goal never reached.

While the gains for women in medicine were most heartening, "microinequalities" continued to exist.[32] At the training level, they included admission committees asking women and not men about their plans for marriage and children, patients mistaking women physicians for nurses, problems in securing on-call rooms for female housestaff, and women physicians and nurses sharing surgical locker rooms. Some specialties such as surgery were less open to women. At the faculty level, women had a harder time rising to the higher academic ranks when contrasted with men because of less mentoring, lower pay, and because promotion was more readily achieved by those who were able to maintain 60- to 70-hour workweeks.[33] Some gains did occur in the 1980s and 1990s, with more liberal policies for maternity leave, shared residency slots, onsite childcare, and gender sensitivity training.[34]

It is worth noting that pediatrics as a specialty was popular among women, with a large number entering pediatric residencies and ultimately obtaining faculty positions. In time, this led to women achieving senior professorial academic ranks as well as senior administrative leadership positions. As we have seen, this important movement began at the Children's Hospital during the encouraging watch of Drs. Janeway and Avery and continued unabated under Drs. Nathan, Pizzo, and Fleisher.

Resident and Residency Stresses

After World War II, residency review committees (RRCs) were developed to review training programs in individual specialties. In addition, reviews by the American Medical Association and the American Association of Medical Colleges led to the recommendation that a single organization have oversight over graduate medical education, and the Liaison Committee on Graduate Medical Education was formed for this purpose. This committee was the forerunner of the Accreditation Council for Graduate Medical Education, which assumed the important role of regular reviews of training programs using the vehicle of the RRCs.

In 1966, the federal government began to support graduate medical education through the Medicare program, with hospital payment dependent on the number of Medicare-eligible patients. This advent of government financing of graduate medical education focused attention on the need to train more physicians in general disciplines, such as internal medicine, family medicine, and pediatrics. By 1970, approximately 26,000 residency positions were filled, and by 1989, that number had grown to 60,000. Simultaneously during that same time period, 38 new subspecialties were approved, and by 1991 the American Board of Medical Specialties had approved 54 subspecialties.

By the mid-1980s, support from Medicare and Medicaid reached $2 billion and support for house officer salaries had grown to 4% of teaching hospital budgets.[35] Control of graduate medical education, its size, and its educational content clearly did not rest with medical schools; rather it rested with the hospitals who paid the residents' salaries, the department chairs who selected the housestaff and hired the faculty, the residency review committees who set the length of training and its content, the specialty boards who certified individuals as "competent" specialists, and the government and private insurers who compensated the hospitals. Clinical learning was increasingly the focus, and research was less and less in evidence during residency as the emphasis on the quality and efficiency of clinical care grew. By the mid-1980s, the duration of residency was simply too short to adequately train a physician for the era of molecular biology; this was left to fellowship training.

The life of a resident in the 1970s and 1980s was far different than in the pre- and post-World War II era.[36] The family atmosphere of the teaching hospital had disappeared. Residencies and fellowships were now very large, and many faculty were less in evidence on the wards, as they became more focused on their labora- tory work and on their own patients, who were followed in outpatient clinics and private offices. The role of the ward attending had, in fact, changed significantly; teaching about the diseases cared for on the wards now took precedence over being the primary responsible caregiver. Most residency training was carried out in the inpatient setting (the domain of the resident staff), while the fellows worked primarily in the outpatient setting. The patients were sicker; there was more use of technology and more tests, and the daily pace was more frenetic. There was also an ever increasing number of mundane duties for housestaff to perform (blood drawing, starting IVs, filling out laboratory slips, contacting referring physicians, dictating discharge summaries), and while the hiring of phlebotomists and technicians helped, there were still far too many chores to be carried out in a day. Overworked, more fatigued, more sleep deprived, and more stressed, some housestaff experienced "burnout" and appeared less caring. Some were also at increased risk of depression, anger, and abuse of alcohol and drugs. Clearly, there was a need for graduate medical education reform, reform that the profession was slow to recognize and to institute.

The Legacy of Libby Zion

These challenges became public with the Libby Zion case in New York City in 1984. The charge of deficient care was brought against the intern and resident involved in the care of Libby Zion.[37] In fact, inadequate faculty supervision and failure of effective communication between the attending physician and the house officer had also taken place. The residents were exonerated by a review committee that had medical and lay representation. Their report was accepted by the New York State Board for Professional Medical Conduct and the com- missioner of public health. The state's board of regents, however, overruled the commissioner and the review committee and voted to "censure and reprimand" the resident physicians for acts of gross negligence.[33] While those involved were never indicted nor their licenses revoked, the incident led to the formation of the Bell Commission in New York and its important recommendations on duty hours and faculty supervision.[25] While New York was the only state to enact and enforce the regulations of the Bell Commission (80-hour workweek, one day off each week, limitations in the frequency of night call, and greater direct faculty supervision), residency review committees responsible to the Accreditation Council for Graduate Medical Education rapidly adopted the new rules throughout the country for the various subspecialties.[38]

Although the need for reform had been great and important progress had been made, the new regulations failed to address many important issues, including: a) continuing house officer stress (ancillary staff were added slowly and housestaff continued to be used as inexpensive labor); b) the need for improvements in housestaff education (the new rules led to a limitation on the ability of housestaff to witness the natural history of disease, and the more frequent turnover of patients resulted in increased opportunities for errors, delay in ordering tests, and more hospital complications); c) the responsibility of the administration and faculty to make residency training more humane through retreats, dinners, advising, counseling, and parental leave.[38]

While shorter house officer hours were a good start, progress was slow and incremental because the needed ancillary personnel were added only very gradually by hospitals due to the serious fiscal constraints of the mid-1990s. In addition, despite the benefits of the new rules, program directors and the residents themselves had great ambivalence about not being able to adequately follow their patients, concerned that the transfer of responsibility for patients from one team to another would lead to underperformance in patient care—as it often did. Duty hours and supervision continued to be a critical issue into the new millennium.

Challenges in Medical Education

Challenges in Clinical Training

By the mid-1980s, significant challenges in residency education at the Children's Hospital had become apparent.[39] The majority of these challenges were created by the remarkable growth in the number, complexity, and serious nature of diseases being cared for in both the inpatient and outpatient settings. The marked proliferation of information and technology contributed to the problem. This complexity was layered upon a structure and system of residency education that had changed relatively little over the preceding 40 years.

The Changing Hospital Environment

Education, which had been heavily inpatient based, was becoming more complex and fast moving. First, patients were admitted less and less frequently to establish a diagnosis. As a result, less emphasis was placed on the skills of physical examination and differential diagnosis. Admissions were increasingly scheduled for specific diagnostic studies or therapeutic interventions, the goals of which were often established without a resident's involvement. Second, although the total number of beds in the hospital had not significantly increased, the number of patients cared for had because of shorter hospital length of stays and more rapid discharge. Length of stay over 14 years at the Children's Hospital had decreased from 10 days for short term admissions and 16 days for long-term admissions in 1970 to seven days in 1984, whereas patient days (per year) and the number of patients treated had significantly increased. In addition, it became more common for the child to be discharged before he or she was fully recovered, resulting in the housestaff's failing to observe the natural history of disease and the beneficial effects of therapy. Thirdly, patients were sicker and their problems were more complex. A higher percentage of the hospital beds were being committed to intensive care and more and more patients were on ventilators and monitors. There was an increasing risk, as Lewis Thomas so aptly stated, of house officers looking after machines rather than patients.[40] Finally, increasingly, children were presenting with illnesses that were more chronic and less curable. Thus, these patients were less often admitted for cure and more often with the goal of improving their medical condition. All of these factors had the overall effect of decreasing the primacy of the role of the resident in the care of their patients.

Proliferation of Information and Technology

Another formidable challenge facing the training program was the proliferation of pediatric information and technology. With an expanding information base and a fixed amount of curricular time, difficult decisions on allotment of time for learning were becoming necessary. The focus in education was shifting to what information a resident *should* learn and *how* they should use that information rather than on the illnesses they were exposed to on the wards.

Simultaneously, there was an additional educational challenge, that of mastering an ever increasing quantity of complex technology. The volume of laboratory tests and radiology examinations was increasing dramatically. The impact of this is best appreciated when one realizes that a house officer must handle each one of these results, interpret them, and then apply them to the patient. Risks, benefits, sensitivity, specificity, and cost analysis were becoming a new language for the resident to learn and understand. An additional adverse effect of too much technology was to pull the resident from the bedside to the classroom, to the X-ray suite and to the catheterization laboratory. The traditional clinical laboratory skills increasingly were transferred from the housestaff to laboratory technicians in the name of accuracy and saving time.

Education and Service—Striking a Balance

The correct balance of education versus service had become a central issue in medical education by the mid-1980s. It would dominate education discussions for the next 25 years. At the heart, was the realization that the hospital's primary mission is to care for patients; the training program's primary mission is to educate house officers. As the clinical care mission grew in size and importance throughout the 1970s and 1980s, the academic hospital came to simulate the tricycle rather than the three-legged stool, with the larger wheel of patient care dominating the smaller wheels of teaching and research.[41] When the wheel of patient care became excessively dominant, the housestaff would voice their concern symbolically through their housestaff show and programmatically through the residency training committee and the housestaff association. Addressing this challenge would become a major focus of the program directors and the residency training committee in the Nathan, Pizzo, and Fleisher eras.

Quality of Life

Issues of quality of life had focused on salary and benefits in the 1960s and 1970s. With these issues now significantly improved, in the 1980s, the focus turned to the quality of life for a house officer—inside and outside of the hospital. The Libby Zion case, as we have seen, focused national attention on the issue of house officer hours while on duty.[42] Housestaff began pressing for a better quality of life, accomplished through more liberal day and night call schedules. In addition, as many as 50% of residents were now married, 10% had children, and many were women, for whom the biological clock ticked loudly.[39] The solutions to these challenges would come only slowly over the next decades, enhanced by an increasing public concern over resident fatigue and the potential for medical error.

Residency Training

Residency Accreditation

The focus of housestaff education during the Avery era was on the quality of the program and the excellence of the residents. The results of these efforts became evident at the time of the program's review by the national certifying body. The pediatric residency review committee of the Accreditation Council for Graduate Medical Education reviewed the residency program in Dr. Janeway's last year of leadership, giving full approval for the requisite two years of training. In mid-1978, the council's liaison committee notified pediatric training programs throughout the U.S. of its intent to only certify three-year residency training programs. The program during Avery's tenure subsequently received the full three-year accreditation in 1978 and again in 1982.

Association of Pediatric Program Directors

In the early 1980s, pediatric program directors at the national level expressed a desire for a forum where issues and concerns pertinent to graduate medical education could be discussed. In the spring of 1984, the American Board of Pediatrics (ABP) approached the American Academy of Pediatrics (AAP) and the Association of Medical School Pediatric Department Chairmen (AMSPDC) requesting the formation of an association of program directors. An ad hoc committee was formed and made a number of recommendations, which included: a) an association of program directors should be formed; b) bylaws should be [and were] drafted; c) the association should be independent of AMSPDC and AAP; d) officers would be apportioned by class of program (medical school, non-medical school, and military); e) membership would be limited to the designated director of the training program or the chair of the department of pediatrics responsible for the program. The first meeting of the association was held on May 9, 1985. The organization has grown progressively in importance and influence over the years. One of its early significant accomplishments was the formalization of the role of the program director, as the individual responsible for the pediatric residents and their curriculum as well as the important task of recommending residents to the ABP to sit for the pediatric certifying examination. Throughout the Avery era, Dr. Avery served as program director, delegating the responsibility for the day-to-day running of the residency to the author. Over time, as the leadership of residency programs became a full-time job, most departmental chairs, including the chair at the Children's Hospital, transferred the total responsibility for administration of the program to the program director.

Intern Selection

Attracting the "best and brightest" into the residency in an increasingly competitive market became a high priority and was accomplished to a significant degree as the result of a hard-working internship selection committee made up of junior and senior faculty and chief residents. In the Janeway era, the stature and length of existence of the training program at the Children's Hospital gave it a competitive advantage over other programs. Serving as a house officer was seen as an honor; the small salary was tolerated. By the Avery era, the program could no longer rest on its laurels. The happiness of the housestaff with the program, salary and benefits, and sufficiently high-quality education relative to the amount of service became important considerations in a fourth-year medical student's selection of one training program over another. The internship selection committee was ably chaired by William Berenberg, whose ability to identify excellent housestaff and future academic leaders was superb. As reflected upon by Dr. Avery's biographer, Bojan Hamlin Jennings, "Meanwhile, at Children's, the residency program in pediatrics was flourishing. Word got around the standards were high, thereby attracting the best and the brightest," with over 500 applicants for 22 to 24 positions.[43] That percentage yield has remained the same over the ensuing 25 years, with both the number of applicants and the number of available positions growing. Dr. Avery's approach to the recruitment of the housestaff for her program was relatively simple and straight forward, to select highly capable people: individuals who were bright, creative, and committed, and who demonstrated initiative and ambition.

An additional indicator of the strength of a residency program is its attractiveness to its own medical students. In the late 1970s and 1980s among a Harvard Medical School class of 160 students, 20 students, or 12% of the class, pursued pediatric residencies nationwide. During the same period of time, approximately one-third, or six to eight, Harvard Medical students joined a class of 22 interns each year at the Children's Hospital.[44] This percentage reflected well on the popularity of the residency. Some of the other medical schools from which the residency program obtained the majority of its interns (in descending order) were: Stanford University School of Medicine, University of Pennsylvania School of Medicine, Yale University School of Medicine, University of Massachusetts Medical School, Columbia University College of Physicians and Surgeons.[44]

Legacies, that is children of pediatricians who had served as house officers in the training program prior to the Avery era, were limited in number to Nathan Talbot (Blackfan era), son of Fritz Talbot (Rotch era), and Richard Goldbloom (Janeway era), son of Alton Goldbloom (Rotch era). The Avery era welcomed an increasing number of legacies to the housestaff: Bill Adams, son of Tom Adams (Janeway era); Jonathan Gitlin, son of David Gitlin (Janeway era); Alan Goldbloom, son of Richard Goldbloom (Janeway era); Colin Rudolph, son of Abraham Rudolph (Janeway era); and Alan Schwartz, son of Robert Schwartz (Janeway era).

The Residents

The nomenclature used throughout the Avery era for the residents was similar to the Janeway era: first year—intern; second year—junior assistant resident; third year—senior assistant resident; and fourth year—chief resident. Similar to training programs throughout the United States and to meet the needs of the increasing volume and complexity of patient care, as shown in Table 1, the residency doubled in size, from 36 residents in the mid- to late 1960s to 68 residents during Avery's tenure (Figures 3–5). A major goal during Avery's tenure was to increase the number of women entering pediatrics as well as her residency. Between 1974 and 1979, among 68 house officers, 17 (25%) were women. For the period from 1981 to 1985, that number had increased to 22 to 26 (or 33% to 38%) of the housestaff (Figures 3–5).

TABLE 1   Medical Housestaff Statistics

	1880s	1890s	1900s	1910s	1920s	1930s	1940–1945	1945–1959	1960s	1970s	1980s
Total	2	3	6	8	13	17	12–17	25–30	30–40	50–60	65–70
Male/ Female	2/0	3/0	6/0	8/0	13/0	17/0	15/1–2	5%*	10%*	25%*	36%*
Chief Residents	0	0	0	0	0	0	0	1–4	2–4	2	1–2

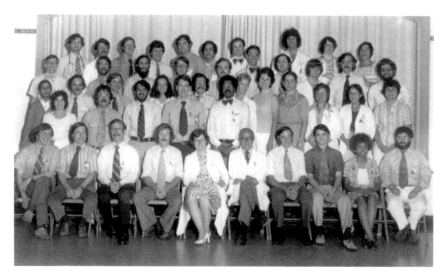

FIGURE 3   The Early Avery Years, 1975–1976

Mary Ellen Avery in the first row center and William Berenberg on her left with her housestaff early in her tenure. Jonathan Bates, second row, fourth from left, served as her chief resident in 1975–1976.

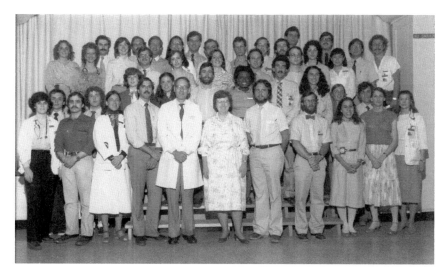

FIGURE 4   The Mid-Avery Years, 1981–1982

Mary Ellen Avery in the first row center with Fred Lovejoy on her right, with her housestaff. Her chief resident in 1981–1982, Alvin Faierman, stands to her left and her chief resident in 1982–1983, David Piccoli, stands to Lovejoy's right.

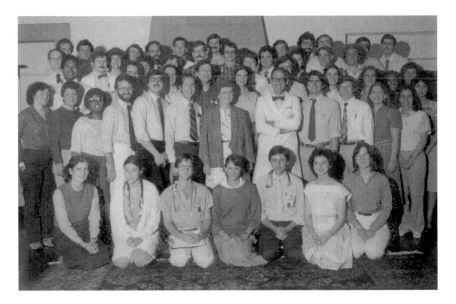

FIGURE 5   The Late Avery Years, 1983–1984

Mary Ellen Avery and Fred Lovejoy in the second row center with her housestaff. Also in the second row are her chief residents that year, Lewis First on her right and George Hoffman on Fred Lovejoy's left.

In contrast to the Janeway era when there were multiple resident tracks, there were only two tracks and two types of residents on the medical service throughout the Avery era. The medical residents in the traditional track made up the majority. Their training and experience took place at the Children's Hospital and the Boston Lying-In and involved rotations on the inpatient and outpatient services. The second track was the ambulatory senior residency, which grew out of the Medical Outpatient Pediatric Department (MOPD) residency of the Janeway era, and involved a year or two of ambulatory-focused training. Many of these residents went on to further fellowship training in the Division of General Pediatrics. The ambulatory residency was popular and launched a number of graduates on distinguished careers in academic general pediatrics. It also stimulated the development of a more sophisticated curriculum in subspecialty outpatient and developmental pediatrics.

Finally in the 1980s, with Avery and Nathan's strong support, the program began to take advantage of the American Board of Pediatrics–sponsored Special Alternative Pathway (SAP) for academic research–oriented residents.[45] The SAP involved two years of residency and three years of fellowship training. Candidates were required to demonstrate significant academic promise and pass a special examination at the end of their intern year with a sufficiently high score to predict success when taking the certifying examination in pediatrics at the end of their fellowship training. One to two residents from the program participated in this special pathway each year. Sixteen residents pursued the Special Alternative Pathway in the Avery era, 16 in the Nathan era, 13 in the Pizzo era, and four in the Fleisher era. The Accelerated Research Pathway and the Integrated Research Pathway replaced the Special Alternative Pathway in popularity among the residents in the Fleisher era. The tradition of active use of the Special Alternative Pathway established during Avery's tenure as chief was thus carried out by all subsequent department chairs.[45]

A succession of excellent chief residents served Dr. Avery during her tenure as chair, as shown in Table 2, one for the inpatient services and one for the outpatient department. In the last two years of her tenure, the two chief residents shared both inpatient and outpatient responsibilities. The chief residents in the Avery era were less involved on the wards and in the clinics when contrasted with the Blackfan, Smith, and Janeway eras. They served less as an extender of the chief in the area of patient care as had occurred in prior eras and more as a leader of their charges, the housestaff.

Three (14%) of Avery's appointees were women.[46] While this represented a better balance of women and men as chief residents, it stands in remarkable contrast (as seen in Chapter 7) to 1996 to 2007 when 29 of 44 medical chief residents, or 66%, were women. Of the 22 chief residents appointed by Avery,

TABLE 2   Mary Ellen Avery's Chief Residents

1974–1975	John Phillips & Judy Lamar
1975–1976	Jonathan Bates & Larry Johnson
1976–1977	Michael Williams & Marc Tanenbaum
1977–1978	Aubrey Katz & Marc Tanenbaum
1978–1979	Martha Magoon & Michael Macknin
1979–1980	Herbert Clegg & Mort Wasserman
1980–1981	Mandel Sher & Marc Lerner
1981–1982	Alvin Faierman & Mariette Murphy
1982–1983	David Piccoli & Robert Wharton
1983–1984	Lewis First & George Hoffman
1984–1985	Norman Rosenblum & Evan Synder

half pursued academic careers, the other half pediatric practice. Jonathan Bates became a distinguished hospital president at the Arkansas Children's Hospital, Lewis First a highly successful pediatric department chair at the University of Vermont College of Medicine and currently one of the longest serving chairs in the country, and Norman Rosenblum and Evan Snyder prominent research leaders (Figure 6). Martha Magoon, a stellar chief resident and neonatologist, commented that she "felt a need to do a superb job to help those women who would come after me . . . I wanted to represent women well." She noted, "Avery . . . served as a role model and mentor and was influential in my career choices as a research fellow with Dr. [John] Clements at the Cardiovascular Research Institute in San Francisco, then as a neonatal fellow with Drs. [Rod] Phibbs and [William] Tooley at Moffit Hospital."[46]

Dr. Avery was, in fact, a committed and constant mentor to her trainees and junior faculty alike. On one occasion, she reflected to the author, "In life, it is less a matter of how smart you are as how much glue there is between the seat of your pants and the seat of your chair." On another occasion, while working on a paper one morning the author rose to greet her. She advised with clear purpose, as she did on several occasions with others, "Don't talk. Write." And

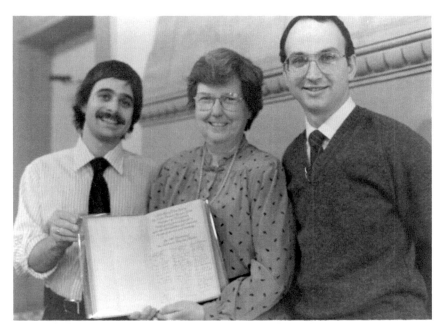

FIGURE 6   Mary Ellen Avery and her Last Chief Residents, 1984–1985
Mary Ellen Avery is shown with Evan Snyder on her right and Norman Rosenblum on her left.

reflecting upon the rich environment of the hospital for the training of residents bound for careers as physician scientists, Norman Rosenblum, one of the last chief residents in the Avery era and later associate dean of the Physician Scientist Training Program and professor of pediatrics at the University of Toronto School of Medicine, noted, "The most important thing is that during your training you meet lots of senior clinician-scientists, and you learn from these people as to what success looks like and what pitfalls look like. I met lots of people [at the Children's Hospital] who were thriving, and I saw other people who were not thriving. I was able to learn from their experiences because I knew them well and could have frank conversations with them."[47]

The residency training committee matured throughout the Avery era as an increasingly effective body for deliberating educational issues faced by the program.[48] The committee was made up of three house officers elected from each year of the program, the chief residents, six to seven faculty members, the chair of the internship selection committee, the residency coordinator (the senior administrator of the residency program), and the department manager. It was chaired by the program director and met monthly, with considerable work done in subcommittees between meetings. The focus of the committee included a) the quality of the housestaff education as experienced on inpatient and outpatient rotations; b) ongoing monitoring and evaluation of rotations and teaching conferences; c) evaluation of the nature and quality of resident evaluation and feedback and monitoring of the process of resident career development; and d) evaluation of quality of life issues.[48] Other issues that deserved high priority were the balance of service and education, intensive care versus general pediatric experiences, and inpatient versus outpatient exposure. Results of resident performance on the American Board of Pediatrics examination as well as success in the yearly internship match were additional important areas of scrutiny. Finally, administrative matters such as resident benefits, sick call, and pregnancy leave fell within the committee's purview. Minutes of the committee's deliberations were circulated to the whole housestaff, and reports were also given regularly to the department chair. Three to four topics were covered during the monthly hour-and-a-half meeting. The committee continues to function today 35 years after its inception, which speaks to its value to the residents, the faculty, and the department chairs.

In May of 1976, a medical service newsletter was first published and appeared each week thereafter.[49] Introduced by Jonathan Bates and Michael Williams, chief residents in 1975–1976 and 1976–1977, it became a much anticipated and enjoyed review of current cases on the medical service. Lessons learned from each case were a particular focus. The number of admissions and most common diagnoses were also carefully tracked and recorded. During the last two years of Avery's tenure, the chief residents, Lewis First and George Hoffman and Norman Rosenblum and Evan Snyder, published this much-appreciated newsletter, now with references and useful figures and diagrams.

The Curriculum

The Janeway era had emphasized different pathways for the training of the housestaff. At the core of his educational philosophy was flexibility in curriculum and rotations to meet the resident's future career needs. While Janeway had clear views on how to optimally train an individual as a resident, an emphasis on goals and objectives of each rotation, the content of each rotation, and formalized evaluation of rotations and residents only began to occur at the end of the Janeway era.

Dr. Avery's view of resident education was less driven by curriculum and was more based on the quality and nature of clinical exposure. She believed residents learned best when they were allowed to "soak up" an environment of rich resources (complex patients and excellent teachers). She believed residents flourished when given responsibility and when pushed to think deeply and carefully. She regularly encouraged her residents to explore widely, always prefaced with the simple question, "What are we missing?"[50] She didn't like the "pat" answer. She believed that one fully understood a topic when one could teach it clearly to a student. She applauded residents who were independent thinkers and learners and went to great lengths to support them in their intellectual pursuits. She depended on her faculty and housestaff to develop the formal curriculum and thus valued deeply and depended greatly on her residency training committee.

When Avery became chair of the Department of Medicine in the fall of 1974, she created an ad hoc faculty–resident curriculum committee chaired by a thoughtful medical educator, Warren Grupe, with two faculty members (Sam Lux, a superior subspecialist, and Fred Mandell, an exceptional, hospital-based practicing pediatrician); four chief residents (Jonathan Bates, Larry Johnson, John Phillips, and Michael Williams); and 11 residents, including Ellis Avner and Paul Dworkin, who, as noted earlier, went on to become pediatric department chairs, and Alan Goldbloom, who became a major hospital administrator, as did Jonathan Bates. The committee was formed in response to a letter in early 1975 signed by many members of the housestaff expressing their concerns with the training program. These ranged from issues related to philosophy and priorities in residency training, to relationships with fellows and specialty divisions, authority in resident decision-making, residency schedules, and elective time. The housestaff members of the committee, themselves products of the turbulent era of the late 1960s and 1970s, and thus activists wishing to achieve curriculum reform, eagerly addressed these perceived inadequacies and needed changes in their program. The subsequent committee report concentrated on three core areas of concern: a) the need for a standardized pedagogical curriculum; b) a set of new principles for program design; and c) a restructured operational design.[51] Once the core elements of change were fully agreed upon, the committee constructed a gradual phase-in approach to the adoption of their recommendations during 1975 and 1976.

The new standardized core curriculum was comprised of exposure to essential aspects of pediatrics offered in the classroom, in conferences, and through patient exposure on the wards and in the outpatient setting. It emphasized an understanding of "growth and development and functional maturation in relation to disease processes."[51] The curriculum focused on integration of education on the clinical service and exposure to the core content of pediatrics over the PL-1 and PL-2 years. Importantly, it pressed for the elimination of a separate ambulatory housestaff, advocated for an ambulatory curriculum presented in a regular and systematic way to all housestaff in the program, provided more continuity clinic exposure for the housestaff, and recommended that housestaff have more flexibility in selecting their ambulatory experiences ("selectives").

The principles of the training program redesign emphasized: a) education and learning reinforced through multiple exposures to a topic in both the inpatient and outpatient setting; b) a gradual increase in responsibility for patient care and decision-making over the three years of training, with PL-1s being supervised by senior residents and ward and clinic attendings, PL-2s being supervised in the subspecialty inpatient setting but more independent in the well-baby, ambulatory, and emergency room settings, and PL-3s supervising in the inpatient and outpatient settings; c) flexibility in the curriculum such that housestaff could emphasize certain areas over others to meet their career goals (or reinforce any areas of perceived weakness); d) integration of the ambulatory and inpatient curriculum into the single training program; e) increased patient care exposure in the outpatient department to general pediatrics, achieved through exposure to the Medical Diagnostic Clinic, certain subspecialty clinics (speech and hearing, early childhood development, learning disabilities, chronic somatic complaints) and resident continuity clinic exposure for a half day to a full day each week (achieved in the Comprehensive Child Health Program, resident continuity clinic, adolescent clinic, neighborhood health center clinics and private pediatrician offices).

Finally, in operational redesign of the program, certain areas were emphasized, including: a) elimination of night and weekend cross coverage on inpatient divisions that had led to a loss of continuity in education and care; b) sufficient length of rotations (approximately six weeks) to allow for competency in one area before moving on to another; c) increased flexibility in the curriculum through more elective time and greater use of ambulatory electives to meet career goals; d) an equal number of housestaff in the PL-1 and PL-2 years; e) elimination of Team C as a geographically diffuse team, with integration of these general pediatric patients into Teams A and B and onto the cardiology and oncology floors.

While not all of the recommendations were accomplished, most were. The housestaff rotations in 1974–1975 on Dr. Avery's arrival and in 1982 at the time of the RRC review and reflecting the residency training committee's recommendations are seen in Table 3.[51,52] In the PL-1 and PL-2 year, the duration of rotations was lengthened, the number decreased, and new assignments, such as behavioral pediatrics, delivery room, well-baby, and night float, were added. In the PL-3 year, the number of rotations was increased, while the length of each was shortened. In addition, new assignments, such as the Clinical Research Center, surgery, and a psychosomatic rotation were added.

Resident Life as a House Officer

The residency in the late 1970s and early 1980s had a distinct flavor. The residents worked hard, being on call during their first two years every third night and during their senior year every fifth to every sixth night. The senior resident (PL-3) was the undisputed leader of the service, thanks to their considerable clinical experience garnered during the prior two years of intensive training. The interns (PL-1) and juniors (PL-2) greatly depended on the seniors, especially for their clinical expertise. The seniors brought the literature from the library that related to clinical cases on the floors. As reflected upon by Leonard Rappaport, a prior resident in the Avery era and future division chief in the Fleisher era, they viewed with considerable skepticism the outsider's view that the Children's Hospital was a "fellow's hospital. They clearly saw it as the senior resident's hospital."[53] They also believed that their role included helping out the interns when their workload was too heavy and teaching medical students.

Assisting and helping fellow residents to complete their work was very much a part of the culture. In the words of Ted Sectish, the future highly experienced

TABLE 3 Resident Rotations

Year	PL-1		PL-2		PL-3	
	1975	1982	1975	1982	1975	1982
Number of Rotations	10	8	12	11	9	13
Length of Rotations	40-41 days	7.4 weeks	33-34 days	4.7 to 7 weeks	40-41 days	28 days
#1	Team A	Team A	Ambulatory	Ambulatory	Team A	Team A
#2	Team B	Team B	Team B or C	Behavioral Pediatrics	Team B	Team B
#3	Team C	Team C	Oncology	Oncology	Team C	Team C
#4	Cardiology	Cardiology	Ambulatory or Night Float	Delivery Room (BLI)	NICU	NICU
#5	BLI	Newborn or MICU	Ambulatory or Night Float	Well Baby	MECL	NICU
#6	MGH/CRC	Ambulatory	NICU	NICU	Teaching Resident	Teaching Resident
#7	Ambulatory/MECL	MICU or CRC	Neurology	Neurology	Elective	Elective or Vacation
#8	Ambulatory	Vacation	MECL	NICU	Elective	Elective
#9	Ambulatory	—	Elective	Elective	Elective or Vacation	Ambulatory or Vacation
#10	Vacation	—	BLI	Night Float	—	Ambulatory
#11	—	—	Elective	Vacation	—	Surgery
#12	—	—	Vacation	—	—	CRC
#13	—	—	—	—	—	Psycho-somatic

Team A—Infants and Toddlers
Team B—Adolescents
Team C—School-age Children

BLI—Boston Lying-In
CRC—Clinical Research Center
MGH—Massachusetts General Hospital

MECL—Medical Emergency Clinic
MICU—Medical Intensive Care Unit
NICU—Neonatal Intensive Care Unit

and respected program director of the Boston Combined Residency Program in the Fleisher era, the residents assumed "complete ownership of their patients."[54] The current concept of the "team's patient" was foreign, and the signing out of the patient for the night was viewed only as a brief interlude in a resident's responsibility for the care of his or her patient.[54] The resident was the "procedure specialist" for the service, acquiring considerable skill with common procedures (intravenous line insertion, bladder catheterization, and lumbar puncture) and to a lesser degree, less common procedures (subdural taps, thoracenteses with chest tube placement, saphenous vein cut downs, and arterial line placement).[54]

The concept of burnout had not yet become part of the nomenclature and culture of the time. Residents worked hard and enjoyed their comrades. Collegiality at a faculty-to-resident level was now replaced by resident-to-resident camaraderie. All residents also worked long hours and in a most collaborative manner with the nurses. Attendings were important as teaching attendings, and also offered oversight and guidance [albeit, often at a distance] in matters of patient care management. They taught about diseases and educated the residents about their field. Moment-to-moment patient care management as well as performance of procedures was the domain of the residents.

The residency structure was pyramidal, with the number of residents in the PL-1 and PL-2 years being equal (22 to 24) and the residents in the PL-3 year numbering approximately 17 or 18 residents (12 as inpatient seniors and five to six as ambulatory senior residents). Those who did not become seniors generally elected to pursue fellowships through the Special Alternative Pathway or specialty residencies such as neurology, anesthesiology, or dermatology. Most residents remained unaware of the competitive nature of the residency for senior positions, a credit to the careful career planning carried out by those in charge of the residency.[53] This system remained in place until 1978, when the American Board of Pediatrics mandated three years of general pediatric training prior to fellowship. At this point, the Special Alternative Pathway ("short tracking"), with two years of residency and three years of fellowship officially began assisting those who wished to pursue academic research-based careers.

The number of women residents grew throughout the Avery era. And although they adapted easily and well to the culture of the residency, they were still aware of the need to "prove themselves especially with the nurses."[55] Marriage during residency remained relatively uncommon and pregnancy even more uncommon. As reflected upon by Alan Leichtner and Maureen Jonas, future stalwarts of the Division of Gastroenterology at the Children's Hospital, a spirit of helping each other out was very much in the culture, with "one senior passing a note to a fellow senior during conference offering to take her call following her delivery."[55,56] For some, not even a new baby was seen as a reason for relinquishing one's patient care responsibilities.

The senior year was the plum of the residency. Residents coveted the opportunity to lead the team, to hone one's teaching skills and to pursue clinical studies and scholarship. The various rotations had a clear pecking order of preference. The ward rotations and specifically the infant toddler rotation (Team A), the school-age child rotation (Team C) and the emergency room rotation were particularly popular. The Clinical Research Center rotation, with its accompanying bone marrow transplants, the oncology rotation, and the emergency room night rotation, staffed by a sole junior resident, were the most demanding. Medical admissions were decided upon ("accepted") by the ward senior resident. The argument for admission delivered by the junior resident in the emergency department was often a challenging task. Asthma, pneumonia, cystic fibrosis, leukemia, diabetes, care of the premature infant, renal diseases such as nephrosis and nephritis, and bronchiolitis were common admissions.

Haemophilus influenzae disease and management of the accompanying epiglottitis, meningitis, and septic arthritis were particularly demanding. The rapid transfer of children with epiglottitis from the emergency room via the "bullet elevator" to the operating room was a long-remembered experience.[53] The medical intensive care unit did not open until 1980, thus acutely ill patients on respirators were handled in two- and four-bed rooms on the general floors with dedicated special nurses. So a house officer might have a Reye syndrome patient on a ventilator with intracranial pressure monitoring next to a chronically ill failure-to-thrive patient, clearly a formidable challenge when it came to offering optimal care to both. Obtaining a CT scan for an emergency department patient was an arduous procedure that involved the transfer by the resident of the patient from the emergency room, through the Bader Building, across the bridge to the Carnegie Building, and into the Jimmy Fund Building. The residents also went out on both neonatal and medical transports, thereby developing their transport skills. This experience was removed in time, taken over by specially trained transport anesthesiologists and nurses.

Education was less formal than today. Senior rounds, which were only for senior residents, were considered a high point in the day with, in the words of Ted Sectish, house officer in the Avery era, the "fresh cases" admitted the night before presented.[54] Grand rounds were generally well attended. A formal lecture series for residents occurred weekly in the Surgical and Radiology Pavilion Building dining room, but in general, the formal didactic curriculum took a backseat to teaching and learning on the floors and clinics. The ambulatory curriculum grew in importance. The ambulatory selective block allowed for exposure to subspecialty patients in the clinics. Time for longitudinal care of patients by residents in continuity clinic was increasingly protected rather than being an add-on as in prior years. Finally, the medical diagnostic clinic, which focused on children with enuresis, encopresis, attention deficit disorder, and school function disorders, while not popular with the residents, was increasingly seen as a critical component of a well-rounded resident education, especially for those entering practice.[53,54]

Triple Threat

Each generation of residents has its giants both at a junior and senior faculty level. The generation of the Avery era was no different. They taught, inspired, and served as important role models for the housestaff. Among the senior faculty were William Berenberg, David Nathan, John Kirkpatrick from radiology, Judah Folkman from surgery, Alexander Nadas, Fred Rosen, Robert Masland, Mary Ellen Wohl, Park Gerald, and John Crigler. Among the junior faculty were Arnold Smith, Dick Grand, Sam Lux, Harvey Cohen, and Donald Goldmann. David Nathan among the faculty epitomized the "triple threat." As remembered by Alan Leichtner: it was not unusual for him to appear on the wards at 11 p.m. asking to see (and teach on) "your sickest patient."[55,56]

An important award, the Charles A. Janeway Award, was established during the Avery era. Spearheaded by Arnold Smith, an infectious disease faculty member and a much revered teacher of the housestaff, the award in honor of Charles A. Janeway was presented annually to the outstanding teacher–clinician at the Children's Hospital and was selected by the vote of the housestaff.[57] The recipients during the Avery years are shown in Table 4. Of the recipients, William Berenberg and the author had been prior Children's Hospital house officers.

The House Officer Experience

The on-call rooms now in the Hunnewell Building (rather than on Longwood Avenue) while not elegant allowed for rapid access to the floors and helped to assure a brief but good sleep. The dress for the day for interns included white pants for males and white skirts or pants for females. The juniors and seniors wore their own dark pants and hospital white coats (with a tie for males). The housestaff library, which had been on Division 37 in the Janeway era, was now on Hunnewell 1. In 1980, the senior residents created the "senior file," a compilation

TABLE 4   Charles A. Janeway Award Recipients

1978	Arnold Smith	Infectious Disease
1979	William Berenberg	Academic Pediatrics
1980	John Kirkpatrick	Radiology
1981	Frederick Lovejoy	Academic Pediatrics
1982	Michael Epstein	Neonatology
1983	Rita Teele	Radiology
1984	Patricia O'Rourke	Medical Intensive Care

of up-to-date references. Each senior assumed responsibility for specific disease areas.[53] This rich resource led to the common practice of the preparation of "handouts" that summarized a topic and were used for teaching rounds.[56] This was an important educational offering for the interns and junior residents, and the senior file was actively used by both fellows and faculty. The housestaff lounge created in 1980, in the words of Leonard Rappaport, was both a "great thing" and a "terrible thing."[53] It fostered camaraderie among the housestaff but no longer would the housestaff share meals with the faculty, thereby depriving them of important opportunities for learning medical lessons as well as acquiring the history and lore of the hospital.

Some housestaff lived in the 25-story apartment tower, located above the Longwood Galleria on Longwood and Brookline Avenues, which had studios and one- or two-bedroom apartments. More, however, lived a short distance from the hospital in neighboring Brookline, Jamaica Plain, and South Boston.

During the Avery years, resident salaries showed a slow but steady increase.[58] Still, to make ends meet, married housestaff had working spouses or partners, and moonlighting, especially in the third year of residency, both inside the hospital (on neonatology and in the emergency room) and outside was extremely common.

The annual housestaff show was a celebrated and enjoyed event for housestaff and faculty alike. In not so subtle ways, the residents were masters at illuminating their current issues and grievances. But they did it with humor clearly emphasizing their central message, for example "What Price Glory" and "Children's at a Le$$er Co$t" and with gentle digs at the faculty, "Dr. Suave Crome" playing Bob Crone, the widely admired director of the medical and surgical intensive care unit; "Dr. Teaberry Beachnut" playing T. Berry Brazelton; and "Dr. Hatesorrow" playing the author. The songs were also poignant, "Cry

Baby Cry" to American Pie, "I've Never Been a Doc Before" to I've Never Been in Love Before, and "Bone Marrow Transplants" to Climb Every Mountain.[59] Other important social events in the life of the housestaff were a very popular intern orientation gathering often held at the Larz Anderson Park in Brookline and the winter dinner dance held at the New England Aquarium or the Museum of Science in Boston.

Resident Reunions

High schools, colleges, and graduate schools celebrate and embrace significant anniversaries of their graduates. Graduates enjoy the opportunity to reunite and reminisce about earlier times. Their institutions, in turn, hope to derive philanthropic support by more closely linking graduates with their schools. This is especially true in the later years of life. Residency classes have not followed this custom because graduates are spread widely geographically, are extremely busy, and many have limited financial resources. Residents mainly come together at academic meetings, rarely by class, rather by discipline and generally coordinated by their departments. Academic hospitals where residents trained are increasingly seeing this as a missed opportunity.

    An early venture into the domain of reunions occurred in 2012 with the 30th reunion of the 1982 residency class from the Avery era (Figure 7). Among a class of 22 seniors, 17 returned for the Margaret Walsh Visiting Professor Grand Rounds (named for their deceased classmate) and a dinner in the home of Elizabeth Woods, a member of the 1982 class who had skillfully organized the reunion. Spread throughout the country and Europe, most had not seen one another in 30 years. They conversed and reunited as if it was 30 years earlier. They reminisced about times in the past and reflected on their careers and their families. When they departed, they promised that five years, not 30 years, would pass before they came together again. Reflecting eloquently and poignantly after the reunion Arthur Lavin spoke for the whole class:

    "The time together Saturday really moved me. It was something to see everyone across a 30-year jump in time. It was sort of fun to play Harvard for a bit, count up accomplishments, and carry the flag of Boston Children's. I have no other experience like this to draw on. I can't think of another group of people I could get together with after 30 years of essentially no, or very little, contact and feel this close to. I walk away from that amazing night, simply grateful. It's almost like a group of vets got together after a long time, discovering that the battles they shared created a bond they didn't know was sitting there all that time. I got that sense from the urgency it seemed we all had, to pull up one more memory, and hear one more too. I found that there were many great, funny moments, but there were also a lot of very painful moments. Perhaps a part of the power of the night was that we had these deeply painful experiences in a moment of great confusion brought on by being completely unprepared for what we were thrown into, not to mention in our 20's—and now had the rare gift of having a night to sort some of it out after 30 years of working in the field of pediatrics, and now being in our 50s or more."[60]

One might predict that in years to come reunions and both struggles and achievements of residents will become more common—a return to the sense of family so present in an earlier era.

Career Directions

A clear goal of the program during the Avery era was to train physician-scientists for academic careers in pediatrics. A review of Avery's graduates (from 1974 to 1986) reveals a superior record in this regard. Of 270 graduates, 224 (83%) took

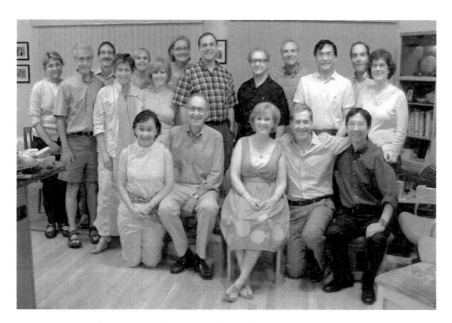

FIGURE 7   30th Reunion of 1982 Residency Class

The author and long-serving residency coordinator Susan Brooks (both seated), join the 1982 residency class in May 2012 at the home of Elizabeth Woods, a member of the 1982 class, for reunion and reminiscence. (Image courtesy of Elizabeth Woods)

a fellowship or did further residency training, while 46 (17%) proceeded directly into practice.[61] This contrasts with two national surveys in pediatrics done at that time in which approximately 60% proceeded into fellowship or further residency and 40% proceeded into practice.[62,63] Among the 224 graduates entering fellowship, neonatology (13%) and hematology/oncology (13%) were selected most frequently, followed by infectious diseases (10%), cardiology (8%), and gastroenterology (8%).[61] When these 224 former house officers were surveyed after fellowship, 66% remained in academic pediatrics, 31% were in practice, and 3% were at the National Institutes of Health, the Centers for Disease Control and Prevention, or in industry or public health.[61] Of those pursuing pediatric practice, a larger percentage were in fee-for-service private practices than in managed care. The figure of 66% pursuing academic careers was much higher than the 23% in academic pediatrics nationwide.[64]

Career Achievements

During the Avery era, a remarkable number of accomplishments were achieved by her graduates. The 16 department chairs trained between 1974 and 1984 are shown in Table 5, with 11 serving as chairs in pediatrics, two in genetics, one in neurology, one in immunology, and one in anesthesiology.

TABLE 5   Department Chairs

Ellis Avner	Case Western Reserve University School of Medicine (Pediatrics)
J. Devn Cornish	Emory University School of Medicine (Pediatrics)
Paul H. Dworkin	University of Connecticut School of Medicine (Pediatrics)
Lewis First	University of Vermont College of Medicine (Pediatrics)
Jonathan D. Gitlin	Vanderbilt University School of Medicine (Pediatrics)
Steven A. Goldstein	University of Chicago School of Medicine (Pediatrics)
George Hoffman	Medical College of Wisconsin (Anesthesiology)
Margaret L. Hostetter	Yale University School of Medicine (Pediatrics); University of Cincinnati School of Medicine (Pediatrics)
Bruce Korf	University of Alabama Medical School at Birmingham (Genetics)
John F. Modlin	Dartmouth Medical School (Pediatrics)

TABLE 5　Department Chairs *(Cont.)*

Scott Pomeroy	Harvard Medical School (Neurology)
David S. Rosenblatt	McGill University School of Medicine (Genetics)
John R. Schreiber	Tufts University School of Medicine (Pediatrics)
Alan L. Schwartz	Washington University School of Medicine (Pediatrics)
Nina F. Schor	University of Rochester School of Medicine and Dentistry (Pediatrics)
Christopher B. Wilson	University of Washington School of Medicine (Immunology)

Five graduates would ultimately go on to serve as presidents of hospitals, healthcare systems, or medical schools. (Table 6).

Other graduates during the Avery era went on to serve as deans (Table 7), lead major national organizations (Table 8), serve as major pediatric program directors (Table 9), become major national leaders in research (Table 10), or assume national clinical leadership positions (Table 11). This diverse list of leadership positions speaks to a heterogeneous set of talents evident among the positions held by graduates from the Avery era, ranging from clinical care to research to administrative roles. In addition, Dr. Avery's support and encouragement of women house officers was now becoming evident in the important leadership roles assumed by her female graduates.

TABLE 6　Presidents of Hospitals, Health Care Systems, or Medical Schools

Steven M. Altschuler	Children's Hospital of Philadelphia
Jonathan R. Bates	Arkansas Children's Hospital
Kathleen Carlson	Toledo Children's Hospital
Raymond S. Greenberg	Medical University of South Carolina
Alan L. Goldbloom	Children's Hospitals and Clinics of Minnesota

TABLE 7　Deans and Provost

S. Bruce Dowton	University of New South Wales Medical School, Australia
Steven A. Goldstein	Provost, Brandeis University
Steven Spielberg	Dartmouth Medical School

TABLE 8   National Organizations

Donald Berwick	Director, U.S. Government Centers for Medicare and Medicaid Services;
Alan E. Guttmacher	Director, National Institute of Child Health and Human Development; Senior Fellow at the Center for American Progress
Alan M. Krensky	Deputy Director, National Institutes of Health
Steven Spielberg	Deputy Commissioner for Medical Devices, Drugs, and Biologics of the Food and Drug Administration
Donald L. Weaver	Assistant Surgeon General and Acting Surgeon General, Department of Health and Human Services

TABLE 9   Pediatric Program Directors

William A. Durbin	University of Massachusetts Medical School
Emmett V. Schmidt	Harvard Medical School (Massachusetts General Hospital)
Edwin Zalneraitis	University of Connecticut School of Medicine
Theodore C. Sectish	Harvard Medical School (Children's Hospital)

TABLE 10   Major Investigators

Diana Bianchi	Vice Chair for Research, Department of Pediatrics, Tufts University School of Medicine
Michael Brownstein	Director of Functional Genomics, J Craig Venter Institute, Maryland; Chief of the Section on Genetics, National Institute of Mental Health
Ira Gewolb	Associate Chair for Research, Michigan State University College of Human Medicine
Lisa Guay-Woodford	Associate Vice President, Clinical and Translational Research, George Washington School of Medicine
Mark A. Israel	Director, Norris Cotton Cancer Center, Dartmouth Medical School
Julie R. Korenberg	Member, Brain Institute and USTAR Professor of Pediatrics at the University of Utah School of Medicine
Stephen Ladish	Scientific Director, Vice Chair for External Affairs, George Washington University School of Medicine
Donald Leung	Head, Division of Pediatric Allergy and Immunology, National Jewish Medical and Research Center, Denver

TABLE 10   Major Investigators *(Cont.)*

Rod McInnes	Director of the Lady Davis Research Institute at the Montreal Jewish General Hospital, McGill University School of Medicine
Stuart H. Orkin	Chair, Department of Pediatric Oncology, Dana-Farber Cancer Institute
Edward V. Prochownik	Director of Oncology Research, University of Pittsburgh School of Medicine
Bonnie W. Ramsey	Director of the Center for Clinical and Translational Research, University of Washington School of Medicine
David S. Rosenblatt	Chair, Department of Genetics, McGill School of Medicine
Norman Rosenblum	Associate Dean, Physician Scientist Training Program, University of Toronto School of Medicine
Alan L Schwartz	Chair, Department of Pediatrics, Washington University School of Medicine
Nina F. Schor	Chair, Department of Pediatrics, University of Rochester School of Medicine and Dentistry
Evan Y. Snyder	Program Director, Stem Cells and Regeneration, Burnham Institute, La Jolla

TABLE 11. CLINICAL LEADERS

Donald Berwick	Emeritus President, Institute for Health Care Improvement, Boston
F. Sessions Cole	Vice-Chair, Department of Pediatrics, Washington University School of Medicine
Holmes Morton	Director, Clinic for Special Children, Strasburg, Penn.
Jane Newburger	Associate Cardiologist-in-Chief and Vice Chair for Academic Affairs, Department of Cardiology, Children's Hospital Boston
David A. Piccoli	Chief, Gastroenterology, Hepatology, and Nutrition, Children's Hospital of Philadelphia
John R. Schreiber	Chair, Department of Pediatrics, Tufts University School of Medicine
Paul H. Wise	Director, Center for Policy, Outcomes and Prevention, Stanford University School of Medicine

While many Avery graduates are still relatively early in their careers, many have achieved prestigious awards in pediatrics, including the Society for Pediatric Research Young Investigator Award (Table 12), the E. Mead Johnson Award (Table 13), president of the Society for Pediatric Research (Table 14), membership in the National Academy of Science and/or the Institute of Medicine (Table 15), and teaching awards given by Harvard Medical School (Table 16). Importantly, two of the three presidents of the Society for Pediatric Research from the Avery era were women, speaking not only to her support of women but in particular, to women pursing academic research careers in pediatrics. Other residents from the Avery era have also achieved important recognition, such as Lewis First, who assumed the role of editor of *Pediatrics* from Jerry Lucey, the latter a neonatology fellowship graduate of the Children's Hospital. In addition, Lewis First received the Joseph W. St. Geme, Jr. Leadership Award from the Federation of Pediatric Organizations in 2014.

TABLE 12   Young Investigator Award of the Society for Pediatric Research

1983	Alan L. Schwartz
1985	Alan M. Krensky
1986	Edward V. Prochownik
1988	Roger E. Breitbart

TABLE 13   E. Mead Johnson Award

1984	John A. Phillips
1987	Stuart H. Orkin
1993	Alan L. Schwartz
1995	Margaret L. Hostetter
1995	Alan M. Krensky
1997	Donald Y.M. Leung
1998	Jonathan D. Gitlin
2001	Steve A. Goldstein

TABLE 14   Presidents of the Society for Pediatric Research

1994	Margaret H. Hostetter
2002	Alan M. Krensky
2005	Lisa Guay-Woodford

TABLE 15   National Academy of Science and/or Institute of Medicine

Donald Berwick
Diana Bianchi
Jonathan Gitlin
Margaret H. Hostetter
Stuart H. Orkin
Alan L. Schwartz

TABLE 16   Harvard Medical School Teaching Awards

1992, 1995	Lewis First
2014	Alan Leichtner

Summation

Deeply committed to medical education, Mary Ellen Avery brought the residency program into the modern era. She was highly successful in attracting women into the pediatric residency and launched the distinguished careers of Margaret Hostetter, Nancy Andrews, Nina Schor, Diana Bianchi, and Lisa Guay-Woodford. Her academic standards were very high and based on an academic meritocracy. She demanded much of herself and of others.

Her second area of great accomplishment was in neonatology. Highly respected for her work on surfactant with Mead, she was able to rejuvenate neonatology, recruit excellent fellows and junior faculty, and build an extremely strong Joint Program in Neonatology. Throughout her tenure, the Division of Neonatology was among the most popular fellowships chosen by the housestaff.

Finally, Mary Ellen Avery was devoted to promoting the health of children around the globe. Following her leadership of the department, and ever the educator, she traveled the globe mentoring, teaching, and advising physicians and nurses in an effort to improve the care of children.

CHAPTER VI

The Nathan Era

*Residency with an Academic Mission
and Impact
1985–1995*

*"Your personal responsibilities for your patients were
strongly emphasized and there was no excuse for not
knowing. You wanted to be a great resident . . ."*

—Jon Finkelstein, reflecting on his time as a house officer in 1992

O N JANUARY 1, 1985, David G. Nathan, the Robert A. Stranahan professor
at Harvard Medical School, became physician-in-chief of the Children's
Hospital, ending a 15-month nationwide search for a successor to Mary Ellen
Avery. The next 10 years would prove to be a time of remarkable growth in academic stature for the Department of Medicine. The hospital had entered a period
of significant physical enhancement, and a close working relationship between
the physician-in-chief and the surgeon-in-chief allowed the medical and surgical departments to flourish. The education programs would also mature greatly
during this halcyon period.

The Children's Hospital and the Department of Medicine

Significant Hospital Events[1]

The learning of medicine in the earlier apprenticeship model occurred through
example. Nowhere was this more evident than in the rich history of Osler,

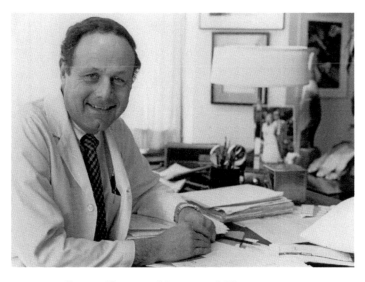

David Gordon Nathan, MD, 1985–1995

Dr. Nathan further enriched the strong academic mission of the Department
of Medicine and the residency program and trained 300 scientifically
oriented housestaff, the majority of whom pursued careers in academic
medicine.

Halsted, and Welch at Johns Hopkins, passed down through the ages in the
written and spoken word. Over the years, the housestaff at the Children's Hospital have watched closely the honoring of past and current medical giants. They
have observed carefully which faculty and which disciplines won national awards
and honors, as well as where the hospital has invested its assets (buildings and
new faculty), thereby reflecting its priorities. And they have basked in the warm
glow of historic moments, as national figures honored their institution. These
events, far removed from care, research, and teaching, served importantly in the
crafting of the culture and lore of the Children's Hospital and thus the soul of its
residents. Important examples in the 10 years of the Nathan era are illustrated
in the following significant hospital events.

In 1985, David Kosowsky was beginning his second year as chair of the board
of trustees and David Weiner his ninth year as president of the hospital. That year
also saw the establishment of a new hospital AIDS committee, a birth defects
service, and an ethics advisory committee. In addition, the hospital received a
large National Institutes of Health (NIH) grant to further its pioneering work
in the study of bone marrow engraftment and a better understanding of graft vs.
host disease. The Massachusetts Regional Poison Center, which had been housed

at the Children's Hospital throughout its history, celebrated its 30th anniversary at the Kennedy Library in Boston. The Clement A. Smith professorship, the first endowed professorship in neonatology in the world, was established to honor Clement Smith, a pioneer in respiratory physiology in the newborn. John Franklin Enders died at age 88. The Research Building, the largest pediatric research facility in the world, had been named the John F. Enders Pediatric Research Laboratories in his honor in 1976.

Construction work on the new inpatient facility, which began in February 1985, was 55% completed by October 1986. The hospital's successful collaboration with the Howard Hughes Medical Institute resulted in Stuart Orkin, associate in hematology/oncology, Samuel Latt, chief of the Division of Genetics, and Bernardo Nadal-Ginard, chief of cardiology, being appointed Hughes investigators. After a six-month nationwide search led by Judy Palfrey and the author, Gary Fleisher, a future physician-in-chief in the new millennium, was appointed chief of the emergency department. Donald Wiley and Steve Harrison were recruited from Harvard College at the suggestion of the Howard Hughes Medical Institute. And the year 1985 saw the deaths of Harry Shwachman, a worldwide authority on the treatment of cystic fibrosis at age 76, and Michael Bresnan, a revered and highly popular teacher of neurology and Janeway Teaching Award recipient at age 47.

Two new named professorships, the Alexander S. Nadas and the William Berenberg professorships in pediatrics at Harvard Medical School, were established in 1987 and 1988, respectively, as a result of the board of trustees' decision to launch a fundraising campaign to honor these two long-serving Children's Hospital physicians. The new inpatient building was dedicated in the fall of 1987, with 600 guests attending the event. Senator Edward M. Kennedy and Mayor Raymond Flynn spoke on this happy occasion. On February 9, 1988, 228 patients were moved in one day into the new building, a remarkable feat accomplished four hours ahead of schedule.

That same year, Fred Rosen, an internationally acclaimed investigator in immunology and loyal faculty member of the Department of Medicine, assumed the presidency of the Center for Blood Research (CBR), a separate institution with its own board of trustees and thus independent from the hospital. Fred Rosen's move to a leadership role proved highly important to the CBR's success over the next 10 to 15 years. This prestigious research program would eventually be incorporated into the Children's Hospital in the Program in Cellular and Molecular Medicine during the Fleisher era. Also in 1988, the *New Child Health Encyclopedia*, with contributions from over 150 Children's Hospital physicians and other health professionals was published by Delacorte Press. Written for the lay public, this book achieved a broad national circulation and wide recognition for the hospital. T. Berry Brazelton, a nationally recognized expert in child development, author of over 17 books and mentor to 60 fellows in child development, stepped down as director of the child development unit in December of 1988. Jeffrey Drazen, in later years the editor of *The New England Journal of Medicine*, assumed directorship of the Ina Sue Perlmutter Cystic Fibrosis Research Laboratories.

In 1989, the Honorable John LeWare, past chairman of the Shawmut Bank in Boston and President Reagan's appointee to the Federal Reserve Board in Washington, assumed chairmanship of the board of trustees from David Kosowsky. Workers began construction on a 12-story expansion of the Enders Building funded by the Howard Hughes Medical Institute. The construction nearly doubled the space for new research laboratories and state-of-the-art equipment. It also included a new, 168-seat auditorium, to be named in the future the Judah Folkman Auditorium, which would house medical and surgical grand rounds, post-graduate seminars, and other important hospital events. A hospital-wide graduate medical education committee was established with Michael Epstein as its chair. Bernardo Nadal-Ginard, a molecular biologist focusing on cardiac muscle cell differentiation and protein expression in muscle cells, assumed the Alexander Nadas professorship in cardiology. The newly created Janeway Service was dedicated in honor of the former physician-in-chief, and Donald Goldmann, an infectious disease expert became its first chief. In addition, Goldmann assumed leadership of the hospital's quality improvement program, and Merton Bernfield, newly recruited from Stanford University School of Medicine, assumed the Clement Smith professorship in neonatology.

In 1990, a number of distinguished honors were bestowed on Children's Hospital physicians. Joseph Murray, chief emeritus of the Division of Plastic Surgery, was the 1990 recipient of a Nobel Prize for his pioneering work at the Peter Bent Brigham Hospital on kidney transplantation; Julius Richmond, who had served as surgeon general of the United States from 1977 to 1981, received the Howland Award from the American Pediatric Society for his public policy accomplishments in addressing the needs of children. David Nathan received the National Medal of Science, the highest scientific honor given by the president of the United States, for his contributions to the diagnosis and treatment of blood disorders and his role in training many of the country's leading pediatric hematologists and oncologists. Mary Ellen Avery assumed the presidency of the American Pediatric Society. The author was appointed secretary of Harvard

Medical School's pediatric executive committee (the committee responsible for academic promotions in pediatrics), succeeding Jack Crawford from the Massachusetts General Hospital, who had served in that capacity from 1968 to 1990.

In February 1990, Children's Hospital scientists moved into the $56 million expansion of the John F. Enders Pediatric Research Laboratories. The hospital's first satellite center staffed by Children's Hospital physicians was opened for outpatient specialty care in Lexington, and their services would be expanded three years later. Nancy Andrews, a Department of Medicine resident, future dean of the Duke University School of Medicine and the first woman to serve as dean of a major research-oriented medical school, received the House Officer Research Award from the Society for Pediatric Research. Gordon Vawter, a revered pathologist and teacher, died in 1990.

In 1991, the board approved plans for a new hospital library and a new archives program. Mary Ellen Avery, physician-in-chief emeritus, was awarded the National Medal of Science for establishing the cause of the respiratory distress syndrome in premature infants. Raif Geha became the first incumbent of the Prince Turki Ben Abdul Aziz Al-Saud of Saudi Arabia professorship for his groundbreaking work in immunology. The author became the first incumbent of the William Berenberg professorship in pediatrics at Harvard Medical School.

George Kidder assumed chairmanship of the board of trustees in 1992. A member of the Children's Hospital community through the Hunnewell family, Kidder had chaired the hospital's successful five-year $40 million campaign. Orah Platt, a member of the Division of Hematology/Oncology, was named director of clinical laboratories with responsibilities for overseeing all of the hospital's clinical laboratories. As a reflection of increasingly successful fundraising efforts, Allan Walker, chief of the Division of Gastroenterology and Nutrition, was named the first Conrad Taff professor of nutrition, and Marian Neutra, master of the Castle Society at Harvard Medical School and director of the gastrointestinal cell biology laboratory, was named the first Ellen and Melvin Gordon professor in medical education.

In 1993, for the fourth year in a row, the Children's Hospital was ranked number one among pediatric hospitals in the country in the *U.S. News and World Report* annual hospital survey. In addition, Harvard Community Health Plan (HCHP) selected the Children's Hospital as its principal hospital for pediatric hospital-based services, and a HCHP pediatric service was established, allowing HCHP physicians to manage the care of their hospitalized patients. This service was led by John Graef, a past chief resident and a longtime Children's

Hospital physician. The hospital began rotating its junior residents to the recently renamed MetroWest Medical Center (Framingham Union Hospital) in July of 1993. Park Gerald, who served most successfully as chief of clinical genetics at the Children's Hospital from 1968 to 1983 and as professor of pediatrics at Harvard Medical School, died at age 72.

125 Years Strong

Children's Hospital celebrated its 125th birthday in 1994 with special exhibits and events recognizing the hospital's distinguished achievements. An anniversary dinner was held at the Copley Plaza Hotel in April, with Senator Edward Kennedy and Mayor Thomas Menino as keynote speakers. Distinguished medical and surgical alumni returned for academic exercises in the Enders Auditorium, a reception at the Harvard Club, and dinner at the Museum of Fine Arts. Additionally in 1994, First Lady Hillary Clinton came to the Children's Hospital, visiting the patients and speaking to the staff.

The new hospital library, located in the Fegan Plaza area, opened in September 1994. Available to staff 24 hours a day and having a modified, reconstructed Gamble Reading Room simulating that in the Blackfan, Smith, and Janeway eras, the library was a much-needed adjunct to the hospital's medical education programs. The Gardner House, on Longwood Avenue opposite the Hunnewell Building, was demolished to make room for a new parking garage for families. Fred Alt, a distinguished immunologist, became the first incumbent of the Charles A. Janeway professorship in pediatrics at Harvard Medical School. And the hospital mourned the passing of John Kirkpatrick at 68 years of age—a revered teacher, department chair of radiology, and hospital leader.

In October 1995, David Nathan stepped down as physician-in-chief after 10 years of distinguished leadership and service to the hospital to assume the position of president and chief executive officer of the Dana-Farber Cancer Institute. Children's Hospital collaborated with 18 other pediatric hospitals in the U.S. in the formation of the Circle of Care and took part in an inaugural conference at the National Institutes of Health, followed by a reception and dinner at the White House hosted by President and Mrs. Clinton. For over 15 years, this organization has continued to offer critical support to freestanding children's hospitals throughout the United States. The Boston Combined Residency Program, the first fully integrated pediatric training program in the U.S. involving two separate medical schools and two separate hospitals, was announced in

October 1995, with plans for the program to admit its first interns on July 1, 1996. F. Roswell Gallagher, emeritus chief and greatly respected founder of the adolescent unit, died at the age of 92.

Construction[2]

The initial construction efforts in the mid-1980s focused on enhancing the infrastructure of the campus. The Farley Building had become outdated. The much anticipated move into the new inpatient hospital occurred in 1988 (Figure 1). This facility, which was to become the housestaff's primary site of work, featured a new main lobby; new rooms for special treatments such as bone marrow transplantation; large parent waiting rooms; and new areas for surgery, radiology, cardiology, cardiac surgery, emergency services, and newborn intensive care; as well as more spacious patient rooms to accommodate larger equipment and rooming-in space for parents. The move into the new Hughes addition to the Enders Laboratories occurred in 1990 (Figure 2). The Children's Hospital in

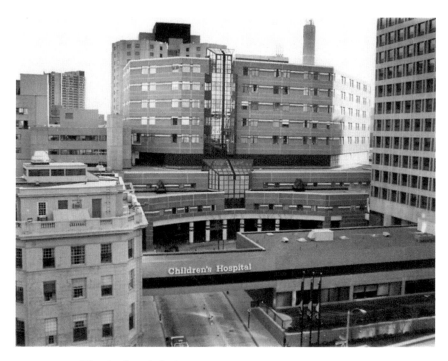

FIGURE 1   The new hospital, circa 1987
The new hospital was a welcome improvement for physicians, nurses, and patients alike.

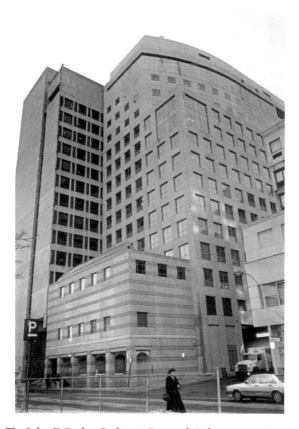

FIGURE 2   The John F. Enders Pediatric Research Laboratories, circa 1989
The Enders Laboratories, enlarged in the late'80s with Howard Hughes Medical Institute
support, as viewed from Longwood Avenue.

1986 and 1987 also saw the development of two new facilities that would benefit
patients, families, and staff, specifically the Longwood Galleria and expansion of
the Children's Inn on the corner of Longwood and Brookline Avenues.

Reconstruction of areas in the Farley, Bader, Hunnewell, and Fegan Buildings continued at a rapid pace, the majority of these changes impacting the housestaff. In 1991, the Department of Laboratory Medicine moved onto the upper
floors of the Farley Building. In 1992, the cardiology department moved onto the
second floor of the Farley and Surgical and Radiology Pavilion Buildings, and
the pathology department relocated to the basement and first floor of the Bader
Building. In 1993, adolescent and young adult medicine moved from the Ida C.
Smith Building to the Hunnewell ground floor, and the Massachusetts Poison
Control Center moved into the vacated quarters in the Ida C. Smith Building.

In September 1994, the new medical library, located between the cafeteria in the Farley Building and the Ida C. Smith Building opened. In the same year, major renovations on Farley 4 occurred, which improved the dialysis unit, the ambulatory treatment center, the General Clinical Research Center (formerly known as the Clinical Research Center and later to be called the Clinical Translational Studies Unit) and the therapeutic aphoresis unit.

The concerning local and national news in 1989 of an unacceptably high infant mortality rate, coupled with inequalities in care in Boston, led the hospital to enhance its primary care services for the children of the City of Boston. These efforts included an enlarged facility for Pediatric Group Associates (a resident-staffed primary care group practice) on Fegan 5 in 1988, new facilities on the ground floor of the Hunnewell Building for the Comprehensive Child Health Program (a faculty-staffed primary care group practice) in 1992, and a new Martha Eliot Health Center for residents of the Bromley–Heath housing complex in Jamaica Plain in 1994.

The need to reach out to the suburban community in an increasingly competitive health care environment led to enhancements in community-oriented facilities surrounding Boston. In 1993, the Children's Hospital and the Beth Israel Hospital collaborated to construct a new facility in Lexington for specialty care of children and adults living north and west of Boston. This was soon followed in the spring of 1995 by a new specialty center in Peabody. These facilities were supplemented by outreach programs for newborn nursery care at Newton Wellesley Hospital and Winchester Hospital and pediatric intensive care services at Boston City Hospital. This burst of construction and addition of programs reflected the new philosophy in health care delivery of extending services to capture "market share" in an increasingly competitive environment while also improving convenience for patients by offering care closer to their communities.

Patient Care[3]

During the Nathan era, the Department of Medicine made a concerted effort to enhance the organization, delivery, and quality of care on the general medical and subspecialty services. This was necessary because of the pressure from payers that began in the 1980s to increase efficiency and lower hospital costs. As the services matured, the census underwent a remarkable change.[3] In 1986, the number of discharges from the general medical inpatient services stood at slightly over 5,000, with an average length of stay of 7.1 days. By 1995, that figured had risen to 7,545 discharges per year (or 45% of all discharges from the hospital), with a length of stay of 3.8 days. The length of stay on the subspecialty services (oncology, bone marrow transplantation, medical intensive care unit, neonatal intensive care unit, and the Clinical Research Center) fell from an average of 8.3 days in 1990 to 5.5 days in 1995. Throughout this 10-year period, the general ward services had a bed occupancy of 85% to 89%, with another 10% to 15% scattered on nonmedical wards throughout the hospital, while the subspecialty units in aggregate had a census of 60% to 65%. The hospital was becoming very busy, and as a consequence so was the housestaff.

Medical outpatient volume experienced considerable growth, from 67,000 patient visits in 1984 (including general pediatric and subspecialty care) to 84,000 visits in 1988, to 108,248 visits in 1994.[4] The latter included 45,700 specialty visits, 42,460 general medicine visits, 10,726 continuity clinic visits, and 9,362 adolescent visits. Emergency room visits increased to 50,000 by 1988 and remained at slightly over that figure throughout the Nathan era. The growth in volume in the emergency department and the continuity clinic predominantly affected the housestaff.

The Service Chief System

David Nathan in 1985 initiated a new system of delivery of care on the general ward services, the service chief system for Teams A, B, and C.[5] A service chief was placed in charge of each geographic unit and a group of attending physicians (approximately 20 to 25 per service) were assigned as permanent members. The services were named after prior physicians-in-chiefs, the Thomas Morgan Rotch Service, the Charles A. Janeway Service, and the Kenneth D. Blackfan Service. The service chiefs Dr. Nathan appointed were seasoned and highly respected faculty members. They were, respectively, for each service Kenneth McIntosh, chief of the Division of Infectious Diseases; Donald Goldmann, director of infection control for the hospital; and Warren Grupe, chief of the Division of Nephrology (Figure 3). They were responsible for developing and delivering the educational curriculum for the residents and students rotating onto their service and carefully coordinating and monitoring the care delivered to the patients. They also guaranteed that the referring physicians were informed about their patients on a regular and timely basis. And they resolved differences of opinion around the care of patients while being careful not to undermine the authority of the senior supervising resident. The effect was dramatic, with important improvements occurring in residency education, efficiency of care, a shortening of length of stay, and better cost control.[6]

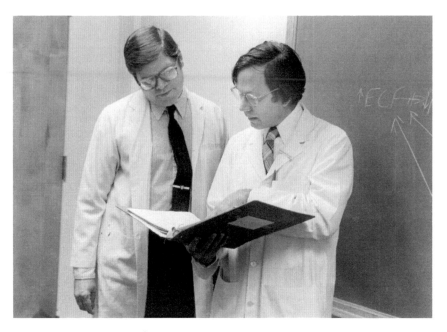

FIGURE 3   Service Chiefs, circa 1986

The first service chiefs included Kenneth McIntosh, on the right, for the Rotch Service and Warren Grupe, on the left, for the Blackfan Service.

With the move into the new hospital, an office was assigned to each chief and administrative assistant. Each chief, in turn, worked closely with his or her counterpart in nursing: Pat Rutherford for the Rotch Service, Sarah Pasternack for the Janeway Service, and Jane Rogers for the Blackfan Service. Jane Tyler served as the senior administrator for all three services. The first Rotch, Janeway, and Blackfan prizes were awarded in the mid-1990s in what would be an annual event of recognition of faculty for excellence in care and teaching.

The service chief system was so successful, both in terms of care and in the teaching of housestaff, that the concept was adopted by the subspecialty inpatient services. The various service chiefs are shown in Table 1. Organizationally, these units were initially part of the inpatient service chief system, but soon joined their subspecialty divisions. This system of care was also adopted by the psychiatry department, with Leslie Rubin and later John Knight, both academic generalist pediatricians, serving as medical chiefs of the inpatient service, which was later named the Richmond Service.

TABLE I   Medical Department Service Chiefs (1985–1995)

Janeway Service	Donald Goldmann
Blackfan Service	Warren Grupe, John Graef, Melanie Kim, Gregory Young
Rotch Service	Kenneth McIntosh, Samir Najjar, Edward O'Rourke
Short-stay Unit Service	Marc Baskin
Oncology Service	Holcombe Grier, Amy Billett
Bone Marrow Transplant Service	Howard Weinstein, Barbara Bierer
Neonatology Service	Michael Epstein, Ann Stark
Medical Intensive Care Service	James Fackler, Robert Truog
General Clinical Research Center	Norman Rosenblum, Kathy Jabs, Alan Ezekowitz
Harvard Community Health Plan Service	John Graef

In addition to the agreement with HCHP, another important change in the delivery of clinical care occurred in the 1990s when the hospital initiated an innovative model of delivery of care for "short-stay" patients on the medical service. John Graef was selected to coordinate the care of HCHP patients at the Children's Hospital and became its service chief. He was ably assisted by James Pert.

The short-stay unit was created because the medical service was increasingly caring for two very distinct groups of patients: chronic, complex long-term patients who needed considerable subspecialty expertise and short-term patients often admitted for brief hospital stays who required less complex care. To meet this demand, a 10-bed unit was established on the Rotch Service for hospitalizations of no longer than 72 hours.[7] The most common admissions to the short-stay unit included asthma, bronchiolitis, cellulitis, R/O (rule out) sepsis, and urinary tract infections. The mean duration of stay was 34 to 36 hours. Marc Baskin, an emergency medicine physician and pioneer in management of the febrile infant, was selected as service chief, with Michael Marks serving as his assistant and Pat Rutherford serving as nurse manager. This system of simplified care proved to be highly efficient and cost effective.[8] Well accepted by the housestaff, it was also a very valuable educational model.[9] The number of admissions to this unit grew dramatically over the ensuing years.

Other valuable innovations in care initiated in the Nathan era included the medical consultation service for the surgical inpatient services, created in 1988. Led by Fred Mandell, an academically oriented practicing pediatrician and expert in sudden infant death syndrome, with the assistance of seasoned senior residents, this service proved to be an important adjunct to the medical care of the surgical patient and a valuable educational experience for the residents.

By the early 1990s, quality improvement initiatives and activities led by Donald Goldmann had begun. Monthly review of quality improvement indicators enhanced patient care. Patient satisfaction indicators were also recorded and monitored. By 1995, quality improvement efforts had further matured, with 25 physician coordinators selected from the divisions and the inpatient and outpatient services. A steering committee was formed and regular quality improvement meetings were held. Finally, the first clinical practice guideline (CPG) for asthma was introduced, designed to serve as a guide for clinical management and to assure high-quality, efficient, cost-effective care. CPGs followed for urinary tract infection, diabetes, osteomyelitis, and septic arthritis, all piloted in the first year of the CPG program. Initially focused to a greater degree on the faculty, over the years, the housestaff became more and more central to the construction and implementation of CPGs.

Medical Education[10]

Education of medical students, which was seen as a highly important pursuit throughout the Blackfan, Janeway, and Avery eras, continued to be a major focus during the Nathan era. As a major pediatric teaching hospital for Harvard medical students, this effort was important not only for the teaching of scientific and clinical knowledge but also for the recruitment of students into pediatrics. The effort spawned a number of future education leaders, who were prior Children's Hospital residents and fellows, as shown in Table 2.

The courses requiring the greatest effort by the faculty included Introduction to Clinical Medicine (later called Patient-Doctor II), the Core Pediatric Clerkship (later called Women and Children's Clerkship), the Advanced Pediatric Clerkship ("Sub I"), the Doctor Patient III course, and the Ambulatory Core Clerkship.[11] These efforts would result in 10% to 12% of a Harvard medical student class entering pediatrics nationwide each year. In addition, the department's numerous subspecialty electives (over 26 by the end of the Nathan era) allowed future intern applicants to directly experience and evaluate the hospital and residency program.

TABLE 2   Medical Student Education Leaders (1985–1995)

Orah Platt	Future Master of the Cannon Society at Harvard Medical School
Norman Rosenblum	Future Associate Dean for Physician Scientists Training at the University of Toronto Faculty of Medicine
Alan Woolf	Future Director of Graduate Medical Education at Children's Hospital
Lewis First	Future Department Chair and Dean for Medical Education at the University of Vermont College of Medicine
Jonathan Gitlin	Future Chairman of Pediatrics at Vanderbilt University School of Medicine

The hospital, in turn, benefited from Harvard Medical School's initiatives in new educational pedagogy and curriculum development, including most specifically the New Pathway for Medical Education(small group, tutorial-based education predicated on adult learning theory), introduced in 1985 and led by Dean Daniel Tostesen and the Resident as Teacher curriculum (a course led by Dean for Medical Education Daniel Federman to enhance the skills of residents in teaching medical students in the hospital setting). In 1992, medical student education was further formalized by the creation of the position of director of medical student education at the Children's Hospital, with Lewis First as the inaugural director. He and a committee coordinated all student courses while offering help with curricular design, course evaluation, and faculty development.

The Introduction to Clinical Medicine course was led by Sessions Cole, a neonatologist and future departmental leader at Washington University School of Medicine in St. Louis, and Jonathan Gitlin, future chair of pediatrics at Vanderbilt University School of Medicine. Later, it was directed by Stephen Sallan, an oncologist and future chief of staff at the Dana-Farber Cancer Institute; Robert Michaels, a practicing pediatrician in Boston; and finally by Shari Nethersole, a medical educator in general pediatrics at the Children's Hospital. This course focused on the teaching of the pediatric history and physical examination to 90 to 100 second-year students in the spring of each year in four to five half-day sessions, carried out in the inpatient, outpatient, and private pediatrician office settings. A remarkable number—over 40 inpatient tutors and over 50 outpatient tutors—were recruited to teach in this effort.

The Core Course in Pediatrics was led by Orah Platt, a much revered teacher of medical students and highly capable director of clinical laboratories at the

Children's Hospital, and Alan Schwartz, future chair of the Department of Pediatrics at Washington University School of Medicine in St. Louis, and upon the latter's departure to St. Louis by Norman Rosenblum, ably assisted by DeWayne Pursley, a neonatologist and future pediatrician-in-chief at the Beth Israel Hospital in Boston. In the mid-1990s, the course was led by Edward O'Rourke, a highly respected member of the infectious disease division; Jonathan Finkelstein, a past chief resident and future associate residency program director; Robert Sundel, a master teacher of rheumatology and physical examination of the pediatric patient; and Ingrid Holm, a past Children's Hospital house officer, as well as a fine geneticist and endocrinologist at the hospital. This flagship course instructed approximately 100 third-year medical students each year. As many as 70 attendings participated annually, teaching students in this course on the three general pediatric services.

The teaching resident (a senior resident–required rotation) made daily walk rounds with the students and offered didactic sessions, a particularly beneficial and popular element of this course. The housestaff on rotation on the various medical services would also prove to be central to the success of the Core course. Feedback to the students was offered twice during each six-week block, with a formal evaluation at the end. The course received very high student ratings throughout the Nathan era.

A number of curricular initiatives were added to the Core Course between 1993 and 1995, including rotation on the short stay unit, with its exposure to common pediatric diseases; the addition of a weekly physical examination skills session focused on the joint, heart, lung, eye, ear, and neurological examinations; a written pediatric examination given at the end of the six-week block; and the addition of multimedia computer-based education modules to enhance learning. The course also gradually moved from being totally located on the inpatient service to two-thirds inpatient and one-third outpatient. This course was supplemented by the Advanced Pediatric Clerkship ("Sub I") for fourth-year Harvard Medical School, as well as non-Harvard, students. The student's role simulated that of the intern but with careful senior resident and faculty supervision. In any given year, half of these students applied to the medical internship at the Children's Hospital, a testimony to the importance of the subinternship as a way for the student to better know the Children's Hospital and for the faculty to appreciate the capabilities of a student as a future resident.

Elective courses were also highly popular and subscribed to by over 100 students each year. These electives were taken in the pediatric subspecialties, with activities occurring predominantly in the outpatient setting. Emergency medicine and adolescent medicine were the most popular, although infectious diseases, endocrinology, and hematology/oncology enjoyed great popularity as well.

A new Ambulatory Core Clerkship course was added in 1994. In this course, the students were closely matched with general pediatricians and general medicine fellows from the Division of General Pediatrics. Didactic sessions were given at the medical school; clinical exposure was offered in the hospitals. The course was carried out at all of Harvard Medical School's teaching hospitals, with Shari Nethersole, a future hospital medical director for community health, leading the effort at the Children's Hospital, together with Margaret Coleman, a faculty member at Cambridge Hospital, and Anita Feins, a practitioner and educator at Harvard Community Health Plan. This course was supplemented by a one-month fourth-year elective in ambulatory pediatrics, which took place in the subspecialty clinics at the Children's Hospital.

Doctor-Patient I and Doctor-Patient III courses were added to the medical school curriculum in the 1990s supplementing the Doctor-Patient II course (known earlier as Introduction to Clinical Medicine). These two courses occurred once a week at Harvard Medical School, the former led by Gordon Harper, the director of the inpatient psychiatry service, and the latter by Fred Mandell, Ralph Earle, and Alan Nauss, all deeply revered and experienced practicing pediatricians in the Boston area. The first-year course focused on introductory issues in medicine, while the third-year course focused on social, cultural, economic, ethical, and health delivery issues.

The service chief system served as the locus for faculty development and educational opportunities for the medical staff and referring physician community. In 1992 in cooperation with the Office of Educational Development at Harvard Medical School, the Department of Medicine set up a series of all-day workshops, initially for physicians on the general medical service, then for the faculty on the subspecialty services, and finally for faculty at the Children's Hospital, the Children's Service at the Massachusetts General Hospital, Cambridge Hospital, and the Harvard Community Health Plan.[12] Five retreats were held over the ensuing three years, with more than 100 participants at each retreat. Small group, bedside, and large group teaching were emphasized as well as principles of active learning and adult learning theory. Professor C. Roland Christensen, a university professor from Harvard Business School and Elizabeth Armstrong from Harvard Medical School were critical to this effort, offering their considerable knowledge and expertise in medical education for the benefit of the faculty.

Finally, between 1985 and 1995, the department continued to offer important education programs for its referring pediatricians. These efforts included the Pediatric Post-Graduate course, run by John Graef; the highly popular "Appreciation Day for New England Pediatricians," led initially by Sherwin Kevy and later by Alan Woolf; the Post-Graduate Seminar series, held each Wednesday followed by medical grand rounds; and finally bimonthly luncheons with David Nathan to discuss concerns of the referring physician community. Grand rounds were taped and made available to the referring physician community. In addition in 1989, *Pediatric News* was initiated to keep referring physicians up to date with recent developments in the Department of Medicine. This proved so successful that it was later taken over by the Public Affairs Department of the Children's Hospital as a hospital-wide publication.

Research[13]

Research flourished in the Department of Medicine during the Nathan years. Basic research, already very strong, was augmented by new initiatives in clinical (translational) research and outcomes research. Nathan further enhanced the basic science capabilities of the department by attracting such distinguished investigators as Stephen Harrison and Donald Wiley and appointing such outstanding Howard Hughes investigators as Fred Alt, Stuart Orkin, and Louis Kunkel.

Research carried out by members of the department exerted a powerful influence on the career direction of residents, as they observed its importance for a successful academic career. In addition, the national reputation garnered by various divisions as a result of their important discoveries significantly influenced residents as they considered their future choices for fellowship training. Clearly, a culture of discovery emanating from the divisions served as a clarion for excellence and future promise for talented young residents in the training program.

Research in infectious diseases, led by Kenneth McIntosh as division chief, focused on respiratory syncytial virus, the most common cause of admission to the hospital, prevention of nosocomial and hospital-acquired infection, and studies of *Staphylococcus epidermidis* as a cause of intravenous catheter infection and E. coli as a cause of neonatal meningitis. The hospital joined eight other centers in the U.S. in testing the drug azidothymidine (AZT) for children with AIDS. AIDS research in the division also focused on immunization for those at highest risk from infection with the AIDS virus due to underlying diseases as well as universal precautions for health workers. By 1989, the study of AZT in mothers with AIDS became a hospital focus.

In genetics, Louis Kunkel achieved acclaim for his research on Duchenne muscular dystrophy. Following his identification of the involved gene in 1986, Kunkel in the next several years identified the involved muscle protein, dystrophin. He noted it to be absent in muscular dystrophy patients and to be of abnormal structure in Becker muscular dystrophy patients (a milder form of the disease). In the 1990s, Diana Bianchi, a prior Children's Hospital resident and future vice chair for pediatric research at Tufts University School of Medicine, demonstrated that a mother's blood could harbor enough fetal cells to make genetic testing possible as an alternative to amniocentesis, and Gail Bruns, a longtime member of the division, in parallel work with others, identified the Wilm's tumor gene (a childhood cancer of the kidney).

In immunology research, the greatly respected Raif Geha, who in time would become the longest serving division chief in the department, identified the molecular binding site for the toxin causing toxic shock syndrome. Jane Newburger and Fred Rosen, both prior Children's Hospital residents, in a three-and-a-half–year clinical trial showed that single high-dose intravenous gamma globulin (IVIG) was as safe and effective as the more commonly used four-day course in the treatment for Kawasaki disease. The division also took the lead in diagnosing and treating primary immunodeficiency diseases and defining the defect in X-linked immunodeficiency syndrome.

The Division of Pulmonary Medicine, under the dedicated leadership of Mary Ellen Wohl, took the lead in clinical trials in cystic fibrosis and in lung transplantation. With Andrew Colin and others, the division carried out trials on DNase (an enzyme that breaks down mucus that accumulates in the lung) and amiloride (which regulates the flow of salt and water in and out of cells) in patients with cystic fibrosis. The division was a collaborator on the first pediatric single-lung transplant in 1990, a double-lung transplant in 1991, and the first pediatric heart–lung transplant in 1993.

The Division of Hematology/Oncology, under the highly talented leadership of Samuel Lux, a prior Children's Hospital resident in the Janeway era, would be the most successful of all divisions in garnering competitive funding support. In the mid- to late 1990s, the division's research focused on the genetics of hemoglobin synthesis and red cell production, basic molecular studies of problems in bone marrow transplantation, the pharmacokinetics of removal of excess iron accumulation in the body (as a result of blood transfusions) in patients with thalassemia, defects in the red cell membrane in sickle cell disease and other hemolytic anemias, mechanisms responsible for the immune destruction of platelets, the use of plasmapheresis to remove antibodies from blood, and finally methods to enhance the effectiveness of storage of blood. Trainees of the program were part of the successful effort that discovered the genes responsible for retinoblastoma (a cancer of the retina), for chronic granulomatous disease (a disorder in which white blood cells inadequately kill invading bacteria and fungi), and the gene mutation in Li-Fraumeni syndrome (a type of familial cancer). Other researchers studied the use of granulocyte macrophage colony stimulating factor (GM-CSF) in immune deficiency diseases and bone marrow failure in aplastic anemia. In the early to mid-1990s, they carried out human trials of recombinant factor VIII in patients with hemophilia (to eliminate the risk from transfusions used to control life-threatening bleeding episodes) and the use of recombinant gamma interferon for chronic granulomatous disease (a disease whose understanding Nathan, Robert Baehner, Alan Ezekowitz, Stuart Orkin, and others at the Children's Hospital had significantly advanced over the years through their research). Finally, in the mid-1990s the Children's Hospital, because of the work of hematologist Orah Platt, became one of four centers in the U.S. participating in clinical trials focused on the use of hydroxyurea for the treatment of sickle cell disease.

In the renal division, William Harmon, the long-serving chief of nephrology, and Cathy Jabs participated in a nationwide study of recombinant human erythropoietin (EPO) in hemodialysis patients, and the endocrine division, led by Joseph Majzoub, studied premature labor and elevated levels of corticotrophin releasing hormone (CRH) and cortisol in the blood of pregnant women during the final weeks of pregnancy. Joseph Majzoub, an internist by training, would go on to build a very large and highly distinguished Division of Endocrinology at the Children's Hospital.

Finally, the department acquired a number of larger institutional grants in support of research. These included in 1991, a Lucille P. Markey Charitable Trust grant to establish a Markey Child Health Research Center to support young physicians in training. In the same year, a Child Health Research Center was established by the National Institute of Child Health and Human Development as one of seven such centers in the U.S. Its support was further enhanced by the hospital's research endowment and the Janeway Fund (an endowed fund in the Department of Medicine in honor of Dr. Janeway). David Nathan was highly instrumental in acquiring this important research funding and Merton Bernfield assumed directorship of the center. Finally in 1995, Isaac Kohane, a prior resident and expert in the application of informatics to clinical medicine, acquired a three-year grant from the National Library of Medicine to develop ways to apply computer technology to enhance patient care.

Finances

The financial trajectory of the hospital and department during the Nathan era was marked by steady growth. The hospital underwent a twofold increase in its operating budget, from $125 million in 1985 to $277 million in 1994, with a slight dropoff during the next two years. The Department of Medicine's operating budget underwent a sevenfold increase, from $2 million in 1985 to nearly $14 million in 1995.[14] In 1985, at the beginning of the Nathan era, the department had 148 research grants, with direct support exceeding $13 million. By 1990, it reached $19 million, and by 1995, direct support for basic and clinical research had grown to over $30 million.

Financial support for the residency came from a number of different sources;[15] the vast majority, approximately 80%, came from the hospital's general funds (the hospital's operating budget). The remainder came from a multiplicity of sources, including the Brigham and Women's Hospital (for resident staffing of the neonatal intensive care units), a primary care grant (for primary care resident support), MetroWest Medical Center (when medical residents began to work in that facility), Boston Medical Center and the Massachusetts General Hospital (when residents from those institutions rotated through the Children's Hospital), and finally the Department of Medicine. While each year was slightly different, the greatest amount of funding came from the hospital, and from 1995 on, the department and the Brigham and Women's Hospital were the next two major sources of funding. Maintaining a modest number of house officers was logical from a financial perspective, but a lean housestaff was also beneficial in assuring close resident-to-resident collegial relationships and allowing the program directors and faculty to direct personalized attention to each house officer. In the face of a growing service load, the housestaff size increased by approximately two positions each year. Comparing 1987 and 1995 is illustrative, as shown in Table 3.

By early 1994, the National Association of Children's Hospitals and Related Institutions in a position statement was taking a firm stand on the need for sound financing for graduate medical education (GME) and the need for an enhanced focus on pediatric education.[16] This was done within the context of strongly supporting comprehensive national health care reform to achieve health care

TABLE 3   The Pediatric Residency Program

	1987 (in FTEs*)	1995 (in FTEs*)
Total Number of Housestaff	63.6	78.5
Funding Source		
Children's Hospital	53.6	64.0
Brigham and Women's Hospital	7.0	8.0
Department of Medicine	—	5.5
MetroWest Medical Center	—	1.0
Boston Medical Center	2.0	—
Massachusetts General Hospital	1.0	—

*FTE: full-time equivalent

coverage for all Americans (adults and children). Funding of pediatric children's hospitals was especially needed to correct the disparity existing between pediatric training programs in general hospitals that received federal GME support and freestanding pediatric institutions that did not. This disparity presented a serious financial challenge for freestanding children's hospitals and their boards of trustees. As the size of residencies grew in an effort to care for a growing number of inpatients and outpatients, significant tension developed between department chairs charged with achieving quality patient care and education of trainees and the hospital administration and trustees acutely aware of their fiduciary responsibilities and maintaining a balanced hospital budget, especially in times of fiscal constraint. This problem would be lessened as a result of federal funding for freestanding children's hospitals in the Philip Pizzo/Gary Fleisher era in the late 1990s and early 2000s.

Departmental Leadership

Eighth Chair of the Department of Medicine

David Nathan (photo, front of chapter) was born in Boston. He attended grammar school and secondary school in Massachusetts and proceeded to Harvard College, where he majored in English. He then crossed the Charles River to Harvard Medical School, receiving his MD in 1955. He entered internship in the Department of Medicine at the Peter Bent Brigham Hospital and went on to the National Cancer Institute. On returning to the Brigham Hospital for senior residency and a faculty appointment, his interest in red cell disorders brought him into contact with Louis K. Diamond and his fellow Frank Oski and the Children's Hospital. On Dr. Diamond's retirement in 1968, Nathan became chief of the Division of Hematology/Oncology, a position he held for 18 years.

In 1985, he was appointed chair of the Department of Pediatrics at Harvard Medical School and physician-in-chief at the Children's Hospital. David Nathan assumed the leadership of the Department of Medicine at a critical time in the hospital's history. Science was in a period of ascendency. A close working relationship with Surgeon-in-Chief Aldo Castenada assured strong physician leadership, and David Weiner's presidency of the hospital assured stability. A dedicated board of trustees had raised the necessary philanthropic support for a new 325-bed clinical facility, and Nathan had generated the necessary funds to increase the size of the John F. Enders Laboratories for Pediatric Research by over 40%.

An internist by training, Nathan had important credentials and a national presence that allowed him to work effectively with the scientific leaders at the NIH, the Howard Hughes Medical Institute, and national foundations. He was supportive of his division chiefs, there when he was needed, but he didn't micromanage. He listened well and could be persuaded to change his mind.

He served with immense distinction in that capacity for 10 years prior his appointment as president of the Dana-Farber Cancer Institute, leading that institution from 1995 to 2000. Nathan's contributions to academic medicine were herculean. He made highly important discoveries in hematology, trained an entire school of pediatric hematologists, and made major contributions to residency training and pediatrics. He built institutions and training programs for physician-scientists. He was a remarkable national leader in academic medicine.

Early Years

David Nathan attended the John D. Runkle School in Brookline, where he was awarded the Good Citizenship badge in 1941. That award rests proudly even today in his office. He had come in second place in the class voting, beaten out by Emily (the vote was 23 to 2) who had won the honor for the three previous years. A fourth time seemed excessive and thus the second place finisher was declared the winner![17] Then it was onto Roxbury Latin School in Boston and Phillips Andover Academy. The war had come to an end so Nathan was not drafted, but instead was admitted to Harvard College. During the summer of his freshman year at Harvard, he was a volunteer in the Marine Corps in Quantico, Virginia;

he was persuaded that a physician's life was preferable to that of a marine. So after college, it was on to Harvard Medical School (the school to which his father had been admitted but never attended on the advice of his grandfather, who did not hold physicians in high esteem).

Following graduation in 1955, he joined 11 other colleagues as an intern at the Peter Bent Brigham Hospital (there were 12 interns, 12 junior residents, six senior residents, and one chief that year). The hours were long (every other night and every other weekend), the salary a modest $25 a month, and the learning curve steep. From Samuel A. Levine, the great cardiologist at the Brigham Hospital, he learned "to worry about my patients all the time."[18] He also learned the practice of medicine: "The average length of stay was endless . . . we learned medicine at the bedside." And "If a patient with renal failure went into pulmonary edema, one performed a phlebotomy and brought the blood to the blood bank, spun it in a venerable centrifuge, squeezed off the plasma, and gave back the red cells."[19]

Academic Training and Leadership

The NIH was transformed during the Truman, Eisenhower, and Kennedy administrations because of the persistence of Senator Lister Hill of Alabama and the superb leadership of NIH Director James Shannon. The Bethesda campus grew rapidly. The budget of $200 million in 1960 grew to $20 billion by the beginning of the new millennium.[20] Nathan, thus, became a clinical associate, was paid a Navy lieutenant's salary, and was "ordered into hematology" by his section chief "because he had four stripes on his sleeve and I had two."[21] In gleaming laboratories with modern equipment and modern research beds, he learned to carry out clinical research as well as to apply modern science at the bedside.[22,23]

He returned to the Brigham Hospital in 1959 and was senior resident when John Riteris was admitted to Ward F in severe renal and secondary cardiac failure; Riteris would soon receive the world's first nonidentical renal transplant. When Riteris was transferred to Joseph Murray's surgical service, Nathan was sure he would never see him again, "but I did—on the cover of *Life* magazine."[24] (As mentioned earlier, Murray went on to win the Nobel Prize for performing the world's first successful organ transplant.) Then it was on to become an attending and carrying out research in his first laboratory, a 100-square-foot room opposite the clinical laboratories at the Peter Bent Brigham Hospital. At that time, the hospital was a "Dickensian" institution with multiple pavilions constructed to isolate patients with infection, the distance to be covered by a house officer placing "a premium on shoe leather."[25] It was at that time that Dr. Diamond began to send Nathan patients upon whom the latter performed red cell survival studies and spleen scans to see if they were suitable for splenectomy. It was also at this time that Nathan began seeing fascinating cases with Diamond's fellow, Frank Oski, and from those encounters sprang a long and close professional association and ultimately a prestigious textbook.

Park Gerald, another talented Diamond fellow, began to send Nathan patients with thalassemia. Charles Janeway then invited Nathan to join the hematology division at the Children's Hospital, with the opportunity to become division chief when Diamond left. This was a significant change of course, and Nathan sought out the advice of one of his three icons, William Castle (the other two being Levine and Janeway), the great hematologist at Boston City Hospital.[26] "Does the idea of going to Children's Hospital make you happy?" Castle asked. "Oh yes . . . but my friends all tell me it's crazy," Nathan replied. "Well, most of the people who come to see me are unhappy. If I were you, I'd go to Children's," Castle drawled. Nathan came to Children's.[27]

His research contributions to pediatric hematology were sustained over time and were far reaching in their national influence. These contributions spanned prenatal diagnostic testing, deferoxamine infusion for iron overload, T cell products as necessary cofactors for red blood cell production, suppression of erythropoiesis by hydroxyurea in sickle cell disease, development of the nitroblue tetrazolium (NBT) test in chronic granulomatous disease, and the first successful bone marrow transplant for Wiscott-Aldrich syndrome. His contributions to pediatric hematology were beautifully captured in his textbook, now in its seventh edition, *Hematology of Infancy and Childhood*, edited initially with Frank Oski, and later with Stuart Orkin[28] and others, and in his book *Genes, Blood and Courage*, which described the history of thalassemia as captured through the life of his longtime patient Dayem Saif (a pseudonym).[29]

His leadership of the training program in hematology/oncology at the Dana-Farber Cancer Institute and the Children's Hospital between 1968 and 1985 led to the training of 88 hematologists and oncologists. Remarkably, 90% remained in academic medicine and biotechnology.[30] Over 40% of the graduates have gone on to become chiefs of hematology/oncology or bone marrow transplantation divisions, and a remarkable number serve or have served as chairs of pediatric departments throughout the United States. Many have also served as presidents of the American Society for Clinical Investigation, the American Society of

Hematology, and the American Society of Pediatric Hematology/Oncology. Additionally, a remarkable number have received the prestigious American Society of Hematology Mentor award.

Pediatric Department Chairman and Hospital President

In January of 1985, he moved to the third floor of the Hunnewell Building as the eighth chair of the Department of Medicine. The managed care revolution was placing serious constraints on the finances of the hospital, and developing the strong scientific underpinning of the department required significant resources to recruit outstanding scientists and division heads and to build modern facilities.[31] He worked with the Howard Hughes Medical Institute, persuading them to strengthen the scientific base of the department by financially supporting the recruitment of Fred Alt, an immunologist and ultimate successor to Fred Rosen as head of the Center for Blood Research; Donald Wiley and Stephen Harrison, top-flight structural biologists from Harvard College; Richard Mulligan, a molecular retrovirologist also from Harvard; Joseph Majzoub, a neuroendocrinologist as chief of the Division of Endocrinology; and Merton Bernfield, a developmental biologist as chief of neonatology.

To develop outcomes and translational research and to improve emergency medicine, he recruited Gary Fleisher, a pediatrician from the Children's Hospital of Philadelphia to lead the emergency medicine division and appointed talented inside faculty members, including Judith Palfrey to lead general pediatrics, Jean Emans to lead adolescent medicine, and William Harmon to lead nephrology. Importantly, he was able to retain other superb scientists already in place, Steven Burakoff and then Stuart Orkin and Samuel Lux as chiefs of hematology/oncology, Louis Kunkel as chief of genetics, and Raif Geha as chief of immunology. Finally, he was able to attract sizable Hughes resources to support new Hughes investigators in the Departments of Medicine and Cardiology.

Nathan was also deeply committed to the training of general pediatricians. In addition to strengthening the inpatient services through the service chief system and the outpatient department through major appointments in Pediatric Group Associates (PGA) and the Children's Comprehensive Health Program (CCHP), he strengthened the housestaff training program with Barry Zuckerman, chief of pediatrics at Boston Medical Center, by conceptualizing the Boston Combined Residency Program.[32] By joining a private, subspecialty-oriented research hospital with a public primary care–oriented inner city hospital to enhance the breadth of house officer training, he created a model of residency training that flourishes today, 19 years after its inception.

It was Nathan's strength of purpose and commitment to academic excellence that made him so widely admired. His words and wisdom to this day ring in the ears and resonate in the memory: "Come to grand rounds"; "Balance your budgets"; "Do the difficult today, the impossible tomorrow"; "It's not a fellow's hospital, it's not even *my* hospital, it's the patient's hospital."[33] And his sense of responsibility and his stewardship shone like a clarion; "Worry constantly about your patients"; "It won't happen on my watch"; "I am the steward of my patients"; "When we give back the life of a child, we gain decades of productive life."[34] When Nathan moved back to Dana-Farber in 1995, his colleagues knew that they had been witness to the likes of Blackfan and the "heroic era"[35] and Janeway, "pediatrician to the world's children."[36]

In the 15 years following his chairmanship of the Department of Medicine, Nathan focused on enlarging the national stature of the Dana-Farber Cancer Institute as its president and enhancing clinical research policy from the prominent national appointments and board memberships that he held. His great influence on research policy bore fruit when he chaired an NIH task force on clinical research, which stimulated a significant number of new research applications to the NIH and led to the passage of the Clinical Research Enhancement Act. Additionally, as noted by Dean Joseph Martin, he played a critical role in facilitating a single federal grant to the Dana-Farber Cancer Institute, Harvard Medical School, and the Massachusetts General Hospital, which led to the formation of the Dana-Farber/Harvard Cancer Center. Without his leadership, generosity, and willingness to step outside the roles he played at the Children's Hospital and Dana-Farber Cancer Institute, this would have never happened.[37]

He received numerous awards and honors, including the National Medal of Science and the Stratton Medal from the American Society of Hematology. He is a past president of the American Society of Hematology and a member of the Institute of Medicine. On his retirement, the trustees of the Dana-Farber Cancer Institute created the David G. Nathan professorship at Harvard Medical School. Stuart Orkin, an early trainee of Nathan's in the '70's and chief of pediatric oncology at Dana-Farber, was the first incumbent of the chair. In 2003, Nathan received the Howland Award from the American Pediatric Society, joining an illustrious group of prior pediatrician recipients from the Harvard faculty, including James Gamble, Bronson Crothers, Louis K. Diamond, Clement Smith, Charles Janeway, Julius Richmond, and Mary Ellen Avery and those who traveled through the Children's Hospital, Allan Butler, Lewis Barness, Abraham Rudolph, Sydney Gellis, Robert Haggerty, Samuel Katz, Richard Johnston, and Philip Pizzo. As reflected upon by David Nathan on a later occasion, his most meaningful recognition was an honorary doctor of science degree from Harvard University received in 2010. The citation read:[38]

> *Wise in the ways of blood*
> *Compassionate in the care of children*
> *Savvy in the guidance of individuals and institutions*
> *Devoted to preserving the finest traditions of his calling*

Division Chiefs[39]

Twelve divisions existed throughout the entire duration of Nathan's leadership. They were adolescent and young adult medicine, general pediatrics, emergency medicine, endocrinology, gastroenterology and nutrition, genetics, hematology and oncology, immunology, infectious disease, nephrology, newborn medicine, and pulmonary medicine. Three divisions were added during his tenure: inpatient medical services in 1988, the Division of Molecular Medicine in 1990, and the General Clinical Research Center in 1991. Judith Palfrey (chief of general pediatrics), Gary Fleisher (chief of emergency medicine), John Crigler (chief of endocrinology), Allan Walker (chief of gastroenterology and nutrition), Samuel Lux and Steve Burakoff (chiefs of hematology and oncology), Raif Geha (chief of immunology), Kenneth McIntosh (chief of infectious disease), and Mary Ellen Wohl (chief of pulmonary medicine) led their divisions throughout Nathan's tenure. Robert Masland directed the Division of Adolescent and Young Adult Medicine until 1993, when Jean Emans and Robert Durant assumed the leadership; Samuel Latt led the Division of Genetics until his untimely death in 1988, when Louis Kunkel became chief of the division; Warren Grupe led the Division of Nephrology until 1987, when William Harmon assumed that role; and Michael Epstein led the Division of Newborn Medicine until 1989, when Merton Bernfield was recruited from Stanford University School of Medicine, to the leadership position.

Nathan led the Division of Laboratory (Molecular) Medicine from 1990 until 1994, when Steve Harrison was appointed to that role. Alan Ezekowitz served as head of the General Clinical Research Center from 1990 until leaving in 1995 to become chair of the Children's Service at the Massachusetts General Hospital. The author led the inpatient medical services from 1988 to 1995.

Nathan recruited from the outside Gary Fleisher, Merton Bernfield, Robert Durant, and Stephen Harrison to their respective positions. Samuel Lux, Raif Geha, Jean Emans, William Harmon, Alan Ezekowitz, and Fred Lovejoy had all grown up in the system, having served as house officers. Nathan also introduced the position of clinical (associate) chief of the divisions, with Samir Najjar holding that role in the Division of Endocrinology, Alan Leichtner in the Division of Gastroenterology, Bruce Korf in the Division of Genetics, and Ann Stark in the Division of Newborn Medicine. Among the 15 divisions, the leadership of each was characterized by remarkable stability throughout the 10 years of Nathan's leadership.

Clinical Programs[40]

A number of programs were formally established during the Nathan era. Many fell under the Division of General Pediatrics and did much to augment clinical care as well as teaching in the department. The first group practice of the department, CCHP, had as its primary mission serving the community surrounding the hospital. William Bithoney moved from the Martha Eliot Health Clinic in the Avery era to run CCHP with great skill for the majority of the Nathan era. His capable associate Joanne Cox took on its leadership in 1994. Lewis First, a leader in ambulatory care in Boston, took on the leadership of the continuity clinic, which had a primary focus on resident education carried out in the context of care of its general pediatric population (PGA) in 1987. The clinic delivered outstanding community care while also serving as the primary site for weekly continuity training of the housestaff. Henry Bernstein, who later led the Division of Ambulatory Pediatrics at Dartmouth Medical School, took on leadership of PGA in 1994 when Lewis First departed to become chair of pediatrics at the University of Vermont College of Medicine. A number of specialty ambulatory leaders supplemented these two important efforts. They included the child development unit, led until 1988 by T. Berry Brazelton and thereafter by Edward Tronik; the developmental evaluation clinic, led by Allen Crocker; the family development study unit, led by Eli Newberger; services to handicapped children, led by William Berenberg; and the medical diagnostic programs, led by Leonard Rappaport. These general pediatric programs were complemented by a number of other specialty programs, including pharmacology/toxicology, led by Alan Woolf; dermatology, led initially by Arthur Rhodes and then in 1988 by Steven Gellis; allergy, led initially by Donald Leung and then by Lynda Schneider; and finally rheumatology, led initially by Fred Rosen and in 1989 by Robert Sundel.

All of these programs were predominantly centered on patient care and thus assumed an important role in the education of the housestaff. As a result, many of these leaders were widely admired by the housestaff.

Academic Promotions[41]

The pediatric executive committee of Harvard Medical School met monthly during the Nathan era to consider and recommend promotions in pediatrics from the Children's Hospital and the Massachusetts General Hospital. The members of the executive committee from the Children's Hospital were David Nathan, Fred Rosen, Harvey Colten, and Fred Lovejoy, and from the Massachusetts General Hospital, Donald Medearis, Jack Crawford, and Allan Walker. Dr. Crawford served for 22 years as the committee's secretary with great wisdom and fairness. In 1995, on the retirement of Dr. Crawford, the author was appointed as the new executive secretary, a position he continues to hold.

The committee considered all promotions and reappointments at the instructor level and above. As many as three to six promotions were reviewed at each meeting prior to their final consideration at the medical school. Reappointments at three- to five-year intervals dependent on rank were also considered. Deliberations were thoughtful and assiduously fair, always with an eye to achieving success for a given individual in the promotion process. Promotions at the full professor level were less frequent. From the Children's Hospital between 1985 and 1995, those promoted to professor were Drs. Lux, Geha, Lovejoy, T. Berry Brazelton, Marian Neutra, Mary Ellen Wohl, Donald Goldmann, James Lock, Marie McCormick, Howard Weinstein, Judith Palfrey, Gary Fleisher, William Harmon, and Orah Platt.

The committee meetings also served as an important gathering for the senior leadership of the departments of pediatrics at Harvard Medical School. Much was accomplished besides promotions. This was to the great credit of the collegial approach that the department chairs, Drs. Nathan and Medearis, brought to the deliberations of the committee. They periodically also invited Dean Daniel Tosteson, Dean for Academic Affairs James Adelstein, and Dean for Medical Education Daniel Federman to attend when medical school input was deemed important. Consideration of teaching of Harvard medical students was a common topic, especially with the introduction of the New Pathway at the medical school and the conversion of the pediatric clerkship to a joint maternal child health clerkship with obstetrics and gynecology. The two departments came together in a wonderfully collaborative manner around this issue much to the benefit of the students. They also considered topics such as current challenges in academic medicine, funding of clinical research, new promotion tracks for teachers and clinicians, and faculty development around teaching skills and educational pedagogy. Additionally, they joined forces at the time of national academic pediatric society meetings for faculty and alumni gatherings.

Finally, early in David Nathan's tenure, he formed a committee led by John Cloherty, a highly respected neonatologist and community pediatrician, to consider all part-time appointments to the Children's Hospital medical staff and to the Harvard Medical School faculty. This appointment structure still exists today, led next by Gregory Young, and currently by Julie Dollinger, both practicing pediatricians and prior housestaff in the department. Each committee chair, as practicing pediatricians with close ties to the hospital, has done much to enhance communication between the department and its referring physician community.

The National Perspective

Prior to the mid-1980s, medicine had lived in a period of abundance, with strong support from the NIH for research, fee-for-service reimbursement, and generous payments from Medicare and Medicaid for care. Hospitals and their faculty had grown rapidly as unrestrained reimbursement for care grew. Pass-through reimbursement also allowed for cross subsidization of medical education and research. But by the mid-'80s, it was clear that fee-for-service reimbursement was going to end, and the next era would be one of fiscal constraint.[42]

Third party payers rose up and demanded lower prices. The insurers rather than the providers now became the drivers of the system. Hospitals would have to adjust. In 1983, prospective payment based on diagnosis related groups (DRGs) became the law of the land. A price was set for the treatment of a given disease. If the hospital could carry out that treatment for less than cost, it kept the profit; if the treatment cost was more expensive, the hospital had to assume the loss. Efficiency of care suddenly mattered as did rapid throughput. Hospitals now began to market their services actively, and strong referral networks became critical. Direct and indirect compensation for graduate medical education assisted hospitals in carrying out their training mission.

Managed care simultaneously grew in response to these changes.[43] It emphasized ambulatory care, less hospitalization, greater use of primary care providers with less dependence on specialists (who were perceived to drive up costs), and preference for patients who had less serious disease. The overall impact of these changes was increasing pressure on the bottom line of hospitals. Nationally, the number of admissions fell and with them, the profit margins.[44] Throughout the first half of the 1990s, the health maintenance organizations (HMOs) grew rapidly in number and in influence. The number of HMO "subscribers" and affiliated primary care providers (physicians) grew, as did network affiliations with hospitals. All of these changes had profound effects on hospitals, medical schools, and medical education.[44]

Effects on the Health Care System

The new order in medicine in the 1980s began to have the following generalized effects:

a. A decrease in the perceived importance of medical education and clinical training in the hospital environment
b. A decrease in the importance of academic values and scholarship
c. An increase in the importance of financial rewards and compensation
d. An augmented importance of the hospital and health care delivery systems over and above medical schools and the university

The forces that brought about these changes were both external and internal to the profession. The public, the business community, the insurers, and Congress were all aligned by the mid-1990s in their determination to control spiraling health care costs. They were, however, less willing to consider the importance of their public responsibility for medical education. Simultaneously, the hospitals and doctors had become too dependent on the unrestrained dollar generated from clinical care and were more vulnerable as a result. They had, in fact, become too comfortable in living in a resource-rich environment with few restrictions.

Emerging Prominence of Clinical Care

The important impact of cost containment and managed care was an acceleration in the growth of the clinical enterprise. The full-time clinical faculty grew significantly in number; hospitals became more responsive to patients' needs, with an emphasis on customer satisfaction; quality improvement and patient safety became increasingly important. While faculty practice revenues grew, profit margins flattened, with fewer dollars available to support the academic mission.

In addition, the atmosphere in the hospitals became less academic.[45] With the push to see more patients, less time was available to devote to research and teaching. New physicians were recruited to the staff of network sites in community hospitals and clinics, their job description being predominately patient care. To recognize clinicians for their contributions, new medical school promotion criteria were adopted, and by 1993, three-fourths of U.S. medical schools had a ladder where teaching and clinical contributions were valued as the primary criteria for academic promotion.[46] Clinical scholar and teacher-clinician tracks that placed less emphasis on investigation and more on clinical care and teaching significantly altered the makeup of medical school faculties.

Sound business practice was increasingly emphasized by business consultants and hospital boards of trustees. Clinicians were expected to generate their own salary, and clinical productivity was measured by dollars generated. Teaching and research were viewed as expenses; care as a revenue. Many recognized these values to be inconsistent with the values of the academy and academic medicine as espoused by the medical school and the university. The medical care system began to look more and more like the proprietary system of the pre-Flexner era, with faculty generating their salary from practice and with teaching being squeezed into the remaining available time.

Marginalization of Education

Medical education is notably different from that of law and business in that the practice of medicine is taught as a part of the medical school curriculum. The hospital thus became essential to the medical school because of its access to patients and its capacity to deliver clinical care. The hospital faculty, in turn, benefited through academic appointment and promotion and access to research and teaching opportunities available through the medical school. But, as the efficiency of clinical care gained importance, the scientific underpinnings of disease tended to be overlooked and the learning environment was eroded. An easy solution was not immediately evident: increasingly medical schools and hospitals struggled to balance the value of the practitioner (who taught the practical aspects of medicine and supplied patients with diseases important for learning) with the traditional values of the academy and academic pursuits.[47] Clearly, the financial well-being of the health center had become more important, while the standards of the academy as well as education and research had become less important.

Finally, the pressures to maximize throughput and efficiency also affected day-to-day care. To provide good care takes time, thought, and strong doctor–patient communication. These values were now being compromised. The brevity of patient visits was taking a toll on physicians, as evidenced by increases in job dissatisfaction, job burnout, and increased anxiety. Concerns also began to surface around the quality of care delivered. The emphasis on throughput was perceived by many as contrary to the goals of quality patient care.

The Children's Hospital Perspective

The initiatives instituted by the hospital and the Department of Medicine during the Nathan era should be considered in light of these changes in medicine and as a response to cost containment and managed care. Hospital initiatives between 1985 and 1995 to increase market share and enhance patient referrals included the opening of the Lexington satellite center, the placement of residents and the staffing of the emergency department at MetroWest Medical Center (Framingham Union Hospital) in Framingham, and the concerted effort to secure the Harvard Community Health Plan contract. Efforts to enhance hospital revenue through philanthropy included an enlarged development office, participation in the previously mentioned nationwide children's hospitals philanthropic effort called the Circle of Care, fundraising for professorships at Harvard Medical School, and support for Howard Hughes investigators. At the departmental level, efforts to increase efficiency and improve education through greater oversight by attending physicians were evident with the service chief system, the short-stay unit, and the expanded emphasis on the quality and efficacy of clinical practice in the inpatient and outpatient settings. Finally, efforts to enhance the education and research missions were reflected in the concerted effort to enlarge the Enders Building through Howard Hughes Medical Institute support, an increased focus on the scientific underpinnings of pediatrics through Saturday morning committee of professor teaching rounds, more scientifically based grand rounds, and support for many new initiatives in medical student, resident, and fellow education.

Trustees and Administration

As we saw in the Rotch and Morse eras, the manager (superintendent) of the Children's Hospital took an active supervisory role over all activities of the house officers. Selection of young men as house officers was also subject to the approval of the board of managers. The hospital rules and regulations of 1894 and 1905 laid out in great detail expectations of the housestaff, which applied to their medical work as well as their daily living. The attendings "visited" only periodically on the wards and thus had limited authority over the housestaff, with the more constant oversight of both the house officers and nurses resting with the superintendent and board of managers.

This would begin to change during Oscar Schloss' brief tenure as chairman and became fully operational during the Blackfan era, with supervision of all medical work and the medical life of the housestaff resting squarely with the chairman of the Department of Medicine. The selection of the housestaff now resided with the faculty and the department. Rules and expectations of house officers as determined by the chief were codified in writing and enforced by the faculty. As we have seen, Harvard Medical School had gradually abdicated its responsibility for housestaff training to the hospital, thereby limiting its educational oversight to medical student and post-doctoral training. The manager of the hospital only heard about housestaff matters when reported by the chair at medical staff executive committee meetings. The board of trustees knew little of the medical education mission of the hospital or the activities of the housestaff. This modus operandi existed throughout the Blackfan, Smith, Janeway, and Avery eras. This was especially significant in light of medical house officer salaries being paid from the hospital's operating budget.

A gradual change began to occur during the Nathan era, stimulated by spiraling medical costs. Cost containment of all expenditures, including housestaff salaries, became a priority. As hospital scrutiny increased, the board of trustees and the hospital's senior leadership became more involved during the Pizzo/Fleisher era, initially with the institution of the role of director of medical education and later with a graduate medical education committee and DIO (designated institutional officer) who had oversight over all residents and fellows at the Children's Hospital. The latter's activities included regulation, certification, education, and financial matters as they related to medical education at the institution. Trustees, administration, and department chairs all worked together to garner graduate medical education federal funding for freestanding children's hospitals as well as philanthropic support for the hospital's medical education mission. Finally, public and private national organizations became more and more involved, especially in the certification process of training programs and their residents and in limiting the growth of residency size.

Thus, this gradual increase in involvement of organizations and individuals external to the departments enhanced the importance of medical education as one of the core missions of the hospital, as laid out by the founding fathers in the hospital's original bylaws of 1869.

TABLE 4 Medical Housestaff Statistics

	1880s	1890s	1900s	1910s	1920s	1930s	1940–1945	1945–1959	1960s	1970s	1980s	1990–1995
Total	2	3	6	8	13	17	12–17	25–30	30–40	50–60	65–70	70–79
Male/Female	2/0	3/0	6/0	8/0	13/0	15/1–2	17/0	5%*	10%*	25%*	36%*	50%*
Chief Residents	0	0	0	0	0	0	0	1–4	2–4	2	1–2	2

Residency Training

The residency grew gradually in size throughout the Nathan era (Figures 4–6). In the early years, the number of residents varied from 65 to 68 with 25 PL-1s, 23 PL-2s, 19 PL-3s, and one PL-4.[48] By 1994, the total number of residents had risen to 79, with 29 PL-1s, 26 PL-2s, 22 PL-3s, and two PL-4s (Table 4).

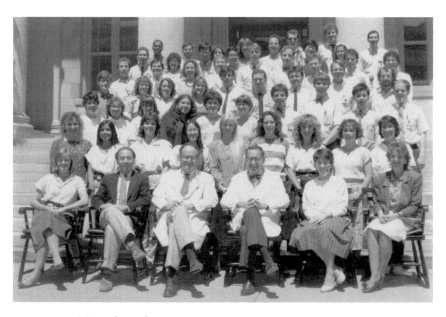

FIGURE 4 The early Nathan era, 1987–1988

The Nathan housestaff. In the front row from left to right: Maribeth Hourihan (chief resident in 1988–1989), Alan Wayne (chief resident in 1987–1988), David Nathan, Fred Lovejoy, Susan Parsons (chief resident in 1989–1990), and Susan Brooks (housestaff coordinator).

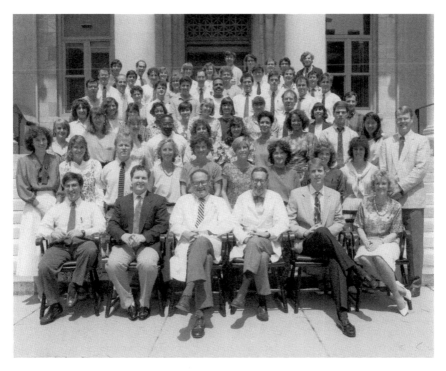

FIGURE 5   The Mid-Nathan era, 1990–1991

The Nathan housestaff. In the front row from left to right: Jonathan Finkelstein and Richard
Bachur (chief residents in 1991–1992), David Nathan, Fred Lovejoy, Gregory Young (chief
resident in 1990–1991), and Susan Brooks (housestaff coordinator).

Most residents remained in the program for three years, although there were
several exceptions. The Special Alternative Pathway, started in the Avery era,
continued to be actively used by one or two residents each year, their pediatric
residency training being shortened by a year so as to enter fellowship.[49] In addition, Nathan started a new pathway called "half tracking," in which a resident
did one-half of the senior year participating in the usual senior resident rotations
and one-half of the year involved in clinical work in a subspecialty. This allowed
them to start their clinical fellowship time six months earlier by shortening the
clinical time of residency, an innovative and flexible approach to residency training that was very popular. Since three months of the usual senior year was taken
in electives, the loss of important senior leadership opportunities was minimal.
For individuals with clear intentions to pursue academic careers, this pathway
allowed them to return to their research training six months earlier. This plan,
however, did not sit well with the American Board of Pediatrics, and in the late

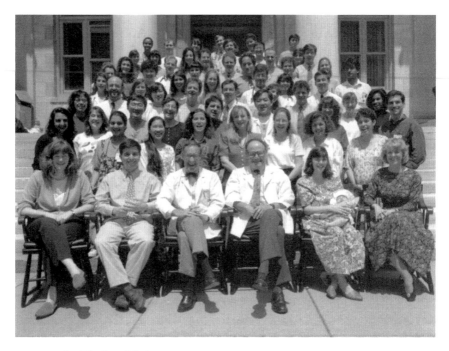

FIGURE 6   The Late Nathan era, 1994–1995

The Nathan housestaff in the front row (from left to right) Monika Woods and David Greenes (chief residents in 1994–1995), Fred Lovejoy, David Nathan, Jessica Kahn and baby (chief resident in 1995–1996), and Susan Brooks (housestaff coordinator).

1990s, the board limited time in any single subspecialty during residency to three months, thereby eliminating this track as an option at the Children's Hospital.

During the early 1990s as part of a growing interest in primary care, the Children's Hospital and the Department of Medicine initiated a joint Medicine–Pediatrics Training Program with the Brigham and Women's Hospital. The program director on the medicine side was a revered internal medicine program director, Marshall Wolf, and on the pediatric side, Robert Masland, who because of his internal medicine training, was an ideal selection as program director. A single slot was reserved for two individuals who alternated sites in six-month block intervals between the two hospitals, thereby completing four years of total training, two years in pediatrics and two years in medicine and board eligibility in both disciplines. This focus on pediatric and adult health was highly popular and after a year, a concerted effort was begun to create a Harvard-wide Medicine–Pediatrics Training Program. This effort would reach fruition in the Pizzo era.

To further strengthen training in outpatient medicine, an ambulatory senior resident year was also offered as an option in the Nathan era. Four residents each year selected this altered senior year rather than participating in the traditional senior year. Some participated as a full ambulatory senior; others split the year, six months spent as an ambulatory senior and six months as a traditional senior. This option was directed by Judith Palfrey and Leonard Rappaport. Daytime responsibilities included a primary care clinic in CCHP, time in the public schools of Boston as a consultant on developmental and behavioral pediatric issues, and finally rotations in the ambulatory specialty clinics (Developmental Consult Program, Preschool Function Program, School Function Program, Adolescent Program, and Pain and Incontinence Program). A robust half-day educational symposium also occurred each week throughout the year. Highly talented subsequent faculty members in the department such as William Barbaresi and Lynn Haynie took advantage of this ambulatory senior resident year.

In addition, each year, several residents pursued one or two years of the traditional pediatric residency and then departed to pursue neurology, genetics, psychiatry, or dermatology residencies. Program flexibility was encouraged, a notable example being made for the highly talented medical writer Perri Klass, who completed her last two years of residency over three years, thereby allowing more time for writing. In addition, a "shared" residency slot was created to be offered to two residents, allowing for a reduced schedule because of family responsibilities. While elongating the total training period, the ability to share childcare responsibilities with one's spouse, especially for the increasing number of women in pediatrics, proved highly successful. Finally, as in any large residency, an occasional resident experienced physical or psychological challenges or wished to pursue a different career. These instances fortunately occurred very infrequently.

Internship Recruitment

Robert Masland led the intern recruitment effort throughout the Nathan era as chair of the internship selection committee (Figure 7). Masland had a magical way with college students, medical students, and house officers. He connected with them on a very personal level. He had a natural ability to pick capable and good people. He enjoyed recruiting young people, and they, in turn, liked and trusted him and flocked to the training program. The internship selection committee during Masland's tenure included clinically oriented faculty and clinical investigators, and among its members were both junior and mid-level faculty. Interview mornings, five each year, were on Saturdays in the late fall and included: introductory talks by the department chair, program director, and chief residents; two to three interviews by members of the faculty; guided tours of the hospital by the housestaff; and lunch for faculty, housestaff, and candidates in the hospital cafeteria. Over 100 faculty participated in the interview process each year; faculty and applicants were carefully matched based on mutual areas of interest. Match day in March was awaited with great anticipation and was seen as an indicator of the popularity and attractiveness of the program. Nathan and Masland after a new group of interns had been selected would hold a celebratory dinner for the selection committee to reflect on and analyze the effort.

Between 1984 and 1995, 600 to 1,000 completed applications were received each year. Not surprisingly, American medical graduates predominated, but the program was also highly attractive to foreign medical graduates. Three hundred to 350 of the applicants were interviewed on Saturday mornings, resulting in 23 to 26 interns per year being matched in the late 1980s and 26 to 29 matched in the early 1990s.[50] Reliable benchmarks of a program's attractiveness are its ability to attract students from its own medical school and the position on the rank list reached to fill the requisite number of available slots. During the Nathan

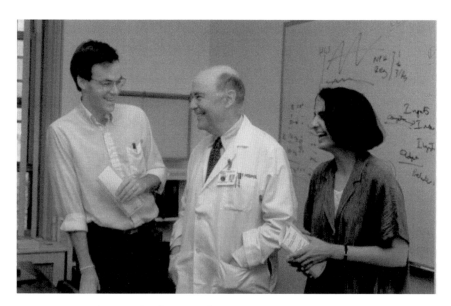

FIGURE 7   Robert Masland, circa early 1990s

Robert Masland, chair of the internship selection committee throughout the Nathan era and program director at the Children's Hospital for the Harvard-wide Medicine–Pediatrics Program, shown with two medicine–pediatrics residents.

years, an average of nine positions, or one-third of the intern class, were filled by Harvard Medical School students.[51] The average rank number over the same period of time to fill 26 slots was 51, it thus taking only two individuals to fill a given slot.[52] Both indices of success were a fine reflection on the popularity of the training program.

The number of women equaled the number of men in an admitted class, and an increasing number held dual degrees (MD/PhD and MD/MPH). Harvard led the list of medical schools filling an internship class, followed in descending order by Stanford, the University of Pennsylvania, Yale, Columbia, Johns Hopkins, Chicago (Pritzker), Case Western Reserve, University of California Los Angeles, and Washington University.[53] East Coast medical schools predominated and each class tended to come from a relatively small number of research-intensive schools. This would change in the Pizzo/Fleisher era when accepted applicants would come from primary care as well as research-oriented medical schools, from lesser known schools, and from schools throughout the U.S. In addition, the number of PhD candidates would increase and the number of accepted women would exceed men.

Finally, lineage continued to be evident in housestaff selection, with William Adams and Jordan Kriedberg, sons of Thomas Adams (a community pediatrician in eastern Massachusetts) and Marshall Kriedberg, (a revered academic pediatrician at Tufts University School of Medicine), both house officers in the Janeway years, being chosen. John Barlow, son of faculty member Charles Barlow, chief of neurology, and Suzanne Shusterman, daughter of faculty member Stephen Shusterman, chief of dentistry, were also chosen to serve as house officers.

Overall, Masland's talents as a recruiter and as an effective chair of the selection committee set a high bar for future recruitment efforts as he successfully attracted many future academic and clinical leaders to the training program.

Philosophy of the Training Program

The residency between the years 1985 and 1995 benefited from constant scrutiny and analysis to be certain that it was achieving its mission and goals. The residency training committee and several ad hoc long-range planning committees were central to this effort.[54] The mission statement in the Nathan years did not change significantly from the Avery years, "to promote the acquisition of knowledge, skills, and attitudes to prepare trainees to care for children in all settings and to assume leadership roles in academic medicine as well as in the practice of pediatrics." The core mission for each of the residency years did not change significantly either. The purpose of the first year was to inculcate core knowledge and skills of general pediatrics, the second year to continue generalist training while also training residents in subspecialty pediatrics, and the third year to foster supervisory skills coupled with sufficient flexibility and time to address individual training goals.

Multiple analyses comparing the Children's Hospital program to other comparable pediatric programs in the U.S. indicated that its size of 70 to 80 residents was equal to the other larger programs.[55] The first and second year were comparable to other large programs, while the third year was comparable in size to programs considered medium sized. Finally, the workload carried out by the residents (based on the number of admissions relative to number of beds) placed the Children's Hospital in the upper ranks. The supervisory role in the third year was deemed to be critical to excellent training and was thus carefully protected in all curriculum planning. The general consensus from these analyses was that the program size was optimal, and if an increase was necessary, it should only be in the first and second year, as the flexibility inherent in the structure of the program was greatly appreciated by residents and faculty. The Special Alternative Pathway, "half-tracking," "shared" residency slots, the ambulatory senior year, and the creation of a medicine–pediatrics track were all well received by residents and faculty. Finally, the resident's career directions in the Nathan years simulated the Avery years and reinforced the view that the residency program's mission of training academic leaders continued to be both emphasized and fulfilled.[56]

As part of a constant analysis of the program, its perceived strengths and weaknesses were clearly identified.[57] The strengths would in fact remain constant over the Avery, Nathan, Pizzo, and Fleisher years. Major strengths included the breadth of the program and its wide exposure to pediatric medicine, the remarkable strength and diversity of the subspecialty faculty, and the high quality and varied interests of the housestaff. The volume and mix of patients at a primary, secondary, and tertiary level resulted in remarkable resident exposure. Additional strengths included the centrality of the program to the department and its divisions and the flexibility of the program, allowing it to meet individual resident's educational needs.

Weaknesses were a reflection of the nature of medical education in the 1980s and 1990s. An insufficient focus on development of critical analysis, problem solving, and independent decision-making skills posed an important pedagogical challenge, exacerbated by a heavy service load and the necessity of increased involvement of the faculty in clinical care responsibilities. A second concern was excessive exposure to technology-intensive subspecialty pediatrics, often with less relevance to general pediatric training, examples being excessive exposure to bone marrow transplantation, cardiac catheterization, and neonatal intensive care. A third concern, felt in all training programs, was the rapid turnover of patients and the shortened length of stay, resulting in house officers failing to observe the natural history of disease, the accuracy of their diagnoses, and the beneficial effects of their therapy. Lastly, other perceived challenges included an insufficient amount of teaching at the bedside and the need for earlier and more electives in the program. The large size of the program offered flexibility, more personnel in times of illness, and more elective time, but large size also risked compromising at times the residency's esprit de corps.

The constant analysis of the program as well as the various committees' recommendations to improve it led to a number of adjustments in rotations and content offerings. In addition, multiple efforts to address more globally the distribution of time in the ambulatory, subspecialty, intensive care, and elective settings were undertaken. Eight adjustments were recommended in 1990 and carried out in subsequent years. They were:[58]

1. A decrease in exposure to intensive care neonatology and bone marrow transplantation
2. An increase in exposure to emergency medicine, neurology, and the general medical services
3. An increased focus on genetics, outcomes assessment, information management, ethics, medical economics, orthopedics, otolaryngology, and general surgery
4. An increase in ambulatory time in the subspecialties (cardiology, neurology, oncology, and the ambulatory "selective" subspecialties)
5. An increase in supervisory time in the second year
6. An increased focus on efficiency of learning, improvements in teaching and in the learning process, attention to the relevance of clinical exposure, and an emphasis on core pediatric exposure
7. A decrease in intensive care time to make room for more training in behavioral and developmental pediatrics, adolescent medicine, and newborn infant care
8. More attention to the critical stages of intellectual development of residents and the timing of introduction of educational information, with core general knowledge introduced in the first year, subspecialty knowledge in the second year, and longitudinal knowledge (often emphasizing social, ethical, and economic issues) in the third year.

Rotations

The number of rotations during the 10 years of Nathan's leadership changed remarkably little. Twelve to 14 rotations existed in each of the three years. The PL-1 year involved general pediatric exposures that included infant/toddler, school age, and adolescent rotations; emergency room, newborn, and developmental and behavioral pediatrics rotations; intensive care training with neonatal and medical intensive care rotations; and a cardiology subspecialty exposure. This first year included leadership by senior residents and the opportunity for interns to work intensively with Harvard Medical School students in the inpatient setting.

In the second year, subspecialty training was emphasized, with rotations in hematology/oncology and neurology as well as ambulatory selectives, a new creation. Residents could choose from endocrinology, nephrology, and gastroenterology; allergy, immunology, rheumatology, and dermatology; genetics and birth defects; cardiology; or primary care and practice, all in the outpatient setting. The opportunity for choice enhanced the popularity of the selectives. Conceptualized and fostered through the residency training committee and led by Leonard Rappaport, later to be named chief of the newly created Division of Developmental and Behavioral Medicine in the Fleisher era, the selectives markedly increased resident exposure to outpatient medicine. The program also encouraged the incorporation of more outpatient exposure in existing rotations that were traditionally inpatient based, such as cardiology, neurology, and hematology/oncology.

In addition, the junior year had considerable emergency room involvement, especially during the evening and night hours when the junior resident supervised interns and worked with them in making important clinical decisions. And during the junior year, residents received considerable neonatal and medical intensive care exposure. In addition to critical care neonatology (NICU), a delivery room rotation was added, where residents attended high-risk deliveries, stabilizing the sick newborn and accompanying the baby to the intensive care unit at the Brigham and Women's Hospital. Finally, electives were increasingly incorporated into the curriculum, with one or two such rotations in the junior year and as many as three or four in the senior year. The junior year had a degree of separation from the general medical residency, as a result of residents working closely with fellows and the subspecialty services. This resulted in a strong educational curriculum for the junior residents but also a degree of isolation from the rest of the residency. This would prove to be an ongoing challenge.

The senior supervisory year was widely considered by the residents to be the plum of the residency. The seniors led the team of interns and students and worked closely with the faculty to create a robust educational curriculum (Figures 8–10). General pediatric rotations, including infant/toddler, school age, adolescent, emergency medicine, and ambulatory selective rotations, were particularly popular and valued. Electives were most plentiful in the senior year, some without night call, allowing for international third world travel or exposure to subspecialties at other academic medical centers in the U.S. The teaching resident rotation involved working closely with the highly talented and popular faculty who served as directors of medical student education. This rotation afforded the opportunity to learn educational pedagogy and improve one's teaching skills. New rotations in the senior year included a night float rotation on the inpatient service. The residents on this rotation admitted patients after midnight, thereby allowing the interns to sleep. They also handled minor medical problems that required immediate attention. A second new rotation was a transport rotation, in which the senior resident accompanied the transport staff as they stabilized sick patients in community hospitals and transported them back to intensive care units at the Children's Hospital. Most transports were from Massachusetts, southern Maine, and southern New Hampshire. Some were from longer distances and even on occasion, from outside the country. Finally, a consult surgical

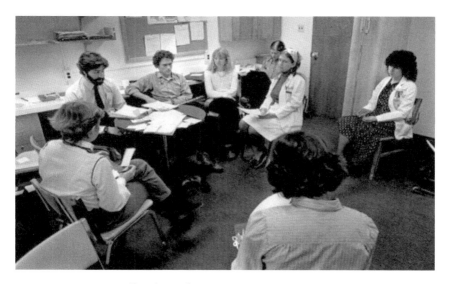

FIGURE 8   Housestaff in the Mid-1980s
Housestaff morning report with ward attending and residents.

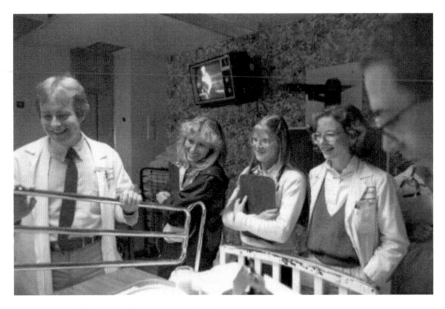

FIGURE 9   Housestaff in the Mid-1980s
Housestaff on walk rounds at the patient's bedside.

rotation was created. Residents on this rotation served as medical consult to patients on the general surgery, orthopedics, and neurosurgery services.

During the senior year, the senior residents reported to the chief residents and their ward attendings and did much to set the tone of the medical service and enhance the success of a given year. The year served as an important stepping stone for residents pursuing subspecialty fellowship positions at the Children's Hospital and beyond. While increasing faculty presence was beginning to encroach on senior residents' autonomy as supervisors in the mid-1990s, the seniors, with the unwavering support of David Nathan, still felt that the service was theirs to lead and the interns theirs to supervise. This would become more and more difficult to achieve during the next 10 to 15 years.

The rotation assignment of residents in aggregate is a reflection of both the service and the educational needs of the program. When the overall distribution of a resident's time over three years in the program in 1993 is considered, 50% of that time was spent on general pediatrics rotations, 30% in subspecialty rotations, 15% on electives, and 5% on vacation.[59] When the location and type of rotation is considered, 54% of a resident's time was spent on inpatient services, while 26% was spent on outpatient rotations, with the remainder on electives and vacation.

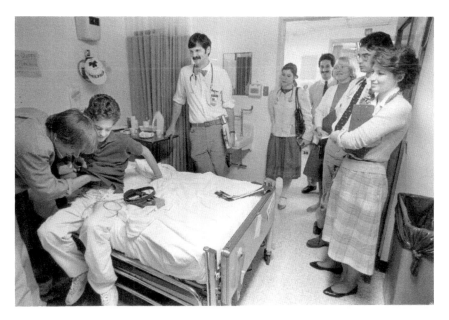

FIGURE 10   Housestaff in the Mid-1980s
Housestaff and medical students at the patient's bedside.

When specific rotations over all three years of training are considered, 20% of a resident's time was spent on the general inpatient wards (Teams A, B, and C), 15% on electives, 14% in the emergency room, 13% in neonatology, 6% on the medical intensive care unit, 5% on oncology and bone marrow transplantation, and 2% to 4% on each of the remaining rotations.[59] Vacation accounted for 5% of the time and continuity clinic for 3% of the total time.

Finally, when the distribution of time by residency year is considered, the greatest amount of time in the intern year was spent on the general pediatric ward teams followed by the emergency room and neonatology, while in the second year, the emergency room occupied the most time, followed by oncology, bone marrow transplantation, and elective time. In the third year, electives occupied the greatest amount of time, followed by the general wards and the emergency department.

Curricular Innovations[60]

The period from 1985 to 1995 saw constant curricular innovation in the residency program. A philosophy that championed change pervaded the program.

The residency training committee (RTC), established in 1980 in the Avery era, now became the vehicle for change. The committee earned a position of trust and respect among both the housestaff and the faculty. David Nathan came to depend on the wisdom of the committee's advice and recommendations. The housestaff were elected yearly by their class to the committee; the seven to 10 faculty members were appointed by the physician-in-chief. Being elected to the committee to represent one's class was considered an honor that was actively sought. The meetings were held monthly from noon to 1:30 p.m. in the board room of the Wolbach Building. The committee depended heavily on the work of its subcommittees, which included faculty and housestaff and were often jointly chaired by both.

In addition to faculty, the RTC consisted of four elected housestaff from each of the PL-1, -2 and -3 years, the president of the housestaff association, and the chief residents. Susan Brooks, the devoted residency coordinator, served as the committee's secretary. Sally Andrews, the Department of Medicine's seasoned administrator, also attended regularly. The program director chaired the meetings. Agenda were prepared for and followed at each meeting. The faculty was essential to the effectiveness of the committee and gave countless hours to its work. Tables 5 and 6 list the faculty who served during the Nathan era. These tables suggest an unusual degree of faculty involvement in resident education and the residency curriculum. Faculty also saw involvement as beneficial to their academic careers as educators. Their selection by the department chair was actively sought after and was noted on their curriculum vitae, this being helpful at the time of promotion. This faculty involvement reflected a national trend and was immensely helpful in establishing the high standards of the program. Election (rather than appointment) of residents to the RTC, charged with the governance of the education program, became the expected process for the residency training committee in the 2000s.

The residency training committee did a large amount of its work between meetings in its subcommittees. Each subcommittee would receive a charge, a committee membership, and a timeline for completing its work. Table 6 shows a partial list of the subcommittees and their area of focus during the Nathan years. The faculty member(s) or chief resident(s) who chaired the committees are also noted. The committees are grouped by area: administration, new curriculum, rotations, and academics and learning. The focus of the committees reflected the desires of the housestaff to address issues important in their education (e.g., rotation evaluations or career planning); the hospital or the medical school's wishes

TABLE 5   Faculty Members of Residency Training Committee (1985–1995)

Faculty	
Grace Caputo	Emergency Medicine
James Ferrera	Oncology
Lewis First	General Pediatrics
Donald Goldmann	Service Chief
William Harmon	Nephrology
Maureen Jonas	Gastroenterology
Fred Lovejoy	Program Director
Fred Mandell	Private Practice
Robert Masland	Adolescent Medicine
Shari Nethersole	General Pediatrics
Edward O'Rourke	Infectious Disease
Leonard Rappaport	General Pediatrics
Steve Ringer	Neonatology
Sarah Schutzman	Emergency Medicine
Philip Spevak	Cardiology
Ann Stark	Neonatology
Administration	
Sally Andrews	Department Administrator
Susan Brooks	Residency Coordinator

TABLE 6   Residency Training Subcommittees (1985–1995)

Administrative Committees	
Long-range Planning Committee	(Chairs—Lovejoy, Finkelstein)
Scheduling Committee	(Chair—First)
Advisor System Committee	(Chairs—Harmon, Kim)
Intern Selection Committee	(Chair—Masland)
Resident/Fellow Committee	(Chairs—Hansen, Chief Residents)
Primary Care Track Committee	(Chairs—Bithoney, Nethersole)
Housestaff Referring Physician Committee	(Chair—Chief Residents)
Harvard Community Health Plan Committee	(Chair—Pert)
Housestaff Retreat Committee	(Chair—Chief Residents)

(continues)

TABLE 6   Residency Training Subcommittees (1985–1995) *(Cont.)*

New Curriculum Committees	
Medicine–Pediatrics Track Committee	(Chairs—Masland, Grier)
MetroWest Hospital Committee	(Chairs—Chief Residents, Mehta)
Ethics Committee	(Chair—Truog)
Procedure Committee	(Chairs—Fackler, Redd)
Managed Care Committee	(Chair—Epstein)
Short-stay Unit Committee	(Chair—Baskin)
Service Chief System Committee	(Chair—Goldmann)
Resident as Teacher Committee	(Chair—Bachur, Hafler)
Rotation Committees	
Oncology Committee	(Chairs—Grier, Ferrara)
Neonatology Committee	(Chairs—Stark, Ringer)
Cardiology Committee	(Chair—Spevak)
Emergency Room Committee	(Chair—Caputo)
Behavioral Pediatrics Committee	(Chairs—Rappaport, Knight)
Continuity Clinic Committee	(Chair—First)
Electives Committee	(Chair—Newburger)
Adolescent Committee	(Chairs—Grace, Emans)
Neurology Committee	(Chair—Volpe)
Selectives Committee	(Chair—Rappaport)
Academics and Learning Committees	
Research Committee	(Chair—Ferrara)
Career Planning Committee	(Chair—Lovejoy)
Resident Evaluation Committee	(Chair—Stark)
Rotation Evaluation Committee	(Chair—Finkelstein)
International Experience Committee	(Chair—Walker)
Clinical Practice Guidelines Committee	(Chair—Goldmann)
Educational Pedagogy Committee	(Chair—Rosenblum)

to address specific issues (e.g., short-stay unit or Resident as Teacher course); or national trends or imperatives (e.g., Medicine–Pediatrics program).

The administrative committees were highly important for the functioning of the program. Some were "standing" committees operating each year, such as the scheduling, advisor system, intern selection, and housestaff retreat committees.

Others met periodically, addressing issues such as the care of Harvard Community Health Plan patients, housestaff referring physician relationships, and interactions of residents and fellows. Both long-range planning committee efforts, one in the late 1980s and the other in the mid-1990s lasted several years and were far reaching in their impact.[61,62]

The new curriculum committees were often in response to national trends (e.g., formation of a Medicine–Pediatrics track or Resident as Teacher curriculum) or local imperatives (e.g., the service chief system, a MetroWest Medical Center rotation, a managed care curriculum) or requirements generated by the Accreditation Council on Graduate Medical Education Residency Review Committee (e.g., procedure monitoring) or the alignment of the hospital's need for increased efficiency with housestaff's educational desires (e.g., the short-stay unit initiative). In the long run, all were innovative in what they accomplished. The Resident as Teacher course, the Medicine–Pediatrics track, and the short-stay unit all exist today. The Resident as Teacher curriculum was well ahead of its time. Its nationwide adoption and current popularity speak to its importance as an innovative educational endeavor.[63] The service chief system gradually morphed into the current hospitalist system used today at the Children's Hospital and throughout the U.S.[64]

The rotation committees were notable for their ability to consider issues raised by the housestaff and were remarkably successful in addressing these concerns. Most involved adjustments in educational emphasis, excessive workload, or scheduling issues. Some of these committees, such as the behavioral pediatrics and selectives committees, created new curricula. The selectives committee created selective options available for the PL-2 year (cardiology or allergy, immunology, rheumatology, and dermatology rotations) and for the PL-3 year (primary care/practice or gastroenterology, endocrinology, and renal rotations). This creative design underwent adjustments over the entire Nathan period but achieved a major educational impact. The electives committee existed well beyond the Nathan era, working on logistics of electives, monitoring their quality, assessing outcomes, and justifying their educational importance in a residency.

Finally, many of the academic and learning committees exist even today in a generally similar form, pointing to their importance in a residency program (e.g., the resident evaluation committee, the rotation evaluation committee and career planning committee). The nascent research committee efforts of the mid-90s grew into a robust initiative in the Boston Combined Residency Program (BCRP). Called the Academic Development Block, it had three months of protected time for focused research and included research faculty mentoring and funding support. The international experience committee efforts are active and effective even today with Schliesman Fund support of residents for third world travel and burgeoning international programs in the BCRP at the Children's Hospital and Boston Medical Center. A formal rotation exists in the BCRP in Tanzania, the Dominican Republic, and Haiti, and a global health track for the program is in place at the Boston Medical Center, supplemented by a close working relationship between the program and Partners in Health at the Brigham and Women's Hospital. The Resident as Teacher initiative is very much alive, with Harvard Medical School and now Department of Medicine funding and with remarkable energy, speaking to its importance in residency training. A final important educational innovation was a study in senior rounds of the use of problem-based learning in resident education, followed by the subsequent application of these new educational principles to many other house officer educational sessions.[65]

Chief Residents

Nathan appointed 17 outstanding chief residents during his tenure (Table 7). Initially, he selected one chief resident each year, feeling that this enhanced clear lines of authority between the physician-in-chief and the residency staff (Gerson and Rome had been selected in Dr. Avery's time), but after 1991, he selected two chief residents, the job having become too large for a single individual to manage. Dr. Nathan continued the precedent established by Dr. Avery at the end of her tenure of a job description that included coverage of both the inpatient and the outpatient services (rather than selection of a separate inpatient and outpatient chief resident, as was the custom in the Janeway era). One-third of those selected were female, a sizeable increase over the 14% of the Avery era.

Of the 17 selected as chief residents, 11 (65%) chose academic careers and six (35%) practice careers. Among those entering academics, the majority are currently affiliated with major academic medical centers; one is affiliated with the National Institutes of Health and another is on staff at a biomedical research institute. All those who entered practice are now affiliated with group practices. The subspecialty fellowships and subsequent careers pursued simulate the residency, with the largest number selecting fellowships in hematology/oncology, followed by an equal number entering cardiology, emergency medicine, and general pediatrics; and one each entering neonatology, infectious disease, adolescent medicine, and endocrinology.

TABLE 7   David Nathan's Chief Residents

1985–1986	William Gerson and Jonathan Rome
1986–1987	DeWayne Pursley
1987–1988	Alan Wayne
1988–1989	Mary Beth Hourihan
1989–1990	Susan Parsons
1990–1991	Gregory Young
1991–1992	Richard Bachur and Jonathan Finkelstein
1992–1993	Victor Nizet and Cedric Priebe
1993–1994	Andria Ruth and Joanne Wolfe
1994–1995	David Greenes and Monika Woods
1995–1996	Jessica Kahn and Mark Palmert

By 2015, 11 of 17 had achieved the rank of associate professor or professor of pediatrics. Palmert and Richard Bachur are division chiefs; Pursley is pediatrician-in-chief at the Beth Israel Hospital in Boston; Nizet is a recipient of the prestigious E. Mead Johnson Award from the Academy of Pediatrics; Finkelstein and Greenes have each served as associate program directors of the residency program at the Children's Hospital; Parsons leads the Health Institute and the Center on Child and Family Outcomes at Tufts Medical Center; and Cedric Priebe is the chief information officer at the Brigham and Women's Hospital.

Awards[66]

The Charles A. Janeway Award, which was established in 1978, with the recipient chosen by vote of the entire housestaff, was given throughout the Nathan era and continues to be awarded annually. Recipients of this prestigious award, bestowed on an outstanding teacher-clinician on the faculty at the Children's Hospital, are shown in Table 8. Lewis First and Norm Rosenblum had been prior Children's Hospital house officers, and Gary Fleisher was to become a future physician-in-chief, while Samir Najjar became dean at the American University of Beirut Medical School. David Greenes and Jeffery Burns, both Nathan residency trainees, were recipients of the prestigious award in 2001 and 20012, respectively. Importantly, this award was given to clinical faculty who had frequent contact with the housestaff.

TABLE 8　　Charles A. Janeway Award (1985–1996)

1985	Howard Weinstein	Oncology
1986	Michael Bresnan	Neurology
1987	Lewis First	Academic Pediatrics
1988	Donald Goldmann	Infectious Disease
1989	Philip Spevak	Cardiology
1990	Samir Najjar	Endocrinology
1991	Grace Caputo	Emergency Medicine
1992	Holcombe Grier	Oncology
1993	Norman Rosenblum	Nephrology
1994	Robert Sundel	Rheumatology
1995	Gary Fleisher	Emergency Medicine
1996	Richard G. Bachur	Emergency Medicine

The Margaret Walsh Visiting Professorship was established in 1984 to honor Margaret (Maggie) Walsh, a beloved house officer, who died in 1984, following a 15-month struggle with leukemia. She was a graduate of Smith College and Duke University School of Medicine and was an outstanding medical resident at the Children's Hospital from 1979 to 1982. She went on to the National Institutes of Health, pursuing laboratory work in virology followed by a Robert Wood Johnson fellowship in general academic pediatrics at Johns Hopkins Hospital. By 2010, 25 consecutive Margaret Walsh Visiting Professors had been chosen to give this prestigious annual lecture, starting with Jerome Klein, a revered infectious disease expert from Boston University School of Medicine (1985) as the first honoree. The selections made during the Nathan years are shown in Table 9. The stature of this visiting professorship is evident when one notes that it includes five pediatric department chairs (Drs. Oski, Gellis, Hockelman, Pizzo, and Feigin), two surgeons general (Drs. Richmond and Elders), the editor of *JAMA* (Dr. DeAngelis) and two deans (Drs. Richmond and Pizzo), as well as three highly admired figures in medicine (Drs. Klein, Weatherall, and Heagarty).

The Paul J. Schliesman Award was first given in 1989 in memory of Paul Schliesman, a Harvard Medical School graduate and a Children's Hospital house officer. Committed to primary care and third world medicine, he died unexpectedly during his senior resident year. "The award is awarded annually to a member of the housestaff who wishes to travel to a third world country to work in primary care. The recipients are chosen by the chief residents, program directors and

TABLE 9   Margaret Walsh Visiting Professors (1985–1995)

1985	Jerome Klein	Boston University School of Medicine
1986	Frank Oski	University of Pennsylvania School of Medicine
1987	Sydney Gellis	Tufts University School of Medicine
1988	Julius Richmond	Surgeon General, U.S. Public Health Service
1989	Margaret Heagarty	Columbia University College of Physicians and Surgeons
1990	Philip Pizzo	National Cancer Institute
1991	Catherine DeAngelis	Johns Hopkins University School of Medicine
1992	Robert Hockelman	University of Rochester School of Medicine and Dentistry
1993	Ralph D. Feigin	Baylor College of Medicine
1994	M. Joycelyn Elders	Surgeon General, U.S. Public Health Service
1995	David J. Weatherall	Oxford University

faculty members, the latter who were members of Paul's residency class." This award assumed increasing relevance and importance in the Pizzo/Fleisher era as international health became more and more engaging and popular among house officers. Recipients in the Nathan years are shown in Table 10.

The Fellow Teaching Award was established in the early 1990s to honor a clinical fellow working at the Children's Hospital who is an outstanding teacher and mentor to the housestaff. Recipients during the Nathan years are shown in Table 11. The honoree is selected by vote of the housestaff. Both Richard Malley

TABLE 10   Paul J. Schliesman Award (1989–1995)

1989	Charles Huskins
1990	William Adams and Claire McCarthy
1991	Mark Schuster
1992	Kim Nichols
1993	Laurie Glader and Richard Malley
1994	Anne Cullen, Catherine Gordon, Michael Rich
1995	James Plews-Ogan, Michelle Weinberg, Anne Wolf

TABLE 11   Fellow Teaching Award (1992–1995)

1992	Nathan Kuppermann	Emergency Medicine
1993	Gregory Toussaint	General Pediatrics
1994	Richard Malley	Infectious Disease
1995	Yao Sun	Neonatology

and Yao Sun had been prior Children's Hospital housestaff. David Greenes and Catherine Gordon, both house officers in the Nathan era, subsequently won the award in 1997 and 2002, respectively.

Career Directions

The career directions of graduates in the Nathan era continued to fulfill the mission of the residency, to prepare residents for leadership roles in academic medicine or the practice of pediatrics, whether in general pediatrics or a subspecialty. Among 275 graduates of the program between 1985 and 1996, 80% pursued fellowship and 20% proceeded into practice or other employment.[67,68] This compared with a Ross survey in 1998 of pediatric residency graduates throughout the United States in which 54% entered fellowship and 46% entered practice. Among the residents at the Children's Hospital in Boston entering fellowship, 78% took their fellowship at Harvard-affiliated hospitals. The Divisions of Hematology/ Oncology attracted the largest number of graduates, followed in descending order by general pediatrics, cardiology, neonatology, emergency medicine, and infectious disease. It is useful to compare this ranking with the Avery era, where the Division of Neonatology led the list, followed by hematology/oncology, infectious disease, cardiology, gastroenterology, and intensive care medicine, and with data from the U.S. as a whole, where neonatology topped the list followed by emergency medicine, hematology/oncology, cardiology, critical care, and gastroenterology.

When those entering practice careers in the Nathan era are surveyed, the majority pursued group private practice. A far smaller percentage entered health maintenance organizations, neighborhood health centers, or school health programs. Approximately 60% elected to stay in Massachusetts, while the remaining 40% distributed themselves throughout the U.S., mainly on the East and West Coasts.

When the graduates of the residency were surveyed upon completion of their residency and fellowship training, two-thirds (68%) were active in academic medicine, 28% in the practice of pediatrics, and 4% in other pursuits (National Institutes of Health, industry, or public health).

Life as a House Officer

Residency Highlights[69]

The first half of the Nathan years witnessed a number of memorable residency moments. The housestaff successfully moved over 200 patients from the Farley Building into the new hospital in one day without mishap. They mourned the loss of their senior resident colleague Paul Schliesman and honored his memory with the establishment of the Schliesman award for international primary care work. The program introduced weekly junior rounds to enhance learning and camaraderie. The housestaff association began to exert an increased influence on resident life, with the winter fling, the housestaff show, class dinners, and gatherings for spouses. The rising chief residents began to attend national workshops instituted to train pediatric chief residents nationwide for their upcoming jobs. The housestaff reached out to the disadvantaged of Boston through work with the homeless, book drives, programs for teen mothers and fathers, and a medical van, "Bridge Over Trouble Waters." Michael R. Epstein, a future cardiology fellow, was the first resident recipient of the hospital's Spirit Award. The housestaff began to present their clinical cases at medical grand rounds to appreciative attendees. Finally, the housestaff made a commitment to electing a representative from the program to attend the resident section of the American Academy of Pediatrics.

The second half of the Nathan years saw a number of lasting changes in the program. James Ogan and Beth Rider were the first to inaugurate a "shared" residency slot. The ambulatory senior year track for four senior residents became a reality, with important educational benefits not only for them but for all residents. A new housestaff team, Team D, was instituted for "off service patients" unable to be admitted to the three general ward medical teams. The strong desire of residents to become better teachers was finalized with a now robust Resident as Teacher curriculum for interns and seniors. The annual winter dances (winter flings) held at local Boston hotels were anxiously anticipated, extremely well attended, and a welcome respite from the rigors of winter. International travel took the housestaff to Pakistan, New Zealand, Bangladesh, Haiti, the Marshall Islands, India, Egypt, Nicaragua, and Guatemala in their primary care pursuits. The chief residents introduced the highly popular "college bowl" rounds, which magically always ended in a tie between the two fiercely competitive teams. Efforts to encourage research during residency were increasingly successful. The prestigious resident research award given by the Society for Pediatric Research was won by Scott Cameron. By 1995, as many as half of the graduating seniors were married and the number of children of housestaff had grown. Vincent Chiang won the hospital's Spirit Award. The efforts of the residency training committee, with enthusiastic support from the housestaff, resulted in a strong primary care presence in the curriculum and program.

Traditions of the Residency

The 1980s and 1990s saw a progressive growth in the number of housestaff traditions. They included the new intern dinner, the Christmas party, housestaff show, housestaff retreats, the housestaff dinners, the senior resident graduation dinner, and graduation.

The new intern dinner came during the week of intern orientation. Large and well attended by the faculty, new interns, and their spouses and significant others, the dinner was held in elaborate settings, such as the Longwood Towers. It was a part of orientation week for the new interns, constructed to allow for a gradual introduction of the newly minted interns to life as resident physicians. The evening also served as the maiden voyage for the rising chief residents, and their performance was scrutinized as closely as their charges. The chief and faculty spoke after dinner, often recalling somewhat nostalgically (but nonetheless happy it was behind them) their first days as an intern.

The Christmas party came at the end of a rigorous fall and halfway through the year. Held at the home of Fred and Jill Lovejoy, it included housestaff, their spouses and significant others; the faculty, and increasingly as the years passed, children of both faculty and housestaff. Well over 100 attended each year, enjoying the approaching holiday season and the much-needed four-day break over Christmas and New Year's. Food was plentiful and spirits always high. This tradition, which started in 1980, would continue for 27 years until 2007.

The housestaff dance (The Christmas Ball, The Winter Fling) generally occurred in February. Planned by the housestaff association, it included a festive dinner followed by dancing. The event was held at a Boston hotel or at one of the museums. Patient care coverage was supplied by the fellows and on occasion the junior faculty. The housestaff and their spouses or significant others were dressed in their finest. As the location and fare became more expensive over the years, the Department of Medicine began to contribute to the support of this event. The occasion always lifted morale and spirits.

The senior resident graduation dinner was part of several events marking the end of the academic year and the soon approaching departure of the seniors to their new jobs. In contrast to earlier years when residents entered the military service, worked at the National Institutes of Health, or trained in two different residency programs, residents tended to stay at the Children's Hospital for all three years of the residency and thereafter for fellowship. This led to many close friendships. This highly impactful period in their training as a doctor was coming to an end and that conclusion deserved to be celebrated. The event included cocktails, followed by dinner and then talks expressing the thanks and the good wishes of the department. Housestaff, spouses and significant others, and the faculty who had meant the most to the seniors were selected to attend. The event offered the opportunity for the physician-in-chief and program director to review the accomplishments of the three years. The evening was always bittersweet. The seniors departed knowing that they had been truly appreciated.

Graduation grew in importance as a hospital-wide event during the Nathan years. Held at grand rounds in June, it involved brief case presentations by the seniors, followed by the presentation of awards (the Janeway, Sidney Farber, and Fellow Teaching awards), followed by the presentation of diplomas to each of the graduating seniors. The event was attended by the hospital-wide community and often by the parents of the graduating seniors. Followed by a luncheon attended by the seniors and their families, it was a fitting conclusion to the year.

Housestaff Retreats[70]

The house officer retreats held each fall and each spring and attended by the housestaff, program directors, and department chair, became a highly important part of the resident's life. The retreats were held at the Endicott House in Dedham in the 1980s and at the Wellesley College Club in Wellesley and the Harvard Club in Boston in the early 1990s. The agenda was set by the chief residents in consultation with the residency training committee. The retreats began between 8 and 9 a.m. following sign-out of patients and lasted generally until 4 or 5 in the afternoon. Attendance was expected, with all services covered by the fellows and attendings. House officer attendance was always high. The faculty included Drs. Nathan and Lovejoy, with other faculty only attending on invitation (generally to present a topic or lead a discussion).

The retreats were most successful and became increasingly important to the effective running of the program. For a day, the housestaff had the full attention of the physician-in-chief and program director. Complaints and suggestions to improve rotations, resident education, and house officer life were welcomed, carefully listened to, and acted on by "the administration." It was understood that retreats were for work, but they were also for fun, with time to relax with walks, exercise, and activities. The agenda was set before the retreat, with subsequent changes implemented by the residency training committee after the retreat. Prior planning of the agenda was most important to assure a successful retreat.

The agenda varied from year to year. The mornings were focused around rotation improvements, challenges to be addressed in the residency, or invited speakers on specific topics. When breakout groups met and formulated suggestions, they reported back to the whole group over lunch or in afternoon discussion sessions. Often the sessions were focused on issues more easily discussed in a retreat format—career planning, financial planning, pediatric practice, acquisition of teaching skills, and stress management. Some retreats were quite specific, with focused outcomes intended (e.g., improvements in specific rotations); others were more global in intent (e.g., balance of education vs. service, success in meeting the goals of the training program). The spring retreats often addressed the schedule for the coming academic year.

Housestaff Shows[71]

The housestaff show became a more prominent part of house officer life during the 1980s and 1990s. The hospital at large was encouraged to attend to enhance revenue from ticket sales. It became an important source of yearly revenue for the housestaff association. Initially held in the Jimmy Fund Auditorium in the basement of the Jimmy Fund Building, it moved to larger auditoriums at the Brigham and Women's Hospital and at the Massachusetts College of Art, and finally by the mid-1990s to the Enders Auditorium. It was often dedicated to departed colleagues, including Paul Schliesman and Joan Tirrell, a Children's Hospital nurse in the mid-1990s. It was also dedicated to the fellows who covered all of the medical services the night of the performance.

Practice sessions became frequent as show night approached. A playbill listing director, musical director, producer, and choreographer as well as others in acting and musical roles was produced. In the mid-1980s, 40 to 50 of the house-staff participated in the production, by the mid-1990s, 60 to 65, three-quarters of the housestaff, were involved. The musical accompaniment was elaborate, drawing on the wide ranging musical talents of housestaff. The instruments included piano, drums, bass, guitar, French horn, and keyboard. The dancing and singing were particularly well done. The carefully written narrative was humorous but purposeful in its construct and intent. The faculty chosen to highlight were those with whom the housestaff had most contact and included the chief (David Nathan), the program director (Fred Lovejoy), and faculty: Gary Fleisher (chief of the emergency department), Lewis First (director of PGA), John Graef (director of the lead clinic), Grace Caputo (associate chief of the emergency department), Mary Ellen Wohl (chief of pulmonary medicine), Michael Epstein (hospital vice president), James Fackler (chief of medical intensive care), and Eli Newberger (director of the child abuse program).

The names of the shows were also carefully chosen, "Central Line" in 1988, "Late Night with David Nathan" in 1992, "Children at a Lesser Cost" in 1993, and "Christmas Carol" in 1995. The musical songs were adopted to current Broadway shows or popular hit tunes: "I've Never Been a Doc Before" to "I've Never Been in Love Before," and "First Night on Call" to "Red Rubber Ball." The topics for each scene depicted a current event or person in the life of the hospital or department in that given year. Frequently highlighted were the MECL (medical emergency clinic), the JPN (Joint Program in Neonatology), the ECMO (extracorporeal membrane oxygenation) unit, Teams A, B and C (general pediatric teams), N-I-C-U (the neonatal intensive care unit), faculty— "Don't Mess with Bill Berenberg" or "Nathan's Planet"—and moments or events of note included "Medical Jeopardy," "Service Chief Beauty Pageant," "Cultural Sensitivity Moment," and "QI Moment."

The major purpose of the shows was to enhance house officer morale during the long dark nights of the winter, and the shows brilliantly succeeded in accomplishing this purpose.

Reflections

The residency in the Nathan era was deeply rooted in the culture of the Black-fan, Janeway, and Avery years. As reflected upon by Jonathan Finkelstein, a future vice chair for quality and outcomes in the Department of Medicine, there was a clear "expectation of excellence."[72] "Your personal responsibility for your patients was strongly emphasized and there was no excuse for not knowing. You wanted to be a great resident and a great senior."[72] As noted by Lisa Diller, a future clinical director of pediatric oncology at the Dana-Farber Cancer Institute, there was also a prevailing view that the "longer you stayed the more you learned."[73] And while residency was very hard work, it bred a resident loyalty and camaraderie. As noted by Betsy Blume, a future transplant cardiologist, the code was to "help each other out. The world outside of residency was the anomaly; residency was all I did. It was hard to explain to non-doctors what residency life was like; I used to say I worked at the GAP so I would appear more normal."[74] But as noted by Jeffery Burns, a future director of the medical intensive care unit, "still the majority of residents loved residency, loved the Children's Hospital and felt deeply that it was a special privilege and honor to be taught by the greats, Nadas, Berenberg, Crigler, Masland, Rosen, Gerald, and Nathan."[75] As reflected upon by Jeffery Burns, to be able to share in the history of the creation of whole fields of pediatrics and to be able to feel these giants' "common passion for understanding a problem and solving it" made for a halcyon period in one's professional life.[75]

Each residency year had its own characteristics. As reflected upon by Anne Stack, a future clinical director of emergency medicine, the intern year was very hard, especially for the first six months, "the hardest year of my life. We had responsibility without the knowledge; we relied heavily on our seniors."[76] And as noted by Michael Rich, a future leader in adolescent medicine, who said that on occasion ". . . we felt like imposters and we worried we would be discovered."[77] In the second year, residents began to feel more confident; they mastered factual and clinical material simultaneously; they began to learn leadership through their supervisory rotations. As noted by Anne Stack, "We were now expected to know the answers and to exhibit good judgement."[76] The senior year was a wonderful year. The senior took the knowledge, synthesized it, and applied it to the patient. Seniors learned to manage up (the attending) and down (the interns and students). Each senior had role models and tried hard to emulate them. As noted by Betsy Blume, "Seniors objected most to the label, 'It's a fellow's hospital.' We felt we did everything; the interns depended on us; we rarely called the fellow. The fellows served very much in a 'consultative role."[74] The well-known college adage also applied to residency:

The intern knows not and knows that he knows not.

The junior knows not and thinks that he knows.

The senior knows but knows that he knows not.

Learning came about as a result of long hours in the hospital, by being the principal caregiver to patients, and by "clinical osmosis" from interaction with seniors and attendings.[73,75] Personal responsibility for one's patients was central to the learning process. Awareness of the exceptional role models who had made a profound impact on medicine set one's sights high.[75] The expectation was to be "forward thinking."[75] Toward the end of the Nathan era, the pedagogy of New Pathway learning espoused by Harvard Medical School entered the residency, instilling "decision by consensus" and less of a "hierarchical approach."[72] The senior was becoming less of a "drill sergeant and more of a facilitator."[77] As reflected upon by Jonathan Finkelstein, "Computerized searches did not exist; people were the resource; you depended on the minds and experiences of your colleagues. You went to the library, Xeroxed reprints and reviews, and digested the information."[72] Learning at senior rounds thus involved bringing your case and the information you had compiled from the library, and then benefiting from the analysis and judgment of your colleagues and the attendings.

David Nathan was deeply invested in the residency program and had a profound influence on it. Teaching residents was central to his leadership of the department as was his deep commitment to launching trainees on successful careers. He (and the program director) traveled less than most department chairs, and this allowed the necessary time to be actively involved on a daily basis with the residents on the floors, in the clinics, in teaching conferences, and in his office. And as wisely recalled by Richard Bachur, a future chief of emergency medicine, "Dr. Nathan's effectiveness was enhanced by his presence, his manner, and his authority."[78] His teaching style was "translational," patient centered and "holistic" in its approach.[76] He moved effortlessly from the patient to the science of disease and back again. On ward rounds the chaos stopped, everyone was prepared to present their cases and discuss them well.[78] At senior rounds he stimulated discussion through insightful questions. His career advice was actively sought after and was offered in a "fatherly" way such that you left the meeting with the confidence that the breadth and depth of his experience was offering the best vision for your future. Thus a formidable residency culture was created in the '80s and '90s as a result of Nathan's constant presence.[78]

Career Achievements

Graduates of the residency program in the 10 years of David Nathan's leadership range in age today from their mid-40s to their mid-50s. Thus their record of accomplishments is still expanding as the years pass and allow for the prestigious

TABLE 12   Hospital Presidents, Deans, Institute Leaders

Nancy C. Andrews	Dean, Duke University School of Medicine (previously Dean for Basic Sciences and Graduate Study, Harvard Medical School)
Kevin B. Churchwell	COO, Children's Hospital; former CEO, Nemours/Alfred I. duPont Hospital for Children
Alan F. Guttmacher	Director, National Institute of Child Health and Human Development, Bethesda, Md.
Jody Heymann	Dean, Fielding School of Public Health, University of California, Los Angeles
DeWayne Pursley	Neonatologist-in-Chief, Beth Israel Deaconess Medical Center, Boston
Cedric Priebe	Chief Information Officer, Brigham and Women's Hospital

honors and leadership roles that come only with time. Still, a number of individuals have already achieved remarkable accomplishments and Tables 12 through 15 offer a picture of their multiple leadership achievements. Of the 45 leadership positions in these four tables, a remarkable 20% are now filled by women. Also, importantly, in addition to faculty pursuing basic and translational research, other faculty are now focusing on outcomes and public health/policy-related research.

TABLE 13   Department Chairs

Alan B. Ezekowitz	Chair of Pediatrics, Massachusetts General Hospital, Harvard Medical School
Steven A. N. Goldstein	Chair of Pediatrics, University of Chicago School of Medicine
Scott Pomeroy	Neurologist-in-Chief and Chair of Neurology, Children's Hospital Boston, Harvard Medical School
Stephen Teach	Chair of Pediatrics, Children's National Medical Center, Washington, D.C.
Alan Wayne	Chair of Pediatrics, Children's Hospital of Los Angeles, University of Southern California School of Medicine

TABLE 14   Division Chiefs

Richard G. Bachur	Pediatric Emergency Medicine, Children's Hospital Boston
Kenneth Alexander	Pediatric Infectious Disease, Comer Children's Hospital, Chicago
Kanwaljeet J.S. Anand	Critical Care Medicine, Le Bonheur Children's Medical Center, Memphis
Jeffery Burns	Critical Care Medicine, Children's Hospital Boston
James J. Filiano	Pediatric Critical Care, Dartmouth-Hitchcock Medical Center
Jin S. Hahn	Pediatric Neurology, Lucile Packard Children's Hospital at Stanford
Barry Kosofsky	Pediatric Neurology, New York Presbyterian Hospital
Tracie Miller	Pediatric Clinical Research, Batchelor Children's Institute, Miami
Clement L. Ren	Pediatric Pulmonology, University of Rochester School of Medicine and Dentistry
Steven J. Roth	Pediatric Cardiology, Lucile Packard Children's Hospital at Stanford
Mark E. Rothenberg	Allergy and Immunology, Cincinnati Children's Hospital Medical Center
David H. Rowitch	Neonatology, UCSF Benioff Children's Hospital, San Francisco
Colin Rudolph	Pediatric Gastroenterology and Nutrition, Children's Hospital of Wisconsin
J. Philip Saul	Pediatric Cardiology, Medical University of South Carolina, Children's Hospital
Mark A. Schuster	General Pediatrics, Children's Hospital Boston
Robert D. Sege	Ambulatory Pediatrics, Boston Medical Center
Gary A. Silverman	Newborn Medicine, Children's Hospital of Pittsburgh
Michael A. Wood	Pediatric Endocrinology, Helen DeVos Children's Hospital

TABLE 15   Clinical and Academic Leaders

William Barbaresi	Associate Chief, Developmental Medicine, Children's Hospital Boston
Lisa R. Diller	Clinical Director of Pediatric Oncology, Dana-Farber Cancer Institute
Todd R. Golub	Director, Cancer Program, Broad Institute of Harvard Medical School and MIT
Jody Heymann	Founding Director, Health and Social Policy, McGill University Medical School; Dean, Fielding School of Public Health, University of California, Los Angeles
Isaac Kohane	Director, Bioinformatics Laboratory for Genetics and Genomics, Harvard Medical School
David Ludwig	Director, Optimal Weight for Life Clinic, Children's Hospital Boston
Louis J. Muglia	Director, Center for Prevention of Preterm Birth, Cincinnati Children's Hospital Medical Center
Ellis Neufeld	Associate Chief, Hematology/Oncology, Children's Hospital Boston
Hans C. Oettgen	Associate Chief, Allergy/Immunology, Children's Hospital Boston
Susan Parsons	Director of the Health Institute and the Center on Child and Family Outcomes, Tufts Medical Center
Thomas N. Robinson	Associate Director, Center for Policy, Outcomes and Prevention, Children's Health Initiatives, Lucile Packard Children's Hospital at Stanford
Jonathan J. Rome	Director, Cardiac Catheterization Laboratory, Children's Hospital of Philadelphia
Joshua Sharfstein	Commissioner of Public Health, City of Baltimore, Secretary of Health and Mental Hygiene, Baltimore
Benjamin L. Schneider	Director, Hepatology Center, Children's Hospital of Pittsburgh
Lauren Smith	Interim Commissioner of Public Health in Massachusetts
Anne M. Stack	Clinical Chief, Emergency Medicine, Children's Hospital Boston
Anne Trontell	Centers for Education and Research on Therapeutics, Agency for Health Care Research and Quality, Washington, D.C.

Tables 16 through 18 offer a glimpse of national as well as local awards and honors compiled by trainees from the Nathan and Pizzo eras. Of particular note there have been a remarkable number of recipients of the highly prestigious E. Mead Johnson Award over its 76 year history who were Children's Hospital residents. From this talented group of graduates will undoubtedly further evolve the future leaders of national organizations, medical schools, hospitals, and departments as well as additional prestigious national honors.

Finally, Nathan's housestaff have also excelled in less traditional avenues of accomplishment, including becoming popular authors and writers or major leaders in biotechnology or business. Tables 19 and 20 offer a glimpse of these achievements.

TABLE 16   Young Investigator Award of the Society for Pediatric Research

1994	Nancy C. Andrews
1997	Todd R. Golub
1999	Louis J. Muglia

TABLE 17   E. Mead Johnson Award

2002	Nancy C. Andrews
2006	David S. Pellman
2007	Mark E. Rothenberg
2008	Todd R. Golub
2008	Victor Nizet
2011	Joel Hirschhorn
2012	Scott Armstrong
2013	William Pu
2014	Atul Butte
2015	Loren Walensky

TABLE 18   Harvard Medical School Teaching Award

2001	Vincent Chiang
2002	Shari Nethersole
2008	Jonathan E. Alpert

TABLE 19   Major Lay Authors

Ari Brown	Author of pediatric-focused material for lay audiences
Perri Klass	President, Reach Out and Read; Professor of Pediatrics and Journalism, New York University
Claire McCarthy	Senior Medical Editor, Harvard Health Publications; Medical Communications Director, Children's Hospital Boston

TABLE 20   Biotech and Business Leaders

Alan B. Ezekowitz	Senior Vice President, Merck Research Laboratories
Roslyn Feder	Senior Vice President, Bristol Myers Squibb
Anula Jayasuriya	Co-founder, Evolvence India Life Science Fund
Linda McKibben	Vice President, The Lewin Group

Summation

Because David Nathan was a fine mentor of bright young people, the residents and residency flourished. His broad knowledge of pediatrics made him a formidable teacher at senior rounds and at the bedside. He wove together brilliantly basic science and clinical medicine in his teaching of the house staff. He was very comfortable and skilled in his strong commitment to scientific excellence and the training of future academic leaders.

A natural leader, who engendered loyalty as well as great credibility, Nathan enabled the department to become cutting-edge and lead scientifically in the modern era. He appointed the largest number of pediatric Howard Hughes investigators nationally and recruited outstanding basic and translational scientists and division chiefs.

Finally, he greatly strengthened clinical care through the creation of the service chief system as well as improvements in ambulatory care and emergency services, all of which benefited both the education and the patient care missions of the department. The reputation of the department soared as a result of his leadership. Nathan was, in fact, the right person for the job at the right time.

CHAPTER VII

The Pizzo/Fleisher Era

The Boston Combined Residency Program in Pediatrics
1996–2007

"The climate of the residency challenges you to ask and answer questions and go to the evidence-based literature . . ."

—Lise Nigrovic, reflecting on her time as a house officer in 2001

"We never forgot it was a privilege to be called a Boston Combined Residency Program resident."

—Rebekah Mannix, reflecting on her time as a house officer in 2003

THE 12 YEARS between 1995 and 2007 saw phenomenal changes in the hospital and department as well as in residency training, both at the Children's Hospital and throughout the country. The long tenure of hospital leadership under David Weiner ended, and a new and equally remarkable stewardship began under James Mandell. The Department of Medicine was led by two chairs, Philip Pizzo for five years, followed by current Chair Gary Fleisher. The department experienced amazing growth, particularly in the 2000s, both on the Longwood campus and at satellite hospital and clinic sites, as the financially constrained times in the latter half of the 1990s gave way to an uplifting period of financial

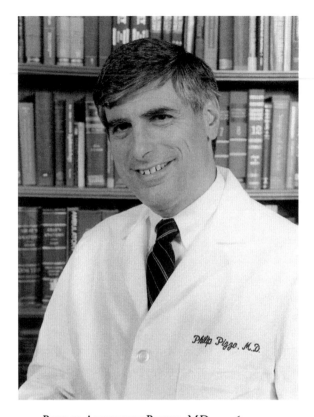

PHILIP ANTHONY PIZZO, MD, 1996–2001

Dr. Pizzo nurtured the Boston Combined Residency Program
in Pediatrics in its early years and melded primary care and
subspecialty training for the over 200 housestaff from the two
participating medical schools and academic hospitals during
his five years of leadership.

and physical growth for the hospital. One of the most significant events in this
period took place in 1996 with the birth of the Boston Combined Residency
Program in Pediatrics. Bringing together the training programs at the Children's
Hospital and Boston Medical Center, it has achieved remarkable success over
the ensuing years.

The Children's Hospital and The Department of Medicine[1]

In 1996, for the seventh year in a row, the hospital was ranked first among
children's hospitals by *U.S. News and World Report*. Philip Pizzo, a resident in

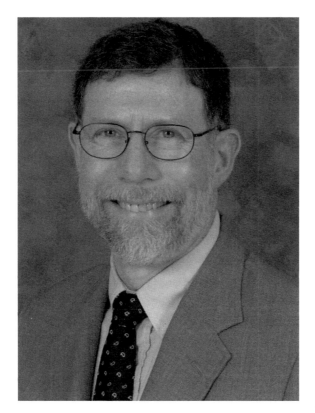

GARY ROBERT FLEISHER, MD, 2002–PRESENT

During his 15 years of leadership of the Department of
Medicine, Dr. Fleisher has trained more than 600 housestaff
in the Boston Combined Residency Program in Pediatrics. He
has served as a superior academic and clinical role model for
trainees during a halcyon era for the department.

the Janeway era, was appointed physician-in-chief, following a national search
chaired by Joseph Volpe, chair of the Department of Neurology. And the hospital welcomed First Lady Hillary Clinton. Accompanied by Senator Edward
Kennedy, she spoke to the staff about health care reform and met with patients
in the entertainment center.

Accomplishments in 1996 included the opening of a new Martha Eliot
Health Center in Jamaica Plain, the acquisition of "night nurse" (an after-hour
triage service for patients of community physicians), and the redesign of the hospital's lobby for retail use, with the inclusion of a CVS pharmacy, Au Bon Pain,
and the Museum of Science shop. The hospital celebrated the 10th anniversary

of its first cardiac transplant and mourned the loss of Leonard Cronkhite, the hospital's president from 1962 to 1977; Paul Gallop, director of the Laboratory of Human Biochemistry; and Lynn Haynie, a much admired and loved pediatric chronic disease specialist.

In 1997, under the wise leadership of George Kidder, chair of the board of trustees, the hospital affirmed its prior decision to remain independent rather than merging with other Boston hospitals. Judith Palfrey was named the T. Berry Brazelton professor of pediatrics. Neonatal medicine was split into two divisions: developmental and newborn biology directed by Merton Bernfield, newly recruited from Stanford University School of Medicine, and newborn medicine, directed by Gary Silverman, a former Department of Medicine resident and fellow.

In 1998, William Boyan, a dedicated trustee and prominent Bostonian, became the new chair of the board of trustees; Stephen Laverty, who had served as senior administrative officer of the Beverly Hospital, arrived as chief operating officer; and David Kirshner arrived as chief financial officer. The Children's Hospital Trust, the development wing of the hospital, was launched under Stephen Karp, a widely admired real estate developer and future chair of the board of trustees, and Janet Cady, senior vice president of development, marketing, and public affairs. Janet Cady had been successfully recruited from the Children's Hospital of Wisconsin, where she was executive vice president of the Children's Hospital Foundation.

Maurice Ziegler was appointed chief of surgery and surgeon-in-chief in 1998 following a national search. Great progress was made in the integration of the multiple clinical departments using the "foundation model" and coordinated by the physicians' organization. It was also a period of significant innovation for the hospital and the Department of Medicine. Advances in clinical care, education, and research took the form of a new system of inpatient and outpatient care (the firm system), faculty retreats throughout the year that focused on student, resident, fellow, faculty and continuing medical education, and a new strategic research plan for the hospital. Robert Haggerty, a former Children's Hospital resident and faculty member, received the Howland Award from the American Pediatric Society. However, all of this positive momentum was offset in part by budgetary constraints and a tightening of the belt.

In 1999, financial challenges continued. The Children's Hospital, once again ranked as the number one pediatric hospital, was joined by Harvard Medical School, ranked number one among graduate medical schools in the country by *U.S. News and World Report*. Mary Ellen Avery gave the Blackfan Lecture and happily received an honorary degree from her alma mater, Johns Hopkins University. Sandra Fenwick, a much-admired administrative leader at the Beth Israel Hospital, was appointed as the hospital's chief operating officer (COO). (In 2008, she would be appointed president, and in 2013, relinquish her COO role to become chief executive officer.) The Community Physician Award for outstanding service by practicing physicians was established. David Weiner announced his intention to retire in October 2000 after a tenure of long and dedicated leadership of the hospital. After a persistent effort on the part of Senator Edward Kennedy, David Weiner, and Philip Pizzo, in November 1999, the United States House and Senate passed the bill for funding resident salaries in freestanding children's hospitals—a herculean accomplishment. Resident salaries at such hospitals prior to that time throughout the country had been funded from each hospital's operating budget.

In 2000, following an extensive search, James Mandell, a past faculty member in the Department of Urology and dean of Albany Medical School, was selected as president and chief executive officer (CEO) of the hospital and assumed his position on October 1. He served as president until 2008 and as CEO until 2013. In 2014, the hospital's new 10-story building on Binney Street was officially named the James Mandell Building, as a tribute to his years of service and commitment to children and families.

The relationship between Harvard Medical School (HMS) and the Children's Hospital was close and highly effective during this period, with Board Chair Bill Boyan and widely admired HMS Dean Joseph Martin co-chairing the search committee that ultimately selected Jim Mandell. This model would be used in many of the other Harvard Medical School–affiliated hospitals in their searches for new CEOs. Michael Wessels, an expert in bacterial pathogenesis at the Channing Laboratory, was selected to replace the deeply respected Kenneth McIntosh as the new chief of the Division of Infectious Diseases, and Stuart Orkin, a superior basic investigator in the genetics of blood disorders, was appointed chair of pediatric oncology at the Dana-Farber Cancer Institute.

David Nathan was recognized by the Society for Pediatric Research with the establishment in 2000 of the David G. Nathan Award for Excellence in Basic Science Research, given to a fellow, and the David G. Nathan professorship was established at Harvard Medical School. Mary Ellen Avery received the Walsh McDermott Medal from the Institute of Medicine, and T. Berry Brazelton was named a "Living Legend" in a ceremony at the Library of Congress. The hospital celebrated the 70th birthday of Fred Rosen, president of the Center for Blood Research, longtime Chief of Immunology, and highly distinguished

James Gamble Professor of Pediatrics at Harvard Medical School. Phil Pizzo announced his decision to leave Children's Hospital to become dean of the medical school at Stanford, commencing in April 2001. During the interim period in 2001 and 2002, the Department of Medicine was led by Gary Fleisher, Joseph Majzoub, and Fred Lovejoy. Gary Fleisher assumed the chairmanship of the department in June of 2002.

James Lock, who had become chief of the Department of Cardiology in 1993, assumed the additional important role of physician-in-chief in 2002, a position he held with distinction until 2008. During the years 2002 and 2003, Gary Fleisher made a number of vice chair and division chief appointments. Jean Emans, Raif Geha, Bill Harmon, and Fred Lovejoy, all past Children's Hospital house officers, were appointed vice chairs for clinical affairs, research, finance, and education, respectively. New division chief appointments were made in pulmonary medicine, emergency medicine, and gastroenterology and nutrition; they were Craig Gerard, Michael Shannon, and Wayne Lencer, respectively. Joseph Majzoub, the highly accomplished chief of the Division of Endocrinology, successfully acquired a $1.6 million physician-scientist training grant for the department from the National Institutes of Health, bringing the total number of training grants in the department to 17. Richard Grand, recently recruited back to Children's Hospital after a distinguished career at Tufts University School of Medicine and the Floating Hospital, led a successful effort to acquire General Clinical Research Center funding. All hospital medical and surgical departments now utilized the foundation model, with a centralized physicians' organization coordinating the financial activities of the physician groups. Leonard Zon became president of the International Stem Cell Society, and in 2004, geneticist Joel Hirschhorn, a prior Harvard medical student and medical house officer, won the Young Investigator Award from the Society for Pediatric Research.

In 2004 and 2005, as part of a hospital-wide strategy to expand clinical services as well as produce more basic science, translational, and outcomes research, a large number of new clinicians and physician–scientists joined the medical department; two-thirds were basic scientists and one-third had been trained at the Children's Hospital. In 2006, the Department of Medicine underwent a highly successful departmental review carried out by Harvard Medical School that encompassed clinical care, teaching and research activities, as well as faculty appointments. These years also saw important new divisional appointments in the Division of Neonatology (Stella Kourembanas) and the Division of Genetics (Christopher Walsh). Important new senior recruitments occurred as well, including Dale Umetsu in allergy and immunology and Charles Nelson in the program in developmental psychology. Umetsu had been a medical house officer at the Children's Hospital and was recruited from the medical school faculty at Stanford.

Inpatient admissions and outpatient visits began to show remarkable increases as a result of a growing hospital pediatric market share. Similar volume increases were also seen at the hospital's satellite sites, which had grown in number and size since the mid-1990s. David Nathan received the prestigious George Kober Medal from the Association of American Physicians, and in 2005, Mary Ellen Avery received the Alfred DuPont Award for Excellence in Children's Health Care and the Howland Award from the American Pediatric Society.

The years 2006 and 2007 continued to be marked by extraordinary department achievements. The department continued to grow in size, and the faculty's clinical work and research achievements led to a most healthy financial picture. Three important new divisional appointments were made in general pediatrics, hematology/oncology, and behavioral and developmental pediatrics, with these superb leadership appointments being assumed by Mark Schuster, David Williams, and Leonard Rappaport, respectively. Both Mark Schuster and Leonard Rappaport had been prior house officers. The author stepped down after 27 years as residency program director, and Ted Sectish was recruited from Stanford University School of Medicine to become the new program director for the Boston Combined Residency Program in Pediatrics (BCRP) while Niraj Sharma was recruited from the University of Miami School of Medicine to be program director for the Brigham and Women's/Boston Children's Hospital Medicine-Pediatric Residency. New Children's Hospital chairs, funded jointly by the hospital and the department (discussed later in this chapter) were established to honor legendary Department of Medicine faculty: Drs. John Crigler, Mary Ellen Beck Wohl, Robert Masland, Warren Grupe, Harry Shwachman, Richard Grand, Park Gerald, and Harvey Levy.

Clinical Care[2]

There was a progressive escalation in the importance of clinical care throughout the Pizzo/Fleisher era. This resulted in new organizational structures, a growing number of new clinical faculty who worked on the wards and clinics in addition to their laboratories, a plethora of new and highly innovative clinical programs, and an increasing number of patients seen in satellite community clinics and hospitals.

In the Pizzo era, the new firm structure which was a further evolution of the service chief system of the Nathan era was the primary means for enhancing clinical care. This model sought to integrate inpatient and outpatient services, break down compartmentalization of care, and allow residents, fellows, and faculty to follow patients in inpatient and outpatient settings. It aligned providers across the continuum of care in order to give families a more seamless experience.

A clinical advisory group (CAG) under Phil Pizzo's watchful guidance began to develop the firm model in the fall of 1996; it was implemented 21 months later in July of 1998. The department had operated with three age-based inpatient units (the service-chief system) from 1986 to 1996, the Rotch, Blackfan, and Janeway Services. In the new firm model, patients were cared for by one of two multispecialty firms that operated in both the inpatient and outpatient settings. The Blackfan Medical Firm (Firm I), often with younger patients, was composed of five services (general pediatrics; hematology; allergy and immunology; gastroenterology; and the development, genetics, and chronic care service). It also included the short-stay unit, which began in the Nathan era. Christopher Frantz, a superior house officer and later an oncologist in the Janeway era, was recruited to lead Firm I. Nursing and patient services were skillfully managed by Patricia Rutherford. Core attendings (an early form of current-day hospitalists) were selected to deliver care and to teach the students and housestaff. A second medical firm (Firm II), the Janeway Medical Firm, often with older patients, was led by Joseph Wolfsdorf, the widely admired clinical director of endocrinology. A highly talented Jayne Rogers was selected to co-manage this firm as nurse manager. Firm II was composed of six services (general pediatrics, adolescent medicine, infectious disease, pulmonary, endocrinology, and nephrology). Each firm and service was also named for a distinguished faculty member, and was led by a service chief and had a group of core attendings who were active in care and teaching. Finally, additional firms were established in oncology, with Stephen Sallan appointed as firm chief, and in newborn medicine, with Gary Silverman similarly appointed. In October of 1999, as a result of further evolution of the firms, Chris Frantz assumed leadership of the inpatient component of Firms I and II, this being his area of clinical expertise, while Joseph Wolfsdorf focused his attention on the outpatient component of these two firms, his clinical strength. The makeup of the firms and their leadership is shown in Table 1.

Over the next two to three years, a number of major accomplishments were achieved, often aided and enhanced by powerful outside forces. The financial constraints of the late 1990s created an important imperative for efficiency in the delivery of care in both the inpatient and outpatient settings. This led to core

TABLE 1   Pizzo Era Firm Model (1998–2001)

Firm	Chief
Kenneth D. Blackfan Medical Firm	Christopher Frantz
David G. Nathan General Pediatric Service	Christopher Frantz
Louis K. Diamond Hematology Service	Ellis Neufeld
Fred S. Rosen Allergy and Immunology Service	Mitchell Lester, Hans Oettgen
Harry Shwachman Gastroenterology Service	Alan Leichtner
Marilyn Hayne/Park S. Gerald Development/ Genetics/Chronic Care Services	Bruce Korf, Mira Irons, Leonard Rappaport
Short Stay Unit	Marc Baskin
Nurse Manager	Patricia Rutherford
Charles A. Janeway Medical Firm	Joseph Wolfsdorf
William Berenberg General Pediatric Service	Joseph Wolfsdorf
F. Rosewell Gallagher Adolescent Medicine Service	Jean Emans
John F. Enders Infectious Disease Service	Sandra Burchett
Mary Ellen Avery Pulmonary Service	Andrew Colin
John F. Crigler Endocrinology Service	Norman Spack
James L. Gamble Nephrology Service	John Herrin
Nurse Manager	Jayne Rogers
Oncology Firm	Stephen Sallan
Nurse Manager	Patricia Branowicki
Newborn Medicine Firm	Gary Silverman
Nurse Manager	Ann Colangelo

attendings committing longer periods of time each day on the wards, adding continuity to both the clinical care and teaching enterprise. A similar trend occurred in the outpatient setting, where new standards and expectations were established for the faculty. This created greater continuity, efficiency, and quality of care. Another significant achievement involved housestaff education. The Residency Review Committee (RRC) for Pediatrics of the Accreditation Council for Graduate Medical Education (ACGME) was requiring that residents spend a greater amount of time in the outpatient setting. The firm system aligned itself well with this goal. Patients cared for on the wards were seen with greater frequency in follow-up by the housestaff in the clinics, a training model that was more in concert with clinical practice. Lastly, a new emphasis was placed on measurement of cost-effectiveness and on the quality of care, along with close monitoring of patient and referring physician satisfaction. These metrics would be increasingly important in the Fleisher era.

The firm system also encountered several challenges. The first involved the establishment of clear lines of authority by the service chiefs in the area of subspecialty care, an arena that had traditionally rested with the division chiefs. This issue was accommodated through negotiation but with decision-making sometimes slowed. A second challenge related to the major domains of care for residents on the wards and for fellows in the clinics. To fulfill the goal of moving residents into the clinics, coverage of the wards by fellows was necessary. For fellows, this was a difficult change and was only partially accomplished. Similarly, the housestaff had difficulty leaving their patients on the wards, with the result being that consistent outpatient follow-up was incompletely realized. Overall, however, implementation of the firm system led to a number of important changes in the culture of the department, the most important being an enhanced emphasis and thoughtfulness about patient care and its delivery. This change laid the organizational structure and framework that would allow both the medical and nursing services to handle subsequent clinical growth in the Fleisher era.

By 1998, admissions to the medical service numbered 8,591; by 2003, 9,380; by 2007, 9,369; and by 2012, 10,659. (These numbers include admissions to general and subspecialty pediatrics, oncology, bone marrow transplantation, intermediate care program, neonatal intensive care, solid organ transplantation, medical intensive care, and the General Clinical Research Center but exclude cardiology, neurology, and medical–surgical intensive care at the Children's Hospital and neonatal intensive care at the Brigham and Women's Hospital and the Beth Israel Hospital.) The services with the most admissions in 2012 included (in descending order) general pediatrics, hematology/oncology/ bone marrow transplantation, medical critical care, gastroenterology/hepatology/nutrition, and pulmonary medicine.

The daily census generally hovered at 90%. Total patient days in 1999 were 25,747, with a length of stay of 3.5 days. In the emergency department, 50,000 visits were recorded in 1999, with another approximately 50,000 visits occurring at the five affiliated emergency medicine programs housed at the hospital's satellite sites: Beverly, MetroWest, Norwood, South Shore, and Winchester Hospitals. Ambulatory visits rose from 83,088 in 1996 to 92,846 in 1998. By 2000, they surpassed 100,000, rising to 111,124, by 2007, to 151,443, and by 2013, to 200,000 ambulatory visits, with the greatest increases seen in adolescent medicine, endocrinology, gastroenterology, hematology/oncology, and immunology (in descending order).

New Clinical Care Services

Three new clinical programs were created in the Fleisher era. The Children's Hospital Inpatient Service (CHIPS) was staffed by hospitalist physicians and run by Vincent Chiang, a seasoned and highly capable emergency medicine physician and residency program leader.[3] This system of care evolved out of the core attending model instituted in the Pizzo era. The staffing included hospitalist physicians often recruited shortly after residency or fellowship as well as subspecialty hospitalists appointed by the divisions. They were responsible for both patient care and teaching. Time taken away from office practice made serving as an attending for a full month increasingly impractical for a community practitioner so that by 2007, the hospitalist system had assumed responsibility for the care of 90% of the patients on the general medical service.

This model of care proved highly successful. Subspecialty and general hospitalists were able to deliver complex general and specialty care efficiently and effectively. Communication between the department's hospitalists and subspecialty faculty and the referring community physicians and various community hospital services improved in the inpatient, outpatient, and out-of-hospital settings. Hospitalist jobs were actively sought, with superior young faculty recruited into this new role. The residents benefited by more consistent and excellent teaching. A fellowship in hospitalist medicine added an important academic and research depth to the hospitalist activities. Started and run by Christopher Landrigan, a recent house officer graduate and emerging clinical investigator who would gain recognition for his work on resident sleep deprivation and patient safety, this fellowship became most attractive and highly desirable. The greatest challenge posed by the 24/7 hospitalist attending model for the faculty was a diminished opportunity to attend and teach on the general ward services, with resultant loss of highly valued contact with the housestaff. A second challenge was some loss of resident autonomy in decision making.

Conceptualized in 2002, the intermediate care unit cared for children too ill to remain on the general pediatric floors but not requiring mechanical ventilatory support and not so ill as to require the medical–surgical intensive care unit.[4] The four-bed unit opened in July 2003, directed by Michael Agus, who had been jointly trained in endocrinology and critical care medicine, and was managed daily by a hospitalist and a senior and junior resident. Nurses from the general ward services were trained to staff the unit. The most common diagnoses included respiratory illnesses (asthma, bronchiolitis, pneumonia, and croup), diabetes mellitus, and toxic ingestions. Initially located on the medicine inpatient unit on 8 East, by 2007, it had grown to 10 beds, and was located on 9 South, with four faculty members (one intensivist and three hospitalists) staffing the unit. It moved to its current home on the 11th floor in 2008. The intermediate care unit has proven to be highly successful, well received by the housestaff (for its strong teaching and resident autonomy), by the nurses (as evidenced by a very high retention rate), and by patients and families, who are highly satisfied with the care received. Important outcome measures, such as a shortened time to clinical improvement of diabetes ketoacidosis (a shorter time to close the anion gap and only one case of cerebral edema over seven years), were also encouraging. Thanks to all of these successes, this unit would become a new division, the Division of Medicine Critical Care, led by Michael Agus.

Under the direction of Baruch Krauss, a third new service, the sedation service, was added to assist in the care of inpatients. Drs. Chiang, Agus, and Krauss had all been trained in the hospital's residency program.

Concerted efforts were thus made throughout the Pizzo/Fleisher era to enhance the clinical services. Simultaneously, Harvard Medical School importantly established new promotion criteria that rewarded clinicians. In the Department of Medicine, an incentivized financial system was instituted, associate division chiefs were appointed, and a greater emphasis on outcomes through hospital policies, standards, and guidelines occurred. Monthly morbidity and mortality conferences also emphasized the importance of clinical care, thereby enhancing the role of the clinician.

Medical Education[5]

The four domains of medical education (student, house officer, fellow, and faculty/practitioner) continued, but both the breadth and the impact of these educational efforts grew throughout the Pizzo/Fleisher era. A new group of highly capable educators was appointed as leaders, educational offerings grew in sophistication, and efforts to evaluate the quality and outcomes of the educational efforts in the Department of Medicine became a primary focus. In addition, at Harvard Medical School, pediatrics assumed a more integral role in the school's educational efforts, carried out at both the Children's Hospital and by colleagues at the Massachusetts General Hospital. During the Pizzo/Fleisher era, many faculty held important positions on the two departmental education committees established by Dr. Pizzo and later by Dr. Fleisher, as shown in Tables 2–4.

TABLE 2   Children's Hospital—Education Steering Committee (1996–2000)

Sally Andrews	
Elizabeth Armstrong	Chair, Faculty Education
Merton Bernfield	Chair, Fellow Education
Jonathan Finkelstein	Chair, Resident Education
Donald Goldmann	
Frederick Lovejoy	Chair
Samuel Lux	
Philip Pizzo	Chair, Department of Medicine
Orah Platt	Chair, Medical Student Education
Alan Woolf	Chair, Continuing Medical Education

TABLE 3   Children's Hospital—Education Leadership Committee (2001–2007)

Vincent Chiang	Director, Medical Student Education
Gary Fleisher	Chair, Department of Medicine
Frederick Lovejoy	Vice Chair for Education; Program Director, Boston Combined Residency Program in Pediatrics
Janet Shahood	Manager, Research and Education
Robert Vinci	Program Director, Boston Combined Residency Program in Pediatrics
Alan Woolf	Director, Continuing Medical Education
Individual Program Directors	13 Subspecialty Fellowship Programs

In the late 1990s, the faculty were recognized for their contributions in education, with 23 individuals selected as members of the newly formed Harvard Medical School Academy (a group of medical educators on the Harvard faculty and residing throughout the teaching hospital system): 17 as scholars, three as distinguished scholars, two as associate members, and one as a fellow. As another example of educational achievement between 1973 and 2007, the medical school awarded 313 prizes for excellence in teaching and mentoring. Twenty-five, or 8%, of these awards were given to Children's Hospital faculty. In the Pizzo/Fleisher era, nine of 25 (or one-third) were recipients, with three (Vincent Chiang, Shari Nethersole, and Isaac Kohane) being former Children's Hospital resident trainees.

TABLE 4   Medical School—Education Leadership Roles (1996–2007)

Nancy Andrews	Dean, Basic Science and Graduate Studies
Gary Fleisher	Chair, Department of Pediatrics, Harvard Medical School
Jean Emans	Director, Office of Faculty Development at Children's Hospital
Isaac Kohane	Director, Countway Library of Medicine
Alan Leichtner	Director, Medical Education, Office of Faculty Development at Children's Hospital
Frederick Lovejoy	Executive Secretary, Harvard Medical School Pediatric Executive Committee
Robert Masland	Associate Master, Cannon Society
Philip Pizzo	Chair, Department of Pediatrics and Faculty Dean, Harvard Medical School
Orah Platt	Master, Castle Society; Council of Academic Deans

Medical Student Education

Children's Hospital faculty participated in all four years of the Harvard Medical School curriculum. In the first and second years, the pediatric faculty taught courses in genetics, gastroenterology, immunology/microbiology/infectious diseases, hematology/oncology, clinical epidemiology, ethics, and mental health. Gordon Harper, a senior Children's Hospital psychiatrist and pediatrician, led the pediatric offering in the first-year Patient/Doctor I course, an introduction to the physician and society. The Patient/Doctor II course (an introductory course in history taking and physical examination) in the second year became a major investment of faculty effort each year. Carried out in both the hospital and the community, during the Pizzo era, this course was initially led by Shari Nethersole, a Harvard Medical School graduate and prior graduate of the residency program at the Children's Hospital. Alan Woolf, former director of the Massachusetts Poison Control System, took over this important course in the Fleisher era. Approximately 100 students participated each year. The number of preceptors was initially large, but with the decision to financially compensate the instructors for their time and effort, the faculty became smaller, with the most dedicated teachers chosen. Greater uniformity in teaching and in course pedagogy was thus achieved.

The Principal Clinical Year (Core) Course in Pediatrics for third-year students was led in the early Pizzo era by Edward O'Rourke, an infectious disease expert, as director. Robert Sundel, an outstanding clinical rheumatologist, and Ingrid Holm, an endocrinologist and geneticist, were associate directors. Later in the Pizzo/Fleisher era, Vincent Chiang served as director, with Richard Malley, Shari Nethersole, and Joshua Nagler as associate directors. Over 100 students each year took this extremely popular course, which became one of the most highly ranked at the medical school. The course was supplemented by an Advanced Pediatric Course (also called the sub-internship), again expertly led by Vincent Chiang and taken by 12 students each year. Both the Core Course and Advanced Course involved concentrated work with the pediatric housestaff on the general and subspecialty inpatient services. The close relationship between housestaff and students, enhanced by a robust Resident as Teacher curriculum and with the active involvement of select pediatric faculty, made these two courses the department's flagship offerings for Harvard medical students. During a six-year period, from 2000 to 2006, among 160 medical students in a class each year, on average, 18, or 11%, pursued a pediatric career and on average, six of 18, or one-third, matched at the Children's Hospital. These results reflected well on the commitment and effort of those involved in medical student education.

Sixteen pediatric electives, in essentially all subspecialties, were offered to fourth-year Harvard medical students as well as students from medical schools throughout the country. The most highly subscribed for the years 2000 to 2007 in descending order are shown in Table 5. On average, 100 medical students each year participated in these electives, demonstrating a robust contribution of subspecialty expertise in support of medical student education.

TABLE 5   Pediatric Electives (2000–2007)

Subject	Course Director	Number of Students/Year
Emergency Medicine	Debra Weiner	25
Endocrinology	Norman Spack	13
Advanced Pediatrics	Vincent Chiang	12
Ambulatory Pediatrics	Shari Nethersole	9
	and Ronald Samuels	8
Gastroenterology	Alan Leichtner	7
Oncology	Holcombe Grier	7

House Officer Training

The Boston Combined Residency Program in Pediatrics and the many and varied aspects of the training of housestaff are covered in greater depth later in this chapter.

Fellowship Training

Thirteen fellowship programs with training in subspecialty medicine existed during the Pizzo/Fleisher era. Eleven resided in the Department of Medicine, while the fellowship in critical care medicine was in the Department of Anesthesiology and the fellowship in cardiology was within that department. Responsibility for these programs lay with the division chiefs (or department in the case of the Departments of Cardiology and Anesthesiology). Fellows were selected by the divisions. Each program was accredited by the RRC for Pediatrics of the ACGME. The 13 fellowships and their program directors are listed in Table 6.

Over a five-year period during the Fleisher era, there were 1,702 applications to 11 fellowships (cardiology and critical care medicine excluded) with 220 selected, an acceptance rate of 13%. The programs admitted one to seven fellows each year. The Division of Emergency Medicine received the most applications, followed by allergy/immunology, hematology/oncology, newborn medicine,

TABLE 6   Fellowship Training Programs and Program Directors (1996–2007)

Subspecialty	Program Director
Adolescent Medicine	Jean Emans
Cardiology	Peter Lang
Critical Care Medicine	Jeffrey Burns
General Pediatrics	Judith Palfrey
Emergency Medicine	Michael Shannon/Richard Bachur
Endocrinology	Joseph Majzoub
Gastroenterology	Wayne Lencer
Hematology/Oncology	Samuel Lux
Immunology/Allergy	Raif Geha/Hans Oettgen
Infectious Disease	Robert Husson
Neonatology	Stella Kourembanas
Nephrology	William Harmon
Pulmonary Medicine	Debra Boyer

pulmonary medicine, and gastroenterology (in descending order). Hematology/ oncology and newborn medicine admitted the largest number of fellows each year, followed by general pediatrics and emergency medicine. Of the 220 selected, 54% were women, 19% were minorities, and 17% were MD/PhDs.

Among 207 graduates over the same five years from the 11 fellowships, an impressive 90% entered faculty positions or pursued further post-doctoral training while 10% entered practice. Of those pursuing academic careers, 55% remained at the Children's Hospital or Harvard Medical School; of those entering subspecialty practice, 53% joined practices in Massachusetts. Thus, the Children's Hospital fellowships, like the residency, were extremely important feeder programs of highly talented individuals for faculty positions at the Children's Hospital and Harvard Medical School.

These data clearly suggest that the Department of Medicine succeeded admirably in achieving its goal of encouraging fellows to pursue academic careers. There was a constant flow of talented young residents into the department's highly coveted and competitive fellowship training positions. The fellowship programs were of very high quality, as assessed by the RRC of the ACGME, and the level of innovation was exceptional. The majority of graduates subsequently pursued highly successful academic careers.

Continuing Medical Education

The department worked closely with the hospital in the Pizzo/Fleisher era to expand its post-graduate education programs to local, regional, national, and international audiences. A remarkable number of courses extended the reach of the hospital, especially throughout New England. Between 2000 and 2006, 15 post-graduate courses were held, with over 2,500 participants. All courses were accredited through Harvard Medical School's continuing education department and all received extremely high ratings. In fact, in a survey of referring physicians carried out by the Children's Hospital, the continuing medical education courses rated highest among services offered by the hospital. The continuing medical education effort was under the overall direction of Alan Woolf. Both Alan Woolf and Jean Emans served on the Harvard Medical School Department of Continuing Education committee. Selected courses and their directors are shown in Table 7.

Hospital-based offerings consisted of medical grand rounds for the hospital community, directed by Gary Fleisher, Fred Lovejoy, and the medical chief residents; Pediatric Practice Seminar for community physicians, directed by Fred

TABLE 7   Post-graduate Courses and Directors (1996–2007)

Courses	Directors
Advances in Pediatric Health Care	Alan Woolf
Adolescent Medicine	Jean Emans
Pediatric and Adolescent Gynecology	Jean Emans and Mark Laufer
Pediatric Infectious Disease	Kenneth McIntosh and Sandra Burchett
Inpatient Medicine	Julie Dollinger
Leadership Development Program for Physicians and Scientists	Elizabeth Armstrong and Jean Emans

Mandell and later by Ben Willwerth; mini grand rounds for the housestaff, directed by Vincent Chiang; and finally, a number of subspecialty conferences. In addition, several post-graduate educational conferences were instituted at the Children's Hospital satellite hospitals, including Beverly Hospital, Winchester Hospital, Brockton Hospital, MetroWest Medical Center, and South Shore Hospital. In the mid-2000s "Current Concepts in Pediatric Medicine" was instituted as a new initiative to foster distance learning. A collaborative effort between the Departments of Medicine and Surgery and the hospital, this effort featured senior faculty teaching specialty topics on cable television via a medical news channel to national audiences.

The continuing education effort had two major goals, the first to educate practicing physicians, nurses, and other caregivers about the many rapid changes in pediatric medicine and the second to allow Children's Hospital physicians and community physicians to know each other better, with the objective of enhancing clinical care.

Research[6]

The influence of the research enterprise on house officers during their residency was indirect. They witnessed it every day through the imposing research buildings (Enders and Karp), the stature of the research faculty, the faculty's papers and national recognition, and the impact of clinical research on their daily activities in patient care. When a prior Children's Hospital resident received national recognition for his or her science and research, it also sent a clear message to the other residents that research was important.

The research greats were part of the hospital lore learned by every resident: Enders, Weller, and Robbins for growing the polio virus in tissue culture; Murray for performing the first kidney transplant; David Smith for the development of the *Haemophilus influenzae* vaccine; and Robert Gross for performing the first successful cardiac surgery at the Children's Hospital—ligation of the patent ductus arteriosus. By 1999, grant funding had risen to $51 million, with $38 million from the NIH and other federal support and $13 million from industry, foundations, and state funding. By 2007, grant support in the department had grown to $86 million, with $79 million from federal, state, foundation, and industry sources and $6.5 million in training grants, and by 2012, the total funding for research grants had reached $135 million, of which $128 million came from federal, state, foundation, and industry sources and $7 million from training grants. By 2014, the total research grant support had reached $172 million. The number of junior faculty with K research awards had increased from 23 in 1998 to 39 in 2001, to 55 in 2006, and 63 in 2012. Meanwhile, the number of T32 training grant awards rose from 12 in 1999 to 18 in 2007 and to 24 in 2012. The increase in research space by 2007 was also remarkable, 88,000 square feet in the Enders and Karp Buildings and 20,000 square feet of office space for clinical research. By 2013, basic research space alone had reached a total of 112,000 square feet. Those divisions and programs most heavily funded included (in descending order): hematology/oncology, followed by the Howard Hughes Medical Institute, immunology, infectious diseases, molecular biology, and genetics.

The remarkable impact of basic and clinical research in the department can be appreciated when one considers the faculty publications record, the E. Mead Johnson Award winners, and memberships in prestigious national societies. A 2006 search of the PubMed database for the prior decade, compiled by Samuel Lux, the outstanding vice chair for basic research and prior chief of the Division of Hematology and Oncology, using the five-year averaged impact factor, netted impressive results. Of 2,266 published articles by Department of Medicine faculty, 177 (7%) were in the top 10 journals, 338 (13.7%) were in the top 20 journals, and 667 (27%) were in the top 35 journals.

Receipt of the E. Mead Johnson Award is another metric of investigator success. Over a 76-year period from 1939 to 2015, with two awards given each year, on 42 occasions, or 27% of the time, a Children's Hospital faculty member was the recipient. The remarkable number of award winners in the Pizzo/Fleisher era who were prior house officers is listed in Table 8.

Additional awards received by housestaff included the Young Investigator Award given by the Society for Pediatric Research and won by Joel Hirschhorn (2004), Brian Feldman (2008), Loren Walensky (2009), Atul Butte (2010), and Kimberly Stegmaier (2012), Sallie Permar (2014) and Vijay Sankaran (2015); the

TABLE 8　　E. Mead Johnson Award (1995–2014)

Alan Krensky and Margaret Hostetter	1995
Donald Leung	1997
Jonathan Gitlin	1998
Steven Goldstein	2001
Nancy Andrews	2002
David Pellman	2005
Marc Rothenberg	2007
Todd Golub	2008
Victor Nizet	2008
Joel Hirschhorn	2011
Scott Armstrong	2012
William Pu	2013
Atul Butte	2014

Presidential Early Career Award, won by Catherine Gordon and Kenneth Mandl in 2004; and the Resident Research Award, given by the Society for Pediatric Research and won by Ofer Levy in 1999, Carey Lumeng in 2003, Sallie Permar in 2007, Alicia Demirjian (2009), Laura McCullough (2009), Joyce Hsu (2011), and Lakshmi Ganapathi (2012).

By the end of 2007, among the department's 827 faculty, 90 had been elected to the Society for Pediatric Research, 40 to the American Pediatric Society, 24 to the American Society for Clinical Investigation, 14 to the American Academy of Arts and Sciences, nine to the Institute of Medicine, five to the National Academy of Sciences, and another eight were appointed as Howard Hughes Investigators. By 2012, 108 faculty had been elected members of the Society for Pediatric Research, and 62 members of the American Pediatric Society, illustrating the prominent position held nationally by the Children's Hospital as a research institution. Past house officers at the Children's Hospital in these prestigious societies include among others Nancy Andrews, Donald Berwick, Raif Geha, Sam Lux, Philip Pizzo, Stuart Orkin, Isaac Kohane, Joel Hirschhorn, Ellis Neufeld, David Pellman, and Dale Umetsu. Those in recent years who have been named Howard Hughes investigators include Fred Alt, George Daley, Stephen Harrison, Friedhelm Hildebrandt, Louis Kunkel, Stuart Orkin, David Pellman, Christopher Walsh, Morris White, Yi Zhang, and Leonard Zon.

Promotions and Recognitions[7]

In the Pizzo/Fleisher era, four tracks for promotion existed at Harvard Medical School. Full-time promotions were made through Investigator, Teacher Clinician, and Longer Service tracks, and part-time promotions were made through the Academic Part-time track. Each track had a different set of criteria dependent on academic rank. Initiated in 1999 by the widely admired dean of Harvard Medical School, Joseph Martin, and implemented by the long-serving and highly effective Dean for Faculty Affairs, Eleanor Shore, the innovative Longer Service track recognized instructors in the Harvard system who had served loyally and well for more than 10 years at that rank with inadequate recognition. In 2008, a new full-time system with areas of excellence (Investigation, Teaching and Educational Leadership, and Clinical Expertise and Innovation) was instituted at Harvard Medical School. The Longer Service and Part-time tracks continue to exist.

The department used two committees for academic promotions, the newly created Children's Hospital Committee on Academic Appointments and Promotions (CAAP) in the Pizzo era and the Harvard Medical School Pediatric Executive Committee (PEC). The CAAP considered all instructor, assistant professor, associate professor, and professor promotions. All successful pediatric promotion applications then went to the PEC, this committee appointed by the dean of Harvard Medical School. It included representatives from the Children's Hospital and the Massachusetts General Hospital for Children and considered pediatric promotions from these two institutions as well as from Cambridge Hospital, Harvard Vanguard Medical Associates, and pediatricians in community practice. Following approval by both committees, assistant and associate professor promotions went to Harvard Medical School's Promotions and Reappointments (P&R) Committee while promotions to full professor were passed on to the Subcommittee of Professors (SOP). Membership on the two pediatric committees is shown in Table 9 for both the Pizzo and Fleisher eras. Philip Pizzo, Gary Fleisher, Alan Ezekowitz, and Ronald Kleinman presented all academic promotions for consideration by the CAAP and PEC. Fred Lovejoy served as executive secretary for each committee and chaired the committee meetings, and Elayne Fournier served administratively and with remarkable effectiveness as faculty coordinator for academic promotions at the Children's Hospital. At any point in time, each committee had eight or nine members.

In the Pizzo era, on average, 20 promotions were carried out each year. From July 1996 through October 1999, of 60 promoted faculty, 51% were promoted

TABLE 9   Membership on the Pediatric Promotions Committees 1996–2007

Pizza Era	Fleisher Era
Committee on Academic Appointments and Promotions	
Philip Pizzo*	Gary Fleisher*
Frederick Lovejoy**	Frederick Lovejoy**
Merton Bernfield	Mary Clark
Gary Fleisher	Steve Colan
Raif Geha	Jean Emans
Donald Goldmann	Raif Geha
Samuel Lux	Donald Goldmann
Kenneth McIntosh	Richard Grand
Marian Neutra	Joseph Majzoub
Jane Newburger	Kenneth McIntosh
Orah Platt	Marian Neutra
Allan Walker	
Mary Ellen Wohl	
Harvard Medical School Pediatric Executive Committee	
Philip Pizzo*	Gary Fleisher*
Alan Ezekowitz***	Alan Ezekowitz***
Frederick Lovejoy**	Ronald Kleinman***
Lewis Holmes	Frederick Lovejoy**
Stuart Orkin	Lewis Holmes
	Samuel Lux
Fred Rosen	Joseph Majzoub
Allan Walker	Jane Newburger
	Fred Rosen
	Allan Walker
	Howard Weinstein

* Chair (Children's Hospital)

** Executive Secretary

*** Chair (Massachusetts General Hospital)

by Investigator criteria, 42% by Clinician Teacher criteria, 3% by Longer Service criteria and 4% by Academic Part-time criteria. Eight were promoted to professor, 18 to associate professor, and 34 to assistant professor.[8]

Throughout the Fleisher era, from 2001 through 2007, on average each year, 36 candidates for assistant, associate, or full professor were promoted. Of these, 62% were male, 38% female. This stands in contrast with two-thirds of the medical residents at the Children's Hospital being female and one-third being male during the same time period, but with the hope that over time, the number of women promoted will equal the number of men. Of the promotions, 48% were by Investigator criteria, 37% Clinician Teacher criteria, 12% Longer Service criteria, and 3% Academic Part-time criteria. Of the promotions, 66% occurred at the assistant professor level, 22% at the associate professor level, and 12% at the full professor level. Three full professors (Kohane, Pellman, and Schuster) had been prior house officers. From 2007 through 2013, an average of 41 candidates were promoted each year, a reflection of the growing size of the faculty. These figures reflect a greater number of total faculty as well as total number of women faculty promoted each year. They also reflect a commitment to promote clinical as well as research faculty.

In the Fleisher era, nine new Harvard Medical School–endowed professorships were added to the 10 already in existence. The 10 professorships in existence were the Berenberg, Brazelton, Enders, Fikes, Gamble, Nadas, Smith, Stranahan, Prince Turki, and Rotch chairs. Those added were the Egan, Grousbeck, Grupe/Merrill, Janeway, Manton, Nathan, Perlmutter, Rosen, and Scott professorships. The 19 Harvard Medical School professorships as of 2007 as well as the incumbents are shown in Table 10. By 2012, a total of 25 Children's Hospital fully funded professorships existed at Harvard Medical School. Included among the 25 is the first endowed pediatric professorship at Harvard Medical School to honor a female faculty member working at the Children's Hospital, Jane Newburger. She currently holds the Commonwealth Professorship in the Field of Cardiovascular Medicine, established in 2008, but, as established by Harvard University policy, the name will be changed to the Jane Newburger Professorship at the time of her retirement.

The Mary Ellen Avery Professorship in Pediatrics in the Field of Newborn Medicine, established in 2014, was the second chair established at Harvard Medical School to recognize the accomplishments of a female faculty member. This professorship is held by Terrie Inder, chair of the Department of Pediatric Newborn Medicine at the Brigham and Women's Hospital. Additionally, the Mary Deming Scott Professorship was established in developmental medicine in the early 2000s to honor Dr. Scott, a community pediatrician. This professorship is held by Leonard Rappaport, chief of the Division of Developmental Medicine at the Children's Hospital.

In addition, in cooperation with the Children's Hospital, 21 newly named hospital-based chairs within the Department of Medicine at the Children's Hospital were created in 2007. These chairs "at the Children's Hospital" recognized important past and current department leaders and supported a portion of the incumbents' salaries. They were funded by the Department of Medicine, with matching funds from the hospital. The various Harvard Medical School professorships and Children's Hospital chairs and their incumbents are shown in Tables 10 and 11.

TABLE 10   Harvard Medical School Endowed Professorships 1996–2007

Professorships	Incumbents
Berenberg	Frederick Lovejoy/Mark Schuster
Brazelton	Judith Palfrey
Egan Family	Gary Fleisher
Enders	Michael Wessels
Fikes	Stuart Orkin/Nancy Andrews/David Williams
Gamble	Fred Rosen/Raif Geha
Grousbeck	Leonard Zon
Grupe/Merrill	Mohammed Sayegh/Friedhelm Hildebrandt
Janeway	Fred Alt
Manton	Alan Beggs
Nadas	James Lock
Nathan	Stuart Orkin
Perlmutter	Craig Gerard
Scott	Leonard Rappaport
Smith	Merton Bernfield/Stella Kourembanas
Stranahan	David Nathan/Samuel Lux
Prince Turki	Raif Geha/Dale Umetsu
Rotch	Philip Pizzo/Gary Fleisher/Joseph Majzoub
Rosen	Klaus Rajewsky/Yi Zhang

TABLE 11   Children's Hospital Chairs (2007)

Chairs	Incumbents
Avery	Scott Armstrong
Berenberg	Ellen Grant
Bernfield	Yang Shi
Blackfan	Ofer Levy
Crigler	David Ludwig
Diamond	Kenneth Mandl
Grand	Alan Leichtner
Grupe	William Harmon
Gerald	Mira Irons
Levy	Gerald Berry
Lux	George Daley
Masland	Jean Emans
McIntosh	Richard Malley
Modell	Luigi Notarangelo
Schwachman	Wayne Lencer
Richard Scott	Charles Nelson
Wohl	Gary Visner
Department of Medicine Chairs	William Barbaresi/Richard Bachur/Isaac Kohane/Louis Kunkel

Harvard Medical School and its Affiliated Hospitals

Central to the issue of promotions is the complex but pivotal relationship between Harvard Medical School and its affiliated teaching hospitals. The core mission of the medical school is education while for a hospital it is patient care. Both consider research to be a central mission. The medical school is ultimately responsible through its dean to the university president and its governing boards, just as the hospital's department chairs and president are responsible to their board of trustees. The governing boards have important fiduciary responsibilities for their respective institutions.

In the current era these two institutions are closely intertwined. The medical school depends on the hospital and its patients for the education of its students. The teaching hospitals, in turn, depend on the medical school for the stature and prestige resulting from their mutual association, thereby enhancing their research, education, clinical care, and fundraising initiatives. In addition, a Harvard Medical School appointment is an important incentive for successful recruitment of faculty. The institutions are thus highly dependent on each other. They are in fact synergistic, although at times, they do compete with each other. The hospitals must also compete with each other for patients and sometimes for faculty, and it is often the medical school and its dean who are critical in lessening this competition.

The faculty have two lines of reporting responsibility, one through the hospital and the other through the medical school. The promotion process is pivotal in this regard. Faculty members derive considerable prestige for their clinical, educational, and research activities as a result of their appointments in the medical school. The promotion process, in turn, serves as a constant stimulus for enhanced faculty productivity and excellence. The importance of a faculty appointment became most apparent in the 1980s when a for-profit hospital chain sought to buy McLean Hospital and terminate medical school faculty appointments. The faculty responded that if this were to occur, they would move to other teaching hospitals, continue their academic appointment, and establish competitive and adversarial relationships. Their action, based primarily on the importance that a Harvard faculty appointment carries, terminated the effort to purchase the McLean Hospital.

The relationship of the Harvard Medical School and its teaching hospitals is critical to the success of the entire medical enterprise. The "power of the appointment" for a faculty member is the outward sign of that relationship. While complex to manage, in this author's opinion, it is central to the remarkable success and stature of Harvard Medical School and its teaching hospitals. During the Pizzo/Fleisher era, the successful nurturing of this relationship can be attributed to the collegial and collaborative leadership of Joseph Martin. During his tenure as dean, Joseph Martin generously joined by highly capable hospital presidents such as David Nathan and Ed Benz at the Dana-Farber Cancer Institute and James Mandell at the Children's Hospital enabled the medical enterprise at Harvard Medical School to grow from strength to strength.

Department Leadership

Ninth Chair of the Department of Medicine

Returning to his roots of early training as a pediatric resident, following a nationwide search, Phil Pizzo (photo, front of chapter) was appointed in the spring of 1996 as chairman of the Department of Medicine, physician-in-chief at the

Children's Hospital, and the Thomas Morgan Rotch professor of pediatrics at Harvard Medical School. He had come from a first-generation immigrant family and was the first in his family to graduate from high school. His rise to important positions came about as a result of high intelligence, a prodigious appetite for work, and a zeal to address new horizons.

He graduated from Fordham University, cum laude, and then matriculated at the University of Rochester School of Medicine and Dentistry, graduating Alpha Omega Alpha with Distinction in Research. This was followed by three years of residency training, from 1970 to 1973, under Charles Janeway at the Children's Hospital. He then departed Boston for the National Institutes of Health and fellowship training as a clinical associate in the Pediatric Oncology Branch of the National Cancer Institute (NCI). His rise to positions of leadership as head of the infectious disease section and as head of pediatrics, both in the Pediatric Branch of the NCI, was rapid. He was also serving as acting scientific director of the Division of Clinical Sciences from 1995 to 1996, when he returned to Harvard Medical School and the Children's Hospital to head the Department of Medicine. He served in this important role for four and a half years prior to departing to become dean of Stanford University School of Medicine.

His research focused on the diagnosis and treatment of infections in children with cancer, pediatric AIDS, and the immunocompromised host. Pizzo's interest in children with infections began with his third published paper, based on work carried out as a resident and describing 100 children with FUO (fever of unknown origin). His scholarship proliferated rapidly and included studies of fever and neutropenia, causes and patterns of fever in cancer patients, empirical antifungal treatment, and the role of compliance in patient outcomes. His publications on pediatric cancer illuminated the treatment of leukemia and solid tumors. His work also clarified the role of Epstein–Barr virus as a contributing factor in lymphomas.

His interest in pediatric AIDS led Pizzo to carry out the first clinical trials involving antiretroviral therapy. These were followed by studies focused on the efficacies of a number of new therapies (AZT and protease inhibitors). His publication record was prolific, with over 500 papers and two books, *Principles and Practice of Pediatric Oncology*, co-edited with David Poplack and now in its sixth edition, and *Pediatric AIDS: HIV Infection in Infants, Children, and Adolescents*, in its third edition, with Catherine Wilfert as co-editor. Both Poplack and Wilfert had been Children's Hospital house officers.

If research was his focus in Washington, innovations in clinical care, medical education, and hospital administration took center stage in Boston. In clinical care, he set about melding the general medical and subspecialty services into a new firm system that cut across the inpatient, outpatient, and out-of-hospital settings, with local administrative control and direction for both care and education. This restructuring of the Department of Medicine led to significant quality of care improvements, greater integration of the specialty services, improved physician and patient satisfaction, and increases in specialty clinic, emergency medicine, and primary care visits.

His administrative talents resulted in important structural changes in the department. A group of newly appointed vice chairs assumed oversight of clinical care, basic research, clinical research, research development and planning, medical education, and finance. A new inpatient service (CHIPS) was formed. The Elizabeth Glaser Center was formed at the hospital (joining other centers nationally) to support clinical and translational research. All of these changes were announced in the weekly *Physician-in-Chief Newsletter* and distributed to full-time physicians, Enders Laboratories research staff, administrative staff, and community physicians.

Deeply interested in education and advising from his earliest days, he mentored over 90 pediatric trainees in oncology and infectious diseases while at the NIH, including a generous number of Children's Hospital residents. Once at the Children's Hospital, he invested great time and effort in medical education at all levels of training. He contributed immeasurably to the maturation of the Boston Combined Residency Program in Pediatrics, which on his arrival was at its earliest stages of development; fostered a robust Resident as Teacher program; and created new research opportunities, especially for residents and fellows. His concern with the disparity between general hospital and freestanding children's hospital graduate medical education (GME) funding led to his strong advocacy for federal support of training in children's hospitals and ultimately, to legislative support for the Children's Hospital GME Support Act. With passage of this act, funding was mandated for pediatric training programs at freestanding children's hospitals throughout the U.S.

His national prominence grew rapidly during his four and a half years in Boston at the Children's Hospital, with membership in the Institute of Medicine of the National Academy of Science, the Association of American Physicians, the American Society for Clinical Investigation, and the American Pediatric Society. He increasingly assumed national leadership roles that included membership on the board of directors of the Infectious Diseases Society of America and the American Society of Clinical Oncology, as well as the presidency of the

International Immunocompromised Host Society. At Harvard Medical School, he became a faculty dean, with oversight of the most senior academic appointments. His remarkable contributions to academic pediatrics were recognized in 2012, when he was awarded the Howland Medal by the American Pediatric Society.

Phil Pizzo always had a strong interest in the big picture of a medical school and its educational mission. After moving in 2001 to become dean at Stanford, many of his innovations had their conceptual roots in Boston. They included integration of basic and patient-oriented science throughout the four-year curriculum, a medical school scholarly project requirement, and joint degree programs (MD and MBA, JD and MA in education) involving Stanford University's several schools.[9,10] As dean, he continued to make clinical rounds in pediatrics, and the *Physician-in-Chief Newsletter* now became *The Dean's Newsletter*.

Dr. Pizzo's tenure as chief was among the briefest of the hospital's 10 physician-in-chiefs (only Oscar Schloss' and Richard Smith's were shorter). It was during his leadership of the department that David Weiner's long and excellent stewardship of the hospital was coming to an end. It would take time before James Mandell and Sandra Fenwick's distinguished leadership would be fully in place. Turnover and some upheaval in a number of critical departments that were essential for the success of the Department of Medicine, including general surgery and radiology, undermined the primacy of the physician leadership seen in the era of Nathan and Surgeon-in-Chief Aldo Castenada. Managed care and cost containment created major hospital operating deficits, with an adjustment downward of the hospital's bond rating. Reduced departmental revenues led to a period of constriction and downsizing.

Yet, as wonderfully described by his friend and Clinical Chief of Endocrinology Joseph Wolfsdorf, " by dent of strong character and armed with moral fortitude, fidelity to ethical precepts, exceptional intelligence, prodigious energy, dogged determination, and personal warmth," his impact was profound.[11]

Tenth Chair of the Department of Medicine

Gary R. Fleisher (photo, front of chapter) received his BS degree from Pennsylvania State University, summa cum laude. This was followed by an MD degree from Jefferson Medical College and pediatric residency and infectious disease fellowship at the Children's Hospital of Philadelphia. He rose rapidly to the rank of associate professor of pediatrics at the University of Pennsylvania School of

Medicine. In 1986, he was recruited to the Children's Hospital as chief of the Division of Emergency Medicine, a position he held until 2002, when he was appointed chairman of the Department of Medicine and pediatrician-in-chief. In 2008, he was also selected to be physician-in-chief.

Among all of the physicians-in-chief in the hospital's history, two have served as residents at the Children's Hospital (Smith and Pizzo), three trained as residents at Johns Hopkins Hospital (Blackfan, Janeway, Avery), one each trained at the Children's Hospital of Philadelphia (Fleisher) and Kings County Hospital in Brooklyn (Schloss), and one trained in medicine at the Boston City Hospital and the Brigham and Women's Hospital (Nathan). Gary Fleisher was promoted to professor of pediatrics at Harvard Medical School in 1997 and was appointed the Thomas Morgan Rotch professor of pediatrics in 2002. In 2005, he accepted the Egan Family Foundation professorship, with Joseph Majzoub assuming the Rotch professorship.

His area of academic focus was emergency medicine. While in Philadelphia, he co-developed the first academic program in pediatric emergency medicine, co-organized the first pediatric emergency medicine fellowship, and co-edited the first textbook as well as the first journal in pediatric emergency medicine. On coming to Boston in 1986, he established the first program in pediatric emergency medicine at Harvard Medical School and acquired the sole NIH training grant in the United States in the discipline of pediatric emergency medicine. He also became editor-in-chief of *Adult and Pediatric Emergency Medicine*, an online textbook, and a section editor of UpToDate, a vast online reference on topics in adult and pediatric medicine and surgery. Nationally, he was one of eight members of the first certification committee of the American Board of Emergency Medicine.

A prolific writer, Fleisher has published over 200 original articles, reviews, and chapters, as well as 10 books and monographs in emergency medicine and infectious diseases. His *Textbook of Pediatric Emergency Medicine*, co-authored with his Children's Hospital of Philadelphia colleague Stephen Ludwig, is in its sixth edition. He developed a translational research program in bacteremia and sepsis that focused on the pathophysiology, diagnosis, and treatment of common infections. Gary Fleisher defined the spectrum of bacteremia, described the evolution of complications, defined the accuracy of clinical and laboratory abnormalities in early diagnosis, pioneered innovations to prevent disease progression, and analyzed the cost effectiveness of clinical approaches. A second area of focus was the development of emergency response to children impacted by disasters. He led the first pediatric disaster team, which became a part of the Department of Homeland Security, and participated in disaster relief around the bombing at the World Trade Center, the earthquake in Bam, Iran, the earthquake in Haiti, and Hurricane Katrina in New Orleans. He assisted in the widely referenced manual *Advanced Disaster Medical Response* in 2003.

As chief of the emergency department, he set a superb example for his faculty, taking his turn on-call, not only as the division chief but later as chair of the Department of Medicine. He recruited a stellar group of fellows to the division and along with hematology/oncology and endocrinology recruited the top residents from the Boston Combined Residency Program in Pediatrics each year. Of the 89 residents recruited during his tenure of leadership of the Division of Emergency Medicine, 27 (30%) were Children's Hospital residents. A superb lecturer, he was a visiting professor at a large number of academic medical institutions. Important teaching awards came his way, including the coveted Charles A. Janeway Award at the Children's Hospital in 1995. He has also served as a member of many editorial boards.

The growth of the Department of Medicine in the Fleisher era has been truly remarkable, as is shown in Table 12.

This growth was a reflection of the strong economic times as well as Gary Fleisher's great capacity to recruit excellent basic and translational research and clinical faculty. It can also be attributed to his skill in managing a very large budget and wisely recruiting outstanding division chiefs. In fact, total revenue including clinical billings, fees, contracts and grants by 2013 had risen to $202 million, reflecting extremely well on the department, its faculty and its chief.

He was elected president of the Society for Pediatric Research in 1996. Remarkably, in the 82-year history of the society, 25% of the presidents have been Children's Hospital trainees or faculty members, and three department chairs (Drs. Janeway, Avery, and Fleisher) have been selected to serve as president.[12] In

TABLE 12   Growth of the Department of Medicine (Fleisher Era)

	2002	2007	Increase
All Revenue (in millions)	$34	$148	4-fold
(Includes medical fees, professional billings, contracts, and salaries from grants)			
Expenses (in millions)	$30	$116	4-fold
(Includes salaries from clinical revenue and grants)			
Gain (in millions)	$4	$32	8-fold
Total Research and Training Awards (in millions)	$59	$86	0.25-fold

2005, he received the Richard D. Wood Distinguished Alumnus Award from the Children's Hospital of Philadelphia, his prior academic institution. He was also made a member of the Institute of Medicine in 2006. In 2010, he became president of the American Pediatric Society, the seventh Children's Hospital physician-in-chief to be so honored (Rotch, Morse, Schloss, Blackfan, Janeway, Avery, and Fleisher). In fact, a remarkable 28 (or 18%) of physicians who have served as president during this society's 123-year history have been Children's Hospital trainees or faculty.

The years 2001 to 2007, the early years of Gary Fleisher's tenure of leadership, were excellent years for the department and hospital. The hospital was in a period of great stability as a result of the leadership of the board of trustees, CEO James Mandell, and COO Sandra Fenwick. Medicine had entered a period of remarkable growth thanks to the favorable economic climate in the country. The hospital and its satellite centers and clinics were proliferating, with the medical staff growing rapidly to care for the patients in these facilities. Gary Fleisher was the right person with the right skills at the right time for the job. He was a skilled manager who understood finances exceedingly well at a time when medicine was becoming big business. A seasoned clinician, he understood what was needed to deliver efficient and effective clinical care. And as a prior division chief, he knew the culture, the needs, and the inclinations of the divisions.

His style of leadership worked superbly. He listened, delegated well, was a colleague, was egalitarian, and saw his leadership as one of stewardship of the department. He built an esprit de corps in the department and enhanced its image. The financial resources of the Department of Medicine foundation formed during his tenure grew remarkably under his careful stewardship. This allowed him to recruit outstanding division chiefs (Williams, Schuster, Gerard, Walsh, and Lencer), and outstanding scientists (Luigi Notarangelo, George Daley, and Dale Umetsu). His outstanding clinical skills as an emergency medicine physician earned him the broad respect of physicians, administrators, and trustees. Finally, he promoted highly qualified and distinguished faculty at senior academic levels at Harvard Medical School and, in addition, developed a number of new Harvard Medical School and Children's Hospital professorships and chairs.

Division Chiefs[13]

The Pizzo/Fleisher era witnessed a maturing and enlarging organizational structure in the Department of Medicine. The faculty had increased to 435 by 2002 at the beginning of the Fleisher era and rose to 827 by 2007, ultimately exceeding 1,000 by 2012 and necessitating a larger administrative structure in each division. Vice chairs, division chiefs, associate chiefs, and other leadership positions are shown in Table 13.

The position of vice chair was created in 1996, with six vice chairs being named in the Pizzo era and five in the Fleisher era. Prior Children's Hospital house officer trainees included Orkin, Geha, Lovejoy, and Lux in the Pizzo era

TABLE 13   Vice Chairs, Division Chiefs, and Associate Chiefs in the Pizzo and Fleisher Eras (1996–2007)

	Pizzo Era	Fleisher Era
Vice Chairs		
Basic Research	Stuart Orkin/Raif Geha	Samuel Lux
Clinical Research and Health Policy	Steve Sallan	Mark Schuster
Education	Frederick Lovejoy	Frederick Lovejoy
Clinical Affairs	Donald Goldmann	Jean Emans
Research Development and Planning	Samuel Lux	
Finance		Bill Harmon
Administration and Strategic Planning	Sally Andrews	
Division Chiefs		
Adolescent Medicine	Robert DuRant/Jean Emans	Jean Emans
Allergy/Immunology	Raif Geha	Raif Geha
Behavioral Developmental Medicine		Leonard Rappaport
Emergency Medicine	Gary Fleisher	Michael Shannon
Endocrinology	Joseph Majzoub	Joseph Majzoub
Gastroenterology and Nutrition	Allan Walker	Wayne Lencer
Genetics/Genomics	Louis Kunkel	Christopher Walsh/Louis Kunkel
General Pediatrics	Judith Palfrey	Judith Palfrey/Mark Schuster

(continues)

TABLE 13   Vice Chairs, Division Chiefs, and Associate Chiefs in the Pizzo and Fleisher Eras (1996–2007) *(Cont.)*

Hematology/Oncology	Samuel Lux/Steve Burakoff	Samuel Lux/David Williams/Stuart Orkin
Infectious Disease	Kenneth McIntosh	Michael Wessels
Nephrology	William Harmon	William Harmon
Newborn Medicine	Gary Silverman	Stella Kourembanas
Developmental and Newborn Biology	Merton Bernfield	
Pulmonary Medicine	Mary Ellen Wohl	Craig Gerard
Associate Chiefs		
Adolescent Medicine	Elizabeth Woods	Elizabeth Woods
Allergy/Immunology	Linda Schneider/Mitchell Lester	Hans Oettgen
Emergency Medicine	Michael Shannon	Richard Bachur
Endocrinology	Joseph Wolfsdorf/Norman Spack	Joseph Wolfsdorf
Gastroenterology	Alan Leichtner	Alan Leichtner
Genetics	Bruce Korf	Mira Irons
General Pediatrics	Leonard Rappaport/Henry Bernstein/Joanne Cox	Henry Bernstein/Joanne Cox
Hematology/Oncology	Amy Billett/Holcombe Grier/Eva Guinan	Ellis Neufeld/Lisa Diller
Infectious Disease	Sandra Burchett	Sandra Burchett
Nephrology	John Herrin	John Herrin
Newborn Medicine	Ann Stark/Steve Ringer/DeWayne Pursley	Ann Stark/Steve Ringer/Anne Hansen/DeWayne Pursley
Pulmonary Medicine	Andrew Colin/Craig Gerard	Andrew Colin/Henry Dorkin
Other		
General Clinical Research Center	Joseph Majzoub/Mary Ellen Wohl	Richard Grand
Harvard Vanguard Medical Associates	John Graef	John Graef
Firm Chiefs/Hospitalist Service	Joseph Wolfsdorf/Christopher Frantz	Vincent Chiang
Molecular Medicine	Stephen Harrison	Stephen Harrison

and Lux, Schuster, Lovejoy, Emans, and Harmon in the Fleisher era. It is notable that all five of Fleisher's vice chairs (Emans, Geha, Harmon, Lovejoy, and Lux) had been trained as residents under Dr. Janeway. Schuster, Sectish, Leichtner, Chiang, and Finkelstein would be appointed as vice chairs in the later Fleisher years. All had been residents at the Children's Hospital.

Thirteen divisions existed in both eras. The Division of Behavioral and Developmental Pediatrics was newly created, and the Division of Developmental and Newborn Biology was incorporated into the Division of Newborn Medicine in the Fleisher era. Pizzo appointed four new division chiefs (Emans, Wessels, Orkin, and Silverman) and Fleisher seven new division chiefs (Shannon, Lencer, Walsh, Kourembanas, Rappaport, Gerard, and Schuster). Five division chiefs (Emans, Geha, Lux, Silverman, and Harmon) in the Pizzo era and six division chiefs (Emans, Geha, Rappaport, Schuster, Lux, and Harmon) in the Fleisher era had been residency trainees at the Children's Hospital.

As the divisions increasingly differentiated along the lines of clinical care, education, and research and to bolster the growing importance of clinical care, associate chiefs were appointed in all 13 divisions. These leaders oversaw the clinical programs on both the wards and in the clinics and in several cases, were also fellowship program directors. They significantly enhanced the breadth of the contributions from each of the divisions.

Finally, important new senior faculty were recruited into the department. In the Pizzo era they included Kathi Kemper to lead the Center for Holistic Pediatric Education and Research and Michael Grady as vice president for managed care. In the Fleisher era, they included Charles Nelson to lead the research program in behavioral and developmental pediatrics, Morris White to lead the effort in diabetes research, Dale Umetsu to focus research efforts on an understanding of the immune basis of asthma, and Luigi Notarangelo to lead the research program in immune deficiency disorders.

Private Practice Pediatricians

Pediatricians in practice have been a highly influential and valued group of teachers of the housestaff over the department's 125-year history. The nature and location of their practices have varied over the years. And all have given their services to the teaching mission for the privilege of admitting their patients to the hospital, for an academic appointment at the medical school, and perhaps most importantly for the opportunity to interact with bright and talented young trainees. All have served as extremely influential role models for the housestaff, modeling the type and nature as well as the joys and challenges of their practices. Initially, they tended to be solo practitioners. Later, they worked in group practices, in neighborhood health centers in Boston, or even in the delivery of care at a global level. Some tended to alternate between practice and academic work in the hospital. All have exerted a powerful influence over the hospital's young trainees.

In the Rotch/Morse/Schloss era, pediatricians in practice were few in number, with their efforts focused on the well-to-do of Boston. They "visited" for several months each year on the wards of the hospital teaching the residents in the context of the care of the patients. Residents, however, rarely if ever observed them treating their patients in their offices. Hospital-based care was the model, and John Lovett Morse and Richard Smith were superior illustrative examples.

The Blackfan/Smith era saw a new example of practice. The practitioners in this era carried out their academic pursuits as well as their private practice in the community and in the hospital. Many were, in fact, early versions of the triple threat, carrying out care, teaching, and doing clinical research simultaneously. Examples included Louis K. Diamond (hematology), Alexander Nadas (cardiology), John Davies (infectious diseases) and William Berenberg (cerebral palsy). Their knowledge of both general and subspecialty pediatrics was a powerful and admired model for all the housestaff to see.

In the Janeway era, the private practice of pediatrics moved into the community. Pediatricians in practice came to the hospital to see their patients and teach, but they were based in their offices in the community, not the hospital. They taught and demonstrated history taking, physical examination, communication, empathy, and concern. They demonstrated the value of knowing their patients and their families over time. The housestaff, in turn, learned the skills of communication with their patient's physician. They learned respect for the referring physician. Early examples of highly influential and effective practitioners include William Winter in Dedham, Julian Pearlman in Lexington, Ralph Earle in Weston, and Tom Adams in Beverly. Later examples include Alan Nauss in Weston, Norman Spack and John Graef in Brookline, Fred Mandell and Pat Vives in Chestnut Hill, and Gerry Hass in Cambridge. All were greatly admired clinicians and highly effective teachers of the housestaff during the Janeway era and for many years after.

The Avery/Nathan years saw a far smaller number of house officers proceeding into practice. Nonetheless, as superior teachers of the students and housestaff, these practitioners remained highly influential. Examples include Leonard Rappaport, Barbara Seagle, Robert Michaels, Richard Reuben, and Ben Scheindlin.

A renewed interest in pediatric primary care and clinical care commencing in the 1990s resulted in a resurgence in the attractiveness of the practice of pediatrics for the housestaff. This culture was synergized by an enhanced emphasis on ambulatory care in general and subspecialty pediatrics, a recognition of the importance of care and teaching in the academic promotion process as well as the realization by academic hospitals that patient care within the walls of the hospital and its satellites was an important source of much-needed revenue. As a result, superb house officers now began to enter practice, thereby serving as important career models for their younger colleagues. Such examples included Gregory Young at Longwood Pediatrics and Ben Willwerth and Heidi Shaff at Milton Pediatrics. This movement was furthered by many highly admired chief residents entering practice; among them were Kate Jin and Mary Beth Gordon in Milton, Margaret Crawford in Framingham, David Greenes in Needham, Elissa Rottenberg in Newton, and Pearl Riney in Cambridge. The fact that they were all highly seasoned and skilled teachers and found great joy in their work consistent with family lifestyles was clearly evident to the housestaff. Some also entered neighborhood health centers and managed care organizations, but most found the group practice model with the opportunity to teach both students and house officers in their practices as well as in the hospital to be most compelling.

The majority of these practitioners had been trained in the residency program at the Children's Hospital. As a result, they had great credibility in the eyes of the housestaff and, importantly, knew and had experienced the culture of the training program. These factors significantly increased their effectiveness as teachers of the housestaff, continuing a tradition that has been of significant benefit to the training program over its 125-year history.

National Perspective

From 1995 to 2007, a number of national issues impacted residency training. Initially, three forces were at work: the strong influence of managed care with the subsequent growth in primary care, a crisis in NIH funding and the training of physician-scientists, and an era of cost containment that led to "right sizing" (downsizing) of residencies. The first decade of the 2000s saw three new initiatives that while nationally driven were carried out by the profession, the accrediting bodies (ACGME), and the residencies themselves: new resident work hours with the subsequent need for redesign of the workforce; a new emphasis on monitoring of the attainment of resident competencies; and finally, an enhanced focus on and concern with professionalism.

Right Sizing in the 1990s and Redesign in the 2000s of Residencies

The optimal size and makeup of residencies became an important issue in the late 1990s and early 2000s. In the 1990s, it was broadly held that the United States had both an oversupply and a mal-distribution of physicians, with inadequate numbers of primary care physicians in the clinical arena, an overabundance of specialists, and a relative lack of primary care physicians in urban areas. This led to GME reform in the Veterans Health Administration (VA) in 1995, a demonstration project in New York state in 1997, and the nation's Balance Budget and Tax Payer Relief Act of 1997, all of which had the purpose of correcting an oversupply of physicians through incentive payment for those hospitals that voluntarily reduced their number of residents by 20% to 25% over a period of five years.[14,15] These initiatives led to concerted efforts to consider having alternate caregivers (hospitalists, nurse practitioners, clinical fellows) as well as nonteaching ward services deliver patient care. Furthermore, hospitals and medical schools began to consider new ways to educate the resident work force.

A more widespread effort to adjust the distribution of residents in their clinical responsibilities appeared in the early 2000s, over a decade after New York state had instituted house officer work-hour regulations as a result of the Libby Zion case. Following up on the New York experience and the Institute of Medicine report (*To Err is Human*) in 2002, the New Jersey State Assembly approved a bill limiting resident work hours. In 2003, duty-hour requirements were created and operationalized by the ACGME. They included an 80-hour work week or less, one day off per week, a maximum of no more than 24 to 36 hours per shift, and 10 hours off between shifts.[16,17] The rationale for these requirements was based on studies that demonstrated that sleep deprivation increased the number of errors in patient care and created an increased risk for physician car accidents.[17] The movement was reinforced by industries with similar responsibilities for the welfare of the public (airline industry), who had already addressed the public's concern over sleep deprivation and fatigue. While not universally accepted, the duty-hour requirements once in place became the law of the land. Acceptance, compliance, and reengineering of education and care became the next steps in the process.[18]

Concerns raised about the new legislation included the potential loss of continuity of care due to an increased number of handoffs from resident to resident; less clinical experience acquired over the course of a residency; an increased number of patients cared for by a resident, potentially adversely affecting the quality of care; less time in the day available for resident education; increased resident indebtedness because of restrictions on moonlighting; and finally, the potential undermining of a young physician's sense of responsibility for his or her patients because of the imperative to be in compliance with work-hour requirements.[19] To all these concerns was added the admonition of Jeffery Drazen, editor of *The New England Journal of Medicine,* "We risk exchanging our sleep-deprived healers for a cadre of wide-awake technicians."[20]

Hospitals and physicians, however, are highly capable of reengineering in order to adapt to a competitive and cost-conscious market. Already a number of innovations in clinical care have been initiated as an adjustment to work-hour constraints. They include alternate caregivers in place of residents, non-teaching services staffed by hospitalists and attending physicians, streamlined clinical services such as short-stay units, elimination of tasks more appropriately undertaken by non-physicians (transporting of specimens and patients, ordering of tests, collecting results), cross covering of patients by compatible specialty services, night float systems, and finally, reengineered care by new evidence-based handoff processes.[20,21] Reengineering has also occurred with the videotaping of lectures, computer-based teaching, simulation modules to better learn clinical care skills, new methods to learn patient care at the bedside, improved patient handoffs by residents, and new pedagogies to learn basic science.[21] Most importantly, however, have been new ways of thinking. Examples include expert modeling of professionalism by physicians, thereby demonstrating the values of the profession; redesign of the system to optimally deliver care rather than just reduce hours; and "fitness for duty" as a far better paradigm of dedication to patients than "work-created exhaustion."[21]

Professionalism

Launched by the American Board of Internal Medicine in 2002 through its Professionalism Charter Project, the new century witnessed an increased focus on professional behavior in medicine. It was stimulated by a broad recognition that unprofessional behavior by physicians was a major detriment to ethical care of patients by residents and a barrier to the education of students.[22,23] If humanism involved a deep-seated obligation of one human being toward another and professionalism required a way of behaving in accordance with expected values, the passion of humanism synergized a deep commitment to professionalism.[24] Today's increased focus on professional behavior is being implemented in many ways: through a formal curriculum, through role modeling by faculty in their treatment of patients, through greater attention to humanistic values in student and resident applicants, and through creation of an institutional culture that requires monitoring and accountability for professional behavior.[25]

These efforts have been enhanced by the ACGME residency review process and the Liaison Committee on Medical Education medical school accreditation process. Many of the current faculty, as depicted in *The House of God*, were trained in the mid-1970s, when it was believed that doctors needed to be hardened (or in the current nomenclature "depersonalized") to meet medicine's challenges.[26] While debate exists to this day as to the wisdom of the past approach of hardening of physicians, there is growing consensus that this approach in fact makes trainees less empathetic and caring. Fostering professionalism in medical education and care is now an important goal of medical educators.

Competencies

Medical education in the latter half of the 20th century has undergone a paradigm shift, from learning that is structure and process driven to learning that is competency based with measurement of outcomes.[27] This shift has occurred gradually, with its foundation being the six core competencies: 1) patient care, 2) medical knowledge, 3) practice-based learning and improvement, 4) interpersonal and communication skills, 5) professionalism, and 6) system-based practice. A joint effort of the Accreditation Council on Graduate Medical Education and the American Board of Medical Specialties, this focus on competencies has been driven by a growing nationwide expectation of accountability of the profession to the public, with the requirement that competencies be used by each RRC in the process of certifying residency programs in their discipline.[28] The RRCs have also been charged with developing discipline-specific learning objectives that include the necessary tools to assess the meeting of these objectives. Programs, in turn, are expected to assess their residents relative to their obtaining expected competency outcomes. Meeting these goals has been a major focus of all residency and fellowship training programs since the mid-1990s.

Three challenges, however, have arisen. First, the development of appropriate assessment tools to reliably measure the attainment of competencies has been a major challenge. Secondly, focusing on individual domains of competence, rather than observing the performance of a resident caring for the patient (what they do, how they translate and integrate knowledge, whether they do the right thing), may not adequately assure that the resident is a competent physician.[28] Thirdly, the increasing use of computers has moved residents away from the bedside, making assessment of competency more difficult. The process in a fundamental way may challenge medicine's traditional apprenticeship model.[29] Clearly, while competency-based evaluation of residencies is the law of the land, it will undoubtedly undergo adjustments and refinements in the future in the process of meeting its intended goals.

The Boston Combined Residency Program in Pediatrics

Creation of the Program

The culture of the 1990s was one of mergers. Mergers of banks, law firms, and hospitals. The globalization of business also led to mergers outside of the United States. Most were driven by the need to reduce costs, enhance market share, and increase leverage with payers.[30] These goals were particularly evident in the mergers of hospitals and the creation of health care systems. Mergers of residencies and departments in the era of cost containment in the mid-1990s offered the promise of downsizing growing residency staffs and reducing redundancies by combining medical services. Few mergers were predominantly for educational purposes; however, those that did have that intent offered residents the educational benefit of enhanced breadth of patient and faculty exposure, experience with differing styles of clinical practice, and the opportunity to work in different medical cultures. Mergers of public with private institutions, primary and secondary care facilities with tertiary care hospitals, and low-income patients with affluent patients were seen as synergistic in an educational sense, thereby enriching the resident experience. Challenges included the need to resolve conflicts between differing institutional cultures and enlarged size of programs with the potential for decreased resident–faculty collegiality.

In the fall of 1994, Barry Zuckerman (chief of pediatrics at Boston University School of Medicine) and David Nathan (chief of pediatrics at Harvard Medical School) began to discuss the opportunities that might emanate from a merger of the two existing pediatric residencies at Boston Medical Center and the Children's Hospital. The residency at Boston Medical Center needed greater exposure to patients and faculty in the pediatric subspecialties. These opportunities were in abundance at the Children's Hospital. The Children's Hospital, for purposes of training, needed greater exposure to primary care pediatrics, neighborhood health centers, and the ambulatory pediatric faculty who specialized in the care of these patients. In addition, while the large subspecialty faculties and robust fellowship programs found at the Children's Hospital assured excellent resident education, they simultaneously limited resident autonomy in decision-making.

These opportunities were more available on the wards at Boston Medical Center. Thus, a joint program involving a municipal hospital (Boston Medical Center) and a private children's hospital (the Children's Hospital) created a broader and more varied clinical experience, more opportunities for independence and autonomy, enriched career opportunities through enhanced subspecialty educational experiences, and a greater capacity to train broadly educated academic leaders. As stated by David Nathan in January 1995, "By amalgamating our training program with Boston City Hospital [as Boston Medical Center was then known], we open doors of experience to our housestaff that will be invaluable. By creating a larger community of urban primary care faculty, we will create a critical care and research mass in that area that is similar to the mass that we have labored to build in basic and clinical investigation in the Enders Building. From that critical mass will flow the new ideas that we badly need as we face the continued challenges of better health care for the children of Boston."[31] And in the astute view of Rebekah Mannix, a highly talented prior chief resident in the combined residency program and an emergency medicine physician, "The Boston Combined Residency Program came to illustrate wonderfully the medical adage 'See one, do one, teach one.' We saw one at Children's Hospital, we did one at Boston Medical Center, and we taught one at both Children's Hospital and at Boston Medical Center."[32]

Nathan and Zuckerman then turned to the residency program directors of the Children's Hospital and Boston Medical Center, the author and Robert Vinci, respectively, to explore whether such a joint program was achievable and would meet the requirements of the national certifying bodies, the RRC for Pediatrics of the ACGME and the American Board of Pediatrics (ABP). Vinci and Lovejoy, in turn, formed a small planning committee. Steve Pelton, a revered pediatric vice chairman at Boston Medical Center and Chief Resident Jodi Wenger represented that institution, while the Children's Hospital was represented by James Ferrara, a rising leader in hematology/oncology; Jon Finkelstein, the experienced associate residency program director; and Chief Resident Lauren Smith. These individuals met intensively for two months to ascertain the feasibility of a combined program.

By March 1995, they determined that such a program was not only feasible but also highly desirable. A larger planning committee made up of faculty members and chief residents from both institutions with the help of a number of smaller subcommittees, then worked intensively during the spring to submit a plan for the joint program to the RRC in Pediatrics during the summer of 1995. The Boston Combined Residency Program in Pediatrics (BCRP) was so created, with the RRC provisionally accrediting the "Children's Hospital/Boston Medical Center Program" in the fall of 1995. The selection process for new interns began that fall, and the first class of interns started in July 1996. The program was formally reviewed by the RRC in 1998 and received full ACGME accreditation.

The merger led to a training program of 117 residents, 86 from the original Children's Hospital program and 31 from the Boston Medical Center program. A leadership structure of two program directors and two associate program directors (one each from the two institutions) responsible to the two department chairs, a single program (BCRP) with two tracks (categorical and primary care), and a fully integrated program of residents (approximately 39 entering the program each year) characterized the program.

Two separate internship selection committees, one from the Children's Hospital to select interns for the categorical track and one from Boston Medical Center to select interns for the primary care track, were created. The first year of the program (1996–1997) included PL-1s admitted to the BCRP and PL-2s and PL-3s continuing as members of the two separate residencies. In 1997–1998, PL-1s and PL-2s were members of the BCRP, and finally in 1998–1999, all three years were fully integrated into the BCRP. The chief residents initially were independently selected, with two chosen by the Children's Hospital and two chosen by Boston Medical Center. For the 1999–2000 year and thereafter, the four chief residents were chosen from the fully integrated combined program by a joint committee of department chairs, program directors, and chief residents.

The combined residency has thrived up to the current day, at the time of this writing, 19 years. From the thoughtful perspective of Larry Rhein, a chief resident in the program, "the birth of the Boston Combined Residency Program was not a matter of a minor tweaking, it was rather a titanic, macro shift. It wasn't like other residencies, a mother ship and its satellite; it was rather two mother ships acting as one."[33] From its inception, it has undergone constant adjustments in its structure, resident rotations, program innovations, and efforts to enhance its educational quality.

The Merger

The Children's Hospital had considered mergers before 1995. Harvard Medical School had initiated discussions with the intent of joining the pediatric services of the Massachusetts General Hospital and the Children's Hospital. Tufts Medical School and its pediatric facility at the Floating Hospital, had been approached as well as a possible partner. While attractive, these mergers were seen as the joining of institutions with very similar educational goals, cultures, and clinical care philosophies. The departments of pediatrics at the Children's Hospital and Boston City Hospital had also considered merging in the 1980s.[34] The joining of these very *different* cultures was seen as mutually beneficial. These discussions, however, did not come to fruition until the Nathan and Zuckerman discussions of 1994 and 1995. The joining of two institutions with different missions, different cultures, different patient populations, different faculty interests, and different residency goals was seen as educationally beneficial.

At a clinical operations level, much was also different at each institution. The Children's Hospital had services run by service chiefs with their assigned faculty, greater patient volume (beds), and more private and subspecialty patients. Boston Medical Center had fewer beds, predominantly general pediatric patients, and more patients who were to a great extent the responsibility of the housestaff. The Children's Hospital outpatient exposure was heavily subspecialty focused. Boston Medical Center outpatient exposure included a vast array of neighborhood health centers and outpatient hospital clinics that focused on the care of asthma, sickle cell disease and trauma, as well as lead and drug poisoning, the sequellae of abuse of drugs, and diseases associated with poverty. Finally, the teaching milieu was different. The Children's Hospital had a very large faculty with many clinical fellows, which created a rich educational environment. Boston Medical Center also had an excellent faculty and fellows but with different interests and expertise that were clearly complementary to that found at the Children's Hospital.

While the residency merger was extremely complicated and arduous to accomplish, it did not involve the merger of departments or their faculty or the hospitals themselves. Departmental divisions did not combine; no one lost their job; no faculty was incorporated into the other hospital. Still, the merger involved a large change in the underlying culture for the faculty, nurses, and hospital administration of both hospitals. The basic vision and reason for the merger, to enhance the educational experience for the residents, became central in everyone's thinking. It was the sustaining force when the voices of the skeptics at times became loud.

One Program

When Nathan and Zuckerman began to explore a merger of the two residency programs, a single program was an expectation of that action. Less clear were the advantages and disadvantages. The melding of the two very different residencies would not be easy. It would take hours of planning, many meetings, and a careful implementation process. It also risked disenchantment among the residents by altering two existing programs that were widely viewed at both institutions as highly successful. Increasing the residency size risked loss of resident camaraderie and collegiality. The faculty and alumni, in turn, perceived that their residency and its excellence were being placed at risk. Finally, it was also broadly recognized by the leadership that the disparate cultures ran deep in the soul of both institutions and would be difficult to meld together in a combined program. The new program needed to be conceptualized rapidly so as to fit in with the upcoming internship selection cycle. Finally, not known until September 1996 was the fact that the program's conceptual architect, David Nathan, with the credibility to push such a major change through, would precipitously leave to become president of the Dana-Farber Cancer Institute at a time of great challenge for that institution. The Children's Hospital would be led by an interim physician-in-chief (the author) throughout the first year of the combined program.

Balanced against these considerable challenges were important advantages, all educational. Both institutions had a common mission: to train their residents to become highly competent clinical and academic leaders. The increased breadth of patient exposure and the strength of both faculties enhanced the likelihood of success in achieving this goal. During rotations, residents could see different teaching styles and approaches to the treatment of diseases, as well as a different emphasis on research. Also, housestaff with widely varying interests would be offered the opportunity for exposure to an alive and enriching educational environment. Further, the commitment to a single program helped the skeptics to see the final product as the BCRP, not the Children's Hospital or Boston Medical Center program. In short, as was often stated by David Nathan, "one plus one equaled three" in an educational sense.

Two Tracks

The question as to whether to have a single track for the program, a hybrid of one track in the PL-1 and PL-2 years and two tracks in the PL-3 year, or a two-track system was a topic of considerable discussion. In a sense, two tracks had existed with the two prior separate programs, one emphasizing subspecialty pediatrics and the other primary care pediatrics.

A single track with all residents entering the program through a single selection process and all sharing in the same rotations and experiences at the Children's Hospital and Boston Medical Center would solidify and affirm the value of one program. It could be phased in over three years, so those already in the program would not be forced into a program much different than the one originally chosen. It would afford patient, faculty, and ancillary staff exposure to all residents. Finally, residents would not have to pick a track prior to being ready to make such a selection. This model would, however, result in less identification with a given hospital. In addition, it represented a more significant departure from the culture of the prior residencies, and thus was thought to be less easily accepted by most of the faculty and residents at both institutions. This was an important disadvantage.

The second option of a single track in the first two years with differentiation in the third year was a model that leveraged the advantages of both the single-track and the two-track system. It simulated the program at the Children's Hospital, where most were in the program for three years but those interested in primary care could participate in a primary care curriculum in their third year of training. It also simulated the Special Alternative Pathway model, where subspecialty fellowship training (rather than general pediatric training) began in the third year. The greatest concern with this model centered on the fear of residents that they would be forced into primary care or subspecialty track slots to meet service requirements. This was felt to be a serious disadvantage.

Finally, a two-track model was carefully considered. It appeared to be the easiest transition for the housestaff entering from their separate programs into a single program. It maintained valued elements of the past. It was felt to be a more acceptable model for the faculty as well who felt a degree of ownership of *their* residents and valued the opportunity to mold the careers of *their* housestaff. If primary care residents were paid by Boston Medical Center and categorical residents by Children's Hospital, the salary process would also be less complicated. The worry of residents being assigned to a track they did not ultimately want was handled with the decision that the residents could switch tracks if they so wished during their training. This, in fact, rarely occurred. The two-track model was felt to offer the greatest number of advantages and the fewest risks. In the end, this system was adopted, with the tracks labeled primary care (later to be called the urban health and advocacy track in the late 2000s) and categorical.

The educational advantage of a two-track system also proved to be persuasive. The two-track model appeared best for emphasizing diversity in resident interests, enriching curricular opportunities in both subspecialty and primary care pediatrics, individualizing learning for residents with varied interests, and enhancing residents' future career plans. This argument carried the day.

There were several disadvantages. The most important revolved around balancing the goals of a single combined program while also honoring and accomplishing the goals of the two tracks and the residents in those tracks. There was, in addition, the possibility of creating inequality in workload and service requirements, patient exposure, and balance of inpatient and outpatient experience—putting the two tracks in competition with each other. Differences suggested inequality and the risk of one track being better or having an easier workload than the other. These challenges would require the careful attention of the program directors and the chief residents in future years.

The Selection Process

Once the two-track model was chosen, the decision as to whether there should be one or two selection committees came into focus. A single committee with faculty representation from both hospitals had the appeal of enhancing the concept of a single program. It would increase the collegiality of the faculty across the two institutions and still allow them to pick housestaff with interests that mirrored their institution's interests. There would be a single match number. The major difficulty with a single match and two tracks was the assignment by the program of the selected residents to tracks that they might not want. This could lead to great unhappiness, making the risk considerable.

Ultimately, the model with two selection committees—and two match numbers was chosen. The one at the Children's Hospital would be chaired by a Children's Hospital faculty member and would include membership predominantly from the Children's Hospital but with several faculty members from Boston Medical Center. The Boston Medical Center selection committee would have the opposite configuration and makeup. This model was felt to empower the Boston Medical Center and the Children's Hospital faculty to pick residents for the primary care track and categorical track, respectively, to take ownership of their training, and to invest in their careers. An additional advantage important to the residents was two match numbers. This was similar to applying to two different programs, allowing a resident to rank one track and institution first and the other second. Having two match numbers thus increased the chances of being matched in Boston and in the BCRP. In the end, the model of two selection committees seemed to assure assignments of residents to the track that they desired for their career trajectory. In the words of Larry Rhein, "The Boston Combined Residency Program allowed the highest quality people to fulfill their dreams while simultaneously enriching the residency. Where else could you have an academic, research-oriented Scott Armstrong [an oncologist and later director of the Leukemia Center at Memorial Sloan Kettering Cancer Center] and Kevin Strauss [a geneticist and metabolic disease expert] coexisting in synergistic harmony with the primary care–oriented Josh Sharfstein [future public health commissioner in Maryland], and Jack Maypole [chronic disease specialist at Boston Medical Center] to the great benefit of the entire housestaff?"[35]

Commencing with the first internship selection year in 1996, two committees existed, one at the Children's Hospital to select the 26 to 28 categorical residents and one at Boston Medical Center to select the 10 to 11 primary care residents. Throughout the Pizzo era, Bob Masland, longtime and seasoned selection committee chair at the Children's Hospital, and Melanie Kim, greatly admired associate program director and selection chair at Boston Medical Center, astutely led the two committees. In the Fleisher era, the committee at the Children's Hospital was chaired by David Greenes, the associate program director, and then by Samuel Lux, who had achieved an enviable record in the selection of fellows during his tenure as division chief of hematology/oncology. Lux was ably assisted by Celeste Wilson, a devoted faculty member in general pediatrics at the Children's Hospital, who served as associate chair. All three did a superior job in building on the remarkable record achieved by Bob Masland. And all three had the very capable administrative support of Rebecca McKernan and later Elayne Fournier in carrying out their important task. On Melanie Kim's departure, the Boston Medical Center committee chair was assumed by Sigmund Kharash. Finally, a committee chaired by David Ting, director of the Harvard-wide Medicine–Pediatrics Program, selected the eight medicine–pediatric residents.

The selection process for the 1997–1998 class is illustrative of the nature of applicants to the categorical track in the Masland era.[36] The combined program interviewed 241 applicants for the 37 positions (27 categorical and 10 primary care). In total, 20 medical schools were represented, with 11 interns having graduated from Harvard, three each from Johns Hopkins and the University of Pennsylvania, and two each from Yale, the University of Chicago, and the University of Massachusetts. The Masland era of selection was very successful in filling the requisite number of slots at a very low rank number.

The selection process for the 2006–2007 class is illustrative of the nature of the applicants to the categorical track in the Lux era.[37] Of the 28 selected in the categorical track, 14 were PhD or "PhD like" (manifesting significant exposure and experience with research) candidates, 16 were men, 24 different medical schools were represented, and three were non–U.S. citizens. As a reflection of their high quality, 11 had USMLE (United States Medical Licensing Examination) scores greater than 250, 14 were junior Alpha Omega Alpha, and five were summa cum laude graduates from college. As noted by Larry Rhein, "Masland and Lux had a different approach to internship selection; Masland saw a great residency emanating from a collegial class obtained from highly prestigious medical schools; Lux saw a great residency emanating from a focus on selecting highly talented individuals."[38] The Lux era of selection thus reflected a proclivity to select residents from a broader range of medical schools and even foreign medical graduates as well as a desire to select a larger percentage of PhD or "PhD like" candidates with a trajectory toward research-based careers.

The overall track record for the BCRP is outstanding. For a five-year period from 2000 to 2005 from an applicant pool of 4,590 candidates, the remarkably small number of 180, or 4%, were ultimately admitted to the program.[39] Of those selected, 71% were women, 14% were minorities, and 17% were PhD or "PhD like." The Department of Medicine went, on average, down to 61 on the rank list to fill the 28 to 29 categorical slots. These figures are illustrative of the competitiveness of the program. They also illustrate the greater number of women than men, the growing number of minorities, and the greater percentage of PhD or "PhD like" residents taken into the program.

Shared Governance and Committee Structure

From its creation, the combined program modeled shared governance, with the program conceptualized by the two department chairs and formulated in terms of structure and content by a small planning committee of faculty and residents from both institutions. This precedent became the model for the governance of the program going forward.

The concept of shared authority helped to engender a culture of trust, fairness, and transparency among the new partners. The single program necessitated a collegial and collaborative approach. All meetings were co-chaired. All committees had balanced membership from both institutions. Program directors, chief residents, and program coordinators from both institutions were in frequent, often daily, contact solving issues together. Built into the fabric was the concept of giving up something to build something better. This approach allowed for the change from "my" residency to "our" residency.

The leadership learned the wisdom of never being split on issues. A culture was established so that issues would be solved together in a transparent manner.

Educational issues *would* be addressed by the residency program training committee (RPTC), administrative issues by the executive committee. Those issues not solved by these two bodies *would* be resolved by the program directors and, when necessary, by the department chairs. Careful attention to process and fairness became a guiding principle. Trust was created; conflicts were resolved.

Most of the committees used to run the combined program had been in existence in prior years. Consequently, these already effective bodies for governance only needed to be slightly altered in form and function to fit into the new governance structure. Still, several new committees were added, such as the executive committee and resident advisor committee (Figure 1).

The RPTC evolved from the prior residency training committee, begun in the early 1980s at the Children's Hospital. Its purview continued to be residency education. Resident representatives included PL-1s, PL-2s, PL-3s, rising chief residents, and current chief residents from both tracks. Five to six faculty members were also selected from each institution by the department chairs. The associate program directors, the residency coordinators, the internship selection chairs, and the president of the housestaff association were also members. Bob Vinci and Fred Lovejoy alternately chaired meetings, which rotated monthly between the two institutions. Agendas were jointly prepared for each meeting. Minutes were distributed to all housestaff after the meeting. The committee relied heavily on the work of subcommittees and three to five topics were covered at each meeting.

Governance Structure

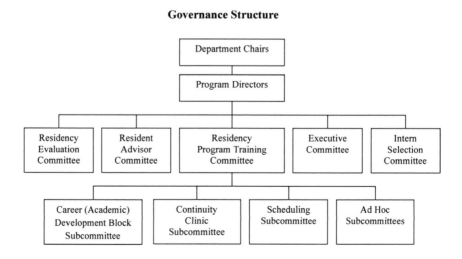

FIGURE I

Subcommittees that persisted over time included the scheduling, continuity clinic, and career development block subcommittees. Ad hoc subcommittees, which were temporary, included among others the work hours, primary care, and competency subcommittees.

The executive committee was established in the first year of the combined program. Its purview was administrative matters, and its membership consisted of the program directors, the chief residents, and the residency coordinators. This committee met monthly, alternating the meeting sites. It used a few standing committees, such as the scheduling subcommittee, to assist in accomplishing its business.

While the resident advisor committee had existed before, the formation of the BCRP program generated a more robust, now combined committee. It was co-chaired by highly respected faculty members from each institution; the chairs from the Children's Hospital were Maureen Jonas, Linda Van Marter, and Betsy Blume and from Boston Medical Center, Elizabeth Barnett. Advisors were selected from both institutions and included clinicians, educators, and clinical and basic science researchers. The 35 to 40 advisors each took on two and three housestaff. They were matched by mutual areas of interest immediately before the start of the internship year. The first meeting occurred during intern orientation and was followed by two or three more meetings spread over the academic year. The role of the advisor was one of counselor and friend, not evaluator. Life as a resident, the balance of work and family life, and career advice were common topics for discussion. Evaluation and feedback were the responsibility of the program directors and the chief residents. Most dyadic relationships were successful. A few were not and necessitated a change of advisors. Each year, an education day for the advisors was held to advance their advising skills.

Evaluations of rotations were completed at the end of the month by the residents, their results aggregated and shared with the rotation directors in an effort to improve the rotations. The aggregated information also proved useful for rotation reviews carried out by the residency program training committee. In addition, the evaluations allowed the residents to evaluate the faculty, offering feedback to improve their instructional style and skills. These important efforts were carefully coordinated by the associate program directors, Melanie Kim and Jon Finkelstein. This information was kept by the department and also proved useful in the promotion process for faculty.

A second type of program evaluation was undertaken once a year through a detailed questionnaire that evaluated educational conferences, clinical rotations, inpatient and outpatient teaching, and the overall strengths and weaknesses of the program. This questionnaire was completed at the spring retreat, the data aggregated and analyzed, and then shared with the residents and faculty. It proved extremely useful for in-depth discussions at RPTC meetings and served as an important information source for long-range planning for the program.

Residents were also evaluated by the faculty at the end of each rotation. The information compiled was viewed as feedback, not as a summative evaluation of their performance. It emphasized resident strengths as well as areas for improvement. These data were filed in each resident's folder (and later online) in the Department of Medicine and were available for review by the residents at meetings with the program directors, which occurred three to four times each year. Each resident had 10 to 12 evaluations each year in his or her folder, offering a reliable analysis of that resident's performance and progress as viewed by multiple faculty. In addition, three times each year a committee of program directors and chief residents reviewed the progress being made by each resident based on these evaluations. These meetings, which were jointly chaired by James Ferrara, an oncologist from the Children's Hospital, and Steven Parker, a child development specialist from Boston Medical Center, proved critical in keeping all of the leadership updated on the progress of each resident. In later years, these meetings were chaired by Susan Parsons and Sandra Burchett on the Children's Hospital side and by Steven Parker, on the Boston Medical Center side. The evaluations for those residents having difficulty were shared with the advisors. If significant problems were encountered of a psychological nature, David DeMaso, a future chair of the Department of Psychiatry, at the Children's Hospital and members of the psychiatry department were called upon for their help.

The evaluation process was serious in its purpose. It required considerable follow-up to be sure that forms were completed, that faculty offered feedback after each rotation, and that a summative evaluation by the program directors occurred on every resident once a year. The data collection mechanism constantly improved during the Pizzo/Fleisher era and was systematized in an important way when computerized data collection became available through the commercially available "New Innovations." The information collected by the evaluation system was also critical for a frank and transparent evaluation of what worked and didn't work in the program. It did much to improve the program.

Appointments, Salaries, and Funding Sources

With all residents in each year working at both hospitals, it was clear that they needed to be appointed and credentialed at both institutions. All residents were also teaching both Harvard Medical School and Boston University School of Medicine students. This led to academic appointments at both medical schools (e.g., teaching fellow in pediatrics at Boston University's medical school and clinical fellow in pediatrics at Harvard Medical School). These medical school appointments afforded many appreciated benefits for the residents, such as the use of the medical school's on-line libraries and physical fitness and athletic facilities.

Once the two-track system was decided on, the source of salary for the residents came into focus, with the conclusion that the primary care–track residents should continue to be paid by Boston Medical Center and categorical track residents by the Children's Hospital. The situation would have been more difficult had a single-payer system been decided on. This was because Boston Medical Center had a well-established housestaff union, which had advocated effectively for resident salaries and benefits over the years. Its considerable credibility had been established in the late 1960s when it successfully staged a "sick in," refusing to discharge patients until union demands of the housestaff were met by the city of Boston. Residents at the Children's Hospital were not part of a union. The decision that the payer of the residents in the combined program would remain as prior to the merger created the challenge of keeping the salary and benefits for all residents equal. Salary levels initially were higher at Boston Medical Center and benefits greater at the Children's Hospital. With concerted effort, the salary and benefits became essentially equal. Maintaining equality of salary and benefits over the subsequent years would, however, continue to be challenging, requiring considerable effort and attention by the program directors at both institutions.

In the early days of the combined program, residents at the Children's Hospital were paid from the hospital's operating budget. This stood in contrast to pediatric services in general hospitals, such as the Children's Service at the Massachusetts General Hospital, where salaries were paid for by Medicare dollars. It was not until 2001 that funding for resident salaries at the Children's Hospital also began to flow from the federal government. Further, the housestaff received a growing number of benefits paid for by each of the departments and hospitals. They included payment for the USMLE examination, one-half of the American Board of Pediatrics certifying examination cost, American Academy of Pediatrics dues, annual hospital bonuses, a travel allowance to attend an academic meeting in the senior year, salary payment during intern orientation, and free pediatric advanced life support, basic life support, and neonatal resuscitation support for these training courses. Additional funding sources from the Children's Hospital for academic pursuits included the Schliesman fund for international travel, Von L. Meyer travel funds, Fred Lovejoy Research and Education Award funds,

Joel Alpert research funds (from Boston Medical Center), and paid travel to a meeting if a resident at any level was presenting his or her work. Finally, by 2007, additional employment benefits included a four-week paid vacation, discounted parking in hospital lots, free weekend parking, discounted public transportation (MBTA) passes, a hospital-based taxi voucher program, and an on-call allowance for the evening meal and post-call breakfast. All of these benefits helped to equalize the salary package (salary and benefits) received by all residents in the program, irrespective of track.

Each department handled the salaries of the program directors and their administrative staff. A final funding question related to ancillary residency costs, for example, retreat costs. It was decided that these costs would be assumed by each department with the split based on the number of residents in each track, a two-thirds to one-third split. Exceptions to this rule were few but included internship selection costs, which were split equally.

It is both remarkable and instructive to consider the growth in housestaff salaries in the relatively short 45-year period since the first such payment occurred in 1961. From an initial intern salary of $10,000 at the Children's Hospital in 1961, this figure increased to $14,000 by the 1970s, to $25,000 by the late 1980s, to $42,000 by the early 2000s, and finally to $50,000 by 2010. Similarly, a senior resident's salary, which had been $12,000 in 1961, rose to $58,000 by 2010, and a chief resident salary, which was $13,500 in 1961, grew to $65,000 by 2010. This progression in salary compensation was critical for attracting bright young students into pediatrics and allowing residents, their spouses, and their families to have a comfortable living style, especially when juxtaposed to long hours and hard work. It also emphasized the necessity of achieving a wise balance between the resident as a student (with a focus on learning) and as an employee (with an adequate salary).

All in all, the payment system arrived at for the combined program, while complicated, proved to be equitable and well accepted by the housestaff. As the hospital's GME office began to exert increased oversight over salaries and benefits in the mid-2000s, even greater attention to the needs of the housestaff came into focus.

Residency Training

Program Leadership

The Boston Combined Residency Program in Pediatrics thrived from 1995 to 2007 under the leadership of Phil Pizzo initially and then Gary Fleisher at the

Children's Hospital and Barry Zuckerman at Boston Medical Center. Barry Zuckerman's wisdom and support as an initial founder of the program was both inspiring and constant. The dedication of Phil Pizzo and Gary Fleisher to the program, having inherited it from their predecessor David Nathan, was truly remarkable. All brought their individual expertise for the betterment of the program: Barry Zuckerman, through his commitment to academic, urban pediatrics, fostered the careers of future primary care leaders; Philip Pizzo, as a medical educator and future dean, fostered important curricular, education, and research innovations; and Gary Fleisher, with his great understanding of how to successfully enhance patient care programs, greatly improved the clinical environment on the wards and clinics to the great benefit of the housestaff. Collectively, these chairs strongly supported educational innovation, research, and scholarship during the residency.

Bob Vinci and Fred Lovejoy served as program directors from 1995 to 2007. Boston Medical Center was Bob Vinci's medical home (Figure 2). He was devoted to the institution and it, in turn, revered and loved him. He had a unique capacity to listen to and connect with housestaff. A former resident and chief resident in the Boston Medical Center pediatric training program, an emergency physician and director of the emergency department, future chair of the Department of Pediatrics at Boston Medical Center and the Joel and Barbara Alpert professor of pediatrics at Boston University School of Medicine, Bob Vinci had a deep understanding of both institutions and the residency program. Fred Lovejoy had served as program director of the pediatric residency program at the Children's Hospital since 1980 and was also deeply committed to its continued success. The two directors formed an inseparable bond at the outset and over the months that followed, developed an operational culture that stood the test of time. In 2007 when Lovejoy stepped down as program director after 27 years at the helm, a search committee was formed to carry out a national search. The committee identified Ted Sectish, a graduate of the Children's Hospital residency program in the late 1970s and a highly respected and successful program director at Stanford as well as a national education leader, to lead the residency program in Boston (Figure 2). He assumed his new responsibilities in April 2007.

Lovejoy, Sectish, and Vinci were fortunate to have highly talented associate program directors, initially Jonathan Finkelstein at the Children's Hospital (Figure 3) and Melanie Kim at Boston Medical Center, and when they stepped down, David Greenes, Vincent Chiang, and Thomas Sandora at the Children's Hospital (Figures 3 and 4) and Richard Goldstein at Boston Medical Center. Jonathan Finkelstein had trained as a resident and served as chief resident in

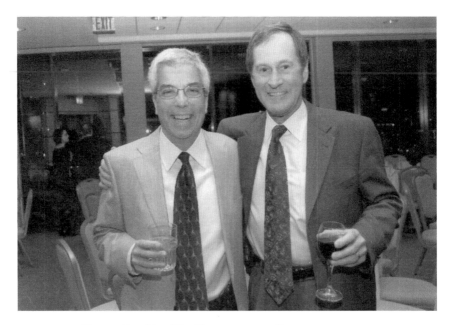

FIGURE 2   Boston Combined Residency program directors
Ted Sectish on the right and Bob Vinci.

the residency program at the Children's Hospital. He was a superior outcomes researcher, and a greatly respected medical educator and future vice chair of the Department of Medicine. Melanie Kim had trained in nephrology at the Children's Hospital and was a highly successful teacher, nephrology faculty member, and service chief prior to moving to Boston Medical Center. In addition to serving as associate program director, she also served as a most successful chair of the internship selection committee at Boston Medical Center. When Jonathan Finkelstein stepped down to assume larger responsibilities at Harvard Medical School and the Department of Ambulatory Care and Prevention, David Greenes was selected to fill this important role. He was a Harvard Medical School graduate, a resident and chief resident at the Children's Hospital, and a highly popular emergency medicine physician. When Greenes left in 2005 to enter private practice, Vincent Chiang, another graduate of the training program, emergency medicine physician, and director of the inpatient services at the Children's Hospital, became associate program director. He brought great expertise in acute-care medicine to the residency, and his leadership of the clinical services in the department served to greatly enhance house officer education. On the Boston Medical Center side, when Melanie Kim moved to UpToDate,

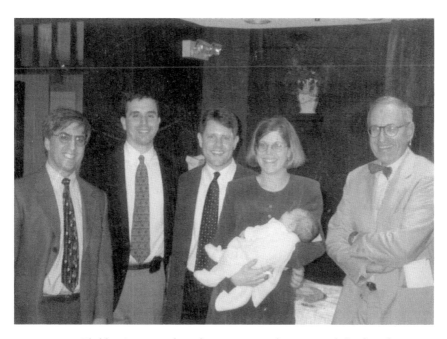

FIGURE 3   Children's Hospital residency program directors and chief residents, circa 2001

From left to right: Program Directors Jonathan Finkelstein and David Greenes; Chief Residents Thomas Sandora and Kelly Cant Wade; and Fred Lovejoy.

an online publication and repository of current medical information, Richard Goldstein was selected by Drs. Zuckerman and Vinci to assume the role of associate program director. Goldstein, a graduate of the residency at the Children's Hospital and an experienced pediatrician with special expertise in behavioral and developmental medicine, wonderfully complemented Bob Vinci's great administrative capacity, interpersonal talents, and acute-care medical skills.

Due to the large size of the program, additional program directors were required. On the Children's Hospital side, Tom Sandora, a Harvard Medical School graduate, resident and chief resident at Children's Hospital, and expert in infection control, became assistant program director with special expertise and responsibility for the house officer's schedule. On the Boston Medical Center side, Bob Vinci recruited James Moses, a University of Chicago School of Medicine graduate, resident and chief resident in the BCRP, and later director of quality and patient safety at Boston Medical Center, to serve as his assistant program director when Richard Goldstein stepped down. The quality of the leadership of the program, the considerable expertise that each brought as medical educators,

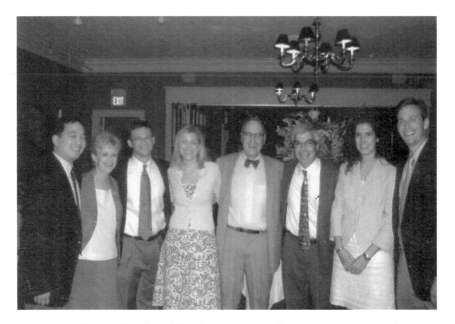

FIGURE 4   Boston Combined Residency program directors, program coordinator, and chief residents, circa 2006

From left to right: Vincent Chiang, Susan Brooks, Chief Residents Michael Gaies and Shaine Morris, Fred Lovejoy, Robert Vinci, and Chief Residents Pearl Riney and James Moses. (Image courtesy of Susan Brooks)

and their love for and deep commitment to the program's success would prove critical.

As the program increased in size and complexity, the need for a talented administrative staff also grew. The program was fortunate to have the highly capable Susan Brooks as residency coordinator on the Children's Hospital side. Susan had assumed her critical role for the Children's Hospital residency 20 years earlier (Figure 4). She brought a deep understanding of the program coupled with an unending energy and commitment to the needs of each and every resident. Maintaining high morale was her domain and she accomplished it brilliantly. Schedules were adjusted to meet family and personal needs. Her door was always open for "her" residents. She was "mother" to the housestaff, with an astute and wise approach that earned her great love and respect. She was joined by a dedicated Shirley Jackson at Boston Medical Center, who similarly knew her institution extremely well and most ably assisted Bob Vinci. Susan and Shirley had very capable help from Lynn Mills at the Children's Hospital and Zandra Spence and Rachael Charles at Boston Medical Center. And behind the scenes at the Children's Hospital making the program run smoothly were Janet Sha-hood for administrative and financial matters, Elayne Fournier for internship selection, and Barbara Roach for resident and program issues. All earned the enduring gratitude of the department chairs and program directors.

Chief Residents

Over the past 50 years, the role of chief resident has undergone significant change.[40] Chief residents in the Blackfan and Janeway eras were the right hand, and the physical presence of the physician-in-chief. They saw the difficult patients for the chief and oversaw the clinical service. As the role of the attending physician grew in importance in the Avery and Nathan eras, this central role of the chief resident gradually changed. The days of the chief resident knowing every admitted patient and roaming the wards at eleven o'clock at night began to disappear. Instead, the chief resident began to take on a larger role in teaching and administration. This role in the Pizzo/Fleisher era would evolve further as more administrative assistants were hired and as the chief resident became a faculty member, assuming attending responsibilities. However, their critical role in education persisted.

Two external forces contributed to changing the role of the chief resident. The first was third-party payment for clinical care (private health insurance, Medicare, Medicaid). This led to the attendings being paid for carrying out their clinical care responsibilities. This trend began in the Avery era and has persisted until today, placing the attending rather than the chief resident in the critical role of supervising and assuring quality of patient care. Secondly, an increasingly active regulatory environment, with its focus on work hours, resident competencies, and a plethora of residency requirements, as promulgated by the RRC of the ACGME and the American Board of Pediatrics, has resulted in the chief resident role becoming highly administrative in nature. Additional support staff helped to lighten these responsibilities, but the growth of administrative and scheduling responsibilities, not always popular, had the risk of reducing the attractiveness of the chief residency position.

The stature of the chief residency has thus changed. In an earlier era, a medical or surgical chief residency was seen as the ticket to an academic career. The chief resident was the "chosen one." Today, while still highly coveted, the perception of its stature is less clear. The department chair and program director view the chief resident's role of educator and clinical leader as more important than the chief residents themselves do.[41] In addition, the department leadership underestimates the amount of time the chief residents spend on administrative matters when contrasted with the chief resident's view. The chief residents generally perceive the acquisition of new skills, the honor of being selected, and the training for an academic carrier as the greatest benefits of the job.

Efforts to correct the deficiencies in the role of the chief resident have led to important improvements, including the hiring of administrative assistants, increasing teaching and clinical time as well as opportunities for research, decreasing the administrative burdens of the job, training rising chief residents in leadership, teaching, and mentoring skills before they assume their new position, and focusing during the chief resident year on skills for future employment as a subspecialty fellow or practitioner. And over the years, the process of selection of chief residents has changed, with less anointing and selection by the department chair, replaced now by encouraging residents to apply for the position and selection by program directors and the current chief residents in addition to the department chair.

Between 1996 and 2007, 44 chief residents were chosen for the Boston Combined Residency Program (Figures 3 and 4) (Table 14).

TABLE 14   Philip Pizzo and Gary Fleisher's Chief Residents (1996–2007)

	Boston Medical Center	Children's Hospital
1996–1997	Christopher DeAngelis, Suzanne Shusterman	Greg Priebe, Lauren Smith
1997–1998	Lisa Scarfo, Jodi Wenger	Laurie Armsby, David Weinstein
1998–1999	Maria Hill, Tram Luu	Ian Davis, Sarah Wood
	Boston Combined Residency Program in Pediatrics	
1999–2000	Robert Graham, John S. Maypole, Andrew Koh, Lawrence Rhein	
2000–2001	Munish Gupta, Elsie Taveras, Thomas Sandora, Kelly Wade	
2001–2002	Lise Nigrovic, Kris Rehm, Joshua Nagler, Paul Lerou	
2002–2003	Elissa Rottenberg, Andrew Shin, Christine Duncan, Rebekah C. Mannix	
2003–2004	Alisa McQueen, Dascha Weir, Katherine Janeway, Katherine Jin	
2004–2005	Jean Raphael, Rebecca Tenney, Margaret Crawford, Mary Beth Son	
2005–2006	James Moses, Pearl Riney, Michael Gaies, Shaine Morris	
2006–2007	Leah Bartsch Mallory, Katherine O'Donnell, Mary Beth Gordon, Amanda Growdon	

For the first three years, the chief residents were selected separately by the Children's Hospital and Boston Medical Center department chairs and program directors. The chief residents worked at the Children's Hospital or Boston Medical Center and assumed primary responsibility for categorical or primary care–track residents, respectively. Commencing in 1999–2000, the chief residents were selected by the leadership from both departments and from the combined program. This process allowed for selection of the chiefs from the entire pool of junior residents and prior to fellowship selection by the subspecialties. The process engendered wide interest in the job and on average, 12 to 13 residents were interviewed each year for the four positions. As reflected upon by Phil Pizzo, "The selection of chief residents was merit based, but we also strove to have a balance of interests and talents among the four chief residents (two each anchored at the Children Hospital and Boston Medical Center). Each of the chief residents I had the pleasure and privilege to work with were remarkable leaders, outstanding educators, thoughtful administrators, and compassionate advocates for the residency program. In fact, more than a third of the residents expressed an interest in becoming a chief resident, which was also a tremendous gift to the program."[42] The selected chief residents then had their senior year to prepare for the job. They watched carefully the leadership characteristics and teaching styles of the chief residents preceding them, gained experience by sitting on the residency program training committee, and often were sent to formal courses of training for chief residency. They began to assume their duties gradually during the several months prior to formally beginning with the new internship class in July of their chief resident year.

Once they began their chief year, they were chief for all the residents in the BCRP, but worked predominately at the Children's Hospital or Boston Medical Center and became institution specific, focusing on rotations and education at their respective hospitals. They divided up their many program responsibilities based on individual areas of interest and expertise. They were in daily contact with each other by phone and met on a regular basis for RPTC, executive committee, and subcommittee meetings. Between 1996 and 2006, four chief residents were selected each year. In 2007 and after, two chief residents were selected by Boston Medical Center and three by the Children's Hospital.

Between 1996 and 2007, of the 44 chief residents selected, 29 (66%) were women and 15 (34%) were men.[43] Remarkably, all chief residents during that 11-year period came from within the program, which speaks to the popularity of the position. Of the 32 (73%) entering fellowship and academic medicine, eight

pursued academic general pediatrics; five, hematology/oncology; four each, neonatology, emergency medicine, and cardiology; two, infectious diseases; and one
each, gastroenterology, toxicology, endocrinology, medical intensive care, and
rheumatology. The number entering academic pediatrics was slightly less than
in the Avery and Nathan years but exceeded the Janeway years. Of the 12 (27%)
entering practice, the majority entered private group practices. All chief residents
served with great distinction and were critical to the success of the program.

The year of chief residency could be demanding. In the words of an astute
Josh Nagler, an emergency medicine physician and chief resident in 2001–2002,
"The plethora of different clinical experiences enriched the menu of opportunities for residents, but it also created significant challenges for the chief residents
in their effort to create equity of clinical experiences among the housestaff."[44]
It could also be most rewarding, as thoughtfully reflected upon by Mary Beth
Son, chief resident in 2004–2005, "Leading senior rounds was certainly one of
the highlights. What an opportunity: complex medical cases discussed by senior
residents and attendings that were so knowledgeable and seemed to have so much
wisdom."[45] In the words of future medical student educator Amanda Growdon,
chief resident in 2006–2007, "The chief residency year was an incredible opportunity for me and I will always reflect warmly on my time as chief. Leading senior
rounds was an unparalleled opportunity to teach, and I learned so much more
than I taught the residents and faculty in attendance. I have taken many lessons
away from the chief year—how to teach a group, how to be an effective leader,
and how to more effectively navigate administrative challenges."[46] And in the
words of Phil Pizzo, "On a very personal basis, each [chief resident] continues to
give me great satisfaction for their personal accomplishments and successes, for
their leadership and charisma, and for their role as present and future leaders."[47]

The Rationale for Rotations

A major challenge for the residency curriculum was how to effectively and
smoothly wed two goals: one, to offer a commonality of inpatient and outpatient rotations experienced by all residents in both tracks, and second, to create
curricular differences such that these differences enriched learning in areas of
interest for residents in each track. This task was made even more challenging
by the need to effectively incorporate new medicine–pediatrics residents with
their specific curricular requirements into the program; to meet the needs of
residents pursuing special programs (Special Alternative Pathway, Accelerated
Research Pathway, Integrated Research Pathway, and neurology, dermatology,

and genetics residencies); and to meet individual curricular and career desires as well as personal needs (part-time residents). This complex agenda required careful balancing of program and individual curricular goals, flexibility among the residents in the achievement of their own goals, and detailed work by the scheduling committee charged with making the program work.

Educational pedagogy suggested the wisdom of differentiation of resident exposure by year of training. It embraced increasing responsibility with each advancing year and strongly supported the value of distributing elective time to enhance individual career goals. Further, the curriculum sought to achieve a more equal percentage of inpatient and outpatient exposure and embraced call-free elective time to allow for international exposure and rotations at other pediatric institutions. The program structure allowed residents to leave after two years of pediatric training to pursue subspecialty interests and saw training juxtaposed to the need to plan families. It fully supported efforts to enhance both in a sensitive and supportive manner. Finally, the program leadership saw the schedule not as a rigid structure that residents had to adapt to but rather, a flexible structure that could bend to meet individual resident career and training goals. "As wisely reflected upon by Josh Nagler, "For a residency training program, standardization is good but excessive rigidity and inflexibility is bad; it stifles creativity."[48]

The program tried to achieve a common core curriculum over the first two years, embracing general pediatrics, neonatology, and emergency room exposure in the first year, subspecialty and more acutely ill patient exposure in the second year, and a more individualized curriculum in the third year, with a heavy concentration of supervisory responsibility and elective exposure. The BCRP sought to achieve differences in the nature of the exposure over three years for each track by requiring one continuity clinic in each of the three years as well as a generous amount of elective time for categorical track residents. For primary care track residents, two continuity clinics in the PL-2 and PL-3 years and a four-month primary care longitudinal block exposure was required. Finally, the program aimed to achieve a relatively equal distribution of time for residents at both hospitals in the first and second year of the program, with the majority of the third year being spent at Boston Medical Center for primary care track residents and at the Children's Hospital for categorical track residents. This was in an effort to enhance a senior resident's supervisory experience as well as the necessary curricular planning and exposure for their future careers.

The combined program sought to increase the richness of the educational experience by emphasizing the strengths of each institution in its rotation offerings. When outstanding strengths existed at both institutions, for example adolescent medicine and behavioral developmental pediatrics, the best educational offerings from each site were kept in the new rotation and the less valuable aspects were eliminated. Movement of residents by day or by week between each site and coordination of the curriculum through joint meetings of the rotation directors were used to enhance the rotation. Evaluations were completed for these rotations by all of the residents in the program, and the rotation directors jointly presented the results to the residency program training committee each year. When different but excellent strengths existed at both institutions—emergency medicine, neonatal intensive care, and general pediatrics—the separate clinical experiences were maintained but coordinated educationally in a complementary way. In some cases, the same experiences were offered but presented at different sites and in a disparate manner, as for example continuity clinic. Finally, when a rotation existed at one site only, for example, endocrinology, cardiology, bone marrow transplantation, oncology, rheumatology, or pulmonary medicine, residents from both tracks were afforded the opportunity for these exposures. This varied use of institutional strengths in fashioning rotations operationalized the rationale for a combined program and significantly enhanced the quality of the rotations offered to the housestaff.

As reflected upon by prior BCRP Chief Resident Rebekah Mannix when considering the nature of the rotations, "But above all, this residency was not a hand holding exercise. Residents were here because they wanted the remarkable experience; they wanted to work hard, be tired, be stressed, and be tested. It also was about the tradition and the legacy of achievement. We didn't want to let down those who had gone before us. We never forgot it was a privilege to be called a Boston Combined Residency Program resident."[49]

The Residents and Rotations

The housestaff size remained stable from 1995 until the mid-2000s, when it began to grow. The number of residents in the categorical track ranged from 77 to a high of 80, with the increase occurring mainly in the PL-3 year to meet residency review committee requirements for supervision. The number of residents in the primary care track remained at 32 until 2006 when it rose to 35. The total number of residents in the four-year Harvard-wide Medicine–Pediatrics Program remained constant at 32 from 1995 to 2007. The overall result, as shown in Table 15, was a stable number of residents in the program at 117 until 2006 when it rose to 123 residents. Residents in the Boston Combined Residency

TABLE 15   Medical Housestaff Statistics

								(Average Number/Year by Decade)						
	1880s	1890s	1900s	1910s	1920s	1930s	1940–1945	1945–1959	1960s	1970s	1980s	1990–1995	1995–2007
Total	2	3	6	8	13	17	12–17	25–30	30–40	50–60	65–70	70–79	117–123*
Male/Female	2/0	3/0	6/0	8/0	13/0	15/1–2	17/0	5%**	10%**	25%**	36%**	50%**	70%**
Chief Residents	0	0	0	0	0	0	0	1–4	2–4	2	1–2	2	4–5

*BCRP excluding eight positions for Medicine–Pediatrics residents

**Percentage of women on the housestaff

335

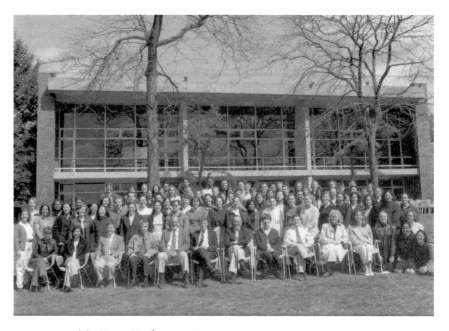

FIGURE 5   The Pizzo/Zuckerman Era, 1998–1999

The Boston Combined Residency Program housestaff. Seated in the front row from left to right: Maria Hill (chief resident), Tram Luu (chief resident), Jonathan Finkelstein, Robert Vinci, Barry Zuckerman, Philip Pizzo, Fred Lovejoy, Melanie Kim, Ian Davis (chief resident) and Sarah Wood (chief resident).

Program are shown in 1998–1999 in the Pizzo era (Figure 5) and in 2004–2005 in the Fleisher era (Figure 6).

The BCRP predominantly used the Children's Hospital and Boston Medical Center for the majority of its housestaff rotations. It used the Brigham and Women's Hospital and Boston Medical Center for the residents' neonatal intensive care and well-baby exposures and the Framingham Union Hospital (later called MetroWest Medical Center) for their community hospital experience. The Beverly Hospital was also used as a second community hospital site for several years. Finally, the Children's Hospital utilized the Martha Eliot Health Center, while Boston Medical Center used as many as 10 neighborhood health centers for continuity clinic training.

The rotations by residency year remained relatively constant throughout the Pizzo and Fleisher years. The PL-1 year rotations offered a sizable exposure to the general pediatric wards, a well-baby rotation, emergency medicine rotations, and subspecialty exposure, including adolescent medicine, cardiology, behavioral and

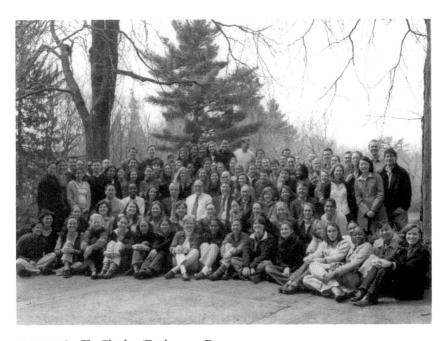

FIGURE 6   The Fleisher/Zuckerman Era, 2004–2005

The Boston Combined Residency Program housestaff. Seated in third row from left to right: Vincent Chiang, Jean Raphael (chief resident), Rebecca Tenney (chief resident), Robert Vinci, Barry Zuckerman, Gary Fleisher, Fred Lovejoy, Margaret Crawford (chief resident), Mary Beth Son (chief resident), and Thomas Sandora.

developmental medicine, and neonatal intensive care rotations. The PL-2 year again saw a generous exposure to the general pediatric wards as well as emergency medicine rotations, intensive care exposure through the pediatric (PICU) and neonatal (NICU) intensive care units, subspecialty inpatient exposure through oncology and bone marrow transplantation rotations, and finally, an ambulatory selective rotation with choice of exposure to endocrinology, gastroenterology, or pulmonary medicine. There was also a community hospital rotation and a month of elective time. The PL-3 year rotations emphasized supervisory exposures on the general pediatric floors, in the emergency department, and the NICU and PICU. Three months were devoted to the Career Development Block, and several months of elective time were also provided. Finally, there were several months devoted to ambulatory subspecialty rotations, including allergy/immunology/dermatology and rheumatology; renal; and neurology exposures. All three years offered a full month of vacation time generally divided into separate two-week blocks.

The Curriculum

Many of the previously constructed teaching sessions at the Children's Hospital remained in place after the BCRP was introduced, and a number of new conferences were also added. They supplemented the daily work rounds and case-based teaching sessions on the wards and in the clinics. The conferences at the Children's Hospital included:

> **General pediatrics teaching conference**—This conference occurred prior to work rounds on the two general pediatric services. Topics covered included general pediatric as well as subspecialty subjects particular to that service (General Pediatrics A—rheumatology, endocrinology, hematology, and toxicology; General Pediatrics B—adolescent medicine, nephrology, infectious disease, and cystic fibrosis). The faculty directed these conferences.
>
> **Grand rounds**—This conference occurred at noon on Wednesdays and was attended by the faculty, fellows, residents, students in the Department of Medicine, and community physicians. This conference provided up-to-date clinical and research information for a large and diverse audience.
>
> **Mini grand rounds**—This weekly discussion at noon on Fridays rotated among the clinical services and focused on recently discharged patients. It was run by the residents and fellows assigned to the services. This conference was highly interactive.
>
> **Core conference**—This didactic conference series occurred weekly and focused on core general pediatric topics. It was attended by residents only and was given by a faculty member.
>
> **Senior rounds**—One of the most popular teaching sessions, this conference was held daily during the week and was attended by junior and senior residents. Different resident-selected faculty members attended each day. The evidence-based discussion was facilitated by the chief residents and focused on the diagnosis and treatment of a recently admitted patient.
>
> **Intern and junior rounds**—These separate weekly conferences specifically focused on the interns and junior residents and were led by the chief residents. General pediatric and subspecialty topics, with an emphasis on decision-making were the focus of these conferences. The rounds were highly interactive.

Basic science journal club—At this monthly conference, a resident selected a basic science article that illustrated a scientific advance with clinical implications and presented it to the housestaff. One or two experts were selected by the resident presenter to contribute to the discussion.

Clinical science journal club—At this monthly conference, a resident selected a clinical research article, discussed issues in study design, and fostered a broad discussion around clinical decision-making. Important lessons learned from the discussion were reinforced by a faculty member.

Ethics conference—This monthly seminar was presented by a resident and focused on ethical issues relevant to pediatric care.

To achieve symmetry in educational offerings for the combined program, Boston Medical Center offered a series of similarly focused conferences, including morning report, core conference lecture series, medical grand rounds, intern rounds, junior rounds, case of the week, and a primary care seminar series.

Another important curricular educational offering was the Resident as Teacher Program. Established by the RPTC in the Nathan era, this program's importance was enhanced with the decision of the Harvard Medical School to formally establish similar programs in each of its affiliated teaching hospitals. The Departments of Pediatrics and Medicine were chosen to lead this effort. The program was further strengthened by financial support from the medical school as salary stipends for the trained faculty teachers. This led to a robust program at the Children's Hospital, with regular teaching exercises involving senior residents instructing interns and interns instructing medical students supplemented by direct faculty observation with immediate feedback. The program was remarkably successful and soon spread with similar but complementary modules to Boston Medical Center and MetroWest Medical Center. Leadership of this program fell to David Greenes and then Josh Nagler, with the assistance of the skilled and talented Janet Hafler, a medical educator from Harvard Medical School.

Housestaff retreats had been offered at the Children's Hospital in an earlier era, focusing on assessment of the program and educational sessions for the housestaff. With the combined program, three retreats were instituted. An intern retreat occurred in September as an overnight affair, away from the hospitals, with the goal of the new housestaff getting to know each other better. This bonding did much to cement camaraderie for an increasingly large intern class (Figure 7). The fall and spring retreats for all three years of the residency used a different format. Planned by the executive committee, they were a day in length, with coverage supplied by the fellows. These retreats had the goal of sharing information with a very large housestaff as well as focusing on ways to improve the program. They were also used to educate the entire housestaff around important skills, such as effective leadership, delivering timely feedback, specific skill certification, and team building activities. Department chairs, program directors, and selected speakers were the only faculty invited to attend, this offering the opportunity for the housestaff to express their concerns frankly at the highest level. They were also an important vehicle for new curricular innovations and change, conceptualized during the retreats but implemented through the work of the RPTC. These retreats did much for morale and were looked forward to greatly each year by the housestaff. Their purpose and value to the housestaff is well reflected in the words of Larry Rhein, "Our retreats were less about solving residency problems; they were all about bonding, listening, appreciating each other and having fun together."[50]

Work-hour restrictions were introduced in 2003. Over the next four years, compliance with the new regulations was taken very seriously. The ACGME residency review process in the mid-2000s emphasized the importance of these requirements. Sporadic monitoring moved to daily monitoring, with the process greatly assisted by computer-based tracking. Rotations that were out of compliance were targeted for corrective action. In addition, the program directors worked with residents who repeatedly exceeded work-hour restrictions. The initial worry was that shortened hours would compromise patient care; this was coupled with the additional concern that resident education would suffer. Adjustments in the rotations and their coverage were the initial approaches taken by the program to address these issues. Over the subsequent years, the program directors would dedicate great effort in accomplishing attitudinal change in the program and the department, specifically that these new rules were the law of the land and the program had to be in full compliance with them. The program also had to adjust and offload some of the residents' less essential tasks so as to be able to both optimally care for their patients and simultaneously be in compliance with the new duty-hour rules.

Gradually, new worries surfaced in the literature and throughout the medical community. Shortened hours with more doctors involved in patient care risked an increase in disjointed care, problems with resident handoffs of information, compromises in continuity of care in the outpatient setting, loss of resident

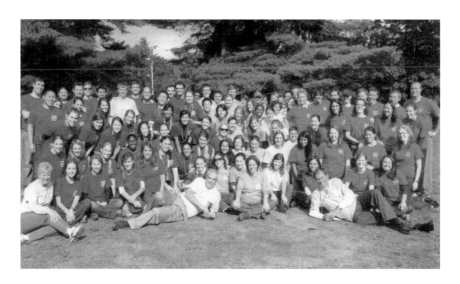

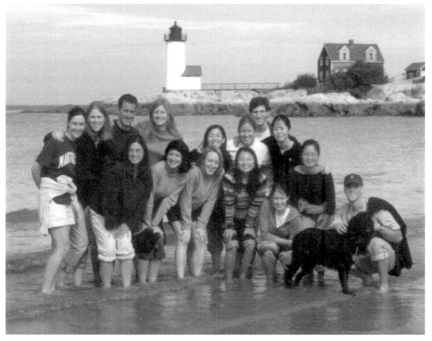

FIGURE 7 Internship retreats

Occurring in September of each year, the retreats were held in Concord and Gloucester (Annisquam), Massachusetts.

autonomy and sense of ownership for one's patient, and finally, an erosion of professionalism.[51] Concerns about adequate time to acquire the knowledge and skills of a competent pediatrician placed a new emphasis on methods and processes involved in resident learning (formal and informal education and resident responsibility for their own learning).[52] While there was some agreement that reduced hours enhanced care by reducing errors, there was also great concern that shortened hours were adversely affecting resident education, with less and less time available to learn an ever growing body of medical information. As the decade came to a close, adjustments in the processes and methods of training residents had become both a local and national focus.[53]

The Medicine–Pediatrics Training Program

The first medicine–pediatrics residency program at Harvard Medical School began in 1991 at the Massachusetts General Hospital (MGH). Soon, a second medicine–pediatrics residency program began in 1994 at the Children's Hospital and the Brigham and Women's Hospital (BWH). A few years later, the two programs merged to form the Harvard-wide Medicine–Pediatrics Program, with 32 residents (Figure 8). Medicine rotations in this program occurred at the MGH and the BWH, and pediatric rotations took place on the Children's Service at the MGH and at the Children's Hospital. This combined program formally began in 1995, with an internship class of eight. Two slots were held for interns rotating at the Children's Hospital in the PL-1 year, four slots in the PL-2 year, and two slots in the PL-3 year. The medicine–pediatrics residents split their first year in pediatrics between MGH and the Children's Hospital, then spent their second year fully at the Children's Hospital, their third year fully at MGH, and their fourth year either at the Children's Hospital or MGH. The program was four years in length and included two full years of pediatric rotations and two full years of medicine rotations, with the acquisition of board certification in both disciplines upon completion.

Lawrence Ronan, a primary care internal medicine physician, was the overall director of the Harvard-wide Medicine–Pediatrics Program with Bob Masland, assisted by Holcombe Grier, a pediatric oncologist trained in medicine and pediatrics, in charge of the pediatric component at the Children's Hospital. When Larry Ronan stepped down in the early 2000s as director, David Ting, a trainee of this same program, was selected to lead it, with Colleen Monaghan (also a former trainee) serving as associate program director and responsible for residents rotating at the Children's Hospital and the BWH.

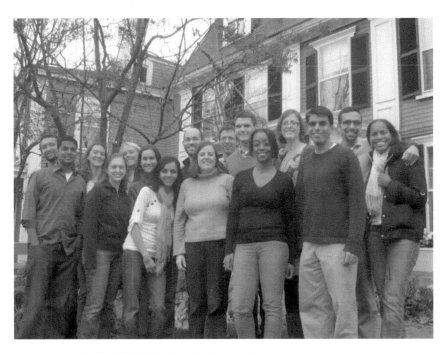

FIGURE 8   BWH/CH Medicine–Pediatrics Program

Medicine–pediatrics residents at the time of a retreat with program directors Niraj Sharma (front row, far right) and Colleen Monaghan (front row, third from right). (Image courtesy of Niraj Sharma)

In 2007, the ACGME required this program to be split into two, a BWH- and Children's Hospital–based program and an MGH-based program. David Ting assumed leadership of the latter, and following a national search, Niraj Sharma, a medicine–pediatrics program director from Miami, was selected as director of the BWH and Children's Hospital (CH) program. And so began the Harvard MGH Medicine–Pediatrics Program and the BWH/CH Medicine–Pediatrics Program.

While complex to integrate from a scheduling perspective, the medicine–pediatrics residents contributed immeasurably to the educational milieu of the residency programs. Their knowledge about adult diseases significantly enhanced the richness of clinical care and conference discussions. In areas of medicine less familiar to pediatric residents, such as anticoagulant therapy and anti-arrhythmia drug therapy, their knowledge was most helpful. The medicine–pediatrics residents, in turn, learned much about pediatric diseases that were increasingly being cared for by internists—inflammatory bowel disease, pediatric oncologic tumors, cystic fibrosis, and congenital heart disease, among others. As reflected upon by Larry Rhein, "The Harvard-wide Medicine–Pediatrics Program joining the Boston Combined Residency Program was a win-win: from them we had learned autonomy, supervisory skills and evidence-based medicine; from us they learned the complexities of pediatric disease and skillful communication."[54]

Medicine–pediatrics programs during this period rode a wave of great popularity, with the result that the residents selected for the Harvard-wide program were of extremely high quality. They also brought a strong interest in primary care as well as international health, synergizing ongoing efforts in both of these areas in the BCRP. The largest challenge for the medicine–pediatrics program was the important requirement to see and care for children and adults simultaneously and at the same site. This was difficult at the adult-oriented BWH and the child-oriented CH, and was partially accomplished at the neighborhood health centers affiliated with both hospitals. Finally, the joint planning around a common mission, involving three different institutions in the Harvard Medical School–affiliated hospital system, did much to enhance a collegial spirit among these intrinsically highly competitive hospitals

Special Pathways of Training

The special pathways of training offered by the American Board of Pediatrics continued throughout the Pizzo/Fleisher era. The Special Alternative Pathway (SAP), which had been used by the residency program most successfully since the late 1970s, continued actively during the Pizzo era but waned rapidly in popularity during the Fleisher era as two new pathways, the Accelerated Research Pathway (ARP) and the Integrated Research Pathway (IRP), began to replace it.[55] Thirteen residents entered the SAP in the Pizzo era. In the Fleisher era from 2001 to 2007, 15 residents pursued the special pathways, four in the SAP, seven in the ARP, and four in the IRP. From 2007 to 2013, two to three residents each year pursued special pathways of training (seven by the ARP, six by the IRP, and three by the SAP).

The ARP was created for residents who wished to pursue academic careers as physician-scientists in a pediatric subspecialty.[56] It involved two years of residency followed by four years of fellowship training. The certifying examination in pediatrics was taken upon completion of two years of residency and one year of fellowship training. Selection of candidates was required to be made by the end of the intern year. The screening examination, used by the SAP, was not a requirement. Rather, selection of candidates by the residency and fellowship program directors based on academic promise and a strong PL-1 ABP In-Training Examination score was necessary. Fellowship directors viewed an additional year of research training as an important and attractive component of this pathway. In the BCRP from 2001 to 2007, three residents pursued the ARP in hematology/oncology, two in neonatology, and one each in endocrinology and in allergy immunology. The ARP proved highly popular with talented young housestaff entering its ranks.

The IRP involved a full year of traditional internship followed by a PL-2 and PL-3 year that was split equally between pediatric residency and research time (usually six months of research and six months of residency time in each year).[57] The candidates, generally residents with MD/PhD degrees, were selected during their internship year. Approval by the ABP was necessary. Candidates for the IRP from the BCRP generally had a prior relationship with a local research mentor and laboratory. In several cases, a laboratory was found during the internship year. The resident's time spent in research was paid for by the involved fellowship or laboratory. Eligibility to sit for the ABP Certifying Examination in Pediatrics required three years of IRP residency and one year of fellowship training. Of the four residents from the BCRP pursuing this pathway from 2001 to 2007, three entered basic research laboratories and one pursued clinical research. Seven publications during training were produced by the four individuals pursuing this pathway. A deep commitment and a track record of success in research coupled with a committed mentor proved to be the most important ingredients for success.

The SAP has been used by the residency at the Children's Hospital to start many house officers on productive academic research careers in pediatric subspecialties. An analysis of 42 residents who pursued the SAP between 1978 and 2000, contrasted with a control group of 97 residents who pursued three years of "traditional" residency training and who were matched by specialty fellowship training during the same time period, demonstrated the success of the program.[58] The characteristics of residents in the SAP included nearly 80% being male and two-thirds having an MD/PhD degree. Two-thirds pursued basic science research during their fellowship. SAP residents achieved assistant and associate professorial rank, their first original paper, their first senior-authored publication, and their first R01 award more rapidly than the traditional residents. In addition, as an indication of quality of scholarship, SAP residents achieved more total original publications, more publications in top subspecialty journals and top laboratory journals, and, finally, more top 10 citations than the traditional residents. Importantly, as judged by "Best Doctor" assignment, there was no difference in perceived excellence as a caregiver between SAP residents with two years of residency training and the traditional residents with three years of training.

Thus, the Children's Hospital residency program prior to 1996 and the BCRP after 1996 used the different pathways offered by the APB both to the advantage of the residents and their careers as well as for the betterment of the residency program. Advantages in the use of special pathways included an earlier return to research for individual residents, the creation of a more dynamic culture of resident-to-resident education because of the diverse scientific interests of the residents, and an enhanced focus on biology and science at all conferences. Minor disadvantages included the missing of the PL-3 year, with its focus on leadership and supervision, and the necessary modification of special pathway resident schedules to meet the requirements of the ABP. In sum, the advantages far outweighed the disadvantages, and the resultant creation of an academic culture during residency training did much to enrich the residency at the Children Hospital.[59]

Research During Residency

A paper in 2003 reviewing the Children's Hospital experience with research carried out during residency suggested the need for research involvement for *all* residents in the program.[60] Similar findings were evident from a survey at a national level, with less than 10% of resident trainees reporting any formal research training or research experience.[61] It might be argued that residency is a time for learning clinical skills. Yet for a program that strives to train future academic leaders, opportunities to learn about and carry out research during the residency years should be fostered. For many who pursued research during medical school, the hiatus of three years of residency without any research exposure was perceived as excessively long and a disadvantage for those committed to research-oriented careers. In the early 2000s, the Accreditation Council of Graduate Medical Education began to require pediatric residency programs to provide a curriculum that fostered residents' knowledge of the basic principles of research while also assuring involvement in scholarly activities by providing resources to support these activities. Simultaneously, the Academy of Pediatrics was advocating education in research methodology for all pediatricians-in-training. Barriers to research during residency were well delineated in the literature and included inadequate protected time, insufficient administrative and financial support, and lack of available mentors.[62] Enhancements had also been clearly described and included a defined, dedicated, mandatory block of time in the curriculum, active support by the departmental leadership, active research mentorship, funding for projects, availability of biostatistical and study design expertise, and informatics resources.[62]

Growing out of a widespread desire among the housestaff for protected time for research and scholarship, the BCRP, in 2003, instituted a three-month required research block in the senior year called the Career Development Block (later called the Academic Development Block).[63] Nine senior residents participated in the block each quarter. The rotation was led by two highly respected senior researchers, Howard Bauchner, who later would become the editor of the prestigious *Journal of the American Medical Association*, from Boston Medical Center and Jonathan Finkelstein from the Children's Hospital. Both had extensive experience in medical education and in clinical research. They were later joined by Sharon Muret-Wagstaff, a quality improvement expert, and still later by Chris Landrigan, an experienced clinical researcher, as associate directors of the rotation. A mandatory curriculum, once a week for three hours (25 hours in total over the rotation) covered such topics as research on human subjects, clinical trial design, literature searches, evidence-based medicine, developing an academic career, preparing a curriculum vitae, writing a grant proposal, issues in health care policy, patient safety and medical errors, and globalization of health care.

The rest of the rotation time was focused on a required scholarly academic project. Residents were also afforded flexibility in elective time to further develop their project. All projects required a faculty member who served as a mentor and development of a project charter with goals for the research endeavor. Residents were encouraged to develop an academic product such as a review article, an educational curriculum, an abstract for presentation at a national meeting, or a manuscript. Rotation evaluation occurred throughout the rotation when residents presented their projects at "works in progress" sessions and at a required final presentation to the rotation directors. Residents had no other responsibilities during the rotation except for continuity clinic and their assigned on-call duties. They emphasized clinical, translational, or outcomes studies and curricular innovations; a smaller number focused on basic science projects. Examples of research projects included protein signaling in malaria, hospitalist management of common pediatric illnesses, use of car seats for newborns, creation of a medical ethics curriculum for residents, and the use of proteomics to discover biomarkers for appendicitis.

The results of these efforts have proven to be quite heartening. A review of seven years of Career Development Block (CDB) experience showed that 50%

of the senior residents completed a clinical project, 25% a project that enhanced their clinical or laboratory skills, 20% an education project, and 5% a basic science project.[64] Overall 36% of the projects met the definition of success, namely a nationally published or presented abstract, a workshop presentation, or a published manuscript. When surveyed, 84% of the seniors rated the rotation as very positive. The strongest components of the rotation included a protected independent learning environment, dedicated research time, and a structured educational experience and curriculum. The factors associated with a successful project included an advanced degree (masters or PhD), an actively involved research mentor, and funding for the project.

As reflected upon by Lise Nigrovic, a clinical investigator and prior chief resident, "What distinguishes this residency program is that it trains a greater proportion of academic leaders. We are well represented at the PAS [pediatric academic society] meetings with resident presentations and resident research awards. CDB, great research mentors, protected time, and research dollars have all helped to create a research climate with an expectation of academic productivity. Exposure to great clinical thinkers helps you to pose the tough questions. The climate of this residency challenges you to ask and answer questions and to go to the evidence-based literature. It is great training for a career as a clinical investigator."[65]

Simultaneously, with the introduction of the Career Development Block, a House Officer Research and Education Endowment was created in 2003 by over 100 alumni of the program, faculty, foundations, and friends of the residency.[66] Led by the department chair, program director, and the hospital's development office, the endowment generates $40,000 to $50,000 of income yearly. Between 2003 and 2010, 68 grants were given, for a total of over $300,000 distributed in aggregate for research projects. Approximately 65% of the submitted projects are funded each year.[67] By 2014, 109 awards had been made with a yearly distribution of $50,000 each year and a total aggregate distribution of $450,000 over 12 years.

Residents apply through a formal application process. All applications require the involvement and support of a mentor. Applications fall into the general areas of clinical, basic, and educational research. A faculty committee reviews and selects the projects to be funded. Supplemental funds from other sources are encouraged. Grants are made in amounts ranging from $2,000 to $6,000. Funds can be spent on laboratory analyses, questionnaires, programmer costs, data analysis, and travel to present at national meetings but cannot be spent for salaries, permanent equipment, or international travel.

When outcomes of the projects that were funded by the House Officer Research and Education Endowment were analyzed, considerable success was evident. Of the 68 research projects carried out between 2003 and 2010, 47 were clinical, 14 basic, and 7 educational in their focus. Mentors were located at the Children's Hospital (44, or 65%), Boston Medical Center (14, or 20%), and other institutions (Massachusetts General Hospital, Harvard Medical School, Dana-Farber Cancer Institute, and Beth Israel Deaconess Medical Center [10, or 15%]). Thirty (44%) of the projects have been published, while an additional 12 (18%) as of this writing were in press.[67] As reflected upon by Lise Nigrovic, "The residents have achieved a remarkably high publication record when contrasted with the size of the funding dollars."[68]

These research projects have garnered a number of awards, including the American Academy of Pediatrics Research Award, The Ambulatory Pediatric Association Young Investigator Award, and the Society for Pediatric Research Resident Award. Additionally, three patents have emanated from projects. A study in 2009 undertaken by Mary Beth Gordon, a former chief resident, found that women resident researchers applying for support from this program tended to ask for less grant money than their male counterparts in applying for research funds. Her results mirrored findings among the women faculty at Harvard Medical School.[69] Once this information was made available to subsequent resident applicants to the fund, the difference between men and women markedly narrowed.

International Health

Since the Janeway era, the residency program has always had a strong interest in international health and the training of physicians from other countries. This interest has its origins in the faculty, specifically with Charles Janeway as a result of his leadership of the International Pediatric Association.[70] The clear intent was to train and send back well-trained young physicians to improve health in both developed and underdeveloped countries. A number of Children's Hospital residents in that era also went on to become outstanding leaders in international health, including Alan Ross, Bob Haggerty, John Rhode, and Stephen Joseph. Distinguished residency graduates of this era included Francisco Tome from Honduras, Mohsen Ziai from Iran, Charlie Phornphutkul from Thailand, and David Lobo from Venezuela.

In the Nathan era, there was a reawakening of interest in international health. By the early 1990s, residents were travelling globally to developing countries on electives to enhance their own education. The electives taken depended on resident interest and often prior exposure during medical school. The death of Paul Schliesman, a house officer in the mid-1980s with strong international interests, resulted in the establishment of the Paul Schliesman Award in 1986, which created travel funds that supported these experiences. These funds were supplemented by the Children's Hospital Von L Meyer Awards for residents and fellows, also in support of travel. These awards are increasingly in demand today.

With the birth of the combined residency program, the international focus further increased with the strong interest and advocacy of the primary care and the medicine–pediatrics residents. Monthly electives used for global travel increased in number. Some residents returned to the same site on multiple occasions during the residency. In addition, group projects were initiated, such as the effort in La Paz, Bolivia, which focused on street children and was led by Chi Huang, a medicine–pediatrics graduate and faculty member at Boston Medical Center. It involved seven to eight members of the intern class each June. A similar opportunity was led by Kim Wilson, a Children's Hospital residency graduate, in the Dominican Republic. A third popular elective was the opportunity to participate in the Indian Health Service in the Southwest with Ship Rock, New Mexico, and Flagstaff, Arizona, being particularly popular. Finally, all these efforts were supplemented by international clinics at the Children's Hospital, Boston Medical Center, and MetroWest Medical Center, where the care of diseases prevalent in foreign countries, such as HIV, tuberculosis, malaria, and typhoid fever was the focus.

During the Fleisher era, the international health effort moved to a new level. In 2004, the Global Child Health Initiative was inaugurated with several important goals, including increasing specialized knowledge, skills, and awareness of global health issues; providing a global health curriculum for all residents; and providing high-quality opportunities for supervised international experiences. Now added were opportunities for research projects and teaching of students and residents facilitated by established partnerships. Such partnership programs, established in Lesotho and Kenya, Africa, were filled monthly by the residents, who provided inpatient, neonatal, and emergency care (Figure 9). Individual residents continued to travel widely to rural primary care sites throughout the world. Continents and countries most commonly frequented included Africa (Liberia, Zambia, Rwanda, Uganda, Malawi, Kenya, Nigeria, Botswana, Lesotho, Zimbabwe, Tanzania), Central and South America (Ecuador, Uruguay, El Salvador, Peru, Guatemala, Honduras, Bolivia), the Caribbean (Haiti, Dominican Republic), and Southeast Asia (Vietnam, Indonesia, Laos).

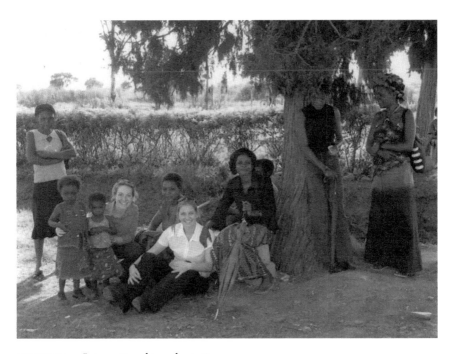

FIGURE 9   International travel rotations

Educationally broadening and highly popular, residents increasingly used electives such as this elective in Kenya, Africa, to supplement their more tradition forms of education in the BCRP. (Image courtesy of Christiana Russ)

Finally, as the result of the leadership of Brett Nelson and Julie Herlihy, primary care residents in the program with extensive experience in global health, the program in 2009 partnered with Boston University to establish the first four-year integrated residency fellowship program. Faculty leadership for all of these international efforts included at Boston Medical Center, Chi Huang, Mark Mirochnick, and Caroline Kistin. Simultaneously at the Children's Hospital, Judith Palfrey, Christiana Russ, and Kim Wilson began a major focus on international health for housestaff, fellows, and faculty with a concentration of effort in partner sites in Haiti, Rwanda, Tanzania, and Liberia.

Evaluation of the Residency

THE PIZZO ERA

As noted before, throughout the Pizzo/Fleisher era, there was a strong focus on the quality of the residency program. This took the form of careful evaluation of the recruitment process, the quality of training during residency, and the achievements of the graduates and alumni of the program.

In 1999 during the Pizzo era, stimulated by budget challenges and the hospital's desire to examine each of its core missions, a working group chaired by Donald Goldmann carefully examined the categorical track and its residents in the Boston Combined Residency Program.[71] The recruitment data showed that the Children's Hospital under Robert Masland selected the best students from the best schools. Among incoming interns, 80% came from the top 10 medical schools in the United States (compared to 40% for other highly competitive residency programs). In addition, 28% of the interns came from Harvard Medical School. Among applicants ranked to match for the 28 available slots in the categorical track, 50% accepted the program's offer, a very strong outcome. The remaining slots were filled by the next 30 or so ranked applicants.

Bright residents would, however, not flourish without an excellent learning environment. Among the program's residents during the Pizzo era, 86% noted the quality of their training to be in the highest category of training: very good or excellent (a similar percentage rated their inpatient and emergency medicine training very good or excellent). Remarkably, 96% of Children's Hospital residents passed the American Board of Pediatrics Certifying Examination on the first try (compared to 82% nationally) achieving a mean score of 560 (contrasted to a score of 500 nationally). Finally 15% of PL-1s, 45% of PL-2s, and 70% of PL-3s exceeded the passing score of 410 on the ABP In-Training Examination *at the beginning* of their PL-1, PL-2 and PL-3 years. The few residents who had difficulty with this examination received careful mentoring and tutoring. Finally, a highly creditable number of residents (32% of the 117 residents) found time to engage in research, this occurring despite an 80- to 90-hour work week. Nearly all indicated they would strongly recommend the program to medical student applicants.

Metrics for retention during the Pizzo era indicated that 97% of incoming interns graduated from the residency, and 80% of a graduating residency class pursued subspecialty fellowships at the Children's Hospital. Remarkably, 50% of the faculty in the Department of Medicine were found to be graduates of the department's residency and fellowship programs. According to data compiled by Don Goldmann's working group, as an example of their outstanding success, although Children's Hospital graduates represent only 1% of all U.S. trainees, among 215 U.S. pediatric departments chairs, 10% had been trained at the Children's Hospital. Additionally, among the top 20–ranked pediatric departments, 30% of the chairs had been trained at the Children's Hospital.

At the same time, the program suffered from a significant degree of physical and psychological stress and sleep deprivation. Notably, in 1998, 94% of residents indicated they had received less than three hours of sleep when on call; 70% felt that lack of sleep compromised patient care; 40% felt that personal relationships outside of the hospital were compromised; and a similar percentage felt that medical errors were potentially due to lack of sleep.[71] These data drew clear attention to work-hour challenges. They highlighted a growing national attention to the need for a limitation in resident work hours.

THE FLEISHER ERA

In the Fleisher era, the faculty and residents continued this focused evaluation of the program.[72] Each year at the spring housestaff retreat, all residents completed a detailed questionnaire with analysis directed by Jonathan Finkelstein. Strengths and weaknesses of rotations, conferences, and the program at large were determined on a yearly basis and a plan for corrective actions formulated to be undertaken by the departments at both institutions and the Residency Program Training Committee.

In open-ended responses to a question asking for the "best things about the program," the most frequently identified assets included (in descending order of frequency): fellow residents, the variety of patients and pathology, and the faculty. Those areas believed most frequently by the residents to be in greatest need of improvement included (in descending order): excessive paper work, difficulty getting to conferences, insufficient opportunities for independent thinking, and supervisory time.

The areas of skill development in the Fleisher era most highly ranked by residents reflected the emphasis on inpatient ward rotations. They included working with ward attendings and consultants, working with patients and families, generating a differential diagnosis, and caring for acutely ill patients. The lowest ranked skill areas, again reflecting the nature of resident exposure during the residency, included interacting with basic scientists, the translation of basic science to clinical care, understanding complementary and alternative medicine, and learning about the care of common orthopedic and surgical conditions. Teaching skills and confidence in one's supervisory capacity improved considerably from the end of the PL-1 year to the end of the PL-3 year, consistent with increased exposure to supervisory roles on clinical rotations.

Those areas of medicine receiving the highest ratings for their quality of training included general inpatient medicine, inpatient specialty medicine, emergency medicine, and critical care medicine. The quality of ambulatory general pediatric and ambulatory subspecialty training was rated somewhat lower. Teaching conferences were generally well-received, particularly senior rounds, intern rounds, firm rounds, core conferences, and team rounds. However, difficulty attending some of these teaching sessions because of clinical responsibilities was a perennial issue.

The mean rating of the overall quality of training, as reported by residents from 2000–2007, was 3.9 [on a scale of 1 (poor) to 5 (excellent)]. The vast majority of residents would recommend the program to an excellent medical student, with a mean response of 3.5 (on a scale of 1 to 4, where 3 indicated "probably yes" and 4 indicated "definitely yes").

Career Directions and Accomplishments[73]

The career direction of trainees from the Boston Combined Residency Program in the Pizzo/Fleisher era clearly met and fulfilled the mission statement of the program, that is to train residents for careers in academic medicine, while also training excellent pediatricians.

When data for the Pizzo period was analyzed, among 109 graduates from 1998 to 2001, 66% entered fellowship while 34% entered practice.[74] When the categorical track residents alone were considered, 72% entered fellowship while 28% entered practice. These data stood in contrast to the Avery, Nathan, and Fleisher eras but not the Janeway era, when practice careers were more common and reflected a nationwide turn towards primary care in the 1990s, only to revert back in the 2000s to numbers more like those seen in the 1970s and 1980s.

When data for the Fleisher period from 2002 to 2009 were analyzed, among 347 graduates, of those pursuing academic careers 80% pursued fellowships or other residencies, 12% became chief residents, and 8% entered the faculty ranks as hospitalists.[75] The remainder (20%) entered private practice, neighborhood health centers, or larger group practices. Of those pursuing fellowship or faculty positions, 80% remained in Boston. The fellowships most commonly chosen (in descending order of frequency selected) included hematology/oncology, emergency medicine, academic general pediatrics, cardiology, neonatology, endocrinology, infectious disease, critical care medicine, and gastroenterology. Of those entering practice careers, a large percentage chose to stay in Massachusetts and New England.

A few differences in these data from previous eras were evident.[76] With the increase in popularity of hospitalist careers in the 2000s, more trainees entered a faculty position prior to pursuing a fellowship or practice. Secondly, several fellowships had become more popular as subspecialty choices, the most notable being emergency medicine. Finally, the national tendency for trainees to stay in the same institution for residency and fellowship training resulted in a large number remaining at the Children's Hospital and in Boston.

While it is less than 20 years since the inception of the Boston Combined Residency Program, its graduates have already achieved significant accomplishments in a diverse number of areas of medicine.[76] To show the breadth of achievement a few illustrative residents will be mentioned. In the area of public health, Joshua Sharfstein was the commissioner of public health in Maryland, Lauren Smith was the medical director of the Massachusetts Department of Public Health, and Patrick Conway was chief medical officer and director of the Office of Clinical Standards and Quality at the Center for Medicare and Medicaid Services. In the area of basic science research, Brian Feldman, Kim Stegmaier, Atul Butte, Joel Hirschhorn, and Loren Walensky were recipients of the Young Investigator Award from the Society for Pediatric Research, and Scott Armstrong and Joel Hirschhorn are recipients of the prestigious E. Mead Johnson Award.

Translational investigation has also thrived, with Kevin Strauss applying genomics to the diagnosis of inherited diseases among Amish children at the Clinic for Special Children in Pennsylvania; David Weinstein has furthered the treatment of glycogen storage disease; Chris Landrigan has importantly advanced our understanding of the association of sleep deprivation and medical errors; and Brian Skotko, through a series of important parental and family questionnaires, has increased our understanding of children with Down syndrome. Peter Weinstock is applying modern concepts of simulation to the care of seriously ill children, and Michael Agus is accomplishing important care innovations in the intermediate care unit at the Children's Hospital.

Tom Sandora and James Moses have applied their education skills to the Boston Combined Residency Program, as associate program directors at the Children's Hospital and Boston Medical Center, respectively. Ellen Rothman continues to apply her considerable literary skills as a thoughtful writer and commentator on health care issues, and Meghan Weir has recorded the life of a pediatric resident in *Between Expectations, Lessons from a Pediatric Residency*.[77] Finally, Gregory Sawicki and Joshua Nagler have achieved recognition as winners of Harvard Medical School teaching awards at graduation.

Residency Life

Highlights of the Residency[78]

The residency program saw many important and memorable events in the 12 years between 1995 and 2007. The Housestaff Association thrived under the leadership of a number of superb leaders, including Ben Willwerth, Sarah Wood, Monica Jones, Nicole House, David Brown, Christine Duncan, Emily Milliken, Christina Ullrich, Christina Miyake, Makia Powers, Stacey Valentine, and Mary Beth Gordon.

The senior resident teaching award was established by the housestaff in 1997 to recognize leadership and educational prowess among each year's senior residents. The housestaff also initiated a number of class projects that served the disadvantaged of Boston, including care for the homeless, a food for hunger program and important work in the public school system. As in prior eras, sons and daughters of past house officers had now became residents in the program, including Larry Rhein, Tanya Geha, Cheryl D'Souza, Christopher Hug, Christopher Landrigan, Cara Pizzo, and Joshua Sharfstein. All had a parent who was a house officer in the Janeway era.

Under the leadership of Larry Rhein, the annual memorial service was first initiated in 1999. Occurring each year in June to remember patients lost in the previous year, it grew from a Department of Medicine initiative to a hospital-wide endeavor under the capable leadership of Kelly Wade, Bryce Binstadt, Christopher Almond, Christina Ullrich, Mary Beth Son, Robyn Byer, and Beth Kaminski. This wonderful program beautifully demonstrates the caring and humane nature of the residents. The housestaff initiated a major effort to renovate the housestaff lounge in 1999 and also worked with the hospital to improve the housestaff sleeping quarters in the Hunnewell Building. The year also ushered in a number of creative educational innovations, including a newsletter and a housestaff manual of instructions relating to the treatment of commonly encountered diseases.

The student teaching awards recognizing both housestaff and faculty were first given in 2000. These awards became a visible acknowledgement of the importance of medical student teaching at the Children's Hospital and also helped to attract intern applicants to a program that truly valued teaching. Educational innovations in that year included a mock code series, a house officer procedure log, and a new emphasis and focus on resident research. Faculty dinners, an important event in past years, were reintroduced in 2001. Led by Monica Jones and in subsequent years by Andrew Shin, Michael Cotter, and Rebecca

Tenney, these dinners included 10 to 15 residents and were held in faculty members' homes. In 2002, housestaff research projects attracted much attention and included the Boston Marathon project (an effort to study fluid and electrolyte imbalance among runners at the end of the event), which resulted in a *New England Journal of Medicine* lead article co-authored by Christopher Almond, Andrew Shin, and Rebekah Mannix and a playground safety project led by Elissa Rottenberg and Martha Perry. Also introduced in 2002 was the house officer publication *Pearls of the Week* as well as the "Intern of the Week" award as morale boosters for PL-1s. Representatives to the Academy of Pediatrics began to fulfill an important liaison role and included Suzette Oyeku in 2001, Joyce Lee in 2003, and Charlotte Moore in 2004. In the early 2000s, the yearly Housestaff Winter Fling continued to be an important part of housestaff life (Figure 10). It featured dinner and dancing with spouses and significant others. Locations utilized for this enjoyable event in Boston included the Harvard Club, the Copley Plaza, and the Lennox Hotel. Leaders in planning the evening included Ann Salerno, Rebekah Mannix, and Catherine Cross.

The year 2003 was notable for the introduction of the Career Development Block, a result of the hard work of Bryce Binstadt and an extremely committed faculty and housestaff education committee. The highly successful basic science journal club, initiated by and under the direction of Samuel Lux, and the clinical journal club, led by Thomas Sandora, were both introduced in 2004. In the same

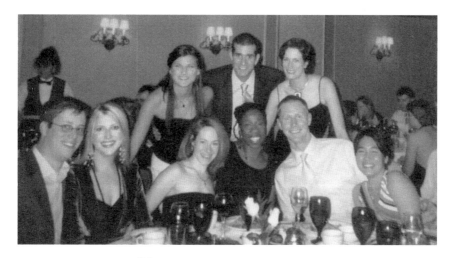

FIGURE 10   Housestaff fling
The Housestaff Winter Fling, an annual and highly popular event. (Image courtesy of the Boston Combined Residency Training Program)

year, the Primary Care Series was introduced by the housestaff. This curricular innovation became extremely popular among both primary care and categorical residents. The first Fred Lovejoy House Officer Research and Education Fund Awards (Table 16) were given in the spring of 2004, synergizing the new research focus and emphasis in the Career Development Block. These efforts resulted in as many as eight to 10 house officer presentations at the Pediatric Academic Society meetings each spring.

Starting in 1999, a robust program of outpatient projects (ACT—Advocacy Clinic Training), emanating out of the continuity clinic experience and

TABLE 16   Fred Lovejoy House Officer Research and Education Fund Award Recipients

2003	Jennifer Cohn, MD
	Patrick Conway, MD
	Amy Fahrenkopf, MD, MPH
	Rani George, MD, PhD
	Christina Ullrich, MD
2004	Manoj Binwale, MD
	Rishi Desai, MD
	Amanda Growdon, MD
	Michael Gaies, MD
	Ward Myers, MD, MPH
	Sallie Permar, MD, PhD
	Lisa Swartz, MD
	Cameron Trenor, MD
	Michael Wei, MD, PhD
2005	Elisabeth Ashley, MD
	Jonathan Brenner, MD
	Andrew Dauber, MD
	Bryan Goldstein, MD
	Farhad Imam, MD, PhD
	Leah Bartsch Mallory, MD
	Andrew Radbill, MD
	Stacey Valentine, MD
	Scott Weiss, MD

TABLE 16   Fred Lovejoy House Officer Research and Education Fund Award
Recipients *(Cont.)*

2006	Samira Brown, MD
	Michael Choma, MD, PhD
	Bryan Goldstein, MD
	Mary Beth Gordon, MD
	David Kantor, MD
	Alex Kentsis, MD, PhD
	Nilesh Mehta, MD
	Allison O'Neill, MD
	Raina Paul, MD
	Sallie Permar, MD, PhD
	Margaret Wolff, MD
2007	Grace Chan, MD
	Michael Choma, MD, PhD
	Amanda Greene, MD
	Alex Kentsis, MD
	Laura McCullough, MD
	Maireade McSweeney, MD
	Tarissa Mitchell, MD
	Leisha Nolen, MD
	Brian Skotko, MD
	Lisa Stutius, MD
	Margaret Wolff, MD

led by Emily Roth, Wanessa Risko, James Moses, and Shaine Morris produced
important experiential learning, individual and group reflection, and resident
involvement in advocacy and community-based activities. ACT projects included
visiting a special needs child, teaching substance abuse prevention, visiting a
legislator on Beacon Hill and special advocacy events such as a voter registration
project and resident and fellow days at the State House. The popular hospitalist
effort under the leadership of Vinny Chiang grew in stature and saw a number
of graduates pursuing a staff attending role after senior residency.

In 2006, the housestaff association introduced the first yearly auction. A
weekend on the Cape, pool parties, and Red Sox and Patriot tickets were all

actively bid on by the hospital community, thereby generating funds for the association. The Frederick H. Lovejoy, Jr. Senior Resident Award, to honor an outstanding graduating senior resident, was established 2006, and the same year saw a number of new education initiatives, including night owl rounds, bedside rounds, and town meetings to both inform housestaff of changes in the program and to capture their input. The very popular housestaff luncheons were also introduced that year.

The housestaff shows continued yearly from 1995 to 2007, with some notable performances, "Gent," "A Reason to Believe," and "Pulp Medicine" (Figure 11). The shows included memorable acts including "Who Wants to be a Pediatric Resident Millionaire," "Send in the Clowns," "Vinci Angels," "Masland Meringue," and "Mock Date." Memorable songs included "Everybody Passes Stool" to "Everybody Plays the Fool" and "Lovejoy Shack" to "Love Shack." Additions to the show's format included the "House Officer Under Appreciated Friend's Award" given to dedicated unit secretaries, page operators, translators, clinical assistants, and cafeteria workers, all individuals who had made house officer life easier. These 12 years clearly had witnessed an important attribute

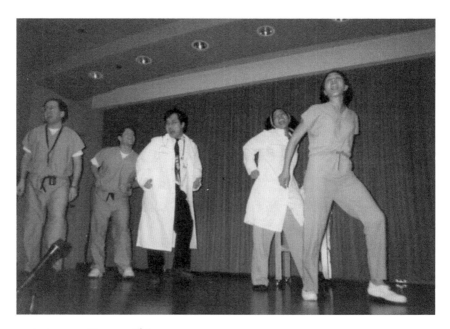

FIGURE 11   Housestaff show

Acting, dancing, and vocal talents on display at the annual housestaff show. (Image courtesy of the Boston Combined Residency Training Program)

of the residents of the Boston Combined Residency Program, the capacity to create and innovate for the training program, for pediatric medicine, for the hospital, and for society.

Awards and Career Achievements

The senior resident dinner (Figure 12), graduation ceremony, and luncheon at the end of each year became an increasingly important event in the life of the hospital and the residency (Figures 12 and 13). Awards were carefully chosen by the housestaff and medical students. They recognized faculty for their teaching contributions and were important in supporting faculty for promotion at Harvard Medical School. To the Farber, Janeway, Margaret Walsh, and Fellow Awards were added the Senior Resident Teaching Award, the Medical Student Teaching Award, and the Frederick H. Lovejoy, Jr. Senior Resident Award. The names of the recipients are inscribed on plaques in the hospital so as to maintain a permanent record of the achievements of the recipients. A description of the various awards listed chronologically from the date of establishment to the present follows.

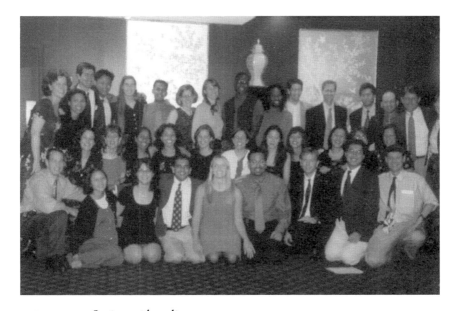

FIGURE 12   Senior resident dinner

Graduates and spouses or significant others gather for a bittersweet evening of memories as they prepare to depart their residency. (Image courtesy of Susan Brooks)

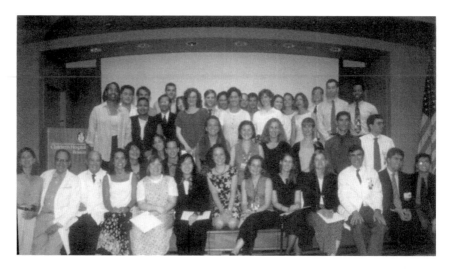

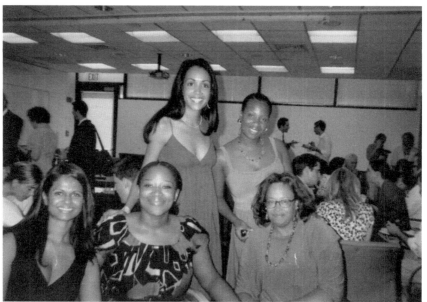

FIGURE 13 Housestaff graduation ceremony and luncheon

Graduation of Boston Combined Residency Program senior residents in the Enders
Auditorium in the Enders Research Building and celebratory luncheon afterward. (Images
courtesy of Susan Brooks)

The Sidney Farber Award continues to be given each year. Established in 1972 to honor Dr. Farber, it "is given each year to a house officer(s) from any department who makes the greatest contribution to the hospital and those principles that Dr. Farber espoused and exemplified." The prize was given until 1992 to any housestaff member in the hospital irrespective of the department in which he or she served. In 1992, the hospital made the decision to give it each year to the chief residents in the Departments of Medicine and Surgery. This approach has been followed from 1996 until the present.

The Charles Janeway Award remains the most prestigious award given to a faculty member. The inscription on the award reads: "The Charles Janeway Award, established in 1978, is presented annually to an outstanding teacher-clinician at the Children's Hospital as selected by the housestaff. The award honors Charles A. Janeway, MD, who served as physician-in-chief at Children's Hospital from 1946 to 1974." Recipients between 1996 and 2007 are shown in Table 17.

This stellar group of clinician-teachers, who were deeply respected for their contributions to the training of residents, included seven past house officers and three past chief residents. Four came from emergency medicine, two each from neonatology, medical intensive care, and hospitalist medicine, and one each from oncology and pulmonary medicine. They also included three division chiefs, four medical educators, and three clinical directors. Forty percent are women; all are predominantly clinicians. The award continues to enjoy the same stature as teaching awards at other Boston institutions, such as the George Thorn Award

TABLE 17   Charles A. Janeway Award Recipients (1996–2007)

1996	Richard Bachur	Emergency Medicine
1997	Steven Ringer	Neonatology
1998	Catherine Perron	Emergency Medicine
1999	Vincent Chiang	Hospital Medicine
2000	Monica Kleinman	Medical Intensive Care
2001	David Greenes	Emergency Medicine
2002	Jeffrey Burns	Medical Intensive Care
2003	Stella Kourembanas	Neonatology
2004	Maureen O'Brien	Oncology
2005	Christopher Landrigan	Hospital Medicine
2006	Debra Boyer	Pulmonary Medicine
2007	Joshua Nagler	Emergency Medicine

TABLE 18   Margaret Walsh Visiting Professor (1996–2007)

1996	Walter Tunnessen
1997	Irwin Redlener
1998	Stephen Ludwig
1999	Harvey Cohen
2000	Paul Wise
2001	Holmes Morton
2002	Frederick Rivara
2003	Robert Blendon
2004	Lewis Goldfrank
2005	Lisa Guay-Woodford
2006	Desmond Bohn
2007	Atul Gawande

at the Brigham and Women's Hospital and the Jerome Klein Award at Boston Medical Center.

The annual Margaret Walsh Visiting Professorship, established in 1985, continues to honor Margaret Walsh, a house officer between 1979 and 1982. Those selected are shown in Table 18.

This group of selected lecturers is remarkable for its diversity of areas of contribution to pediatrics. They all share the ability to teach and mentor residents wisely. Five (Cohen, Wise, Morton, Rivara, and Guay-Woodford) were previous house officers at the Children's Hospital. All had achieved national recognition. Barry Zuckerman, the chair of pediatrics and co-founder of the Boston Combined Residency Program, was selected as the 2008 recipient. In recent years, this lectureship has become an opportunity around which to bring back to the hospital reunioning residency classes.

The Fellow Teaching Award was established in 1992 and "is presented annually by the housestaff to a Children's Hospital fellow who has been an outstanding teacher and mentor." Chosen from among 120 clinical fellows, this prestigious award recognizes not only teaching skills but also commitment to the training of residents. The recipients and their subspecialty focus are shown in Table 19. The list includes six past Children's Hospital house officers, two past chief residents, and two future BCRP residency program directors. Eight different subspecialties are represented.

TABLE 19   Fellow Teaching Award (1996–2007)

1996	Catherine Gordon	Endocrinology
1997	David Greenes	Emergency Medicine
1998	Amy Woodward	Rheumatology
1999	Vincent Wang	Emergency Medicine
2000	Deborah Boyer	Pulmonary Medicine
2001	Peter Nigrovic	Rheumatology
2002	Oscar Benavidez	Cardiology
2003	Bryce Binstadt	Immunology and Rheumatology
2004	Eman Al-Khadra	Medical Intensive Care
2005	Joshua Nagler	Emergency Medicine
	Nilesh Mehta	Medical Intensive Care
2006	Michael Ferguson	Nephrology
2007	Brian Hershenfield	Nephrology

The Senior Resident Teaching Award was established in 1997. "It is presented annually by the internship class to two senior residents who have exhibited outstanding dedication and competence in the education of their interns." The recipients between 1997 and 2007 are shown in Table 20. The explicit intent of this award is to recognize and thank outstanding teachers among the senior

TABLE 20   Senior Resident Teaching Award (1997–2007)

1997	Scott Bateman and Laurie Armsby
1998	Jocelyn Joseph and Stephen Huang
1999	Andrew Koh and Megan Sandel
2000	Grace Lee and Thomas Sandora
2001	James Chattra and Kevin Strauss
2002	Bryce Binstadt and Katie Daley
2003	Maureen O'Brien and Daniel O'Connor
2004	Jean Raphael and Sarah Teele
2005	Patrick Conway and Jennifer Litzow
2006	James LaBelle
2007	Andrew Dauber and Carl Eriksson

residents; the implicit intent is to honor and enhance the stature and importance of teaching within the training program.

The Medical Student Teaching Award, given to residents and faculty, was "established in 2000 to recognized teachers who have excelled in medical student teaching at the Children's Hospital. Each year Harvard Medical School students select the award recipients from among members of the housestaff and faculty." The recipients of this award are shown in Table 21.

This award emphasizes the importance of teaching medical students rotating at the Children's Hospital, whether from Harvard Medical School or medical schools throughout the United States. Boston Medical Center established a similar award in the 1980s; it was renamed to honor Benjamin Siegel, a revered teacher of medical students at Boston University School of Medicine. The first recipient of this award in 1983 was BCRP director Bob Vinci. Recipients of this award from 1996 to 2007 are shown in Table 22. These awards from the two hospitals say much about the importance of medical student education.

TABLE 21   Medical Student Teaching Award Recipients (2000–2007)

	Faculty	Housestaff
2000	Richard Bachur	Christine Duncan
	Clifford Lo	Elliot Melendez
2001	Wanessa Risko	Katherine Janeway
	Christopher Landrigan	Kevin Strauss
2002	Kimberly Lee	Andrew Shin
	Julie Dollinger	Rebekah Mannix
	Peter Lio	
2003	John Watkins	Jennifer Sussman
	Jeffery Lasker	Heather McLauchlan
2004	Samuel Lux	Shaine Morris
	Estherann Grace	Nicole St. Clair
2005	John Cloherty	William Meehan
	Allen Goorin	Melissa McKirdy
2006	Judith Palfrey	Sarah Kim
	Katherine Jin	Emily Willner
2007	Carmon Davis	Nilesh Mehta
	Christopher Duggan	Catherine Humikowski

TABLE 22 Benjamin Siegel Student Teaching Award (1996–2007)

1996	Lisa Scarfo
1997	Jack Maypole
1998	David Brown
1999	Kimberly Stegmaier
2000	Rosandra Kaplan
2001	James Chattra
2002	Peter Lio
2003	Michael Cotter
2004	Pearl Riney
2005	Rishi Desai
2006	Jonathan Brenner
2007	Stacy Cook and Dimitry Dukhovny

In 2006, the Frederick H. Lovejoy, Jr., Senior Resident Award was established. "The award is given yearly at graduation to the outstanding graduating senior resident who has excelled in clinical care, exemplified a commitment to scholarship, demonstrated a compassion and concern for his or her patients and fellow residents, and aspires to be a true leader in academic pediatrics. The award is selected each year by the chief residents in consultation with the Program Directors." The winner in 2006 was Matthew Jolley and in 2007 Sarah Pitts.

Prestigious national awards won by resident trainees in the Pizzo/Fleisher era are shown in Table 23. They predict much about future academic leadership roles for the recipients.

TABLE 23 Young Investigator Award of the Society for Pediatric Research (1996–2015)

2004	Joel N. Hirschhorn
2008	Brian J. Feldman
2009	Loren Walensky
2010	Atul Butte
2012	Kimberly Stegmaier
2014	Sallie Permar
2015	Vijay Sankaran

The constant effort of the Department of Medicine to inspire resident excellence and achievement is best reflected upon by Josh Nagler, "The department asked much of us and they went to great lengths to show their appreciation of our work. They built our self-confidence through housestaff awards, research funds, protected elective time, funds for third world travel, and the year-end graduation dinner."[79]

Summation

In the face of challenging times in academic medicine, Phil Pizzo's accomplishments were significant. First, he was a highly effective advocate and communicator for the hospital and the field of pediatrics in general in Washington. Secondly, he moved the department in new and important ways as a clinical enterprise. This was manifested most visibly in the firm system, which converted wards from age basing to specialty basing and resulted in the introduction of the current hospitalist system and productivity metrics, all of which benefited the education mission of the department. It also placed clinical care on equal footing with research and education in importance. Finally, he became an effective leader of the housestaff, recruiting excellent intern classes and chief residents and strengthening the new BCRP at a critical time in its history. At the time of his departure in 2001 to Stanford as dean, to his great credit, the Boston Combined Residency Program had achieved great stability and respect.

Although this chapter covers events through 2007, as of this writing, Gary Fleisher continues to lead the department with confidence and a steady hand. Among his many achievements, his success with the house staff is particularly notable. A skilled clinician who loves clinical medicine, he has focused assiduously on helping his residents to become excellent pediatricians. With sleeves rolled up, working alongside the house staff, Dr. Fleisher deftly teaches diagnostic assessment and procedural skills. With his vast clinical knowledge of the literature, he is able to offer highly pertinent evidence-based information. He has a fine ability to assess the level of knowledge of his learners and adjusts his teaching to meet their educational needs. Finally, with his residency leaders, Ted Sectish and Sam Lux, he has enabled the Boston Combined Residency Program to continue to grow and flourish.

CHAPTER VIII

Lessons Learned from History

"It was the pervasive understanding—not spoken or overtly
expressed, but somehow understood, that we were being trained to
become pediatricians for sure, but pediatricians who would leave the
field better than we found it. . . . That we were being empowered
from this residency experience to move pediatric medicine forward
in some significant way—no matter what that might mean."

—Jeffrey Burns, reflecting on being a house officer in 1991

IF ONE CANNOT REMEMBER the lessons of the past, one is likely to make the same mistakes in the future.[1] The evolution of the residency at the Children's Hospital, as we have seen, was very much a product of the growth and maturation of both the Department of Medicine and the hospital itself. It was also heavily influenced by professional and public forces external to the hospital. Through its evolution over 125 years, not only is a rich medical history portrayed, but important lessons are learned as well.[2]

Lessons Learned from Each of the Eras

Residency as an Apprenticeship

Residency in the Rotch/Morse/Schloss era (1882–1923) was an extension of the apprenticeship model used in the practice setting and now carried out in the hospital. As we have seen in the 18th and most of the 19th century, trainees learned their trade from physicians by working in their practices. The Children's Hospital, its patients, and the physicians and nurses who cared for the patients from 1882 to 1923 were clearly a further extension of this system. Hospitals saw the residents as useful to the delivery of care. Trainees saw hospitals as valuable for acquiring clinical skills. Learning was predominantly a byproduct of the process of caring for patients. Only in the Schloss era, with the influence of the Johns Hopkins model, did education begin to become a more central part of the patient care process.

Formalized Training and an Educational Curriculum

The Blackfan/Smith era (1923–1946) witnessed an enhanced educational focus in residency training. The faculty grew in number, now with a focus on both research and education as well as care. The number of new illnesses and methods for their treatment also increased. As a result, the number of housestaff grew and their educational needs, the responsibility of the department and its chairman, became increasingly important. These changes augmented the need for a formalized curricular approach to resident education. Expanding knowledge and skills, increasing resident responsibility, and external regulatory forces requiring resident board certification based on their acquisition of knowledge and competency all synergized an enhanced educational focus during the Blackfan/Smith era. The residency model, as we know it today, was fully developed by the end of this era.

Residency with a National and International Impact

The Janeway era (1946–1974) saw a significantly enlarged influence of the Children's Hospital residency, first at the national level and later at the international level. As the number of pediatric departments and residencies grew, the need for new departmental leaders increased as well, a need that the Janeway era admirably filled. In addition, national bodies such as the American Academy of Pediatrics, the Society for Pediatric Research, the American Pediatric Society, and subspecialty pediatric societies facilitated greater interaction across departments and programs. All of these movements enhanced the influence of the Department of Medicine and its trainees.

The Janeway era became known for its remarkable flexibility in the training of residents and its creativity in the designing of tracks to train a very heterogeneous group of house officers. The goal of training now extended from a focus on care and training locally to a national responsibility. To train residents to assume leadership roles throughout the country became a clear goal and as a consequence, the number of residents pursuing an academic focus in their professional careers grew. Janeway, seeing the "world as flat," brought foreign residents to the Children's Hospital for training and then facilitated their return to their countries of origin, thereby allowing for an extension of the influence of the hospital and residency at an international level. In later years, Children's Hospital–trained residents would assume important positions of medical leadership in countries throughout the world.

Residency Program Development with an Academic Mission and Impact

The Avery and Nathan eras (1975–1995) witnessed a new and greatly increased influence of external forces on hospitals, departments, and residencies. The Department of Medicine and the pediatric residency were no exception. The residency during this period defined with remarkable clarity its mission: to train highly competent, research-oriented pediatricians and future academic leaders. The period also saw remarkable growth in the clinical care enterprise, increases in the clinical as well as research faculty, and an enhanced emphasis on patient care—at times at the expense of teaching and academic values. While the size of the residency grew to meet these needs, increases in the number of subspecialty and critical care patients severely taxed residency programs. This challenge augmented an abiding struggle in residency training, that of creating the correct balance between service and education. Simultaneously, scientific research with increased federal funding was fueling the academic enterprise generally to the benefit of the residency program at the Children's Hospital. The enhanced pursuit of subspecialty fellowships and increased use of short-tracking during residency into subspecialties moved the program's graduates increasingly to academic/research careers.

The Avery and Nathan eras would be known for their strong focus on a residency that developed and refined the intake, training, and output of future academic pediatricians. The Avery era, in particular, was remarkably successful in attracting women into the field of pediatrics and enabling research-oriented women to achieve success. The Nathan era, in turn, enabled the residency to become a model for training research-oriented physicians. Its singular focus on a robust curriculum that trained academic leaders became a national model.

Finally, the activism of the 1970s and 1980s laid the foundation for a new focus on the adverse effects of excessive work hours, inadequate pay, and increasing resident stress. In addition, as more and more women entered pediatrics, the clicking biologic clock became a growing issue. Thus, the Avery and Nathan eras clearly signaled a new reality, that no longer could residency training exist in isolation, rather it would be subject to the influences and demands of the broader society.

The Boston Combined Residency Program in Pediatrics

The Pizzo/Fleisher era (1995–2007) of residency training was impacted both by forces external to the hospital and the residency as well as by forces originating within the department and its desire for excellence in the training program. At a national level, optimizing quality of care had become a strong driving force. This was operationalized in residency training through the Accreditation Council for Graduate Medical Education (ACGME) residency review process and through a new emphasis on competency-based training and professionalism. In addition, the long hours a resident was on call had become a national issue leading to shortened work hours and the necessity of redesign of the residency to adequately meet the demands of patient care and resident education. Finally, with medical costs skyrocketing and becoming a national issue, constraints on hospital, medical department, and residency costs became a major factor with which to contend. Clearly, residency training no longer existed in isolation. It had become a national issue.

Internal to the department, forces focused on optimizing the training of a pediatric resident created the Boston Combined Residency Program. This program, to a remarkable extent, was successful in creating the structures necessary to optimally train both the research-oriented academic physician as well as the physician wishing to pursue a primary care career in academic medicine, in practice, in the public health arena, or on the global stage. This multifaceted curricular approach coupled with the diverse interests and passions of the residents it trained served to make the program one of the most sought after of any in the United States. The fact that the program exists today 19 years since its inception offers strong evidence that change based on a sound educational rationale will thrive even in the face of many strong challenges.

Core Elements of Training Program Excellence

The intern match process begun in the 1950s created a powerful incentive for excellence in residency training. The success that a department achieved in the selection process was a clear indication of its relative standing, as measured against other training programs nationally. The selection process also offered choice for applicants; it became an important yard stick of success for hospitals and departments. Attractiveness of the program, excellence in training, and resident success in pursuit of a future career, as a result, assumed great importance for department chairs and program directors as they labored to create an outstanding program. Eight core elements of program excellence will be highlighted in this section.

Clear Vision of the Training Program

Clearly articulated goals are essential for success of a training program. They serve as the compass for the housestaff, the faculty, and the program directors as they fashion the curriculum. They become a guide for day-to-day program decision-making and a means for measurement of a program's success. They strongly influence the type of resident chosen in the selection process and, as a result, the career directions of the housestaff upon graduation.

Breadth of Patients and Faculty

A broad array of patient diseases and a balanced inpatient and outpatient mix, both public and private, advantaged and disadvantaged, and national and international patients, all serve as the critical substrate for educational breadth. With such diversity comes a large and heterogeneous faculty with the expertise and commitment to care for a broad range of patients. A faculty in the aggregate with expertise in clinical care, medical education, clinical and basic research, advocacy, health care policy, and global health all enhance the resident's educational experience, the breadth of their choice of mentors, and their career opportunities. Talented and ambitious young housestaff anxious to learn take full advantage of such rich opportunities.

A Diverse, Talented, and Committed Housestaff

Much education and learning occurs at a peer level, often late in the day or evening when the faculty has gone home. More and more learning occurs in the small group setting in an interactive format where residents teach each other. Diversity of housestaff interest and extraordinary passion and commitment become essential to a great training program, forming the essential substrate for a rich educational experience. A great program should strive to attract future scientists, academic clinicians, educators, and practitioners, all with a deep passion for their areas of interest. Different perspectives and different areas of expertise all synergize the learning process.

A Hospital and Department that Values Education

An academic department rests tenuously balanced on the three-legged stool of care, research, and education. At times, they compete with each other, and external forces often determine whether the stool looks more like a tricycle with one area predominating over the other two. In times of cost constraint, revenue-generating areas are emphasized by the hospital and its trustees. Research-oriented schools will emphasize research and scholarship in their promotion process, with the result being that less time is available for teaching. While medical student teaching is funded through medical schools, and fellowships are funded by federal grants, pediatric resident education does not have as large and reliable a funding source. In addition, high efficiency in patient care can be the enemy of education because resident education is inherently inefficient.

Department heads who are willing to advocate strongly for resident education are essential for a successful program. Their influence on the department is profound. The divisional leadership takes the lead from their chair as to the relative importance that they and their division should place on resident education. The housestaff, while depending on the day-to-day involvement of their program director, value greatly the direction and counsel of their chair in large decisions involving the program as well as their own personal career decisions. Department heads, mobilizing sufficient resources to support program directors and program coordinators in addition to funds for educational programs, resident research projects, and social events, will help to assure a superb educational program while simultaneously enhancing housestaff morale. Finally, resident education being valued at the trustee and hospital administration level is essential for the availability of the necessary hospital resources for training. All will help to assure that resident education is not undervalued.

An Emphasis on Team Care

In an earlier era, the doctor and the nurse worked alongside each other. Each worked in their defined professional area, with the doctor directing most of the decisions. There was a lack of true collaboration. Today, medical care is more complicated and requires a multiplicity of caregivers: physicians, nurses, social workers, pharmacists, and child life specialists. Nursing has, in fact, become so complex that there are nurses with special expertise in emergency care, neonatal and medical intensive care, medical and surgical cardiac care, oncologic and neurological care, and bone marrow and solid organ transplant care. Similarly, not only do the medical residents, subspecialty fellows, and attendings have defined roles, but staff physicians are now highly specialized—oncologist, radiation therapist, surgical oncologist, etc. Each of these players has an important role to play, all working together as a team. No one physician directs all the decisions; it is a shared process.

Clearly, to be well trained, the residents must be exposed to these multiple caregivers. They must learn the team approach in the care of the patient. They must learn communication skills, flexibility in both leading and participating as part of a group process, and skills in coordinating very complex care carried out by multiple caregivers. A training program that emphasizes these important skills will train its housestaff to be competent for medical care in the coming decades.

The faculty in an excellent training program will need to shift their teaching style from one that is predominantly Socratic to one that is more holistic, family centered, patient rather than disease oriented, and mutually respectful of all caregivers. As responsibilities that used to rest with residents are now carried out by other caregivers and as responsibility is owned by the team, residency programs will need to work diligently to maintain a strong sense of house officer responsibility for the care of their patients.

Empowered Implementation and Oversight over Residency Education

The residency review process of the ACGME has led to uniform requirements for program accreditation. The American Board of Pediatrics has similarly defined standards leading to certification of individual residents. To meet these requirements, a residency program must have a clear mechanism for carrying out organized conferences and effective service-based curriculae. The process used to put the curriculum in place will include the active and persistent involvement of the program director(s) and a structure that involves faculty and residents. The program director must be given the authority to create a robust educational curriculum and evaluation system for rotations, the residents, and the faculty. The housestaff and faculty must be actively involved in this process both for their expertise as well as their buy-in. A committee that meets regularly is the best way to carry this out. The committee must have the full backing of the department chair to objectively evaluate what is working and what is not. The committee must also have the authority, in collaboration with the program director, to make the necessary changes to strengthen every aspect of residency education. This process of attentive and timely oversight over all educational aspects of the residency program will help to assure true excellence in residency training.

Residency Program Flexibility and a "Personalized" Curriculum

To accomplish excellence in the training of a pediatrician, a common curriculum in general pediatrics as well as a strong subspecialty focus is necessary. The residency review process is the best vehicle for assuring that this goal is accomplished. But different career directions among residents also strongly argue for diversity and flexibility in the residency curriculum, thereby allowing for resident choice. Currently, this is accomplished by the American Board of Pediatrics' Special Alternative Pathway, Accelerated Research Pathway, and Integrated Research Pathway. It is also evidenced in combined programs such as the medicine–pediatrics training programs and joint programs for training in neurology, genetics, and anesthesiology. Greater flexibility within the three years of training also enables residents to have concentrated exposure to research and international health. Such a "personalized" curricular approach to residency training enhances the residency years and engenders a commitment and passion for work that is enriching both for the individual and the program.[3] Thus, a residency program with a common curriculum for all residents coupled with curricular opportunities focused on a "personalized training" approach will assure a comprehensive and academically productive residency program.

Robust Mentoring

Residency is part of a journey that begins with college and medical school and culminates in professional work as a physician. Selection of one's career deserves the same attention from residents and faculty as does the acquisition of knowledge and skills. As a program is evaluated for its success in the intake process (intern selection) and the quality of the training (the curriculum), it is also judged by its success in placing its residents successfully and happily in their future roles, whether it be in academics, practice, global health, or further training.

A vigorous mentoring program is an essential part of a successful residency program. Residents expect and appreciate it. The faculty increasingly sees advising and mentoring as a part of their job description. Further, while time consuming, advising becomes one of the joyful responsibilities of being a faculty member. Often advising also leads to the salutary result of housestaff entering the mentor's field.

A successful mentoring program will optimally include the involvement of the department chair, the program directors, and a variety of faculty representing as diverse an array of disciplines as possible. Generally, program directors focus their attention on both resident evaluation as well as the process of choice of a future career. Meeting regularly with the housestaff throughout the year becomes an important and fulfilling part of the job. A busy department chair has less time to devote to this task. The chair's involvement, however, in areas of his or her expertise, as well as wisdom gained over the years, is invaluable to residents. The faculty, through thoughtful questioning, gentle probing, and wise advice serve an important role in career choice. They can also be helpful in assisting residents as they address challenges in their professional and personal life during residency. Finally, in a practical way, faculty advisors help with letters of recommendation for fellowship and practice, by suggesting funding sources and mentors for research projects, and by helping residents as they consider their future careers. Advisor weeks offer specific times and opportunities for advisors and advisees to meet. Continuing education for all faculty can be immensely helpful in teaching the skills of advising and mentoring.

An effective program for advising residents takes the full attention of the program and program directors. Program directors must assume the lion's share of responsibility for the process. Building advising into the culture of the hospital and the department is a critical objective and goal of an excellent residency program. The effort required can be great—so too the rewards.

Abiding Dilemmas in Residency Training

A number of lessons have been learned as a result of the opportunity to consider and reflect on the challenges that inevitably arise during residency training. These dilemmas rarely involve a choice of one over another but rather require a careful balancing of *both* to optimally fulfill excellence in residency training. Five central dilemmas in residency training and the issues emanating from their consideration will be discussed.

Service versus Education

One of the most critical and constant of these dilemmas is the correct balance between service and education. Caring for the patient is essential for the effective learning of medicine. It is, in fact, unique in the educational process. However, if carried to an extreme, where care of the patient excessively dominates, it can marginalize the learning that comes from the lecture, small group learning, bedside teaching, and time for reading and study. And while education is central to learning, if it becomes excessive in time and focus, thereby preventing learning through contact with patients, this imbalance will be similarly detrimental.

The wise balancing of service and education is critical for an effective training program. Both must co-exist but be carefully calibrated.

As we have seen over the 125-year history of the Children's Hospital, this challenge has persisted. Service predominated in the early years, a better balance existed in the middle years, and today, there is the risk that the hospital's use of house officers for service and an excessive emphasis on efficiency will marginalize the educational process. The ACGME institutional and program review process has served as an important counterbalance as has the current empowerment of program directors in their educational role by the American Association of Pediatric Program Directors.

Constant refinement of the balance of service and education throughout the three years of residency is also critically important for a thoughtful educational process. The post-graduate year of training, the stage of clinical development of a given resident, and the rotation site where learning occurs require frequent adjustments. The pediatric residency appropriately emphasizes service in the first two years of training with exposure to a broad array of general and subspecialty pediatric diseases, while the third year emphasizes an education and supervisory role to a greater degree accompanied by a focus on teaching, elective exposures for learning, opportunities for research experience, and third world exposure. Similarly, the first year emphasizes general pediatric, emergency medicine, and outpatient clinic exposure. The second year focuses on serious and more complex diseases as seen on the subspecialty services and the intensive care units, and the third year focuses on supervision and imparting knowledge to those less experienced. All are consistent with the developmental stage of the resident. While no simple formula exists for the correct balance of service and education, awareness of its importance and prevention of dominance of one over the other is an important goal for all training programs.

Supervision versus Autonomy

The correct balance of resident supervision and resident autonomy is essential to the education process during residency.[4] Early in training being carefully supervised is critical. To acquire knowledge takes time, to acquire clinical judgment takes even longer. The public demands adequate supervision of interns, and young trainees need it. Later on in training, making decisions on one's own (under the watchful eye of the attending physician) is equally critical to the maturation process. The capacity to make wise and correct decisions is what is expected on completion of residency. Training programs must assure both adequate supervision early in residency and the opportunity for autonomous decision-making with judicious oversight later in residency. Programs and program directors must evaluate both of these processes carefully and know when the correct time for transition from being supervised to supervising should occur.

Training programs must foster this process with attendings who have the capacity to wisely oversee the resident and the care of the patient and who are able to adjust supervision and autonomous decision-making based on the experience and developmental stage of the resident and the severity of the disease being treated. This process is facilitated by a faculty that works closely with residents and therefore know their stage of development as a physician. Excessive supervision when greater autonomy is appropriate is deleterious to a resident's educational growth. Inadequate supervision and excessive resident autonomy at too early a stage is equally deleterious to the care of the patients.

The 125-year history of the Children's Hospital residency possibly suggests an excessive degree of autonomy and autonomous decision-making in the early and middle years. Today, there is a risk of an excessive amount of supervision of residents, with inadequate opportunities for supervised autonomous decision-making, potentially to the detriment of the development of the resident as a physician.

A Required versus Flexible Curriculum

A required curriculum for all residents in a training program has many advantages.[5] It ensures that all areas and topics are systematically covered. Those who teach in a required curriculum become highly proficient in their pedagogy. It is clear which subjects are covered. Residency Review Committee requirements are met. Evaluation can be undertaken so as to be assured that educational goals are met. But flexibility in the residency curriculum is also important, offering many advantages. It allows residents' choice and time to focus on areas of interest. It allows for a diversity of exposure, from clinical care to research to educational opportunities. It optimizes the professional development of individual residents. Choice is also accomplished through the establishment of tracks for groups of residents, as seen with the primary care, research, and global health tracks. For programs with residents who have many different areas of interest, this approach has great appeal.

Flexibility in the use of tracks clearly enhances the "personalized" training of residents. It has the risk, however, of creating inequality in service requirements. "Personalized" training also risks an excessive focus on individual needs rather than the needs of the residency as a whole. These risks are juxtaposed to excessive rigidity in a curriculum that is the same for all. This approach risks failing to enhance the house officers' professional growth during residency.

The correct balance of rigidity and flexibility is an important challenge in the construction of a residency program. Both are needed to create a superior program. Neither should dominate. Awareness of the risks and benefits of both will allow for the wisest approach to this important issue.

So Much to Learn, So Little Time

The amount of new information to be learned by a house officer has increased exponentially over the last three decades. This growth has occurred in both clinical medicine as well as the basic sciences. And this does not include all of the information emerging from laboratory medicine, radiology, and genetics, as well as many other fields—plus the proliferation of biostatistical and epidemiologic information necessary to correctly interpret the literature.

A similar growth has occurred in the care of patients. The number and complexity of patients cared for has increased dramatically over recent years. The plethora of tests to be ordered and interpreted, the amount of documentation to be included in the record, and the necessity of coordination among multiple physicians and consultants caring for complex patients has made the house officer's life remarkably complex and hectic.

As the work to be done and the amount to be learned have grown, with work hour reform, the number of hours available has progressively decreased. This has necessitated the housestaff forcing more and more into a shorter period of time. This basic dilemma will continually force a residency program to make choices in what it presents to a house officer to learn during training. Some knowledge and skills may need to be moved to fellowship. Undoubtedly, what a program offers in medical education as well as the format of its presentation will become an increasingly important area of focus for all residency training programs.

Mind and Soul

The "making of a physician" during the residency years appropriately should focus on both the mind and the soul.[5] The formal curriculum addressing the development of the mind involves acquisition of new medical knowledge, incorporation of research and clinical skills, and the application of a constantly growing body of information emanating from the genomic and informatics revolutions to the care of the patient. It also involves a focus on how to think critically and independently, to understand deeply, and to pursue excellence in thought and action.[6] This curriculum is front and center. It is what we strive daily to inculcate into our learners. It is the core substrate of all of our teaching, our research, and our clinical care.

But there is a second imperative in the making of a physician—the development of the soul. This curriculum is less obvious, more hidden. It impacts the resident on a daily basis influencing their maturation as a physician in subtle ways. This "hidden curriculum" may be beneficial or it may be deleterious. For certain, however, it is central to the process of inculcation of attributes that make up the character and admirable qualities of a physician. The young physician, in fact, is surrounded daily with examples of beneficial and deleterious influences on their ethical and moral development. Examples of the latter include the subtle influences at times of drug representatives, instances of unprofessional behavior of teachers in the treatment of patients or students, or the more complex dilemma of shortened work hours and its impact on a resident's sense of responsibility for his or her patients.

Francis W. Peabody, the revered chief of medicine at the Boston City Hospital in the 1920s, wrote a short book that would be admired by generations of Harvard faculty and students alike. He wrote, "The secret of the care of the patient is in caring for the patient."[7] Characteristics of deep concern, kindness, sensitivity, and profound respect for one's patient, all attributes of Peabody's caring physician, are learned through careful observation of one's instructors during residency, and are subsequently incorporated into the care of one's own patients. When reflected upon years later, the facts presented by the great clinical teachers are often forgotten but those attributes of style and approach are always remembered. Elements of the "hidden curriculum" that are deleterious to the formation of the caring physician must be recognized and corrected. Those elements that are beneficial must be rewarded and celebrated.

The development of the best personal qualities of a physician is a second component of the "hidden curriculum." An abiding responsibility for one's patient, persistent hard work in caring for the sick, total honesty in all professional dealings, and a constant pursuit of professional excellence are critical attributes to be learned by residents during their training. In the aggregate, they make up the best of human qualities of a physician. Some of these qualities are innate and inherent in the human makeup of the resident; others are learned through careful observation and practice in a resident's daily work and life. They need to be modeled by instructors and evaluated, rewarded, and celebrated when achieved. Their development is as important as the development of the mind. These two, mind and soul, go hand in hand in the process of the "making of a physician."

Final Reflections

The residency at the Children's Hospital over its 125 years has achieved a remarkable record of success. This has come about as a result of a sustained ability to attract the best and the brightest coupled with a deep commitment to the mission of producing the future leaders in pediatrics and academic medicine. This objective has been synergized by the training program being deeply embedded in a great academic department with departmental leaders and faculty whose commitment to the program and relentless pursuit of excellence have been an inspiration and powerful role model for young trainees. The end result has been a program that today continues to stand among the very best in the country.

Residency is a pivotal and all-encompassing time in the formation of a physician. This book has tried to create a tapestry of the training and the life of a young physician going through that process. It has focused on one hospital and one training program as well as the local and national imperatives that have influenced that process over its 125-year history.

The Children's Hospital has been my professional home since the mid-1960s. Each of these years has been a joy and a privilege because of the importance of the work carried out in the service of sick children and because of the faithful dedication of all who have labored in the vineyards of healing of this hospital. Each has been able to accomplish more and stand taller because they have stood on the shoulders of those who have gone before. It is a history of which one can be humbly proud and grateful.

Three years of residency, when placed alongside a 40-year career, seems remarkably brief. Yet the impact of those years in molding the mind and the soul of the young physician is immense. Skills, character, and professional aspirations are formed and embedded for a lifetime. Memories of the experience run deep and their influence is present throughout a career. Thus it is perhaps not an exaggeration to reflect that in years to come, many will take note of their most important accomplishments as a physician, while others, house officers who trained in this residency program in Boston, with pride and humility will simply say, "I was a resident at the Children's Hospital."[8]

Bibliography

Alpert, J. J., and Zuckerman, B. "A History of Caring: The Pediatric Service at Boston University School of Medicine, Boston City Hospital and Boston Medical Center." Unpublished, 2014.

Beecher, H. K., and Altschule, M. D. *Medicine at Harvard, the First Three Hundred Years*. The University Press of New England, 1977.

Bull, W., and Bull, M. *Something in the Ether, a Bicentennial History of the Massachusetts General Hospital: 1811 to 2011*. Memoirs Unlimited, 2011.

Cone, Jr., T. E. *History of American Pediatrics*. Little, Brown and Company, 1979.

Finberg, L., and Stiehm, E. R. *The American Pediatric Society: History of Pediatric Subspecialties*. Wolters Kluwer/Lippincott Williams and Wilkins, 2006.

Flexner, A. *Medical Education*. The MacMillan Company, 1925.

Fyler, D. A. *The History of Cardiology at Boston Children's Hospital, the First 50 Years*. Children's Hospital Boston, 2001.

Garland, J. E. *Every Man Our Neighbor, a Brief History of the Massachusetts General Hospital, 1811–1861*. Little, Brown and Company, 1961.

Goostray, S. *Fifty Years, a History of the School of Nursing, the Children's Hospital Boston*. The Alumnae Association of the Children's Hospital School of Nursing, Boston, Massachusetts, 1940.

Haggerty, R. J. *Respectable Rebel: The Autobiography of Robert J. Haggerty, M.D.* Pixel Preserve, Volume 1, 2012; Volume 2, 2013.

Haggerty, R. J., and Lovejoy, Jr., F. H. *Charles A. Janeway: Pediatrician to the World's Children*. Children's Hospital Boston, distributed by Harvard University Press, 2007.

Imber, G. *Genius on the Edge, the Bizarre Double Life of Dr. William Stuart Halsted.* Kaplan Publishing, 2010.

Jennings, B. H. *Mel, a Biography of Dr. Mary Ellen Avery.* Book Surge, 2010.

Larson, J. T., Rockoff, M. A., Breakstone, D. R., Bibbins, P., Davis, M., Taylor, P., and Lovejoy, Jr., F. H. *Children's Hospital Boston.* Arcadia Publishing, 2005.

Lovejoy, Jr, F. H. *A Century of Service, a Celebration of the 100th Anniversary of the Children's Hospital Alumni Association and the 50th Blackfan Lecture.* Harvard University Printing and Publishing, 2003.

Ludmerer, K. M. *Learning to Heal: The Development of American Medical Education.* Basic Books, 1985.

Ludmerer, K. M. *Time to Heal: American Medical Education from the Turn of the Century to the Era of Managed Care.* Oxford University Press, 1999.

Osler, W. *The Evolution of Modern Medicine, a Series of Lectures Delivered at Yale University on the Silliman Foundation in April 1913.* Yale University, 1921.

Park, E. A., Littlefield, J. W., Seidel, H. M., and Wissow, L. S. *The Harriet Lane Home, a Model and a Gem.* The Johns Hopkins University, 2006.

Pearson, H. A. *The American Board of Pediatrics: 1933–2008.* American Board of Pediatrics, 2008.

Pearson, H. A. *The Centennial of the American Pediatric Society: 1888–1988.* American Pediatric Society, distributed by Yale University Printing Service, 1988.

Rosenberg, C. E. *The Care of Strangers: The Rise of America's Hospital System.* Basic Books, 1987.

Scriver, J. B. *The Montreal Children's Hospital, Years of Growth.* McGill-Queen's University Press, 1979.

Smith, C. A. *The Children's Hospital of Boston, "Built Better Than They Knew."* Little, Brown and Company, 1983.

Snedeker, L. *One Hundred Years at Children's.* Children's Hospital, 1969.

Starr, P. *The Social Transformation of American Medicine.* Basic Books, 1982.

The Children's Hospital of Boston, 1869–1951, Eighty-Two Years of Service to the Community and to the Nation. Children's Hospital Medical Center Report, 1946–1951.

Vogel, M. J. *The Invention of the Modern Hospital, Boston: 1870–1930.* The University of Chicago Press, 1980.

Notes

CHAPTER I

1. Material for "Medical House Officer Reflections from 1905" comes from diaries, letters, and publications from housestaff of that era.
2. Material for "Medical House Officer Reflections from 1966" comes from interviews with housestaff from that era.
3. Material for "Medical House Officer Reflections from 2005" comes from interviews with housestaff from that era.

CHAPTER II

1. Data for this section, "National Perspective," come from K. M. Ludmerer, *Time to Heal: American Medical Education from the Turn of the Century to the Era of Managed Care* (Oxford University Press, 1999), Chapters 3 and 4; M. J. Vogel, *The Invention of the Modern Hospital: Boston, 1870–1930* (The University of Chicago Press, 1980), Chapters 1 and 3; P. Starr, *The Social Transformation of American Medicine* (Basic Books, 1982), Chapters 3 and 4; C. E. Rosenberg, *The Care of Strangers: The Rise of America's Hospital System* (Basic Books, 1987), Chapters 6–8.
2. M. J. Vogel, *The Invention of the Modern Hospital: Boston, 1870–1930* (The University of Chicago Press, 1980), Chapter 1.
3. P. Starr, *The Social Transformation of American Medicine* (Basic Books, 1982), Chapter 3.
4. K. M. Ludmerer, *Time to Heal: American Medical Education from the Turn of the Century to the Era of Managed Care* (Oxford University Press, 1999), p. 20.
5. J. A. Curren, "Internships and Residencies: Historical Background and Current Trends," *Journal of Medical Education* 1959;34(9):873–884, p. 874.
6. Note 5, pp. 875–876.
7. Note 5, pp. 873–884.
8. J. E. Garland, *Every Man Our Neighbor, a Brief History of the Massachusetts General Hospital, 1811–1861* (Little, Brown and Company, 1961), pp. 49–52.

9. Note 5, p. 879.
10. *Transactions of the American Medical Association* 1873;24:314–333.
11. C. E. Rosenberg, *The Care of Strangers* (Basic Books, 1987), pp. 175–177.
12. Data for this section come from the Medical Department section of the Children's Hospital annual reports, numbers 1 through 54, 1870–1922.
13. J. T. Larson, M. A. Rockoff, D. R. Breakstone, P. Bibbins, M. Davis, P. Taylor, and F. H. Lovejoy, Jr., *Children's Hospital Boston* (Arcadia Publishing, 2005), pp. 9 and 15.
14. C. A. Smith, *The Children's Hospital of Boston, "Built Better Than They Knew"* (Little, Brown and Company, 1983), pp. 12–21.
15. Note 2, Chapter 1, pp. 22–23.
16. Note 2, Chapter 1, p. 20.
17. Note 2, Chapter 1, p. 20.
18. Note 2, Chapter 3, p. 63.
19. Note 2, Chapter 3, p. 64.
20. Addresses delivered at the Children's Hospital, February 27, 1942, during the memorial exercises for Kenneth D. Blackfan, *Supplement to Harvard Medical Alumni Bulletin* 1942(April);16(3):3–17.
21. F. B. Talbot, "Pediatric Profiles—Thomas Morgan Rotch (1849–1914)," *Journal of Pediatrics* 1956;49:109–112.
22. L. W. Hill, "Pediatric Profiles—John Lovett Morse (1865–1940)," *Journal of Pediatrics* 1954;45:615–619.
23. H. H. Gordon, "Pediatric Profiles—Oscar Menderson Schloss (1882–1952)," *Journal of Pediatrics* 1955;47:373–381.
24. Note 12.
25. "Children's Hospital Rules of 1894," Children's Hospital Boston, Children's Hospital Boston Archives, p. 9.
26. *The Children's Hospital Annual Report and By-Laws*, 1869, p. 1.
27. Note 26, p. 14.
28. S. Goostray, *Fifty Years, a History of the School of Nursing, the Children's Hospital Boston* (The Alumnae Association of the Children's School of Nursing, 1940), p. 10.
29. "By-laws of the Corporation," March 22, 1869, Article 13, Children's Hospital Boston, Children's Hospital Boston Archives.
30. Note 25, pp. 2, 10, 11.
31. "By-laws for Housestaff," 1905, Children's Hospital Boston, Children's Hospital Boston Archives.
32. J. L. Gamble, *Harvard Medical Alumni Bulletin*, January 1954, pp. 9–13.
33. Note 14, p. 83.
34. J. L. Morse, "The History of Pediatrics in Massachusetts," *New England Journal of Medicine* 1931;205:169–180.
35. American Pediatric Society, "Charles Hunter Dunn," *Semi-Centennial Volume of the American Pediatric Society, 1888–1938* (George Banta Publishing Co., 1938), p. 440.

36. Note 35, "Fritz Bradley Talbot," p. 251.
37. Note 35, "Richard Mason Smith," p. 241.
38. Note 35, "Bronson Crothers," p. 115.
39. Note 35, "James Lawler Gamble," p. 137.
40. Note 35, "Edwin Theodore Wyman," p. 277.
41. Note 35, "Lewis Webb Hill," p. 159.
42. Note 35, "Samuel Zachary Levine," p. 175.

CHAPTER III

1. Data for this section come from the Medical Department section of Children's Hospital annual reports, numbers 57, 59, and 62, 1925–1930.
2. Letter from Donald Fyler to James Lock dated March 8, 1992, "Housestaff History," Children's Hospital Boston Archives.
3. Data for this section come from the Medical Department section of Children's Hospital annual reports, numbers 55 through 76, 1923–1945.
4. C. A. Smith, *The Children's Hospital of Boston, "Built Better Than They Knew"* (Little, Brown and Company, 1983), p. 143.
5. J. L. Wilson, "Kenneth D. Blackfan (1883–1941)," *Journal of Pediatrics* 1955;47:261–267, p. 266.
6. E. A. Park, "The History of the Harriet Lane Home," presented by Dr. Park, May 14, 1964, Children's Hospital Boston Archives.
7. K. D. Blackfan and L.K. Diamond, *Atlas of the Blood of Children* (Commonwealth Fund, 1944).
8. Note 5, p. 266.
9. Note 5, p. 263.
10. J. L. Gamble, "In Memoriam, Kenneth Daniel Blackfan (1883–1941)," *Journal of Pediatrics* 1942;20:140–142, p. 141.
11. Note 5, p. 263.
12. Note 10, pp. 140–142.
13. Note 5, p. 263.
14. Note 5, p. 261.
15. Note 5, p. 264.
16. Note 5, p. 265.
17. Note 10, p. 141.
18. Note 5, p. 267.
19. Note 5, p. 267.
20. Note 10, p. 140.
21. R. N. Ganz, "In Memoriam, Richard M. Smith (1881–1981)," *Harvard Medical Magazine*, 1981, p. 68.
22. R. A. Stevens, "Graduate Medical Education: A Continuing History," *Journal of Medical Education* 1978;53:1–18.
23. K. M. Ludmerer, *Time to Heal: American Medical Education from the Turn*

of the Century to the Era of Managed Care (Oxford University Press, 1999), Chapter 4, pp. 79–101.

24. Note 22, p. 7.
25. Note 23, p. 81.
26. J. A. Curran, "Internships and Residencies, Historical Backgrounds and Current Trends," *Journal of Medical Education* 1959;34(9):873–884, p. 878.
27. Note 26, pp. 876–878.
28. Note 23, p. 84–86.
29. Note 23, p. 85.
30. Note 22, p. 9.
31. Note 22, p. 9.
32. Note 26, p. 879.
33. Note 3.
34. "Rules for House Officers," publication of Children's Hospital Boston, 1928, Children's Hospital Boston Archives, pp. 1–8.
35. "Pediatric Service, Infants and Children's Hospital (1935)," Children's Hospital Boston, Children's Hospital Boston Archives, pp. 1–31.
36. Note 35.
37. Excerpt of letter from Clifford S. Grulee, Jr., to Dr. Chester C. d'Autremont, president, Children's Hospital Alumni Association, June 2, 1992, Children's Hospital Boston Archives.
38. Note 3.
39. Note 35, pp. 1–31.
40. *Children's Hospital Medical Center News*, 1963, pp. 1, 2, 11, Children's Hospital Boston Archives.
41. Reflections of Louis K. Diamond, written to Frank Gardner, January 6, 1971, Children's Hospital Boston Archives.
42. C. F. Barlow, "In Memoriam, Randolph K. Byers (1986–1988)," *Harvard Medical Alumni Bulletin*, 1988, pp. 67–68.
43. John McMackin, "Reminiscence," oral history, Children's Hospital Boston Archives.
44. Note 35, p. 9.
45. Note 40, pp. 1, 2, 11.

CHAPTER IV

1. C. A. Janeway, Department of Medicine section of the 1962 annual report of the Children's Hospital Medical Center, Children's Hospital Boston Archives, p. 35.
2. C. A. Janeway, Department of Medicine section of the 1970 annual report of the Children's Hospital Medical Center, Children's Hospital Boston Archives, p. 16.
3. Note 2, p. 18.
4. Note 2, p. 16.
5. D. A. Fyler, "The History of Cardiology at Boston Children's Hospital, The

First 50 Years," 2001; author's files, "Housestaff History," Children's Hospital Boston Archives, pp. 3–8.

6. Note 2, p. 15.
7. G. Imber, *Genius on the Edge, the Bizarre Double Life of Dr. William Stewart Halsted* (Kaplan Publishing, 2010), p. 108.
8. The Children's Hospital of Boston, 1869–1951, *The Children's Hospital Medical Center Report*, 1946–1951, Children's Hospital Boston Archives, pp. 17–20.
9. C. A Smith, *The Children's Hospital of Boston, "Built Better Than They Knew"* (Little, Brown and Company, 1983), pp. 223–224.
10. Note 9, pp. 223–225.
11. Note 9, pp. 253–254.
12. Note 9, pp. 226–228.
13. Communication with David Peck, August 20, 2009; author's files, "Housestaff History," Children's Hospital Boston Archives.
14. Note 9, pp. 244–245.
15. W. Berenberg, W. Castle, J. Enders, R. Haggerty, D. Nathan, F. Rosen, and A. S. Nadas, "Physician to Children, Charles Alderson Janeway, May 26, 1909–May 28, 1981," *Memorial Minute*, Harvard Medical School, Boston, p. 119.
16. R. J. Haggerty and F. H. Lovejoy, Jr., *Charles A. Janeway: Pediatrician to the World's Children* (Children's Hospital Boston, distributed by Harvard University Press, 2007), pp. 7–10, Chapter 3 (pp. 50–66), Chapter 4 (pp. 67–108), Chapter 5 (pp. 109–130), and Chapter 11 (pp. 279–301).
17. Note 16, p. 115.
18. F. S. Rosen, "A Brief History of Immunodeficiency Disease," *Immunological Reviews* 2000;178:8–12.
19. Note 16, p. 281.
20. Note 2, p. 19.
21. Note 16, pp. 283–284.
22. C. A. Janeway, "Medical Education After Medical School," *Journal of Medical Education* 1965;4(2):1–4.
23. Note 16, pp. 282–284.
24. Note 16, p. 121.
25. H. A. Pearson, "History of Pediatric Hematology Oncology," *The American Pediatric Society, History of Pediatric Subspecialties* (Wolters Kluwer/Lippincott, Williams and Wilkins, 2002), pp. 115–139.
26. Note 16, p. 68.
27. Note 2, p. 16.
28. Note 16, pp. 67–72.
29. B. F. Massell, *Rheumatic Fever and Streptococcal Infections: Unraveling the Mysteries of a Dread Disease* (Harvard University Press, 1997), pp. 1–3.
30. D. E. Greydanus and V. C. Strasburger, "Adolescent Medicine," *Primary Care Clinic Office Practice* 2006;33:16.
31. E. M. Alderman, J. Rieder, and M. I. Cohen, "The History of Adolescent Medicine," *Pediatric Research* 2003;54:143.

32. R. J. Haggerty, *Respectable Rebel: The Autobiography of Robert J. Haggerty, M.D.* (Pixel Preserve, 2012), pp. 185–193.

33. S. Ashwal and R. Rust, "Child Neurology in the 20th Century," *The American Pediatric Society, History of Pediatric Subspecialties*; note 25, pp. 262–291.

34. K. M. Ludmerer, *Time to Heal: American Medical Education from the Turn of the Century to the Era of Managed Care* (Oxford University Press, 1990), p. 192.

35. R. G. Harmon, "Intern and Resident Organizations in the United States: 1934–1977," *Milbank Memorial Fund Quarterly* 1978;56(4):506–516.

36. Communication with Richard B. Johnston, Jr., August 27, 2011; author's files, "Housestaff History," Children's Hospital Boston Archives.

37. Communication with John Graef, February 8, 2010; author's files, "Housestaff History," Children's Hospital Boston Archives.

38. Communication with John Graef and Mary Beth Gordon, October 13, 2011; author's files, "Housestaff History," Children's Hospital Boston Archives.

39. C. A. Janeway, Department of Medicine section of the 1964 annual report of the Children's Hospital Medical Center, Children's Hospital Boston Archives, p. 45.

40. T. Lissauer, *50th Anniversary, Boston Children's/St. Mary's Paediatric Exchange 1952–1978* and *15th Anniversary Duke/Oxford Exchange 1986–2001*, April 10–12, 2002; author's files, "Housestaff History," Children's Hospital Boston Archives, p. 5.

41. J. J. Alpert, "A View from the USA," note 40, p. 3.

42. T. Lissauer, "A View from the UK," note 40, p. 2.

43. A. Bergman, note 40, p. 25.

44. M. F. Pendleton, note 40, p. 52.

45. S. Katz, "The Duke/Oxford Exchange," note 40, p. 6.

46. Note 40, p. 12.

47. Note 39, p. 46.

48. Note 39, p. 47.

49. C. A. Janeway, Department of Medicine section of the 1966 annual report of the Children's Hospital Medical Center, Children's Hospital Boston Archives, p. 53.

50. Note 2, pp. 20–21.

51. Note 16, p. 288.

52. I. Grant, W. Dorus, T. McGlashan, S. Perry, and R. Sherman, "The Chief Resident in Psychiatry," *Archives of General Psychiatry* 1974;30:503–507, p. 503.

53. Note 52, p. 503.

54. Note 16, p. 288.

55. Communication with James McKay, June 2009; author's files, "Housestaff History," Children's Hospital Boston Archives.

56. Note 16, pp. 295–298.

57. Communication with Fred Mandell, March 15, 2010; author's files, "Housestaff History," Children's Hospital Boston Archives.

58. Communication with Suzanne Boulter, November 1, 2010; author's files, "Housestaff History," Children's Hospital Boston Archives.
59. Communication with Norman Spack, February 2, 2010; author's files, "Housestaff History," Children's Hospital Boston Archives.
60. Note 36.
61. Note 16, pp. 109–113.
62. Communication with Sherwin Kevy, September 15, 2009; author's files, "Housestaff History," Children's Hospital Boston Archives.
63. Note 2, p. 21.
64. Communication with William Cochran, September 2009; author's files, "Housestaff History," Children's Hospital Boston Archives.
65. Communication with Daniel Cohen, November 2013; author's files, "Housestaff History," Children's Hospital Boston Archives.

CHAPTER V

1. "New Release," October 2, 1973; author's files, "Housestaff History," Children's Hospital Boston Archives.
2. Data for this section, "Significant Hospital Events," come from *Children's World, Year in Review*, inclusive of years 1978 through 1984, and the Department of Medicine section of the Children's Hospital Medical Center annual reports, 1975–1984, by Mary Ellen Avery, Children's Hospital Boston Archives.
3. R. J. Haggerty, *Respectable Rebel: The Autobiography of Robert J. Haggerty, M.D.* (Pixel Preserve, 2012), pp. 228–231.
4. Note 2.
5. Note 2.
6. "The Breath of Life: The Extraordinary Career of Dr. Mary Ellen Avery '48," *Wheaton Quarterly*, Spring 1999, p. 7.
7. M. E. Avery and J. Mead, "Surface Properties in Relation to Atelectasis and Hyaline Membrane Disease," *American Journal of Diseases of Children* 1959;97:517–523.
8. B. H. Jennings, *Mel: A Biography of Dr. Mary Ellen Avery* (Book Surge, 2010), pp. 143–158.
9. Note 8, pp. 320–321.
10. M. E. Avery, Department of Medicine section of the Children's Hospital Medical Center annual reports, including years 1975–1976, 1976–1977, 1978–1979, 1979–1980, 1980–1981, 1981–1982, 1983–1984, 1984–1985, Children's Hospital Boston Archives.
11. M. K. Hostetter, "Introduction of the American Pediatric Society's 2005 John Howland Award Recipient, Mary Ellen Avery, M.D.," *Pediatric Research* 2005;58:1311–1313.
12. Note 8, p. 393.
13. Honorary degree citation, Wheaton College, June 8, 1974; author's files, "Housestaff History," Children's Hospital Boston Archives.

14. "Times Are Changing: The Public Expects Communication with the Physician," *Harvard Magazine*, September/October 1977, p. 57.

15. Mary Ellen Avery, "Pediatrics: The Practice of Preventive Medicine," Rockefeller Archive Center Conference, May 25–27, 1982.

16. "A Memorial Tribute and Celebration, Mary Ellen Avery," The Children's Hospital, February 4, 2012, Children's Hospital Boston Archives, pp. 3–42.

17. *Children's World, Year in Review*, Children's Hospital Medical Center, Boston, including years 1978, 1979, 1980, 1981, 1982, 1983, 1984, Children's Hospital Boston Archives.

18. *Harvard Medical School Pediatric Executive Committee Minutes, 1968–1990*, by J. D. Crawford, Secretary of the Pediatric Executive Committee, Department of Pediatrics, Children's Hospital, Boston; author's files, "Housestaff History," Children's Hospital Boston Archives.

19. Data for this section come from "Brief History of the Department of Medicine, Children's Hospital Boston," by Mary Ellen Avery, March 1997, Children's Hospital Boston Archives.

20. D. C. Fyler, *The History of Cardiology at Boston Children's Hospital, The First 50 Years*, 2001; author's files, "Housestaff History," Children's Hospital Boston Archives, p. 19.

21. H. R. Colten, *A Child Is Dead, A Future Lost* (private printing, 2007); author's files, "Housestaff History," Children's Hospital Boston Archives.

22. D. A. Fisher, "A Short History of Pediatric Endocrinology in North America," *The American Pediatric Society, History of Pediatric Subspecialties* (Wolters Kluwer/Lippincott, Williams and Wilkins, 2006), p. 180.

23. "Medical Service Data Sheet," Department of Medicine, Children's Hospital Boston;. author's files, "Housestaff History," Children's Hospital Boston Archives.

24. J. H. Goldberg, "A New Look at House Officers' Incomes," *Hospital Physician*, March 1968, pp. 34–39.

25. R. G. Harmon, "Intern and Resident Organizations in the United States: 1934–1977," *Milbank Memorial Fund Quarterly* 1978;56(4):500–530.

26. R. Caffaro, "Annual Wage and Education Survey," *Hospital Physician*, January 1978, p. 25.

27. C. Lopate, *Women in Medicine* (Johns Hopkins University Press, 1968), p. 30.

28. K. M. Ludmerer, *Time to Heal: American Medical Education from the Turn of the Century to the Era of Managed Care* (Oxford University Press, 1999), pp. 249–259.

29. S. Shea and M. T. Fullilove, "Entry of Black and Other Minority Students into U.S. Medical Schools, Historical Perspective and Recent Trends," *New England Journal of Medicine* 1985;313(15):933–940, p. 935.

30. Note 28, p. 256.

31. H. W. Nickens, T. P. Ready, and R. G. Petersdorf, "Project 3000 by 2000—Racial and Ethnic Diversity in U.S. Medical Schools," *New England Journal of Medicine* 1994;331:472–476, p. 473.

32. J. Bickel, "Scenarios for Success—Enhancing Women Physicians' Professional Advancement," *Western Journal of Medicine* 1995;162:165–169, p. 166.

33. P. L. Carr, R. H. Friedman, M. A. Moskowitz, and L. E. Kazis, "Comparing the Status of Women and Men in Academic Medicine," *Annals of Internal Medicine* 1993;119:908–913.

34. F. K. Conley, "Toward a More Perfect World—Eliminating Sexual Bias in Academic Medicine," *New England Journal of Medicine* 1993;328:351–352.

35. Note 28, p. 317.

36. J. W. Smith, W. F. Denny, and D. B. Witzke, "Emotional Improvement in Internal Medical House Staff," *Journal of the American Medical Association* 1996;255:1155–1158, p. 1158.

37. N. Spritz, "Oversight of Physicians' Conduct by State Licensing Agencies, Lessons from New York's Libby Zion Case," *Annals of Internal Medicine* 1991;115:219–220.

38. Note 28, pp. 320–324.

39. F. H. Lovejoy, Jr., "Current Challenges in House-Officer Training," *Southern Medical Journal* 1990;83:315–319.

40. M. T. Rabkin, "The Teaching Hospital and Medical Education, One Room Schoolhouse, Multiversity Dinosaur," *Journal of Medical Education* 1985;60:92–97, p. 95.

41. J. H. Grossman, "Perspectives: A Teaching Hospital Executive," *Health Affairs* 1988;7:70–77.

42. J. S. Alpert and R. Coles, "Resident Reform, an Urgent Necessity," *Archives of Internal Medicine* 1988;148:1507–1508, p. 1507.

43. Note 8, pp. 354–355.

44. "Internship Application Statistics," Department of Medicine, Children's Hospital, 1983;. author's files, "Housestaff History," Children's Hospital Boston Archives.

45. V. Chiang, F. H. Lovejoy, S. Lux, and V. Osganian, "Use and Results of the Special Alternative Pathway at Children's Hospital Boston" (unpublished); author's files, "Housestaff History," Children's Hospital Boston Archives.

46. "Children's Hospital Boston, Female Chief Residents, 1970–2007," Children's Hospital Boston Archives, 2008.

47. Gregory R. Handrigan, "An Interview with Dr. Norman Rosenblum: Reflections on a Career as a Physician Scientist and Advice for Trainees," *University of Toronto Medical Journal* 2011;88:167–170.

48. F. H. Lovejoy, Jr. and L. R. First, "Ten Years of a Residency Training Committee," *Academic Medicine* 1990;66:602–603.

49. *Medical Service Newsletters*, inclusive of years 1976–1984; author's files, "Housestaff History," Children's Hospital Boston Archives.

50. Communication with Norman Rosenblum, January 10, 2012; author's files, "Housestaff History," Children's Hospital Boston Archives.

51. "Report of the Residency Training Committee, Children's Hospital Medical

Center," May 1976; author's files, "Housestaff History," Children's Hospital Boston Archives.

52. Children's Hospital Pediatric Residency Program, submission to the American College of Graduate Medical Education, Residency Review Committee, 1981; author's files, "Housestaff History," Children's Hospital Boston Archives.

53. Communication from Leonard Rappaport to the author, February 27, 2010; author's files, "Housestaff History," Children's Hospital Boston Archives.

54. Communication with Ted Sectish, February 28, 2010; author's files, "Housestaff History," Children's Hospital Boston Archives.

55. Communication with Maureen Jonas, February 26, 2010; author's files, "Housestaff History," Children's Hospital Boston Archives.

56. Communication with Alan Leichtner, March 5, 2010; author's files, "Housestaff History," Children's Hospital Boston Archives.

57. "The Charles A. Janeway Award," graduation brochure, June 20, 2007; author's files, "Housestaff History," Children's Hospital Boston Archives.

58. Children's Hospital Medical Staff Executive Committee minutes, 1985, Children's Hospital Boston, Children's Hospital Boston Archives.

59. Housestaff shows, 1980–1986; author's files, 'Housestaff History,' Children's Hospital Boston Archives.

60. A. Lavin, remarks made at 1982 Residency Class Reunion, May 2012; author's files, "Housestaff History," Children's Hospital Boston Archives.

61. F. H. Lovejoy, Jr. and D. G. Nathan, "Careers Chosen by Graduates of a Major Pediatric Residency Program, 1974–1986," *Academic Medicine* 1992;67:272–274.

62. *USA PL4 Pediatric Resident Survey* (Ross Laboratories, 1990).

63. T. K. Oliver, Jr., "Presidential Address to the Association of Medical School Pediatric Department Chairmen," Point Clear, Alabama, 1985 (unpublished); author's files, "Housestaff History," Children's Hospital Boston Archives.

64. American Academy of Pediatrics Committee on Manpower, "Projecting Pediatric Patterns: A Survey of Pediatrics," *Pediatrics* 1978;62:625–665, p. 627.

CHAPTER VI

1. Data for this section, "Significant Hospital Events," come from *Children's World, Year in Review*, inclusive of years 1985–1995, and annual reports of the Department of Medicine, inclusive of years 1985–1995, by David G. Nathan, Children's Hospital Boston Archives.

2. Data for this section, "Construction," come from *Children's World, Year in Review*, inclusive of years 1985–1995, and annual reports of the Department of Medicine, inclusive of years 1985–1995, by David G. Nathan, Children's Hospital Boston Archives.

3. David G. Nathan, annual reports of the Department Medicine, inclusive of years 1985–1986 through 1994–1995, Children's Hospital Boston Archives.

4. Note 3, inclusive of years 1984–1985 through 1994–1995.

5. D. A. Goldmann, S. M. Andrews, S. Pasternack, D. G. Nathan, and F. H.

Lovejoy, Jr., "A Service Chief Model for General Pediatric Inpatient Care and Residency Training," *Pediatrics* 1992;89:601–607.

6. Note 5, pp. 604–605.

7. M. K. Marks, F. H. Lovejoy, Jr., P. A. Rutherford, and M. N. Baskin, "Impact of a Short Stay Unit on Asthma Patients Admitted to a Tertiary Pediatric Hospital," *Quality Management in Health Care* 1997;6(1):14–22.

8. Note 7, pp. 14–22.

9. M. K. Marks, M. N. Baskin, F. H. Lovejoy, Jr., and J. P. Hafler, "Intern Learning and Education on a Short Stay Unit: A Qualitative Study," *Archive of Pediatrics and Adolescent Medicine* 1997;151:193–198, p. 194.

10. Data for this section, "Medical Education," come from the Department of Medicine section of Children's Hospital Boston annual reports, inclusive of years 1985–1995, by David G. Nathan, Children's Hospital Boston Archives.

11. Note 3, inclusive of years 1985–1995, Children's Hospital Boston Archives.

12. E. G. Armstrong and F. H. Lovejoy, Jr., "Pediatric Faculty Development Handbook: Harvard Medical School," Office of Educational Development, Harvard Medical School, 1996.

13. Data for this section, "Research," come from *Children's World, Year in Review*, inclusive of years 1985–1995, and the Department of Medicine section of Children's Hospital Boston annual reports, inclusive of years 1985–1995, by David G. Nathan, Children's Hospital Boston Archives.

14. Note 3, inclusive of years 1985–1995, Children's Hospital Boston Archives.

15. Sally Andrews, "The Department of Medicine Housestaff," inclusive of years 1981–2000; author's files, "Housestaff History," Children's Hospital Boston Archives.

16. "NACHRI Position Statement: Financing Graduate Medical Education in the Context of Healthcare Reform Based on Managed Competition," September 27, 1993, pp. 1–4; author's files, "Housestaff History," Children's Hospital Boston Archives.

17. Communication with David Nathan, March 26, 2002; author's files, "Housestaff History," Children's Hospital Boston Archives.

18. D. G. Nathan, "A Journey in Clinical Research," Howland Award presentation, May 4, 2003; author's files, "Housestaff History," Children's Hospital Boston Archives, p. 4.

19. D. G. Nathan, "Tribute to Joseph E. Murray and E. Donnell Thomas"; author's files, "Housestaff History," Children's Hospital Boston Archives, p. 1.

20. D. G. Nathan, "The Kenneth Blackfan Lecture," June 5, 2002; author's files, "Housestaff History," Children's Hospital Boston Archives, p. 4.

21. Note 18, p. 4.

22. D. G. Nathan, "AOA Lecture," University of California Medical School; 9 May 1991. Author's files, "Housestaff History," Children's Hospital Boston Archives, pp. 6–8.

23. Note 18, p. 5.

24. Note 19, p. 2.

25. Note 22, p. 3.
26. Note 18, pp. 6–7.
27. Note 18, p. 6.
28. S. H. Orkin, D. G. Nathan, D. Ginsburg, A. T. Look, D. E. Fisher, and S. E. Lux, Eds., *Nathan and Oski's Hematology of Infancy and Childhood*, 7th edition (Saunders Elsevier, 2009).
29. D. G. Nathan, *Genes, Blood and Courage, a Boy Called Immortal Sword* (The Belknap Press of Harvard University Press, 1995).
30. S. E. Lux IV, "David G. Nathan Hematology/Oncology Trainees," September 18, 2001; author's files, "Housestaff History," Children's Hospital Boston Archives.
31. F. H. Lovejoy, Jr., "D. G. Nathan and the 2003 Howland Award," *Pediatric Research* 2004;56:167–168.
32. F. H. Lovejoy, Jr., D. G. Nathan, B. S. Zuckerman, P. A. Pizzo, G. R. Fleisher, and R. J. Vinci, "The Merger of Two Pediatric Residency Programs: Lessons Learned," *Pediatrics* 2008;153:731–732.
33. F. H. Lovejoy, Jr., "Celebratory Dinner in Honor of David Nathan," July 1996; author's files, "Housestaff History," Children's Hospital Boston Archives, pp. 6–7.
34. Note 33, pp. 7–8.
35. C. A. Smith, *The Children's Hospital of Boston, "Built Better Than They Knew"* (Little, Brown and Company, 1983).
36. R. J. Haggerty and F. H. Lovejoy, Jr., *Charles A. Janeway: Pediatrician to the World's Children* (Children's Hospital Boston, distributed by Harvard University Press, 2007).
37. Communication with Joseph Martin, September 16, 2012; author's files, "Housestaff History," Children's Hospital Boston Archives.
38. Harvard University commencement exercises, May 27, 2010, delivered by the president of Harvard University.
39. Data for this section, "Division Chiefs," come from *Children's World, Year in Review*, inclusive of years 1985–1995, and the Department of Medicine section of Children's Hospital Boston annual reports, inclusive of years 1985–1995, by David G. Nathan, Children's Hospital Boston Archives.
40. Data for this section, "Clinical Programs," come from Executive Committee minutes, Department of Pediatrics, inclusive of years 1985 to 1995; author's files, "Housestaff History," Children's Hospital Boston Archives.
41. Data for this section, "Academic Programs," come from Department of Pediatrics Executive Committee minutes, inclusive of years 1985 to 1995; author's files, "Housestaff History," Children's Hospital Boston Archives.
42. K. M. Ludmerer, *Time to Heal: American Medical Education from the Turn of the Century to the Era of Managed Care* (Oxford University Press, 1999), pp. 349–350.
43. J. K. Iglehart, "The American Health Care System: Teaching Hospitals," *New England Journal of Medicine* 1993;329:1052–1056, p. 1054.

44. J. P. Kassirer, "Academic Medical Centers Under Siege," *New England Journal of Medicine* 1994;331:1370.
45. L. S. Schlesinger and C. M. Helms, "Cost-Conscious Care, Housestaff Training and the Academic Health Center," *Academic Medicine* 1995;70:561–562.
46. F. H. Lovejoy, Jr. and M. B. Clark, "A Promotion Ladder for Teachers: Experiences and Challenges," *Academic Medicine* 1995;70:1079–1086, p. 1079.
47. D. A. Blake, "Whither Academic Values During the Transition from Academic Medical Centers to Integrated Health Delivery Systems," *Academic Medicine* 1996;71:818–819.
48. "Intern Rank List, 1973–2001," Department of Medicine; author's files, "Housestaff History," Children's Hospital Boston Archives.
49. V. Chiang, F. H. Lovejoy, Jr., S. Lux IV, and V. Osganian, "Use and Results of the Special Alternative Pathway at Children's Hospital Boston" (unpublished); author's files, "Housestaff History," Children's Hospital Boston Archives.
50. "Internship Application Statistics: 1986–1998," Department of Medicine; author's files, "Housestaff History," Children's Hospital Boston Archives.
51. Note 50.
52. Note 50.
53. Note 50.
54. "Long Range Planning Committee Report, The Children's Hospital Residency Training Program," March 15, 1990;.author's files, "Housestaff History," Children's Hospital Boston Archives.
55. Note 54, pp. 6–7.
56. Note 54, p. 5.
57. Note 54, pp. 3–5.
58. Note 54, pp. 10–11.
59. "Residency Training Program 1994–1995, Schedule Distribution over Three Years"; author's files, "Housestaff History," Children's Hospital Boston Archives.
60. Data for this section, "Residency Curricular Innovations," come from Residency Training Committee minutes, inclusive of years 1985–1995, recorded by Susan Brooks; author's files, 'Housestaff History,' Children's Hospital Boston Archives.
61. Note 54.
62. "Long Range Planning Committee Report," September 15, 1995;.author's files, 'Housestaff History,' Children's Hospital Boston Archives.
63. C. E. Johnson, R. Bachur, C. Priebe, F. H. Lovejoy, Jr., and J. P. Hafler, "Developing Residents as Teachers—Process and Content," *Pediatrics* 1996;97:907–916.
64. C. P. Landrigan, P. Conway, S. Edwards, and R. Scrivasta, "Pediatric Hospitalist: A Systematic Review of the Literature," *Pediatrics* 2006;117:1736–1744.
65. N. D. Rosenblum, J. Nagler, F. H. Lovejoy, Jr., and J. P. Hafler, "The Pedagogical Characteristics of a Clinical Conference for Senior Pediatric Residents and Faculty," *Archives of Pediatric Adolescent Medicine* 1995;149:1023–1028.

66. Data for this section, "Awards," come from graduation brochures of the Department of Medicine, inclusive of years 1985–1995; author's files, "Housestaff History," Children's Hospital Boston Archives.
67. "Career Directions of Children's Hospital Housestaff, 1985–1995"; author's files,
68. "Housestaff History," Children's Hospital Boston Archives.
69. "What Are Our Housestaff Doing—Implications for Hospital and Training Program"; author's files, "Housestaff History," Children's Hospital Boston Archives.
70. Data for this section, "Residency Highlights," come from senior resident dinner speeches, written by the author; author's files, "Housestaff History," Children's Hospital Boston Archives.
71. Data for this section, "House Officer Retreats," come from Residency Training Committee minutes, inclusive of dates 1985–1995, recorded by Susan Brooks; author's files, "Housestaff History," Children's Hospital Boston Archives.
72. Data for this section, "Housestaff Shows," come from playbills for the Children's Hospital housestaff shows, inclusive of the years 1986, 1987, 1988, 1991, 1993, 1995; author's files, "Housestaff History," Children's Hospital Boston Archives.
73. Communication with Jonathan Finkelstein, September 24, 2010; author's files, "Housestaff History," Children's Hospital Boston Archives.
74. Communication with Lisa Diller, September 30, 2010; author's files, "Housestaff History," Children's Hospital Boston Archives.
75. Communication with Betsy Blume, September 15, 2010; author's files, "Housestaff History," Children's Hospital Boston Archives.
76. Communication with Jeffery Burns, October 13, 2010; author's files, "Housestaff History," Children's Hospital Boston Archives.
77. Communication with Anne Stack, September 12, 2010; author's files, "Housestaff History," Children's Hospital Boston Archives.
78. Communication with Michael Rich, September 20, 2010; author's files, "Housestaff History," Children's Hospital Boston Archives.
79. Communication with Richard Bachur, September 13, 2010; author's files, "Housestaff History," Children's Hospital Boston Archives.

CHAPTER VII

1. Data for this section, "The Children's Hospital and The Department of Medicine," come from *Children's Hospital News*; the *Physician-in-Chief Newsletter* by Philip A. Pizzo; *Harvard Medical School Dean's Review*; and the Department of Medicine section of Children's Hospital Boston annual reports, by Gary R. Fleisher.
2. Data for this section, "Clinical Care," come from *Children's Hospital News*, March 1998; the *Physician-in-Chief Newsletter*, 1998–2000, by Philip A. Pizzo; *Harvard Medical School Dean's Review*; and the Department of Medicine

section of Children's Hospital Boston annual reports, 2006 and 2010, by Gary R. Fleisher.

3. Communication with Vincent Chiang, February 25, 2011; author's files, "Housestaff History," Children's Hospital Boston Archives.

4. Communication with Michael Agus, February 28, 2011; author's files, "Housestaff History," Children's Hospital Boston Archives.

5. Data for this section, "Medical Education," come from the *Physician-in-Chief Newsletter*, 1998–2000, by Philip A. Pizzo; *Harvard Medical School Dean's Review*, Department of Medicine section, June 2006, by Gary R. Fleisher; and the Department of Medicine section of Children's Hospital Boston annual reports 2001–2007, by Gary R. Fleisher.

6. Data for this section, "Research," come from the *Physician-in-Chief Newsletter*, 1998–2000, by Philip A. Pizzo; *Harvard Medical School Dean's Review*; the Department of Medicine section of Children's Hospital Boston annual reports 2006 and 2012, by Gary R. Fleisher; and the Harvard Medical School Five-year Clinical Department Review 2014, by Gary R. Fleisher.

7. Data for this section, "Promotions and Recognitions," come from Department of Medicine Executive Committee minutes, inclusive of years 1996–2007, by Frederick H. Lovejoy, Jr.; *Physician-in-Chief Newsletter*, 1998–2000, by Philip A. Pizzo; the Department of Medicine section of Children's Hospital Boston annual reports 2006 and 2012, by Gary R. Fleisher; and the Harvard Medical School Five-year Clinical Department Review 2014, by Gary R. Fleisher.

8. *Physician-in-Chief Newsletter*, December 1999, by Philip A. Pizzo; author's files, "Housestaff History," Children's Hospital Boston Archives.

9. Charles G. Prober, letter of nomination to the Association of American Medical Colleges, Awards Selection Committee, May 3, 2010; author's files, "Housestaff History," Children's Hospital Boston Archives, pp. 3–6.

10. David K. Stevenson, letter of nomination to the American Pediatric Society, Nomination Award Committee, May 26, 2010; author's files, "Housestaff History," Children's Hospital Boston Archives, pp. 4–6.

11. Joseph Wolfsdorf, remarks at the farewell dinner for Philip A. Pizzo, February 27, 2001; author's files, "Housestaff History," Children's Hospital Boston Archives.

12. American Pediatric Society, http://www.aps-spr-org/APS/Pres.htm

13. Data from this section, "Division Chiefs," come from the *Physician-in-Chief Newsletter*, 1998–2000, by Philip A. Pizzo; *Harvard Medical School Dean's Review*; and the Department of Medicine section of the Children's Hospital Boston annual report, June 2006, by Gary R. Fleisher.

14. D. P. Stevens, "GME Reform Needs Visionary Academic Leadership," *Academic Medicine* 1997;72(11):986–987.

15. J. J. Cohen, "A Little Help for Right Sizing Residencies," *Academic Medicine* 1997;72:984.

16. D. M. Gaba and S. K. Howard, "Fatigue Among Clinicians and the Safety of Patients," *New England Journal of Medicine* 2002;347(16):1249–1255, p. 1253.

17. C. P. Landrigan, J. M. Rothschild, J. W. Cronin, R. Kaushal, E. Burdick, J. T. Katz, C. M. Lilly, P. H. Stone, S. W. Lockley, D. W. Bates, and C. A. Czeisler, "Effects of Reducing Intern's Work Hours on Serious Medical Errors in Intensive Care Units," *New England Journal of Medicine* 2004;351:1838–1848, p. 1838.

18. J. E. Barone and M. E. Ivy, "Resident Work Hours: The Five Stages of Grief," *Academic Medicine* 2004;79:379–380.

19. J. E. Fischer, "Continuity of Care: A Casualty of the 80-Hour Work Week," *Academic Medicine* 2004;79:381–383.

20. J. M. Drazen and A. M. Epstein, "Rethinking Medical Training—Critical Work Ahead," *New England Journal of Medicine* 2002;347:1271–1272.

21. D. F. Weinstein, "Duty Hours for Resident Physicians—Tough Choices for Teaching Hospitals," *New England Journal of Medicine* 2002;347:1275–1277.

22. K. L. Smith, R. Saavedra, J. L. Roeke, and A. A. O'Donell, "The Journey to Creating a Campus-wide Culture of Professionalism," *Academic Medicine* 2007;82(11):1015–1021.

23. M. E. Witcomb, "Professionalism in Medicine," *Academic Medicine* 2007;82:1009.

24. J. J. Cohen, "Linking Professionalism to Humanism: What It Means, Whether It Matters," *Academic Medicine* 2007;82:1029–1032, p. 1029.

25. A. A. Brainard and H. C. Breslen, "Learning Professionalism: A View from the Trenches," *Academic Medicine* 2007;82:1010–1013, pp. 1012–1013.

26. M. E. Whitcomb, "Fostering an Evaluating Professionalism in Medical Education," *Academic Medicine* 2002;77:473–474.

27. C. Carraccio, S. D. Wolfsthal, R. Englander, K. Ferentz, and C. Martin, "Shifting Paradigms: From Flexner to Competencies," *Academic Medicine* 2002;77:361–366, pp. 362–363.

28. M. Whitcomb, "More on Competency-Based Education," *Academic Medicine* 2004;79:493–494.

29. T. Huddle and G. R. Heudebert, "Taking Apart the Art: The Risk of Anatomizing Clinical Competence," *Academic Medicine* 2007;82:536–541.

30. F. H. Lovejoy, Jr., D. G. Nathan, B. S. Zuckerman, P. A. Pizzo, G. R. Fleisher, and R. J. Vinci, "The Merger of Two Pediatric Residency Programs: Lessons Learned," *Journal of Pediatrics* 2008;153:731–732.

31. D. G. Nathan, "Proposed BCH Consolidation," January 25, 1995; author's files, "Housestaff History," Children's Hospital Boston Archives.

32. Communication with Rebekah Mannix, April 4, 2011; author's files, "Housestaff History," Children's Hospital Boston Archives.

33. Communication with Larry Rhein, April 6, 2011; author's files, "Housestaff History," Children's Hospital Boston Archives.

34. J. J. Alpert and B. Zuckerman, "History of Caring: The Pediatric Service at Boston University School of Medicine, Boston City Hospital, Boston Medical Center" (unpublished); author's files, "Housestaff History," Children's Hospital Boston Archives, p. 122.

35. Communication with Larry Rhein, April 6, 2011; author's files, "Housestaff History," Children's Hospital Boston Archives.

36. R. Masland, "Report of the Boston Combined Residency Program Selection Committee for the Year 1998"; author's files, "Housestaff History," Children's Hospital Boston Archives.

37. F. H. Lovejoy, Jr., "Medical Education Report for the Department of Medicine," in the Department of Medicine annual report, 2005–2006, by Gary R. Fleisher, Children's Hospital Boston Archives.

38. Communication with Larry Rhein, April 6, 2011; author's files, "Housestaff History," Children's Hospital Boston Archives.

39. F. H. Lovejoy, Jr., "Medical Education Report for the Department of Medicine, 2000–2005," in the Department of Medicine annual report, 2006–2007, by Gary R. Fleisher, Children's Hospital Boston Archives.

40. J. S. Bomalaski and G. J. Martin, "The Medical Chief Resident in the 1980s," *American Journal of Medicine* 1983;74:737–740.

41. T. E. Norris, J. L. Susman, and C. S. Gilbert, "Do Program Directors and Their Chief Residents View the Role of Chief Residents Similarly?" *Family Medicine* 1996;28:343–345.

42. P. A. Pizzo, "Reflections on Chief Residents at Children's Hospital Boston," 2005; author's files, "Housestaff History," Children's Hospital Boston Archives.

43. T. C. Sectish, F. H. Lovejoy, Jr., and R. J. Vinci, "Chief Residents at Children's Hospital Boston" (unpublished); author's files, "Housestaff History," Children's Hospital Boston Archives.

44. Communication with Joshua Nagler, April 4, 2011; author's files, "Housestaff History," Children's Hospital Boston Archives.

45. M. B. Son, "Reflections on Chief Residents at Children's Hospital Boston," 2005; author's files, "Housestaff History," Children's Hospital Boston Archives.

46. A. Growdon, "Reflections on Chief Residents at Children's Hospital Boston," 2005; author's files, "Housestaff History," Children's Hospital Boston Archives.

47. P. A. Pizzo, "Reflections on Chief Residents at Children's Hospital Boston," 2005; author's files, "Housestaff History," Children's Hospital Boston Archives.

48. Communication with Josh Nagler, April 4, 2011; author's files, "Housestaff History," Children's Hospital Boston Archives.

49. Communication with Rebekah Mannix, April 4, 2011; author's files, "Housestaff History," Children's Hospital Boston Archives.

50. Communication with Larry Rhein, April 6, 2011; author's files, "Housestaff History," Children's Hospital Boston Archives.

51. Communication with James Moses, April 15, 2011; author's files, "Housestaff History," Children's Hospital Boston Archives.

52. Communication with Amanda Growdon, April 20, 2011; author's files, "Housestaff History," Children's Hospital Boston Archives.

53. Gary R. Fleisher, "Earthquakes, Tectonic Shifts in Graduate Medical Education, and the Role of the APS in Finding Solid Ground," American Pediatric Society,

President's Address to the Pediatric Academic Society, Denver, Colorado, May 1, 2011.

54. Communication with Larry Rhein, April 6, 2011; author's files, "Housestaff History," Children's Hospital Boston Archives.

55. American Board of Pediatrics, "General Pediatric Special Pathways, Special Alterative Pathway (SAP)," February 6, 2008, www.abp.org/ABPwebsite/certinfo/genpeds/sappolicy.htm

56. Note 55, "Accelerated Research Pathway (ARP)."

57. Note 55, "Integrated Research Pathway (IRP)."

58. V. W. Chiang, V. K. Osganian, S. V. Lux IV, and F. H. Lovejoy, Jr., "The Special Alternative Pathway: Results from a 25 Year Experience" (unpublished); "Housestaff History," Children's Hospital Boston Archives.

59. F. H. Lovejoy, Jr., B. S. Zuckerman, G. R. Fleisher, and R. J. Vinci, "Creating an Academic Culture During Residency," *Journal of Pediatrics* 2008;152:599–600.

60. N. Ullrich, C. A. Botelho, P. Hibberd, and H. H. Bernstein, "Research During Pediatric Residency: Predictors and Resident Determined Influences," *Academic Medicine* 2003;78:1253–1258.

61. W. Cull, B. K. Yudowsky, D. J. Schonfeld, C. Berkowitz, and R. J. Pan, "Research Exposure During Pediatric Residency: Influences on Career Expectations," *Journal of Pediatrics* 2003;143:564–569, p. 564.

62. Note 59, pp. 599–600.

63. Note 59, p. 599.

64. R. J. Vinci, H. Bauchner, J. Finkelstein, P. K. Newby, S. Muret-Wagstaff, and F. H. Lovejoy, Jr., "Research During Pediatric Residency Training: Outcome of a Senior Resident Block Rotation," *Pediatrics* 2009;124:1126–1134, pp. 1128–1129.

65. Communication with Lise Nigrovic, April 7, 2011; author's files, "Housestaff History," Children's Hospital Boston Archives.

66. Note 59, p. 600.

67. F. H. Lovejoy, Jr., "Summative Data on Fred Lovejoy Resident Research and Education Fund Awards from 2003 to 2010"; author's files, "Housestaff History," Children's Hospital Boston Archives.

68. Communication with Lise Nigrovic, April 7, 2011; author's files, "Housestaff History," Children's Hospital Boston Archives.

69. M. B. Gordon, S. K. Osganian, J. S. Emans, and F. H. Lovejoy, Jr., "Gender Differences in Research Grant Applications for Pediatric Residents," *Pediatrics* 2009;124:e355-e361.

70. *Physician-in-Chief Newsletter*, August 17, 1998, by Philip A. Pizzo; author's files, "Housestaff History," Children's Hospital Boston Archives.

71. *Report of Working Group on Quality of Graduate Medical Education*, by Donald Goldmann, August 12, 1998; author's files, "Housestaff History," Children's Hospital Boston Archives.

72. "Program Evaluation," inclusive of years 2002–2005, by Jonathan Finkelstein; author's files, "Housestaff History," Children's Hospital Boston Archives.

73. Data for this section, "Career Directions and Accomplishments," come from Children's Hospital, Department of Medicine, graduation brochures, inclusive of years 1996–2009.

74. F. H. Lovejoy, Jr., "Career Directions 1998–2001"; author's files, "Housestaff History," Children's Hospital Boston Archives.

75. F. H. Lovejoy, Jr. and T. Sectish, "Residency Education Programs," in the Department of Medicine annual report, 2008–2009, by Gary R. Fleisher, Children's Hospital Boston Archives.

76. Senior dinner speeches, inclusive of years 1995–2007, by Frederick H. Lovejoy, Jr.; author's files, "Housestaff History," Children's Hospital Boston Archives.

77. Meghan M. Weir, *Between Expectations, Lessons from a Pediatric Residency* (Free Press, a Division of Simon and Shuster, 2011).

78. Data for this section, "Highlights of the Residency," come from senior resident graduation speeches, inclusive of years 1995–2007, by Frederick H. Lovejoy, Jr.; author's files, "Housestaff History," Children's Hospital Boston Archives.

79. Communication with Joshua Nagler, April 4, 2011; author's files, "Housestaff History," Children's Hospital Boston Archives.

CHAPTER VIII

1. George Santanya, *The Life of Reason*, Vol. 1, (C. Scribner's Sons, 1905).

2. Joseph B. Martin, *Alfalfa to Ivy: Memoir of a Harvard Medical School Dean* (The University of Alberta Press, 2011), p. 372.

3. Communication with Bob Vinci, October 17, 2011; author's files, "Housestaff History," Children's Hospital Boston Archives.

4. Robert H. Ebert, "The Dilemma of Medical Teaching," in John Knowles, Ed., *The Teaching Hospital* (Harvard University Press, 1966), p. 77.

5. Harry R. Lewis, *Excellence Without a Soul* (Public Affairs, a member of the Perseus Books Group, 2006), pp. 21–43, 49–51.

6. Richard C. Levin, *The Work of the University* (Yale University Press, 2003), pp. 30–31, 52–53.

7. Francis W. Peabody, *Doctor and Patient* (The MacMillian Company, 1930), p. 57.

8. Lynne Olson, *Citizens of London* (Random House, 2010), p. 394.

Index

ArtScroll Mesorah Series®

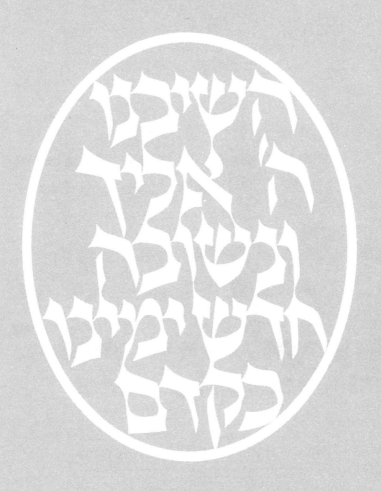

Rabbi Nosson Scherman / Rabbi Meir Zlotowitz
General Editors

זכור לאברהם

קינות ותפלות

לתשעה באב

NUSACH ASHKENAZ — נוסח אשכנז

Published by

Mesorah Publications, ltd

Cantor David S. Levine

A PROJECT OF THE

Mesorah Heritage Foundation

The Complete
tishah b'av service

A new translation and anthologized commentary

composed by

Rabbi Avrohom Chaim Feuer
and Rabbi Avie Gold

Designed by

Rabbi Sheah Brander

FIRST EDITION
First Impression . . . June, 1991

Published and Distributed by
MESORAH PUBLICATIONS, Ltd.
Brooklyn, New York 11232

Distributed in Israel by
MESORAH MAFITZIM / J. GROSSMAN
Rechov Harav Uziel 117
Jerusalem, Israel

Distributed in Europe by
J. LEHMANN HEBREW BOOKSELLERS
20 Cambridge Terrace
Gateshead, Tyne and Wear
England NE8 1RP

Distributed in Australia & New Zealand by
GOLD'S BOOK & GIFT CO.
36 William Street
Balaclava 3183, Vic., Australia

Distributed in South Africa by
KOLLEL BOOKSHOP
22 Muller Street
Yeoville 2198
Johannesburg, South Africa

THE ARTSCROLL MESORAH SERIES ®
"ZECHOR L'AVRAHAM / The Complete Tishah B'Av Service"
Nusach Ashkenaz
© Copyright 1989, by MESORAH PUBLICATIONS, Ltd.
4401 Second Avenue / Brooklyn, N.Y. 11232 / (718) 921-9000

ISBN: 0-89906-878-2 (hard cover)
ISBN: 0-89906-879-0 (paper back)

Typography by CompuScribe at ArtScroll Studios, Ltd., Brooklyn, NY
Bound by **Sefercraft, Inc.,** Brooklyn, NY

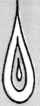

כָּל שֶׁרוּחַ הַבְּרִיּוֹת נוֹחָה הֵימֶנּוּ רוּחַ הַמָּקוֹם נוֹחָה הֵימֶנּוּ

If the spirit of one's fellows is pleased with him, the spirit of the Omnipresent is pleased with him (Avos 3:13)

This volume is dedicated
to the memory of

אברהם אלטר בן משה ע״ה

Abraham Vegh ע״ה

May 7, 1991 / נפטר כ״ג אייר תשנ״א

Abraham Vegh was born and raised in Apsha, and grew to manhood in Kashau. All his life he remained loyal to the teachings and teachers of those towns that are revered in Jewish memory. After surviving Auschwitz he came to Boston where he established himself as a skilled and sought after tailor.

But he worried about raising his children in the spirit of "der heim." So he moved to Williamsburg and then to Boro Park, and started all over again. For twenty-five years, his cleaning and tailoring store was a temple of honesty. He would not accept a job if it was not in the customer's best interest, and whatever he did, he did well — so well that customers requested that he do their work in his apartment after he retired.

When it seemed "impossible" in the early 50's to be a Shomer Shabbos, to wear a yarmulka at work in the store, or to daven with a minyan three times a day — he did it. He would leave the store to go to shul, because obligation came first, to his Maker as to his customers.

Chumash, Tehillim, Pirkei Avos — these were his life and he became their living embodiment.

To the people with whom he davened at the Sfardishe Shul for close to 30 years and the Apsha Beis Medrash during the last several years, he was known as an exceptional baal tefillah, with his heart and with his voice.

All his life, he fought to be true to Torah and Middos. In his resting place in Beit Shemesh, near Jerusalem, his memory remains a monument to the eternity of the Jew.

תנצב״ה

Lovingly Dedicated by,

Mrs. Serena Vegh

Mutty and Shoshy Vegh, Chani, Tova and Yaffa

Robby and Rozzy Vegh, David Jeffrey, Shalom and Ariella

Hy and Ruthy Kislak, Golde and Yitzy

⧫§ Publisher's Preface

Tishah B'Av is a day of tragedy and hope: a day of tragedy because, as Maimonides calls it, it is "the day that was designated for punishment," and day on which both Temples destroyed and many other misfortunes occurred; and a day of hope because it is the day on which the Redemption will be — or has been — spawned. The Book of Eichah/Lamentations and the Kinnos of Tishah B'Av consume the major parts of the evening and morning services but, to say the least, they are complex and difficult. And because they are, it is quite understandable that so many people find it difficult to attain the level of inspiration that is so essential to the day. The Sages teach that those who grieve over Jerusalem will be privileged to see its consolation; that being so, it is important that the sacred and meaning — laden words of the Kinnos be made comprehensible so that they can fulfill their portentous mission. That is the reason for this Siddur for Tishah B'Av. It is meant to be a volume that will guide the supplicant from the first moment of the day until the last word of Kiddush Levanah. In addition to the translation and commentary, this volume contains the necessary directions and laws, so that the reader will spend less time on searching and groping, and more on understanding and feeling the day's services.

The volume also includes two contemporary Kinnos, memorializing Churban Europe, the destruction of European Jewry in World War II. The authors, the Bobover Rav, שליט״א and HaGaon HaRav Shimon Schwab of K'hal Adas Jeshurun, respectively, composed them for recitation by their communities and they have since been adopted by others. (See introductions to both Kinnos).

⧫§ **Contents** This Siddur is as complete as possible. It includes translations of all the prayers and Torah readings, and translations and commentaries on Eichah and the Kinnos. The services for the full day are self-contained so that the reader will be spared the annoying chore of turning back and forth. The Overview provides a perspective on Tishah B'Av.

Although the Kinnos are standard in both Nusach Ashkenaz and Nusach Sefard, there are minor variations among the texts. Some of these are obviously the work of Christian censors, who removed or altered stanzas, phrases, or words they found offensive. The authors and editors of this work consulted many different editions of the Kinnos in order to arrive at the text that seemed to be correct. We emphasize, however, that the variations are relatively Jew.

⧫§ **Translation** The translation seeks to balance the lofty beauty of the heavily nuanced text and a readily understood English rendering. Where a choice had to be made, we generally preferred fidelity to the text over inaccurate simplicity, but occasionally, we had to stray from the literal translation in order to capture the essence of a phrase in an accessible English idiom. Especially in the Kinnos we had to go beyond a strictly literal translation, and sometimes rely on the commentary to clarify the meaning of the text.

⧫§ **Commentary** Because ordinary Torah study is forbidden on Tishah B'Av, this volume contains no commentary on the regular prayer order or the Torah readings. There is commentary, however, on Eichah and the Kinnos, for their saddening content makes it permissible to study as well as recite them. In addition, each kinnah/lamentation is provided with an introduction giving its background and historical context.

◆§ **Laws and Instructions** *Clear instructions are provided throughout. More complex or lengthy halachos are discussed at the end of the Siddur in the 'Laws' section, which the reader will find to be a very helpful guide. This section includes general halachos that are relevant to the regular prayer service. Throughout the volume, we refer to these laws by paragraph (§) number.*

◆§ **Layout and Typography** *We have followed the pattern of the ArtScroll Siddur and Machzorim, which have been greatly praised for their ease of use and clarity of layout. With its clear instructions, copious subtitles, and precise page headings, this Siddur was designed to make the service easy for everyone to follow: The first and last phrases of the translation on each page parallel the first and last phrases of the Hebrew text; paragraphs begin with bold-type words to facilitate the individual tefillos; each paragraph in the translation is introduced with the parallel Hebrew word to ease cross-checking; portions said aloud by the chazzan are indicated by either the symbol * or the word 'chazzan.' An asterisk (*) after a word indicates that that word or phrase is treated in the commentary. Numbered footnotes give the Scriptural sources of countless verses that have been melded into the prayers, as well as variant readings. A footnote beginning 'Cf.' indicates that the Scriptural source is paraphrased.*

◆§ **Hebrew Grammar** *As a general rule in the Hebrew language, the accent is on the last syllable. Where the accent is on an earlier syllable, it is indicated with a messeg, a vertical line below the accented letter: שִׁירוּ. In the case of the Shema and the Song at the Sea, which are given with the cantillation [trop], the accent follows the trop. A שְׁוָא נָע [sh'va na] is indicated by a hyphen mark above the letter: בָּרְכוּ; except for a sh'va on the first letter of a word, which is always a sh'va na. In identifying a sh'va na, we have followed the rules of the Vilna Gaon and Rabbi Yaakov Emden.*

Acknowledgments

The ArtScroll Series has been privileged to benefit from the advice and support of the venerable Torah leaders of the previous and present generations. MARAN HAGAON HARAV MOSHE FEINSTEIN, MARAN HAGAON HARAV YAAKOV KAMINETSKY, MARAN HAGAON HARAV GEDALIA SCHORR and HARAV HAGAON HARAV SHNEUR KOTLER, זצ״ל. Among today's gedolei Yisrael להבחל״ח MARAN HAGAON HARAV MORDECHAI GIFTER שליט״א has been a father and mentor from the start, and MARAN HAGAON HARAV ZELIK EPSTEIN שליט״א is a treasured counselor.

We are deeply grateful to Maranan HaGeonim HARAV DAVID FEINSTEIN, HARAV DAVID COHEN and HARAV HILLEL DAVID שליט״א for their involvement and for placing their encyclopedic scholarship at our disposal.

We are proud that the outstanding Torah scholar, HARAV HERSH GOLDWURM שליט״א, has been associated with the ArtScroll Series virtually since its inception. In this volume Rabbi Goldwurm has contributed the 'Laws,' reviewed most of the instructions, and been available for research and guidance.

The authors of this work, RABBI AVROHOM CHAIM FEUER and RABBI AVIE GOLD are familiar to ArtScroll readers. Here they have collaborated in a work that, we are confident, will place countless Jews further in their debt. Praise is superfluous; their words speak for themselves. We are proud to be associated with them.

Among those whose guidance was invaluable are such leaders of organizational and rabbinic life as RABBI MOSHE SHERER, RABBI PINCHAS STOLPER, RABBI BORUCH B. BORCHARDT, RABBI JOSHUA FISHMAN, RABBI FABIAN SCHONFELD, RABBI BENJAMIN WALFISH, MR. DAVID H. SCHWARTZ, RABBI YISRAEL H. EIDELMAN, RABBI BURTON JAFFA, and RABBI MICHOEL LEVI.

This work was conceived by our very dear friend, RABBI RAPHAEL BUTLER, whose heroic efforts on behalf of Torah propagation have earned him many admirers — and, more importantly, have brought thousands of people close to their heritage.

Special recognition and gratitude is due to the trustees of the MESORAH HERITAGE FOUNDATION, which sponsors this and other projects that bring the classics of our heritage to English-speaking Jews.

We are also grateful to the good and loyal friends who dedicated the various editions of the ArtScroll Siddur (in order of their publication): MR. and MRS. ZALMAN MARGULIES; MR. and MRS. JOSEPH BERLINER; MR. and MRS. AARON L. HEIMOWITZ; MRS. MALA WASSNER; MR. and MRS. HIRSH WOLF; MR. and MRS. BEREL TENNENBAUM, MR. and MRS. SOLLY KROK; MR. and MRS. DAN SUKENIK, and MR. and MRS. MOSHE SUKENIK; those who have dedicated the Ashkenaz Machzorim (in order of publication): MRS. EMOMA GLICK and her sons YITZCHAK (EDWARD) and NAFTALI (NORMAN); MRS. TILLIE FEDER and her children NORMAN and MARUEEN; the KUSHNER and LAULICT families; the sons of ARNOLD and HELEN LEE; MR. AND MRS. MICHAEL GROSS; and MRS. ROCHELLE SORSCHER; and to MR. AND MRS. ELI STERN and MR. AND MRS. JOSEPH STERN, who dedicated all five Nusach Sefard Machzorim.

Many other people have provided the assistance needed to produce such Torah projects. In addition to those mentioned in previous editions of the Siddur and other ArtScroll works, we are grateful to MR. and MRS. LOUIS GLICK, whose sponsorship of the ArtScroll Mishnah Series with the YAD AVRAHAM commentary is a jewel in the crown of Torah dissemination; and MR. and MRS. IRVING STONE and MR. and MRS. MORRY WEISS, who are sponsoring the forthcoming one-volume STONE EDITION of the Chumash.

We are proud and grateful that MR. AND MRS. JEROME SCHOTTENSTEIN and MRS. AND MRS. JAY SCHOTTENSTEIN and their families have undertaken to sponsor the monumental elucidation of the Talmud, which will henceforth be known as the SCHOTTENSTEIN EDITION. In the course of the work on the Talmud we have been privileged to gain the friendship and patronage of DAVID BERNSTEIN, PAUL PEYSER, and MICKEY SCHLISSER.

The following people have been particularly helpful in making possible the publication of this Siddur: MR. ABRAHAM FRUCHTHANDLER; RABBI CHAIM LEIBEL; RABBI YEHUDAH LEVI; MR. SHLOMO PERL; MR. ALBERT REICHMANN; MR. SHMUEL RIEDER; MR. ELLIS SAFDEYE; MR. LAURENCE A. TISCH; MR. WILLY WIESNER; MR. JUDAH SEPTIMUS; and MR. NATHAN SILBERMAN.

Only a fellow craftsman can perceive the excruciating hours that REB SHEAH BRANDER expended in designing the Siddur for the mispallel's maximum ease. In this project he has outdone even his own standard of excellence. Moreover, his learned and incisive comments improved every aspect of this work.

The eminent scholar RABBI AVROHOM YOSEIF ROSENBERG reviewed the vowelization of the Kinnos. We are honored and proud to have a talmid chacham of his stature associated with this work.

MRS. ESTIE DICKER, MRS. ESTHER FEIERSTEIN, MRS. YAFFA DANZIGER, BASSIE GOLDSTEIN, NICHIE FENDRICH, and YEHUDA GORDON typed the manuscript diligently and conscientiously. RABBI YOSEF GESSER and MRS. FAYGIE WEINBAUM carefully proofread the entire work; and MRS. JUDI DICK assisted in compiling sources.

The entire staff has a share in our service to the community, each in his or her area of responsibility: SHMUEL BLITZ, SHIMON GOLDING, SHEILA TENNEN-BAUM, and AVROHOM BIDERMAN, of the sales staff; ELI KROEN, YITZCHAK SAFTLAS, EPHRAIM ROSENSTOCK, YOSEF TIMINSKY, MICHAEL ZIVITZ, SAID KOHAN FOLAD, LEA FREIER, MRS. LIBBY GLUSTEIN, MRS. FAIGIE PERLOWITZ, ESTIE KUSHNER and RAIZY BRANDER. We conclude with gratitude to Hashem Yisborach for His infinite blessings and for the opportunity to have been the quill that records His word. May He guide our work in the future for the benefit of His people.

Rosh Chodesh Av 5751
Brooklyn, NY

Rabbis Meir Zlotowitz/Nosson Scherman

✦§ An Overview
Kinnos: A Trail of Tears —
From Tragedy to Triumph!

I. Tears: The Essence of the Soul

אָמַר ר׳ יוֹחָנָן: אוֹתוֹ הַיּוֹם [שֶׁחָזְרוּ הַמְרַגְּלִים] עֶרֶב תִּשְׁעָה בְּאָב הָיָה. אָמַר הקב״ה, אַתֶּם בְּכִיתֶם בְּכִיָּה שֶׁל חִנָּם, וַאֲנִי קוֹבֵעַ לָכֶם בְּכִיָּה לְדוֹרוֹת.

Rabbi Yochanan said that this day [when the spies returned and delivered their derogatory report about Eretz Yisrael] was Tishah B'Av eve. The Holy One, Blessed is He, said, 'You wept in vain. I will establish this date for you as a time of real weeping for all generations' (Taanis 29a).

Tears are uniquely suited to Tishah B'Av. Special dates in the Jewish calendar have their own tangible means to convey their essence. Rosh Hashanah has its *shofar*, Pesach has its *matzoh*, and so on. The *mitzvah* of Tishah B'Av is tears.

On the afternoon before Tishah B'Av, the *Chasam Sofer* would already be sobbing bitterly in anticipation of this day of misfortune. He collected every tear in a cup, and, when he ate his final meal before the fast, he would dip his bread into his tears and into ashes, as a sign of intense mourning. Thus would he fulfill the verse כִּי אֵפֶר כַּלֶּחֶם אָכָלְתִּי וְשִׁקֻּוַי בִּבְכִי מָסָכְתִּי, *For I have eaten ashes like bread, and mixed my drink with tears* (Psalms 102:10).

What is the significance of tears? Real tears, meaningful tears that are shed out of deep and sincere feelings, are the most genuine expression of the essence of the human personality. *Rav Hirsch* describes tears as 'the sweat of the soul.' When man is honestly moved or agitated, he sheds tears.

Maharal (Netzach Yisrael ch. 8) explains that when the Jews were redeemed from Egypt, God was actually submitting them to a new process of creation, whereby a new national entity called 'Israel' was being fashioned — a nation whose collective soul would be inextricably bound up with the teachings of the Torah and with the land of the Torah, *Eretz Yisrael*. When the Jewish people accepted the negative reports of the spies, however, they dramatically transformed their essential nature and ripped the Land of Israel out of the core of their being. They didn't merely accept the spies' report intellectually; rather, they shed real tears. Thereby they expressed the depths of their soul's antipathy for *Eretz Yisrael* — and thereby they severed their soul-bond with the Holy Land.

In order to forge a new soul-bond with the holy soil, the same tears that once·

dissolved our link to the Land of Israel must now be shed in love and yearning for our homeland. Once our souls are merged with the Land, the return of our bodies will follow.

II: My Soul Weeps in Secret

בְּמִסְתָּרִים תִּבְכֶּה נַפְשִׁי מִפְּנֵי גֵוָה.

My soul shall weep in secrecy for your pride (Jeremiah 13:17).

This teaches that God has a concealed place called מִסְתָּרִים, *secrecy, where He weeps over the pride of Israel that was stripped from them and given to the nations of the World . . . Some say that God weeps over the Divine glory which has been concealed from this world . . .*

But how can we say God weeps, are we not told that עֹז *וְחֶדְוָה בִּמְקֹמוֹ, strength and rejoicing are in His Presence? (I Chronicles 16:27).*

No, this is not a contradiction! On the inside [in secret], God weeps; on the outside, He appears to rejoice (Chagigah 5b).

Perceiving the Real Loss

MAHARAL (NETZACH YISRAEL CHAPTER 9) reveals the location of God's secret hideaway — it is within the soul of every Jew. For the soul is really an aspect of God concealed within man, and that fundamental soul of man cries incessantly over the Destruction of the Temple. The average person is not in touch with his inner soul, with his real self, so he is oblivious to its weeping. The average person is aware only of his external facade, the outer world of the body, where everything appears to be fine and growing better — with abundant '*strength and rejoicing.*'

The chassidic master, Reb Bunim of P'shis'cha, illustrated this concept with a parable of a king who amassed tremendous treasures and hid them in a secret storage room, deep inside his palace. One day the palace caught fire and burned down to the ground. The entire nation and the royal court cried over the loss of the beautiful palace, but the king cried more bitterly than any of them, for he alone knew the true extent of the loss. Only he knew of the enormous hidden treasure that went up in smoke.

Similarly, a person who is out of touch with his inner soul hardly appreciates the spiritual loss suffered with the Temple's destruction.

Rav Elya Lopian זצ״ל illustrated this with the following incident (see *Lev Eliahu I, Shevivei Or* 155):

Rav Moshe Isserles, the *Rama*, wrote in *Toras HaOlah*, that when King Nebuchadnezzar came to destroy the First Temple, the Greek philosopher Plato accompanied him. After the Destruction, Plato met the prophet Jeremiah near the Temple Mount, weeping and wailing bitterly over the Temple ruins. Plato asked him two questions: 1) 'Behold, you are the preeminent sage in Israel, is it befitting a man of your intellectual stature to cry over a building, which is really no more than a pile of sticks and stones?' 2) 'This building is already in ruins; what good will your tears do now? Why cry over the past?'

Jeremiah responded, 'Plato, as a world-renowned philosopher, you surely have many perplexing questions.'

The Greek recited his long list of complicated problems. Humbly and quietly, Jeremiah solved them all in a few brief sentences. Plato was dumbfounded. 'I can't believe that any mortal man can be so wise!'

Jeremiah pointed sadly to the Temple ruins and said, 'All of this profound wisdom I derived from those "sticks and stones," and that is why I am crying. As for your second question, "Why do I cry over the past," this I cannot tell you because you will not be able to understand the answer.'

Rav Elya Lopian related that Rav Simcha Zissel of Kelm explained Jeremiah's answer. Our tears are not for the past; rather, we cry for the future, because even though all the gateways to heaven were sealed at the time of the *Churban* [Destruction], the gateway of tears always remains open (*Berachos* 32b). Every tear we shed is collected in heaven and contributes to the reconstruction of the next Temple. This concept, which is so simple for any Jew to understand, is beyond the comprehension of a 'rational,' world-renowned Plato.

❧ ❧ ❧

JEREMIAH BEGAN OUR TRAIL of tears twenty-five centuries ago. Since then, tragically, the trail has been enlarged into an expanding stream, a mighty river,

Transcending Sadness

a surging torrent — and the tears continue to flow even in our days.

Jeremiah poured all of his tears into *Eichah*, the Book of *Lamentations*, wherein he painfully predicted the travails of his tormented people. In his commentary to the *Rambam*, *Yad Hamelech* asks: The rule is that our Holy Scriptures, the *Tanach*, must be written by a proven prophet while he is under the influence and inspiration of רוּחַ הַקּוֹדֶשׁ, *the Divine spirit*. The Talmud (*Shabbos* 30b) clearly teaches, however, that this holy spirit cannot envelop a person while he is in a state of sorrow, because it settles only on a person whose spirit enjoys the ecstasy of performing a *mitzvah*. If so, how could Jeremiah write the Book of *Lamentations* while he was shrouded in mourning?

Yad Hamelech explains that the spirit of prophecy rests upon men of greatness, who demonstrate nobility of character and generosity of spirit. Ordinarily, people who wallow in self-pity and are consumed by their personal woes lead narrow, self-centered lives, and are remote from the qualities of a prophet. Conversely, people who exult in performing God's commandments display a purity of character. But there is another proof of sterling character, one that is valid even in the vail of tears.

Jeremiah was not sad about himself or his plight; his personal situation concerned him not at all. Rather, his tears were over the miserable plight of his fellow Jews, and over the pain of God's Presence, which had been forced into exile. Consequently, Jeremiah's sorrow proved the greatness of his selfless personality, thus making him fit for prophetic inspiration.

III: A Tear Is Never Wasted

> *Rabbi Eliezer said: Since the day the Temple was destroyed, the heavenly gates of prayer have been shut, as it is written, 'Though I cry out and I plead, He shuts out my prayer' (Lam. 3:8); nevertheless, the gates of tears have not been sealed, as it is written, Hear my prayer, HASHEM, listen to my outcry, be not mute to my tears (Psalms 39:13) (Berachos 32b).*

THE QUESTION HAS been asked: If the gates of tears are never locked, why did God make them in the first place? The Gerrer Rebbe explained that although **Power** sincere tears always gain admission above, the gates are needed to **of Tears** shut out *false* tears, which are abominable to God. We might add that although these gates are never locked, they are closed and can be opened only as far as the flow of tears will push them! Indeed, Yaaros Devash (II:11) observes that the numerical value of בְּכִי, weeping, equals that of לֵב, heart, because tears are meaningful only if they are sincere expressions of the heart. Such tears are truly priceless.

Rav Aryeh Levin of Jerusalem was a man of rare compassion and sensitivity. Once, a distraught, recently widowed woman came to his home and cried uncontrollably. All of his efforts to offer solace were to no avail, until the widow said, 'Rabbi, I will accept your words of consolation on one condition. Please tell me what happened to all of my tears? I prayed and prayed for my late husband, I recited chapter after chapter of Tehillim, and shed thousands upon thousands of tears. My very soul flowed into those tears. Were they all wasted?'

Gently, Rav Aryeh replied, 'After a hundred and twenty years, when you will leave this world and ascend to the heavenly tribunal, you will see how meaningful and precious your tears were. You will discover that God himself gathered them in and counted every single teardrop and treasured it like a priceless gem. And you will discover that, whenever some harsh and evil decree was looming over the Jewish people, one of your tears came and washed the evil away, making it null and void. Even one sincere tear is a source of salvation!'

Hearing, this the woman burst into a fresh flow of tears — not tears of sorrow and grief, but tears of courage and hope.

Sometime later she came back to Reb Aryeh and said, 'Rabbi, you remember what you told me? Please tell me again.'

THE JEW WHO sheds tears for his personal concerns does so as the external, physical person. Deep inside the secret recesses of his soul, however, the Godly **For the** portion within him cries over one thing only, the loss of **Nation's Sake** the Divine Presence, for that is the source of all other tragedies and the underlying reason for Jewish suffering.

Our personal suffering is a direct offshoot of the collective, national suffering of the Jewish people in exile. The Midrash (*Eichah Rabbasi* 1:25, see also *Sanhedrin* 104b) tells of a widow in Rabban Gamliel's neighborhood, who would weep bitterly over her plight. When Rabban Gamliel heard her cries in the night, he would arise and cry over the destruction of the Temple and the Jewish exile. HaRav Mordechai Gifter explains that Rabban Gamliel knew that her personal woes were an outgrowth of Israel's general misfortune. When Israel is delivered collectively, all personal problems will be resolved as well.

For many years, Rabbi Yoel Sirkis, known as the *Bach*, could not arrange for the publication of *Bais Chadash*, his commentary on the *Tur Shulchan Aruch*. Whenever it was about to go to print, an unforeseen circumstance would arise and delay the printing. After many years of frustration, the *Bach* was heartbroken. One midnight, as he grieved over his personal misfortune, he stopped and berated himself: 'How selfish of me to weep over my personal problems when there is a far greater tragedy in the world, the calamity of Israel in Exile!' So he took off his shoes like a mourner and recited *Tikkun Chatzos*, the midnight prayer for the Redemption of Israel.

Eventually, fatigue overcame the *Bach* and he fell asleep. A heavenly voice addressed him in a dream: 'Know that for many years they have been displeased with you in heaven, because you became so engrossed in writing *Bais Chadash* that you neglected the recitation of *Tikkun Chatzos*. As great as Torah study is, one must never lose sight of the plight of the Jewish people. Tonight, for the first time in years, you cried over the collective misery of God and Israel — so you have regained favor in heaven.'

TODAY'S JERUSALEM IS A beautiful urban complex, replete with every type of structure and institution necessary for modern life. The rebuilt Jerusalem of our times serves all the physical and spiritual needs of her citizens. If so, why do we continue to plead for the 'rebuilding' of Jerusalem?

Heart of Our Nation

This question can be answered with an analogy to the patient who receives a heart transplant. The patient is up and around and appears to be healthy, but he is filled with anxiety lest his new heart be rejected or malfunction. He is extremely vulnerable to infection, and distressingly susceptible to unexpected, side effects. As advanced as technology may be, the new heart is not his own.

Similarly, the heart of mankind in general and the Jews in particular is the *Beis HaMikdash*, the Holy Temple. In that location, Adam was created and there God breathed life into his nostrils. God continued to pump vitality into mankind through the Temple until it was destroyed. Now, we are still maintained, but it is not the same. We are weak and fragile, susceptible to spiritual and moral contamination and disease. We are easily worn out. The whole system can collapse at any time.

The Temple and the Holy City are the heart of our nation; when they were destroyed we suffered a national cardiac arrest. If we are crippled as a nation, how can any individual be fully healthy? Only when Jerusalem is rebuilt will Israel be healed: As King David said, *The Builder of Jerusalem is HASHEM, He will gather in the outcasts of Israel. He is the Healer of the broken-hearted and the One Who binds up their sorrows (Psalms 147:2,3).*

IV: Jeremiah the Prophet: Fighting Fire With Tears

Jeremiah cursed the ninth day of Av, Tishah B'Av, the day of his birth (Midrash Iyov).

Every time Jeremiah admonished the Jewish people, they mocked, scorned, and humiliated him (Mishlei Rabbasi 1).

JEREMIAH WAS PROBABLY the most unpopular prophet in history. For forty years he fearlessly hammered away at the people of Israel and warned them of **Unbridled** God's impending retribution. Everything he said, he said **Brazenness** publicly, in the marketplace, for all to hear. The people despised him for his prophecies. He was not just unpopular — he was scorned, hated, threatened, and persecuted. But he was never intimidated or silenced, because he spoke the word of God — and the word of God must be heard.

The one who detested Jeremiah most was King Yehoyakim. The height of King Yehoyakim's brazen defiance is described in chapter 36 of the Book of *Jeremiah*.

In the fourth year of his reign, eighteen years before the *Churban*, God commanded Jeremiah to prepare a scroll upon which he would record God's prediction of the evil that would befall the land during the future *Churban*. Our Rabbis teach that Jeremiah, who was then in prison because of his intrepid prophecies, recorded the basic text of the Book of *Lamentations* (chapters 1,2, and 4). Because he was incarcerated, Jeremiah sent his devoted disciple Baruch ben Neriyah to the king's palace to read this prophetic warning to him. This took place on the eighth day of Kislev while the king was in his winter palace, which was warmed by a roaring fire. One of the king's officers began to read:

'Alas — she (Jerusalem) *sits in solitude!' (Lam.* 1:1). 'Who cares,' responded Yehoyakim, 'as long as I remain king!'

'She weeps bitterly in the night' (ibid. 1:2). 'Who cares,' he shrugged, 'as long as I remain king!'

'Judah has gone into exile because of suffering' (ibid. 1:3). 'Who cares! I am still king!' *'The roads of Zion are in mourning!'* (ibid. 1:4). 'Who cares! I am still king!'

'Her adversaries have become her ruling monarch' (ibid. 1:5).

'That I will never accept! I must remain king!' (*Moed Katan* 26a).

Enraged Yehoyakim seized a sharp razor, and cut out every Name of God from the scroll, and then threw God's Names and the holy scroll into the roaring fire — where it burnt until everything turned to ashes.

After the king committed this sacrilege, neither he nor any of his retinue felt any remorse or fear whatsoever. Ordinarily, when a sacred Torah scroll goes up in flames and God's Name is obliterated, it is considered a calamity of the highest order, and one must tear his clothing in mourning, and fast and repent. Not so Yehoyakim and his court; they rejoiced over the conflagration of the Torah.

For this, Yehoyakim was doomed to die a terrible death, with his remains treated like an animal's carcass, unburied and left to rot in the street. And his subjects, who tolerated his wickedness, were doomed to destruction by sword and fire.

GOD TOLD JEREMIAH to take up the prophet's pen once again to rewrite the Book of *Lamentations* to which was now added chapter three, the longest and

Jeremiah's Mission
most tragic chapter of all. It begins: *I am the man who has seen affliction by the rod of His anger (Lam. 3:1).*
This was Jeremiah's sorrowful destiny. He saw the destruction looming closer and closer, yet he could do nothing to prevent it, because the people and their leaders refused to listen. He tried with all his might to get the people to cry, because he knew that nothing would extinguish the flame of God's fury like sincere tears of penitence; but their hearts were hardened and not a tear would they shed.

After the destruction of the Temple, Jeremiah resolved to follow the multitude of Jews who were led into captivity. When he found a blood-drenched trail, he knew he was in the right direction. All too soon, he came across dead bodies, severed limbs, and the pitiful corpses of tiny sucklings and babes. When he finally caught up with the captives, he hugged and kissed them, clung to them in warm embrace, and accompanied them all the way to the shores of the Euphrates River, in Babylonia, where he bid them farewell saying, 'I must return to comfort the remnants of Israel who remain on the holy soil.'

When the captives realized that the prophet was leaving them, they burst into tears, 'Our dear father Jeremiah, how can you leave us?' they wept. With deep compassion, Jeremiah responded, 'I hereby bring heaven and earth to testify that I tell you the absolute truth; if only you had cried sincerely but once while you were still in Zion, you never would have been exiled.' With that, Jeremiah turned toward the Holy Land, shedding bitter tears (*Pesikta Rabbasi* 26).

THE TEARS OF KINNOS are a never-ending stream. When I began to translate and elucidate the *Kinnos* on the day after Succos, I called my rebbe, HaRav

A Cry For All Seasons
Mordechai Gifter, and asked, 'How can I get into the mood of writing about *Kinnos* just a day after Simchas Torah, while the happy tunes of joy still resonate in my ears and Tishah B'Av is still so far off in the future? Who can think of *Kinnos* now?'

He replied: 'You are mistaken. *Kinnos* are not only for Tishah B'Av, they are for the entire year, except that throughout the year we recite *Kinnos* in a whisper, while on Tishah B'Av we shout them out loud! Whoever neglects *Kinnos* all year long and attempts to start reciting them on Tishah B'Av will not succeed in saying them even then, because he will recite the verses without any feeling and he will become bored. We must cry and mourn over the *Churban* all year long, in every season, and then our *Kinnos* will reach their climax of pain on Tishah B'Av!'

This concept of regular mourning over the *Churban* is codified in the very first chapter of *Shulchan Aruch (Orach Chaim* 1:3): *It is proper for every God-fearing person to feel and anguish over the destruction of the Holy Temple.*

The *Sfas Emes* was once asked: 'And what should someone do if he feels no anguish over the *Churban* of the Temple?' The Rebbi replied, 'Then he should be consumed with pain and anguish over his own personal *Churban*. If a Jew doesn't feel real pain over the *Churban*, it shows that his soul is in a wretched, abysmal state!'

True, *kinnos* are for all year round — but when does one begin to develop a feeling for them? On Tishah B'Av. If one truly comprehends and feels the *Kinnos* he recites on this day, he will be inspired to refer back to them throughout the year. For this reason the halachah places special emphasis on understanding the meaning of every word in the *Kinnos*:

> ... the entire congregation should understand them — including the women and children — because women are obligated to hear the *Kinnos* like the men — and undoubtedly we must make certain that the young boys understand (*Tur Shulchan Aruch, Orach Chaim* §559).

V: Tishah B'Av: The Birthday of Mashiach

> כֵּיָן שֶׁחָרַב בֵּית הַמִּקְדָּשׁ נוֹלַד הַמָּשִׁיחַ.
> *From the moment the Temple was destroyed Mashiach was born (Midrash Abba Gorion).*
>
> What is the name of the Messiah? Rav Yehudah said in the name of Rav Iva, 'His name is Menachem, as it is written: עַל אֵלֶּה אֲנִי בוֹכִיָּה עֵינִי עֵינִי יֹרְדָה מַּיִם כִּי רָחַק מִמֶּנִּי מְנַחֵם מֵשִׁיב נַפְשִׁי, *Over these things I weep; my eyes run with water because a comforter (Menachem) to revive my spirit is far from me (Lam. 1:16).*
> ... On the day the Temple was destroyed the Messianic Savior of Israel was born. What is his name? Menachem (comforter) (*Midrash Eichah Rabbasi* 1:57).

ON TISHAH B'AV we recite over forty *kinnos* expressing our pain and misery over the destruction of our Temple and the exile of the Jewish people. Scores of

No Contradiction major Jewish themes are interwoven into the rich and complex tapestry of the *kinnos*, yet one fundamental concept is missing. There is no mention of *Mashiach!* This deletion is particularly puzzling since, according to many Rabbinic sources, *Mashiach's* birthday is on this very day of Tishah B'Av!

Perhaps the solution to this enigma may be found in the Redeemer's identity. He is מָשִׁיחַ בֶּן דָּוִד, *Messiah the son of David*, an extension and an amplification of the life and accomplishments of King David, 'The Sweet Singer of Israel' (see Overview to *ArtScroll Tehillim*). The Psalmist was uniquely able to sing God's praises under even the most adverse circumstances. Indeed, the more David suffered, the more he praised God. The more intense the pain, the more intense the passion, because David extracted the precious nugget of goodness from within every grief.

For David and for the Messiah, his scion, there are no bleak, mournful *kinnos*/lamentations, there are only exultant *mizmorim*/songs. Indeed, this is precisely how *Mashiach* will redeem Israel from her travails, by teaching Jews how to discern the positive, productive forces that are encased within every negative experience. In all of the Scriptures, no one was as afflicted as David. No one was so misunderstood, no one had so many enemies. Job's suffering was unbearable, but it lasted for relatively a short while. But David's entire life was an endless succession of misfortune.

This is the wondrous secret of *Tehillim*. David cries out in pain, yet songs of joy pour forth from his lips. His words are those of melancholy and despair, yet a spirit of happiness saturates every syllable.

David could cry out, '*Every night my bed I drench, with my tears I soak my couch*' — and still he could exult, '*HASHEM has heard my plea, HASHEM will accept my prayer*' (*Psalms* 6:7,10). There was no contradiction, because David understood that his affliction and his acceptance were one (*Tzidkas HaTzaddik* 129).

One of David's greatest misfortunes was the rebellion of Absalom, his son.

מִזְמוֹר לְדָוִד בְּבָרְחוֹ מִפְּנֵי אַבְשָׁלוֹם בְּנוֹ ה׳ מָה רַבּוּ צָרָי רַבִּים קָמִים עָלָי.

A song of David, as he fled from Absalom his son. HASHEM, how many are my tormentors! The great rise up against me! (*Psalms* 3:1,2).

IN VIEW OF THE tragic circumstances under which this psalm was composed — a revolution led by the son over whom he had doted! — the title 'A **song** of

To Cope With Heartbreak

David,' seems to be incongruous. As the Talmud asserts, it should have been called a **kinnah/lament**! Said Rabbi Shimon ben Avishalom, this be likened to a person in debt. Before he pays, he is worried and sad, but after he pays, he rejoices. So too with David. Since God had warned him, *I will raise up evil against you from out of your own house*' (*II Samuel* 12:11), he was saddened. Perhaps a merciless slave or an illegitimate child would rise up in vengeance, without any mercy. Now that he saw that he was menaced by his own son, who, despite his treachery, indeed hesitated to follow Ahitophel's counsel that he pursue and slaughter his father, David sang in gratitude to God (*Berachos* 7b).

Similarly we read in Psalms how the Psalmist took a different view of the destruction of the Temple. Even in this catastrophe, he found cause to sing.

מִזְמוֹר לְאָסָף אֱלֹהִים בָּאוּ גוֹיִם בְּנַחֲלָתֶךָ טִמְּאוּ אֶת הֵיכַל קָדְשֶׁךָ שָׂמוּ אֶת יְרוּשָׁלַ͏ִם לְעִיִּים.

A song of Assaf, O God! The nations have entered into Your estate, they defiled the Sanctuary of Your holiness, they turned Jerusalem into a heap of rubble (*Psalms* 79:1).

Since this woeful composition describes the Temple's destruction, the *Midrash* asks here too: מִזְמוֹר? קִינָה מִיבָּעֵי לֵהּ׳, *A song? This should be titled, a* קִינָה, *a kinnah!*

The *Midrash* answers with a parable. A king once erected a beautiful bridal canopy for his son's nuptials. The son, however, was so stubborn and rude that he infuriated his father. The king stormed into the wedding hall and vented his rage on the gorgeous canopy, ripping it to shreds.

So too did the stubbornness of Israel exceedingly anger God. However, He was merciful, and directed His anger at the stones and beams of the Holy Temple rather than at the Jews themselves. Although the people of Israel were severely punished, only the Temple was destroyed; the nation survived.

Clearly, David/Messiah is able to transform every *kinnah* into a *mizmor*, song. Thus, it is impossible to include the concept of the hopeful, optimistic *Mashiach* in the despairing, despondent *kinnos* of Tishah B'Av. Where there is Mashiach, there can be no *kinnos!*

Jeremiah, the prophet who was born on Tishah B'Av, said: *'Cursed be the day on which I was born, let not the day on which my mother gave birth to me have any blessing* (Jeremiah 20:14). But this very tragedy shall lead us to our ultimate triumph. Because the very fact that for thousands of years Jews the world over have forgotten the woes of the present and plunged themselves into an ocean of tears over a Holy Temple that they and their parents never saw, and lamented over a Holy Land upon which their feet never trod — this is Israel's supreme merit. The very fact that we return to our lament every Tishah B'Av, year after year, shows that we remember what was and lament what was lost, that we *do* have hope and that our faith *is* strong. Thus, as the *Kinnos* end, Jeremiah's accursed birthday is transformed into *Moshiach's* blessed birthday. Once again the *kinnah* is exchanged for a *mizmor.*

VI: Rabbi Elazar HaKalir: A Balm for Burning Eyes

PIYUT, LITURGICAL POETRY, has been a hallowed and time-honored component of our prayer service for many centuries. Rabbi Elazar HaKalir is universally

Master Paytan accepted as 'the Father of the *Paytanim'* [liturgical poets], having achieved an unsurpassed degree of excellence in language and style, combined with a superior level of Torah scholarship.

Magen Avraham (*Orach Chaim* 68:1) quotes *Shibbolei Haleket* who writes: 'I heard from my father who heard from his teachers that when the Kalir composed the piyut "And the fiery angels face the celestial Throne," a heavenly fire encircled him. This is what my father heard from his teachers. Indeed, Rabbi Shimon HaGadol, who was a miracle-worker, would recite that *piyut* every day.'

THE GREATEST MYSTERY surrounding the Kalir is his identity. Who was this awesome person? When and where did he live?

Who Was He? Some scholars claim that the Kalir lived in the era of *Rav Saadya Gaon* (882-942 C.E.). Another school of thought, based on the Midrash and the Pesikta, maintains that the Kalir was a Tannaitic scholar who lived in *Eretz Yisrael.* Indeed the *Tosafos* (*Chagigah* 13a s.v. *Veragli*) and *Rabbeinu Asher* (*Berachos* 3:21) cite an opinion that the Kalir was no less than the renowned Tanna, Rabbi Elazar the son of Rabbi Shimon bar Yochai, who studied Torah in a cave for thirteen years, during which the Kabbalistic mysteries of the holy *Zohar* were revealed to them.

What is the meaning of the name *Kalir?* There are various opinions. I would humbly suggest the word *Kalir* is derived from קילורין [killorin,] which means 'a balm for the eyes' (see *Shabbos* 108b and *Yalkut Shimoni, Tehillim* §675). Incessant weeping and bitter tears had burned and reddened the eyes of the Jewish people. Rabbi Elazar the Kalir composed his beautiful, soul-stirring poems in order to soothe and cool the feverish eyes and hearts of his suffering brethren.

THE TALMUD (SHABBOS 33B) relates that when the Roman government condemned Rabbi Shimon to death, he and his son Rabbi Elazar fled and hid in **The World** a cave for twelve years. When they emerged they were on such a lofty spiritual plane that they couldn't tolerate common folk **Survives** pursuing such mundane endeavors as plowing a field. 'How can people ignore the Eternal World and pursue this world?' Everyone upon whom they focused their eyes critically was immediately consumed by fire.

A Heavenly voice thundered at them, 'Did you leave the cave in order to destroy My world?'

They returned to the cave for one more year. When they emerged a second time, Rabbi Elazar remained as zealous as ever, and his eyes continued to set things afire, while his father Rabbi Shimon had mellowed, and his eyes healed and restored everything that his son's eyes had destroyed.

The Talmud does not tell us the outcome. Perhaps Rabbi Elazar finally calmed his seething emotions and soothed his fiery eyes by composing the *piyutim*, *selichos*, and *Kinnos* that expressed the passion and feelings of his great soul.

Generations upon generations of Jews have found an expression of their innermost spiritual pain and yearning in these *Kinnos* composed by those who expanded upon the original elegies and dirges of Jeremiah the Prophet. Surely the Holy One, Blessed is He, listens carefully as He collects and cherishes our tears. Surely the treasury of tears has already been filled to overflowing by countless years of Jewish suffering. Surely the time has come to call a halt to the flow of tears and to replace our weeping with laughter.

May the tears we shed this Tishah B'Av be the last tears for all time, and may we witness the fulfillment of the Talmudic blessing: כָּל הַמִּתְאַבֵּל עַל יְרוּשָׁלַיִם זוֹכֶה וְרוֹאֶה בְּשִׂמְחָתָה, Whoever mourns over Jerusalem is deserving to witness her joy! (*Megillah* 30b).

✑§ Prologue

The All-Encompassing Aleph-Beis:
From Aleph to Tav, and Back Again

(based on The Wisdom in the Hebrew Alphabet,
by Rabbi Michael F. Munk)

I n Jewish thought, the *Aleph Beis* is unlike any other alphabet; it is not merely a haphazard collection of consonants whose order was determined by convention, but that could have been — or still could be — changed without loss of content. The individual letter, their names, graphic forms, *gematrios* [numerical equivalents], and respective positions in the *Aleph Beis* are Divinely ordained. [See Overview of the Artscroll The *Wisdom in the Hebrew Alphabet* for a discussion of the Divine forces represented by the letters and their various combinations.] A corollary of this principle is the halachic requirement that every letter in a Torah scroll, *mezuzah*, and *tefillin* must be written perfectly. No part of a letter may be omitted or distorted, nor may its individual integrity be compromised by contact with any other letter. Every word must be spelled correctly; a missing, extra, transposed, or blemished letter can invalidate the entire scroll.

In Scripture, as in our prayers and *kinnos*, we often find verses or phrases progressing through the Hebrew alphabet from *aleph* to *tav*; conversely, there are passages that reverse the order, beginning with *tav* and going back to *aleph*. What is the significance of these letter progressions?

is said to be covered מֵאָלֶף וְעַד תָּיו, *from aleph to tav*. Since the very order of the

Aleph to Tav: Completion letters represents profound halachic and philosophic concepts, this expression is far more encompassing than the idiomatic "from A to Z" or from "*alpha* to *omega*."

The use of an alphabetical sequence to praise God, or describe a person or concept, denotes totality and perfection. For example, the אֵשֶׁת חַיִל, *An Accomplished Woman*, is described in *Proverbs* (31:10-31) in twenty-two verses beginning with the respective letters of the *Aleph-Beis*. The twenty-two alphabetical verses of "An Accomplished Woman" [אֵשֶׁת חַיִל] express the entire range of the woman's virtues in following the ways of Torah, which was translated into human expression by means of the twenty-two letters.

THE DEFINITE ARTICLE *the* is expressed in Hebrew by prefixing the letter ה to a word. Often, for extra emphasis, the word אֶת (or אֵת) is employed in addition

Complete Blessing and Tempered Curse to the prefix. Because it is spelled with the first and last letters of the *Aleph Beis*, אֶת alludes to completion and perfection. Thus the Torah uses this emphatic article in describing the beginning of Creation: בְּרֵאשִׁית בָּרָא אֱלֹהִים אֵת הַשָּׁמַיִם וְאֵת הָאָרֶץ, *In the beginning of God's creating the heavens and the earth* (*Genesis* 1:1). This usage indicates that the universe was created in complete perfection, "from *aleph* to *tav*."

The detailed blessings promised those who observe the entire Torah begin with the א of אִם [*If you follow My decrees...*] (*Leviticus* 26:3) and end with the ת of קוֹמְמִיּוּת, (*upright* ibid. v. 13). This indicates that the commandments are as perfect as the universe in which they are to be fulfilled (*Maharal, Netzach*), and that the blessings bestowed as a reward for *mitzvah* observance are complete and all-encompassing.

IN A LESS HAPPY USE, alphabetic acrostics are employed to symbolize totality of destruction and transgression. In the period before the destruction of the First

Consolation Amid Tragedy

Temple when Israel no longer deserved blessings, the prophet Jeremiah composed the Book of *Eichah* [*Lamentations*], which contains a series of lamentations. Its verses begin, respectively, with the twenty-two letters of the *Aleph-Beis*, in order to indicate that God's *full* fury was unleashed against the people of Israel, because "they transgressed the Torah, which was given them with the twenty-two letters" (*Sanhedrin* 104a).

But there is consolation even amid tragedy. Although the Temple has not been rebuilt, the Torah, symbolizing the completion and perfection of the full *Aleph-Beis*, remains the legacy of Israel. The month of tragedy, is called מְנַחֵם אָב, or *consolation of the Aleph Beis* (*Kotzker*).

THE ENTIRE ALEPH-BEIS is a single unit in which all the letters are interrelated. Just as every part of the universe was created by God and is totally dependent on

The Universal Cycle of Return: From Tav to Aleph

His mercy at all times, so too the *aleph* — symbol of God's uniqueness and primacy — is the root and leader of all the sacred letters. The letters can be compared to a flame; though tongues and sparks of fire spring out in many directions, they all originate from and are part of the same flame, because all forces emanate from the One God and are connected by an underlying unity.

Accordingly, Kabbalistic literature teaches that the *Aleph-Beis* — representing all Divine forces — does not culminate with the *tav*, but turns around to reunite again with the *aleph*, which symbolizes the יְחִידוֹ שֶׁל עוֹלָם, *the Unique One of the universe*, Who is אֵין סוֹף, *Infinite*. Having attained the level of *aleph* to *tav* by making his way to completion, one has not completed his task. The achievement has elevated him, given him new insights. From the vantage point of his *tav*, one looks back at his previous insights — and begins anew — because he now sees the *aleph*, the very beginning, with new eyes. He begins again, because the ladder climaxing in the *tav* has given him a new perspective on the *aleph*, which in turn leads him to ever higher levels of perfection as he ascends from letter to letter, from teaching to teaching, from aspiration to aspiration.

THE FORCE THAT DRAWS the holy letters back to the *aleph* reflects the spiritual cycle of the universe. At the beginning of Creation, nothing stood in opposition

The Spiritual Cycle in the Universe

to the will of God. Heaven and earth, from the mightiest galaxies to the tiniest microbe, reflected only His will. They existed as testimony to the revelation of His Oneness. But this sublime era ceased with the creation of man. Only man has free will. Only he can accept powers other than the Divine; only he can disobey God's will. Adam and Eve did so when they let the serpent entice them into eating from the forbidden fruit in the Garden of Eden. Ever since, sin has been part of man's nature, with the result that God's Oneness is concealed [הֶסְתֵּר יְחוּדוֹ]. But man's aberration is not permanent; eventually the cycle will return to its starting point, when — in Messianic times — Hashem will be acknowledged by all mankind as the exclusive and absolute Ruler (*R' Moshe Chaim Luzatto*).

Every individual human being is challenged in his own life to make a spiritual cycle that will return him to his lofty origin. Thus, the cycle of striving for the *tav* and then of reinvigorating one's personal *aleph* is the mission of mankind as a whole and of every individual Jew.

KING SOLOMON DERIVES FROM the cycles in the universe an allegoric illustration of man's fate, which can change from darkness to light. In the words

The Continuous Cycle of Generations

the sun rises and the sun sets (*Koheles* 1:5), Solomon expresses the idea of continuity. Before the "sun" of a righteous man sets, Providence causes the sun of another righteous man to rise. Before the sun of Moses set, God caused the sun of Joshua to rise. Before Sarah's sun set, Rebeccah's rose. On the day R' Akiva died, R' Yehudah HaNassi was born. And so, on and on, generations perish and new generations are born.

Jewish history is filled with the recurring phenomenon that periods of darkness and oppression are followed by periods of light and relief. In the midst of the Egyptian exile and slavery, Pharaoh learned from his astrologers of the imminent birth of Israel's redeemer. The king tried to prevent Moses' emergence by ordering the murder of all newborn males, but in that tragic hour of Israel's history Moses was born (*Rashi, Exodus* 1:16). Divine Providence decreed that Israel's first redeemer — the very person the Egyptian ruler wanted to annihilate — was saved by Pharaoh's own daughter and raised in the royal palace. Indeed, light emerged from darkness!

Divine Providence has assured Israel that the greater the affliction, the closer and surer the redemption (*Sotah* 11a). Thus on the darkest day of the year, Tishah B'Av [the Ninth of Av], when the Jew mourns the destruction of both Holy Temples, he is consoled by the knowledge that the Messiah will be born on this very day, and Tishah B'Av will eventually become a joyous festival (*Midrash Abba Gurion*).

Imrei Emes finds an allusion to this thought in the fact that Tishah B'Av always falls on the same day of the week as the first day of the preceding Pesach. This indicates that the day inaugurating the redemption (from Egypt) also marks its end (the destruction of the Temple). However, in the life-cycle of Israel, as well as in the letter-cycle of the *Aleph-Beis*, "the beginning is anchored in the end and the end in its beginning." Thus our Sages assure us that Tishah B'Av contains in itself the spark of the final redemption, although we cannot see it in the present darkness.

This change from pain to joy is anticipated in *Eichah* (1:15), which calls the Ninth of Av a מוֹעֵד, *festival*. Hence, even during the exile, on that day Jews do not recite *Tachanun*, the weekday plea for salvation (*Orach Chaim* 559:4).

Even the stones that were retrieved from the debris of *Eretz Yisrael's* destruction and transported to Babylonia to erect new houses of worship and study will complete the cycle of Divine Providence. The synagogues and study halls of Babylonia — and, by extension, of Israel's every sojourn during the long exile — will, in the future, be established in *Eretz Yisrael* (*Megillah* 29a). *Maharsha* explains that the Third Temple will be as large as the entire city of Jerusalem because it will have to accommodate all the Jews returning from the Diaspora. For this purpose their synagogues and study halls will accompany them on their return to the land. These edifices will become merged with the Temple so that their combined area will cover the whole city. Thus we may conclude that spiritual intentions are never lost; they transcend all destruction and become the foundation of future redemptions.

IN THE TIMELESS REALM before Creation, the letters existed in a sequence opposite that of the *aleph-beis*. They began with *tav* and proceeded in the

The Celestial Order of the Holy Letters and Man's Aspiration for It

backward order of ת,ש,ר,ק and so on, concluding with *aleph*. Those letters represented the pure Divine Spirit of the Almighty and were engraved with flaming fire in the כֶּתֶר, *Crown* of God (*Sefer Yetzirah*).

When the Almighty intended to create the world through the Divine letters, He did so in the order of ת,ש,ר,ק . . . Accordingly, the Midrash (*Yalkut* 1:1) relates: When the letters descended from the Crown of the Almighty and appeared before Him in order, each one to plead that the world should be created with it, the procession began with *tav* and continued until the plea of the *beis* was accepted.

THE ONLY DIVINE NAME FOUND in the first chapter of *Genesis* is אֱלֹהִים, *God [of Judgment]*. This teaches us that God intended the universe to be ruled by the

א''ב for Mercy; תשר''ק for Judgment

scales of justice. Then He tempered Justice with Mercy, and this new process was indicated by the Torah in *Genesis* 2:4, where it begins to refer to God as ה' אֱלֹהִים, combining His Name of Mercy [י-ה-ו-ה] with His Name of Judgment [אֱלֹהִים].

The Midrash compares this to a king who wanted a warm drink, but had only very expensive and delicate stemware. The king thought, "If I pour in the hot water first, the thin glass will expand and crack. But if I pour in the cold water first, the thin glass will contract and snap." So he mixed the hot water with the cold and filled his glass with the warm water.

Similarly, God said, "If I create the world on the basis of Divine Mercy alone (represented by the Name Hashem) its sins will abound; on the basis of Divine

Judgment alone [Elohim] it cannot endure. Therefore, I will create it on the basis of both Judgment and Mercy, and may it then stand! "Hence, the combined expression: Hashem, Elohim.

Thus, in telling of the Creation of the universe as a whole, Elohim is used and heaven is mentioned first, for, indeed, only the celestial beings can endure governance by Justice alone. But when man entered the scene, "earth" is mentioned first and the added use of Hashem signifies that His justice must be tempered with mercy (*Kli Yakar*).

The association of Mercy with Judgment at the creation of mankind did not effect the *essence* of the celestial letters. What changed was the *order* of the letters. By reversing their order — to begin with an *aleph* instead of *tav* — God mercifully indicated that the scheme of Creation was not intended to include only the celestial beings but was planned especially for the sake of man (*Maharal*).

The *Aleph-Beis* is a ladder and a link. It binds us to the spiritual origin of creation and life. It enables us to aspire to heights and to infuse all areas of existence with the celestial summit. It illuminates us with renewed aspiration for new life and redemption. It teaches us to pull ourselves from the *alpeh* of potential life to the *tav* of achievement — and then to begin again to attain ever new levels of accomplishment until our aspirations for the Messianic times will be fulfilled.

⊷§ Erev Tishah B'Av

Although the fast does not begin until sundown, the mourning of Tishah B'Av is manifested in many laws and customs that are observed during the afternoon before the fast. The last meal before the fast — the *seudah hamafsekes* — is governed by many restrictions that limit the types of foods that may be eaten and the beverages that may be drunk (see *Halachos* pp. 470-481). Therefore it is customary to eat a full meal before *Minchah* to prepare oneself for the fast, and to eat the *seudah hamafsekes* after *Minchah*. That final meal customarily consists of bread, some of which is dipped in ashes, and a hard boiled egg. One sits on the ground while eating this meal. Regarding food after the *seudah hamafsekes*, see *Halachos* §17-20.

It is also customary to restrict one's learning on the afternoon before the fast to sad subject matter, i.e. laws pertaining to Tishah B'Av and mourning, and matters relevant to the destruction of the Holy Temple. See *Halachos* §2. Regarding learning on Tishah B'Av or its eve when they fall on a Sabbath, see *Halachos* §29. Concerning the *seudah hamafsekes* in such a case, see *Halachos* §23-24.

Just before sunset, one must remove his leather shoes for the duration of Tishah B'Av, and commence the fast. If *Maariv* is recited before sundown, the shoes must be removed before *barchu*. If Tishah B'Av or its eve fall on the Sabbath, the congregants recite the formula בָּרוּךְ הַמַּבְדִּיל בֵּין קוֹדֶשׁ לְחוֹל, and remove their shoes after *barchu*, but the *chazzan* removes his shoes before *barchu*. For a short summary of activities that are prohibited because of the fast day aspect of Tishah B'Av, see *Halachos* §31-41.

There are many laws and customs that reflect the special mourning aspect of this day. E.g., it is customary to sit on the ground or on a low stool until noon of *Tishah* B'Av, one does not greet his fellows throughout the day, *tefillin* and *talis* are not donned for *Shacharis* prayer, and so on. For a fuller treatment of these subjects, see the *Halachos* section at the end of this volume (pp. 470-481).

FOR LAWS PERTAINING TO THE EVE OF TISHAH B'AV, SEE PAGE 1.

﴾ **מעריב** ﴿

On Saturday night the following is recited before *Maariv*:

בָּרוּךְ הַמַּבְדִּיל בֵּין קֹדֶשׁ לְחוֹל.

On Saturday night the *chazzan* removes his shoes at this point.

Congregation, then *chazzan*:

וְהוּא רַחוּם יְכַפֵּר עָוֹן וְלֹא יַשְׁחִית, וְהִרְבָּה לְהָשִׁיב אַפּוֹ,
וְלֹא יָעִיר כָּל חֲמָתוֹ.¹ יהוה הוֹשִׁיעָה, הַמֶּלֶךְ
יַעֲנֵנוּ בְיוֹם קָרְאֵנוּ.²

In some congregations the *chazzan* chants a melody during his recitation of בָּרְכוּ,
so that the congregation can then recite יִתְבָּרֵךְ.

Chazzan bows at בָּרְכוּ and straightens up at 'ה.

יִתְבָּרַךְ וְיִשְׁתַּבַּח וְיִתְפָּאַר
וְיִתְרוֹמַם וְיִתְנַשֵּׂא שְׁמוֹ שֶׁל
מֶלֶךְ מַלְכֵי הַמְּלָכִים, הַקָּדוֹשׁ
בָּרוּךְ הוּא. שֶׁהוּא רִאשׁוֹן
וְהוּא אַחֲרוֹן, וּמִבַּלְעָדָיו אֵין
אֱלֹהִים.³　　　סֶלוּ,　　　לָרֹכֵב

בָּרְכוּ אֶת יהוה הַמְבֹרָךְ ·

Congregation, followed by *chazzan*, responds,
bowing at בָּרוּךְ and straightening up at 'ה.

בָּרוּךְ יהוה הַמְבֹרָךְ לְעוֹלָם וָעֶד ·

בָּעֲרָבוֹת, בְּיָהּ שְׁמוֹ, וְעִלְזוּ לְפָנָיו.⁴ וּשְׁמוֹ מְרוֹמַם עַל כָּל בְּרָכָה וּתְהִלָּה.⁵ בָּרוּךְ שֵׁם כְּבוֹד מַלְכוּתוֹ
לְעוֹלָם וָעֶד. יְהִי שֵׁם יהוה מְבֹרָךְ, מֵעַתָּה וְעַד עוֹלָם.⁶

On Saturday night the congregants remove their shoes at this point.

ברכות קריאת שמע

בָּרוּךְ אַתָּה יהוה אֱלֹהֵינוּ מֶלֶךְ הָעוֹלָם, אֲשֶׁר בִּדְבָרוֹ מַעֲרִיב
עֲרָבִים, בְּחָכְמָה פּוֹתֵחַ שְׁעָרִים, וּבִתְבוּנָה מְשַׁנֶּה עִתִּים,
וּמַחֲלִיף אֶת הַזְּמַנִּים, וּמְסַדֵּר אֶת הַכּוֹכָבִים בְּמִשְׁמְרוֹתֵיהֶם
בָּרָקִיעַ כִּרְצוֹנוֹ. בּוֹרֵא יוֹם וָלָיְלָה, גּוֹלֵל אוֹר מִפְּנֵי חֹשֶׁךְ וְחֹשֶׁךְ
מִפְּנֵי אוֹר. וּמַעֲבִיר יוֹם וּמֵבִיא לָיְלָה, וּמַבְדִּיל בֵּין יוֹם וּבֵין לָיְלָה,
יהוה צְבָאוֹת שְׁמוֹ. ٭ אֵל חַי וְקַיָּם, תָּמִיד יִמְלוֹךְ עָלֵינוּ, לְעוֹלָם
וָעֶד. בָּרוּךְ אַתָּה יהוה, הַמַּעֲרִיב עֲרָבִים. (Cong.— אָמֵן.)

אַהֲבַת עוֹלָם בֵּית יִשְׂרָאֵל עַמְּךָ אָהָבְתָּ. תּוֹרָה וּמִצְוֹת,
חֻקִּים וּמִשְׁפָּטִים, אוֹתָנוּ לִמַּדְתָּ. עַל כֵּן יהוה
אֱלֹהֵינוּ, בְּשָׁכְבֵנוּ וּבְקוּמֵנוּ נָשִׂיחַ בְּחֻקֶּיךָ, וְנִשְׂמַח בְּדִבְרֵי

---

(1) *Psalms* 78:38. (2) 20:10. (3) Cf. *Isaiah* 44:6. (4) *Psalms* 68:5.
(5) Cf. *Nehemiah* 9:5. (6) *Psalms* 113:2.

FOR LAWS PERTAINING TO THE EVE OF TISHAH B'AV, SEE PAGE 1.

⊰{ **MAARIV** }⊱

On Saturday night the following is recited before *Maariv*:
Blessed is He Who separates between holy and secular.
On Saturday night the *chazzan* removes his shoes at this point.

Congregation, then *chazzan*:

וְהוּא *He, the Merciful One, is forgiving of iniquity and does not destroy. Frequently He withdraws His anger, not arousing His entire rage.[1] HASHEM, save! May the King answer us on the day we call.[2]*

In some congregations the *chazzan* chants a melody during his recitation of *Borchu*, so that the congregation can then recite 'Blessed, praised . . .'

Chazzan bows at 'Bless' and straightens up at 'HASHEM.'

Bless HASHEM, the blessed One.

Congregation, followed by *chazzan*, responds, bowing at 'Blessed' and straightening up at 'HASHEM.'

Blessed is HASHEM, the blessed One, for all eternity.

Blessed, praised, glorified, exalted and upraised is the Name of the King Who rules over kings — the Holy One, Blessed is He. For He is the First and He is the Last and aside from Him there is no god.[3] Extol Him — Who rides the highest heavens — with His Name, YAH, and exult before Him.[4] His Name is exalted beyond every blessing and praise.[5] Blessed is the Name of His glorious kingdom for all eternity. Blessed be the Name of HASHEM from this time and forever.[6]

On Saturday night the congregants remove their shoes at this point.

BLESSINGS OF THE SHEMA

בָּרוּךְ *Blessed are You, HASHEM, our God, King of the universe, Who by His word brings on evenings, with wisdom opens gates, with understanding alters periods, changes the seasons, and orders the stars in their heavenly constellations as He wills. He creates day and night, removing light before darkness and darkness before light. He causes day to pass and brings night, and separates between day and night —* HASHEM, *Master of Legions, is His Name.* Chazzan— *May the living and enduring God continuously reign over us, for all eternity. Blessed are You, HASHEM, Who brings on evenings.*   (Cong.— *Amen.*)

אַהֲבַת *With an eternal love have You loved the House of Israel, Your nation. Torah and commandments, decrees and ordinances have You taught us. Therefore HASHEM, our God, upon our retiring and arising, we will discuss Your decrees and we will rejoice with the words*

⊰§ **Laws of Maariv** (see also *Laws* §95-109 for the laws of *Shema*)

The ideal time for *Maariv* is after dark. However, if one recited *Maariv* earlier he must repeat the three chapters of *Shema* after dark.

As a general rule, no אָמֵן, *Amen,* or other prayer response may be recited between *Borchu* and *Shemoneh Esrei*, but there are exceptions. The main exception is 'between chapters' [בֵּין הַפְּרָקִים] of the *Shema Blessings* — i.e., after each of the blessings, and between the three chapters of *Shema*. At those points, אָמֵן (but not בָּרוּךְ הוּא וּבָרוּךְ שְׁמוֹ) may be said in response to any blessing. Some responses, however, are so important that they are permitted at any point in the *Shema* blessings. They are: (a) In *Kaddish,* עָלְמַיָּא ... אָמֵן יְהֵא שְׁמֵהּ רַבָּא and the אָמֵן after דַּאֲמִירָן בְּעָלְמָא; and (b) the response to בָּרְכוּ.

No interruptions whatever are permitted during the two verses of שְׁמַע and בָּרוּךְ שֵׁם.

תוֹרָתֶךָ, וּבְמִצְוֹתֶיךָ לְעוֹלָם וָעֶד. ∵ כִּי הֵם חַיֵּינוּ, וְאֹרֶךְ יָמֵינוּ, וּבָהֶם נֶהְגֶּה יוֹמָם וָלָיְלָה. וְאַהֲבָתְךָ, אַל תָּסִיר מִמֶּנּוּ לְעוֹלָמִים. בָּרוּךְ אַתָּה יהוה, אוֹהֵב עַמּוֹ יִשְׂרָאֵל. (Cong.– אָמֵן.)

שמע

Immediately before its recitation, concentrate on fulfilling the positive commandment of reciting the *Shema* twice daily. It is important to enunciate each word clearly and not to run words together. For this reason, vertical lines have been placed between two words that are prone to be slurred into one and are not separated by a comma or a hyphen. See *Laws* §95-109.

When praying without a *minyan,* begin with the following three-word formula:

אֵל מֶלֶךְ נֶאֱמָן.

Recite the first verse aloud, with the right hand covering the eyes, and concentrate intently upon accepting God's absolute sovereignty.

שְׁמַע | יִשְׂרָאֵל, יהוה | אֱלֹהֵינוּ, יהוה | אֶחָד:¹

In an undertone – בָּרוּךְ שֵׁם כְּבוֹד מַלְכוּתוֹ לְעוֹלָם וָעֶד.

While reciting the first paragraph (דברים ו:ה-ט), concentrate on accepting the commandment to love God.

וְאָהַבְתָּ אֵת | יהוה | אֱלֹהֶיךָ, בְּכָל־לְבָבְךָ, וּבְכָל־נַפְשְׁךָ, וּבְכָל־מְאֹדֶךָ: וְהָיוּ הַדְּבָרִים הָאֵלֶּה, אֲשֶׁר | אָנֹכִי מְצַוְּךָ הַיּוֹם, עַל־לְבָבֶךָ: וְשִׁנַּנְתָּם לְבָנֶיךָ, וְדִבַּרְתָּ בָּם, בְּשִׁבְתְּךָ בְּבֵיתֶךָ, וּבְלֶכְתְּךָ בַדֶּרֶךְ, וּבְשָׁכְבְּךָ וּבְקוּמֶךָ: וּקְשַׁרְתָּם לְאוֹת | עַל־יָדֶךָ, וְהָיוּ לְטֹטָפֹת בֵּין | עֵינֶיךָ: וּכְתַבְתָּם | עַל־מְזֻזוֹת בֵּיתֶךָ, וּבִשְׁעָרֶיךָ:

While reciting the second paragraph (דברים יא:יג-כא), concentrate on accepting all the commandments and the concept of reward and punishment.

וְהָיָה, אִם־שָׁמֹעַ תִּשְׁמְעוּ אֶל־מִצְוֹתַי, אֲשֶׁר | אָנֹכִי מְצַוֶּה | אֶתְכֶם הַיּוֹם, לְאַהֲבָה אֶת־יהוה | אֱלֹהֵיכֶם וּלְעָבְדוֹ, בְּכָל־לְבַבְכֶם, וּבְכָל־נַפְשְׁכֶם: וְנָתַתִּי מְטַר־אַרְצְכֶם בְּעִתּוֹ, יוֹרֶה וּמַלְקוֹשׁ, וְאָסַפְתָּ דְגָנֶךָ וְתִירֹשְׁךָ וְיִצְהָרֶךָ: וְנָתַתִּי | עֵשֶׂב | בְּשָׂדְךָ לִבְהֶמְתֶּךָ, וְאָכַלְתָּ וְשָׂבָעְתָּ: הִשָּׁמְרוּ לָכֶם, פֶּן־יִפְתֶּה לְבַבְכֶם, וְסַרְתֶּם וַעֲבַדְתֶּם | אֱלֹהִים | אֲחֵרִים, וְהִשְׁתַּחֲוִיתֶם לָהֶם: וְחָרָה | אַף־יהוה בָּכֶם, וְעָצַר | אֶת־הַשָּׁמַיִם, וְלֹא־יִהְיֶה מָטָר, וְהָאֲדָמָה

◂§ שְׁמַע / The Shema

The recitation of the three passages of *Shema* is required by the Torah, and one must have in mind that he is about to fulfill this *mitzvah*. Although one should try to concentrate on the meaning of all three passages, he must concentrate at least on the first (שְׁמַע, *Hear* ...) and the second verses (בָּרוּךְ שֵׁם, *Blessed* ...) because the recitation of *Shema* represents fulfillment of the paramount commandment of acceptance of

God's absolute sovereignty [קַבָּלַת עוֹל מַלְכוּת שָׁמַיִם]. By declaring that God is One, Unique, and Indivisible, we subordinate every facet of our lives to His will.

We have included cantillation symbols (*trop*) for those who recite שְׁמַע as it is read from the Torah. To enable those unfamiliar with *trop* to group the words properly, we inserted commas.

◂§ שְׁמַע יִשְׂרָאֵל — *Hear, O Israel.* Although many layers of profound meaning lie in this seminal

of Your Torah and with Your commandments for all eternity. *Chazzan—* For they are our life and the length of our days and about them we will meditate day and night. May You not remove Your love from us forever. Blessed are You, HASHEM, Who loves His nation Israel. (*Cong.—* Amen.)

THE SHEMA

Immediately before its recitation, concentrate on fulfilling the positive commandment of reciting the Shema twice daily. It is important to enunciate each word clearly and not to run words together. See Laws §§95-109.

When praying without a minyan, begin with the following three-word formula:

God, trustworthy King.

Recite the first verse aloud, with the right hand covering the eyes, and concentrate intently upon accepting God's absolute sovereignty.

Hear, O Israel: HASHEM is our God, HASHEM, the One and Only.¹

In an undertone— *Blessed is the Name of His glorious Kingdom for all eternity.*

While reciting the first paragraph (Deuteronomy 6:5-9), concentrate on accepting the commandment to love God.

You shall love HASHEM, your God, with all your heart, with all your soul and with all your resources. Let these matters that I command you today be upon your heart. Teach them thoroughly to your children and speak of them while you sit in your home, while you walk on the way, when you retire and when you arise. Bind them as a sign upon your arm and let them be tefillin between your eyes. And write them on the doorposts of your house and upon your gates.

While reciting the second paragraph (Deuteronomy 11:13-21), concentrate on accepting all the commandments and the concept of reward and punishment.

And it will come to pass that if you continually hearken to My commandments that I command you today, to love HASHEM, your God, and to serve Him, with all your heart and with all your soul — then I will provide rain for your land in its proper time, the early and late rains, that you may gather in your grain, your wine, and your oil. I will provide grass in your field for your cattle and you will eat and be satisfied. Beware lest your heart be seduced and you turn astray and serve gods of others and bow to them. Then the wrath of HASHEM will blaze against you. He will restrain the heaven so there will be no rain and the ground will

---

(1) *Deuteronomy 6:4.* [When reciting this] verse, one should have at least the following points in mind during its recitation:

□ At this point in history, 'ה, HASHEM, is only אֱלֹקֵינוּ, our God, for He is not acknowledged universally. Ultimately, however, all will recognize Him as אֶחָד, *the One and Only God*

□ ה — HASHEM, God is the Eternal One, Who was, is, and always will be (הָיָה הֹוֶה וְיִהְיֶה), and He is אֱלֹקֵינוּ, *our Master,* of all.

□ אֱלֹקֵינוּ — *Our God,* He is all-Powerful (*Orach Chaim* 5).

אֶחָד — *The One and Only.* This has two connotations: (a) There is no God other than HASHEM (*Rashbam*); and, (b) though we perceive God in many roles — kind, angry, merciful, wise, judging, etc. — they are not contradictory, even though human intelligence does not comprehend their harmony.

While saying אֶחָד, draw out the ח a bit and emphasize the final ד. While drawing out the ח — a letter with the numerical value of eight — bear in mind that God is Master of the earth and the seven heavens. While clearly enunciating the final ד — which has the numerical value of four — bear in mind that God is Master in all four directions, meaning everywhere.

לְשָׁנָה ...

...

וְאָהַבְתָּ ...

— Chazzan repeats

.וַיֹּאמֶר יהוה אֱלֹהֵיכֶם אֱמֶת.

Although the word מֵאָז belongs to the next paragraph,
it is appended to the conclusion of the previous one.

— אֱמֶת ׀ וֶאֱמוּנָה ׀ יהוה ׀ אֱלֹהֵינוּ ׀ הוּא

Concentrate on fulfilling the
commandment of remember-
ing the Exodus from Egypt.

...

וְיַצֵּב ׀ יהוה ׀ אֱלֹהֵינוּ ׀ הוּא ...

...

וְאָהַבְתָּ ...

ברכת השכיבנו

...

9 / ערבית   סדר קריאת שמע

not yield its produce. And you will swiftly be banished from the goodly land which HASHEM gives you. Place these words of Mine upon your heart and upon your soul; bind them for a sign upon your arm and let them be tefillin between your eyes. Teach them to your children, to discuss them, while you sit in your home, while you walk on the way, when you retire and when you arise. And write them on the doorposts of your house and upon your gates. In order to prolong your days and the days of your children upon the ground that HASHEM has sworn to your ancestors to give them, like the days of the heaven on the earth.

Numbers 15:37-41

וַיֹּאמֶר And HASHEM said to Moses saying: Speak to the Children of Israel and say to them that they are to make themselves tzitzis on the corners of their garments, throughout their generations. And they are to place upon the tzitzis of each corner a thread of techeiles. And it shall constitute tzitzis for you, that you may see it and remember all the commandments of HASHEM and perform them; and not explore after your heart and after your eyes after which you stray. So that you may remember and perform all My commandments; and be holy to your God. I am HASHEM, your God, Who has removed you from the land of Egypt to be a God to you; I am HASHEM your God — it is true —

Concentrate on fulfilling the commandment of remembering the Exodus from Egypt.

Although the word אֱמֶת, 'it is true,' belongs to the next paragraph, it is appended to the conclusion of the previous one.

Chazzan repeats: **HASHEM, your God, is true.**

וֶאֱמוּנָה And faithful is all this, and it is firmly established for us that He is HASHEM our God, and there is none but Him, and we are Israel, His nation. He redeems us from the power of kings, our King Who delivers us from the hand of all the cruel tyrants. He is the God Who exacts vengeance for us from our foes and Who brings just retribution upon all enemies of our soul; Who performs great deeds that are beyond comprehension, and wonders beyond number.[1] Who set our soul in life and did not allow our foot to falter.[2] Who led us upon the heights of our enemies and raised our pride above all who hate us; Who wrought for us miracles and vengeance upon Pharaoh; signs and wonders on the land of the offspring of Ham; Who struck with His anger all the firstborn of Egypt and removed His nation Israel from their midst to eternal freedom; Who brought His children through the split parts of the Sea of Reeds while those who pursued them and hated them He caused to sink into the depths. When His children perceived His power, they lauded and gave grateful praise to His Name. Chazzan — And His Kingship they accepted upon themselves willingly. Moses and the Children of Israel raised their voices to You in song with abundant gladness — and said unanimously:

(1) *Job 9:10.* (2) *Psalms 66:9.*

Some congregations omit the following prayers and continue with Half-Kaddish (p. 12).

(‏קהל – Cong.)

(‏קהל – Cong.)

מִי כָמְכָה **Who** is like You among the heavenly powers, HASHEM! Who is like You, mighty in holiness, too awesome for praise, doing wonders![1] Chazzan– Your children beheld Your majesty, as You split the sea before Moses: 'This is my God!'[2] they exclaimed, then they said:

יהוה **'HASHEM** shall reign for all eternity!'[3] Chazzan– And it is further said: 'For HASHEM has redeemed Jacob and delivered him from a power mightier than he.'[4] Blessed are You, HASHEM, Who redeemed Israel.
(Cong.– Amen.)

הַשְׁכִּיבֵנוּ **Lay** us down to sleep, HASHEM our God, in peace, raise us erect, our King, to life; and spread over us the shelter of Your peace. Set us aright with good counsel from before Your Presence, and save us for Your Name's sake. Shield us, remove from us foe, plague, sword, famine, and woe; and remove spiritual impediment from before us and behind us, and in the shadow of Your wings shelter us[5] — for God Who protects and rescues us are You; for God, the Gracious and Compassionate King, are You.[6] Chazzan– Safeguard our going and coming, for life and for peace from now to eternity.[7] Blessed are You, HASHEM, Who protects His people Israel forever.   (Cong.– Amen.)

Some congregations omit the following prayers and continue with Half-*Kaddish* (p. 12).

בָּרוּךְ **Blessed** is HASHEM forever, Amen and Amen.[8] Blessed is HASHEM from Zion, Who dwells in Jerusalem, Halleluyah![9] Blessed is HASHEM, God, the God of Israel, Who alone does wondrous things. Blessed is His glorious Name forever, and may all the earth be filled with His glory, Amen and Amen.[10] May the glory of HASHEM endure forever, let HASHEM rejoice in His works.[11] Blessed be the Name of HASHEM from this time and forever.[12] For HASHEM will not cast off His nation for the sake of His Great Name, for HASHEM has vowed to make you His own people.[13] Then the entire nation saw and fell on their faces and said, 'HASHEM — only He is God! HASHEM — only He is God!'[14] Then HASHEM will be King over all the world, on that day HASHEM will be One and His Name will be One.[15] May Your kindness, HASHEM, be upon us, just as we awaited You.[16] Save us, HASHEM, our God, gather us from the nations, to thank Your Holy Name and to glory in Your praise![17] All the nations that You made will come and bow before You, My Lord, and shall glorify Your Name. For You are great and work wonders; You alone, O God.[18] Then we, Your nation and the sheep of Your pasture, shall thank You forever; for generation after generation we will relate Your praise.[19] Blessed is HASHEM by day; Blessed is HASHEM by night; Blessed is HASHEM when we retire; Blessed is HASHEM when we arise. For in Your hand are the souls of the living and the dead. He in Whose hand is the soul of all the living and the spirit of every

(1) *Exodus* 15:11. (2) 15:2. (3) 15:18. (4) *Jeremiah* 31:10. (5) Cf. *Psalms* 17:8.
(6) Cf. *Nehemiah* 9:31. (7) Cf. *Psalms* 121:8. (8) 89:53. (9) 135:21.
(10) 72:18-19. (11) 104:31. (12) 113:2. (13) *I Samuel* 12:22. (14) *I Kings* 18:39.
(15) *Zechariah* 14:9. (16) *Psalms* 33:22. (17) 106:47. (18) 86:9-10. (19) 79:13.

בָּשָׂר אִישׁ. בְּיָדְךָ אַפְקִיד רוּחִי, פָּדִיתָה אוֹתִי, יהוה אֵל אֱמֶת.²
אֱלֹהֵינוּ שֶׁבַּשָּׁמַיִם יַחֵד שִׁמְךָ, וְקַיֵּם מַלְכוּתְךָ תָּמִיד, וּמְלוֹךְ
עָלֵינוּ לְעוֹלָם וָעֶד.

יִרְאוּ עֵינֵינוּ וְיִשְׂמַח לִבֵּנוּ וְתָגֵל נַפְשֵׁנוּ בִּישׁוּעָתְךָ בֶּאֱמֶת,
בֶּאֱמֹר לְצִיּוֹן מָלַךְ אֱלֹהָיִךְ.³ יהוה מֶלֶךְ,⁴ יהוה מָלָךְ,⁵
יהוה יִמְלֹךְ לְעֹלָם וָעֶד.⁶ ּ∴כִּי הַמַּלְכוּת שֶׁלְּךָ הִיא, וּלְעוֹלְמֵי עַד
תִּמְלוֹךְ בְּכָבוֹד, כִּי אֵין לָנוּ מֶלֶךְ אֶלָּא אָתָּה. בָּרוּךְ אַתָּה יהוה,
הַמֶּלֶךְ בִּכְבוֹדוֹ תָּמִיד יִמְלוֹךְ עָלֵינוּ לְעוֹלָם וָעֶד, וְעַל כָּל
מַעֲשָׂיו. (אָמֵן. —Cong.)

חֲצִי קַדִּישׁ The chazzan recites.

יִתְגַּדַּל וְיִתְקַדַּשׁ שְׁמֵהּ רַבָּא. (אָמֵן. —Cong.) בְּעָלְמָא דִּי בְרָא כִרְעוּתֵהּ,
וְיַמְלִיךְ מַלְכוּתֵהּ, בְּחַיֵּיכוֹן וּבְיוֹמֵיכוֹן וּבְחַיֵּי דְכָל בֵּית יִשְׂרָאֵל,
בַּעֲגָלָא וּבִזְמַן קָרִיב. וְאִמְרוּ: אָמֵן.
(אָמֵן. יְהֵא שְׁמֵהּ רַבָּא מְבָרַךְ לְעָלַם וּלְעָלְמֵי עָלְמַיָּא. —Cong.)
יְהֵא שְׁמֵהּ רַבָּא מְבָרַךְ לְעָלַם וּלְעָלְמֵי עָלְמַיָּא.
יִתְבָּרַךְ וְיִשְׁתַּבַּח וְיִתְפָּאַר וְיִתְרוֹמַם וְיִתְנַשֵּׂא וְיִתְהַדָּר וְיִתְעַלֶּה וְיִתְהַלָּל
שְׁמֵהּ דְּקֻדְשָׁא בְּרִיךְ הוּא (בְּרִיךְ הוּא —Cong.) — לְעֵלָּא מִן כָּל בִּרְכָתָא
וְשִׁירָתָא תֻּשְׁבְּחָתָא וְנֶחֱמָתָא, דַּאֲמִירָן בְּעָלְמָא, וְאִמְרוּ: אָמֵן. (אָמֵן. —Cong.)

שמונה עשרה – עמידה }∗

Take three steps backward, then three steps forward. Remain standing with the feet together while
reciting *Shemoneh Esrei*. Recite it with quiet devotion and without interruption, verbal or otherwise.
Although its recitation should not be audible to others, one must pray loudly enough to hear himself.

אֲדֹנָי שְׂפָתַי תִּפְתָּח, וּפִי יַגִּיד תְּהִלָּתֶךָ.⁷

אבות

Bend the knees at בָּרוּךְ; bow at אַתָּה; straighten up at ה'.

בָּרוּךְ אַתָּה יהוה אֱלֹהֵינוּ וֵאלֹהֵי אֲבוֹתֵינוּ, אֱלֹהֵי אַבְרָהָם, אֱלֹהֵי
יִצְחָק, וֵאלֹהֵי יַעֲקֹב, הָאֵל הַגָּדוֹל הַגִּבּוֹר וְהַנּוֹרָא, אֵל
עֶלְיוֹן, גּוֹמֵל חֲסָדִים טוֹבִים וְקוֹנֵה הַכֹּל, וְזוֹכֵר חַסְדֵי אָבוֹת, וּמֵבִיא
גוֹאֵל לִבְנֵי בְנֵיהֶם, לְמַעַן שְׁמוֹ בְּאַהֲבָה. מֶלֶךְ עוֹזֵר וּמוֹשִׁיעַ וּמָגֵן.

Bend the knees at בָּרוּךְ; bow at אַתָּה; straighten up at ה'.

בָּרוּךְ אַתָּה יהוה, מָגֵן אַבְרָהָם.

גבורות

אַתָּה גִּבּוֹר לְעוֹלָם אֲדֹנָי, מְחַיֵּה מֵתִים אַתָּה, רַב לְהוֹשִׁיעַ.
מְכַלְכֵּל חַיִּים בְּחֶסֶד, מְחַיֵּה מֵתִים בְּרַחֲמִים רַבִּים,

human being.[1] In Your hand I shall entrust my spirit, You redeemed me, HASHEM, God of truth.[2] Our God, Who is in heaven, bring unity to Your Name; establish Your kingdom forever and reign over us for all eternity.

יִרְאוּ May our eyes see, our heart rejoice and our soul exult in Your salvation in truth, when Zion is told, 'Your God has reigned!'[3] HASHEM reigns,[4] HASHEM has reigned,[5] HASHEM will reign for all eternity.[6] Chazzan— For the kingdom is Yours and for all eternity You will reign in glory, for we have no King but You. Blessed are You, HASHEM, the King in His glory — He shall constantly reign over us forever and ever, and over all His creatures.   (Cong.— Amen.)

The chazzan recites Half-*Kaddish.*

יִתְגַּדַּל May His great Name grow exalted and sanctified (Cong.— Amen.) in the world that He created as He willed. May He give reign to His kingship in your lifetimes and in your days, and in the lifetimes of the entire Family of Israel, swiftly and soon. Now respond: Amen.

(Cong.— Amen. May His great Name be blessed forever and ever.)
May His great Name be blessed forever and ever.

Blessed, praised, glorified, exalted, extolled, mighty, upraised, and lauded be the Name of the Holy One, Blessed is He (Cong.— Blessed is He) — beyond any blessing and song, praise and consolation that are uttered in the world. Now respond: Amen. (Cong.— Amen.)

⋇ SHEMONEH ESREI – AMIDAH ⋇

Take three steps backward, then three steps forward. Remain standing with the feet together while reciting Shemoneh Esrei. Recite it with quiet devotion and without interruption, verbal or otherwise. Although its recitation should not be audible to others, one must pray loudly enough to hear himself.

My Lord, open my lips, that my mouth may declare Your praise.[7]

PATRIARCHS

Bend the knees at 'Blessed'; bow at 'You'; straighten up at 'HASHEM.'

בָּרוּךְ Blessed are You, HASHEM, our God and the God of our fore-fathers, God of Abraham, God of Isaac, and God of Jacob; the great, mighty, and awesome God, the supreme God, Who bestows beneficial kindnesses and creates everything, Who recalls the kindnesses of the Patriarchs and brings a Redeemer to their children's children, for His Name's sake, with love. O King, Helper, Savior, and Shield.

Bend the knees at 'Blessed'; bow at 'You'; straighten up at 'HASHEM.'

Blessed are You, HASHEM, Shield of Abraham.

GOD'S MIGHT

אַתָּה You are eternally mighty, my Lord, the Resuscitator of the dead are You; abundantly able to save. He sustains the living with kindness, resuscitates the dead with abundant mercy,

---

(1) Job 12:10. (2) Psalms 31:6. (3) Cf. Isaiah 52:7. (4) Psalms 10:16.
(5) 93:1 et al. (6) Exodus 15:18. (7) Psalms 51:17.

סוֹמֵךְ נוֹפְלִים, וְרוֹפֵא חוֹלִים, וּמַתִּיר אֲסוּרִים, וּמְקַיֵּם אֱמוּנָתוֹ לִישֵׁנֵי עָפָר. מִי כָמוֹךָ בַּעַל גְּבוּרוֹת, וּמִי דוֹמֶה לָּךְ, מֶלֶךְ מֵמִית וּמְחַיֶּה וּמַצְמִיחַ יְשׁוּעָה. וְנֶאֱמָן אַתָּה לְהַחֲיוֹת מֵתִים. בָּרוּךְ אַתָּה יהוה, מְחַיֵּה הַמֵּתִים.

קדושת השם

אַתָּה קָדוֹשׁ וְשִׁמְךָ קָדוֹשׁ, וּקְדוֹשִׁים בְּכָל יוֹם יְהַלְלוּךָ סֶּלָה. בָּרוּךְ אַתָּה יהוה, הָאֵל הַקָּדוֹשׁ.

בינה

אַתָּה חוֹנֵן לְאָדָם דַּעַת, וּמְלַמֵּד לֶאֱנוֹשׁ בִּינָה.

After the Sabbath add [if forgotten do not repeat Shemoneh Esrei].

אַתָּה חוֹנַנְתָּנוּ לְמַדַּע תּוֹרָתֶךָ, וַתְּלַמְּדֵנוּ לַעֲשׂוֹת חֻקֵּי רְצוֹנֶךָ וַתַּבְדֵּל יהוה אֱלֹהֵינוּ בֵּין קֹדֶשׁ לְחוֹל בֵּין אוֹר לְחֹשֶׁךְ, בֵּין יִשְׂרָאֵל לָעַמִּים בֵּין יוֹם הַשְּׁבִיעִי לְשֵׁשֶׁת יְמֵי הַמַּעֲשֶׂה. אָבִינוּ מַלְכֵּנוּ הָחֵל עָלֵינוּ הַיָּמִים הַבָּאִים לִקְרָאתֵנוּ לְשָׁלוֹם חֲשׂוּכִים מִכָּל חֵטְא וּמְנֻקִּים מִכָּל עָוֹן וּמְדֻבָּקִים בְּיִרְאָתֶךָ. וְ ...

חָנֵּנוּ מֵאִתְּךָ דֵּעָה בִּינָה וְהַשְׂכֵּל. בָּרוּךְ אַתָּה יהוה, חוֹנֵן הַדָּעַת.

תשובה

הֲשִׁיבֵנוּ אָבִינוּ לְתוֹרָתֶךָ, וְקָרְבֵנוּ מַלְכֵּנוּ לַעֲבוֹדָתֶךָ, וְהַחֲזִירֵנוּ בִּתְשׁוּבָה שְׁלֵמָה לְפָנֶיךָ. בָּרוּךְ אַתָּה יהוה, הָרוֹצֶה בִּתְשׁוּבָה.

סליחה

Strike the left side of the chest with the right fist while reciting the words פָּשָׁעְנוּ *and* חָטָאנוּ.

סְלַח לָנוּ אָבִינוּ כִּי חָטָאנוּ, מְחַל לָנוּ מַלְכֵּנוּ כִּי פָשָׁעְנוּ, כִּי מוֹחֵל וְסוֹלֵחַ אָתָּה. בָּרוּךְ אַתָּה יהוה, חַנּוּן הַמַּרְבֶּה לִסְלֹחַ.

גאולה

רְאֵה בְעָנְיֵנוּ, וְרִיבָה רִיבֵנוּ, וּגְאָלֵנוּ[1] מְהֵרָה לְמַעַן שְׁמֶךָ, כִּי גּוֹאֵל חָזָק אָתָּה. בָּרוּךְ אַתָּה יהוה, גּוֹאֵל יִשְׂרָאֵל.

רפואה

רְפָאֵנוּ יהוה וְנֵרָפֵא, הוֹשִׁיעֵנוּ וְנִוָּשֵׁעָה, כִּי תְהִלָּתֵנוּ אָתָּה,[2]

supports the fallen, heals the sick, releases the confined, and maintains His faith to those asleep in the dust. Who is like You, O Master of mighty deeds, and who is comparable to You, O King Who causes death and restores life and makes salvation sprout! And You are faithful to resuscitate the dead. Blessed are You, HASHEM, Who resuscitates the dead.

HOLINESS OF GOD'S NAME

אַתָּה You are holy and Your Name is holy, and holy ones praise You every day, forever. Blessed are You, HASHEM, the holy God.

INSIGHT

אַתָּה You graciously endow man with wisdom and teach insight to a frail mortal.

After the Sabbath add [if forgotten do not repeat Shemoneh Esrei].

אַתָּה You have graced us with intelligence to study Your Torah and You have taught us to perform the decrees You have willed. HASHEM, our God, You have distinguished between the sacred and the secular, between light and darkness, between Israel and the peoples, between the seventh day and the six days of labor. Our Father, our King, begin for us the days approaching us for peace, free from all sin, cleansed from all iniquity and attached to fear of You. And . . .

Endow us graciously from Yourself with wisdom, insight, and discernment. Blessed are You, HASHEM, gracious Giver of wisdom.

REPENTANCE

הֲשִׁיבֵנוּ Bring us back, our Father, to Your Torah, and bring us near, our King, to Your service, and influence us to return in perfect repentance before You. Blessed are You, HASHEM, Who desires repentance.

FORGIVENESS

Strike the left side of the chest with the right fist while reciting the words 'erred' and 'sinned.'

סְלַח Forgive us, our Father, for we have erred; pardon us, our King, for we have willfully sinned; for You pardon and forgive. Blessed are You, HASHEM, the gracious One Who pardons abundantly.

REDEMPTION

רְאֵה Behold our affliction, take up our grievance, and redeem us[1] speedily for Your Name's sake, for You are a powerful Redeemer. Blessed are You, HASHEM, Redeemer of Israel.

HEALTH AND HEALING

רְפָאֵנוּ Heal us, HASHEM — then we will be healed; save us — then we will be saved, for You are our praise.[2] Bring

---

(1) Cf. Psalms 119:153-154. (2) Cf. Jeremiah 17:14.

וְהַעֲלֵה רְפוּאָה שְׁלֵמָה לְכָל מַכּוֹתֵינוּ, °°כִּי אֵל מֶלֶךְ רוֹפֵא נֶאֱמָן וְרַחֲמָן אָתָּה. בָּרוּךְ אַתָּה יהוה, רוֹפֵא חוֹלֵי עַמּוֹ יִשְׂרָאֵל.

ברכת השנים

בָּרֵךְ עָלֵינוּ יהוה אֱלֹהֵינוּ אֶת הַשָּׁנָה הַזֹּאת וְאֶת כָּל מִינֵי תְבוּאָתָהּ לְטוֹבָה, וְתֵן בְּרָכָה עַל פְּנֵי הָאֲדָמָה, וְשַׂבְּעֵנוּ מִטּוּבֶךְ, וּבָרֵךְ שְׁנָתֵנוּ כַּשָּׁנִים הַטּוֹבוֹת. בָּרוּךְ אַתָּה יהוה, מְבָרֵךְ הַשָּׁנִים.

קיבוץ גליות

תְּקַע בְּשׁוֹפָר גָּדוֹל לְחֵרוּתֵנוּ, וְשָׂא נֵס לְקַבֵּץ גָּלֻיּוֹתֵינוּ, וְקַבְּצֵנוּ יַחַד מֵאַרְבַּע כַּנְפוֹת הָאָרֶץ.[1] בָּרוּךְ אַתָּה יהוה, מְקַבֵּץ נִדְחֵי עַמּוֹ יִשְׂרָאֵל.

דין

הָשִׁיבָה שׁוֹפְטֵינוּ כְּבָרִאשׁוֹנָה, וְיוֹעֲצֵינוּ כְּבַתְּחִלָּה,[2] וְהָסֵר מִמֶּנּוּ יָגוֹן וַאֲנָחָה, וּמְלוֹךְ עָלֵינוּ אַתָּה יהוה לְבַדְּךָ בְּחֶסֶד וּבְרַחֲמִים, וְצַדְּקֵנוּ בַּמִּשְׁפָּט. בָּרוּךְ אַתָּה יהוה, מֶלֶךְ אוֹהֵב צְדָקָה וּמִשְׁפָּט.

ברכת המינים

וְלַמַּלְשִׁינִים אַל תְּהִי תִקְוָה, וְכָל הָרִשְׁעָה כְּרֶגַע תֹּאבֵד, וְכָל אֹיְבֶיךָ מְהֵרָה יִכָּרֵתוּ, וְהַזֵּדִים מְהֵרָה תְעַקֵּר וּתְשַׁבֵּר וּתְמַגֵּר וְתַכְנִיעַ בִּמְהֵרָה בְיָמֵינוּ. בָּרוּךְ אַתָּה יהוה, שׁוֹבֵר אֹיְבִים וּמַכְנִיעַ זֵדִים.

צדיקים

עַל הַצַּדִּיקִים וְעַל הַחֲסִידִים, וְעַל זִקְנֵי עַמְּךָ בֵּית יִשְׂרָאֵל, וְעַל פְּלֵיטַת סוֹפְרֵיהֶם, וְעַל גֵּרֵי הַצֶּדֶק וְעָלֵינוּ, יֶהֱמוּ רַחֲמֶיךָ יהוה אֱלֹהֵינוּ, וְתֵן שָׂכָר טוֹב לְכָל הַבּוֹטְחִים בְּשִׁמְךָ בֶּאֱמֶת, וְשִׂים חֶלְקֵנוּ עִמָּהֶם לְעוֹלָם, וְלֹא נֵבוֹשׁ כִּי בְךָ בָּטָחְנוּ. בָּרוּךְ אַתָּה יהוה, מִשְׁעָן וּמִבְטָח לַצַּדִּיקִים.

°°At this point one may interject a prayer for one who is ill:

יְהִי רָצוֹן מִלְּפָנֶיךָ יהוה אֱלֹהַי וֵאלֹהֵי אֲבוֹתַי, שֶׁתִּשְׁלַח מְהֵרָה רְפוּאָה שְׁלֵמָה מִן הַשָּׁמַיִם, רְפוּאַת הַנֶּפֶשׁ וּרְפוּאַת הַגּוּף

לַחוֹלֶה (patient's name) בֶּן (mother's name) בְּתוֹךְ שְׁאָר חוֹלֵי יִשְׂרָאֵל.—for a male

לַחוֹלָה (patient's name) בַּת (mother's name) בְּתוֹךְ שְׁאָר חוֹלֵי יִשְׂרָאֵל.—for a female

כִּי אֵל ...—continue

complete recovery for all our ailments, °°for You are God, King, the faithful and compassionate Healer. Blessed are You, HASHEM, Who heals the sick of His people Israel.

YEAR OF PROSPERITY

בָּרֵךְ Bless on our behalf — O HASHEM, our God — this year and all its kinds of crops for the best, and give a blessing on the face of the earth, and satisfy us from Your bounty, and bless our year like the best years. Blessed are You, HASHEM, Who blesses the years.

INGATHERING OF EXILES

תְּקַע Sound the great shofar for our freedom, raise the banner to gather our exiles and gather us together from the four corners of the earth.[1] Blessed are You, HASHEM, Who gathers in the dispersed of His people Israel.

RESTORATION OF JUSTICE

הָשִׁיבָה Restore our judges as in earliest times and our counselors as at first;[2] remove from us sorrow and groan; and reign over us — You, HASHEM, alone — with kindness and compassion, and justify us through judgment. Blessed are You, HASHEM, the King Who loves righteousness and judgment.

AGAINST HERETICS

וְלַמַּלְשִׁינִים And for slanderers let there be no hope; and may all wickedness perish in an instant; and may all Your enemies be cut down speedily. May You speedily uproot, smash, cast down, and humble the wanton sinners — speedily in our days. Blessed are You, HASHEM, Who breaks enemies and humbles wanton sinners.

THE RIGHTEOUS

עַל הַצַּדִּיקִים On the righteous, on the devout, on the elders of Your people the Family of Israel, on the remnant of their scholars, on the righteous converts and on ourselves — may Your compassion be aroused, HASHEM, our God, and give goodly reward to all who sincerely believe in Your Name. Put our lot with them forever, and we will not feel ashamed, for we trust in You. Blessed are You, HASHEM, Mainstay and Assurance of the righteous.

°°At this point one may interject a prayer for one who is ill:

May it be Your will, HASHEM, my God, and the God of my forefathers, that You quickly send a complete recovery from heaven, spiritual healing and physical healing to the patient (name) son/daughter of (mother's name) among the other patients of Israel.   Continue: For You are God ...

---

(1) Cf. *Isaiah* 11:12. (2) Cf. 1:26.

בנין ירושלים

וְלִירוּשָׁלַיִם עִירְךָ בְּרַחֲמִים תָּשׁוּב, וְתִשְׁכּוֹן בְּתוֹכָהּ כַּאֲשֶׁר דִּבַּרְתָּ, וּבְנֵה אוֹתָהּ בְּקָרוֹב בְּיָמֵינוּ בִּנְיַן עוֹלָם, וְכִסֵּא דָוִד מְהֵרָה לְתוֹכָהּ תָּכִין. בָּרוּךְ אַתָּה יהוה, בּוֹנֵה יְרוּשָׁלָיִם.

מלכות בית דוד

אֶת צֶמַח דָּוִד עַבְדְּךָ מְהֵרָה תַצְמִיחַ, וְקַרְנוֹ תָּרוּם בִּישׁוּעָתֶךָ, כִּי לִישׁוּעָתְךָ קִוִּינוּ כָּל הַיּוֹם. בָּרוּךְ אַתָּה יהוה, מַצְמִיחַ קֶרֶן יְשׁוּעָה.

קבלת תפלה

שְׁמַע קוֹלֵנוּ יהוה אֱלֹהֵינוּ, חוּס וְרַחֵם עָלֵינוּ, וְקַבֵּל בְּרַחֲמִים וּבְרָצוֹן אֶת תְּפִלָּתֵנוּ, כִּי אֵל שׁוֹמֵעַ תְּפִלּוֹת וְתַחֲנוּנִים אָתָּה. וּמִלְּפָנֶיךָ מַלְכֵּנוּ רֵיקָם אַל תְּשִׁיבֵנוּ, °°כִּי אַתָּה שׁוֹמֵעַ תְּפִלַּת עַמְּךָ יִשְׂרָאֵל בְּרַחֲמִים. בָּרוּךְ אַתָּה יהוה, שׁוֹמֵעַ תְּפִלָּה.

עבודה

רְצֵה יהוה אֱלֹהֵינוּ בְּעַמְּךָ יִשְׂרָאֵל וּבִתְפִלָּתָם, וְהָשֵׁב אֶת הָעֲבוֹדָה לִדְבִיר בֵּיתֶךָ. וְאִשֵּׁי יִשְׂרָאֵל וּתְפִלָּתָם בְּאַהֲבָה תְקַבֵּל בְּרָצוֹן, וּתְהִי לְרָצוֹן תָּמִיד עֲבוֹדַת יִשְׂרָאֵל עַמֶּךָ.

°°During the silent *Shemoneh Esrei* one may insert either or both of these personal prayers.

For livelihood:	For forgiveness:

For forgiveness:

אָנָּא יהוה, חָטָאתִי עָוִיתִי וּפָשַׁעְתִּי לְפָנֶיךָ, מִיּוֹם הֱיוֹתִי עַל הָאֲדָמָה עַד הַיּוֹם הַזֶּה (וּבִפְרָט בַּחֵטְא ....). אָנָּא יהוה, עֲשֵׂה לְמַעַן שִׁמְךָ הַגָּדוֹל, וּתְכַפֵּר לִי עַל עֲוֹנִי וַחֲטָאַי וּפְשָׁעַי שֶׁחָטָאתִי וְשֶׁעָוִיתִי וְשֶׁפָּשַׁעְתִּי לְפָנֶיךָ, מִנְּעוּרַי עַד הַיּוֹם הַזֶּה. וּתְמַלֵּא כָּל הַשֵּׁמוֹת שֶׁפָּגַמְתִּי בְּשִׁמְךָ הַגָּדוֹל.

For livelihood:

אַתָּה הוּא יהוה הָאֱלֹהִים, הַזָּן וּמְפַרְנֵס וּמְכַלְכֵּל מִקַּרְנֵי רְאֵמִים עַד בֵּיצֵי כִנִּים. הַטְרִיפֵנִי לֶחֶם חֻקִּי, וְהַמְצֵא לִי וּלְכָל בְּנֵי בֵיתִי מְזוֹנוֹתַי קוֹדֶם שֶׁאֶצְטָרֵךְ לָהֶם, בְּנַחַת וְלֹא בְצַעַר, בְּהֶתֵּר וְלֹא בְאִסּוּר, בְּכָבוֹד וְלֹא בְבִזָּיוֹן, לְחַיִּים וּלְשָׁלוֹם, מִשֶּׁפַע בְּרָכָה וְהַצְלָחָה, וּמִשֶּׁפַע בְּרָכָה עֶלְיוֹנָה, כְּדֵי שֶׁאוּכַל לַעֲשׂוֹת רְצוֹנֶךָ וְלַעֲסוֹק בְּתוֹרָתֶךָ וּלְקַיֵּם מִצְוֹתֶיךָ. וְאַל תַּצְרִיכֵנִי לִידֵי מַתְּנַת בָּשָׂר וָדָם. וִיקֻיַּם בִּי מִקְרָא שֶׁכָּתוּב: פּוֹתֵחַ אֶת יָדֶךָ, וּמַשְׂבִּיעַ לְכָל חַי רָצוֹן.[1] וְכָתוּב: הַשְׁלֵךְ עַל יהוה יְהָבְךָ וְהוּא יְכַלְכְּלֶךָ.[2]

Continue— *כִּי אַתָּה* ...

REBUILDING JERUSALEM

וְלִירוּשָׁלַיִם *And to Jerusalem, Your city, may You return in compassion, and may You rest within it, as You have spoken. May You rebuild it soon in our days as an eternal structure, and may You speedily establish the throne of David within it. Blessed are You, HASHEM, the Builder of Jerusalem.*

DAVIDIC REIGN

אֶת צֶמַח *The offspring of Your servant David may You speedily cause to flourish, and enhance his pride through Your salvation, for we hope for Your salvation all day long. Blessed are You, HASHEM, Who causes the pride of salvation to flourish.*

ACCEPTANCE OF PRAYER

שְׁמַע *Hear our voice, HASHEM our God, pity and be compassionate to us, and accept — with compassion and favor — our prayer, for God Who hears prayers and supplications are You. From before Yourself, our King, turn us not away empty-handed,* ∞ *for You hear the prayer of Your people Israel with compassion. Blessed are You, HASHEM, Who hears prayer.*

TEMPLE SERVICE

רְצֵה *Be favorable, HASHEM, our God, toward Your people Israel and their prayer and restore the service to the Holy of Holies of Your Temple. The fire-offerings of Israel and their prayer accept with love and favor, and may the service of Your people Israel always be favorable to You.*

∞ During the silent *Shemoneh Esrei* one may insert either or both of these personal prayers.

For forgiveness:

אָנָא *Please, O HASHEM, I have erred, been iniquitous, and willfully sinned before You, from the day I have existed on earth until this very day (and especially with the sin of . . .). Please, HASHEM, act for the sake of Your Great Name and grant me atonement for my iniquities, my errors, and my willful sins through which I have erred, been iniquitous, and willfully sinned before You, from my youth until this day. And make whole all the Names that I have blemished in Your Great Name.*

For livelihood:

אַתָּה *It is You, HASHEM the God, Who nourishes, sustains, and supports, from the horns of re'eimim to the eggs of lice. Provide me with my allotment of bread; and bring forth for me and all members of my household, my food, before I have need for it; in contentment but not in pain, in a permissible but not a forbidden manner, in honor but not in disgrace, for life and for peace; from the flow of blessing and success and from the flow of the Heavenly spring, so that I be enabled to do Your will and engage in Your Torah and fulfill Your commandments. Make me not needful of people's largesse; and may there be fulfilled in me the verse that states, 'You open Your hand and satisfy the desire of every living thing'[1] and that states, 'Cast Your burden upon HASHEM and He will support you.'[2]*

Continue: *For You hear the prayer . . .*

---

(1) *Psalms* 145:16. (2) 55:23.

וְתֶחֱזֶינָה עֵינֵינוּ בְּשׁוּבְךָ לְצִיּוֹן בְּרַחֲמִים. בָּרוּךְ אַתָּה יהוה,
הַמַּחֲזִיר שְׁכִינָתוֹ לְצִיּוֹן.

הודאה

Bow at מוֹדִים; straighten up at 'ה.

מוֹדִים אֲנַחְנוּ לָךְ שָׁאַתָּה הוּא יהוה אֱלֹהֵינוּ וֵאלֹהֵי אֲבוֹתֵינוּ
לְעוֹלָם וָעֶד. צוּר חַיֵּינוּ, מָגֵן יִשְׁעֵנוּ אַתָּה הוּא לְדוֹר
וָדוֹר. נוֹדֶה לְּךָ וּנְסַפֵּר תְּהִלָּתֶךָ עַל חַיֵּינוּ הַמְּסוּרִים בְּיָדֶךָ, וְעַל
נִשְׁמוֹתֵינוּ הַפְּקוּדוֹת לָךְ, וְעַל נִסֶּיךָ שֶׁבְּכָל יוֹם עִמָּנוּ, וְעַל
נִפְלְאוֹתֶיךָ וְטוֹבוֹתֶיךָ שֶׁבְּכָל עֵת, עֶרֶב וָבֹקֶר וְצָהֳרָיִם. הַטּוֹב כִּי
לֹא כָלוּ רַחֲמֶיךָ, וְהַמְרַחֵם כִּי לֹא תַמּוּ חֲסָדֶיךָ,² מֵעוֹלָם קִוִּינוּ לָךְ.
וְעַל כֻּלָּם יִתְבָּרַךְ וְיִתְרוֹמַם שִׁמְךָ מַלְכֵּנוּ תָּמִיד לְעוֹלָם וָעֶד.

Bend the knees at בָּרוּךְ; bow at אַתָּה; straighten up at 'ה.

וְכֹל הַחַיִּים יוֹדוּךָ סֶּלָה, וִיהַלְלוּ אֶת שִׁמְךָ בֶּאֱמֶת, הָאֵל
יְשׁוּעָתֵנוּ וְעֶזְרָתֵנוּ סֶלָה. בָּרוּךְ אַתָּה יהוה, הַטּוֹב שִׁמְךָ וּלְךָ נָאֶה
לְהוֹדוֹת.

שלום

שָׁלוֹם רָב עַל יִשְׂרָאֵל עַמְּךָ תָּשִׂים לְעוֹלָם, כִּי אַתָּה הוּא מֶלֶךְ
אָדוֹן לְכָל הַשָּׁלוֹם. וְטוֹב בְּעֵינֶיךָ לְבָרֵךְ אֶת עַמְּךָ
יִשְׂרָאֵל, בְּכָל עֵת וּבְכָל שָׁעָה בִּשְׁלוֹמֶךָ. בָּרוּךְ אַתָּה יהוה,
הַמְבָרֵךְ אֶת עַמּוֹ יִשְׂרָאֵל בַּשָּׁלוֹם.

יִהְיוּ לְרָצוֹן אִמְרֵי פִי וְהֶגְיוֹן לִבִּי לְפָנֶיךָ, יהוה צוּרִי וְגֹאֲלִי.³

אֱלֹהַי, נְצוֹר לְשׁוֹנִי מֵרָע, וּשְׂפָתַי מִדַּבֵּר מִרְמָה,⁴ וְלִמְקַלְלַי נַפְשִׁי
תִדֹּם, וְנַפְשִׁי כֶּעָפָר לַכֹּל תִּהְיֶה. פְּתַח לִבִּי בְּתוֹרָתֶךָ,
וּבְמִצְוֹתֶיךָ תִּרְדּוֹף נַפְשִׁי. וְכֹל הַחוֹשְׁבִים עָלַי רָעָה, מְהֵרָה הָפֵר
עֲצָתָם וְקַלְקֵל מַחֲשַׁבְתָּם. עֲשֵׂה לְמַעַן שְׁמֶךָ, עֲשֵׂה לְמַעַן יְמִינֶךָ,
עֲשֵׂה לְמַעַן קְדֻשָּׁתֶךָ, עֲשֵׂה לְמַעַן תּוֹרָתֶךָ. לְמַעַן יֵחָלְצוּן יְדִידֶיךָ,
הוֹשִׁיעָה יְמִינְךָ וַעֲנֵנִי.⁵

Some recite verses pertaining to their names here. See page 482.

יִהְיוּ לְרָצוֹן אִמְרֵי פִי וְהֶגְיוֹן לִבִּי לְפָנֶיךָ, יהוה צוּרִי וְגֹאֲלִי.³

עֹשֶׂה שָׁלוֹם בִּמְרוֹמָיו, הוּא יַעֲשֶׂה
שָׁלוֹם עָלֵינוּ, וְעַל כָּל יִשְׂרָאֵל. וְאִמְרוּ:
אָמֵן.

Bow and take three steps back. Bow left and say ... עֹשֶׂה; bow right and say ... הוּא יַעֲשֶׂה; bow forward and say וְעַל כָּל ... אָמֵן.

וְתֶחֱזֶינָה   May our eyes behold Your return to Zion in compassion. Blessed are You, HASHEM, Who restores His Presence to Zion.

THANKSGIVING [MODIM]

Bow at 'We gratefully thank You'; straighten up at 'HASHEM.'

מוֹדִים   We gratefully thank You, for it is You Who are HASHEM, our God and the God of our forefathers for all eternity; Rock of our lives, Shield of our salvation are You from generation to generation. We shall thank You and relate Your praise[1] — for our lives, which are committed to Your power and for our souls that are entrusted to You; for Your miracles that are with us every day; and for Your wonders and favors in every season — evening, morning, and afternoon. The Beneficent One, for Your compassions were never exhausted, and the Compassionate One, for Your kindnesses never ended[2] — always have we put our hope in You.

For all these, may Your Name be blessed and exalted, our King, continually forever and ever.

Bend the knees at 'Blessed'; bow at 'You'; straighten up at 'HASHEM.'

Everything alive will gratefully acknowledge You, Selah! and praise Your Name sincerely, O God of our salvation and help, Selah! Blessed are You, HASHEM, Your Name is 'The Beneficent One' and to You it is fitting to give thanks.

PEACE

שָׁלוֹם   Establish abundant peace upon Your people Israel forever, for You are King, Master of all peace. May it be good in Your eyes to bless Your people Israel at every time and every hour with Your peace. Blessed are You, HASHEM, Who blesses His people Israel with peace.

May the expressions of my mouth and the thoughts of my heart find favor before You, HASHEM, my Rock and my Redeemer.[3]

אֱלֹהַי   My God, guard my tongue from evil and my lips from speaking deceitfully.[4] To those who curse me, let my soul be silent; and let my soul be like dust to everyone. Open my heart to Your Torah, then my soul will pursue Your commandments. As for all those who design evil against me, speedily nullify their counsel and disrupt their design. Act for Your Name's sake; act for Your right hand's sake; act for Your sanctity's sake; act for Your Torah's sake. That Your beloved ones may be given rest; let Your right hand save, and respond to me.[5]

Some recite verses pertaining to their names at this point. See page 482. May the expressions of my mouth and the thoughts of my heart find favor before You, HASHEM, my Rock and my Redeemer.[3] He Who makes peace in His heights, may He make peace upon us, and upon all Israel. Now respond: Amen.

Bow and take three steps back. Bow left and say, 'He Who makes peace ...'; bow right and say, 'may He make peace ...'; bow forward and say, 'and upon ... Amen.'

---

(1) Cf. *Psalms* 79:13. (2) Cf. *Lam.* 3:22. (3) *Psalms* 19:15. (4) Cf. 34:14. (5) 60:7;108:7.

יְהִי רָצוֹן מִלְּפָנֶיךָ יהוה אֱלֹהֵינוּ וֵאלֹהֵי אֲבוֹתֵינוּ, שֶׁיִּבָּנֶה בֵּית הַמִּקְדָּשׁ בִּמְהֵרָה בְיָמֵינוּ, וְתֵן חֶלְקֵנוּ בְּתוֹרָתֶךָ. וְשָׁם נַעֲבָדְךָ בְּיִרְאָה, כִּימֵי עוֹלָם וּכְשָׁנִים קַדְמוֹנִיּוֹת. וְעָרְבָה לַיהוה מִנְחַת יְהוּדָה וִירוּשָׁלָיִם, כִּימֵי עוֹלָם וּכְשָׁנִים קַדְמוֹנִיּוֹת.¹

SHEMONEH ESREI ENDS HERE.

Remain standing in place for at least a few moments before taking three steps forward.

קדיש שלם

.קַדִּישׁ שָׁלֵם *The chazzan recites*

יִתְגַּדַּל וְיִתְקַדַּשׁ שְׁמֵהּ רַבָּא. (.Cong – אָמֵן.) בְּעָלְמָא דִּי בְרָא כִרְעוּתֵהּ. וְיַמְלִיךְ מַלְכוּתֵהּ, בְּחַיֵּיכוֹן וּבְיוֹמֵיכוֹן וּבְחַיֵּי דְכָל בֵּית יִשְׂרָאֵל, בַּעֲגָלָא וּבִזְמַן קָרִיב. וְאִמְרוּ: אָמֵן.

(.Cong – אָמֵן. יְהֵא שְׁמֵהּ רַבָּא מְבָרַךְ לְעָלַם וּלְעָלְמֵי עָלְמַיָּא.)

יְהֵא שְׁמֵהּ רַבָּא מְבָרַךְ לְעָלַם וּלְעָלְמֵי עָלְמַיָּא.

יִתְבָּרַךְ וְיִשְׁתַּבַּח וְיִתְפָּאַר וְיִתְרוֹמַם וְיִתְנַשֵּׂא וְיִתְהַדָּר וְיִתְעַלֶּה וְיִתְהַלָּל שְׁמֵהּ דְּקֻדְשָׁא בְּרִיךְ הוּא (.Cong – בְּרִיךְ הוּא) – לְעֵלָּא מִן כָּל בִּרְכָתָא וְשִׁירָתָא תֻּשְׁבְּחָתָא וְנֶחֱמָתָא, דַּאֲמִירָן בְּעָלְמָא. וְאִמְרוּ: אָמֵן. (.Cong–אָמֵן.)

(.Cong – קַבֵּל בְּרַחֲמִים וּבְרָצוֹן אֶת תְּפִלָּתֵנוּ.)

תִּתְקַבֵּל צְלוֹתְהוֹן וּבָעוּתְהוֹן דְּכָל בֵּית יִשְׂרָאֵל קֳדָם אֲבוּהוֹן דִּי בִשְׁמַיָּא. וְאִמְרוּ: אָמֵן. (.Cong – אָמֵן.)

(.Cong – יְהִי שֵׁם יהוה מְבֹרָךְ, מֵעַתָּה וְעַד עוֹלָם.²)

יְהֵא שְׁלָמָא רַבָּא מִן שְׁמַיָּא, וְחַיִּים עָלֵינוּ וְעַל כָּל יִשְׂרָאֵל. וְאִמְרוּ: אָמֵן. (.Cong – אָמֵן.)

(.Cong – עֶזְרִי מֵעִם יהוה, עֹשֵׂה שָׁמַיִם וָאָרֶץ.³)

Take three steps back. Bow left and say . . . עֹשֶׂה; bow right and say . . . הוּא; bow forward and say אָמֵן . . . וְעַל כָּל. Remain standing in place for a few moments, then take three steps forward.

עֹשֶׂה שָׁלוֹם בִּמְרוֹמָיו, הוּא יַעֲשֶׂה שָׁלוֹם עָלֵינוּ, וְעַל כָּל יִשְׂרָאֵל. וְאִמְרוּ: אָמֵן. (.Cong – אָמֵן.)

On Saturday night a lit multi-wicked candle or two ordinary candles with flames touching each other are held up and the following blessing is recited.
After the blessing the fingers are held up to the flame to see the reflected light:

בָּרוּךְ אַתָּה יהוה אֱלֹהֵינוּ מֶלֶךְ הָעוֹלָם, בּוֹרֵא מְאוֹרֵי הָאֵשׁ.

יְהִי רָצוֹן May it be Your will, HASHEM, our God and the God of our forefathers, that the Holy Temple be rebuilt, speedily in our days. Grant us our share in Your Torah, and may we serve You there with reverence, as in days of old and in former years. Then the offering of Judah and Jerusalem will be pleasing to HASHEM, as in days of old and in former years.[1]

SHEMONEH ESREI ENDS HERE.

Remain standing in place for at least a few moments before taking three steps forward.

FULL KADDISH

The chazzan recites the Full Kaddish.

יִתְגַּדַּל May His great Name grow exalted and sanctified (Cong.— Amen.) in the world that He created as He willed. May He give reign to His kingship in your lifetimes and in your days, and in the lifetimes of the entire Family of Israel, swiftly and soon. Now respond: Amen.

(Cong.— Amen. May His great Name be blessed forever and ever.)

May His great Name be blessed forever and ever.

Blessed, praised, glorified, exalted, extolled, mighty, upraised, and lauded be the Name of the Holy One, Blessed is He (Cong.— Blessed is He) — beyond any blessing and song, praise and consolation that are uttered in the world. Now respond: Amen. (Cong.— Amen.)

(Cong.— Accept our prayers with mercy and favor.)

May the prayers and supplications of the entire Family of Israel be accepted before their Father Who is in Heaven. Now respond: Amen. (Cong.— Amen.)

(Cong.— Blessed be the Name of HASHEM, from this time and forever.[2])

May there be abundant peace from Heaven, and life, upon us and upon all Israel. Now respond: Amen. (Cong.— Amen.)

(Cong.— My help is from HASHEM, Maker of heaven and earth.[3])

Take three steps back. Bow left and say, 'He Who makes peace . . .';
bow right and say, 'may He . . .'; bow forward and say, 'and upon all Israel . . .'
Remain standing in place for a few moments, then take three steps forward.

He Who makes peace in His heights, may He make peace upon us, and upon all Israel. Now respond: Amen. (Cong.— Amen.)

On Saturday night a lit multi-wicked candle or two ordinary candles with flames touching each other are held up and the following blessing is recited.
After the blessing the fingers are held up to the flame to see the reflected light:

בָּרוּךְ Blessed are You, HASHEM, our God, King of the universe, Who creates the illuminations of the fire.

(1) Malachi 3:4. (2) Psalms 113:2. (3) 121:2.

❖ מגילת איכה ❖

פרק ראשון

א אֵיכָה* | יָשְׁבָה בָדָד* הָעִיר רַבָּתִי עָם הָיְתָה כְּאַלְמָנָה* רַבָּתִי
בַגּוֹיִם שָׂרָתִי בַּמְּדִינוֹת הָיְתָה לָמַס: ב בָּכוֹ תִבְכֶּה* בַּלַּיְלָה וְדִמְעָתָהּ
עַל לֶחֱיָהּ אֵין לָהּ מְנַחֵם מִכָּל אֹהֲבֶיהָ כָּל רֵעֶיהָ בָּגְדוּ בָהּ הָיוּ לָהּ
לְאֹיְבִים: ג גָּלְתָה יְהוּדָה* מֵעֹנִי וּמֵרֹב עֲבֹדָה הִיא יָשְׁבָה בַגּוֹיִם לֹא
מָצְאָה מָנוֹחַ כָּל רֹדְפֶיהָ הִשִּׂיגוּהָ בֵּין הַמְּצָרִים:* ד דַּרְכֵי צִיּוֹן
אֲבֵלוֹת מִבְּלִי בָּאֵי מוֹעֵד כָּל שְׁעָרֶיהָ שׁוֹמֵמִין כֹּהֲנֶיהָ נֶאֱנָחִים
בְּתוּלֹתֶיהָ נוּגוֹת וְהִיא מַר לָהּ: ה הָיוּ צָרֶיהָ לְרֹאשׁ אֹיְבֶיהָ שָׁלוּ כִּי
יהוה הוֹגָהּ עַל רֹב פְּשָׁעֶיהָ* עוֹלָלֶיהָ הָלְכוּ שְׁבִי* לִפְנֵי צָר* וַיֵּצֵא
מִבַּת* צִיּוֹן כָּל הֲדָרָהּ הָיוּ שָׂרֶיהָ כְּאַיָּלִים לֹא מָצְאוּ מִרְעֶה וַיֵּלְכוּ

°מן בת כ'

[This commentary to *Eichah* has been abridged from that volume
in the ArtScroll Tanach Series, by Rabbi Meir Zlotowitz.]

CHAPTER ONE

1. אֵיכָה — *Alas.* The prophet, Jeremiah, wrote סֵפֶר
קִינוֹת, the *Book of Lamentations.* This is the Scroll
which Yehoyakim burned *on the fire that was in
the brazier* [Jeremiah 36:23].

[The book laments the fall of the Jews and
Jerusalem after the חֻרְבָּן, *Destruction,* of the
First Temple. Originally the book consisted of 3
acrostic chapters [1,2 and 4] which Jeremiah
rewrote after the burning. He later added chapter
3 consisting of three additional acrostics, as well
as chapter 5 (*Rashi; Moed Katan* 26a).

According to *Tzemach David,* the Destruction
took place during the reign of King Zedekiah in
the year 3338 from Creation [422 B.C.E.]. Judah
was then exiled from the Land by Nebuchadnezzar. (The ten tribes had been exiled 133 years
earlier.)

For a period of 52 years after the Destruction,
Eretz Yisrael lay desolate: the roads and villages
were uninhabited; not even cattle or birds
inhabited the Land (*Yoma* 54a).

The Exile lasted 70 years until 3408, when
Darius, son of Queen Esther and King
Ahasuerus, permitted the rebuilding of the
Temple. The Destruction of the Second Temple
took place in the days of Rabban Yochanan ben
Zakkai in the year 3828 (*Tzemach David*).

אֵיכָה יָשְׁבָה בָדָד — *Alas — She sits in solitude!*
Three people uttered prophecies using the word
אֵיכָה, *Eichah:* Moses, Isaiah, and Jeremiah. . . Rav
Levi said: It is comparable to a nation that had
three groomsmen: The first beheld her in her
happiness; the second beheld her in her infidelity,
and the third beheld her in her disgrace. Similarly, Moses beheld the Jews in their glory and
happiness, and exclaimed: אֵיכָה אֶשָּׂא לְבַדִּי טָרְחֲכֶם,

How can I alone bear your cumbrance? (Deut.
1:12) [they presented all the difficulties of a large,
growing, and flourishing nation]. Isaiah beheld
them in their infidelity and exclaimed: אֵיכָה הָיְתָה
לְזוֹנָה, *How has the faithful city become a harlot*
(Isaiah 1:21)? Jeremiah beheld them in their
disgrace and said: אֵיכָה יָשְׁבָה בָדָד, *Alas — She sits
in solitude!* (*Midrash*).

The Book of *Lamentations* is written in a series
of alphabetical acrostics. The *Talmud* notes: Why
was Israel smitten with an alphabetical dirge? —
Because they transgressed the Torah from *Alef* to
Tav, i.e., from the first to the last letter of the
alphabet (*Sanhedrin* 104b).

יָשְׁבָה בָדָד — *She sits in solitude.* Bereft of her
inhabitants (*Rashi*) [*she* — i.e., Jerusalem personified as a woman].

הָיְתָה כְּאַלְמָנָה — *Has become like a widow.* The
Talmud stresses the prefix כְּ, *as:* Jerusalem's
widow-hood was not total, but temporary — she
is like a woman whose husband went to a foreign
country, but with the intention of returning to
her (*Sanhedrin* 104b).

Another interpretation: She *is* a widow — she
is bereft of the ten tribes, but not of the tribes of
Judah and Benjamin. . . The Rabbis said: She was
widowed of *all* the tribes [all the tribes —
including Judah and Benjamin were exiled, and
Jerusalem was bereft of them] but she was never
deserted by God (*Midrash*).

2. בָּכוֹ תִבְכֶּה — *She weeps bitterly* [lit., *weeping
she weeps.*] Many interpretations are offered for
the use of בָּכוֹ תִבְכֶּה, the double form of the verb
בכה, *weep:*

According to the *Talmud:* Why this 'double
weeping'? — Once for the First Temple; once for
the Second (*Sanhedrin* 104b).

⊰{ THE BOOK OF EICHAH }⊱

CHAPTER ONE

¹ **A**las* — she sits in solitude!* The city that was great with people has become like a widow.* The greatest among nations, the princess among provinces, has become a tributary. ² She weeps bitterly* in the night and her tear is on her cheek. She has no comforter from all her lovers; all her friends have betrayed her, they have become her enemies. ³ Judah has gone into exile* because of suffering and harsh toil. She dwelt among the nations, but found no rest; all her pursuers overtook her in narrow straits.* ⁴ The roads of Zion are in mourning for lack of festival pilgrims. All her gates are desolate, her priests sigh; her maidens are aggrieved, and she herself is embittered. ⁵ Her adversaries have become her master, her enemies are at ease, for HASHEM has aggrieved her for her abundant transgressions.* Her young children have gone into captivity* before the enemy. ⁶ Gone from the daughter of Zion is all her splendor. Her leaders were like deer that found no pasture, but walked on

---

Other explanations of the 'double weeping' are: On account of Judah, and of Zion and Jerusalem; on account of the exile of the ten tribes, and of Judah and Benjamin.

Another interpretation: בָּכוֹ וּתְבְכֶּה, she weeps and makes others weep with her (*Midrash*).

The word בַּלַּיְלָה, *in the night*, refers to the specific night of Tishah B'Av, which, from the time of the מְרַגְּלִים, spies, has been mournfully observed as a night of weeping and meditation (*Lechem Dim'ah*)...

As the *Talmud* (*Sanhedrin* 104b) relates: When the מְרַגְּלִים (the spies sent by Moses to investigate the land of Canaan) returned with discouraging news, the *people wept that night* (*Numbers* 14:1). That night was the ninth of Av, and God said to Israel: You have wept without cause; therefore will I appoint [this date as a time of] weeping for you in future generations.

3. גָּלְתָה יְהוּדָה — *Judah has gone into exile* — from its land (*Rashi*).

Judah is a general term encompassing both the male and female members of the tribe of Judah (*Ibn Ezra*). [The term *Judah* also includes the tribe of Benjamin who was exiled together with Judah.]

The *Midrash* compares the exile of other nations to that of Israel:

Heathen nations also go into exile, however, since they eat the bread and drink the wine [of their enemies], they do not experience real exile [i.e., they do not experience privation]. For Israel, however, which is forbidden to eat their bread or drink their wine, the exile is real.

בֵּין הַמְּצָרִים — *In narrow straits*, i.e., by cornering them (*Rashi*).

Some understand this literally, but the *Midrash* understands the phrase בֵּין הַמְּצָרִים as *within the days of distress*, i.e., all who pursued her overtook her during the period between the 17th

of Tammuz when the first breach in Jerusalem's walls was made and the 9th of Av [exactly 3 weeks later, when the Temple was destroyed].

[This phrase בֵּין הַמְּצָרִים, *within the days of distress*, is used today in halachic literature as well as in common Hebrew usage to refer to the period between the 17th of Tammuz and the 9th of Av.]

5. כִּי־יְ־הֹ־וָ־ה הוֹגָהּ עַל־רֹב פְּשָׁעֶיהָ — *For HASHEM has aggrieved her for her abundant transgressions.* The *Midrash*, as interpreted by the commentaries, notes that God's punishment was in direct proportion to Israel's many transgressions. Even הָיוּ צָרֶיהָ לְרֹאשׁ, *her enemies have become her master*, was part of the punishment.

[The word רֹב, *many*, can also mean *majority*, *most*. Since the phrase is רֹב פְּשָׁעֶיהָ, *her many sins*, instead of כָּל פְּשָׁעֶיהָ, *all of her sins*, it is, perhaps, possible to translate the verse: *for God has aggrieved her for the majority of her transgressions.* In the final analysis, God *was* compassionate, for had He exacted punishment at that time for *all* her transgressions, *no one* would have survived.]

Harav David Cohen points out that *Rambam* in *Hilchos Teshuvah* 2:2 discusses the evaluation of iniquities and merits and concludes: *This valuation takes into account not the number but the magnitude* [i.e., *qualitative rather than quantitative*] *of merits and iniquities. There may be a single merit that outweighs many iniquities... and there may be one iniquity that offsets many merits... God alone makes this evaluation; He alone knows how to set off merit against iniquities.*

עוֹלָלֶיהָ הָלְכוּ שְׁבִי — *Her young children have gone into captivity.* The *Midrash* stresses that the children are the most beloved to God. According to this view, the Sanhedrin did not go into exile with them; the priestly watches were exiled, but

בְּלֹא־כֹחַ לִפְנֵי רוֹדֵף:* ז זָכְרָה יְרוּשָׁלַם* יְמֵי עָנְיָהּ* וּמְרוּדֶיהָ כֹּל מַחֲמֻדֶיהָ אֲשֶׁר הָיוּ מִימֵי קֶדֶם בִּנְפֹל עַמָּהּ בְּיַד־צָר וְאֵין עוֹזֵר לָהּ רָאוּהָ צָרִים שָׂחֲקוּ עַל־מִשְׁבַּתֶּהָ: ח חֵטְא חָטְאָה יְרוּשָׁלַם עַל־כֵּן לְנִידָה הָיָתָה כָּל־מְכַבְּדֶיהָ הִזִּילוּהָ כִּי־רָאוּ עֶרְוָתָהּ גַּם־הִיא נֶאֶנְחָה וַתָּשָׁב אָחוֹר: ט טֻמְאָתָהּ בְּשׁוּלֶיהָ לֹא זָכְרָה אַחֲרִיתָהּ וַתֵּרֶד פְּלָאִים אֵין מְנַחֵם לָהּ רְאֵה יהוה אֶת־עָנְיִי כִּי הִגְדִּיל אוֹיֵב: י יָדוֹ פָּרַשׂ צָר עַל כָּל־מַחֲמַדֶּיהָ כִּי־רָאֲתָה גוֹיִם בָּאוּ מִקְדָּשָׁהּ אֲשֶׁר צִוִּיתָה לֹא־יָבֹאוּ בַקָּהָל לָךְ:* יא כָּל־עַמָּהּ נֶאֱנָחִים מְבַקְשִׁים לֶחֶם נָתְנוּ °מַחֲמַדֵּיהֶם בְּאֹכֶל לְהָשִׁיב נָפֶשׁ רְאֵה יהוה וְהַבִּיטָה כִּי הָיִיתִי זוֹלֵלָה: יב לוֹא אֲלֵיכֶם כָּל־עֹבְרֵי דֶרֶךְ הַבִּיטוּ וּרְאוּ אִם־יֵשׁ מַכְאוֹב כְּמַכְאֹבִי אֲשֶׁר עוֹלַל לִי אֲשֶׁר הוֹגָה יהוה בְּיוֹם חֲרוֹן אַפּוֹ:* יג מִמָּרוֹם שָׁלַח־אֵשׁ בְּעַצְמֹתַי* וַיִּרְדֶּנָּה פָּרַשׂ רֶשֶׁת לְרַגְלַי הֱשִׁיבַנִי אָחוֹר נְתָנַנִי שֹׁמֵמָה כָּל־הַיּוֹם דָּוָה: יד נִשְׂקַד עֹל פְּשָׁעַי בְּיָדוֹ יִשְׂתָּרְגוּ עָלוּ עַל־צַוָּארִי הִכְשִׁיל כֹּחִי נְתָנַנִי אֲדֹנָי בִּידֵי לֹא־אוּכַל קוּם: טו סִלָּה כָל־אַבִּירַי* אֲדֹנָי בְּקִרְבִּי קָרָא עָלַי מוֹעֵד* לִשְׁבֹּר בַּחוּרָי גַּת דָּרַךְ אֲדֹנָי לִבְתוּלַת בַּת־יְהוּדָה:* טז עַל־אֵלֶּה אֲנִי בוֹכִיָּה* עֵינִי עֵינִי יֹרְדָה מַּיִם כִּי־רָחַק מִמֶּנִּי מְנַחֵם מֵשִׁיב נַפְשִׁי

°מחמודיהם כ'

---

the *Shechinah* [God's Presence] did not go into exile with them. However, when the children were exiled, the *Shechinah* went into exile with them. Therefore, it is written: *Her young children have gone into captivity before the enemy.* This is immediately followed by, *Gone from the daughter of Zion is all her splendor* [i.e., the *Shechinah*].

6. לִפְנֵי רוֹדֵף — *Before the pursuer. Rashi* observes that wherever else in Scripture the word רוֹדֵף appears it is spelled רֹדֵף, *defectively* — i.e., without the ו, *vav*. In our verse, however, the full spelling is used to imply that the Jews were pursued vigorously and fully.

7. זָכְרָה יְרוּשָׁלַם — *Jerusalem recalled.* While in exile (*Rashi*).

יְמֵי עָנְיָהּ — *The days of her affliction* i.e., the Destruction which was the cause of her affliction (*Rashi*).

8. [The author now attributes all of the suffering described in verses 1-7 to Divine retribution for Jerusalem's grievous sins.]

The *Midrash*, commenting on the use of the double verb, חָטְא חָטְאָה, *sinned a sin,* explains: They sinned doubly and were punished doubly,

as it is written: כִּי לָקְחָה מִיַּד ה' כִּפְלַיִם בְּכָל־חַטֹּאתֶיהָ — *She received from God's hand double for all her sins* (Isaiah 40:2); and they were comforted doubly, as it is written: נַחֲמוּ נַחֲמוּ עַמִּי, *Comfort My people, comfort* (Isaiah 40:1).

Meshech Chachmah interprets the double verb: *Jerusalem sinned repeatedly* and grew accustomed to the fact, viewing it naturally, and feeling no remorse. . .

[As the *Talmud* (*Moed Katan* 27b) remarks: *As soon as a person has committed a sinful act and has repeated it* — נַעֲשֵׂית לוֹ כְּהֶיתֵּר, it has become to him as though it were something permissible (see *Overview*).]

According to the Talmud, a sin consists of two parts: the sinful act itself and the thoughts and satisfaction surrounding it. Each part of the sin is evaluated separately and punished separately (*Kiddushin* 40a). Therefore, the verse uses a twin expression of sin. In the same way, the thought leading up to a good deed and the satisfaction one derives from having performed it are rewarded by God along with the good deed itself (*Hagaon Rav Moshe Feinstein*).

10. אֲשֶׁר צִוִּיתָה לֹא־יָבֹאוּ בַקָּהָל לָךְ — *About whom You had commanded that they should not enter* *without strength before the pursuer.* ⁷ Jerusalem recalled* the days of her affliction* and sorrow — all the treasures that were hers in the days of old. With the fall of her people into the enemy's hand and none to help her, her enemies saw her and gloated at her downfall. ⁸ Jerusalem sinned greatly, she has therefore become a wanderer. All who once respected her disparage her, for they have seen her disgrace. She herself sighs and turns away. ⁹ Her impurity is on her hems, she was heedless of the consequences. She has sunk astonishingly, there is no one to comfort her. 'Look, HASHEM, at my misery, for the enemy has acted prodigiously!' ¹⁰ The enemy spread out his hand on all her treasures; indeed, she saw nations invade her sanctuary — about whom You had commanded that they should not enter Your congregation.* ¹¹ All her people are sighing, searching for bread. They traded their enemies for food to keep alive. 'Look, HASHEM,* and behold what a glutton I have become!' ¹² May it not befall you — all who pass by this road. Behold and see, if there is any pain like my pain which befell me; which HASHEM has afflicted me on the day of His wrath.* ¹³ From on high He sent a fire into my bones,* and it crushed them. he spread a net for my feet hurling me backward. He made me desolate; in constant misery. ¹⁴ The burden of my transgressions was accumulated in His hand; they were knit* together and thrust upon my neck — He sapped my strength. The Lord has delivered me into the hands of those I cannot withstand. ¹⁵ The Lord has trampled all my heroes in my midst; He proclaimed a set time against me* to crush my young men. As in a winepress the Lord has trodden the maiden daughter of Judah.* ¹⁶ Over these things I weep;* my eyes run with water because a comforter to revive my spirit is far from me.*

Your congregation. When the enemies entered the Temple, Ammonites and Moabites entered among them. While the others ran to plunder the silver and gold, the Ammonites and Moabites ran to plunder the Torah itself to expunge the verse (Deut. 23:4): לֹא־יָבֹא עַמּוֹנִי וּמוֹאָבִי בִּקְהַל ה׳, *An Ammonite or Moabite shall not enter the Assembly of HASHEM* (Midrash).

11. רְאֵה ה׳ — *'Look, HASHEM.'* An impassioned plea. From this point on, Jerusalem, itself, laments. The Community of Israel says to the nations of the world: May there not occur to you what has occurred to me.

12. בְּיוֹם חֲרוֹן אַפּוֹ — *On the day of His wrath,* i.e., the Ninth of Av when so many tragedies befell Israel throughout its history (Shaar Bas Rabim).

The *Midrash* stresses *the day,* i.e., that particular day upon which God's fierce anger was kindled: Had Israel repented that very day they could have cooled [i.e., averted] His anger.

13. מִמָּרוֹם שָׁלַח אֵשׁ־בְּעַצְמֹתַי — *From on high He sent a fire into my bones.* The Midrash understands this literally: God Himself sent a fire to burn the Temple so the heathens could not boast

that they themselves destroyed it.

14. נִשְׂקַד...יִשְׂתָּרְגוּ — *Was accumulated... were knit.* Instead of constantly doling out small, proportioned punishment for every one of Zion's sins whenever she transgressed, God collected all her transgressions, noting and remembering them. He then metaphorically knit them together into a heavy garment which he thrust upon her neck in one heavy, cumulative load, effectively weighing her down, and sapping her strength until she was unable to withstand the enemy.

15. קָרָא עָלַי מוֹעֵד — *He proclaimed a set time against me,* i.e., the Ninth of Av (Taanis 29a). [See comm. to verse 2, s.v. בַּלַּיְלָה].

[Since Tishah B'Av is referred to as מוֹעֵד, *set time, festival,* the Sages state that halachically, as on a holiday, *Tachanun* is not said during *Minchah* services on *Erev Tishah B'Av* (Shulchan Aruch, Orach Chaim 552).

לִבְתוּלַת בַּת־יְהוּדָה — The *maiden daughter of Judah,* i.e., Jerusalem (Rashi).

16. עַל־אֵלֶּה אֲנִי בוֹכִיָּה — *Over these things I weep.* The verb בוֹכִיָּה implies a constant action: *I*

הָיוּ בָנַי שׁוֹמֵמִים כִּי גָבַר אוֹיֵב: יז פֵּרְשָׂה צִיּוֹן בְּיָדֶיהָ אֵין מְנַחֵם לָהּ
צִוָּה יהוה לְיַעֲקֹב סְבִיבָיו צָרָיו הָיְתָה יְרוּשָׁלַ͏ִם לְנִדָּה בֵּינֵיהֶם:
יח צַדִּיק הוּא יהוה כִּי פִיהוּ מָרִיתִי שִׁמְעוּ־נָא °כָל־הָעַמִּים וּרְאוּ
מַכְאֹבִי בְּתוּלֹתַי וּבַחוּרַי הָלְכוּ בַשֶּׁבִי: יט קָרָאתִי לַמְאַהֲבַי הֵמָּה
רִמּוּנִי* כֹּהֲנַי וּזְקֵנַי בָּעִיר גָּוָעוּ כִּי־בִקְשׁוּ אֹכֶל לָמוֹ וְיָשִׁיבוּ
אֶת־נַפְשָׁם: כ רְאֵה יהוה* כִּי־צַר־לִי* מֵעַי חֳמַרְמָרוּ נֶהְפַּךְ לִבִּי
בְּקִרְבִּי כִּי מָרוֹ מָרִיתִי מִחוּץ שִׁכְּלָה־חֶרֶב בַּבַּיִת כַּמָּוֶת: כא שָׁמְעוּ
כִּי נֶאֱנָחָה אָנִי* אֵין מְנַחֵם לִי כָּל־אֹיְבַי שָׁמְעוּ רָעָתִי שָׂשׂוּ כִּי
אַתָּה עָשִׂיתָ* הֵבֵאתָ יוֹם־קָרָאתָ וְיִהְיוּ כָמֹנִי: כב תָּבֹא כָל־רָעָתָם
לְפָנֶיךָ וְעוֹלֵל לָמוֹ כַּאֲשֶׁר עוֹלַלְתָּ לִי עַל כָּל־פְּשָׁעָי כִּי־רַבּוֹת
אַנְחֹתַי וְלִבִּי דַוָּי:

פרק שני

א אֵיכָה יָעִיב בְּאַפּוֹ | אֲדֹנָי אֶת־בַּת־צִיּוֹן* הִשְׁלִיךְ מִשָּׁמַיִם אֶרֶץ
תִּפְאֶרֶת יִשְׂרָאֵל* וְלֹא־זָכַר הֲדֹם־רַגְלָיו* בְּיוֹם אַפּוֹ: ב בִּלַּע אֲדֹנָי
°וְלֹא חָמַל אֵת כָּל־נְאוֹת יַעֲקֹב* הָרַס בְּעֶבְרָתוֹ מִבְצְרֵי
בַת־יְהוּדָה הִגִּיעַ לָאָרֶץ חִלֵּל מַמְלָכָה וְשָׂרֶיהָ: ג גָּדַע* בָּחֳרִי־אַף
כֹּל קֶרֶן יִשְׂרָאֵל הֵשִׁיב אָחוֹר יְמִינוֹ מִפְּנֵי אוֹיֵב וַיִּבְעַר בְּיַעֲקֹב*
כְּאֵשׁ לֶהָבָה אָכְלָה סָבִיב: ד דָּרַךְ קַשְׁתּוֹ כְּאוֹיֵב נִצָּב יְמִינוֹ כְּצָר

°כָל־עַמִּים כ'   °לֹא־חָמַל כ'

---

weep incessantly; or I have become known as a
habitual weeper (Lechem Dim'ah). Various
causes for her weeping are offered in the
Midrash, which relates many harrowing inci-
dents of barbarous atrocities which befell the
Jews at the time of the Destruction (1:16). [The
post-Holocaust generation understands only too
well how the Jewish people can suffer at the
hands of cruel and bestial people. Indeed, the
atrocities of the Nazis are also foreshadowed in
the lament of Jeremiah.]

18. Zion itself resumes the lament, and confesses
publicly and without reservation that God is
righteous and justified in what He has done.

19. קָרָאתִי לַמְאַהֲבַי הֵמָּה רִמּוּנִי — I called for my
lovers but they deceived me. Lovers — i.e., those
who feigned friendship (Rashi) [i.e., the neighboring countries — Egypt, Moab, Ammon, with
whom Judea had hoped to form an alliance].

The Rabbis interpret this verse as an allusion to
the false prophets who made me love their idol
worship. הֵמָּה רִמּוּנִי, they deceived me, by
incessantly uttering false prophecies of reassurance decrying Jeremiah's calls for repentance,

until they caused me to go into exile.

20. רְאֵה ה׳. — See, HASHEM. [This verse begins
with a supplication to God to bear witness to the
extent of Zion's affliction, and culminates with
an appeal (verse 22) for Divine retribution
against the enemy.]

21. שָׁמְעוּ כִּי נֶאֱנָחָה אָנִי —They heard how I sighed,
i.e., my lovers [referred to above in verses 2 and
19] heard me sigh and did not even comfort me;
my real enemies, on the other hand, actually
rejoiced upon hearing my plight, knowing You
have caused it (Ibn Ezra).

כִּי אַתָּה עָשִׂיתָ —For it was You Who did it [i.e., my
misfortune emanated from Your will]. You are
the cause of their hating us because You prohibited us from eating their food or marrying their
children. Had we socialized and intermarried
with them, would they not have compassion
upon us and on their offspring? (Midrash; Rashi).

Lechem Dim'ah notes that here [unlike verse
12] Zion prays that the enemies be punished for
rejoicing at her downfall. And lest anyone think
that Zion might then rejoice at her enemies'

My children have become forlorn, because the enemy has prevailed.
¹⁷ Zion spread out her hands; there was none to comfort her. HASHEM
commanded against Jacob that his enemies should surround him;
Jerusalem has become as one unclean in their midst. ¹⁸ It is HASHEM Who
is righteous, for I disobeyed His utterance. Listen, all you peoples and
behold my pain: My maidens and my youths have gone into captivity.
¹⁹ I called for my lovers but they deceived me.* My priests and my elders
perished in the city as they sought food for themselves to keep alive.
²⁰ See, HASHEM,* how distressed I am; my insides churn! My heart is
turned over inside me for I rebelled grievously. Outside the sword
bereaved, inside was death-like. ²¹ They heard how I sighed,* there was
none to comfort me. All my enemies heard of my plight and rejoiced, for
it was You Who did it.* O bring on the day You proclaimed and let them
be like me! ²² Let all their wickedness come before You, and inflict them
as You inflicted me for all my transgressions. For my groans are many,
and my heart is sick.

CHAPTER TWO

¹ Alas — the Lord in His anger has clouded the daughter of Zion.* He
cast down from heaven to earth the glory of Israel.* He did not
remember His footstool* on the day of His wrath. ² The Lord consumed
without pity all the dwellings of Jacob;* in His anger He razed the
fortresses of the daughter of Judah down to the ground; He profaned the
kingdom and its leaders.* ³ He cut down,* in fierce anger, all the dignity
of Israel; He withdrew His right hand in the presence of the enemy.
He burned through Jacob* like a flaming fire, consuming on all sides.
⁴ He bent His bow like an enemy. His right hand poised like a foe,

---

downfall, the verse concludes: No, there is no room for rejoicing! *My groans are many, and my heart is sick.*

CHAPTER TWO

1. בַּת־צִיּוֹן — *Daughter of Zion.* A poetic form, used to denote Jerusalem; its populace.

הִשְׁלִיךְ מִשָּׁמַיִם אֶרֶץ תִּפְאֶרֶת יִשְׂרָאֵל — *He cast down from heaven to earth the glory of Israel.* After having raised up the Jews to the uppermost heavens, He cast them down to the nethermost depths — not gradually, but in one thrust (*Rashi*).

וְלֹא־זָכַר הֲדֹם־רַגְלָיו — *He did not remember His footstool,* i.e., the בֵּית הַמִּקְדָּשׁ, *the Holy Temple* (*Midrash; Rashi*).

The *Midrash* notes, homiletically, that הֲדֹם, *footstool,* has the same spelling as הַדָּם, *the blood,* i.e., God in His anger preferred not to remember Abraham's blood of circumcision or the blood in which they wallowed in Egypt, and which they put on the doorposts there (II:1).

2. אֵת כָּל־נְאוֹת יַעֲקֹב — *All the dwellings of Jacob.* The *Midrash* homiletically translates נְאוֹת יַעֲקֹב, *the beauty of Jacob* — referring to the Torah

Sages who were martyred during the Destruction.

חִלֵּל מַמְלָכָה וְשָׂרֶיהָ — *He profaned the kingdom and its leaders.* This refers to Israel which is called מַמְלֶכֶת כֹּהֲנִים, *a kingdom of priests* (*Rashi*); also, to Zedekiah, King of Judah (*Midrash*).

3. גָּדַע — *He cut down,* i.e., the branches only, leaving the root intact so it could eventually grow back (*Lechem Dim'ah*).

The *Midrash* notes that when the enemy entered Jerusalem, they took the mighty men of Israel and bound their hands behind them. The Holy One, Blessed is He, saw their distress, so He, too — anthropomorphically — *withdrew His right hand behind Him* [i.e., symbolizing His endurance of the many indignities heaped upon His glory by the heathens, as if His hands, so to speak, were behind His back, powerless to avenge] (*Yefe Anaf*).

וַיִּבְעַר בְּיַעֲקֹב — *He burned through Jacob.* The *Midrash* comments: When punishment comes into the world, no one feels it as much as [the patriarch] Jacob; and when there is good in the world, no one rejoices as much as Jacob, i.e., Jacob feels it more keenly than the other patriarchs

וַיַּהֲרֹג כֹּל מַחֲמַדֵּי־עָיִן* בְּאֹהֶל בַּת־צִיּוֹן שָׁפַךְ כָּאֵשׁ חֲמָתוֹ: ה הָיָה
אֲדֹנָי | כְּאוֹיֵב* בִּלַּע יִשְׂרָאֵל בִּלַּע כָּל־אַרְמְנוֹתֶיהָ שִׁחֵת מִבְצָרָיו
וַיֶּרֶב בְּבַת־יְהוּדָה תַּאֲנִיָּה וַאֲנִיָּה: וּ וַיַּחְמֹס כַּגַּן* שֻׂכּוֹ* שִׁחֵת
מֹעֲדוֹ* שִׁכַּח יְהוָה | בְּצִיּוֹן מוֹעֵד וְשַׁבָּת וַיִּנְאַץ בְּזַעַם־אַפּוֹ מֶלֶךְ
וְכֹהֵן: ז זָנַח אֲדֹנָי | מִזְבְּחוֹ* נִאֵר מִקְדָּשׁוֹ הִסְגִּיר בְּיַד־אוֹיֵב
חוֹמֹת אַרְמְנוֹתֶיהָ קוֹל נָתְנוּ בְּבֵית־יְהוָה כְּיוֹם מוֹעֵד:* ח חָשַׁב
יְהוָה | לְהַשְׁחִית* חוֹמַת בַּת־צִיּוֹן נָטָה קָו לֹא־הֵשִׁיב יָדוֹ
מִבַּלֵּעַ וַיַּאֲבֶל־חֵל וְחוֹמָה יַחְדָּו אֻמְלָלוּ: ט טָבְעוּ בָאָרֶץ שְׁעָרֶיהָ*
אִבַּד וְשִׁבַּר בְּרִיחֶיהָ מַלְכָּהּ וְשָׂרֶיהָ בַגּוֹיִם אֵין תּוֹרָה* גַּם־נְבִיאֶיהָ
לֹא־מָצְאוּ חָזוֹן מֵיְהוָה: יֵשְׁבוּ לָאָרֶץ יִדְּמוּ* זִקְנֵי בַת־צִיּוֹן
הֶעֱלוּ עָפָר עַל־רֹאשָׁם חָגְרוּ שַׂקִּים הוֹרִידוּ לָאָרֶץ רֹאשָׁן בְּתוּלֹת
יְרוּשָׁלִָם: יא כָּלוּ בַדְּמָעוֹת עֵינַי חֳמַרְמְרוּ מֵעַי נִשְׁפַּךְ לָאָרֶץ
כְּבֵדִי עַל־שֶׁבֶר בַּת־עַמִּי בֵּעָטֵף עוֹלֵל* וְיוֹנֵק בִּרְחֹבוֹת קִרְיָה:
יב לְאִמֹּתָם יֹאמְרוּ* אַיֵּה דָּגָן וָיָיִן* בְּהִתְעַטְּפָם כֶּחָלָל בִּרְחֹבוֹת

---

because he experienced the most tribulations in raising his family (*Torah Temimah*).

4. In this verse Hashem is depicted, not only in His passive role as One who withdrew His support, but as One who actively participated in Israel's destruction.

וַיַּהֲרֹג כֹּל מַחֲמַדֵּי־עָיִן — *He slew all who were of pleasant appearance.*

Rav Tanchum ben Yirmiyah said this refers to the children who were as dear to their parents as the apple of their eye. The Rabbis said this refers to the members of the Sanhedrin who were as dear to Israel as the apple of their eye (*Midrash*).

5. . . . הָיָה ה' כְּאוֹיֵב — *The Lord became like an enemy. . .* After all of the above, the Jews did not repent. Still, God restrained Himself. The verse likens His anger to that of an enemy, but He did not become an enemy. Also, בִּלַּע, *He consumed Israel,* but not כָּל יִשְׂרָאֵל, *all of Israel;* בִּלַּע כָּל אַרְמְנוֹתֶיהָ, *He consumed all her citadels;* and thus vented His anger by directing His actions עַל עֵצִים וַאֲבָנִים, *on wood and stone* [i.e., on inanimate objects, rather than on human lives], so as to avoid the total slaughter of the Jews themselves (*Palgei Mayim*).

6. וַיַּחְמֹס כַּגַּן שֻׂכּוֹ — *He stripped His Booth like a garden. His Booth,* related to סֻכָּה, *sukkah* (Ibn Ezra), i.e., His dwelling place (*Rashi*) — the קֹדֶשׁ קֳדָשִׁים, *Holy of Holies* (*Palgei Mayim*).

The *Midrash* notes that the word for booth, שֻׂכּוֹ [*sukko*], can be read שְׂכּוֹ [*shukko*], *His appeasement,* i.e., when He stripped [Jerusalem] as one strips a garden, שֶׁכָּכָה חֲמָתוֹ שֶׁל הקב"ה,

God's wrath was appeased [having vented His anger on wood and stone].

כַּגַּן — *Like a garden.* I.e., as one cuts vegetables in a garden. Jerusalem became like a garden which had been deprived of its water (*Midrash*) [and nothing looks as desolate as a garden stripped of its plants].

שִׁחֵת מֹעֲדוֹ — *He destroyed His place of assembly,* i.e., the קֹדֶשׁ קֳדָשִׁים, *the Holy of Holies,* where God presents Himself [נוֹעַד] to His children [*Exodus* 25:22] (*Rashi*).

שִׁכַּח ה' בְּצִיּוֹן מוֹעֵד וְשַׁבָּת — *HASHEM made Zion oblivious of festival and Sabbath* [i.e., as a result of God's destruction of the Temple and sacrifices, it was as if the festivals and Sabbath were forgotten].

7. זָנַח ה' מִזְבְּחוֹ — *The Lord rejected His altar.* The Holy One, Blessed is He, said to Israel: Do you provoke Me because you rely on the sacrifices which you offer to Me? Here, have them! They are thrown in your face (*Midrash*).

כְּיוֹם מוֹעֵד — *As though it were a festival* i.e., the heathens clamored joyously at the destruction of the Temple, matching the fervor of Israel's joyous chants on its holiday (*Alshich; Rashi*).

8. חָשַׁב ה' לְהַשְׁחִית — *HASHEM resolved to destroy.* The *Midrash* explains that the resolve was not new — but an old one, as it is written: כִּי עַל אַפִּי וְעַל חֲמָתִי הָיְתָה לִּי הָעִיר הַזֹּאת לְמִן הַיּוֹם אֲשֶׁר בָּנוּ אוֹתָהּ, *For this city [Jerusalem] has been to Me a provocation of My fury and My anger from the day that they built it [Jer. 32:31] [and God, in a*

He slew all who were of pleasant appearance.* In the tent of the daughter of Zion He poured out His wrath like fire. ⁵ The Lord became like an enemy.* He consumed Israel; He consumed all her citadels, He destroyed its fortresses. He increased within the daughter of Judah moaning and mourning. ⁶ He stripped His Booth like a garden,* He destroyed His place of assembly.* HASHEM made Zion oblivious of festival and Sabbath,* and in His fierce anger He spurned king and priest. ⁷ The Lord rejected His altar,* abolished His Sanctuary; He handed over to the enemy the walls of her citadels. They raised a clamor in the House of HASHEM as though it were a festival.* ⁸ HASHEM resolved to destroy* the wall of the daughter of Zion. He stretched out the line and did not relent from devouring. Indeed, He made rampart and wall mourn; together they languished. ⁹ Her gates have sunk into the earth,* He has utterly shattered her bars; her king and officers are among the heathen, there is no Torah;* her prophets, too, find no vision from HASHEM. ¹⁰ The elders of the daughter of Zion sit on the ground in silence;* they have strewn ashes on their heads, and wear sackcloth. The maidens of Jerusalem have bowed their heads to the ground. ¹¹ My eyes fail with tears, my insides churn; my liver spills on the ground at the shattering of my people, while babes and sucklings swoon in the streets of the city. ¹² They say to their mothers,* 'Where is bread and wine?'* as they swoon like a dying man in the streets

---

sense, restrained Himself until then].

9. טָבְעוּ בָאָרֶץ שְׁעָרֶיהָ — *Her gates have sunk into the earth.* According to the *Midrash* the gates sunk into the ground [i.e., miraculously, and were not destroyed by the enemy], because when Solomon brought the אֲרוֹן הַבְּרִית, *Ark of the Covenant,* into Jerusalem, the gates paid honor to the Ark by rising to allow the Ark to enter [*Shabbos* 30a]. *Rashi* adds that the gates were invulnerable to the enemy because they were the handiwork of King David [*Sotah* 9a].

Minchas Shay explains that the ט, *Tes,* of טָבְעוּ, *sunk,* is small to allude to ט, *the Ninth,* of Av when the Temple was destroyed.

אֵין תּוֹרָה — *There is no Torah,* i.e., no one to provide religious instruction (*Rashi*). [All the most important people — king, princes, priests — in whose hands lay the religious administration of the country are either gone or not functioning.]

Most commentators and the *Midrash* attach this clause to the preceding and translate: *Her king and her officers are among the heathen where there is no Torah.* Hence, the *Midrash* concludes: Should a person tell you there is חָכְמָה, *wisdom,* among the nations, believe it; but if he tells you there is Torah among the nations, do not believe it.

10. In this verse, the prophet depicts the elders — who no longer have a worldly occupation to keep them occupied, and who have suffered and endured so much — mourning for Zion. They

have no words, no prayers, only silent resignation. Note also the poetic contrast between the זְקֵנִים, *elders,* and בְּתוּלוֹת, *maidens,* as depicting the extremes of the population spectrum (*Kol Yaakov; Lechem Dim'ah*).

יֵשְׁבוּ לָאָרֶץ יִדְּמוּ — *Sit on the ground in silence.* [The Biblical classic form of mourning includes strewing dust on the head, wearing sackcloth, and bowing the head.]

This verse is cited as a basis for the halachic custom of sitting on the ground on *Tishah B'Av.* The 12th-century *Sefer HaEshkol* says: After the final meal, we go to the synagogue without shoes and sit on the ground, as it is written: *sit on the ground in silence.*

11. [In a personal interjection of special grief, the prophet laments the tragic sight of children languishing from hunger in the streets.]

12. לְאִמֹּתָם יֹאמְרוּ — *They* [i.e., the swooning children mentioned in the last verse] *say to their mothers.*

אַיֵּה דָּגָן וָיָיִן — *Where is bread* [lit., *grain*] *and wine?* (The translation 'bread' follows the *Midrash.*)

It is obvious that fine bread and good wine were not available during the siege, and the verse could not be suggesting that the children seriously expected to receive these foods during the famine; the children would have been satisfied with any morsels of food to still their hunger pangs. Rather, as they swooned from hunger,

עִ֗יר בְּהִשְׁתַּפֵּ֤ךְ נַפְשָׁם֙ אֶל־חֵ֣יק אִמֹּתָֽם: יג מָֽה־אֲעִידֵ֞ךְ מָ֣ה אֲדַמֶּה־
לָּ֗ךְ הַבַּת֙ יְר֣וּשָׁלִַ֔ם מָ֤ה אַשְׁוֶה־לָּךְ֙ וַאֲנַֽחֲמֵ֔ךְ* בְּתוּלַ֖ת בַּת־צִיּ֑וֹן
כִּֽי־גָד֥וֹל כַּיָּ֛ם שִׁבְרֵ֖ךְ מִ֥י יִרְפָּא־לָֽךְ: יד נְבִיאַ֗יִךְ* חָ֤זוּ לָךְ֙ שָׁ֣וְא וְתָפֵ֔ל
וְלֹֽא־גִלּ֥וּ עַל־עֲוֺנֵ֖ךְ לְהָשִׁ֣יב שְׁבוּתֵ֑ךְ* וַיֶּ֣חֱזוּ לָ֔ךְ מַשְׂא֥וֹת שָׁ֖וְא
וּמַדּוּחִֽם: טו סָֽפְק֨וּ עָלַ֤יִךְ כַּפַּ֙יִם֙ כָּל־עֹ֣בְרֵי דֶ֔רֶךְ שָֽׁרְקוּ֙ וַיָּנִ֣עוּ רֹאשָׁ֔ם*
עַל־בַּ֖ת יְרוּשָׁלָ֑͏ִם הֲזֹ֣את הָעִ֗יר* שֶׁיֹּֽאמְרוּ֙ כְּלִ֣ילַת יֹ֔פִי מָשׂ֖וֹשׂ
לְכָל־הָאָֽרֶץ: טז פָּצ֨וּ* עָלַ֤יִךְ פִּיהֶם֙ כָּל־אֹ֣יְבַ֔יִךְ שָֽׁרְקוּ֙ וַיַּֽחַרְקוּ־שֵׁ֔ן
אָֽמְר֖וּ בִּלָּ֑עְנוּ אַ֣ךְ זֶ֥ה הַיּ֛וֹם שֶׁקִּוִּינֻ֖הוּ מָצָ֥אנוּ רָאִֽינוּ:* יז עָשָׂ֨ה יְהֹוָ֜ה
אֲשֶׁ֣ר זָמָ֗ם בִּצַּ֤ע אֶמְרָתוֹ֙ אֲשֶׁ֣ר צִוָּ֣ה מִֽימֵי־קֶ֔דֶם* הָרַ֖ס וְלֹ֣א חָמָ֑ל
וַיְשַׂמַּ֤ח עָלַ֙יִךְ֙ אוֹיֵ֔ב* הֵרִ֖ים קֶ֥רֶן צָרָֽיִךְ: יח צָעַ֥ק לִבָּ֖ם אֶל־אֲדֹנָ֑י
חוֹמַ֣ת בַּת־צִ֠יּוֹן הוֹרִ֨ידִי כַנַּ֤חַל דִּמְעָה֙ יוֹמָ֣ם וָלַ֔יְלָה אַֽל־תִּתְּנִ֤י פוּגַת֙
לָ֔ךְ אַל־תִּדֹּ֖ם בַּת־עֵינֵֽךְ:* יט ק֣וּמִי ׀ רֹ֣נִּי בליל֗ה* לְרֹאשׁ֙ אַשְׁמֻר֔וֹת*
שִׁפְכִ֤י כַמַּ֙יִם֙ לִבֵּ֔ךְ* נֹ֖כַח פְּנֵ֣י אֲדֹנָ֑י שְׂאִ֧י אֵלָ֣יו כַּפַּ֗יִךְ עַל־נֶ֙פֶשׁ֙

°מָה־אֲעוֹדֵךְ כ'   °שְׁבִיתֵךְ כ'   °בְּלִיל כ'

---

they beseeched their mothers, remembering their past comforts, and saying, 'What happened to the fine food which you used to feed us?' (Lechem Dim'ah).

13. מָֽה־אֲעִידֵךְ מָה אֲדַמֶּה־לָּךְ — *With what shall I bear witness for you? To what can I compare you?* I.e., what instance can I cite of any other nation that suffered a calamity equal to yours? (*Zohar; Alshich*).

The *Midrash*, interpreting the verb אֲעִידֵךְ, *witness*, by its other meaning, *warn*, translates: [God said:] How many prophets did I send to *warn* you [of the consequences of your evil ways]? I.e., what more could I have done for you? (*Torah Temimah*).

מָה אַשְׁוֶה־לָּךְ וַאֲנַחֲמֵךְ — *To what can I liken you to comfort you?* I.e., whose suffering and circumstances can be likened to yours, so that you can be comforted by the comparison? (*Lechem Dim'ah*).

Human nature is such that in times of trouble one finds comfort in hearing of others who experienced similar tribulations (*Rashi*) (II:12).

14. נְבִיאַיִךְ — *Your prophets,* i.e., those prophets — whom you believed to have the most spiritual and moral insight — prophesied falsely, and whitewashed your iniquities, soothing you into self-righteousness by indulging in deceptive oracles (*Rav Arama*).

Alshich concludes: Not only did your prophets not reprimand you for your transgressions — they actually led you astray from God with their vain and deceptive prophecies. Indeed, who can heal such a nation? And if you expect to derive comfort from passersby who see your

suffering and commiserate with you, you are sadly mistaken . . . [see *Alshich* next verse].

15. סָפְקוּ עָלַיִךְ כַּפַּיִם . . . שָׁרְקוּ וַיָּנִעוּ רֹאשָׁם — *Clap hands at you; they hiss and wag their head* — upon witnessing your disaster (*Kiflayim L'Sushiyah*).

. . .In mock and derision, not over your loss, Jerusalem, but for themselves, as the Sages proclaimed: Had the heathens known how much they would lose by destroying the Temple, they would not have done it. The Divine blessing that had rested upon the entire world left with the Destruction (*Alshich*).

[*Rashi* implies that this verse refers to a sincere manifestation of grief which one naturally expresses upon seeing such a precipitous decline in someone who was once great. Perhaps, in this light, we can differentiate between this verse and the next. In this verse the prophet laments the fact that Zion's state is so lamentable that *all* neutral *passersby* will be sincerely moved to commiserate at the great loss. The next verse, however, speaks of the confirmed אוֹיֵב, *enemy*, who jeers and gnashes his teeth, openly displaying *joy* at her present condition.]

הֲזֹאת הָעִיר — *Could this be the city. . .?* [This is what the passersby are moved to say, remembering her past glory, and seeing her in her present state of destruction.]

16. פָּצוּ — *(They) jeered.* [*Lamentations* is written in the form of an alphabetical acrostic, but in this chapter, and also in chapters 3 and 4, the verse beginning with פ precedes that of ע. The name of the letter פ means *mouth*; the name of the letter ע

of the town; as their soul ebbs away in their mothers' laps. [13] *With what shall I bear witness for you? To what can I compare you,* O daughter of Jerusalem? To what can I liken you to comfort you,* O maiden daughter of Zion? — Your ruin is as vast as the sea; who can heal you?* [14] *Your prophets* envisioned for you vanity and foolishness, and they did not expose your iniquity to bring you back in repentance; they prophesied to you oracles of vanity and deception.* [15] *All who pass along the way clap hands at you; they hiss and wag their head* at the daughter of Jerusalem: 'Could this be the city* that was called Perfect in Beauty, Joy of All the Earth?'* [16] *All your enemies jeered* at you; they hiss and gnash their teeth. They say: 'We have devoured her! Indeed, this is the day we longed for; we have actually seen it!'** [17] *HASHEM has done what He planned;* He carried out His decree which He ordained long ago;* He devastated without pity. He let the enemy rejoice over you;* He raised the pride of your foes.* [18] *Their heart cried out to the Lord. O wall of the daughter of Zion: Shed tears like a river, day and night; give yourself no respite, do not let your eyes be still.** [19] *Arise, cry out at night* in the beginning of the watches!* Pour out your heart like water* in the Presence of the Lord; lift up your hands to Him for the life of*

---

means eye.] Rashi notes: Why did he place the פ before the ע? Because they [i.e., the Spies — (Sanhedrin 104b; see also comm. to 1:2)] spoke with their mouths what they had not seen with their eyes [thus putting one before the other].

According to *Lechem Dim'ah*, Rashi is referring [not to the Spies as in *Sanhedrin*, 104b, but] to the enemies who cast diatribes at Israel long before the actual Destruction took place. Hence, the sequence of the verses: First, צָצַף, *All your enemies jeered at you,* then, עָשָׂה ה' . . . הָרַס, *HASHEM has done. . .has devasted.*

מָצָאנוּ רָאִינוּ — *We have actually seen it* [lit., *we have found, we have seen*]. The *Arizal* explains that the enemy had hoped for the day when they could burn the Temple themselves. They were disappointed because *'we found, we saw,'* i.e., they found that God had already sent down the fire that burned the Temple [see commentary 1:13].

17. עָשָׂה ה' אֲשֶׁר זָמָם — *HASHEM has done what He planned.*

Although most human plans are never executed, God's resolve was carried through in its entirety (*Lechem Dim'ah*).

אֲשֶׁר צִוָּה מִימֵי־קֶדֶם — *Which He ordained long ago* [lit. *which He commanded from ancient days*]. According to *Rashi* this refers to the warnings in the Torah of the dire results of disobedience (e.g., *Leviticus* 26:27).

וַיְשַׂמַּח עָלַיִךְ אוֹיֵב — *He let the enemy rejoice over you.* God Himself rejoices with Israel when good befalls them; but when anything bad befalls them, He lets others do the rejoicing (*Midrash*).

18. אַל־תִּתְּנִי פוּגַת לָךְ אַל־תִּדֹּם בַּת־עֵינֵךְ — *Give*

yourself no respite, do not let your eyes [lit., *pupils*] *be still.*

'The greatest sin of all is that we, in our time, stopped mourning properly for Jerusalem. I am convinced that, in punishment for this, our exile has lasted so long, we have never been able to find rest, and we are always being persecuted. Historically, whenever we found some security in any of the lands of our exile, we forgot Jerusalem and did not place it at the foremost place in our minds' (*Rav Yaakov Emden*).

19. [This verse is a continuation of the last, in which the prophet exhorts the sufferers to pray unrestrainedly to God].

בַּלַּיְלָה — *At night.* [See Commentary on 1:2.]

Midrash Lekach Tov comments that *night* refers to the night of *Tishah B'Av* which should be observed annually as an eve of weeping and lamentation.

The כְּתִיב, *written form,* of the *night* is לֵיל, and refers to the earlier part of the evening, which is the רֹאשׁ אַשְׁמֻרוֹת, *beginning of the first two watches,* and is the most effective time (*Lechem Dim'ah*).

לְרֹאשׁ אַשְׁמֻרוֹת — *In the beginning of the watches,* the night being divided into three equal *watches* (*Rashi*).

שִׁפְכִי כַמַּיִם לִבֵּךְ נֹכַח פְּנֵי ה' — *Pour out your heart like water in the Presence of the Lord.* And confess your guilt (*Ibn Yachya*).

Wherever *Hashem's* name appears as אֲדֹנָי, it refers to the *Shechinah*. Therefore, first *pour out your heart* like water at the 'departure' of the *Shechinah*, and then pray for the *life of your infants,* i.e., for your own needs (*Lechem Dim'ah*).

עוֹלָלַיִךְ* הָעֲטוּפִים בְּרָעָב בְּרֹאשׁ כָּל־חוּצוֹת: כִּרְאֵה יהוה
וְהַבִּיטָה לְמִי עוֹלַלְתָּ כֹּה אִם־תֹּאכַלְנָה נָשִׁים פִּרְיָם* עֹלְלֵי
טִפֻּחִים* אִם־יֵהָרֵג בְּמִקְדַּשׁ אֲדֹנָי כֹּהֵן וְנָבִיא: כא שָׁכְבוּ לָאָרֶץ
חוּצוֹת נַעַר וְזָקֵן בְּתוּלֹתַי וּבַחוּרַי נָפְלוּ בֶחָרֶב הָרַגְתָּ בְּיוֹם
אַפֶּךָ טָבַחְתָּ לֹא חָמָלְתָּ: כב תִּקְרָא כְיוֹם מוֹעֵד* מְגוּרַי מִסָּבִיב
וְלֹא הָיָה בְּיוֹם אַף־יהוה פָּלִיט וְשָׂרִיד אֲשֶׁר־טִפַּחְתִּי וְרִבִּיתִי
אֹיְבִי כִלָּם:

פרק שלישי

א אֲנִי הַגֶּבֶר* רָאָה עֳנִי בְּשֵׁבֶט עֶבְרָתוֹ: ב אוֹתִי נָהַג וַיֹּלַךְ חֹשֶׁךְ
וְלֹא־אוֹר: ג אַךְ בִּי יָשֻׁב יַהֲפֹךְ יָדוֹ* כָּל־הַיּוֹם: ד בִּלָּה בְשָׂרִי
וְעוֹרִי* שִׁבַּר עַצְמוֹתָי: ה בָּנָה עָלַי וַיַּקַּף רֹאשׁ וּתְלָאָה: ו בְּמַחֲשַׁכִּים
הוֹשִׁיבַנִי כְּמֵתֵי עוֹלָם: ז גָּדַר בַּעֲדִי* וְלֹא אֵצֵא הִכְבִּיד נְחָשְׁתִּי:
ח גַּם כִּי אֶזְעַק וַאֲשַׁוֵּעַ* שָׂתַם תְּפִלָּתִי:* ט גָּדַר דְּרָכַי בְּגָזִית

Since the שַׁעֲרֵי דְמָעוֹת, *gates of weeping*, were never closed [*Berachos* 32b], the prophet assured them that sincere weeping would reach פְּנֵי ה׳, the *Presence of the Lord* (*Yismach Moshe*).

עַל־נֶפֶשׁ עוֹלָלָיִךְ — *For the life* [lit., *soul*] *of your young children.* Most commentators understand 'children' literally, referring to the starving children in verses 11 and 12. *Midrash Lekach Tov* seems to understand it as the swooning children [i.e., citizens] of personified Jerusalem — who had been exiled בְּרֹאשׁ כָּל־חוּצוֹת, in foreign heathen countries [בְּחוּץ לָאָרֶץ] throughout the world.

Lechem Dim'ah interprets the verse: *Pour out your heart like water in the Presence of the Lord,* and if that is ineffective because your merits are insufficient, then *lift up your hands to Him as if you were praying for the life of your innocent infants who swoon* etc.

20. [In this verse, the thoughts of the prophet revert to Hashem.]

אִם־תֹּאכַלְנָה נָשִׁים פִּרְיָם — *Should women eat their own offspring?* An incredulous question: Has it ever happened to any other nation that their afflictions should result in the ghastly extreme of mothers eating their own offspring, עֹלְלֵי טִפֻּחִים, *babes of their care* — whom they previously fondled and cared for like all compassionate mothers? Is such a thing right? (*Alshich; Palgei Mayim*).

Wouldn't it have been sufficient to let them die from starvation without having their mothers eat them? (*Ibn Yachya*).

[Apparently, not only mothers were reduced to such a state of cruelty:] Rav Yochanan said: Fathers, too, ate the flesh of their sons and

daughters at the Destruction of both the First and Second Temples. Jeremiah lamented this horror by crying, '*Therefore shall fathers eat the sons in your midst, and the sons shall eat their fathers*' [*Ezek.* 5:10] (*Pesikta Rabbasi*).

עֹלְלֵי טִפֻּחִים — *Babes of their care,* i.e., objects of their fondling, caressing (*Ibn Ezra*).

The *Talmud* relates the incident of a child, Doeg ben Yosef, whose father died and he was left in his mother's care. Everyday she would lovingly measure him בְּטִפְחָה, *with her hand-breadth,* and give his [extra] weight in gold to the Temple. When the enemy prevailed, however, she slaughtered him and ate him. It was to her that Jeremiah referred when he lamented to God: *Shall women eat their own offspring,* עֹלְלֵי טִפֻּחִים, *the babes they measured by handbreadths.?* [A play on *tipuchim* — *of their care; fondled* — read as *tefuchim* — *measured by handbreadths* — as a sign of love, as in this story] (*Yoma* 38b; *Midrash; Rashi*).

21. הָרַגְתָּ בְּיוֹם אַפֶּךָ טָבַחְתָּ לֹא חָמָלְתָּ — *You slew them on the day of Your wrath; You slaughtered and showed no mercy.*

Had the Destruction come on a day other than *the day of Your wrath,* i.e., Tishah B'Av, it would have been tempered with mercy and restraint. Having come on the day You specifically set aside for display of Your anger, it was untempered and complete (*Lechem Dim'ah*).

22. כְיוֹם מוֹעֵד — *As though at festival time.* The enemy so swarmed over Jerusalem and the Temple that it was reminiscent of the throngs of Jewish pilgrims who used to swarm into Jerusalem on the festivals (*Ibn Shuib*).

your young children,* who swoon from hunger at every street corner.
²⁰ *Look, HASHEM, and behold, whom You have treated so. Should women
eat their own offspring,* the babes of their care?* Should priest and
prophet be slain in the Sanctuary of the Lord? ²¹ Out on the ground, in
the streets they lie, young and old; my maidens and my young men have
fallen by the sword. You slew them on the day of Your wrath; You
slaughtered them and showed no mercy.* ²² You invited, as though at
festival time,* my evil neighbors round about. So that, at the day of
HASHEM's wrath, there were none who survived or escaped. Those who
I cherished and brought up, my enemy has wiped out.*

CHAPTER THREE

¹ **I** *am the man* who has seen affliction by the rod of His anger. ² He
has driven me on and on into unrelieved darkness. ³ Only against
me* did He turn His hand repeatedly* all day long. ⁴ He has worn away
my flesh and skin;* He broke my bones. ⁵ He besieged and encircled me
with bitterness and travail. ⁶ He has placed me in darkness like the
eternally dead. ⁷ He has walled me in* so I cannot escape; He has
weighed me down with chains. ⁸ Though I would cry out and plead,* He
shut out my prayer.* ⁹ He has walled up my roads with hewn stones;*

CHAPTER THREE

1. אֲנִי הַגֶּבֶר — *I am the man.* Jeremiah, in a
personal statement, laments that he saw more
affliction than all the other prophets who
foretold the Destruction of the Temple. For it was
destroyed not in their days, but in his (*Rashi*). (It
had been noted that the numerical value of אֲנִי
הַגֶּבֶר, *I am the man* [=271], equals יִרְמְיָהוּ,
Jeremiah [*Tzfunos Yisrael*]).

[Chapter 3 is composed of a triple acrostic. It is
written in the form of three-verse units, each
verse beginning with the same letter.]

2. [In the verses 2-16 the sufferer proceeds to
describe his suffering figuratively in a series of
more or less isolated pictures. The translation,
which already incorporates much of the exegesis
of the Sages, makes the verses, for the most part,
readily understandable. The commentary, in this
chapter, has therefore been intended mainly to
remove surface difficulties.]

3. אַךְ בִּי — *Only against me* — i.e., I alone am the
constant recipient of His punishment (*Rashi*).

Sifsei Chachamim personifies the phrase as
referring specifically to Jeremiah: *On no prophet
but me* [see comm. 3:1].

All nations sin but toward no other nation is
God so zealous in exacting retribution as toward
Israel (*Rav Yosef Kara*).

יָשֻׁב יַהֲפֹךְ יָדוֹ — *Turn His hand repeatedly.* In
punishment, anthropomorphically, as if — so to
speak — He wants the punishment to be
constant; when one hand 'tires,' He uses the other
(*Toras Chesed*).

Alshich translates: He removed His compas-

sionate hand [i.e., His protection] from me.

4. [The verse speaks of man's total physical
suffering:]

בִּלָּה בְשָׂרִי וְעוֹרִי — *He has worn away my flesh
and skin.* The flesh and skin — which are
sensitive to pain — He wore away. The bones —
which have no tactile sensation — He crushed
(*Ibn Ezra*).

7. גָּדַר בַּעֲדִי — *He has walled* [lit., hedged] *me in.*
The prophet alludes to our long exile. God has, in
effect, walled us in — so that the dark exile
imprisons us. The verses continue that he
weighed us down with oppression and closed the
door to our prayers (*Lechem Dim'ah*).

8. גַּם כִּי אֶזְעַק וַאֲשַׁוֵּעַ — *Though I would cry out
and plead.* Rav Eliezer said: From the day the
Temple was destroyed, the gates of prayer
have been shut, as it is written: *Though I would
cry out and plead, He shut out my prayer*
(*Berachos* 32b).

This refers to insincere private prayer; public
prayer or sincere private prayer is always accepted (*Torah Temimah*).

שָׂתַם תְּפִלָּתִי — *He shut out my prayer* by closing
the 'windows' of Heaven (*Rashi*); and by placing
an 'iron barrier' between Him and Israel (*Mik-
dash Lechak Tov*).

The *Midrash* notes that prayers said with a
congregation are more acceptable than those said
alone or after the congregation has finished.
[This is suggested by the fact that the word
תְּפִלָּתִי, my *prayer*, is in the singular; this
indicating that, had a quorum prayed, their
supplication would have been heard (*Torah*

נְתִיבֹתַי עִוָּה: יֹדֹב אֹרֵב הוּא לִי* °אֲרִי בְּמִסְתָּרִים: יֹא דְּרָכַי סוֹרֵר
וַיְפַשְּׁחֵנִי שָׂמַנִי שֹׁמֵם: יֹב דָּרַךְ קַשְׁתוֹ וַיַּצִּיבֵנִי* כַּמַּטָּרָא לַחֵץ:
יֹג הֵבִיא בְּכִלְיֹתָי בְּנֵי אַשְׁפָּתוֹ:* יֹד הָיִיתִי שְּׂחֹק לְכָל־עַמִּי* נְגִינָתָם
כָּל־הַיּוֹם:* טֹו הִשְׂבִּיעַנִי בַמְּרוֹרִים הִרְוַנִי לַעֲנָה: טֹז וַיַּגְרֵס בֶּחָצָץ
שִׁנָּי הִכְפִּישַׁנִי בָּאֵפֶר:* יֹז וַתִּזְנַח מִשָּׁלוֹם נַפְשִׁי נָשִׁיתִי טוֹבָה:
יֹח וָאֹמַר אָבַד נִצְחִי וְתוֹחַלְתִּי מֵיהוה: יֹט זְכָר־עָנְיִי וּמְרוּדִי לַעֲנָה
וָרֹאשׁ: כֹ זָכוֹר תִּזְכּוֹר* °וְתָשׁוֹחַ עָלַי נַפְשִׁי: כֹא זֹאת אָשִׁיב אֶל־לִבִּי*
עַל־כֵּן אוֹחִיל: כֹב חַסְדֵי יהוה כִּי לֹא־תָמְנוּ* כִּי לֹא־כָלוּ רַחֲמָיו:
כֹג חֲדָשִׁים לַבְּקָרִים* רַבָּה אֱמוּנָתֶךָ:* כֹד חֶלְקִי יהוה אָמְרָה נַפְשִׁי
עַל־כֵּן אוֹחִיל לוֹ: כֹה טוֹב יהוה לְקֹוָו לְנֶפֶשׁ תִּדְרְשֶׁנּוּ: כֹו טוֹב וְיָחִיל
וְדוּמָם לִתְשׁוּעַת יהוה: כֹז טוֹב לַגֶּבֶר כִּי־יִשָּׂא עֹל בִּנְעוּרָיו: כֹח יֵשֵׁב
בָּדָד וְיִדֹּם כִּי נָטַל עָלָיו: כֹט יִתֵּן בֶּעָפָר פִּיהוּ אוּלַי יֵשׁ תִּקְוָה:

<hr>

°אריה כ'   °ותשיח כ'

Temimah).] If ten righteous men pray and a wicked person joins them, would Hashem say, 'I refuse to hear their prayers because of this single wicked person'? But if a person comes after the congregation is finished, and stands alone in prayer, his every deed and thought is scrutinized.

10. דֹב אֹרֵב הוּא לִי — *He is a lurking bear to me.* [The verse does not make it clear who is referred to: God; or His delegate — the enemy.]

According to *Rashi*, the subject is the Holy One, Blessed is He, Who has become like a lurking bear.

The *Midrash* however, interprets *bear* as referring to Nebuchadnezzar or, prophetically, to Vespasian. *Lion* refers to Nebuzaradan [the general who made the final attack during the First Destruction], or to Trajan [the conquering general during the Second Destruction].

According to many commentators (*Alshich; Ibn Yachya; Kol Yehudah*), the verse refers to the enemy who lay in hiding ready to pounce upon Israel without warning.

12. דָּרַךְ קַשְׁתוֹ וַיַּצִּיבֵנִי — *He bent his bow and set me up. Lechem Dim'ah* notes that the order is reversed. Usually one first sets up his target and then takes aim. The verse implies the enemy kept him in constant terror by keeping his bow bent and aimed at him.

[Being 'walled in without escape' and 'weighed down with chains' as described in verses 7-9, he was certainly an easy target!]

14. הָיִיתִי שְּׂחֹק לְכָל־עַמִּי — *I have become a laughingstock to all my people* [i.e., an object of derision]. עַמִּי, *my people*, is explained as: The people in whose midst I dwell (*Lechem Dim'ah*).

The *Targum* translates: פְּרִיצֵי, *the impudent* (*scorners*) *of my nation.*

The *Midrash* explains this as referring to 'the nations of the world who sit in theaters and circuses. After they eat and drink and become intoxicated, they sit and discuss me, scoffing at me.'

According to *Palgei Mayim*, Jeremiah is lamenting how, whenever he prophesied oracles of reproof and impending disaster, the Jews would laugh and taunt him. Because of their inattentiveness to his prophecies, disaster fell.

נְגִינָתָם כָּל־הַיּוֹם — *Their jibes* [lit., *songs*] *all day long* [i.e., I became the theme of their satirical songs].

15. The *Midrash*, linking בַמְּרוֹרִים, *bitterness*, with מָרוֹר, *the bitter herbs*, eaten at the Passover *Seder*, notes that the night of the week on which the first day of Passover occurs is always the same as the night on which Tishah B'Av falls.

16. הִכְפִּישַׁנִי בָּאֵפֶר — *He made me cower in ashes,* i.e., He covered me with ashes (*Rashi*).

The *Talmud* relates that on the eve of Tishah B'Av, after Rav would complete his regular meal, he would dip a morsel of bread into ashes and say, 'This is the essence of the Erev Tishah B'Av meal, in fulfillment of the verse:. . .*He made me cower in ashes*' (*Yerushalmi Taanis 4:6*).

20. The *Midrash* translates: זָכוֹר תִּזְכּוֹר, *You will surely remember* [O God,] the nations of the world and will punish them for oppressing me, but while waiting for the vengeance, תָשׁוֹחַ עָלַי נַפְשִׁי, *my soul is despondent* [i.e., I haven't the patience to wait any longer]. A proverb declares: While the fat one grows lean, the lean one expires.

He tangled up my paths. [10] *He is a lurking bear to me,* a lion in hiding.* [11] *He has strewn my paths with thorns and made me tread carefully; He made me desolate.* [12] *He bent his bow and set me up* as a target for the arrow.* [13] *He shot into my vitals the arrows of His quiver.* [14] *I have become a laughingstock to all my people;* object of their jibes all day long.* [15] *He filled me with bitterness, sated me with wormwood.* [16] *He ground my teeth on gravel, He made me cower in ashes.* [17] *My soul despaired of having peace, I have forgotten goodness.* [18] *And I said, 'Gone is my strength and my expectation from* HASHEM.' [19] *Remember my afflictions and my sorrow; the wormwood and bitterness.* [20] *My soul remembers well — and makes me despondent.* [21] *Yet, this I bear in mind;* therefore I still hope:* [22] HASHEM's *kindness surely has not ended,* nor are His mercies exhausted.* [23] *They are new every morning;* great is Your faithfulness!* [24] '*HASHEM is my portion,' says my soul, therefore I have hope in Him.* [25] HASHEM *is good to those who trust in Him;* to the soul that seeks Him.* [26] *It is good to hope submissively for* HASHEM's *salvation, for He has laid it upon him.* [27] *It is good for a man that he bear a yoke in his youth.* [28] *Let one sit in solitude and he submissive, for He has laid it upon him.* [29] *Let him put his mouth to the dust — there may yet be hope.**

---

21. וזאת אָשִׁיב אֶל־לִבִּי — [Yet,] *this I bear in mind.* After my heart told me that it *'lost its expectation from* HASHEM' [verse 18], I bore this in mind and thus restored my faith (*Rashi*).

[Verses 19-21 represent the transition from the despair (which culminates in verse 18) and the doctrine of hope which is achieved by recalling God's mercy in verses 22-38.]

In the time to come when the era of redemption arrives, God will say to Israel, 'My sons, I wonder how you waited for Me all these years.' And they will answer, 'Lord of the universe, had it not been for Your Torah which You gave us, the heathen peoples would long ago have caused us to perish.'

Therefore, it is stated: וזאת אָשִׁיב אֶל־לִבִּי, *this I bear in mind,* and וזאת, *this,* indicates nothing else than the Torah, as it is said וְזֹאת הַתּוֹרָה, *And this is the Torah* [*Deut.* 4:44] (*Midrash*).

22. [This verse begins the expression of faith and hope alluded to in the previous verse and continues through verse 38.]

חַסְדֵי ה' כִּי לֹא־תָמְנוּ — HASHEM's *kindness surely has not ended* [i.e., is inexhaustible]. *Rashi,* whose translation we followed, gives an alternate translation: חַסְדֵי ה', *it is due to* HASHEM's *kindness,* כִּי לֹא־תָמְנוּ, *that we were not annihilated for our transgressions,* כִּי לֹא־כָלוּ רַחֲמָיו — *because His mercies are not exhausted* [see *Numbers* 17-28].

23. חֲדָשִׁים לַבְּקָרִים — *They are new every morning* [i.e., Your kindnesses are renewed from day to day (*Rashi*)]. *Alshich* interprets the subject of this verse as the soul of man: *God renews man's life every morning, and I have faith that He will continue to do so in the future and redeem us.*

The *Talmud* interprets esoterically that each day God creates a band of new angels who utter a song before Him and then pass away (*Chagigah* 14a).

רַבָּה אֱמוּנָתֶךָ — *Great is your faithfulness,* i.e., great is Your promise; and it is great to believe in Your fulfilling and guarding whatever You promised (*Rashi*).

One earns great merit by believing in You (*Lechem Dim'ah*).

25. טוֹב ה' לְקֹוָו — HASHEM *is good to those who trust in Him.* The *Midrash* cites an apparent contradiction between this verse and the verse in *Psalms* 145:9 stating that Hashem is good to all, not only to those who trust in Him. The *Midrash* explains with a parable: When one waters his orchard, he waters all of it. When one hoes, however, he hoes only the better plants. [So, too, in normal times, God provides for everyone equally, but in a time of punishment and destruction, only those who hope in Him are worthy of individual intervention (*Torah Temimah*).]

26⁻27. Since we are certain that God will not eternally neglect us, the prudent thing to do is to accept God's afflictions submissively, in quiet resignation, and silently anticipate God's ultimate salvation. As for the suffering he inflicts upon us in the interim... *It is better to bear the yoke in one's youth* — while one is young and has the vigor to withstand the tribulations, rather than when old and lacking the stamina (*Alshich*).

29. אוּלַי יֵשׁ תִּקְוָה — *There may yet be hope* — that God will forgive him (*Alshich*).

When Rabbi [the compiler of the *Mishnah*] reached these verses [29-31], he wept (*Midrash*),

ל יִתֵּן לְמַכֵּהוּ לֶחִי יִשְׂבַּע בְּחֶרְפָּה:* לא כִּי לֹא יִזְנַח לְעוֹלָם אֲדֹנָי:*
לב כִּי אִם־הוֹגָה וְרִחַם כְּרֹב חֲסָדָו: לג כִּי לֹא עִנָּה מִלִּבּוֹ* וַיַּגֶּה
בְנֵי־אִישׁ: לד לְדַכֵּא תַּחַת רַגְלָיו כֹּל אֲסִירֵי אָרֶץ:* לה לְהַטּוֹת
מִשְׁפַּט־גָּבֶר* נֶגֶד פְּנֵי עֶלְיוֹן: לו לְעַוֵּת אָדָם בְּרִיבוֹ אֲדֹנָי לֹא רָאָה:
לז מִי זֶה אָמַר וַתֶּהִי אֲדֹנָי לֹא צִוָּה: לח מִפִּי עֶלְיוֹן לֹא תֵצֵא הָרָעוֹת
וְהַטּוֹב:* לט מַה־יִּתְאוֹנֵן אָדָם חָי גֶּבֶר עַל־חֲטָאָו:* מ נַחְפְּשָׂה
דְרָכֵינוּ וְנַחְקֹרָה וְנָשׁוּבָה עַד־יהוה:* מא נִשָּׂא לְבָבֵנוּ אֶל־כַּפָּיִם*
אֶל־אֵל בַּשָּׁמָיִם: מב נַחְנוּ פָשַׁעְנוּ* וּמָרִינוּ אַתָּה לֹא סָלָחְתָּ:
מג סַכֹּתָה בָאַף וַתִּרְדְּפֵנוּ הָרַגְתָּ לֹא חָמָלְתָּ: מד סַכֹּתָה בֶעָנָן לָךְ
מֵעֲבוֹר תְּפִלָּה:* מה סְחִי וּמָאוֹס תְּשִׂימֵנוּ בְּקֶרֶב הָעַמִּים: מו פָּצוּ
עָלֵינוּ פִּיהֶם* כָּל־אֹיְבֵינוּ: מז פַּחַד וָפַחַת הָיָה לָנוּ הַשֵּׁאת וְהַשָּׁבֶר:

because even after all the indignities which were heaped upon Israel, the prophet still said אוּלַי, *perhaps,* as if hope was still doubtful (*Torah Temimah*).

31. [In the last several verses, the prophet exhorted man to completely debase himself in resignation before God. Now, he justifies his advice by extolling the compassion of God.]

כִּי לֹא יִזְנַח לְעוֹלָם ה' — *For the Lord does not reject forever,* [i.e., His anger is of limited duration] and it is therefore good to be submissive [silent] (*Rashi*).

God waits for man to repent (*Alshich*).

33. כִּי לֹא עִנָּה מִלִּבּוֹ — *For He does not torment capriciously,* i.e., He has no desire to punish capriciously; everything is in retribution for one's sins (*Rashi; Alshich*).

34. כֹּל אֲסִירֵי אָרֶץ — *All the prisoners of the earth.* This phrase is a poetic description referring to all mankind. Are we not all *prisoners on God's earth* with no way to escape His providence? (*Alshich*).

35. לְהַטּוֹת מִשְׁפַּט־גָּבֶר — *Nor deny a man justice.* According to *Rashi,* this verse, too, continues the theme begun in verse 33, enumerating what Hashem does not capriciously do or allow.

37-40. *Rashi* groups together three verses and explains: One should never ascribe his suffering to chance, because from whom else but from God does good and evil emanate? Therefore, why should a man complain? Let everyone put the blame on his own sins! — and [verse 40] search his ways and repent.

הָרָעוֹת וְהַטּוֹב — *Evil and good. Palgei Mayim,* in contrast to *Rashi,* takes this phrase as a statement and explains that although everything *does* emanate from God, the choice of man's actions — good or bad — is not Divine, but human...

Thus, the *Rambam* [in his *Hilchos Teshuvah* and *Eight Chapters*] writes that man is mistaken in ascribing to God his evil ways — as if they were Divinely forced upon him. When justice is meted out to him, why should someone complain that he was coerced? גֶּבֶר עַל־חֲטָאָו, he is a *strong man* over his sins! Let him conquer his evil ways! Where there is knowledge of God there is free choice.

מַה־יִּתְאוֹנֵן אָדָם חַי גֶּבֶר עַל־חֲטָאָו — *Of what shall a living man complain? A strong man for his sins!* Let him be thankful that he is alive! Rav Levi said: The Holy One, Blessed is He, declared: Your existence is in My hand, and, being alive, you complain! Rav Huna said: Let him stand up like a brave man, acknowledge his sins, and not complain. Rav Berachiah explained the verse: Why does man complain against Him who lives eternally? If a man wishes to complain, let it be about his own sins! (*Midrash*).

This כְּתִיב, *written form,* is חֶטְאוֹ, *his sin* [in the singular], while the קְרִי, *reading,* is חֲטָאָיו, *his sins. Shaar Bas Rabim* points out that someone should be particularly concerned about his *first* sin. He dare not overlook it, or take it lightly, because עֲבֵירָה גּוֹרֶרֶת עֲבֵירָה, *one sin leads to another* (*Avos* 4:2), and his entire future might very well depend upon how he reacted to that first sin.

Similarly, *Rav Yonasan Eyebescheutz* points out that one should not overlook even a single transgression — however minor it appears — rather, *man should complain about every single sin.*

40. נַחְפְּשָׂה דְרָכֵינוּ וְנַחְקֹרָה — *Let us search and examine our ways.* This is the climax of the previous verses. Since man has only his own sins to blame for any misfortunes emanating from God, he should not grumble and recriminate. Instead, let us search our conduct to find the cause of our suffering — and

³⁰ *Let one offer his cheek to his smiter, let him be filled with disgrace.*
³¹ *— For the Lord does not reject forever;** ³² *He first afflicts, then pities
according to His abundant kindness.* ³³ *For He does not torment
capriciously, nor afflict man.* ³⁴ *Nor crush under His feet all the
prisoners of the earth;** ³⁵ *nor deny a man justice* in the presence of the
Most High.* ³⁶ *To wrong a man in his conflict — the Lord does not
approve.* ³⁷ *Whose decree was ever fulfilled unless the Lord ordained
it?* ³⁸ *It is not from the mouth of the Most High that evil and good*
emanate?* ³⁹ *Of what shall a living man complain? A strong man for his
sins!** ⁴⁰ *Let us search and examine our ways* and return to HASHEM.**
⁴¹ *Let us lift our hearts with our hands* to God in heaven:* ⁴² *We have
transgressed* and rebelled — You have not forgiven.* ⁴³ *You have
enveloped Yourself in anger and pursued us; You have slain mercilessly.* ⁴⁴ *You wrapped Yourself in a cloud that no prayer can pierce.**
⁴⁵ *You made us a filth and refuse among the nations.'* ⁴⁶ *All our
enemies jeered at us;** ⁴⁷ *panic and pitiful were ours, ravage and ruin.*

then repent (*Kiflayim LeSushiyah*).

As the *Talmud* advises: If a man sees that pain
and suffering visit him, let him examine his
conduct, as it says: *Let us examine our ways and
return to HASHEM* (*Berachos* 5a).

This verse is reminiscent of *Zephaniah* 1:12: *I
will search Jerusalem with candles.* One should
search his ways so that his repentance will reach
up to HASHEM — to His Throne of Glory
(*Midrash Lekach Tov*).

Rav Galanti elaborates that this soul-searching
must be accomplished in a manner similar to
meticulous searching with the light of a candle —
in every nook and crevice — as required when
searching for *chametz* before Passover. The
simile here refers to the soul which is likened to
light [נֵר ה׳ נִשְׁמַת אָדָם, *the light of God is the soul
of man*]. When one is guided by his soul and
conducts the search properly throughout every
nook and cranny of his being even in areas where
he least suspects it — he will inevitably discover
some *chametz*, the symbol of sin and improper
behavior. When he removes the *chametz*, his
repentance will surely reach '*up to HASHEM's
Throne of Glory.*'

וְנָשׁוּבָה עַד־ה׳ — *And return* [or: *and repent*]
to *HASHEM.* The *Midrash* and commentators
explain the use of the more forceful עַד, *until; up
to,* rather than the more direct אֶל, *to,* by quoting
the Talmudic dictum [*Yoma* 86b]: גְּדוֹלָה תְּשׁוּבָה
שֶׁמַּגַּעַת עַד כִּסֵּא הַכָּבוֹד, *Great is repentance for
it reaches* [עַד] *up to the Throne of Glory.* Thus,
the verse alludes to a concept often stressed
by our Sages: A repenter rises above the status
of a sinner who falls short of the ideal. Repentance raises one to the level of the most
righteous.

41. נִשָּׂא לְבָבֵנוּ אֶל־כַּפָּיִם — *Let us lift our hearts
with* [lit., *to*] *our hands.* The translation follows
the first of *Rashi's* two interpretations: When we

lift our hands [in prayer] to God, let us lift our
hearts along with him [i.e., in utmost sincerity]
broken-heartedly — before God.

Prayer is efficacious only when the external
lifting of the hands is accompanied by the
internal lifting of the heart (*Alshich*).

As the *Talmud* explains: A man's prayer is
answered only if he takes his heart in his hands
[i.e., is sincere] (*Taanis* 8a).

42. נַחְנוּ פָשַׁעְנוּ — *We have transgressed... You
have not forgiven,* i.e., in transgressing, *we* have
been true to *our* nature and Evil Inclination; but
You have not conformed to Your Merciful ways
— You did not forgive (*Midrash; Rashi; Alshich*).

Ibn Ezra views this verse as a separate lament:
We have transgressed — and did not repent.
Therefore, *You have not forgiven.*

44. סַכֹּתָה... מֵעֲבוֹר תְּפִלָּה — *You wrapped
Yourself in a cloud that no prayer can pierce.*

Cloud is used here allegorically, as if the cloud
formed a barrier between our prayers and
Hashem (*Ibn Ezra*).

The *Talmud* relates that Raba would not
proclaim a fast on a cloudy day because 'God
wrapped Himself *in a cloud that no prayer can
pierce*' (*Berachos* 32b).

46. [Verses 46-48 which begin with פ precede,
rather than follow, verses 49-51 which begin
with the earlier Hebrew letter ע. (See *comm.* to
2:16).]

פָּצוּ עָלֵינוּ פִּיהֶם — *(They) jeered at us.* Instead of
completely ignoring us — as one would normally
ignore *filth and refuse* — our enemies taunted
and jeered at us, giving us no peace; not even
allowing us to wallow, undisturbed, in our
misery (*Ibn Yachya*).

Ibn Ezra relates שַׁאת to שׁוֹאָה, *sudden catastrophe.*

מח פַּלְגֵי־מַיִם תֵּרַד עֵינִי* עַל־שֶׁבֶר בַּת־עַמִּי: מט עֵינִי נִגְּרָה וְלֹא
תִדְמֶה מֵאֵין הֲפֻגוֹת: נ עַד־יַשְׁקִיף וְיֵרֶא יהוה מִשָּׁמָיִם: נא עֵינִי
עוֹלְלָה לְנַפְשִׁי מִכֹּל בְּנוֹת עִירִי: נב צוֹד צָדוּנִי כַּצִּפּוֹר אֹיְבַי חִנָּם:
נג צָמְתוּ בַבּוֹר חַיָּי וַיַּדּוּ־אֶבֶן בִּי: נד צָפוּ־מַיִם עַל־רֹאשִׁי* אָמַרְתִּי
נִגְזָרְתִּי: נה קָרָאתִי שִׁמְךָ יהוה* מִבּוֹר תַּחְתִּיּוֹת: נו קוֹלִי שָׁמָעְתָּ
אַל־תַּעְלֵם אָזְנְךָ לְרַוְחָתִי לְשַׁוְעָתִי: נז קָרַבְתָּ בְּיוֹם אֶקְרָאֶךָ
אָמַרְתָּ אַל־תִּירָא:* נח רַבְתָּ אֲדֹנָי רִיבֵי נַפְשִׁי גָּאַלְתָּ חַיָּי:
נט רָאִיתָה יהוה עַוָּתָתִי שָׁפְטָה מִשְׁפָּטִי: ס רָאִיתָה כָּל־נִקְמָתָם
כָּל־מַחְשְׁבֹתָם לִי: סא שָׁמַעְתָּ חֶרְפָּתָם יהוה* כָּל־מַחְשְׁבֹתָם עָלָי:
סב שִׂפְתֵי קָמַי וְהֶגְיוֹנָם עָלַי כָּל־הַיּוֹם:* סג שִׁבְתָּם וְקִימָתָם הַבִּיטָה
אֲנִי מַנְגִּינָתָם: סד תָּשִׁיב לָהֶם גְּמוּל יהוה כְּמַעֲשֵׂה יְדֵיהֶם:*
סה תִּתֵּן לָהֶם מְגִנַּת־לֵב תַּאֲלָתְךָ לָהֶם: סו תִּרְדֹּף בְּאַף וְתַשְׁמִידֵם
מִתַּחַת שְׁמֵי יהוה:*

פרק רביעי

א אֵיכָה יוּעַם זָהָב* יִשְׁנֶא הַכֶּתֶם הַטּוֹב תִּשְׁתַּפֵּכְנָה אַבְנֵי־
קֹדֶשׁ בְּרֹאשׁ כָּל־חוּצוֹת: ב בְּנֵי צִיּוֹן הַיְקָרִים* הַמְסֻלָּאִים בַּפָּז
אֵיכָה נֶחְשְׁבוּ לְנִבְלֵי־חֶרֶשׂ מַעֲשֵׂה יְדֵי יוֹצֵר: ג גַּם־°תַּנִּים חָלְצוּ

°תנין כ'

---

48. פַּלְגֵי־מַיִם תֵּרַד עֵינִי — *My eye shed streams of water.* Eye is singular. If only one eye produces such streams of water, how much more so both eyes! (*Alshich*).

51. This is a personal lament of Jeremiah who was of an aristocratic, priestly family. He anguished that his weeping eye figuratively contorted his face and aggrieved his spirit more than any inhabitant of the city. His family was particularly affected, and suffered more than others because, as priests, they had been selected for holiness and the service of God (*Rashi*).

54. . . . צָפוּ־מַיִם עַל־רֹאשִׁי — *Waters flowed over my head; I thought: 'I am doomed!'* When a man is in water up to his hips, there is still hope, but when water — here allegorically referring to the heathen nations — flows *over* one's head, one gives up all hope. Rather, קָרָאתִי שִׁמְךָ ה׳, *I called on Your Name, HASHEM* (*Rashi*).

55־56. שִׁמְךָ ה׳ — *Your Name, HASHEM.* When one is in great anguish, drained of strength, he merely calls out the name of a passerby with such anguish that the hearer immediately discerns the gravity of the situation and responds. Here, too, he simply called God's Name hoping

that קוֹלִי שָׁמָעְתָּ, *You heard my voice,* and therefore אַל־תַּעְלֵם אָזְנְךָ לְרַוְחָתִי לְשַׁוְעָתִי, *You would not turn Your ear from my prayer for my relief when I cry out* (*Kiflayim LeSushiyah*).

As Jonah called upon You from inside the fish and from the depths of the sea, so does Israel call upon You from its exile among the nations — likened to the depths of a pit — to hear their prayers and deliver them (*Midrash Lekach Tov*).

57. אַל־תִּירָא — *Fear not!* [The utterance, *Do not be afraid!*, is a constant refrain throughout Scripture — and was said not only on segregated occasions but to virtually every one of the fathers of our people; it is a Divine promise that Israel need not fear. To mention several: *Fear not, Avram, I am your shield* (Gen. 15:1); *Fear not,* (Isaac) (Gen. 26:24); *Fear not,* (Jacob) *to go down to Egypt* (Gen. 46:3); *Fear him not,* (Moses). . . (Numbers 21:34); *Fear not,* (Children of Israel,) *nor be discouraged* (Deut. 1:21); *Fear not,* (Joshua,) *nor be dismayed* (Josh. 8:1); to Gideon (Judges 6:23); to Elijah (II Kings 1:15); to Hezekiah (II Kings 19:6); to Isaiah (Isaiah 7:4); to Jeremiah (Jeremiah 1:8); Servant Yaakov (Jeremiah 30:10); to Daniel (Daniel 10:12)].

⁴⁸ My eye shed streams of water* at the shattering of my people. ⁴⁹ My eye will flow and will not cease — without relief — ⁵⁰ until HASHEM looks down and takes notice from heaven. ⁵¹ My eyes have brought me grief over all the daughters of my city. ⁵² I have been constantly ensnared like a bird by my enemies without cause. ⁵³ They cut off my life in a pit and threw stones at me. ⁵⁴ Waters flowed over my head;* I thought, 'I am doomed!' ⁵⁵ I called on Your name, HASHEM,* from the depths of the pit. ⁵⁶ You have heard my voice; do not shut your ear from my prayer for my relief when I cry out. ⁵⁷ You always drew near on the day I would call You; You said, 'Fear not!'* ⁵⁸ You always championed my cause, O Lord, you redeemed my life. ⁵⁹ You have seen, HASHEM, the injustices I suffer; judge my cause. ⁶⁰ You have seen all their vengeance, all their designs against me. ⁶¹ You have heard their insults, HASHEM;* all their designs regarding me. ⁶² The speech and thoughts of my enemies are against me all day long.* ⁶³ Look, in everything they do, I am the butt of their taunts. ⁶⁴ Pay them back their due, HASHEM, as they have done.* ⁶⁵ Give them a broken heart; may Your curse be upon them! ⁶⁶ Pursue them in anger and destroy them from under the heavens of HASHEM.*

CHAPTER FOUR

¹ Alas — the gold is dimmed!* The finest gold is changed! Sacred stones are scattered at every street corner! ² The precious children of Zion,* who are comparable to fine gold — alas, are now treated like earthen jugs, work of a potter. ³ Even tanim will offer

---

61⁻63. שָׁמַעְתָּ חֶרְפָּתָם — *You have heard their insults, HASHEM.* Alshich translates the verse as referring to their blasphemies against Hashem, i.e., *You have heard how they reviled You, HASHEM, and how they designed against me.*

Most commentators, however, see *Israel* as being the object of their insults, and explain verses 61-63 as referring to designs of the enemy — in thought, word and action.

כָּל־הַיּוֹם — *All day long.* Even though my enemies already accomplished many of their evil plans, their mind is not at ease. They continue to plan and talk about me incessantly *all day long,* as if their power of speech was given them just to deride me (*Lechem Dim'ah*).

64⁻66. [In the verses that follow, Hashem is asked to mete out retribution to Israel's enemies, in kind, for all their evil.]

כְּמַעֲשֵׂה יְדֵיהֶם — *As they have done.* I.e., for having acted in consonance with, and as emissaries of, God's will in bringing about punishment to Israel — for that they are absolved. However, כְּמַעֲשֵׂה יְדֵיהֶם, for what they added *of their own hands,* i.e., of their viciousness and overzealousness beyond the bounds expected of them — for that Hashem is asked to

punish them (*Lechem Dim'ah*).

וְתַשְׁמִידֵם מִתַּחַת שְׁמֵי ה׳ — *And destroy them from under the heavens of HASHEM* — Don't punish them with exile, as You punished us. Destroy them from the face of the earth (*Rav Galanti*).

The obliteration should be so complete that they should have no descendants, and that no one will be able to say, 'This tree, or camel, or lamb belongs to him' [i.e., there will be no trace of identity left] (*Midrash*).

[Thus, with the plea that God utterly wipe out the enemy, the chapter closes.]

CHAPTER FOUR

1. אֵיכָה יוּעַם זָהָב — *Alas — the gold is dimmed!* The *gold* figuratively refers to the people of Jerusalem. It has become covered over, i.e., dull only in its external appearance and brilliance, but not in substance (*Midrash; Rashi; Ibn Yachya*).

Rashi comments that this elegy was originally pronounced over יֹאשִׁיָּהוּ, King Josiah, as mentioned in *II Chronicles* 35:25. Jeremiah also incorporated within it the references to Zion.

2. בְּנֵי צִיּוֹן הַיְקָרִים — *The precious children of Zion.* [The verse laments how Zion's precious inhabitants, once greatly esteemed, are now

שַׁד* הֵינִיקוּ גּוּרֵיהֶן בַּת־עַמִּי לְאַכְזָר °כַּיְעֵנִים בַּמִּדְבָּר: ד דָּבַק
לְשׁוֹן יוֹנֵק אֶל־חִכּוֹ בַּצָּמָא* עוֹלָלִים שָׁאֲלוּ לֶחֶם פֹּרֵשׂ אֵין לָהֶם:
ה הָאֹכְלִים לְמַעֲדַנִּים נָשַׁמּוּ בַּחוּצוֹת הָאֱמֻנִים עֲלֵי תוֹלָע חִבְּקוּ
אַשְׁפַּתּוֹת: ו וַיִּגְדַּל עֲוֹן בַּת־עַמִּי מֵחַטַּאת סְדֹם* הַהֲפוּכָה
כְמוֹ־רָגַע* וְלֹא־חָלוּ בָהּ יָדָיִם: ז זַכּוּ נְזִירֶיהָ מִשֶּׁלֶג צַחוּ מֵחָלָב
אָדְמוּ עֶצֶם מִפְּנִינִים סַפִּיר גִּזְרָתָם: ח חָשַׁךְ מִשְּׁחוֹר תָּאֳרָם לֹא
נִכְּרוּ בַּחוּצוֹת* צָפַד עוֹרָם עַל־עַצְמָם יָבֵשׁ הָיָה כָעֵץ: ט טוֹבִים
הָיוּ חַלְלֵי־חֶרֶב* מֵחַלְלֵי רָעָב שֶׁהֵם יָזֻבוּ מְדֻקָּרִים מִתְּנוּבֹת שָׂדָי:
י יְדֵי נָשִׁים רַחֲמָנִיּוֹת בִּשְּׁלוּ יַלְדֵיהֶן הָיוּ לְבָרוֹת לָמוֹ בְּשֶׁבֶר
בַּת־עַמִּי: יא כִּלָּה יהוה אֶת־חֲמָתוֹ שָׁפַךְ חֲרוֹן אַפּוֹ וַיַּצֶּת־אֵשׁ
בְּצִיּוֹן וַתֹּאכַל יְסֹדֹתֶיהָ: יב לֹא הֶאֱמִינוּ מַלְכֵי־אֶרֶץ* °כֹּל יֹשְׁבֵי
תֵבֵל כִּי יָבֹא צַר וְאוֹיֵב בְּשַׁעֲרֵי יְרוּשָׁלָ͏ִם: יג מֵחַטֹּאת נְבִיאֶיהָ*

°כי ענים כ'   °וכל כ'

---

treated like common clay.]

Midrash Lekach Tov, commenting on the precious character of the people of Jerusalem, notes that when residents of Jerusalem sat down to eat they would hang a cloth over their door as a signal to the poor that they might come to share their meal [see also *Bava Basra* 93b].

3. גַּם־תַּנִּים חָלְצוּ שַׁד — *Even tanim will offer the breast.* [The word תַּנִּים, *tanim*, refers to a wild animal but its exact identity is unknown. The word usually means *reptile* or *fish* and in modern Hebrew, תַּן means *jackal*. Since the specific guidance of Talmudic sources is lacking, we have left the word untranslated.]

Although *tanim* are vicious, they display warmth and kindness to their young by nursing them. Jeremiah laments how, as a result of the ravages and stress of famine, the usually compassionate Jewish mothers became cruel and placed their own lives before their children's. They consumed whatever food was available, and allowed their children to go hungry, ignoring their cries for food (*Rashi*).

According to many commentators, *tanim* figuratively refers to the vicious enemy who חָלְצוּ שַׁד, *bared the breast*, i.e., forced Jewish women to nurse their enemy's children with the tragic result that the nursing mothers had no milk left for their own children. The Jewish daughters, unable to respond to the needs of their children who cried *like ostriches in the desert*, seemed to be אַכְזָר, *cruel* (*Alshich, Palgei Mayim*).

At very least, the Jews could expect that the enemy's children who were nursed by Jewish women should display some compassion for the women who reared them. This, too, was not forthcoming. They were as cruel as ostriches in the desert (*Lechem Dim'ah*).

4. לְשׁוֹן יוֹנֵק ... בַּצָּמָא — *The tongue of the suckling ... for thirst.* Since, in the previous verse, *the daughter of my people has become cruel,* the sucklings who depend on their mothers for milk are described as dying of thirst, whereas the עוֹלָלִים, *the young children,* beg for bread (*Kiflayim LeSushiyah*).

The *Midrash* relates how the enemy also destroyed the conduits which carried water through the land. Even when a father took his thirsty child to the conduit, he found no water.

5. In this verse Jeremiah further laments the fall of the people from their previous heights to the nethermost depths to which they have fallen. People, who were brought up eating *only* the finest delicacies and dressed *only* in the most luxurious clothing, lay faint from hunger in the streets, and scrounged through garbage heaps for the most meager scraps of food (*Lechem Dim'ah*).

6. וַיִּגְדַּל עֲוֹן ... מֵחַטַּאת סְדֹם — *The iniquity is greater ... than the sin of Sodom.* The punishment of Zion, greater than that of Sodom [see next comm.], proves that their iniquity was greater than Sodom's (*Rashi*).

הַהֲפוּכָה כְמוֹ־רָגַע — *Which was overturned in a moment,* i.e., Sodom was destroyed instantly — without the suffering of a prolonged siege. Hence its sin is considered not as grave as *the breast* and suckle their young; the daughter of my people has become cruel, like ostriches in the desert.* ⁴ *The tongue of the suckling cleaves to its palate for thirst;* young children beg for bread, no one extends it to them.* ⁵ *Those who feasted extravagantly lie destitute in the streets; those who were brought up in scarlet clothing wallow garbage.* ⁶ *The iniquity of the daughter of my people is greater than the sin of Sodom,* which was overturned in a moment* without mortal hands being laid on her.* ⁷ *Her princes were purer than snow, whiter than milk; their appearance was ruddier than rubies, their outside was like sapphire.* ⁸ *Their appearance has become blacker than soot, they are not recognized in the streets;* their skin has shriveled on their bones, it became dry as wood.* ⁹ *More fortunate were the victims of the sword* than the victims of famine, for they pine away, stricken, lacking the fruits of the field.* ¹⁰ *Hands of compassionate women have boiled their own children;* they became their food when the daughter of my people was shattered.* ¹¹ HASHEM *vented His fury,* He poured out His fierce anger; He kindled a fire in Zion which consumed its foundations.* ¹² *The kings of the earth did not believe,* nor did any of the world's inhabitants, that the adversary or enemy could enter the gates of Jerusalem.* ¹³ *It was for the sins of her prophets,**

Jerusalem's, which was punished with famine, sieges, war — and an exile which still endures! (Rashi; Lechem Dim'ah).

7-8. [The dramatic 'then and now' comparisons demonstrate the ravages of famine and war upon the nobility. Formerly they were prince-like figures of grace and nobility, while now they are *blacker than soot*.]

8. לֹא נִכְּרוּ בַּחוּצוֹת — *They are not recognized in the streets.* The *Midrash* relates of Rav Zadok that the ravages of the Destruction bore so hard upon him that his body never returned to normal although he lived for many years after the Destruction.

9. טוֹבִים הָיוּ חַלְלֵי־חֶרֶב — *More fortunate were the victims of the sword* or: *The good* [people] *were the victims of the sword* because they died a swift death, one preferable to the slow agony of famine (*Alshich*).

10. [The extent of the depravity is described. (See also 2:20.)]

יְדֵי נָשִׁים רַחֲמָנִיּוֹת בִּשְּׁלוּ יַלְדֵיהֶן — *Hands of compassionate women have boiled their own children.*

The impending Destruction and the ravages and famine of war caused compassionate mothers to become so depraved that *with their own hands they boiled their children* and they consumed them without even leaving flesh for other members of the family (*Alshich*).

Rav Almosnino comments that they boiled

their own *dead* children — but did not murder them.

The *Shelah* comments that this phrase also contains moralistic criticism of overly compassionate and over-indulgent mothers who, for example, let their children sleep late rather than go to synagogue or to school. With this 'misplaced compassion' they 'roast' and destroy their children's souls.

11. כָּלָה ה׳ אֶת חֲמָתוֹ — HASHEM *vented His fury.* The fury, pent up within Him for many years [see comm. to 2:8], was vented when He exacted vengeance upon them.

12. לֹא הֶאֱמִינוּ מַלְכֵי־אָרֶץ — *The kings of the earth did not* [or *could not*] *believe.* The miraculous defeat of Sennacherib [*II Chronicles 32*] created the impression that Jerusalem was impregnable (*Midrash Lekach Tov*).

They didn't realize that because its sanctity had been defiled, it had become vulnerable (*Alshich*).

13. מֵחַטֹּאת נְבִיאֶיהָ — *It was for the sins of her prophets,* i.e., she became vulnerable to such calamity because of the sins of her false prophets (*Rashi*).

[These prophets gave her false security by indulging in deceptive oracles, and did not exhort her to repent. Compare *Jeremiah 8:10-12: From prophet to priest everyone deals falsely, for they have healed the hurt of my people superficially by saying, 'Peace, peace,' when there is no peace... Therefore they shall fall*

עוֹנֹת כֹּהֲנֶיהָ הַשֹּׁפְכִים בְּקִרְבָּהּ דַּם צַדִּיקִים: יד נָעוּ עִוְרִים
בַּחוּצוֹת* נְגֹאֲלוּ בַּדָּם בְּלֹא יוּכְלוּ יִגְּעוּ בִּלְבֻשֵׁיהֶם: טו סוּרוּ
טָמֵא קָרְאוּ לָמוֹ סוּרוּ סוּרוּ אַל־תִּגָּעוּ כִּי נָצוּ גַּם־נָעוּ אָמְרוּ
בַּגּוֹיִם לֹא יוֹסִפוּ לָגוּר:* טז פְּנֵי יהוה חִלְּקָם לֹא יוֹסִיף לְהַבִּיטָם
פְּנֵי כֹהֲנִים לֹא נָשָׂאוּ* °וּזְקֵנִים לֹא חָנָנוּ: יז °עוֹדֵינוּ תִּכְלֶינָה
עֵינֵינוּ אֶל־עֶזְרָתֵנוּ הָבֶל* בְּצִפִּיָּתֵנוּ צִפִּינוּ אֶל־גּוֹי לֹא יוֹשִׁעַ:
יח צָדוּ צְעָדֵינוּ* מִלֶּכֶת בִּרְחֹבֹתֵינוּ קָרַב קִצֵּנוּ מָלְאוּ יָמֵינוּ כִּי־בָא
קִצֵּנוּ: יט קַלִּים הָיוּ רֹדְפֵינוּ מִנִּשְׁרֵי שָׁמָיִם עַל־הֶהָרִים דְּלָקֻנוּ
בַּמִּדְבָּר אָרְבוּ לָנוּ: כ רוּחַ אַפֵּינוּ מְשִׁיחַ יהוה* נִלְכַּד בִּשְׁחִיתוֹתָם
אֲשֶׁר אָמַרְנוּ בְּצִלּוֹ נִחְיֶה בַגּוֹיִם: כא שִׂישִׂי וְשִׂמְחִי בַּת־אֱדוֹם*
°יוֹשַׁבְתִּ בְּאֶרֶץ עוּץ* גַּם־עָלַיִךְ תַּעֲבָר־כּוֹס* תִּשְׁכְּרִי וְתִתְעָרִי:*
כב תַּם־עֲוֹנֵךְ בַּת־צִיּוֹן לֹא יוֹסִיף לְהַגְלוֹתֵךְ* פָּקַד עֲוֹנֵךְ בַּת־
אֱדוֹם גִּלָּה עַל־חַטֹּאתָיִךְ:

°וּזְקֵנִים כ'   °עֹדֵינָה כ'   °יוֹשַׁבְתִּי כ'

---

among the fallen. This caused the blood of the righteous to be shed in their midst.]

A different approach is taken by *Rav Alkabetz* in interpreting verses 12-13: The priests and prophets of Israel were renowned throughout the world for their holiness and sincerity. Therefore: *The kings of the earth could not believe that Jerusalem would be made vulnerable* as a result of any sins, and if it were to become subject to conquest, it could be *on the fault of her priests and prophets.*

14-15. נָעוּ עִוְרִים בַּחוּצוֹת — *The blind wandered through the streets.* This translation follows *Rashi* who explains: When the blind wandered through the streets, their feet slipped in the blood of the murdered Jews who lay throughout the city.

Ibn Ezra interprets עִוְרִים as an adverb and translates: they wandered through the streets *blindly.*

אָמְרוּ בַּגּוֹיִם לֹא יוֹסִפוּ לָגוּר — *The nations had said: 'They will not sojourn again.'* The nations predicted that the Jews will never again return to their land to dwell as before (*Ibn Ezra; Akeidas Yitzchak*) because [next verse] God is the One Who exiled them (*Alshich*).

Other commentators translate: For the nations resolved — after seeing Israel's defilement — that they will not allow her to dwell [peacefully] in their lands, and they will compel her to wander about (*Lechem Dim'ah*).

[In this chapter, too, the verse beginning with פ precedes the verse beginning with ע. See

comm. to 2:16.]

16. פְּנֵי כֹהֲנִים לֹא נָשָׂאוּ — *They showed no regard for the priests.* The end of the verse gives the reason that God dispersed the Jews and avoided looking after them: Because they showed no regard for the priests and elders, God showed no regard, as it were, for them (*Alshich*).

17. עוֹדֵינוּ תִּכְלֶינָה עֵינֵינוּ אֶל־עֶזְרָתֵנוּ הָבֶל — *Our eyes still strained in vain for our deliverance.* [The verse reproduces the state of mind that prevailed in the last days of the siege, when nearly everyone sustained the hope that outside help would arrive. From *Jeremiah 37:5-11* we know that the advance of the Egyptian army caused the Babylonians to retreat from Jerusalem, but as Jeremiah predicted, the relief was only temporary. The Egyptians never came to save them, and the Babylonians returned as Jeremiah predicted.]

18. These verses describe the miserable state of the Jews who remained in Judea under Chaldean rule (*Ibn Shuib*).

צָדוּ צְעָדֵינוּ — *They dogged our steps so we could not walk in our streets,* i.e, they ambushed us (*Rashi*), so that when a Jew went to market they would pounce upon him screaming, 'There goes a Jew!' (*Lekach Tov*).

20. רוּחַ אַפֵּינוּ מְשִׁיחַ ה' — *The breath of our nostrils, HASHEM's anointed.* [The expression רוּחַ אַפֵּינוּ, *the breath of our nostrils,* occurs only here, and poetically expresses the very essence of national hope and identity — its very survival *the iniquities of her priests, who had shed in her midst the blood of the righteous.* ¹⁴ *The blind wandered through the streets,* defiled with blood, so that none could touch their garments.* ¹⁵ *'Away, unclean one!' people shouted at them; 'Away! Away! Don't touch! For they are loathsome and wander about.' The nations had said: 'They will not sojourn again.'** ¹⁶ *The anger of* HASHEM *has divided them, caring for them no longer; they showed no regard for the priests* nor favor for the elders.* ¹⁷ *Our eyes still strained in vain for our deliverance;* in our expectations we watched for a nation that could not save.* ¹⁸ *They dogged our steps* so we could not walk in our streets; our end drew near, out days are done, for our end has come.* ¹⁹ *Our pursuers were swifter than eagles in the sky; they chased us in the mountains, ambushed us in the desert.* ²⁰ *The breath of our nostrils,* HASHEM's *anointed,* was caught in their traps; he, under whose protection, we had thought, we would live among the nations.* ²¹ *Rejoice and exult, O daughter of Edom,* who dwells in the land of Uz;* to you, too, will the cup pass,* you will be drunk and will vomit.** ²² *Your iniquity is expiated, O daughter of Zion,* He will not exile you again;* He remembers your iniquity, daughter of Edom, He will uncover your sins.*

---

and 'breath of life' — which focused on the monarch, God's anointed.]

21. שִׂישִׂי וְשִׂמְחִי בַּת־אֱדוֹם — *Rejoice and exult, O daughter of Edom.* These words are spoken sarcastically, as if to say: Rejoice while you can, because you will not escape punishment for your sins (*Midrash Lekach Tov*).

Ibn Ezra explains that Edom is referred to here because of its implacable hatred for Israel. They rejoiced at Jerusalem's downfall, as it is written (*Psalms* 137:7): *Remember,* HASHEM, *for the sons of Edom, the day of Jerusalem, for those who say, 'Destroy it, destroy it, unto its very foundation!'* [See also *Ovadiah* 1:10-14 for a description of the malice which Edom demonstrated on the day of Jerusalem's disaster.]

According to *Rashi* and the *Midrash*, this verse refers not to contemporary Edom but prophetically to the Romans [whom the Sages identify with Biblical Edom] who Jeremiah foresaw would destroy the Second Temple.

יוֹשֶׁבֶת בְּאֶרֶץ עוּץ — *Who dwells in the land of Uz.* [The Arameans' land bordering upon Edom (see *Jeremiah* 25:20) and named after its early Edomite settler, Uz, son of Seir (*Gen.* 36:28).]

גַּם־עָלַיִךְ תַּעֲבָר־כּוֹס — *To* [lit., *upon*] *you, too, will the cup pass,* i.e., the cup of punishment (*Rashi*).

תִּשְׁכְּרִי וְתִתְעָרִי — *You will be drunk and will vomit* [i.e., you will drink so much from the cup of punishment and wrath that you will get intoxicated from its abundance, and, like a drunken man, will vomit].

Rav Yonasan Eyebesheutz notes that the curse of vomiting is that as a result of vomiting she will have room to drink more from the cup of punishment.

[It is perhaps possible to relate תִתְעָרִי to the Edomite outcry against Jerusalem (*Psalms* 137:7: עָרוּ עָרוּ, *'destroy it! destroy it!'*). Just as you Edomites called excessively for Jerusalem's destruction, so will you drink excessively from the cup of destruction and be destroyed.]

22. תַּם־עֲוֹנֵךְ בַּת־צִיּוֹן — *Your iniquity is expiated, O daughter of Zion,* i.e., you have been punished for all your sins (*Rashi*).

You have been punished in one blow for the accumulation of all your iniquity (*Alshich*).

The *Midrash* notes that [the miseries and calamities related in] the Book of *Lamentations* were better for Israel than the forty years during which Jeremiah exhorted and prophesied. Because of the Destruction of the Temple, all Israel's sins were expiated that very day.

לֹא יוֹסִיף לְהַגְלוֹתֵךְ — *He will not exile you again,* beyond the Edomite [Roman, i.e., current] exile (*Rashi*).

[*Rashi* thus understands the subject *He* as referring to God.]

Ibn Ezra suggests that the subject is *your iniquity* [i.e., your iniquity will never again cause you to be exiled].

[The verse closes this chapter with the prophetic consolation that the worst of God's wrath upon the Jews has passed, and that now it is time for Edom's Day of Judgment.]

פרק חמישי

א זְכֹר יהוה מֶה־הָיָה לָנוּ °הַבִּיטָה וּרְאֵה אֶת־חֶרְפָּתֵנוּ:°
ב נַחֲלָתֵנוּ נֶהֶפְכָה לְזָרִים בָּתֵּינוּ לְנָכְרִים: ג יְתוֹמִים הָיִינוּ °וְאֵין
אָב° אִמֹּתֵינוּ כְּאַלְמָנוֹת: ד מֵימֵינוּ בְּכֶסֶף שָׁתִינוּ° עֵצֵינוּ בִּמְחִיר
יָבֹאוּ: ה עַל צַוָּארֵנוּ נִרְדָּפְנוּ יָגַעְנוּ °וְלֹא הוּנַח־לָנוּ:° ו מִצְרַיִם
נָתַנּוּ יָד° אַשּׁוּר לִשְׂבֹּעַ לָחֶם: ז אֲבֹתֵינוּ חָטְאוּ °וְאֵינָם °וַאֲנַחְנוּ
עֲוֹנֹתֵיהֶם סָבָלְנוּ:° ח עֲבָדִים מָשְׁלוּ בָנוּ פֹּרֵק אֵין מִיָּדָם: ט בְּנַפְשֵׁנוּ
נָבִיא לַחְמֵנוּ מִפְּנֵי חֶרֶב הַמִּדְבָּר: י עוֹרֵנוּ כְּתַנּוּר נִכְמָרוּ מִפְּנֵי
זַלְעֲפוֹת רָעָב: יא נָשִׁים בְּצִיּוֹן עִנּוּ בְּתֻלֹת בְּעָרֵי יְהוּדָה:° יב שָׂרִים
בְּיָדָם נִתְלוּ פְּנֵי זְקֵנִים לֹא נֶהְדָּרוּ: יג בַּחוּרִים טְחוֹן נָשָׂאוּ וּנְעָרִים

°הַבִּיט כ' °אֵין כ' °לֹא כ' °אֵינָם כ' °אֲנַחְנוּ כ'

CHAPTER FIVE

[Chapter five is composed of 22 verses like chapters 1, 2, and 4 — it differs from the previous four chapters in that it is not alphabetically arranged.]

1. זְכֹר ה' מֶה־הָיָה לָנוּ — *Remember, HASHEM, what has befallen us* [lit., *what we have been to us*], i.e., Remember the sufferings we endured before the Destruction, as well as our present disgraceful condition (*Ibn Ezra*).

Israel spoke before the Holy One, Blessed is He: We are subject to forgetfulness, but You are not. Since there is no forgetfulness before You, please remember... (*Midrash*).

Alshich interprets this as alluding not to former *suffering*, but to former *glory* (see below).

הַבִּיטָה וּרְאֵה אֶת־חֶרְפָּתֵנוּ — *Look and see our disgrace.* Remember, God, those who died at the hands of our enemies, and *look and see* the disgrace which we survivors suffer (*Lechem Dim'ah*).

Alshich explains that the suffering of a poor man who has never seen wealth cannot be compared with the greater suffering of a wealthy man who has been reduced to pauperdom — who is now publicly disgraced at having to beg for his very sustenance. Thus the exiles, who were thrust from the heights of glory to the lowest conditions of servility, commiserated over their fate and lamented: זְכֹר ה' מֶה־הָיָה לָנוּ, *Remember, HASHEM, what we have been* — during our time of royalty. And as You remember our former grandeur, הַבִּיט, *look*, at our present condition in exile, וּרְאֵה אֶת־חֶרְפָּתֵנוּ, *see our disgrace* now, compared with our former glory.

3. יְתוֹמִים הָיִינוּ וְאֵין אָב — *We have become orphans, fatherless. Fatherless* refers to our relationship with God who is called *our Father* — i.e. God has, in a sense, removed Himself from us, leaving us *fatherless* (*Alshich*).

Lechem Dim'ah [who also interprets *father* as God] notes that the כְּתִיב, written text, has אֵין אָב, *there is no father*, without the connecting prefix ו, *and*. It is therefore intended to be understood as a separate clause: The ravages of war made us *become orphans* from our natural father; in addition to that calamity, אֵין אָב, *there is no father*, because God has hidden Himself, so to speak, from us. But this verse is not to be understood as suggesting that God is no longer the Father of Israel, ח"ו, but that *He is not there*, in the sense that He maintains a distance instead of being available and paternal to His children.

4. מֵימֵינוּ בְּכֶסֶף שָׁתִינוּ — *We pay money to drink our own water* [lit., *our water for silver we drank*]. Because, due to the enemy, they were afraid to fetch it from the river. Instead, they were forced to purchase it at a high price from the enemy (*Rashi*) who had taken possession of their wells (*Alshich*).

Even the wells and trees which had been common property were sold at exorbitant prices due to the siege (*Ibn Ezra*).

5. וְלֹא הוּנַח־לָנוּ — *But nothing is left us.* They acquired everything we had by imposing taxes and levies (*Rashi*).

The *Midrash* translates וְלֹא הוּנַח־לָנוּ, *and we were given no rest.*

6. מִצְרַיִם נָתַנּוּ יָד — *We stretched out a hand to Egypt.* The *Midrash* relates that the Jews had traded their oil with Egypt for foodstuff which they then sent to Assyria in the hope that, if the enemy were to advance, Egypt and Assyria would come to their assistance. Ultimately the pact was fruitless — when the attack came, her 'allies' ignored her [see also 4:17]. The futility of

CHAPTER FIVE

¹ Remember, HASHEM, what has befallen us;* look and see our disgrace.* ² Our inheritance has been turned over to strangers; our houses to foreigners. ³ We have become orphans, fatherless;* our mothers are like widows. ⁴ We pay money to drink our own water,* obtain our wood at a price. ⁵ Upon our necks we are pursued; we toil, but nothing is left us.* ⁶ We stretched out a hand to Egypt,* and to Assyria to be satisfied with bread. ⁷ Our fathers have sinned and are no more, and we have suffered for their iniquities.* ⁸ Slaves ruled us, there is no rescuer from their hands. ⁹ In mortal danger we bring out bread, because of the sword of the wilderness. ¹⁰ Our skin was scorched like an oven, with the fever of famine. ¹¹ They ravaged women in Zion; maidens in the towns of Judah.* ¹² Leaders were hanged by their hand, elders were shown no respect. ¹³ Young men drag the millstone, and youths

---

this ill-fated arrangement is now lamented by the prophet (Torah Temimah).

7. אֲבֹתֵינוּ חָטְאוּ וְאֵינָם וַאֲנַחְנוּ עֲוֹנֹתֵיהֶם סָבָלְנוּ — *Our fathers have sinned and are no more, and we have suffered for their iniquities.* Several interpretations are given for this important verse. A comprehensive selection follows:

Ibn Ezra comments that our misfortune is the result of our sins which intermingled with the sins of our ancestors for which they were not punished according to the doctrine of פֹּקֵד עֲוֹן אָבֹת עַל־בָּנִים . . . [לְשֹׂנְאָי], *punishing the iniquity of the fathers upon the children. . .[of those that hate Me]* (Exodus 20:5). [Ramban, quoting the Talmud (Sanhedrin 27b), explains that God punishes children for the sins of the fathers only if the children persist in committing those sins.]

The *Arizal* offers an interpretation to harmonize the apparent contradiction between the verses *punishing the* עֲוֹן, *inquity, of the fathers upon the children* (Exodus 20:5), and אִישׁ בְּחֶטְאוֹ יוּמָתוּ, *Each man will die for his own sin* (Deut. 24:16). He points out — in addition to the Talmudic explanation above that the verse in *Exodus* applies only when the children persist in their fathers' ways — that there is also a distinction between עֲוֹן, *iniquity,* and חֵטְא, *sin.* Iniquity [referring to the verse in *Exodus*] applies to מֵזִיד, *willful* transgressions, for which, according to the Torah, children share the guilt. The verse in *Deuteronomy*, however, refers to חֵטְא, *unintentional* transgressions, for which children are not punished. Thus, the *Arizal* explains our verse [as does *Ibn Yachya, Lechem Dim'ah*]: Our fathers חָטְאוּ, sinned unintentionally, וְאֵינָם, and they are not — i.e. we are not being held accountable for them; וַאֲנַחְנוּ עֲוֹנֹתֵיהֶם סָבָלְנוּ, but for עֲוֹנֹתֵיהֶם, their intentional transgressions — for these we do suffer.

[It must be stressed that the Jews were *not* suggesting that their suffering was *wholly* the

result of their fathers' sins. They admitted complicity, too, as evidenced by the outcry in verse 16: אוֹי־נָא לָנוּ כִּי חָטָאנוּ, *woe to us, for we have sinned.* Rather, as suggested by *Ibn Ezra* (above), they acknowledged their share of the iniquity. Added together with the sins of their ancestors, the cumulative guilt was the cause of their present predicament.]

Lechem Dim'ah explains that it would be more appropriate for the fathers to receive their own punishment. But since אֵינָם, *they are no more,* it is only just their children — who according to halachah are enjoined to say after a father's death, אֲנִי כַּפָּרַת מִשְׁכָּבוֹ, *'I am the atonement for his repose'* — who should accept responsibility. As the *Alshich* notes, no atonement is necessary for חֲטָאִים, *the unintentional sins* of parents, because death atones for them. For עֲוֹנוֹת, *intentional trangressions,* however, death does not suffice — suffering is a required part of the atonement. Children, therefore, should accept the obligation to atone for the sins of their parents.

11. נָשִׁים בְּצִיּוֹן עִנּוּ בְּתֻלֹת בְּעָרֵי יְהוּדָה — *They ravaged women in Zion; maidens in the town of Judah.* As if the sufferings of famine were not punishment enough, the slaves [verse 8] ravaged our wives (Ibn Ezra).

The greater the sanctity of the place, the more heinous their sins. In Judah, the enemy limited himself to ravaging בְּתֻלֹת, *unmarried maidens;* in the higher sanctity of Zion, the environs of Jerusalem and the Temple, he was brazen and defiant enough toward God to show his comtempt and ravage נָשִׁים, *married women* (Kiflayim LeSushiyah).

Lechem Dim'ah explains that when the Babylonian soldiers marched on Zion, they first passed through the towns of Judah. Not yet being sure of their own strength, they limited their ravages to unmarried maidens. But by the time they reached Jerusalem, the tide of war was

בָּעֵץ כָּשָׁלוּ:* יד זְקֵנִים מִשַּׁעַר שָׁבָתוּ בַּחוּרִים מִנְּגִינָתָם:* טו שָׁבַת מְשׂוֹשׂ לִבֵּנוּ נֶהְפַּךְ לְאֵבֶל מְחֹלֵנוּ: טז נָפְלָה עֲטֶרֶת רֹאשֵׁנוּ אוֹי־נָא לָנוּ כִּי חָטָאנוּ:* יז עַל־זֶה הָיָה דָוֶה לִבֵּנוּ עַל־אֵלֶּה חָשְׁכוּ עֵינֵינוּ:* יח עַל הַר־צִיּוֹן שֶׁשָּׁמֵם שׁוּעָלִים הִלְּכוּ־בוֹ: יט אַתָּה יהוה לְעוֹלָם תֵּשֵׁב כִּסְאֲךָ לְדֹר וָדוֹר: כ לָמָּה לָנֶצַח תִּשְׁכָּחֵנוּ תַּעַזְבֵנוּ לְאֹרֶךְ יָמִים: כא הֲשִׁיבֵנוּ יהוה ׀ אֵלֶיךָ °וְנָשׁוּבָה* חַדֵּשׁ יָמֵינוּ כְּקֶדֶם:* כב כִּי אִם־מָאֹס מְאַסְתָּנוּ קָצַפְתָּ עָלֵינוּ עַד־מְאֹד:

The following verse is recited aloud by the congregation, then repeated by the reader:

הֲשִׁיבֵנוּ יהוה* ׀ אֵלֶיךָ וְנָשׁוּבָה חַדֵּשׁ יָמֵינוּ כְּקֶדֶם:

°וְנָשׁוּב כ'

---

going with them and they were fully confident of victory. Then they stopped at nothing, even ravaging married women.

The *Targum* translates: Married women in Zion were ravaged by Arameans [Edomites; *Ibn Yachya* and *Lechem Dim'ah* version of *Targum* reads *Romans*]; *maidens in the towns of Judah* by Chaldeans (Babylonians).

13. וּנְעָרִים בָּעֵץ כָּשָׁלוּ — *And youths stumble under* [lit., *in* or *with*] *the wood.* Rav Yehoshua ben Levi said: Three hundred children were found hung by the enemy on one branch (*Midrash*).

According to *Alshich*: The children grew so weak that they would stumble over a branch lying on the road.

14. זְקֵנִים מִשַּׁעַר שָׁבָתוּ בַּחוּרִים מִנְּגִינָתָם — *The elders are gone from the gate; the young men* [ceased] *from their music.* [It had been the custom for elders to station themselves at the gates (see *Ruth* 4:1; *Esther* 2:21). Now the gates lie desolate (see above 1:4).]

Elders here refer to the wise men, as the *Talmud* states: כִּי אֵין זָקֵן אֶלָּא מִי שֶׁקָּנָה חָכְמָה — For זָקֵן, *elder,* means only one who has acquired wisdom [*Kiddushin* 32b]. They have departed from the *gates of Halachah.* Similarly, *young men* refers to the young students who would study Mishnah by heart, and put the words to a melody as an aid to memorization. They, too, sang no longer (*Lechem Dim'ah*).

In verses 11-14, we have a description of how the enemy attacked every segment of the population in every social strata: married women and maidens; officers and elders; young men and children (*Rav Almosnino*).

16. אוֹי־נָא לָנוּ כִּי חָטָאנוּ — *Woe to us, for we have sinned.* Now that the Temple is destroyed, how will we atone for our sins? Previously, a sinner would offer a sacrifice to atone for his sins. Now

there is no longer a Temple. Woe to us! (*Lechem Dim'ah*).

[This is an obvious confession, a recognition that everything that has befallen them is the result — and just reward — for their sinful ways (see comm. to verse 7).]

17-18. עַל־זֶה הָיָה דָוֶה לִבֵּנוּ — *For this our heart was faint* [or *sick,*] etc. For what is described in the next verse (the desolation of Mount Zion with foxes prowling it) (*Rashi*).

Alshich interprets the first half of this verse as referring to remorse over her sins which were the cause of Destruction; the second half of the verse to the desolation of Mount Zion.

The *Midrash* comments: Just as a woman who separates from her husband for a few days because of impurity is called דָּוָה, *sick* [*Leviticus* 15:33], how much more should we be called דָּוֶה, *sick,* for being separated from the 'house of our life,' the Temple, for these many years!

עַל־אֵלֶּה חָשְׁכוּ עֵינֵינוּ — *For these our eyes dimmed* from excessive weeping (*Ibn Ezra*).

For none of our other catastrophes and suffering did our hearts grow so faint or did we weep so much, as for '*Mount Zion which lies desolate, foxes prowled over it*' (*Rav Yosef Kara; Palgei Mayim*).

עַל הַר־צִיּוֹן שֶׁשָּׁמֵם... — *For Mount Zion which lies desolate, foxes prowled over it.* Its desolation is so utter, that foxes, which usually dwell in ruins, prowl freely and undisturbed over it (*Alshich; Ibn Ezra*).

[In this context *Mount Zion* is used poetically in place of Mount Moriah — the actual site of the Temple.]

19-20. אַתָּה ה' לְעוֹלָם תֵּשֵׁב — *Yet You, HASHEM, are enthroned forever.* Although the manifestation of Your Kingship on earth is in ruins, nevertheless, Your dominion will never cease. You are enthroned forever. So if Your incorporeality is undiminished, and our sins *stumble under the wood.** [14] *The elders are gone from the gate, the young men from their music.** [15] *Gone is the joy of our hearts, our dancing has turned into mourning.* [16] *The crown of our head has fallen; woe to us, for we have sinned.** [17] *For this our heart was faint, for these our eyes dimmed:** [18] *for Mount Zion which lies desolate, foxes prowled over it.* [19] *Yet You, HASHEM, are enthroned forever, Your throne is ageless.* [20] *Why do You ignore us eternally, forsake us for so long?* [21] *Bring us back to You, HASHEM, and we shall return,** *renew our days as of old.** [22] *For even if You had utterly rejected us, You have already raged sufficiently against us.*

The following verse is recited aloud by the congregation, then repeated by the reader:

Bring us back to You, HASHEM,* and we shall return,
renew our days as of old.

---

only affect material manifestations of Your holiness, *why do You ignore us eternally?* (*Alshich*).

[It follows that since Hashem's Kingship *is* ageless, His throne itself will ultimately be restored.] Is there enthronement without a throne; a king without a consort? [Jerusalem is the throne; Israel the consort (*Torah Temimah*)] (*Midrash*).

21. הֲשִׁיבֵנוּ ה' אֵלֶיךָ וְנָשׁוּבָה — *Bring us back to You, HASHEM, and we shall return* [or *repent*]. Israel addresses God: All we ask is for some Divine assistance. If You initiate the action, and draw us near to You, then we will repent our sins and return to You wholeheartedly (*Lechem Dim'ah*).

The *Midrash* relates that there is a constant dispute, so to speak, between Hashem and Israel. God insists: שׁוּבוּ אֵלַי וְאָשׁוּבָה אֲלֵיכֶם, [First] *return to Me and* [then] *I will return to you* (*Malachi* 3:7); and Israel answers: הֲשִׁיבֵנוּ ה' אֵלֶיךָ, [First] *bring us back to You and* [then] *we shall return.* Neither side gives in and thus the dispute, as to who will take the initiative, continues. . .

. . .The *Maggid of Kozhnitz* explains homiletically that this is why we face the Master of the universe and say: לָמָּה לָנֶצַח תִּשְׁכָּחֵנוּ, *why for the sake of* נִצָּחוֹן, *victory, do You forget us,* Your children? Whom are you defeating — Your foolish stubborn children? Concede, O Merciful God, this one time! הֲשִׁיבֵנוּ ה' אֵלֶיךָ וְנָשׁוּבָה, *Bring us back to You, HASHEM, and we shall return!*

Ibn Ezra translates הֲשִׁיבֵנוּ, *bring us back,* in the physical sense: *Bring us back* to the city of the Dwelling Place of Your Name, [Jerusalem,] and we will resume serving You as before.

חַדֵּשׁ יָמֵינוּ כְּקֶדֶם — *Renew our days as of old.* As it is written (*Malachi* 3:4): *Then shall the offering of Judah and Jerusalem be pleasant to*

HASHEM, כִּימֵי עוֹלָם, *as in the days of old,* וּכְשָׁנִים קַדְמוֹנִיּוֹת, *and as in ancient years* (*Midrash*) — Renew our days as You did when You took us out of Egypt (*Ibn Shuib*).

22. כִּי אִם־מָאֹס מְאַסְתָּנוּ — *For even if You had utterly rejected us* [lit., *reject You rejected us*], *You have already raged sufficiently against us.* Although we sinned, You did not have to increase rage against us as much as You did (*Rashi*).

The use of the double verb מָאֹס מְאַסְתָּנוּ, *Reject You rejected us,* is interpreted as referring prophetically to both Temples (*Alshich*).

Pesikta d'Rav Kahana translates: *If it is 'rejection,' then You completely rejected us; but You are very 'wroth' against us.* That is, if God has *rejected* Israel, then there is no hope. If, however, He is no more than *wrathful,* then there is hope, for He Who is angered is likely to become reconciled.

Rav Levi Yitzchak of Berditchev explains these verses as follows:

Someone may divorce his wife for one of two reasons: for having found in her עֶרְוַת דָּבָר, an immorality; or because she no longer finds favor in his eyes. If he divorces her for the former reason, he may never remarry her; if for the latter, he may remarry her. This is how these verses הֲשִׁיבֵנוּ, *Bring us back,* are to be understood. You did not divorce us because of עֶרְוַת דָּבָר, that our behavior was so improper that You cannot ever take us back. Rather, You divorced us, כִּי אִם־מָאֹס מְאַסְתָּנוּ, because You utterly rejected us; i.e. we no longer found favor in Your eyes. As such You may bring us back to You.

הֲשִׁיבֵנוּ ה' — *Bring us back . . . HASHEM.* It is customary to repeat verse 21 rather than end with the words of rebuke in verse 22. We act similarly at the conclusion of *Isaiah, Malachi,* and *Ecclesiastes* [and thus end these books on a comforting note] (*Rashi*).

◄§ קינות §►

א.

זְכֹר יהוה* מֶה הָיָה לָנוּ,   אוֹי,

הַבִּיטָה וּרְאֵה אֶת חֶרְפָּתֵנוּ,   אוֹי, מֶה הָיָה לָנוּ.

נַחֲלָתֵנוּ נֶהֶפְכָה לְזָרִים,   אוֹי,

בָּתֵּינוּ לְנָכְרִים,   אוֹי, מֶה הָיָה לָנוּ.

יְתוֹמִים הָיִינוּ וְאֵין אָב,   אוֹי,

אִמּוֹתֵינוּ מְקוֹנְנוֹת בְּחֹדֶשׁ אָב,   אוֹי, מֶה הָיָה לָנוּ.

מֵימֵינוּ בְּכֶסֶף שָׁתִינוּ,   אוֹי,

כִּי נִסּוּךְ הַמַּיִם בָּזִינוּ,*   אוֹי, מֶה הָיָה לָנוּ.

עַל צַוָּארֵנוּ נִרְדָּפְנוּ,   אוֹי,

כִּי שִׂנְאַת חִנָּם רָדָפְנוּ,   אוֹי, מֶה הָיָה לָנוּ.

מִצְרַיִם נָתַנּוּ יָד,   אוֹי,

וְאַשּׁוּר צָדֽוֹנוּ כְּצֵידָךְ,   אוֹי, מֶה הָיָה לָנוּ.

אֲבוֹתֵינוּ חָטְאוּ וְאֵינָם,   אוֹי,

וַאֲנַחְנוּ סוֹבְלִים אֶת עֲוֺנָם,   אוֹי מֶה הָיָה לָנוּ.

עֲבָדִים מָשְׁלוּ בָנוּ,   אוֹי,

כִּי שִׁלּוּחַ עֲבָדִים בָּטַלְנוּ,[1]   אוֹי, מֶה הָיָה לָנוּ.

בְּנַפְשֵׁנוּ נָבִיא לַחְמֵנוּ,   אוֹי,

כִּי קִפַּצְנוּ מֵעֲנִי יָדֵינוּ,[2]   אוֹי, מֶה הָיָה לָנוּ.

עוֹרֵנוּ כְּתַנּוּר נִכְמָרוּ,   אוֹי,

כִּי כְבוֹדָם בְּקָלוֹן הֵמִירוּ,[3]   אוֹי, מֶה הָיָה לָנוּ.

נָשִׁים בְּצִיּוֹן עִנּוּ,   אוֹי,

כִּי אִישׁ אֶת אֵשֶׁת רֵעֵהוּ טִמְּאוּ וְזָנוּ,[4]   אוֹי, מֶה הָיָה לָנוּ.

◄§ זְכֹר ה'* — *Remember, HASHEM*. Many of the *kinnos* are arranged according to the verses of one or more chapters of *Eichah* (the Book of Lamentations). This first *kinnah* is based on the fifth chapter. Each stanza contains two lines. The first stich is the opening phrase of the corresponding verse in *Eichah*, followed by the word אוֹי, *O woe!* The second stich rhymes with the first and is either the *paytan's* extension of

the verse's lament, or his explanation of why the tragedy described in the first stich occurred. The phrase, 'אוֹי מֶה הָיָה לָנוּ, *O woe! What has befallen us!*' is inserted at the end of the stanza. This format allows us to focus carefully on each tragedy and to respond with a personal sigh of grief, אוֹי, *O woe . . .'* The last four verses of *Eichah* appear at the end of the *kinnah* in their entirety, without the added phrases.

֎ KINNOS ֍

1.

זְכֹר Remember, HASHEM, what has befallen us,   O woe!
    Look and see our disgrace —   O woe! What has befallen us!

Our inheritance has been turned over to strangers,   O woe!
    Our homes to foreigners —   O woe! What has befallen us!

We have become orphans, fatherless,   O woe!
    Our mothers lament in the month of Av — O woe! What has befallen us!

We pay money to drink our own water,   O woe!
    Because we scorned the water libations ceremony* —

                  O woe! What has befallen us!

Upon our necks we are pursued,   O woe!
    Because we pursued purposeless hatred — O woe! What has befallen us!

We stretched out a hand to Egypt,   O woe!
    While Assyria trapped us like a hunter — O woe! What has befallen us!

Our fathers have sinned and are no more,   O woe!
    And we [who continue in their ways]
    bear the burden of their iniquities —   O woe! What has befallen us!

Slaves rule over us,   O woe!
    Because we discontinued the liberation of the [Hebrew] slaves[1] —

                  O woe! What has befallen us!

In mortal danger we bring our bread,   O woe!
    Because we have clamped our hands tightly against the poor[2] —

                  O woe! What has befallen us!

Our skin was scorched like an oven,   O woe!
    Because they have exchanged their dignity for degradation[3] —

                  O woe! What has befallen us!

They ravaged women in Zion,   O woe!
    Because they sullied and seduced their neighbor's wives[4] —

                  O woe! What has befallen us!

---

(1) See *Exodus* 21:2 and *Jeremiah* 34:8ff.
(2) Cf. *Deuteronomy* 15:7. (3) Cf. *Hosea* 4:7. (4) Cf. *Ezekiel* 18:11.

In some early editions of *Kinnos* this *kinnah* does not appear. Instead, there is an instruction that reads: 'The *chazzan* repeats [the chapter beginning] זכר ה', *Remember, HASHEM*, and inserts אוי, *O woe!*, in the middle of each verse, and אוי מה הָיָה לָנוּ, *O woe! What has befallen us!*, at the end. From the verse אַתָּה ה', *Yet You, HASHEM*, he omits the insertions ... but recites the verses as they appear in *Eichah* ...'

Whether this *kinnah* is recited in the words of *Eichah* or in the words of the *paytan*, the repetition of the last chapter of Jeremiah's lament emphasizes that the Destruction of the Temples did not bring an end to Jewish suffering and tragedy; on the contrary, it marked the beginning of what seems like an interminable series of exiles and massacres. Nevertheless, if we return to *Hashem*, He will return us to Him and to His Land.

כִּי נָסוֹךְ הַמַּיִם בָּזִינוּ — *Because we scorned the water libations ceremony*. It is axiomatic that

שָׂרִים בְּיָדָם נִתְלוּ, אוֹי,

כִּי גְזֵלַת הֶעָנִי חָמְסוּ וְגָזְלוּ,[1] אוֹי, מֶה הָיָה לָנוּ.

בַּחוּרִים טְחוֹן נָשָׂאוּ, אוֹי,

כִּי בְּבֵית זוֹנָה* נִמְצָאוּ, אוֹי, מֶה הָיָה לָנוּ.

זְקֵנִים מִשַּׁעַר שָׁבָתוּ, אוֹי,

כִּי מִשְׁפַּט יָתוֹם וְאַלְמָנָה עִוְּתוּ, אוֹי, מֶה הָיָה לָנוּ.

שָׁבַת מְשׂוֹשׂ לִבֵּנוּ, אוֹי,

כִּי נִבְטְלוּ עוֹלֵי רְגָלֵינוּ, אוֹי, מֶה הָיָה לָנוּ.

נָפְלָה עֲטֶרֶת רֹאשֵׁנוּ, אוֹי,

כִּי נִשְׂרַף בֵּית מִקְדָּשֵׁנוּ,[2] אוֹי, מֶה הָיָה לָנוּ.

עַל זֶה הָיָה דָוֶה לִבֵּנוּ, אוֹי,

כִּי נִבְטַל כְּבוֹד בֵּית מַאֲוַיֵּנוּ, אוֹי, מֶה הָיָה לָנוּ.

עַל הַר צִיּוֹן שֶׁשָּׁמֵם, אוֹי,

כִּי הַר הַבַּיִת מְשׁוֹמֵם, אוֹי, מֶה הָיָה לָנוּ.

אַתָּה יהוה לְעוֹלָם תֵּשֵׁב כִּסְאֲךָ לְדוֹר וָדוֹר.

לָמָּה לָנֶצַח תִּשְׁכָּחֵנוּ תַּעַזְבֵנוּ לְאֹרֶךְ יָמִים.

הֲשִׁיבֵנוּ יהוה אֵלֶיךָ וְנָשׁוּבָה חַדֵּשׁ יָמֵינוּ כְּקֶדֶם.

כִּי אִם מָאֹס מְאַסְתָּנוּ קָצַפְתָּ עָלֵינוּ עַד מְאֹד.

הֲשִׁיבֵנוּ יהוה אֵלֶיךָ וְנָשׁוּבָה חַדֵּשׁ יָמֵינוּ כְּקֶדֶם.

_____

(1) Cf. *Isaiah* 3:14. (2) Cf. 64:10.

Leaders were hanged by their hand,   *O woe!*
  Because they plundered and robbed the loot of the poor[1] —
                              O woe! What has befallen us!

Young men bear the millstone,   *O woe!*
  Because they were found in the harlot's house* —
                              O woe! What has befallen us!

The elders are gone from the gate,   *O woe!*
  Because they twisted the judgment of the orphan and the widow —
                              O woe! What has befallen us!

Gone is the joy of our hearts,   *O woe!*
  Because the festival pilgrimage has been discontinued —
                              O woe! What has befallen us!

The crown of our head has fallen,   *O woe!*
  Because our Holy Temple has been burnt down[2] —
                              O woe! What has befallen us!

For this our heart was faint,   *O woe!*
  Because the glory has ceased from the House of our Aspirations —
                              O woe! What has befallen us!

For Mount Zion which lies desolate,   *O woe!*
  Because the Temple Mount is in ruins —   *O woe! What has befallen us!*

Yet You, HASHEM, are enthroned forever, Your throne is ageless.
Why do You ignore us eternally, forsake us for so long?
Bring us back to You, HASHEM, and we shall return,
  renew our days as of old.
For even if You had utterly rejected us,
  You have already raged sufficiently against us.
Bring us back to You, HASHEM, and we shall return,
  renew our days as of old.

God rewards and punishes מִדָּה כְּנֶגֶד מִדָּה, *measure for measure.* Therefore, when retribution is visited upon the nation, there must be a cause and effect relationship between the deed in whose wake that retribution comes and the specific form it takes. In thirteen of the next fifteen stanzas, the *paytan* traces these relationships.

טְחוּן ... בְּבֵית זוֹנָה — *The millstone ... in the harlot's house.* The Sages understand the root טחן, literally, *grind*, as a euphemism for adultery (*Sotah* 10a; *Eichah Rabbah* 5:13). Hence, the burden of carrying a heavy millstone is apt punishment for frequenting the harlot's house.

ON SATURDAY NIGHT:

ב.

אֵיךְ מִפִּי בֶן וּבַת, הֶגוֹת קִינוֹת רַבַּת,

תְּמוּר שִׁירִים וַחֲדָוַת,

וַיְהִי נֹעַם' נִשְׁבַּת,* בְּמוֹצָאֵי שַׁבָּת.

אוֹי, כִּי נִגְזְרָה גְזֵרָה, בָּחֳרִי אַף וְגַם עֶבְרָה,

וְאַפּוֹ בָנוּ חָרָה, וּבָעֲרָה חֲמָתוֹ כָּלַבַּת,²

וַיְהִי נֹעַם נִשְׁבַּת, בְּמוֹצָאֵי שַׁבָּת.

אוֹי, כִּי בָתֵּינוּ שֻׁנּוּ,³ וּבְתוּלוֹתֵינוּ עֻנּוּ,⁴

וּפָנֵינוּ נִשְׁתַּנּוּ, וְגַם הוּשְׁחָרוּ⁵ כְּמַחֲבַת,

וַיְהִי נֹעַם נִשְׁבַּת, בְּמוֹצָאֵי שַׁבָּת.

אוֹי, כִּי שֻׁדּוּנוּ צָרִים, וְגַם הִפִּילוּ בָנוּ פְגָרִים,

בְּנֵי צִיּוֹן הַיְקָרִים,⁶ הָיוּ נְצוּרִים כְּבָבַת,

וַיְהִי נֹעַם נִשְׁבַּת, בְּמוֹצָאֵי שַׁבָּת.

אוֹי, כִּי נָפְלָה עֲטֶרֶת,⁷ וְגָבְרָה כָתֵף סוֹרֶרֶת,⁸

וְחָדַל הוֹד וְתִפְאֶרֶת, צֻמְּתוּם שְׁכֶן חִבַּת,

וַיְהִי נֹעַם נִשְׁבַּת, בְּמוֹצָאֵי שַׁבָּת.

אוֹי, כִּי נִטְּלָה מְנוֹרָה, וּקְטֹרֶת לְבוֹנָה הַטְּהוֹרָה,

וְנִבְזֶה גָזִית מִיָּקְרָה, אָבְלָה אֶרֶץ זָבַת,

וַיְהִי נֹעַם נִשְׁבַּת, בְּמוֹצָאֵי שַׁבָּת.

נֹעַם נִשְׁבַּת וַיְהִי — *The [prayer]'May the Pleasantness' is omitted.* Although this prayer (*Psalms*
90:17-91:16) is usually recited at the departure of
the Sabbath, it is omitted when Tishah B'Av
follows immediately after the Sabbath. This is
because the prayer was composed by Moses in
honor of the completion of the מִשְׁכָּן [*Mishkan*],

Tabernacle, in the Wilderness (*Midrash
Tehillim*). Since the *Mishkan* served the same
function as the *Beis HaMikdash*, it would be
unseemly to recite this prayer on the anniversary
of the Destruction (*Matteh Moshe 729*, cited in
Taamei HaMinhagim).

ON SATURDAY NIGHT:

2.

אֵיךְ *O how from the mouth of son and daughter*
   many lamentations resound, instead of songs and jubilation.
The [prayer] 'May the pleasantness'[1] is omitted,*
   as the Sabbath departs.

O woe! For the decree was issued
   with blazing anger and with wrath;
His anger blazed against us and His fury burned like a flame![2]
      The [prayer] 'May the pleasantness' is omitted, as the Sabbath departs.

O woe! For they turned over our homes [to strangers][3]
   and ravished our virgins;[4]
our faces are distorted and blackened[5]
   like [the bottom of] a frying pan.
      The [prayer] 'May the pleasantness' is omitted, as the Sabbath departs.

O woe! For enemies have plundered us
   and caused corpses to fall among us,
the precious children of Zion,[6]
   who had been protected like the pupil [of the eye].
      The [prayer] 'May the pleasantness' is omitted, as the Sabbath departs.

O woe! For the crown[-like Temple] has fallen,[7]
   because the shoulder turned away[8]
   [from God's service] has prevailed;
splendor and majesty have ceased, [from the Beis HaMikdash
   in which He] constricted His loving Presence.
      The [prayer] 'May the pleasantness' is omitted, as the Sabbath departs.

O woe! For the Menorah has been taken,
   along with the pure frankincense offering;
the [Sanhedrin's] cherished hewn-stone [chamber] has been degraded;
   and the land overflowing [with milk and honey]
   has been consumed.
      The [prayer] 'May the pleasantness' is omitted, as the Sabbath departs.

---

(1) *Psalms* 90:17-91:16. (2) Cf. *Eichah* 2:3. (3) Cf. 5:2. (4) Cf. 5:11. (5) Cf. 4:8.
(6) 4:2. (7) Cf. *Eichah* 5:16. (8) Cf. *Zechariah* 7:11; *Nehemiah* 9:29.

ג.

בְּלֵיל זֶה יִבְכָּיוּן וְיֵילִילוּ בָנַי. . .

בְּלֵיל זֶה חָרַב בֵּית קָדְשִׁי וְנִשְׂרְפוּ אַרְמוֹנַי,[1]

וְכָל בֵּית יִשְׂרָאֵל יֶהְגּוּ בִיגוֹנַי,

וְיִבְכּוּ אֶת הַשְּׂרֵפָה אֲשֶׁר שָׂרַף יהוה.[2]

בְּלֵיל זֶה תְּיַלֵּל מַר עֲנִיָּה נֶחֱדֶלֶת,

וּמִבֵּית אָבִיהָ בַּחַיִּים מֻבְדֶּלֶת,

וְיָצְאָה מִבֵּיתוֹ וְנִסְגַּר הַדֶּלֶת,

וְהָלְכָה בַּשִּׁבְיָה בְּכָל פֶּה נֶאֱכֶלֶת,

בְּיוֹם שָׁלְחָה בָאֵשׁ בּוֹעֶרֶת וְאוֹכֶלֶת,

וְאֵשׁ עִם גַּחֶלֶת יָצְאָה מֵאֵת יהוה,[3]

בְּלֵיל זֶה יִבְכָּיוּן וְיֵילִילוּ בָנַי.

בְּלֵיל זֶה הַגַּלְגַּל סָבֵב הַחוֹבָה,*

רִאשׁוֹן גַּם שֵׁנִי בֵּיתִי נֶחֱרָבָה,

וְעוֹד לֹא רֻחָמָה בַּת הַשּׁוֹבֵבָה,*[4]

הִשְׁקַתָּה מֵי רוֹשׁ[5] וְאֶת בִּטְנָה צָבָה,*

וְשָׁלְחָה מִבֵּיתוֹ וְגַם נָשְׁתָה טוֹבָה,[6]

גְּדוֹלָה הַשִּׂנְאָה מֵאֵת אֲשֶׁר אַהֲבָה,[7]

∫**בְּלֵיל זֶה** — *On this night.* When the Spies returned after forty days of reconnoitering the Land of Canaan, they produced a terribly slanderous report about the Land. Rather than have faith in God's promise to bring them to a land flowing with milk and honey where they would live under Divine protection, the nation chose to believe the Spies' discouraging word, and they wept that night (*Numbers* 13:25 - 14:1). God was infuriated at Israel's treachery and declared, 'Since you shed tears on this night for no reason, I shall give you many reasons to cry on this night!' (*Taanis* 29a).

Thus, the date of Tishah B'Av became a day of repeated tragedies, throughout Jewish history. The Mishnah enumerates five of these dire events: (a) Because the nation believed the Spies' malicious report, the guilty ones were sentenced to die in the wilderness, before the nation would enter the Land; (b-c) the First and Second Temples were destroyed; (d) Bar Kochba's revolt was crushed and his stronghold at Beitar was captured by the Romans [so many Jews were slain at that time that the non-Jews fertilized their vineyards for seven years with the blood of the Jews killed at Beitar (*Gittin* 57a)]; and (e) the Roman governor Turnus Rufus had the city of Jerusalem razed and plowed under (*Taanis* 26b).

The *paytan* places this lament into the mouth of either Jerusalem (which *Eichah* describes as a widow) or the nation as a whole lamenting to her children (the exiles) about the bitter tragedies which have befallen her. Alternatively, the narrator of the *kinnah* is addressing his own children to explain the reasons for the sadness of the day.

הַגַּלְגַּל סָבֵב הַחוֹבָה — *The calendrical cycle turned to an inauspicious date.* The Mishnah states that both the First and Second Temples were destroyed on the Ninth of Av (*Taanis* 26b). The Talmud adduces verses that verify this date for the First Temple, then seeks proof that the second Destruction also occurred on Tishah B'Av. The following *baraisa* is cited: מִגַּלְגְּלִין

3.

בְּלֵיל זֶה *On this night,* weep and wail, my children,*
  for on this night my Holy Temple was destroyed
and my palaces were burnt down;[1]
the entire House of Israel shall lament over my agony,
and they shall bewail the conflagration
  that HASHEM has ignited.[2]

On this night, the impoverished,
  abandoned one [Israel] shall wail bitterly;
she who was estranged from her Father's Temple
  even while He is alive;
she went forth from his house and the door
  [to redemption] was sealed;
she went into captivity
  where she was devoured by every mouth,
on that day she was exiled by a flaming, consuming fire —
the fire and the flaming coal that went forth from HASHEM.[3]

  On this night, weep and wail, my children. . .

On this night, the calendrical cycle
  turned to an inauspicious date;*
my First and my Second Temple were both destroyed;
the rebellious daughter[4]
  is still unworthy of compassion;*
she was forced to drink bitter waters[5]
  and her belly was bloated;*
she was exiled from His House
  and has forgotten what good is;[6]
greater is [God's] hatred [now]
  than [His] love for her had been;[7]

---

(1) Cf. *II Chronicles* 36:19. (2) *Leviticus* 10:6. (3) Cf. *Numbers* 16:35.
(4) *Jeremiah* 31:21, 49:4. (5) Cf. 9:14. (6) Cf. *Eichah* 3:17. (7) Cf. *II Samuel* 13:15.

זְכוּת לְיוֹם וַכַּאי וְחוֹבָה לְיוֹם חַיָּיב, *They [the Heavenly Court] make a good event occur on an auspicious date, and a bad event on an inauspicious date* (ibid. 29a; *Arachin* 11b).

וְעוֹד לֹא רְחָמָה בַּת הַשּׁוֹבֵבָה — *The rebellious daughter is still unworthy of compassion.* God appeared to the prophet Hosea in a vision and ordered him to concretize Israel's wayward lust for idolatry in a most dramatic manner: '*Take a harlot unto yourself and bear children of adultery, for the land has been adulterous in turning away from HASHEM* ' (Hosea 1:2). The prophet did so and three children were born to him. God told him what to name each baby — names that describe His displeasure with the nation.

The second child, a daughter, was to be called לֹא רְחָמָה, *Lo-Ruchamah* [lit., *unworthy of compassion* or *unpitied*] (ibid. 1:6). When the nation will be exiled, learn its lesson and return to God's service, her name will be changed to רֻחָמָה, *Ruchamah*, i.e., *worthy of compassion* (ibid. 2:3).

הִשְׁקָתָה מֵי רוֹשׁ וְאֶת בִּטְנָה צָבָה — *She was forced to drink bitter waters and her belly was bloated.* Although *Rashi* (Jeremiah 9:14) renders מֵי רֹאשׁ as *snake venom* and *Radak* translates *bitter grass*, from the context of the *kinnah* it is obvious that the *paytan* alludes to the ordeal and degradation of the סוֹטָה, *wayward wife*, as described in Scripture (*Numbers* 5:11-31).

וּכְאַלְמְנוּת חַיּוֹת כְּאִשָּׁה נֶעֱזָבָה,
וַתֹּאמֶר צִיּוֹן עֲזָבַנִי יהוה,[1]

בְּלֵיל זֶה יִבְכָּיוֹן וְיֵילִילוּ בָנָי.

בְּלֵיל זֶה קָדַרְתִּי וְחָשְׁכוּ הַמְּאוֹרוֹת,
לְחָרְבַּן בֵּית קָדְשִׁי וּבְטוּל מִשְׁמָרוֹת,[2]
בְּלֵיל זֶה סַבּוּנִי אֲפָפוּנִי צָרוֹת,
וְגַם קָרָא מוֹעֵד[3] בְּדִין חָמֵשׁ גְּזֵרוֹת,
בְּכִי חִנָּם בָּכוּ וְנִקְבַּע לַדּוֹרוֹת,
יַעַן כִּי הָיְתָה סִבָּה מֵעִם יהוה,[4]

בְּלֵיל זֶה יִבְכָּיוֹן וְיֵילִילוּ בָנָי.

בְּלֵיל זֶה אֵרְעוּ בּוֹ חָמֵשׁ מְאֹרָעוֹת,
גָּזַר עַל אָבוֹת בִּפְרוֹעַ פְּרָעוֹת,[5]
וְדָבְקוּ בוֹ צָרוֹת רַבּוֹת וְרָעוֹת,[6]
יוֹם מוּכָן הָיָה בִּפְגוֹעַ פְּגָעוֹת,
וְהֶעֱמִיד הָאוֹיֵב* וְהֵרִים קוֹל זְוָעוֹת,
קוּם כִּי זֶה הַיּוֹם אֲשֶׁר אָמַר יהוה,[7]

בְּלֵיל זֶה יִבְכָּיוֹן וְיֵילִילוּ בָנָי.

וְהֶעֱמִיד הָאוֹיֵב — *[God] set the enemy [against us].* Some commentaries understand 'the enemy' as the subject of the verb and render: *The enemy set up [an idol in the Temple].* This interpretation is difficult because the Mishnah (*Taanis* 4:6) lists that event as one of the five tragedies of the Seventeenth of Tammuz, while this stanza of the *kinnah* recounts the tragic events of Tishah B'Av.

she is like a widow of the living, like an abandoned woman.
*And Zion said: H*ASHEM *has forsaken me.*[1]

On this night, weep and wail, my children. . .

On this night, I was blackened
　　and the luminaries turned dark,
because of the destruction of my Holy Temple
and the discontinuation of the [priestly] watches.[2]
On this night, troubles encircled and surrounded me,
and He proclaimed this date as a fixed time[3]
　　for five [harsh] decrees.
[On this night,] they cried without cause, so it was designated
[a night of weeping] for all generations;
*therefore H*ASHEM *caused it to happen so.*[4]

On this night, weep and wail, my children. . .

On this night, five tragedies occurred:
He decreed against [our] ancestors
　　when they rebelled wantonly,[5]
and many terrible troubles[6] *cleaved to them this [day],*
a day destined for dreadful visitations.
[God] set the enemy [against us],* and he raised a terrifying cry:
*'Arise! For this is the day of which H*ASHEM *has said*[7]
[that we should destroy His Temple]!'

On this night, weep and wail, My children. . .

---

(1) *Isaiah* 49:14. (2) See prefatory remarks to *kinnah* 10. (3) Cf. *Eichah* 1:15. (4) *I Kings* 12:15.
(5) *Judges* 5:2; see commentaries there for various other interpretations of this phrase.
(6) Some editions read מְצָרוֹת וְנֶם רָעוֹת, but the meaning is the same. (7) Cf. *Judges* 4:14.

ד.

שׁוֹמְרוֹן קוֹל תִּתֵּן מְצָאוּנִי עוֹנִי,[1]

לְאֶרֶץ אַחֶרֶת יְצָאוּנִי בָנַי,[2]

וְאָהֳלִיבָה תִּזְעַק נִשְׂרְפוּ אַרְמוֹנַי,[3]

וַתֹּאמֶר צִיּוֹן עֲזָבַנִי יהוה.[4]

לֹא לָךְ אָהֳלִיבָה חֲשֹׁב עָנְיֵךְ כְּעָנְיִי,

הֲתַמְשִׁילִי חָלְיֵךְ לְשִׁבְרִי וּלְחָלְיִי,

אֲנִי אָהֳלָה סוּרָה בָּגַדְתִּי בְקַשְׁיִי,

וְקָם עָלַי כַּחֲשִׁי וְעָנָה בִי מֶרְיִי,[5]

וּלְמִקְצַת הַיָּמִים שְׁלַמְתִּי נִשְׁיִי,

וְתִגְלַת פִּלְאֶסֶר[6] אָכַל אֶת פִּרְיִי,

חֲמַדְתִּי פָּשַׁט וְהִצִּיל אֶת עֶדְיִי,[7]*

וְלַחֲלַח וְחָבוֹר[8] נָשָׂא אֶת שִׁבְיִי,

דְּמִי אָהֳלִיבָה וְאַל תִּבְכִּי כִּבְכְיִי,

שְׁנוֹתַיִךְ אָרְכוּ וְלֹא אָרְכוּ שָׁנָי.*

וְאָהֳלִיבָה תִּזְעַק נִשְׂרְפוּ אַרְמוֹנִי,
וַתֹּאמֶר צִיּוֹן עֲזָבַנִי יהוה.

מְשִׁיבָה אָהֳלִיבָה אֲנִי כֵן נֶעֱקַשְׁתִּי,

וּבְאַלּוּף נְעוּרַי[9] כְּאָהֳלָה בָּגַדְתִּי,

דְּמִי אָהֳלָה כִּי יְגוֹנִי זָכַרְתִּי,

נָדַדְתְּ אַתְּ אַחַת וְרַבּוֹת נָדַדְתִּי,

הִנֵּה בְּיַד הַכַּשְׂדִּים פְּעָמִים נִלְכַּדְתִּי,

וּשְׁבִיָּה עֲנִיָּה לְבָבֶל יָרַדְתִּי,

שׁוֹמְרוֹן — *Shomron.* This *kinnah* is based on chapter 23 of *Ezekiel*, where God bids the prophet to expose the sins of the Jewish people. Then unfolds the shocking parable of two faithless wives who seek fulfillment of their unnatural lusts through numerous lovers. Ezekiel tells of two sisters, אָהֳלָה, *Oholah*, and אָהֳלִיבָה, *Oholivah*, who are both married to the same man. Oholah is identified as Shomron [Samaria, capital of the Northern Kingdom, also called the Kingdom of Israel, which comprised ten of the tribes] and Oholivah as Jerusalem [capital of the Southern Kingdom, also called the Kingdom of Judah, which comprised Judah and Benjamin]. Both are 'wed' to one 'husband', God, but both brazenly betray Him.

The names, אָהֳלָה, *Oholah*, and אָהֳלִיבָה, *Oholivah*, are both derived from אֹהֶל, *a tent* or *dwelling place.* However, אָהֳלָה, is a contraction of הָאֹהֶל שֶׁלָּה, *her tent*, because God had no part in the tabernacles of Shomron. They were 'her own tents' which she had dedicated to the golden calves Jeroboam ben Nevat had erected (see *I Kings* 12:28). On the other hand, אָהֳלִיבָה is

4.

שׁוֹמְרוֹן Shomron gives forth [her] voice,
'The deserts of my sins have found me![1]
My children have gone forth from me[2] to another land!'
Then Oholivah screams, 'My palaces were burnt down!'[3]
And Zion says, 'HASHEM has abandoned me!'[4]

ל [Oholah:] 'It is not right for you, Oholivah,
to consider your suffering as mine!
Can you compare your sickness to my fracture and sickness?
I, Oholah, [am now] displaced, I have rebelled in my stubbornness,
but now my deceitfulness has risen against me,[5]
and my defiance has testified against me,
and after a short time I paid my debts [for my sins].
[The Assyrian king] Tiglath-pileser[6] devoured my [womb's] fruits,
he stripped away my precious possessions
and confiscated my jewelry,[7]*
then [his successor Shalmaneser] carried away my captives
to Halah and Habor.[8]
[Therefore,] Oholivah be silent and weep not as I weep!
Your years [in the Land] were prolonged,
but my years were not prolonged!*

Then Oholivah screams, 'My palaces were burnt down!'
And Zion says, 'HASHEM has abandoned me!'

מ Oholivah responds: 'I too deviated,
and like Oholah, I betrayed [God,] the Mentor of my youth![9]
Be still, Oholah, for I remember my agony.
You were exiled but once, while I was exiled repeatedly.
Behold, by the hands of the Chaldeans I was taken twice;
as a miserable captive I descended to Babylon;

---

(1) Cf. II Kings 7:9. (2) Cf. Jeremiah 10:20. (3) Cf. II Chronicles 36:19. (4) Isaiah 49:14.
(5) Cf. Job 16:8. (6) II Kings 15:29. (7) Cf. Exodus 33:6. (8) See II Kings 17:3-6. (9) Cf. Jeremiah 3:4.

a contraction of הָאֹהֶל שֶׁלִּי בָהּ, My Tent is within her, i.e., the Tent of God, the Beis HaMikdash. These names place Judah, in which God's Temple stood, in sharp contrast to Shomron.

The wicked city of Shomron, with the abominations of its citizens, epitomizes all of the evil of the Ten Tribes. That segment of Israel became so corrupted that to this day those tribes are lost in exile and the possibility of their ultimate return remains the subject of considerable Talmudic debate (see Sanhedrin 110b and Ramban, Sefer HaGeulah, shaar I).

In this kinnah, the author compares the tragedies which befell both Judah and Samaria by means of a debate raging between the two. Each capital claims — and vehemently defends

its claim — that it suffered more at the hand of the marauding enemy.

The composer of the kinnah, R' Shlomo ibn Gabirol (11th-century Spain), used the letters of his name שְׁלֹמֹה to begin the respective stanzas.

חֲמַדְתִּי ... עֶדְיִי — My precious possessions ... my jewelry. Some commentators understand these expressions as allusions to the two Temples. We have rejected that interpretation because Oholah is the speaker, but the Temples had stood in Oholivah's estate.

שְׁנוֹתַיִךְ אָרְכוּ וְלֹא אָרְכוּ שָׁנַי — Your years [in the Land] were prolonged, but my years were not prolonged! Oholah, the Northern Kingdom of Samaria, was exiled more than one hundred

וְנִשְׂרַף הַהֵיכָל אֲשֶׁר בּוֹ נִכְבַּדְתִּי,

וּלְשִׁבְעִים שָׁנָה בְּבָבֶל נִפְקַדְתִּי,

וְשַׁבְתִּי לְצִיּוֹן עוֹד וְהֵיכָל יָסַדְתִּי,

גַם זֹאת הַפַּעַם מְעַט לֹא עָמָדְתִּי,

עַד לְקָחַנִי אֱדוֹם וְכִמְעַט אָבָדְתִּי,

וְעַל כָּל הָאֲרָצוֹת נָפְצוּ הֲמוֹנִי,

וְאָהֳלִיבָה תִּזְעַק נִשְׂרְפוּ אַרְמוֹנַי,

וַתֹּאמֶר צִיּוֹן עֲזָבַנִי יהוה.

הַחוֹמֵל עַל דַּל חֲמוֹל עַל דַּלּוּתָם,*

וּרְאֵה שְׁמָמוֹתָם[1] וְאָרֶךְ גָּלוּתָם,

אַל תִּקְצוֹף עַד מְאֹד[2] וּרְאֵה שִׁפְלוּתָם,

וְאַל לָעַד תִּזְכּוֹר עֲוֹנָם[2] וְסִכְלוּתָם,

רְפָא נָא אֶת שִׁבְרָם[3] וְנַחֵם אֲבֵלוּתָם,

כִּי אַתָּה סִבְרָם וְאַתָּה אֱיָלוּתָם,

חַדֵּשׁ יָמֵינוּ כִּימֵי קַדְמוֹנָי,[4]

כְּנַאֲמֶךָ בּוֹנֵה יְרוּשָׁלַיִם יהוה.[5]

(1) Cf. *Daniel* 9:18. (2) Cf. *Isaiah* 64:8. (3) Cf. *Psalms* 60:4. (4) Cf. *Eichah* 5:21. (5) *Psalms* 147:2.

*and the Sanctuary by which I was honored
    was burnt down.
After seventy years in Babylon I was recalled [by God];
I returned once again to Zion
    and established the [Second] Temple.
This time, too, I did not last long
before Edom seized me and I was all but annihilated.
Through all the lands were my multitudes dispersed.'*

> *Then Oholivah screams, 'My palaces were burnt down!'*
> *And Zion says, 'HASHEM has abandoned me!'*

ה *O You Who takes pity on the pauper,
    take pity on their poverty.**
See their desolation[1] and the length of their exile.
Do not be overly angered,[2] rather take note of their degradation.
Do not eternally remember their sins[2] and their foolishness.
Please heal their wounds[3] and assuage their mourning;
for You are their Hope and You are their Strength.*

> *Renew our days as the days of my youth;[4]
> as You have said: 'The Builder of Jerusalem is HASHEM.'[5]*

---

thirty years before Oholivah, the Southern
Kingdom of Judah.

דַּלּוּתָם — *Their poverty.* Until this point, the
kinnah has been a one-on-one debate between
Oholah and Oholivah. Thus, the statements
are all in first or second person singular. The
last stanza, however, is the *paytan's* supplication for the restitution of both, and consequently is couched in third person plural.
Finally, the last line prays for the reunification
of the two Kingdoms with Jerusalem as
the focal point as it was in 'the days of my
youth.'

ה.

עַד אָנָה בְּכִיָּה בְצִיּוֹן וּמִסְפֵּד בִּירוּשָׁלָיִם,
תְּרַחֵם צִיּוֹן וְתִבְנֶה חוֹמוֹת יְרוּשָׁלָיִם.²

אָז בַּחֲטָאֵינוּ חָרַב מִקְדָּשׁ, וּבַעֲוֹנוֹתֵינוּ נִשְׂרַף הֵיכָל.
בָּאָרֶץ חֶבְרָה לָהּ³ קָשְׁרָה מִסְפֵּד,* וּצְבָא הַשָּׁמַיִם נָשְׂאוּ קִינָה.
עַד אָנָה בְּכִיָּה בְצִיּוֹן וּמִסְפֵּד בִּירוּשָׁלָיִם, תְּרַחֵם צִיּוֹן וְתִבְנֶה חוֹמוֹת יְרוּשָׁלָיִם.

גַּם בָּכוּ בְמָרֵר שִׁבְטֵי יַעֲקֹב, וְאַף מַזָּלוֹת יִזְּלוּ דִמְעָה.
דִּגְלֵי יְשֻׁרוּן חָפוּ רֹאשָׁם,⁴ וְכִימָה וּכְסִיל⁵ קָדְרוּ פְּנֵיהֶם.
עַד אָנָה בְּכִיָּה בְצִיּוֹן וּמִסְפֵּד בִּירוּשָׁלָיִם, תְּרַחֵם צִיּוֹן וְתִבְנֶה חוֹמוֹת יְרוּשָׁלָיִם.

הֶעְתִּירוּ אָבוֹת וְלֹא שָׁמַע אֵל, צָעֲקוּ בָנִים וְלֹא עָנָה אָב.⁶
וְקוֹל הַתּוֹר* נִשְׁמַע בַּמָּרוֹם, וְרוֹעֶה נֶאֱמָן לֹא הִטָּה אָזֶן.
עַד אָנָה בְּכִיָּה בְצִיּוֹן וּמִסְפֵּד בִּירוּשָׁלָיִם, תְּרַחֵם צִיּוֹן וְתִבְנֶה חוֹמוֹת יְרוּשָׁלָיִם.

זֶרַע קֹדֶשׁ לָבְשׁוּ שַׂקִּים,⁸ וּצְבָא הַשָּׁמַיִם גַּם הֵם שַׂק הוּשַׂם כְּסוּתָם.
חָשַׁךְ הַשֶּׁמֶשׁ וְיָרֵחַ קָדַר,⁹ וְכוֹכָבִים וּמַזָּלוֹת אָסְפוּ נָגְהָם.¹⁰
עַד אָנָה בְּכִיָּה בְצִיּוֹן וּמִסְפֵּד בִּירוּשָׁלָיִם, תְּרַחֵם צִיּוֹן וְתִבְנֶה חוֹמוֹת יְרוּשָׁלָיִם.

טָלֶה רִאשׁוֹן* בָּכָה בְמַר נֶפֶשׁ, עַל כִּי כְבָשָׂיו לַטֶּבַח הוּבָלוּ.¹¹
וְלַיְלָה הִשְׁמִיעַ שׁוֹר בַּמָּרוֹמִים, כִּי עַל צַוָּארֵנוּ¹² נִרְדָּפְנוּ כֻּלָּנוּ.
עַד אָנָה בְּכִיָּה בְצִיּוֹן וּמִסְפֵּד בִּירוּשָׁלָיִם, תְּרַחֵם צִיּוֹן וְתִבְנֶה חוֹמוֹת יְרוּשָׁלָיִם.

(1) Psalms 102:14. (2) Cf. 51:20. (3) Cf. 122:3. (4) Cf. Jeremiah 14:3. (5) See Ibn Ezra to Amos 5:8 for the identifications and locations of these star clusters. (6) Cf. Exodus 22:22. (7) Song of Songs 2:12. (8) Cf. Isaiah 50:3. (9) Cf. 13:10. (10) Cf. Joel 2:10. (11) Cf. Isaiah 53:7. (12) Cf. Eichah 5:5.

עַד אָנָה — *How long?* The theme of this *kinnah* is derived from the *Midrash* which teaches that at the time of the Temple's destruction the celestial star formations called מַזָּלוֹת [*mazalos*], *constellations*, joined in Israel's mourning (*Yalkut Shimoni* II:1008). The Rabbis teach that the term מַזָּל is cognate with נוֹזֵל, *flow*, because God causes His blessings to flow to earth, with the *mazalos* acting as conduits and transformers that bring His infinite beneficence down to the finite world. The varying positions of the *mazalos* with relation to both time and earth will affect this heavenly flow in such manner that it can be said that mankind is under the influence or control of the *mazalos*. Nevertheless, the Talmud (*Shabbos* 156a) teaches that אֵין מַזָּל לְיִשְׂרָאֵל, *Mazal does not control Israel*. Rashi explains that since *mazal* is nothing more than a tool in God's hands, a Jew can overcome his *mazal* by appealing to *Hashem* through prayer or righteous deeds and He will rearrange the *mazalos* to be favorable to the petitioner. This *kinnah* describes how, on Tishah B'Av, God aligned all of the *mazalos* against

Israel, so that they were all positioned in a way that would cause a negative, harmful flow upon Israel. The *paytan* records how each of the *mazalos* cried because it had a hand in this terrible tragedy.

בָּאָרֶץ חֶבְרָה לָהּ קָשְׁרָה מִסְפֵּד — *On earth, the people attached to it joined in eulogy.* Just as 'the angels of the multitude above join Your people Israel who are assembled below' to crown God with praises (as stated in the Kedushah of Mussaf according to the Sefardic rite), so after the Destruction, did Israel on earth and the legions of angels in heaven unite in lamenting the *Beis HaMikdash.*

Some editions read בְּעִיר שֶׁחֻבְּרָה לָהּ, *in the city joined to it* [i.e., to Jerusalem], and refers to celestial Jerusalem which, as the Talmud (*Taanis* 5a) teaches, is joined to the terrestrial Jerusalem. Accordingly, the *paytan* tells us that the Heavenly City united with the angels in mourning the destruction of its earthly counterpart. (See also Rashi to Psalms 122:3.)

וְקוֹל הַתּוֹר — *The voice of the turtledove.* This is

5.

How long must there be weeping in Zion and eulogy in Jerusalem?
Show Zion mercy[1] and rebuild the walls of Jerusalem![2]

א *At that time, through our sins, the [Beis Ha]Mikdash was destroyed,*
and through our iniquities the Temple was burnt down.

ב *On earth, the people attached to it[3] joined in eulogy,**
while the celestial legions raised a lament.

> *How long must there be weeping in Zion and eulogy in Jerusalem?*
> *Show Zion mercy and rebuild the walls of Jerusalem!*

ג *The tribes of Jacob also cried bitterly,*
and even the constellations shed tears.

> *How long must there be weeping in Zion and eulogy in Jerusalem?*
> *Show Zion mercy and rebuild the walls of Jerusalem!*

ד *The bannered tribes of Yeshurun [Israel] hid their heads [in shame];[4]*
the countenance of Pleiades and Orion[5] blackened.

> *How long must there be weeping in Zion and eulogy in Jerusalem?*
> *Show Zion mercy and rebuild the walls of Jerusalem!*

ה *The Patriarchs pleaded but God did not listen;*
the children screamed, but the Father did not respond.[6]

ו *The voice of the turtledove[7]* was heard on High,*
yet the Faithful Shepherd [God] did not bend an ear.

> *How long must there be weeping in Zion and eulogy in Jerusalem?*
> *Show Zion mercy and rebuild the walls of Jerusalem!*

ז *The sacred progeny garbed themselves in sackcloth,*
and the celestial legions made their garments of sackcloth.[8]

> *How long must there be weeping in Zion and eulogy in Jerusalem?*
> *Show Zion mercy and rebuild the walls of Jerusalem!*

ח *The sun darkened and the moon blackened,[9]*
the stars and constellations held back their gleam.[10]

> *How long must there be weeping in Zion and eulogy in Jerusalem?*
> *Show Zion mercy and rebuild the walls of Jerusalem!*

ט *The Ram, the first* [constellation], bleated with bitterness of soul,*
because his lambs were led to the slaughter.[11]

י *The Bull made [its] wailing heard in the heavens,*
because we were all pursued upon our necks.[12]*

> *How long must there be weeping in Zion and eulogy in Jerusalem?*
> *Show Zion mercy and rebuild the walls of Jerusalem!*

---

variously explained as an allusion to Moses (*Shir HaShirim Rabbah* 2:12), Israel (see *Psalms* 74:19 with *Rashi*), or the Torah (some editions even read וְקוֹל הַתּוֹרָה צוֹעֵק בְּמָרָה, *the voice of the Torah cries out bitterly*).

טָלֶה רֹאשׁוֹן — *The Ram, the first* ... Each of the *mazalos*, whose plaints the *paytan* now enumerates, corresponds to another month of the Hebrew calendar (*Sefer Yetzirah* 5:2). The Ram which corresponds to the first month, Nissan, is called רֹאשׁוֹן, *the first*.

The *paytan* reversed the order of the tenth and eleventh constellations. Perhaps he did this to juxtapose the verses of the Rainbow and the

Bucket, both of which speak of water. The chart on the following page enumerates the twelve constellations.

עַל צַוָּארֵנוּ — *Upon our necks*, i.e., with the yoke of heavy labor (*Rashi* to *Eichah* 5:5). According to the Midrash, this refers to a decree issued by the wicked Adrianus: Every Jew must shave himself bald; any Jew found with a single hair on his head or neck would be beheaded (*Eichah Rabbah* 5:5).

Others note that in another context the word צַוָּאר, *neck*, alludes to the *Beis HaMikdash* (*Megillah* 16b). Thus, the verse means that we were pursued because we acted treacherously to the Temple.

כּוֹכַב **תְּאוֹמִים** נִרְאָה חָלוּק, כִּי דַם אַחִים נִשְׁפַּךְ כַּמָּיִם.
לָאָרֶץ בְּקֵשׁ לִנְפּוֹל **סַרְטָן**, כִּי נִתְעַלַּפְנוּ מִפְּנֵי צָמָא.[1]

עַד אָנָה בְּכִיָּה בְצִיּוֹן וּמִסְפֵּד בִּירוּשָׁלָיִם, תְּרַחֵם צִיּוֹן וְתִבְנֶה חוֹמוֹת יְרוּשָׁלָיִם.

מָרוֹם נִבְעַת מִקּוֹל **אַרְיֵה**, כִּי שַׁאֲגָתֵנוּ לֹא עָלְתָה לַמָּרוֹם.[2]
נֶהֶרְגוּ בְתוּלוֹת וְגַם בַּחוּרִים,[3] כִּי עַל כֵּן **בְּתוּלָה** קָדְרָה פָנֶיהָ.

עַד אָנָה בְּכִיָּה בְצִיּוֹן וּמִסְפֵּד בִּירוּשָׁלָיִם, תְּרַחֵם צִיּוֹן וְתִבְנֶה חוֹמוֹת יְרוּשָׁלָיִם.

סָבֵב **מֹאזְנַיִם** וּבַקֵּשׁ תְּחִנָּה, כִּי נִבְחַר לָמוֹ מָוֶת מֵחַיִּים.[4]
עַקְרָב לָבַשׁ פַּחַד וּרְעָדָה, כִּי בְּחֶרֶב וּבְרָעָב שְׁפָטָנוּ צוּרֵנוּ.

עַד אָנָה בְּכִיָּה בְצִיּוֹן וּמִסְפֵּד בִּירוּשָׁלָיִם, תְּרַחֵם צִיּוֹן וְתִבְנֶה חוֹמוֹת יְרוּשָׁלָיִם.

פַּלְגֵי מַיִם[5] הוֹרִידוּ דִמְעָה כַּנַּחַל,[6] כִּי אוֹת **בַּקֶּשֶׁת** לֹא נִתַּן לָנוּ.*
צָפוּ מַיִם עַל רֹאשֵׁנוּ,[7] **וּבִדְלִי** מָלֵא חִכֵּנוּ יָבֵשׁ.

עַד אָנָה בְּכִיָּה בְצִיּוֹן וּמִסְפֵּד בִּירוּשָׁלָיִם, תְּרַחֵם צִיּוֹן וְתִבְנֶה חוֹמוֹת יְרוּשָׁלָיִם.

קָרְבָּנוּ קָרְבָּן וְלֹא נִתְקַבֵּל, **וּגְדִי** פָּסַק שְׂעִיר חַטֹּאתֵנוּ.
רַחֲמָנִיּוֹת בִּשְּׁלוּ יַלְדֵיהֶן,[8] וּמַזַּל **דָּגִים** הֶעֱלִים עֵינָיו.

עַד אָנָה בְּכִיָּה בְצִיּוֹן וּמִסְפֵּד בִּירוּשָׁלָיִם, תְּרַחֵם צִיּוֹן וְתִבְנֶה חוֹמוֹת יְרוּשָׁלָיִם.

שָׁכַחְנוּ שַׁבָּת בְּלִבּוֹת שׁוֹבְבִים, שַׁדַּי שִׁכַּח כָּל צִדְקוֹתֵינוּ.
תְּקַנֵּא לְצִיּוֹן קִנְאָה גְדוֹלָה,[9] וְתָאִיר לְרַבָּתִי עָם[10] מְאוֹר נָגְהֶךָ.

תְּרַחֵם צִיּוֹן כַּאֲשֶׁר אָמַרְתָּ, וּתְכוֹנְנֶהָ כַּאֲשֶׁר דִּבַּרְתָּ, תְּמַהֵר יְשׁוּעָה וְתָחִישׁ גְּאֻלָּה, וְתָשׁוּב לִירוּשָׁלַיִם בְּרַחֲמִים רַבִּים.

כַּכָּתוּב עַל יַד נְבִיאֶךָ, לָכֵן כֹּה אָמַר יְהוָה, שַׁבְתִּי לִירוּשָׁלַיִם בְּרַחֲמִים, בֵּיתִי יִבָּנֶה בָּהּ, נְאֻם יְהוָה צְבָאוֹת, וְקָו יִנָּטֶה עַל יְרוּשָׁלָיִם.[11]

HEBREW NAME	ASTRONOMICAL NAME	MONTH
טָלֶה / RAM OR LAMB	ARIES (THE RAM)	NISSAN
שׁוֹר / BULL	TAURUS (THE BULL)	IYAR
תְּאוֹמִים / TWINS	GEMINI (THE TWINS)	SIVAN
סַרְטָן / CRAB	CANCER (THE CRAB)	TAMMUZ
אַרְיֵה / LION	LEO (THE LION)	AV
בְּתוּלָה / MAIDEN	VIRGO (THE VIRGIN)	ELUL
מֹאזְנַיִם / SCALES	LIBRA (THE SCALES)	TISHREI
עַקְרָב / SCORPION	SCORPIO (THE SCORPION)	CHESHVAN
קֶשֶׁת / RAINBOW	SAGITTARIUS (THE ARCHER)	KISLEV
גְּדִי / GOAT OR KID	CAPRICORN (THE GOAT)	TEVES
דְּלִי / BUCKET	AQUARIUS (THE WATER BEARER)	SHEVAT
דָּגִים / FISH	PISCES (THE FISH)	ADAR

ב The constellation of the Twins appeared separated,
  because the blood of brothers was spilled like water.
ל The Crab was ready to fall to the earth
  because we swooned with thirst.[1]

> How long must there be weeping in Zion and eulogy in Jerusalem?
> Show Zion mercy and rebuild the walls of Jerusalem!

מ The heavens were terrified by the Lion's voice,
  because our roaring did not ascend on high.[2]
נ Maidens and also young men were slain,[3]
  therefore the Maiden's face blackened.

> How long must there be weeping in Zion and eulogy in Jerusalem?
> Show Zion mercy and rebuild the walls of Jerusalem!

ס The Scales caused themselves to tilt [in our favor]
  and pleaded in supplication,
  because, for them [Israel], death had become preferable to life.[4]
ע The Scorpion garbed itself in fear and trepidation,
  because with sword and hunger did our Creator condemn us.

> How long must there be weeping in Zion and eulogy in Jerusalem?
> Show Zion mercy and rebuild the walls of Jerusalem!

פ [Like] streams of water,[5] they shed tears like a river,[6]
  because the omen of the Rainbow was not bestowed upon us.*
צ [Endless suffering] flowed over our heads like water[7]
  and while the Bucket was full, our palate was parched.

> How long must there be weeping in Zion and eulogy in Jerusalem?
> Show Zion mercy and rebuild the walls of Jerusalem!

ק We brought an offering, but it was not accepted, and
  the Goat [mourned] the discontinuation of the he-goat sin-offering.
ר Compassionate women boiled their own children,[8]
  and the Fish constellation averted his eyes.

> How long must there be weeping in Zion and eulogy in Jerusalem?
> Show Zion mercy and rebuild the walls of Jerusalem!

ש We have neglected the Sabbath, with hearts gone astray,
  so the Almighty has made all our righteousness to be forgotten.
ת Avenge Zion with great vengeance,[9]
  illuminate [the city] 'great with people'[10] with Your shining light.

Show Zion mercy as You have said, and establish her as You have spoken.
Hasten salvation and speed redemption and return to Jerusalem with abundant compassion.

As it is written by the hand of Your prophet: Therefore, thus says HASHEM,
'I shall return to Jerusalem with compassion, My House shall be rebuilt
within it,' says HASHEM, Master of Legions, 'and a [measuring] string shall be
stretched over Jerusalem.' [11]

---

(1) Cf. *Amos* 8:13. (2) Some editions read כִּי שַׁאֲגָתֵנוּ עָלְתָה לַמָּרוֹם, *when our roaring ascended on high*.
(3) Cf. *Eichah* 2:21. (4) Cf. *Jeremiah* 8:3; some editions read לָנוּ, *for us*, instead of לָמוֹ, *for them*;
some read כִּי נִכְרַע לָנוּ כַּף מָוֶת מֵחַיִּים, *because the scale of death outweighed that of life for us.*
(5) Cf. *Eichah* 3:48; *Psalms* 119:136. (6) Cf. *Eichah* 2:18. (7) Cf. 3:54. (8) Cf. 4:10.
(9) Cf. *Zechariah* 1:14. (10) *Eichah* 1:1. (11) *Zechariah* 1:16.

כִּי אוֹת בְּקֶשֶׁת לֹא נִתַּן לָנוּ — *Because the omen of the*
Rainbow was not bestowed upon us. As indicated
by the chart, the constellation קֶשֶׁת may be

rendered either *Rainbow* or *Archer's Bow*; the
paytan uses the former. The sign of the rainbow
was given to Noah as an omen that (a) the people

וְנֶאֱמַר, עוֹד קְרָא לֵאמֹר, כֹּה אָמַר יהוה צְבָאוֹת, עוֹד תְּפוּצֶנָה
עָרַי מִטּוֹב, וְנִחַם יהוה עוֹד אֶת צִיּוֹן, וּבָחַר עוֹד בִּירוּשָׁלָיִם.[1] וְנֶאֱמַר,
כִּי נִחַם יהוה צִיּוֹן, נִחַם כָּל חָרְבֹתֶיהָ, וַיָּשֶׂם מִדְבָּרָהּ כְּעֵדֶן,
וְעַרְבָתָהּ כְּגַן יהוה, שָׂשׂוֹן וְשִׂמְחָה יִמָּצֵא בָהּ, תּוֹדָה וְקוֹל זִמְרָה.[2]

At this point, some congregations have introduced the custom of reciting a *kinnah*
lamenting the tragedy of the six million Jews murdered during the Holocaust.
Two *kinnos* of this genre appear on pages 382-391.

וַיְהִי נֹעַם, USUALLY RECITED ON SATURDAY NIGHT, IS NOT RECITED ON TISHAH B'AV;
וְאַתָּה קָדוֹשׁ IS RECITED EVEN ON WEEKNIGHTS.

The primary part of וְאַתָּה קָדוֹשׁ is the *Kedushah* recited by the angels. These verses are presented in
bold type and it is preferable that the congregation recite them aloud and in unison. However, the
interpretive translation in Aramaic (which follows the verses in bold type) should be recited softly.

וְאַתָּה קָדוֹשׁ יוֹשֵׁב תְּהִלּוֹת יִשְׂרָאֵל.[3]

וְקָרָא זֶה אֶל זֶה וְאָמַר:

קָדוֹשׁ, קָדוֹשׁ, קָדוֹשׁ יהוה צְבָאוֹת, מְלֹא כָל הָאָרֶץ כְּבוֹדוֹ.[4]

וּמְקַבְּלִין דֵּין מִן דֵּין וְאָמְרִין:

קַדִּישׁ בִּשְׁמֵי מְרוֹמָא עִלָּאָה בֵּית שְׁכִינְתֵּהּ,

קַדִּישׁ עַל אַרְעָא עוֹבַד גְּבוּרְתֵּהּ,

קַדִּישׁ לְעָלַם וּלְעָלְמֵי עָלְמַיָּא, יהוה צְבָאוֹת,

מַלְיָא כָל אַרְעָא זִיו יְקָרֵהּ.[5]

⋄ וַתִּשָּׂאֵנִי רוּחַ, וָאֶשְׁמַע אַחֲרַי קוֹל רַעַשׁ גָּדוֹל:

בָּרוּךְ כְּבוֹד יהוה מִמְּקוֹמוֹ.[6]

וּנְטָלַתְנִי רוּחָא, וְשִׁמְעֵת בַּתְרַי קָל זִיעַ סַגִּיא דִּמְשַׁבְּחִין וְאָמְרִין:

בְּרִיךְ יְקָרָא דַיהוה מֵאֲתַר בֵּית שְׁכִינְתֵּהּ.[7]

יהוה יִמְלֹךְ לְעֹלָם וָעֶד.[8]

יהוה מַלְכוּתֵהּ קָאֵם לְעָלַם וּלְעָלְמֵי עָלְמַיָּא.[9]

יהוה אֱלֹהֵי אַבְרָהָם יִצְחָק וְיִשְׂרָאֵל אֲבֹתֵינוּ, שָׁמְרָה זֹּאת
לְעוֹלָם, לְיֵצֶר מַחְשְׁבוֹת לְבַב עַמֶּךָ, וְהָכֵן לְבָבָם אֵלֶיךָ.[10] וְהוּא
רַחוּם, יְכַפֵּר עָוֹן וְלֹא יַשְׁחִית, וְהִרְבָּה לְהָשִׁיב אַפּוֹ, וְלֹא יָעִיר כָּל
חֲמָתוֹ.[11] כִּי אַתָּה אֲדֹנָי טוֹב וְסַלָּח, וְרַב חֶסֶד לְכָל קֹרְאֶיךָ.[12]
צִדְקָתְךָ צֶדֶק לְעוֹלָם, וְתוֹרָתְךָ אֱמֶת.[13] תִּתֵּן אֱמֶת לְיַעֲקֹב, חֶסֶד
לְאַבְרָהָם, אֲשֶׁר נִשְׁבַּעְתָּ לַאֲבֹתֵינוּ מִימֵי קֶדֶם.[14] בָּרוּךְ אֲדֹנָי יוֹם
יוֹם יַעֲמָס לָנוּ, הָאֵל יְשׁוּעָתֵנוּ סֶלָה.[15] יהוה צְבָאוֹת עִמָּנוּ, מִשְׂגָּב
לָנוּ אֱלֹהֵי יַעֲקֹב סֶלָה.[16] יהוה צְבָאוֹת, אַשְׁרֵי אָדָם בֹּטֵחַ בָּךְ.[17]
יהוה הוֹשִׁיעָה, הַמֶּלֶךְ יַעֲנֵנוּ בְיוֹם קָרְאֵנוּ.[18]

And it is said: Call out again, saying, Thus says HASHEM, Master of Legions, 'My cities shall again overflow with beneficence, and again HASHEM will assuage Zion and again He will choose Jerusalem.'[1]

And it is said: For HASHEM comforts Zion, He comforts her ruins, and He will make her wilderness like Eden, and her wastes like a garden of HASHEM; gladness and joy shall be found there, thanksgiving and the sound of music.[2]

At this point, some congregations have introduced the custom of reciting a *kinnah* lamenting the tragedy of the six million Jews murdered during the Holocaust. Two *kinnos* of this genre appear on pages 382-391.

וַיְהִי נֹעַם, USUALLY RECITED ON SATURDAY NIGHT, IS NOT RECITED ON TISHAH B'AV; וְאַתָּה קָדוֹשׁ IS RECITED EVEN ON WEEKNIGHTS.

The primary part of וְאַתָּה קָדוֹשׁ is the *Kedushah* recited by the angels. These verses are presented in bold type and it is preferable that the congregation recite them aloud and in unison. However, the interpretive translation in Aramaic (which follows the verses in bold type) should be recited softly.

וְאַתָּה קָדוֹשׁ *You are the Holy One, enthroned upon the praises of Israel.*[3]
And one [angel] will call another and say:

'Holy, holy, holy is HASHEM, Master of Legions, the whole world is filled with His glory.'[4]

And they receive permission from one another and say: 'Holy in the most exalted heaven, the abode of His Presence; holy on earth, product of His strength; holy forever and ever is HASHEM, Master of Legions — the entire world is filled with the radiance of His glory.'[5]

❖ *And a wind lifted me; and I heard behind me the sound of a great noise:*

'Blessed is the glory of HASHEM from His place.'[6]

And a wind lifted me and I heard behind me the sound of the powerful movement of those who praised saying: 'Blessed is the honor of HASHEM from the place of the abode of His Presence.'[7]

HASHEM shall reign for all eternity.[8]

HASHEM — His kingdom is established forever and ever.[9]

HASHEM, God of Abraham, Isaac, and Israel, our forefathers, may You preserve this forever as the realization of the thoughts in Your people's heart, and may You direct their heart to You.[10] *He, the Merciful One, is forgiving of iniquity and does not destroy; frequently He withdraws His anger, not arousing His entire rage.*[11] *For You, my Lord, are good and forgiving, and abundantly kind to all who call upon You.*[12] *Your righteousness remains righteous forever, and Your Torah is truth.*[13] *Grant truth to Jacob, kindness to Abraham, as You swore to our forefathers from ancient times.*[14] *Blessed is my Lord for every single day, He burdens us with blessings, the God of our salvation, Selah.*[15] *HASHEM, Master of Legions, is with us, a stronghold for us is the God of Jacob, Selah.*[16] *HASHEM, Master of Legions, praiseworthy is the man who trusts in You.*[17] *HASHEM, save! May the King answer us on the day we call.*[18]

---

(1) *Zechariah* 1:17. (2) *Isaiah* 51:3. (3) *Psalms* 22:4. (4) *Isaiah* 6:3. (5) *Targum Yonasan* to *Isaiah* 6:3. (6) *Ezekiel* 3:12. (7) *Targum Yonasan* to *Ezekiel* 3:12. (8) *Exodus* 15:18. (9) *Targum Onkelos* to *Exodus* 15:18. (10) *I Chronicles* 29:18. (11) *Psalms* 78:38. (12) 86:5. (13) 119:142. (14) *Micah* 7:20. (15) *Psalms* 68:20. (16) 46:8. (17) 84:13. (18) 20:10.

---

have lapsed into sinfulness, and (b) even though the world deserves another Flood, it will not come because of God's promise to Noah (see *Genesis* 9:12-16). We lament because the rainbow was not sent to stop the flood of our tears.

בָּרוּךְ הוּא אֱלֹהֵינוּ שֶׁבְּרָאָנוּ לִכְבוֹדוֹ, וְהִבְדִּילָנוּ מִן הַתּוֹעִים, וְנָתַן לָנוּ תּוֹרַת אֱמֶת, וְחַיֵּי עוֹלָם נָטַע בְּתוֹכֵנוּ. הוּא יִפְתַּח לִבֵּנוּ בְּתוֹרָתוֹ, וְיָשֵׂם בְּלִבֵּנוּ אַהֲבָתוֹ וְיִרְאָתוֹ וְלַעֲשׂוֹת רְצוֹנוֹ וּלְעָבְדוֹ בְּלֵבָב שָׁלֵם, לְמַעַן לֹא נִיגַע לָרִיק, וְלֹא נֵלֵד לַבֶּהָלָה.[1]

יְהִי רָצוֹן מִלְּפָנֶיךָ יהוה אֱלֹהֵינוּ וֵאלֹהֵי אֲבוֹתֵינוּ, שֶׁנִּשְׁמֹר חֻקֶּיךָ בָּעוֹלָם הַזֶּה, וְנִזְכֶּה וְנִחְיֶה וְנִרְאֶה וְנִירַשׁ טוֹבָה וּבְרָכָה לִשְׁנֵי יְמוֹת הַמָּשִׁיחַ וּלְחַיֵּי הָעוֹלָם הַבָּא. לְמַעַן יְזַמֶּרְךָ כָבוֹד וְלֹא יִדֹּם, יהוה אֱלֹהַי לְעוֹלָם אוֹדֶךָּ.[2] בָּרוּךְ הַגֶּבֶר אֲשֶׁר יִבְטַח בַּיהוה, וְהָיָה יהוה מִבְטַחוֹ.[3] בִּטְחוּ בַיהוה עֲדֵי עַד, כִּי בְּיָהּ יהוה צוּר עוֹלָמִים.[4] ❖ וְיִבְטְחוּ בְךָ יוֹדְעֵי שְׁמֶךָ, כִּי לֹא עָזַבְתָּ דֹרְשֶׁיךָ, יהוה.[5] יהוה חָפֵץ לְמַעַן צִדְקוֹ, יַגְדִּיל תּוֹרָה וְיַאְדִּיר.[6]

קַדִּישׁ שָׁלֵם בְּלֹא תִּתְקַבַּל. The chazzan recites

יִתְגַּדַּל וְיִתְקַדַּשׁ שְׁמֵהּ רַבָּא. (.Cong – אָמֵן.) בְּעָלְמָא דִּי בְרָא כִרְעוּתֵהּ. וְיַמְלִיךְ מַלְכוּתֵהּ, בְּחַיֵּיכוֹן וּבְיוֹמֵיכוֹן וּבְחַיֵּי דְכָל בֵּית יִשְׂרָאֵל, בַּעֲגָלָא וּבִזְמַן קָרִיב. וְאִמְרוּ: אָמֵן.

(.Cong – אָמֵן. יְהֵא שְׁמֵהּ רַבָּא מְבָרַךְ לְעָלַם וּלְעָלְמֵי עָלְמַיָּא.)

יְהֵא שְׁמֵהּ רַבָּא מְבָרַךְ לְעָלַם וּלְעָלְמֵי עָלְמַיָּא.

יִתְבָּרַךְ וְיִשְׁתַּבַּח וְיִתְפָּאַר וְיִתְרוֹמַם וְיִתְנַשֵּׂא וְיִתְהַדָּר וְיִתְעַלֶּה וְיִתְהַלָּל שְׁמֵהּ דְּקֻדְשָׁא בְּרִיךְ הוּא (.Cong – בְּרִיךְ הוּא) – לְעֵלָּא מִן כָּל בִּרְכָתָא וְשִׁירָתָא תֻּשְׁבְּחָתָא וְנֶחֱמָתָא, דַּאֲמִירָן בְּעָלְמָא. וְאִמְרוּ: אָמֵן. (.Cong – אָמֵן.)

יְהֵא שְׁלָמָא רַבָּא מִן שְׁמַיָּא, וְחַיִּים עָלֵינוּ וְעַל כָּל יִשְׂרָאֵל. וְאִמְרוּ: אָמֵן. (.Cong – אָמֵן.)

Take three steps back. Bow left and say . . . עֹשֶׂה; bow right and say . . . הוּא; bow forward and say וְעַל כָּל . . . אָמֵן. Remain standing in place for a few moments, then take three steps forward.

עֹשֶׂה שָׁלוֹם בִּמְרוֹמָיו, הוּא יַעֲשֶׂה שָׁלוֹם עָלֵינוּ, וְעַל כָּל יִשְׂרָאֵל. וְאִמְרוּ: אָמֵן. (.Cong – אָמֵן.)

Stand while reciting עָלֵינוּ.

עָלֵינוּ לְשַׁבֵּחַ לַאֲדוֹן הַכֹּל, לָתֵת גְּדֻלָּה לְיוֹצֵר בְּרֵאשִׁית, שֶׁלֹּא עָשָׂנוּ כְּגוֹיֵי הָאֲרָצוֹת, וְלֹא שָׂמָנוּ כְּמִשְׁפְּחוֹת הָאֲדָמָה. שֶׁלֹּא שָׂם חֶלְקֵנוּ כָּהֶם, וְגוֹרָלֵנוּ כְּכָל הֲמוֹנָם. (שֶׁהֵם מִשְׁתַּחֲוִים לְהֶבֶל וָרִיק, וּמִתְפַּלְלִים אֶל אֵל לֹא יוֹשִׁיעַ.[7]) וַאֲנַחְנוּ

Bow while reciting
וַאֲנַחְנוּ כּוֹרְעִים וּמִשְׁתַּחֲוִים

כּוֹרְעִים וּמִשְׁתַּחֲוִים וּמוֹדִים, לִפְנֵי מֶלֶךְ מַלְכֵי הַמְּלָכִים הַקָּדוֹשׁ בָּרוּךְ הוּא. שֶׁהוּא נוֹטֶה שָׁמַיִם וְיֹסֵד אָרֶץ,[8]

Blessed is He, our God, Who created us for His glory, separated us from those who stray, gave us the Torah of truth and implanted eternal life within us. May He open our heart through His Torah and imbue our heart with love and awe of Him and that we may do His will and serve Him wholeheartedly, so that we do not struggle in vain nor produce for futility.[1]

May it be Your will, HASHEM, our God and the God of our forefathers, that we observe Your decrees in This World, and merit that we live and see and inherit goodness and blessing in the years of Messianic times and for the life of the World to Come. So that my soul might sing to You and not be stilled, HASHEM, my God, forever will I thank You.[2] *Blessed is the man who trusts in HASHEM, then HASHEM will be his security.*[3] *Trust in HASHEM forever, for in God, HASHEM, is the strength of the worlds.*[4] Chazzan— *Those knowing Your Name will trust in You, and You forsake not those Who seek You, HASHEM.*[5] *HASHEM desired, for the sake of its [Israel's] righteousness, that the Torah be made great and glorious.*[6]

The *chazzan* recites the following *Kaddish*.

יִתְגַּדֵּל *May His great Name grow exalted and sanctified* (Cong.— *Amen.*) *in the world that He created as He willed. May He give reign to His kingship in your lifetimes and in your days, and in the lifetimes of the entire Family of Israel, swiftly and soon. Now respond: Amen.*

(Cong.— *Amen. May His great Name be blessed forever and ever.*)

May His great Name be blessed forever and ever.

Blessed, praised, glorified, exalted, extolled, mighty, upraised, and lauded be the Name of the Holy One, Blessed is He (Cong.— *Blessed is He*) — *beyond any blessing and song, praise and consolation that are uttered in the world. Now respond: Amen.* (Cong.— *Amen.*)

May there be abundant peace from Heaven, and life, upon us and upon all Israel. Now respond: Amen. (Cong.— *Amen.*)

Take three steps back. Bow left and say, 'He Who makes peace . . .';
bow right and say, 'may He . . .'; bow forward and say, 'and upon all Israel . . .'
Remain standing in place for a few moments, then take three steps forward.

He Who makes peace in His heights, may He make peace upon us, and upon all Israel. Now respond: Amen. (Cong.— *Amen.*)

Stand while reciting עָלֵינוּ, 'It is our duty . . .'

עָלֵינוּ *It is our duty to praise the Master of all, to ascribe greatness to the Molder of primeval creation, for He has not made us like the nations of the lands, and has not emplaced us like the families of the earth; for He has not assigned our portion like theirs nor our lot like all their multitudes. (For they bow to vanity and emptiness and*

Bow while reciting
'But we bend our knees.'

pray to a god which helps not.[7]*) But we bend our knees, bow, and acknowledge our thanks before the King Who reigns over kings, the Holy One, Blessed is He. He stretches out heaven and establishes earth's foundation,*[8] *the*

---

(1) Cf. *Isaiah* 65:23. (2) *Psalms* 30:13. (3) *Jeremiah* 17:7. (4) *Isaiah* 26:4.
(5) *Psalms* 9:11. (6) *Isaiah* 42:21. (7) *Isaiah* 45:20. (8) 51:13.

וּמוֹשַׁב יְקָרוֹ בַּשָּׁמַיִם מִמַּעַל, וּשְׁכִינַת עֻזּוֹ בְּגָבְהֵי מְרוֹמִים. הוּא אֱלֹהֵינוּ, אֵין עוֹד. אֱמֶת מַלְכֵּנוּ, אֶפֶס זוּלָתוֹ, כַּכָּתוּב בְּתוֹרָתוֹ: וְיָדַעְתָּ הַיּוֹם וַהֲשֵׁבֹתָ אֶל לְבָבֶךָ, כִּי יהוה הוּא הָאֱלֹהִים בַּשָּׁמַיִם מִמַּעַל וְעַל הָאָרֶץ מִתָּחַת, אֵין עוֹד.¹

עַל כֵּן נְקַוֶּה לְּךָ יהוה אֱלֹהֵינוּ לִרְאוֹת מְהֵרָה בְּתִפְאֶרֶת עֻזֶּךָ, לְהַעֲבִיר גִּלּוּלִים מִן הָאָרֶץ, וְהָאֱלִילִים כָּרוֹת יִכָּרֵתוּן, לְתַקֵּן עוֹלָם בְּמַלְכוּת שַׁדַּי. וְכָל בְּנֵי בָשָׂר יִקְרְאוּ בִשְׁמֶךָ, לְהַפְנוֹת אֵלֶיךָ כָּל רִשְׁעֵי אָרֶץ. יַכִּירוּ וְיֵדְעוּ כָּל יוֹשְׁבֵי תֵבֵל, כִּי לְךָ תִּכְרַע כָּל בֶּרֶךְ, תִּשָּׁבַע כָּל לָשׁוֹן.² לְפָנֶיךָ יהוה אֱלֹהֵינוּ יִכְרְעוּ וְיִפֹּלוּ, וְלִכְבוֹד שִׁמְךָ יְקָר יִתֵּנוּ. וִיקַבְּלוּ כֻלָּם אֶת עוֹל מַלְכוּתֶךָ, וְתִמְלֹךְ עֲלֵיהֶם מְהֵרָה לְעוֹלָם וָעֶד. כִּי הַמַּלְכוּת שֶׁלְּךָ הִיא וּלְעוֹלְמֵי עַד תִּמְלוֹךְ בְּכָבוֹד, כַּכָּתוּב בְּתוֹרָתֶךָ: יהוה יִמְלֹךְ לְעֹלָם וָעֶד.³ ✧ וְנֶאֱמַר: וְהָיָה יהוה לְמֶלֶךְ עַל כָּל הָאָרֶץ, בַּיּוֹם הַהוּא יִהְיֶה יהוה אֶחָד וּשְׁמוֹ אֶחָד.⁴

Some congregations recite the following after עלינו.

אַל תִּירָא מִפַּחַד פִּתְאֹם, וּמִשֹּׁאַת רְשָׁעִים כִּי תָבֹא.⁵ עֻצוּ עֵצָה וְתֻפָר, דַּבְּרוּ דָבָר וְלֹא יָקוּם, כִּי עִמָּנוּ אֵל.⁶ וְעַד זִקְנָה אֲנִי הוּא, וְעַד שֵׂיבָה אֲנִי אֶסְבֹּל, אֲנִי עָשִׂיתִי וַאֲנִי אֶשָּׂא, וַאֲנִי אֶסְבֹּל וַאֲמַלֵּט.⁷

קדיש יתום

In the presence of a minyan, mourners recite קַדִּישׁ יָתוֹם, the Mourner's Kaddish (see Laws §132-134).

יִתְגַּדַּל וְיִתְקַדַּשׁ שְׁמֵהּ רַבָּא. (.Cong – אָמֵן.) בְּעָלְמָא דִּי בְרָא כִרְעוּתֵהּ, וְיַמְלִיךְ מַלְכוּתֵהּ, בְּחַיֵּיכוֹן וּבְיוֹמֵיכוֹן וּבְחַיֵּי דְכָל בֵּית יִשְׂרָאֵל, בַּעֲגָלָא וּבִזְמַן קָרִיב. וְאִמְרוּ: אָמֵן.

(.Cong – אָמֵן. יְהֵא שְׁמֵהּ רַבָּא מְבָרַךְ לְעָלַם וּלְעָלְמֵי עָלְמַיָּא.)

יְהֵא שְׁמֵהּ רַבָּא מְבָרַךְ לְעָלַם וּלְעָלְמֵי עָלְמַיָּא.

יִתְבָּרַךְ וְיִשְׁתַּבַּח וְיִתְפָּאַר וְיִתְרוֹמַם וְיִתְנַשֵּׂא וְיִתְהַדָּר וְיִתְעַלֶּה וְיִתְהַלָּל שְׁמֵהּ דְּקֻדְשָׁא בְּרִיךְ הוּא (.Cong – בְּרִיךְ הוּא) – לְעֵלָּא מִן כָּל בִּרְכָתָא וְשִׁירָתָא תֻּשְׁבְּחָתָא וְנֶחֱמָתָא, דַּאֲמִירָן בְּעָלְמָא. וְאִמְרוּ: אָמֵן. (.Cong – אָמֵן.)

יְהֵא שְׁלָמָא רַבָּא מִן שְׁמַיָּא, וְחַיִּים עָלֵינוּ וְעַל כָּל יִשְׂרָאֵל. וְאִמְרוּ: אָמֵן. (.Cong – אָמֵן.)

Take three steps back. Bow left and say . . . עֹשֶׂה; bow right and say . . . הוּא; bow forward and say וְעַל כָּל . . . אָמֵן. Remain standing in place for a few moments, then take three steps forward.

עֹשֶׂה שָׁלוֹם בִּמְרוֹמָיו, הוּא יַעֲשֶׂה שָׁלוֹם עָלֵינוּ, וְעַל כָּל יִשְׂרָאֵל. וְאִמְרוּ: אָמֵן. (.Cong – אָמֵן.)

seat of His homage is in the heavens above and His powerful Presence is in the loftiest heights. He is our God and there is none other. True is our King, there is nothing beside Him, as it is written in His Torah: 'You are to know this day and take to your heart that HASHEM is the only God — in heaven above and on the earth below — there is none other.'[1]

עַל כֵּן *Therefore we put our hope in You, HASHEM, our God, that we may soon see Your mighty splendor, to remove detestable idolatry from the earth, and false gods will be utterly cut off, to perfect the universe through the Almighty's sovereignty. Then all humanity will call upon Your Name, to turn all the earth's wicked toward You. All the world's inhabitants will recognize and know that to You every knee should bend, every tongue should swear.[2] Before You, HASHEM, our God, they will bend every knee and cast themselves down and to the glory of Your Name they will render homage, and they will all accept upon themselves the yoke of Your kingship that You may reign over them soon and eternally. For the kingdom is Yours and You will reign for all eternity in glory as it is written in Your Torah: HASHEM shall reign for all eternity.[3]* Chazzan— *And it is said: HASHEM will be King over all the world — on that day HASHEM will be One and His Name will be One.[4]*

Some congregations recite the following after *Aleinu.*

אַל תִּירָא *Do not fear sudden terror, or the holocaust of the wicked when it comes.[5] Plan a conspiracy and it will be annulled; speak your piece and it shall not stand, for God is with us.[6] Even till your seniority, I remain unchanged; and even till your ripe old age, I shall endure. I created you and I shall bear you; I shall endure and rescue.[7]*

MOURNER'S KADDISH

In the presence of a *minyan*, mourners recite קַדִּישׁ יָתוֹם, the Mourner's *Kaddish* (see *Laws* 132-134).
[A transliteration of this *Kaddish* appears on page 486.]

יִתְגַּדַּל *May His great Name grow exalted and sanctified* (Cong.— *Amen.*) *in the world that He created as He willed. May He give reign to His kingship in your lifetimes and in your days, and in the lifetimes of the entire Family of Israel, swiftly and soon. Now respond: Amen.*

(Cong.— *Amen. May His great Name be blessed forever and ever.*)

May His great Name be blessed forever and ever.

Blessed, praised, glorified, exalted, extolled, mighty, upraised, and lauded be the Name of the Holy One, Blessed is He (Cong.— *Blessed is He*) — *beyond any blessing and song, praise and consolation that are uttered in the world. Now respond: Amen.* (Cong.— *Amen*).

May there be abundant peace from Heaven, and life, upon us and upon all Israel. Now respond: Amen. (Cong.— *Amen.*)

Take three steps back. Bow left and say, 'He Who makes peace . . .';
bow right and say, 'may He . . .'; bow forward and say, 'and upon all Israel . . .'
Remain standing in place for a few moments, then take three steps forward.

He Who makes peace in His heights, may He make peace upon us, and upon all Israel. Now respond: Amen. (Cong.— *Amen.*)

---

(1) *Deuteronomy* 4:39. (2) Cf. *Isaiah* 45:23. (3) *Exodus* 15:18.
(4) *Zechariah* 14:9. (5) *Proverbs* 3:25. (6) *Isaiah* 8:10. (7) 46:4.

‮❧ השכמת הבוקר ❧‬

A Jew should wake up with gratitude to God for having restored his faculties and with a lionlike resolve to serve his Creator. Before getting off the bed or commencing any other conversation or activity, he declares his gratitude:

מוֹדֶה אֲנִי לְפָנֶיךָ, מֶלֶךְ חַי וְקַיָּם, שֶׁהֶחֱזַרְתָּ בִּי נִשְׁמָתִי בְּחֶמְלָה – רַבָּה אֱמוּנָתֶךָ.

Wash the fingers, but not the palms, according to the ritual procedure: Pick up the vessel of water with the right hand, pass it to the left, and pour water over the right. Then with the right hand pour over the left. Follow this procedure until water has been poured over each hand three times. (When the fingers are still damp, they may be used to remove mucus from the eyes.) Then, recite:

רֵאשִׁית חָכְמָה יִרְאַת יהוה, שֵׂכֶל טוֹב לְכָל עֹשֵׂיהֶם, תְּהִלָּתוֹ עֹמֶדֶת לָעַד.[1] בָּרוּךְ שֵׁם כְּבוֹד מַלְכוּתוֹ לְעוֹלָם וָעֶד.

‮❧ ציצית, טלית, ותפילין ❧‬

The *tallis kattan* (tzitzis) is worn, but the blessing is omitted.
The *tallis* and *tefillin* are not worn at *Shacharis*, but are worn at *Minchah*.

SOME CONGREGATIONS OMIT CERTAIN PASSAGES OF THE PRAYERS PRECEEDING *PESUKEI D'ZIMRAH*. CUSTOMS REGARDING WHETHER AND WHICH PASSAGES ARE OMITTED VARY GREATLY. THEREFORE WE HAVE NOT OMITTED ANY PASSAGES. EACH CONGREGATION SHOULD FOLLOW ITS ESTABLISHED CUSTOM.

‮❧ ברכות השחר ❧‬

Recite the following collection of verses upon entering the synagogue:

מַה טֹּבוּ אֹהָלֶיךָ יַעֲקֹב, מִשְׁכְּנֹתֶיךָ יִשְׂרָאֵל.[2] וַאֲנִי בְּרֹב חַסְדְּךָ אָבוֹא בֵיתֶךָ, אֶשְׁתַּחֲוֶה אֶל הֵיכַל קָדְשְׁךָ בְּיִרְאָתֶךָ.[3] יהוה אָהַבְתִּי מְעוֹן בֵּיתֶךָ, וּמְקוֹם מִשְׁכַּן כְּבוֹדֶךָ.[4] וַאֲנִי אֶשְׁתַּחֲוֶה וְאֶכְרָעָה, אֶבְרְכָה לִפְנֵי יהוה עֹשִׂי.[5] וַאֲנִי, תְפִלָּתִי לְךָ יהוה, עֵת רָצוֹן, אֱלֹהִים בְּרָב חַסְדֶּךָ, עֲנֵנִי בֶּאֱמֶת יִשְׁעֶךָ.[6]

אֲדוֹן עוֹלָם אֲשֶׁר מָלַךְ, בְּטֶרֶם כָּל יְצִיר נִבְרָא.

לְעֵת נַעֲשָׂה בְחֶפְצוֹ כֹּל, אֲזַי מֶלֶךְ שְׁמוֹ נִקְרָא.

וְאַחֲרֵי כִּכְלוֹת הַכֹּל, לְבַדּוֹ יִמְלוֹךְ נוֹרָא.

וְהוּא הָיָה וְהוּא הֹוֶה, וְהוּא יִהְיֶה בְּתִפְאָרָה.

וְהוּא אֶחָד וְאֵין שֵׁנִי, לְהַמְשִׁיל לוֹ לְהַחְבִּירָה.

בְּלִי רֵאשִׁית בְּלִי תַכְלִית, וְלוֹ הָעֹז וְהַמִּשְׂרָה.

וְהוּא אֵלִי וְחַי גֹּאֲלִי, וְצוּר חֶבְלִי בְּעֵת צָרָה.

וְהוּא נִסִּי וּמָנוֹס לִי, מְנָת כּוֹסִי בְּיוֹם אֶקְרָא.

---

(1) *Psalms* 111:10. (2) *Numbers* 24:5. (3) *Psalms* 5:8. (4) 26:8. (5) Cf. 95:6. (6) 69:14.

⅏ UPON ARISING ⅏

A Jew should wake up with gratitude to God for having restored his faculties and with a lionlike
resolve to serve his Creator. Before getting off the bed or commencing any other conversation or
activity, he declares his gratitude:

מוֹדֶה אֲנִי *I gratefully thank You, O living and eternal King, for You*
have returned my soul within me with compassion —
abundant is Your faithfulness!

Wash the fingers, but not the palms, according to the ritual procedure: Pick up the vessel of water
with the right hand, pass it to the left, and pour water over the right. Then with the right hand
pour over the left. Follow this procedure until water has been poured over each hand three times.
(When the fingers are still damp, they may be used to remove mucus from the eyes.) Then, recite:

רֵאשִׁית חָכְמָה *The beginning of wisdom is the fear of HASHEM —*
good understanding to all their practitioners; His
praise endures forever.[1] *Blessed is the Name of His glorious kingdom for*
all eternity.

⅏ TZITZIS, TALLIS, AND TEFILLIN ⅏

The *tallis kattan (tzitzis)* is worn, but the blessing is omitted.
The *tallis* and *tefillin* are not worn at *Shacharis,* but are worn at *Minchah.*

SOME CONGREGATIONS OMIT CERTAIN PASSAGES OF THE PRAYERS PRECEEDING
PESUKEI D'ZIMRAH. CUSTOMS REGARDING WHETHER AND WHICH PASSAGES
ARE OMITTED VARY GREATLY. THEREFORE WE HAVE NOT OMITTED ANY PASSAGES.
EACH CONGREGATION SHOULD FOLLOW ITS ESTABLISHED CUSTOM.

⅏ MORNING BLESSINGS ⅏

Recite the following collection of verses upon entering the synagogue:

מַה טֹּבוּ *How goodly are your tents, O Jacob, your dwelling places, O*
Israel.[2] *As for me, through Your abundant kindness I will*
enter Your House; I will prostrate myself toward Your Holy Sanctuary
in awe of You.[3] *O HASHEM, I love the House where You dwell, and the*
place where Your glory resides.[4] *I shall prostrate myself and bow, I shall*
kneel before HASHEM my Maker.[5] *As for me, may my prayer to You,*
HASHEM, be at an opportune time; O God, in Your abundant kindness,
answer me with the truth of Your salvation.[6]

אֲדוֹן עוֹלָם *Master of the universe, Who reigned*
before any form was created,
At the time when His will brought all into being —
then as 'King' was His Name proclaimed.
After all has ceased to be, He, the Awesome One, will reign alone.
It is He Who was, He Who is, and He Who shall remain, in splendor.
He is One — there is no second to compare to Him,
to declare as His equal.
Without beginning, without conclusion —
His is the power and dominion.
He is my God, my living Redeemer, Rock of my pain in time of distress.
He is my banner, a refuge for me, the portion in my cup on the day I call.

בְּעֵת אִישַׁן וְאָעִירָה,   בְּיָדוֹ אַפְקִיד רוּחִי,

יהוה לִי וְלֹא אִירָא.   וְעִם רוּחִי גְּוִיָּתִי,

נִמְצָא וְאֵין עֵת אֶל מְצִיאוּתוֹ.   **יִגְדַּל** אֱלֹהִים חַי וְיִשְׁתַּבַּח,

נֶעְלָם וְגַם אֵין סוֹף לְאַחְדּוּתוֹ.   אֶחָד וְאֵין יָחִיד כְּיִחוּדוֹ,

לֹא נַעֲרוֹךְ אֵלָיו קְדֻשָּׁתוֹ.   אֵין לוֹ דְּמוּת הַגּוּף וְאֵינוֹ גוּף,

רִאשׁוֹן וְאֵין רֵאשִׁית לְרֵאשִׁיתוֹ.   קַדְמוֹן לְכָל דָּבָר אֲשֶׁר נִבְרָא,

יוֹרֶה גְדֻלָּתוֹ וּמַלְכוּתוֹ.   הִנּוֹ אֲדוֹן עוֹלָם לְכָל נוֹצָר,

אֶל אַנְשֵׁי סְגֻלָּתוֹ וְתִפְאַרְתּוֹ.   שֶׁפַע נְבוּאָתוֹ נְתָנוֹ,

נָבִיא וּמַבִּיט אֶת תְּמוּנָתוֹ.   לֹא קָם בְּיִשְׂרָאֵל כְּמשֶׁה עוֹד,

עַל יַד נְבִיאוֹ נֶאֱמַן בֵּיתוֹ.   תּוֹרַת אֱמֶת נָתַן לְעַמּוֹ אֵל,

לְעוֹלָמִים לְזוּלָתוֹ.   לֹא יַחֲלִיף הָאֵל וְלֹא יָמִיר דָּתוֹ,

מַבִּיט לְסוֹף דָּבָר בְּקַדְמָתוֹ.   צוֹפֶה וְיוֹדֵעַ סְתָרֵינוּ,

נוֹתֵן לְרָשָׁע רָע כְּרִשְׁעָתוֹ.   גּוֹמֵל לְאִישׁ חֶסֶד כְּמִפְעָלוֹ,

לִפְדּוֹת מְחַכֵּי קֵץ יְשׁוּעָתוֹ.   יִשְׁלַח לְקֵץ הַיָּמִין מְשִׁיחֵנוּ,

בָּרוּךְ עֲדֵי עַד שֵׁם תְּהִלָּתוֹ.   מֵתִים יְחַיֶּה אֵל בְּרֹב חַסְדּוֹ,

﴾ ברכות השחר ﴿

Although many hold that the blessing עַל נְטִילַת יָדַיִם should be recited immediately after the ritual washing of the hands upon arising, others customarily recite it at this point. Similarly, some recite אֲשֶׁר יָצַר immediately after relieving themselves in the morning, while others recite it here.

בָּרוּךְ אַתָּה יהוה אֱלֹהֵינוּ מֶלֶךְ הָעוֹלָם, אֲשֶׁר קִדְּשָׁנוּ בְּמִצְוֹתָיו, וְצִוָּנוּ עַל נְטִילַת יָדָיִם.

בָּרוּךְ אַתָּה יהוה אֱלֹהֵינוּ מֶלֶךְ הָעוֹלָם, אֲשֶׁר יָצַר אֶת הָאָדָם בְּחָכְמָה, וּבָרָא בוֹ נְקָבִים נְקָבִים, חֲלוּלִים חֲלוּלִים. גָּלוּי וְיָדוּעַ לִפְנֵי כִסֵּא כְבוֹדֶךָ, שֶׁאִם יִפָּתֵחַ אֶחָד מֵהֶם, אוֹ יִסָּתֵם אֶחָד מֵהֶם, אִי אֶפְשָׁר לְהִתְקַיֵּם וְלַעֲמוֹד לְפָנֶיךָ. בָּרוּךְ אַתָּה יהוה, רוֹפֵא כָל בָּשָׂר וּמַפְלִיא לַעֲשׂוֹת.

At this point, some recite אֱלֹהַי נְשָׁמָה (p. 74).

Into His hand I shall entrust my spirit when I go to sleep —
  and I shall awaken!
With my spirit shall my body remain. HASHEM is with me,
  I shall not fear.

יִגְדַּל *Exalted be the Living God and praised,*
    He exists — unbounded by time is His existence.
He is One — and there is no unity like His Oneness.
    Inscrutable and infinite is His Oneness.
He has no semblance of a body nor is He corporeal;
    nor has His holiness any comparison.
He preceded every being that was created —
    the First, and nothing precedes His precedence.
Behold! He is Master of the universe to every creature,
    He demonstrates His greatness and His sovereignty.
He granted His flow of prophecy
    to His treasured splendrous people.
In Israel none like Moses arose again —
    a prophet who perceived His vision clearly.
God gave His people a Torah of truth,
    by means of His prophet, the most trusted of His household.
God will never amend nor exchange His law
    for any other one, for all eternity.
He scrutinizes and knows our hiddenmost secrets;
    He perceives a matter's outcome at its inception.
He recompenses man with kindness according to his deed;
    He places evil on the wicked according to his wickedness.
By the End of Days He will send our Messiah,
    to redeem those longing for His final salvation.
God will revive the dead in His abundant kindness —
    Blessed forever is His praised Name.

◈ MORNING BLESSINGS ◈

Although many hold that the blessing עַל נְטִילַת יָדַיִם, '...*regarding washing the hands,*' should be recited immediately after the ritual washing of the hands upon arising, others customarily recite it at this point. Similarly, some recite אֲשֶׁר יָצַר, '*Who fashioned* . . .,' immediately after relieving themselves in the morning, while others recite it here.

בָּרוּךְ *Blessed are You, HASHEM, our God, King of the universe, Who*
    has sanctified us with His commandments and has commanded
us regarding washing the hands.

בָּרוּךְ *Blessed are You, HASHEM, our God, King of the universe, Who*
    fashioned man with wisdom and created within him many
openings and many cavities. It is obvious and known before Your Throne
of Glory that if but one of them were to be ruptured or but one of them
were to be blocked it would be impossible to survive and to stand before
You. Blessed are You, HASHEM, Who heals all flesh and acts wondrously.

At this point, some recite אֱלֹהַי נְשָׁמָה, '*My God, the soul* . . .' (p. 74).

ברכות התורה

It is forbidden to study or recite Torah passages before reciting the following blessings. Since the commandment to study Torah is in effect all day long, these blessings need not be repeated if one studies at various times of the day. Although many *siddurim* begin a new paragraph at וְהַעֲרֶב נָא, according to the vast majority of commentators the first blessing does not end until לְעַמּוֹ יִשְׂרָאֵל.

בָּרוּךְ אַתָּה יהוה אֱלֹהֵינוּ מֶלֶךְ הָעוֹלָם, אֲשֶׁר קִדְּשָׁנוּ בְּמִצְוֹתָיו, וְצִוָּנוּ לַעֲסוֹק בְּדִבְרֵי תוֹרָה. וְהַעֲרֶב נָא יהוה אֱלֹהֵינוּ אֶת דִּבְרֵי תוֹרָתְךָ בְּפִינוּ וּבְפִי עַמְּךָ בֵּית יִשְׂרָאֵל. וְנִהְיֶה אֲנַחְנוּ וְצֶאֱצָאֵינוּ וְצֶאֱצָאֵי עַמְּךָ בֵּית יִשְׂרָאֵל, כֻּלָּנוּ יוֹדְעֵי שְׁמֶךָ וְלוֹמְדֵי תוֹרָתֶךָ לִשְׁמָהּ. בָּרוּךְ אַתָּה יהוה, הַמְלַמֵּד תּוֹרָה לְעַמּוֹ יִשְׂרָאֵל.

בָּרוּךְ אַתָּה יהוה אֱלֹהֵינוּ מֶלֶךְ הָעוֹלָם, אֲשֶׁר בָּחַר בָּנוּ מִכָּל הָעַמִּים וְנָתַן לָנוּ אֶת תּוֹרָתוֹ. בָּרוּךְ אַתָּה יהוה, נוֹתֵן הַתּוֹרָה.

במדבר ו:כד-כו

יְבָרֶכְךָ יהוה וְיִשְׁמְרֶךָ. יָאֵר יהוה פָּנָיו אֵלֶיךָ וִיחֻנֶּךָּ. יִשָּׂא יהוה פָּנָיו אֵלֶיךָ, וְיָשֵׂם לְךָ שָׁלוֹם.

משנה, פאה א:א

אֵלּוּ דְבָרִים שֶׁאֵין לָהֶם שִׁעוּר: הַפֵּאָה וְהַבִּכּוּרִים וְהָרַאְיוֹן וּגְמִילוּת חֲסָדִים וְתַלְמוּד תּוֹרָה.

שבת קכז.

אֵלּוּ דְבָרִים שֶׁאָדָם אוֹכֵל פֵּרוֹתֵיהֶם בָּעוֹלָם הַזֶּה וְהַקֶּרֶן קַיֶּמֶת לוֹ לָעוֹלָם הַבָּא. וְאֵלּוּ הֵן: כִּבּוּד אָב וָאֵם, וּגְמִילוּת חֲסָדִים, וְהַשְׁכָּמַת בֵּית הַמִּדְרָשׁ שַׁחֲרִית וְעַרְבִית, וְהַכְנָסַת אוֹרְחִים, וּבִקּוּר חוֹלִים, וְהַכְנָסַת כַּלָּה, וּלְוָיַת הַמֵּת, וְעִיּוּן תְּפִלָּה, וַהֲבָאַת שָׁלוֹם בֵּין אָדָם לַחֲבֵרוֹ — וְתַלְמוּד תּוֹרָה כְּנֶגֶד כֻּלָּם.

אֱלֹהַי, נְשָׁמָה שֶׁנָּתַתָּ בִּי טְהוֹרָה הִיא. אַתָּה בְרָאתָהּ אַתָּה יְצַרְתָּהּ, אַתָּה נְפַחְתָּהּ בִּי, וְאַתָּה מְשַׁמְּרָהּ בְּקִרְבִּי, וְאַתָּה עָתִיד לִטְּלָהּ מִמֶּנִּי, וּלְהַחֲזִירָהּ בִּי לֶעָתִיד לָבֹא. כָּל זְמַן שֶׁהַנְּשָׁמָה בְקִרְבִּי, מוֹדֶה אֲנִי לְפָנֶיךָ, יהוה אֱלֹהַי וֵאלֹהֵי אֲבוֹתַי, רִבּוֹן כָּל הַמַּעֲשִׂים, אֲדוֹן כָּל הַנְּשָׁמוֹת. בָּרוּךְ אַתָּה יהוה, הַמַּחֲזִיר נְשָׁמוֹת לִפְגָרִים מֵתִים.

BLESSINGS OF THE TORAH

It is forbidden to study or recite Torah passages before reciting the following blessings. Since the commandment to study Torah is in effect all day long, these blessings need not be repeated if one studies at various times of the day. Although many *siddurim* begin a new paragraph at וְהַעֲרֶב נָא, 'Please, HASHEM,' according to the vast majority of commentators the first blessing does not end until לְעַמּוֹ יִשְׂרָאֵל, '. . . His people Israel.'

בָּרוּךְ   *Blessed are You, HASHEM, our God, King of the universe, Who has sanctified us with His commandments and has commanded us to engross ourselves in the words of Torah. Please, HASHEM, our God, sweeten the words of Your Torah in our mouth and in the mouth of Your people, the family of Israel. May we and our offspring and the offspring of Your people, the House of Israel — all of us — know Your Name and study Your Torah for its own sake. Blessed are You, HASHEM, Who teaches Torah to His people Israel.*

בָּרוּךְ   *Blessed are You, HASHEM, our God, King of the universe, Who selected us from all the peoples and gave us His Torah. Blessed are You, HASHEM, Giver of the Torah.*

Numbers 6:24-26

יְבָרֶכְךָ   *May HASHEM bless you and safeguard you. May HASHEM illuminate His countenance for you and be gracious to you. May HASHEM turn His countenance to you and establish peace for you.*

Mishnah, Peah 1:1

אֵלּוּ דְבָרִים   *These are the precepts that have no prescribed measure: the corner of a field [which must be left for the poor], the first-fruit offering, the pilgrimage, acts of kindness, and Torah study.*

Talmud, Shabbos 127a

אֵלּוּ דְבָרִים   *These are the precepts whose fruits a person enjoys in This World but whose principal remains intact for him in the World to Come. They are: the honor due to father and mother, acts of kindness, early attendance at the house of study morning and evening, hospitality to guests, visiting the sick, providing for a bride, escorting the dead, absorption in prayer, bringing peace between man and his fellow — and the study of Torah is equivalent to them all.*

אֱלֹהַי   *My God, the soul You placed within me is pure. You created it, You fashioned it, You breathed it into me, You safeguard it within me, and eventually You will take it from me, and restore it to me in Time to Come. As long as the soul is within me, I gratefully thank You, HASHEM, my God and the God of my forefathers, Master of all works, Lord of all souls. Blessed are You, HASHEM, Who restores souls to dead bodies.*

The *chazzan* recites the following blessings aloud, and the congregation responds אָמֵן to each blessing. Nevertheless, each person must recite these blessings for himself. Some people recite the blessings aloud for one another so that each one can have the merit of responding אָמֵן many times.

בָּרוּךְ אַתָּה יהוה אֱלֹהֵינוּ מֶלֶךְ הָעוֹלָם, אֲשֶׁר נָתַן לַשֶּׂכְוִי בִינָה¹ לְהַבְחִין בֵּין יוֹם וּבֵין לָיְלָה.

בָּרוּךְ אַתָּה יהוה אֱלֹהֵינוּ מֶלֶךְ הָעוֹלָם, שֶׁלֹּא עָשַׂנִי גּוֹי.

בָּרוּךְ אַתָּה יהוה אֱלֹהֵינוּ מֶלֶךְ הָעוֹלָם, שֶׁלֹּא עָשַׂנִי עָבֶד.

Women say:	*Men say:*
בָּרוּךְ אַתָּה יהוה אֱלֹהֵינוּ מֶלֶךְ הָעוֹלָם, שֶׁלֹּא עָשַׂנִי אִשָּׁה.	בָּרוּךְ אַתָּה יהוה אֱלֹהֵינוּ מֶלֶךְ הָעוֹלָם, שֶׁעָשַׂנִי כִּרְצוֹנוֹ.

בָּרוּךְ אַתָּה יהוה אֱלֹהֵינוּ מֶלֶךְ הָעוֹלָם, פּוֹקֵחַ עִוְרִים.²

בָּרוּךְ אַתָּה יהוה אֱלֹהֵינוּ מֶלֶךְ הָעוֹלָם, מַלְבִּישׁ עֲרֻמִּים.

בָּרוּךְ אַתָּה יהוה אֱלֹהֵינוּ מֶלֶךְ הָעוֹלָם, מַתִּיר אֲסוּרִים.³

בָּרוּךְ אַתָּה יהוה אֱלֹהֵינוּ מֶלֶךְ הָעוֹלָם, זוֹקֵף כְּפוּפִים.²

בָּרוּךְ אַתָּה יהוה אֱלֹהֵינוּ מֶלֶךְ הָעוֹלָם, רוֹקַע הָאָרֶץ עַל הַמָּיִם.⁴

Some postpone the recital of this blessing until they don leather shoes after the fast has ended.

בָּרוּךְ אַתָּה יהוה אֱלֹהֵינוּ מֶלֶךְ הָעוֹלָם, שֶׁעָשָׂה לִי כָּל צָרְכִּי.

בָּרוּךְ אַתָּה יהוה אֱלֹהֵינוּ מֶלֶךְ הָעוֹלָם, הַמֵּכִין מִצְעֲדֵי גָבֶר.⁵

בָּרוּךְ אַתָּה יהוה אֱלֹהֵינוּ מֶלֶךְ הָעוֹלָם, אוֹזֵר יִשְׂרָאֵל בִּגְבוּרָה.

בָּרוּךְ אַתָּה יהוה אֱלֹהֵינוּ מֶלֶךְ הָעוֹלָם, עוֹטֵר יִשְׂרָאֵל בְּתִפְאָרָה.

בָּרוּךְ אַתָּה יהוה אֱלֹהֵינוּ מֶלֶךְ הָעוֹלָם, הַנּוֹתֵן לַיָּעֵף כֹּחַ.⁶

Although many *siddurim* begin a new paragraph at וִיהִי רָצוֹן, the following is one long blessing that ends at לְעַמּוֹ יִשְׂרָאֵל.

בָּרוּךְ אַתָּה יהוה אֱלֹהֵינוּ מֶלֶךְ הָעוֹלָם, הַמַּעֲבִיר שֵׁנָה מֵעֵינַי וּתְנוּמָה מֵעַפְעַפָּי. וִיהִי רָצוֹן מִלְּפָנֶיךָ, יהוה אֱלֹהֵינוּ וֵאלֹהֵי אֲבוֹתֵינוּ, שֶׁתַּרְגִּילֵנוּ בְּתוֹרָתֶךָ וְדַבְּקֵנוּ בְּמִצְוֹתֶיךָ, וְאַל תְּבִיאֵנוּ לֹא לִידֵי חֵטְא, וְלֹא לִידֵי עֲבֵרָה וְעָוֹן, וְלֹא לִידֵי נִסָּיוֹן, וְלֹא לִידֵי בִזָּיוֹן, וְאַל תַּשְׁלֶט בָּנוּ יֵצֶר הָרָע. וְהַרְחִיקֵנוּ מֵאָדָם רָע וּמֵחָבֵר רָע. וְדַבְּקֵנוּ בְּיֵצֶר הַטּוֹב וּבְמַעֲשִׂים טוֹבִים, וְכוֹף אֶת יִצְרֵנוּ לְהִשְׁתַּעְבֶּד לָךְ. וּתְנֵנוּ הַיּוֹם וּבְכָל יוֹם לְחֵן וּלְחֶסֶד וּלְרַחֲמִים בְּעֵינֶיךָ, וּבְעֵינֵי כָל רוֹאֵינוּ, וְתִגְמְלֵנוּ חֲסָדִים טוֹבִים. בָּרוּךְ אַתָּה יהוה, גּוֹמֵל חֲסָדִים טוֹבִים לְעַמּוֹ יִשְׂרָאֵל.

---

(1) Cf. *Job* 38:36. (2) *Psalms* 146:8. (3) v. 7. (4) Cf. 136:6. (5) Cf. 37:23. (6) *Isaiah* 40:29.

The *chazzan* recites the following blessings aloud, and the congregation responds *'Amen'* to each blessing. Nevertheless, each person must recite these blessings for himself. Some people recite the blessings aloud for one another so that each one can have the merit of responding *Amen* many times.

בָּרוּךְ Blessed are You, HASHEM, our God, King of the universe, Who gave the heart understanding[1] to distinguish between day and night.

Blessed are You, HASHEM, our God, King of the universe, for not having made me a gentile.

Blessed are You, HASHEM, our God, King of the universe, for not having made me a slave.

Men say:	Women say:
Blessed are You, HASHEM, our God, King of the universe, for not having made me a woman.	Blessed are You, HASHEM, our God, King of the universe, for having made me according to His will.

Blessed are You, HASHEM, our God, King of the universe, Who gives sight to the blind.[2]

Blessed are You, HASHEM, our God, King of the universe, Who clothes the naked.

Blessed are You, HASHEM, our God, King of the universe, Who releases the bound.[3]

Blessed are You, HASHEM, our God, King of the universe, Who straightens the bent.[2]

Blessed are You, HASHEM, our God, King of the universe, Who spreads out the earth upon the waters.[4]

Some postpone the recital of this blessing until they don leather shoes after the fast has ended.

Blessed are You, HASHEM, our God, King of the universe, Who has provided me my every need.

Blessed are You, HASHEM, our God, King of the universe, Who firms man's footsteps.[5]

Blessed are You, HASHEM, our God, King of the universe, Who girds Israel with strength.

Blessed are You, HASHEM, our God, King of the universe, Who crowns Israel with splendor.

Blessed are You, HASHEM, our God, King of the universe, Who gives strength to the weary.[6]

בָּרוּךְ Blessed are You, HASHEM, our God, King of the universe, Who removes sleep from my eyes and slumber from my eyelids. And may it be Your will, HASHEM, our God, and the God of our forefathers, that You accustom us to [study] Your Torah and attach us to Your commandments. Do not bring us into the power of error, nor into the power of transgression and sin, nor into the power of challenge, nor into the power of scorn. Let not the Evil Inclination dominate us. Distance us from an evil person and an evil companion. Attach us to the Good Inclination and to good deeds and compel our Evil Inclination to be subservient to You. Grant us today and every day grace, kindness, and mercy in Your eyes and in the eyes of all who see us, and bestow beneficent kindnesses upon us. Blessed are You, HASHEM, Who bestows beneficent kindnesses upon His people Israel.

יְהִי רָצוֹן מִלְּפָנֶיךָ, יהוה אֱלֹהַי וֵאלֹהֵי אֲבוֹתַי, שֶׁתַּצִּילֵנִי הַיּוֹם וּבְכָל יוֹם מֵעַזֵּי פָנִים וּמֵעַזּוּת פָּנִים, מֵאָדָם רָע, וּמֵחָבֵר רָע, וּמִשָּׁכֵן רָע, וּמִפֶּגַע רָע, וּמִשָּׂטָן הַמַּשְׁחִית, מִדִּין קָשֶׁה וּמִבַּעַל דִּין קָשֶׁה, בֵּין שֶׁהוּא בֶן בְּרִית, וּבֵין שֶׁאֵינוֹ בֶן בְּרִית.

⦑ עקדה ⦒

אֱלֹהֵינוּ וֵאלֹהֵי אֲבוֹתֵינוּ, זָכְרֵנוּ בְּזִכָּרוֹן טוֹב לְפָנֶיךָ, וּפָקְדֵנוּ בִּפְקֻדַּת יְשׁוּעָה וְרַחֲמִים מִשְּׁמֵי שְׁמֵי קֶדֶם. וּזְכָר לָנוּ יהוה אֱלֹהֵינוּ אַהֲבַת הַקַּדְמוֹנִים אַבְרָהָם יִצְחָק וְיִשְׂרָאֵל עֲבָדֶיךָ, אֶת הַבְּרִית וְאֶת הַחֶסֶד וְאֶת הַשְּׁבוּעָה שֶׁנִּשְׁבַּעְתָּ לְאַבְרָהָם אָבִינוּ בְּהַר הַמּוֹרִיָּה, וְאֶת הָעֲקֵדָה שֶׁעָקַד אֶת יִצְחָק בְּנוֹ עַל גַּבֵּי הַמִּזְבֵּחַ, כַּכָּתוּב בְּתוֹרָתֶךָ:

בראשית כב:א-יט

וַיְהִי אַחַר הַדְּבָרִים הָאֵלֶּה, וְהָאֱלֹהִים נִסָּה אֶת אַבְרָהָם, וַיֹּאמֶר אֵלָיו, אַבְרָהָם, וַיֹּאמֶר, הִנֵּנִי. וַיֹּאמֶר, קַח נָא אֶת בִּנְךָ, אֶת יְחִידְךָ, אֲשֶׁר אָהַבְתָּ, אֶת יִצְחָק, וְלֶךְ לְךָ אֶל אֶרֶץ הַמֹּרִיָּה, וְהַעֲלֵהוּ שָׁם לְעֹלָה עַל אַחַד הֶהָרִים אֲשֶׁר אֹמַר אֵלֶיךָ. וַיַּשְׁכֵּם אַבְרָהָם בַּבֹּקֶר, וַיַּחֲבֹשׁ אֶת חֲמֹרוֹ, וַיִּקַּח אֶת שְׁנֵי נְעָרָיו אִתּוֹ, וְאֵת יִצְחָק בְּנוֹ, וַיְבַקַּע עֲצֵי עֹלָה, וַיָּקָם וַיֵּלֶךְ אֶל הַמָּקוֹם אֲשֶׁר אָמַר לוֹ הָאֱלֹהִים. בַּיּוֹם הַשְּׁלִישִׁי, וַיִּשָּׂא אַבְרָהָם אֶת עֵינָיו, וַיַּרְא אֶת הַמָּקוֹם מֵרָחֹק. וַיֹּאמֶר אַבְרָהָם אֶל נְעָרָיו, שְׁבוּ לָכֶם פֹּה עִם הַחֲמוֹר, וַאֲנִי וְהַנַּעַר נֵלְכָה עַד כֹּה, וְנִשְׁתַּחֲוֶה וְנָשׁוּבָה אֲלֵיכֶם. וַיִּקַּח אַבְרָהָם אֶת עֲצֵי הָעֹלָה, וַיָּשֶׂם עַל יִצְחָק בְּנוֹ, וַיִּקַּח בְּיָדוֹ אֶת הָאֵשׁ וְאֶת הַמַּאֲכֶלֶת, וַיֵּלְכוּ שְׁנֵיהֶם יַחְדָּו. וַיֹּאמֶר יִצְחָק אֶל אַבְרָהָם אָבִיו, וַיֹּאמֶר, אָבִי, וַיֹּאמֶר, הִנֶּנִּי בְנִי, וַיֹּאמֶר, הִנֵּה הָאֵשׁ וְהָעֵצִים, וְאַיֵּה הַשֶּׂה לְעֹלָה. וַיֹּאמֶר אַבְרָהָם, אֱלֹהִים יִרְאֶה לּוֹ הַשֶּׂה לְעֹלָה, בְּנִי, וַיֵּלְכוּ שְׁנֵיהֶם יַחְדָּו. וַיָּבֹאוּ אֶל הַמָּקוֹם אֲשֶׁר אָמַר לוֹ הָאֱלֹהִים, וַיִּבֶן שָׁם אַבְרָהָם אֶת הַמִּזְבֵּחַ, וַיַּעֲרֹךְ אֶת הָעֵצִים, וַיַּעֲקֹד אֶת יִצְחָק בְּנוֹ, וַיָּשֶׂם אֹתוֹ עַל הַמִּזְבֵּחַ מִמַּעַל לָעֵצִים. וַיִּשְׁלַח אַבְרָהָם אֶת יָדוֹ, וַיִּקַּח אֶת הַמַּאֲכֶלֶת לִשְׁחֹט אֶת בְּנוֹ. וַיִּקְרָא אֵלָיו מַלְאַךְ יהוה מִן הַשָּׁמַיִם, וַיֹּאמֶר, אַבְרָהָם, אַבְרָהָם, וַיֹּאמֶר, הִנֵּנִי. וַיֹּאמֶר, אַל תִּשְׁלַח יָדְךָ אֶל הַנַּעַר, וְאַל תַּעַשׂ לוֹ מְאוּמָה, כִּי עַתָּה יָדַעְתִּי כִּי

יְהִי רָצוֹן   May it be Your will, HASHEM, my God, and the God of my
forefathers, that You rescue me today and every day from
brazen men and from brazenness, from an evil man, an evil companion, an
evil neighbor, an evil mishap, the destructive spiritual impediment, a harsh
trial and a harsh opponent, whether he is a member of the covenant or
whether he is not a member of the covenant.

◆❧ THE AKEIDAH ❧◆

אֱלֹהֵינוּ   Our God and the God of our forefathers, remember us with a favorable
memory before You, and recall us with a recollection of salvation and
mercy from the primeval loftiest heavens. Remember on our behalf — O HASHEM,
our God — the love of the Patriarchs, Abraham, Isaac and Israel, Your servants;
the covenant, the kindness, and the oath that You swore to our father Abraham
at Mount Moriah, and the Akeidah, when he bound his son Isaac atop the altar,
as it is written in Your Torah:

Genesis 22:1-19

וַיְהִי   And it happened after these things that God tested Abraham
and said to him, 'Abraham.'

And he replied, 'Here I am.'

And He said, 'Please take your son, your only one, whom you love —
Isaac — and get yourself to the Land of Moriah; bring him up there as an
offering, upon one of the mountains which I shall indicate to you.'

So Abraham awoke early in the morning and he saddled his donkey; he
took his two young men with him, and Isaac, his son. He split the wood for
the offering, and rose and went toward the place which God had indicated
to him.

On the third day, Abraham looked up, and perceived the place from
afar. And Abraham said to his young men, 'Stay here by yourselves with
the donkey, while I and the lad will go yonder; we will prostrate ourselves
and we will return to you.'

And Abraham took the wood for the offering, and placed it on Isaac, his
son. He took in his hand the fire and the knife, and the two of them went
together. Then Isaac spoke to Abraham his father and said, 'Father — '

And he said, 'Here I am, my son.'

And he said, 'Here are the fire and the wood, but where is the lamb for
the offering?'

And Abraham said, 'God will seek out for Himself the lamb for the
offering, my son.' And the two of them went together.

They arrived at the place which God indicated to him. Abraham built the
altar there, and arranged the wood; he bound Isaac, his son, and he placed
him on the altar atop the wood. Abraham stretched out his hand, and took
the knife to slaughter his son.

And an angel of HASHEM called to him from heaven, and said, 'Abraham!
Abraham!'

And he said, 'Here I am.'

And he [the angel quoting HASHEM] said, 'Do not stretch out your hand
against the lad nor do anything to him, for now I know that you are a

יְרֵא אֱלֹהִים אַתָּה, וְלֹא חָשַׂכְתָּ אֶת בִּנְךָ אֶת יְחִידְךָ מִמֶּנִּי. וַיִּשָּׂא אַבְרָהָם אֶת עֵינָיו וַיַּרְא, וְהִנֵּה אַיִל, אַחַר, נֶאֱחַז בַּסְּבַךְ בְּקַרְנָיו, וַיֵּלֶךְ אַבְרָהָם וַיִּקַּח אֶת הָאַיִל, וַיַּעֲלֵהוּ לְעֹלָה תַּחַת בְּנוֹ. וַיִּקְרָא אַבְרָהָם שֵׁם הַמָּקוֹם הַהוּא יְהוָה יִרְאֶה, אֲשֶׁר יֵאָמֵר הַיּוֹם, בְּהַר יְהוָה יֵרָאֶה. וַיִּקְרָא מַלְאַךְ יְהוָה אֶל אַבְרָהָם, שֵׁנִית מִן הַשָּׁמָיִם. וַיֹּאמֶר, בִּי נִשְׁבַּעְתִּי נְאֻם יְהוָה, כִּי יַעַן אֲשֶׁר עָשִׂיתָ אֶת הַדָּבָר הַזֶּה, וְלֹא חָשַׂכְתָּ אֶת בִּנְךָ אֶת יְחִידֶךָ. כִּי בָרֵךְ אֲבָרֶכְךָ, וְהַרְבָּה אַרְבֶּה אֶת זַרְעֲךָ כְּכוֹכְבֵי הַשָּׁמַיִם, וְכַחוֹל אֲשֶׁר עַל שְׂפַת הַיָּם, וְיִרַשׁ זַרְעֲךָ אֵת שַׁעַר אֹיְבָיו. וְהִתְבָּרְכוּ בְזַרְעֲךָ כֹּל גּוֹיֵי הָאָרֶץ, עֵקֶב אֲשֶׁר שָׁמַעְתָּ בְּקֹלִי. וַיָּשָׁב אַבְרָהָם אֶל נְעָרָיו, וַיָּקֻמוּ וַיֵּלְכוּ יַחְדָּו אֶל בְּאֵר שָׁבַע, וַיֵּשֶׁב אַבְרָהָם בִּבְאֵר שָׁבַע.

רִבּוֹנוֹ שֶׁל עוֹלָם, יְהִי רָצוֹן מִלְּפָנֶיךָ, יְהוָה אֱלֹהֵינוּ וֵאלֹהֵי אֲבוֹתֵינוּ, שֶׁתִּזְכָּר לָנוּ בְּרִית אֲבוֹתֵינוּ. כְּמוֹ שֶׁכָּבַשׁ אַבְרָהָם אָבִינוּ אֶת רַחֲמָיו מִבֶּן יְחִידוֹ, וְרָצָה לִשְׁחוֹט אוֹתוֹ כְּדֵי לַעֲשׂוֹת רְצוֹנֶךָ, כֵּן יִכְבְּשׁוּ רַחֲמֶיךָ אֶת כַּעַסְךָ מֵעָלֵינוּ, וְיָגֹלּוּ רַחֲמֶיךָ עַל מִדּוֹתֶיךָ, וְתִכָּנֵס אִתָּנוּ לִפְנִים מִשּׁוּרַת דִּינֶךָ, וְתִתְנַהֵג עִמָּנוּ, יְהוָה אֱלֹהֵינוּ, בְּמִדַּת הַחֶסֶד וּבְמִדַּת הָרַחֲמִים. וּבְטוּבְךָ הַגָּדוֹל, יָשׁוּב חֲרוֹן אַפְּךָ מֵעַמְּךָ וּמֵעִירְךָ וּמֵאַרְצְךָ וּמִנַּחֲלָתֶךָ. וְקַיֶּם לָנוּ, יְהוָה אֱלֹהֵינוּ, אֶת הַדָּבָר שֶׁהִבְטַחְתָּנוּ עַל יְדֵי מֹשֶׁה עַבְדֶּךָ, כָּאָמוּר: וְזָכַרְתִּי אֶת בְּרִיתִי יַעֲקוֹב, וְאַף אֶת בְּרִיתִי יִצְחָק, וְאַף אֶת בְּרִיתִי אַבְרָהָם אֶזְכֹּר, וְהָאָרֶץ אֶזְכֹּר.[1]

לְעוֹלָם יְהֵא אָדָם יְרֵא שָׁמַיִם בְּסֵתֶר וּבְגָלוּי, וּמוֹדֶה עַל הָאֱמֶת, וְדוֹבֵר אֱמֶת בִּלְבָבוֹ, וְיַשְׁכֵּם וְיֹאמַר:

רִבּוֹן כָּל הָעוֹלָמִים, לֹא עַל צִדְקוֹתֵינוּ אֲנַחְנוּ מַפִּילִים תַּחֲנוּנֵינוּ לְפָנֶיךָ, כִּי עַל רַחֲמֶיךָ הָרַבִּים. מָה אֲנַחְנוּ, מֶה חַיֵּינוּ, מֶה חַסְדֵּנוּ, מַה צִּדְקוֹתֵינוּ, מַה יְשׁוּעָתֵנוּ, מַה כֹּחֵנוּ, מַה גְּבוּרָתֵנוּ. מַה נֹּאמַר לְפָנֶיךָ, יְהוָה אֱלֹהֵינוּ וֵאלֹהֵי אֲבוֹתֵינוּ, הֲלֹא כָּל הַגִּבּוֹרִים כְּאַיִן לְפָנֶיךָ, וְאַנְשֵׁי הַשֵּׁם כְּלֹא הָיוּ, וַחֲכָמִים כִּבְלִי מַדָּע, וּנְבוֹנִים כִּבְלִי הַשְׂכֵּל. כִּי רוֹב מַעֲשֵׂיהֶם תֹּהוּ, וִימֵי חַיֵּיהֶם הֶבֶל לְפָנֶיךָ, וּמוֹתַר הָאָדָם מִן הַבְּהֵמָה אָיִן, כִּי הַכֹּל הָבֶל.[2]

אֲבָל אֲנַחְנוּ עַמְּךָ, בְּנֵי בְרִיתֶךָ, בְּנֵי אַבְרָהָם אֹהַבְךָ שֶׁנִּשְׁבַּעְתָּ לּוֹ בְּהַר הַמּוֹרִיָּה, זֶרַע יִצְחָק יְחִידוֹ שֶׁנֶּעֱקַד עַל גַּב הַמִּזְבֵּחַ,

God-fearing man, since you have not withheld your son, your only one, from Me.'

And Abraham looked up and saw — behold a ram! — after it had been caught in the thicket by its horns. So Abraham went and took the ram and brought it as an offering instead of his son. And Abraham named that site 'HASHEM Yireh,' as it is said this day: On the mountain HASHEM is seen.

The angel of HASHEM called to Abraham, a second time from heaven, and said, " 'By Myself I swear,' declared HASHEM, 'that since you have done this thing, and have not withheld your son, your only one, I shall surely bless you and greatly increase your offspring like the stars of the heavens and like the sand on the seashore; and your offspring shall inherit the gate of its enemy; and all the nations of the earth shall bless themselves by your offspring, because you have listened to My voice.' "

Abraham returned to his young men, and they rose and went together to Beer Sheba, and Abraham stayed at Beer Sheba.

רִבּוֹנוֹ שֶׁל עוֹלָם Master of the universe! May it be Your will, HASHEM, our God, and the God of our forefathers, that You remember for our sake the covenant of our forefathers. Just as Abraham our forefather suppressed his mercy for his only son and wished to slaughter him in order to do Your will, so may Your mercy suppress Your anger from upon us and may Your mercy overwhelm Your attributes. May You overstep with us the line of Your law and deal with us — O HASHEM, our God — with the attribute of kindness and the attribute of mercy. In Your great goodness may You turn aside Your burning wrath from Your people, Your city, Your land, and Your heritage. Fulfill for us, HASHEM, our God, the word You pledged through Moses, Your servant, as it is said: 'I shall remember My covenant with Jacob; also My covenant with Isaac, and also My covenant with Abraham shall I remember; and the land shall I remember.'[1]

לְעוֹלָם Always let a person be God-fearing privately and publicly, acknowledge the truth, speak the truth within his heart, and arise early and proclaim:

Master of all worlds! Not in the merit of our righteousness do we cast our supplications before You, but in the merit of Your abundant mercy. What are we? What is our life? What is our kindness? What is our righteousness? What is our salvation? What is our strength? What is our might? What can we say before You, HASHEM, our God, and the God of our forefathers — are not all the heroes like nothing before You, the famous as if they had never existed, the wise as if devoid of wisdom and the perceptive as if devoid of intelligence? For most of their deeds are desolate and the days of their lives are empty before You. The pre-eminence of man over beast is non-existent for all is vain.[2]

But we are Your people, members of Your covenant, children of Abraham, Your beloved, to whom You took an oath at Mount Moriah; the offspring of Isaac, his only son, who was bound atop the altar;

(1) Leviticus 26:42. (2) Ecclesiastes 3:19.

עֲדַת יַעֲקֹב בִּנְךָ בְּכוֹרֶךָ, שֶׁמֵּאַהֲבָתְךָ שֶׁאָהַבְתָּ אוֹתוֹ וּמִשִּׂמְחָתְךָ שֶׁשָּׂמַחְתָּ בּוֹ, קָרָאתָ אֶת שְׁמוֹ יִשְׂרָאֵל וִישֻׁרוּן.

לְפִיכָךְ אֲנַחְנוּ חַיָּבִים לְהוֹדוֹת לְךָ, וּלְשַׁבֵּחֲךָ, וּלְפָאֶרְךָ, וּלְבָרֵךְ וּלְקַדֵּשׁ וְלָתֵת שֶׁבַח וְהוֹדָיָה לִשְׁמֶךָ. אַשְׁרֵינוּ, מַה טּוֹב חֶלְקֵנוּ, וּמַה נָּעִים גּוֹרָלֵנוּ, וּמַה יָּפָה יְרֻשָּׁתֵנוּ. ✧ אַשְׁרֵינוּ, שֶׁאֲנַחְנוּ מַשְׁכִּימִים וּמַעֲרִיבִים, עֶרֶב וָבֹקֶר וְאוֹמְרִים פַּעֲמַיִם בְּכָל יוֹם:

שְׁמַע יִשְׂרָאֵל, יהוה אֱלֹהֵינוּ, יהוה אֶחָד. [1]
בָּרוּךְ שֵׁם כְּבוֹד מַלְכוּתוֹ לְעוֹלָם וָעֶד. — In an undertone

Some congregations complete the first chapter of the *Shema* (following paragraph) at this point, although most omit it. However if you fear that you will not recite the full *Shema* later in *Shacharis* before the prescribed time has elapsed, recite all three chapters of *Shema* (p. 118-120) here.

דברים ו:ה-ט

וְאָהַבְתָּ אֵת יהוה אֱלֹהֶיךָ, בְּכָל לְבָבְךָ, וּבְכָל נַפְשְׁךָ, וּבְכָל מְאֹדֶךָ. וְהָיוּ הַדְּבָרִים הָאֵלֶּה, אֲשֶׁר אָנֹכִי מְצַוְּךָ הַיּוֹם, עַל לְבָבֶךָ. וְשִׁנַּנְתָּם לְבָנֶיךָ, וְדִבַּרְתָּ בָּם, בְּשִׁבְתְּךָ בְּבֵיתֶךָ, וּבְלֶכְתְּךָ בַדֶּרֶךְ, וּבְשָׁכְבְּךָ וּבְקוּמֶךָ. וּקְשַׁרְתָּם לְאוֹת עַל יָדֶךָ, וְהָיוּ לְטֹטָפֹת בֵּין עֵינֶיךָ. וּכְתַבְתָּם עַל מְזֻזוֹת בֵּיתֶךָ וּבִשְׁעָרֶיךָ.

אַתָּה הוּא עַד שֶׁלֹּא נִבְרָא הָעוֹלָם, אַתָּה הוּא מִשֶּׁנִּבְרָא הָעוֹלָם, אַתָּה הוּא בָּעוֹלָם הַזֶּה, וְאַתָּה הוּא לָעוֹלָם הַבָּא. ✧ קַדֵּשׁ אֶת שִׁמְךָ עַל מַקְדִּישֵׁי שְׁמֶךָ, וְקַדֵּשׁ אֶת שִׁמְךָ בְּעוֹלָמֶךָ. וּבִישׁוּעָתְךָ תָּרִים וְתַגְבִּיהַּ קַרְנֵנוּ. בָּרוּךְ אַתָּה יהוה, מְקַדֵּשׁ אֶת שִׁמְךָ בָּרַבִּים. (אָמֵן. —Cong.)

אַתָּה הוּא יהוה אֱלֹהֵינוּ, בַּשָּׁמַיִם וּבָאָרֶץ וּבִשְׁמֵי הַשָּׁמַיִם הָעֶלְיוֹנִים. אֱמֶת, אַתָּה הוּא רִאשׁוֹן, וְאַתָּה הוּא אַחֲרוֹן, וּמִבַּלְעָדֶיךָ אֵין אֱלֹהִים. [2] קַבֵּץ קוֹיֶךָ מֵאַרְבַּע כַּנְפוֹת הָאָרֶץ. יַכִּירוּ וְיֵדְעוּ כָּל בָּאֵי עוֹלָם כִּי אַתָּה הוּא הָאֱלֹהִים לְבַדְּךָ לְכָל מַמְלְכוֹת הָאָרֶץ. אַתָּה עָשִׂיתָ אֶת הַשָּׁמַיִם וְאֶת הָאָרֶץ, [3] אֶת הַיָּם, וְאֶת כָּל אֲשֶׁר בָּם. וּמִי בְּכָל מַעֲשֵׂה יָדֶיךָ בָּעֶלְיוֹנִים אוֹ בַתַּחְתּוֹנִים שֶׁיֹּאמַר לְךָ, מַה תַּעֲשֶׂה. אָבִינוּ שֶׁבַּשָּׁמַיִם, עֲשֵׂה עִמָּנוּ חֶסֶד בַּעֲבוּר שִׁמְךָ הַגָּדוֹל שֶׁנִּקְרָא עָלֵינוּ, וְקַיֶּם לָנוּ יהוה אֱלֹהֵינוּ מַה שֶּׁכָּתוּב: בָּעֵת הַהִיא אָבִיא אֶתְכֶם, וּבָעֵת קַבְּצִי אֶתְכֶם, כִּי אֶתֵּן אֶתְכֶם לְשֵׁם וְלִתְהִלָּה בְּכֹל עַמֵּי הָאָרֶץ, בְּשׁוּבִי אֶת שְׁבוּתֵיכֶם לְעֵינֵיכֶם, אָמַר יהוה. [4]

the community of Jacob, Your firstborn son, whom — because of the love with which You adored him and the joy with which You delighted in him — You named Israel and Jeshurun.

לְפִיכָךְ Therefore, we are obliged to thank You, praise You, glorify You, bless, sanctify, and offer praise and thanks to Your Name. We are fortunate — how good is our portion, how pleasant our lot, and how beautiful our heritage! Chazzan— We are fortunate for we come early and stay late, evening and morning, and proclaim twice each day:

Hear, O Israel: Hashem is our God, Hashem, the One and Only.[1]

In an undertone— *Blessed is the Name of His glorious kingdom for all eternity.*

Some congregations complete the first chapter of the *Shema* (following paragraph) at this point, although most omit it. However if you fear that you will not recite the full *Shema* later in *Shacharis* before the prescribed time has elapsed, recite all three chapters of *Shema* (p. 118-120) here.

Deuteronomy 6:5-9

וְאָהַבְתָּ You shall love Hashem, your God, with all your heart, with all your soul and with all your resources. Let these matters, which I command you today, be upon your heart. Teach them thoroughly to your children and speak of them while you sit in your home, while you walk on the way, when you retire and when you arise. Bind them as a sign upon your arm and let them be tefillin between your eyes. And write them on the doorposts of your house and upon your gates.

אַתָּה It was You before the world was created, it is You since the world was created, it is You in This World, and it is You in the World to Come. Chazzan— Sanctify Your Name through those who sanctify Your Name, and sanctify Your Name in Your universe. Through Your salvation may You exalt and raise our pride. Blessed are You, Hashem, Who sanctifies Your Name among the multitudes.

(*Cong.*— *Amen.*)

אַתָּה It is You Who are Hashem, our God, in heaven and on earth and in the loftiest heavens. True — You are the First and You are the Last, and other than You there is no God.[2] Gather in those who yearn for You, from the four corners of the earth. Let all who walk the earth recognize and know that You alone are the God over all the kingdoms of the earth. You have made the heavens, the earth,[3] the sea, and all that is in them. Who among all Your handiwork, those above and those below, can say to You, 'What are You doing?' Our Father in Heaven, do kindness with us for the sake of Your great Name that has been proclaimed upon us. Fulfill for us, Hashem, our God, what is written: 'At that time I will bring you and at that time I will gather you in, for I will set you up for renown and praise among all the peoples of the earth, when I bring back your captivity, before your own eyes,' said Hashem.[4]

(1) Deuteronomy 6:4. (2) Cf. Isaiah 44:6. (3) II Kings 19:15. (4) Zephaniah 3:20.

SOME CONGREGATIONS OMIT CERTAIN PASSAGES OF THE PRAYERS PRECEDING *PESUKEI D'ZIMRAH*. CUSTOMS REGARDING WHETHER AND WHICH PASSAGES ARE OMITTED VARY GREATLY. THEREFORE WE HAVE NOT OMITTED ANY PASSAGES. EACH CONGREGATION SHOULD FOLLOW ITS ESTABLISHED CUSTOM.

﷽ קרבנות ﷽

הכיור

שמות ל:י״ז-כ״א

וַיְדַבֵּר יהוה אֶל מֹשֶׁה לֵּאמֹר. וְעָשִׂיתָ כִּיּוֹר נְחֹשֶׁת, וְכַנּוֹ נְחֹשֶׁת, לְרָחְצָה, וְנָתַתָּ אֹתוֹ בֵּין אֹהֶל מוֹעֵד וּבֵין הַמִּזְבֵּחַ, וְנָתַתָּ שָׁמָּה מָיִם. וְרָחֲצוּ אַהֲרֹן וּבָנָיו מִמֶּנּוּ, אֶת יְדֵיהֶם וְאֶת רַגְלֵיהֶם. בְּבֹאָם אֶל אֹהֶל מוֹעֵד יִרְחֲצוּ מַיִם וְלֹא יָמֻתוּ, אוֹ בְגִשְׁתָּם אֶל הַמִּזְבֵּחַ לְשָׁרֵת לְהַקְטִיר אִשֶּׁה לַיהוה. וְרָחֲצוּ יְדֵיהֶם וְרַגְלֵיהֶם וְלֹא יָמֻתוּ, וְהָיְתָה לָהֶם חָק עוֹלָם, לוֹ וּלְזַרְעוֹ לְדֹרֹתָם.

תרומת הדשן

ויקרא ו:א-ו

וַיְדַבֵּר יהוה אֶל מֹשֶׁה לֵּאמֹר. צַו אֶת אַהֲרֹן וְאֶת בָּנָיו לֵאמֹר, זֹאת תּוֹרַת הָעֹלָה, הִוא הָעֹלָה עַל מוֹקְדָה עַל הַמִּזְבֵּחַ כָּל הַלַּיְלָה עַד הַבֹּקֶר, וְאֵשׁ הַמִּזְבֵּחַ תּוּקַד בּוֹ. וְלָבַשׁ הַכֹּהֵן מִדּוֹ בַד, וּמִכְנְסֵי בַד יִלְבַּשׁ עַל בְּשָׂרוֹ, וְהֵרִים אֶת הַדֶּשֶׁן אֲשֶׁר תֹּאכַל הָאֵשׁ אֶת הָעֹלָה עַל הַמִּזְבֵּחַ, וְשָׂמוֹ אֵצֶל הַמִּזְבֵּחַ. וּפָשַׁט אֶת בְּגָדָיו, וְלָבַשׁ בְּגָדִים אֲחֵרִים, וְהוֹצִיא אֶת הַדֶּשֶׁן אֶל מִחוּץ לַמַּחֲנֶה, אֶל מָקוֹם טָהוֹר. וְהָאֵשׁ עַל הַמִּזְבֵּחַ תּוּקַד בּוֹ, לֹא תִכְבֶּה, וּבִעֵר עָלֶיהָ הַכֹּהֵן עֵצִים בַּבֹּקֶר בַּבֹּקֶר, וְעָרַךְ עָלֶיהָ הָעֹלָה, וְהִקְטִיר עָלֶיהָ חֶלְבֵי הַשְּׁלָמִים. אֵשׁ תָּמִיד תּוּקַד עַל הַמִּזְבֵּחַ, לֹא תִכְבֶּה.

קרבן התמיד

Some authorities hold that the following (until קְטֹרֶת) should be recited standing.

יְהִי רָצוֹן מִלְּפָנֶיךָ, יהוה אֱלֹהֵינוּ וֵאלֹהֵי אֲבוֹתֵינוּ, שֶׁתְּרַחֵם עָלֵינוּ וְתִמְחָל לָנוּ עַל כָּל חַטֹּאתֵינוּ, וּתְכַפֵּר לָנוּ אֶת כָּל עֲוֹנוֹתֵינוּ, וְתִסְלַח לְכָל פְּשָׁעֵינוּ, וְתִבְנֶה בֵּית הַמִּקְדָּשׁ בִּמְהֵרָה בְיָמֵינוּ, וְנַקְרִיב לְפָנֶיךָ קָרְבַּן הַתָּמִיד שֶׁיְּכַפֵּר בַּעֲדֵנוּ, כְּמוֹ שֶׁכָּתַבְתָּ עָלֵינוּ בְּתוֹרָתֶךָ עַל יְדֵי מֹשֶׁה עַבְדֶּךָ, מִפִּי כְבוֹדֶךָ, כָּאָמוּר:

במדבר כח:א-ח

וַיְדַבֵּר יהוה אֶל מֹשֶׁה לֵּאמֹר. צַו אֶת בְּנֵי יִשְׂרָאֵל וְאָמַרְתָּ אֲלֵהֶם, אֶת קָרְבָּנִי לַחְמִי לְאִשַּׁי, רֵיחַ נִיחֹחִי, תִּשְׁמְרוּ לְהַקְרִיב לִי בְּמוֹעֲדוֹ. וְאָמַרְתָּ לָהֶם, זֶה הָאִשֶּׁה אֲשֶׁר תַּקְרִיבוּ

SOME CONGREGATIONS OMIT CERTAIN PASSAGES OF THE PRAYERS PRECEDING *PESUKEI D'ZIMRAH*. CUSTOMS REGARDING WHETHER AND WHICH PASSAGES ARE OMITTED VARY GREATLY. THEREFORE WE HAVE NOT OMITTED ANY PASSAGES. EACH CONGREGATION SHOULD FOLLOW ITS ESTABLISHED CUSTOM.

⋇⦃ OFFERINGS ⦄⋇

THE LAVER

Exodus 30:17-21

וַיְדַבֵּר HASHEM spoke to Moses, saying: Make a laver of copper, and its base of copper, for washing; and place it between the Tent of Appointment and the Altar and put water there. Aaron and his sons are to wash their hands and feet from it. When they arrive at the Tent of Appointment they are to wash with water so that they not die, or when they approach the Altar to serve, to burn a fire-offering to HASHEM. They are to wash their hands and feet so that they not die; and this shall be an eternal decree for them — for him and for his offspring — throughout their generations.

THE TAKING OF ASHES

Leviticus 6:1-6

וַיְדַבֵּר HASHEM spoke to Moses saying: Instruct Aaron and his sons saying: This is the teaching of the elevation-offering, it is the elevation-offering that stays on the pyre on the Altar all night until morning, and the fire of the Altar should be kept burning on it. The Kohen should don his linen garment, and he is to don linen breeches upon his flesh; he is to pick up the ashes of what the fire consumed of the elevation-offering upon the Altar and place it next to the Altar. Then he should remove his garments and don other garments; then he should remove the ashes to the outside of the camp to a pure place. The fire on the Altar shall be kept burning on it, it may not be extinguished, and the Kohen shall burn wood upon it every morning. He is to prepare the elevation-offering upon it and burn upon it the fats of the peace-offerings. A permanent fire should remain burning on the Altar; it may not be extinguished.

THE TAMID OFFERING

Some authorities hold that the following (until קְטֹרֶת /Incense) should be recited standing.

יְהִי רָצוֹן May it be Your will, HASHEM, our God, and the God of our forefathers, that You have mercy on us and pardon us for all our errors, atone for us all our iniquities, forgive all our willful sins; and that You rebuild the Holy Temple speedily, in our days, so that we may offer to You the continual offering that it may atone for us, as You have prescribed for us in Your Torah through Moses, Your servant, from Your glorious mouth, as it is said:

Numbers 28:1-8

וַיְדַבֵּר HASHEM spoke to Moses, saying: Command the Children of Israel and tell them: My offering, My food for My fires, My sat-isfying aroma, you are to be scrupulous to offer Me in its appointed time. And you are to tell them: 'This is the fire-offering that you are to bring

לַיהוה, כְּבָשִׂים בְּנֵי שָׁנָה תְמִימִם, שְׁנַיִם לַיּוֹם, עֹלָה תָמִיד. אֶת
הַכֶּבֶשׂ אֶחָד תַּעֲשֶׂה בַבֹּקֶר, וְאֵת הַכֶּבֶשׂ הַשֵּׁנִי תַּעֲשֶׂה בֵּין
הָעַרְבָּיִם. וַעֲשִׂירִית הָאֵיפָה סֹלֶת לְמִנְחָה, בְּלוּלָה בְּשֶׁמֶן כָּתִית
רְבִיעִת הַהִין. עֹלַת תָּמִיד, הָעֲשֻׂיָה בְּהַר סִינַי, לְרֵיחַ נִיחֹחַ, אִשֶּׁה
לַיהוה. וְנִסְכּוֹ רְבִיעִת הַהִין לַכֶּבֶשׂ הָאֶחָד, בַּקֹּדֶשׁ הַסֵּךְ נֶסֶךְ שֵׁכָר
לַיהוה. וְאֵת הַכֶּבֶשׂ הַשֵּׁנִי תַּעֲשֶׂה בֵּין הָעַרְבָּיִם, כְּמִנְחַת הַבֹּקֶר
וּכְנִסְכּוֹ תַּעֲשֶׂה, אִשֵּׁה רֵיחַ נִיחֹחַ לַיהוה.

וְשָׁחַט אֹתוֹ עַל יֶרֶךְ הַמִּזְבֵּחַ צָפֹנָה לִפְנֵי יהוה, וְזָרְקוּ בְּנֵי
אַהֲרֹן הַכֹּהֲנִים אֶת דָּמוֹ עַל הַמִּזְבֵּחַ סָבִיב.[1]

יְהִי רָצוֹן מִלְּפָנֶיךָ, יהוה אֱלֹהֵינוּ וֵאלֹהֵי אֲבוֹתֵינוּ, שֶׁתְּהֵא אֲמִירָה זוֹ
חֲשׁוּבָה וּמְקֻבֶּלֶת וּמְרֻצָּה לְפָנֶיךָ כְּאִלּוּ הִקְרַבְנוּ קָרְבַּן
הַתָּמִיד בְּמוֹעֲדוֹ וּבִמְקוֹמוֹ וּכְהִלְכָתוֹ.

﷽ קטרת ﷽

אַתָּה הוּא יהוה אֱלֹהֵינוּ שֶׁהִקְטִירוּ אֲבוֹתֵינוּ לְפָנֶיךָ אֶת קְטֹרֶת הַסַּמִּים
בִּזְמַן שֶׁבֵּית הַמִּקְדָּשׁ קַיָּם, כַּאֲשֶׁר צִוִּיתָ אוֹתָם עַל יְדֵי מֹשֶׁה
נְבִיאֶךָ, כַּכָּתוּב בְּתוֹרָתֶךָ:

שמות ל:לד-לו, ז:ח

וַיֹּאמֶר יהוה אֶל מֹשֶׁה, קַח לְךָ סַמִּים, נָטָף וּשְׁחֵלֶת וְחֶלְבְּנָה,
סַמִּים וּלְבֹנָה זַכָּה, בַּד בְּבַד יִהְיֶה. וְעָשִׂיתָ אֹתָהּ קְטֹרֶת,
רֹקַח, מַעֲשֵׂה רוֹקֵחַ, מְמֻלָּח, טָהוֹר, קֹדֶשׁ. וְשָׁחַקְתָּ מִמֶּנָּה הָדֵק,
וְנָתַתָּה מִמֶּנָּה לִפְנֵי הָעֵדֻת בְּאֹהֶל מוֹעֵד אֲשֶׁר אִוָּעֵד לְךָ שָׁמָּה,
קֹדֶשׁ קָדָשִׁים תִּהְיֶה לָכֶם.

וְנֶאֱמַר: וְהִקְטִיר עָלָיו אַהֲרֹן קְטֹרֶת סַמִּים, בַּבֹּקֶר בַּבֹּקֶר,
בְּהֵיטִיבוֹ אֶת הַנֵּרֹת יַקְטִירֶנָּה. וּבְהַעֲלֹת אַהֲרֹן אֶת הַנֵּרֹת בֵּין
הָעַרְבַּיִם, יַקְטִירֶנָּה, קְטֹרֶת תָּמִיד לִפְנֵי יהוה לְדֹרֹתֵיכֶם.

כריתות ו., ירושלמי יומא ד:ה

תָּנוּ רַבָּנָן, פִּטּוּם הַקְּטֹרֶת כֵּיצַד. שְׁלֹשׁ מֵאוֹת וְשִׁשִּׁים וּשְׁמוֹנָה
מָנִים הָיוּ בָהּ. שְׁלֹשׁ מֵאוֹת וְשִׁשִּׁים וַחֲמִשָּׁה
כְּמִנְיַן יְמוֹת הַחַמָּה — מָנֶה לְכָל יוֹם, פְּרָס בְּשַׁחֲרִית וּפְרָס בֵּין
הָעַרְבָּיִם; וּשְׁלֹשָׁה מָנִים יְתֵרִים, שֶׁמֵּהֶם מַכְנִיס כֹּהֵן גָּדוֹל מְלֹא
חָפְנָיו בְּיוֹם הַכִּפּוּרִים. וּמַחֲזִירָם לְמַכְתֶּשֶׁת בְּעֶרֶב יוֹם הַכִּפּוּרִים,
וְשׁוֹחֲקָן יָפֶה יָפֶה כְּדֵי שֶׁתְּהֵא דַקָּה מִן הַדַּקָּה. וְאַחַד עָשָׂר סַמָּנִים

to HASHEM: [male] first-year lambs, unblemished, two a day, as a continual elevation-offering. One lamb-service you are to perform in the morning and the second lamb-service you are to perform in the afternoon; with a tenth-ephah of fine flour as a meal-offering, mixed with a quarter-hin of crushed olive oil. It is the continual elevation-offering that was done at Mount Sinai, for a satisfying aroma, a fire-offering to HASHEM. And its libation is a quarter-hin for each lamb, to be poured on the Holy [Altar], a fermented libation to HASHEM. And the second lamb-service you are to perform in the afternoon, like the meal-offering of the morning and its libation are you to make, a fire-offering for a satisfying aroma to HASHEM.'

He is to slaughter it on the north side of the Altar before HASHEM, and Aaron's sons the Kohanim are to dash its blood upon the Altar, all around.[1]

יְהִי רָצוֹן May it be Your will, HASHEM, our God and the God of our forefathers, that this recital be worthy and acceptable, and favorable before You as if we had offered the continual offering in its set time, in its place, and according to its requirement.

⊰{ INCENSE }⊱

אַתָּה It is You, HASHEM, our God, before Whom our forefathers burned the incense-spices in the time when the Holy Temple stood, as You commanded them through Moses Your prophet, as is written in Your Torah:

Exodus 30:34-36, 7-8

וַיֹּאמֶר HASHEM said to Moses: Take yourself spices — stacte, onycha, and galbanum — spices and pure frankincense; they are all to be of equal weight. You are to make it into incense, a spice-compound, the handiwork of an expert spice-compounder, thoroughly mixed, pure and holy. You are to grind some of it finely and place some of it before the Testimony in the Tent of Appointment, where I shall designate a time to meet you; it shall be a holy of holies for you.

It is also written: Aaron shall burn upon it the incense-spices every morning; when he cleans the lamps he is to burn it. And when Aaron ignites the lamps in the afternoon, he is to burn it, as continual incense before HASHEM throughout your generations.

Talmud, Kereisos 6a, Yerushalmi Yoma 4:5

תָּנוּ רַבָּנָן The Rabbis taught: How is the incense mixture formulated? Three hundred sixty-eight maneh were in it: three hundred sixty-five corresponding to the days of the solar year — a maneh for each day, half in the morning and half in the afternoon; and three extra maneh, from which the Kohen Gadol would bring both his handfuls [into the Holy of Holies] on Yom Kippur. He would return them to the mortar on the day before Yom Kippur, and grind them very thoroughly so that it would be exceptionally fine. Eleven kinds of spices

---

(1) *Leviticus* 1:11.

הָיוּ בָהּ, וְאֵלוּ הֵן: (א) הַצֵּרִי, (ב) וְהַצִּפֹּרֶן, (ג) הַחֶלְבְּנָה, (ד) וְהַלְּבוֹנָה, מִשְׁקַל שִׁבְעִים שִׁבְעִים מָנֶה; (ה) מוֹר, (ו) וּקְצִיעָה, (ז) שִׁבֹּלֶת נֵרְדְּ, (ח) וְכַרְכֹּם, מִשְׁקַל שִׁשָּׁה עָשָׂר שִׁשָּׁה עָשָׂר מָנֶה; (ט) הַקֹּשְׁטְ שְׁנֵים עָשָׂר, (י) וְקִלּוּפָה שְׁלֹשָׁה, (יא) וְקִנָּמוֹן תִּשְׁעָה. בֹּרִית כַּרְשִׁינָה תִּשְׁעָה קַבִּין, יֵין קַפְרִיסִין סְאִין תְּלָתָא וְקַבִּין תְּלָתָא, וְאִם אֵין לוֹ יֵין קַפְרִיסִין, מֵבִיא חֲמַר חִוַּרְיָן עַתִּיק, מֶלַח סְדוֹמִית רֹבַע הַקַּב; מַעֲלֶה עָשָׁן כָּל שֶׁהוּא. רַבִּי נָתָן הַבַּבְלִי אוֹמֵר: אַף כִּפַּת הַיַּרְדֵּן כָּל שֶׁהוּא. וְאִם נָתַן בָּהּ דְּבַשׁ, פְּסָלָהּ. וְאִם חִסַּר אַחַת מִכָּל סַמָּנֶיהָ, חַיָּב מִיתָה.

רַבָּן שִׁמְעוֹן בֶּן גַּמְלִיאֵל אוֹמֵר: הַצֵּרִי אֵינוֹ אֶלָּא שְׂרָף הַנּוֹטֵף מֵעֲצֵי הַקְּטָף. בֹּרִית כַּרְשִׁינָה לָמָּה הִיא בָאָה, כְּדֵי לְיַפּוֹת בָּהּ אֶת הַצִּפֹּרֶן, כְּדֵי שֶׁתְּהֵא נָאָה. יֵין קַפְרִיסִין לָמָּה הוּא בָא, כְּדֵי לִשְׁרוֹת בּוֹ אֶת הַצִּפֹּרֶן, כְּדֵי שֶׁתְּהֵא עַזָּה. וַהֲלֹא מֵי רַגְלַיִם יָפִין לָהּ, אֶלָּא שֶׁאֵין מַכְנִיסִין מֵי רַגְלַיִם בַּמִּקְדָּשׁ מִפְּנֵי הַכָּבוֹד.

תַּנְיָא, רַבִּי נָתָן אוֹמֵר: כְּשֶׁהוּא שׁוֹחֵק, אוֹמֵר הָדֵק הֵיטֵב, הֵיטֵב הָדֵק, מִפְּנֵי שֶׁהַקּוֹל יָפֶה לַבְּשָׂמִים. פִּטְּמָה לַחֲצָאִין, כְּשֵׁרָה; לִשְׁלִישׁ וְלִרְבִיעַ, לֹא שָׁמֵעְנוּ. אָמַר רַבִּי יְהוּדָה: זֶה הַכְּלָל – אִם כְּמִדָּתָהּ, כְּשֵׁרָה לַחֲצָאִין; וְאִם חִסַּר אַחַת מִכָּל סַמָּנֶיהָ, חַיָּב מִיתָה.

תַּנְיָא, בַּר קַפָּרָא אוֹמֵר: אַחַת לְשִׁשִּׁים אוֹ לְשִׁבְעִים שָׁנָה הָיְתָה בָאָה שֶׁל שִׁירַיִם לַחֲצָאִין. וְעוֹד תָּנֵי בַּר קַפָּרָא: אִלּוּ הָיָה נוֹתֵן בָּהּ קוֹרְטוֹב שֶׁל דְּבַשׁ, אֵין אָדָם יָכוֹל לַעֲמֹד מִפְּנֵי רֵיחָהּ. וְלָמָּה אֵין מְעָרְבִין בָּהּ דְּבַשׁ, מִפְּנֵי שֶׁהַתּוֹרָה אָמְרָה: כִּי כָל שְׂאֹר וְכָל דְּבַשׁ לֹא תַקְטִירוּ מִמֶּנּוּ אִשֶּׁה לַיהוה.[1]

The next three verses, each beginning 'ה, are recited three times each.

יהוה צְבָאוֹת עִמָּנוּ, מִשְׂגָּב לָנוּ אֱלֹהֵי יַעֲקֹב, סֶלָה.[2]
יהוה צְבָאוֹת, אַשְׁרֵי אָדָם בֹּטֵחַ בָּךְ.[3]
יהוה הוֹשִׁיעָה, הַמֶּלֶךְ יַעֲנֵנוּ בְיוֹם קָרְאֵנוּ.[4]

אַתָּה סֵתֶר לִי, מִצַּר תִּצְּרֵנִי, רָנֵּי פַלֵּט, תְּסוֹבְבֵנִי, סֶלָה.[5] וְעָרְבָה לַיהוה מִנְחַת יְהוּדָה וִירוּשָׁלָיִם, כִּימֵי עוֹלָם וּכְשָׁנִים קַדְמֹנִיּוֹת.[6]

were in it, as follows: (1) stacte, (2) onycha, (3) galbanum, (4) frank-incense — each weighing seventy maneh; (5) myrrh, (6) cassia, (7) spikenard, (8) saffron — each weighing sixteen maneh; (9) costus — twelve maneh; (10) aromatic bark — three; and (11) cinnamon — nine. [Additionally] Carshina lye, nine kab; Cyprus wine, three se'ah and three kab — if he has no Cyprus wine, he brings old white wine; Sodom salt, a quarter-kab; and a minute amount of a smoke-raising herb. Rabbi Nassan the Babylonian says: Also a minute amount of Jordan amber. If he placed fruit-honey into it, he invalidated it. But if he left out any of its spices, he is liable to the death penalty.

רַבָּן שִׁמְעוֹן Rabban Shimon ben Gamliel says: The stacte is simply the sap that drips from balsam trees. Why is Carshina lye used? To bleach the onycha, to make it pleasing. Why is Cyprus wine used? So that the onycha could be soaked in it, to make it pungent. Even though urine is more suitable for that, nevertheless they do not bring urine into the Temple out of respect.

תַּנְיָא It is taught, Rabbi Nassan says: As one would grind [the incense] another would say, 'Grind thoroughly, thoroughly grind,' because the sound is beneficial for the spices. If one mixed it in half-quantities, it was fit for use, but as to a third or a quarter — we have not heard the law. Rabbi Yehudah said: This is the general rule — In its proper proportion, it is fit for use in half the full amount; but if he left out any one of its spices, he is liable to the death penalty.

תַּנְיָא It is taught, Bar Kappara says: Once every sixty or seventy years, the accumulated leftovers reached half the yearly quantity. Bar Kappara taught further: Had one put a kortov of fruit-honey into it, no person could have resisted its scent. Why did they not mix fruit-honey into it? — because the Torah says: 'For any leaven or any fruit-honey, you are not to burn from them a fire-offering to HASHEM.'[1]

The next three verses, each beginning 'HASHEM,' are recited three times each.

HASHEM, Master of Legions, is with us,
a stronghold for us is the God of Jacob, Selah![2]
HASHEM, Master of Legions,
praiseworthy is the person who trusts in You.[3]
HASHEM, save! May the King answer us on the day we call![4]

You are a shelter for me; from distress You preserve me; with glad song of rescue, You envelop me, Selah![5] May the offering of Judah and Jerusalem be pleasing to HASHEM, as in days of old and in former years.[6]

---

(1) Leviticus 2:11. (2) Psalms 46:8. (3) 84:13. (4) 20:10. (5) 32:7. (6) Malachi 3:4.

יומא לג.

אַבַּיֵי הֲוָה מְסַדֵּר סֵדֶר הַמַּעֲרָכָה מִשְּׁמָא דִּגְמָרָא וְאַלִּבָּא דְּאַבָּא
שָׁאוּל: מַעֲרָכָה גְדוֹלָה קוֹדֶמֶת לְמַעֲרָכָה שְׁנִיָּה שֶׁל
קְטֹרֶת; וּמַעֲרָכָה שְׁנִיָּה שֶׁל קְטֹרֶת קוֹדֶמֶת לְסִדּוּר שְׁנֵי גִזְרֵי עֵצִים;
וְסִדּוּר שְׁנֵי גִזְרֵי עֵצִים קוֹדֵם לְדִשּׁוּן מִזְבֵּחַ הַפְּנִימִי; וְדִשּׁוּן מִזְבֵּחַ
הַפְּנִימִי קוֹדֵם לַהֲטָבַת חָמֵשׁ נֵרוֹת; וַהֲטָבַת חָמֵשׁ נֵרוֹת קוֹדֶמֶת
לְדַם הַתָּמִיד; וְדַם הַתָּמִיד קוֹדֵם לַהֲטָבַת שְׁתֵּי נֵרוֹת; וַהֲטָבַת שְׁתֵּי
נֵרוֹת קוֹדֶמֶת לִקְטֹרֶת; וּקְטֹרֶת קוֹדֶמֶת לְאֵבָרִים; וְאֵבָרִים לְמִנְחָה;
וּמִנְחָה לַחֲבִתִּין; וַחֲבִתִּין לִנְסָכִין; וּנְסָכִין לְמוּסָפִין; וּמוּסָפִין
לְבָזִיכִין; וּבָזִיכִין קוֹדְמִין לְתָמִיד שֶׁל בֵּין הָעַרְבָּיִם, שֶׁנֶּאֱמַר: וְעָרַךְ
עָלֶיהָ הָעֹלָה, וְהִקְטִיר עָלֶיהָ חֶלְבֵי הַשְּׁלָמִים.[1] עָלֶיהָ הַשְׁלֵם כָּל
הַקָּרְבָּנוֹת כֻּלָּם.

אב״ג ית״ץ	**אָנָּא בְּכֹחַ** גְּדֻלַּת יְמִינְךָ תַּתִּיר צְרוּרָה.
קר״ע שט״ן	קַבֵּל רִנַּת עַמְּךָ שַׂגְּבֵנוּ טַהֲרֵנוּ נוֹרָא.
נג״ד יכ״ש	נָא גִבּוֹר דּוֹרְשֵׁי יִחוּדְךָ כְּבָבַת שָׁמְרֵם.
בט״ר צת״ג	בָּרְכֵם טַהֲרֵם רַחֲמֵם צִדְקָתְךָ תָּמִיד גָּמְלֵם.
חק״ב טנ״ע	חֲסִין קָדוֹשׁ בְּרוֹב טוּבְךָ נַהֵל עֲדָתֶךָ.
יג״ל פז״ק	יָחִיד גֵּאֶה לְעַמְּךָ פְּנֵה זוֹכְרֵי קְדֻשָּׁתֶךָ.
שק״ו צי״ת	שַׁוְעָתֵנוּ קַבֵּל וּשְׁמַע צַעֲקָתֵנוּ יוֹדֵעַ תַּעֲלֻמוֹת.
	בָּרוּךְ שֵׁם כְּבוֹד מַלְכוּתוֹ לְעוֹלָם וָעֶד.

רִבּוֹן הָעוֹלָמִים, אַתָּה צִוִּיתָנוּ לְהַקְרִיב קָרְבַּן הַתָּמִיד בְּמוֹעֲדוֹ,
וְלִהְיוֹת כֹּהֲנִים בַּעֲבוֹדָתָם, וּלְוִיִּם בְּדוּכָנָם, וְיִשְׂרָאֵל
בְּמַעֲמָדָם. וְעַתָּה בַּעֲוֹנוֹתֵינוּ חָרַב בֵּית הַמִּקְדָּשׁ וּבָטֵל הַתָּמִיד, וְאֵין לָנוּ
לֹא כֹהֵן בַּעֲבוֹדָתוֹ, וְלֹא לֵוִי בְּדוּכָנוֹ, וְלֹא יִשְׂרָאֵל בְּמַעֲמָדוֹ. וְאַתָּה אָמַרְתָּ:
וּנְשַׁלְּמָה פָרִים שְׂפָתֵינוּ.[1] לָכֵן יְהִי רָצוֹן מִלְּפָנֶיךָ, יְהוָה אֱלֹהֵינוּ וֵאלֹהֵי
אֲבוֹתֵינוּ, שֶׁיְּהֵא שִׂיחַ שִׂפְתוֹתֵינוּ חָשׁוּב וּמְקֻבָּל וּמְרֻצֶּה לְפָנֶיךָ, כְּאִלּוּ
הִקְרַבְנוּ קָרְבַּן הַתָּמִיד בְּמוֹעֲדוֹ, וְעָמַדְנוּ עַל מַעֲמָדוֹ.

משנה, זבחים פרק ה

[א] **אֵיזֶהוּ** מְקוֹמָן שֶׁל זְבָחִים. קָדְשֵׁי קָדָשִׁים שְׁחִיטָתָן בַּצָּפוֹן.
פָּר וְשָׂעִיר שֶׁל יוֹם הַכִּפּוּרִים שְׁחִיטָתָן בַּצָּפוֹן,
וְקִבּוּל דָּמָן בִּכְלִי שָׁרֵת בַּצָּפוֹן. וְדָמָן טָעוּן הַזָּיָה עַל בֵּין הַבַּדִּים, וְעַל
הַפָּרֹכֶת, וְעַל מִזְבַּח הַזָּהָב. מַתָּנָה אַחַת מֵהֶן מְעַכָּבֶת. שְׁיָרֵי הַדָּם

---

(1) *Leviticus* 6:5.

Talmud, Yoma 33a

אַבַּיֵי   *Abaye listed the order of the Altar service based on the tradition and according to Abba Shaul: The arrangement of the large pyre precedes that of the secondary pyre for the incense-offering; the secondary pyre for the incense-offering precedes the placement of two logs; the placement of two logs precedes the removal of ashes from the Inner Altar; the removal of ashes from the Inner Altar precedes the cleaning of five lamps [of the Menorah]; the cleaning of the five lamps precedes the [dashing of the] blood of the continual offering; the blood of the continual offering precedes the cleaning of the [other]two lamps; the cleaning of the two lamps precedes the incense; the incense precedes the [burning of the] limbs; the [burning of the] limbs [precedes] the meal-offering; the meal-offering [precedes] the pancakes; the pancakes [precede] the wine-libations; the wine-libations [precede] the mussaf-offering; the mussaf-offering [precedes] the bowls [of frankincense]; the bowls [precede] the afternoon continual offering, for it is said: 'And he is to arrange the elevation-offering upon it and burn the fats of the peace-offerings upon it,'[1] — 'upon it' [the elevation-offering] you are to complete all the [day's] offerings.*

אָנָּא בְּכֹחַ   *We beg You! With the strength of Your right hand's greatness, untie the bundled sins. Accept the prayer of Your nation; strengthen us, purify us, O Awesome One. Please, O Strong One — those who foster Your Oneness, guard them like the pupil of an eye. Bless them, purify them, show them pity, may Your righteousness always recompense them. Powerful Holy One, with Your abundant goodness guide Your congregation. One and only Exalted One, turn to Your nation, which proclaims Your holiness. Accept our entreaty and hear our cry, O Knower of mysteries.*
   Blessed is the Name of His glorious Kingdom for all eternity.

רִבּוֹן הָעוֹלָמִים   *Master of the worlds, You commanded us to bring the continual offering at its set time, and that the Kohanim be at their assigned service, the Levites on their platform, and the Israelites at their station. But now, through our sins, the Holy Temple is destroyed, the continual offering is discontinued, and we have neither Kohen at his service, nor Levite on his platform, nor Israelite at his station. But You said: 'Let our lips compensate for the bulls'[1] — therefore may it be Your will, HASHEM, our God and the God of our forefathers, that the prayer of our lips be worthy, acceptable and favorable before You, as if we had brought the continual offering at its set time and we had stood at its station.*

Mishnah, Zevachim Chapter 5

[1] אֵיזֶהוּ   *What is the location of the offerings? [Regarding] the most holy offerings, their slaughter is in the north. The slaughter of the bull and the he-goat of Yom Kippur is in the north and the reception of their blood in a service-vessel is in the north. Their blood requires sprinkling between the poles [of the Holy Ark], and toward the Curtain [of the Holy of Holies] and upon the Golden Altar. Every one of these applications [of blood] is essential. The leftover blood*

הָיָה שׁוֹפֵךְ עַל יְסוֹד מַעֲרָבִי שֶׁל מִזְבֵּחַ הַחִיצוֹן; אִם לֹא נָתַן, לֹא עִכֵּב.

[ב] **פָּרִים** הַנִּשְׂרָפִים וּשְׂעִירִים הַנִּשְׂרָפִים שְׁחִיטָתָן בַּצָּפוֹן, וְקִבּוּל דָּמָן בִּכְלִי שָׁרֵת בַּצָּפוֹן. וְדָמָן טָעוּן הַזָּיָה עַל הַפָּרֹכֶת וְעַל מִזְבַּח הַזָּהָב. מַתָּנָה אַחַת מֵהֶן מְעַכֶּבֶת. שְׁיָרֵי הַדָּם הָיָה שׁוֹפֵךְ עַל יְסוֹד מַעֲרָבִי שֶׁל מִזְבֵּחַ הַחִיצוֹן; אִם לֹא נָתַן, לֹא עִכֵּב. אֵלּוּ וָאֵלּוּ נִשְׂרָפִין בְּבֵית הַדֶּשֶׁן.

[ג] **חַטָּאת** הַצִּבּוּר וְהַיָּחִיד – אֵלּוּ הֵן חַטֹּאת הַצִּבּוּר, שְׂעִירֵי רָאשֵׁי חֳדָשִׁים וְשֶׁל מוֹעֲדוֹת – שְׁחִיטָתָן בַּצָּפוֹן, וְקִבּוּל דָּמָן בִּכְלִי שָׁרֵת בַּצָּפוֹן. וְדָמָן טָעוּן אַרְבַּע מַתָּנוֹת עַל אַרְבַּע קְרָנוֹת. כֵּיצַד, עָלָה בַכֶּבֶשׁ, וּפָנָה לַסּוֹבֵב וּבָא לוֹ לְקֶרֶן דְּרוֹמִית מִזְרָחִית, מִזְרָחִית צְפוֹנִית, צְפוֹנִית מַעֲרָבִית, מַעֲרָבִית דְּרוֹמִית. שְׁיָרֵי הַדָּם הָיָה שׁוֹפֵךְ עַל יְסוֹד דְּרוֹמִי. וְנֶאֱכָלִין לִפְנִים מִן הַקְּלָעִים, לְזִכְרֵי כְהֻנָּה, בְּכָל מַאֲכָל, לְיוֹם וָלַיְלָה, עַד חֲצוֹת.

[ד] **הָעוֹלָה** קֹדֶשׁ קָדָשִׁים. שְׁחִיטָתָהּ בַּצָּפוֹן, וְקִבּוּל דָּמָהּ בִּכְלִי שָׁרֵת בַּצָּפוֹן. וְדָמָהּ טָעוּן שְׁתֵּי מַתָּנוֹת שֶׁהֵן אַרְבַּע; וּטְעוּנָה הֶפְשֵׁט וְנִתּוּחַ, וְכָלִיל לָאִשִּׁים.

[ה] **זִבְחֵי** שַׁלְמֵי צִבּוּר וַאֲשָׁמוֹת, אֵלּוּ הֵן אֲשָׁמוֹת: אֲשַׁם גְּזֵלוֹת, אֲשַׁם מְעִילוֹת, אֲשַׁם שִׁפְחָה חֲרוּפָה, אֲשַׁם נָזִיר, אֲשַׁם מְצוֹרָע, אֲשַׁם תָּלוּי. שְׁחִיטָתָן בַּצָּפוֹן, וְקִבּוּל דָּמָן בִּכְלִי שָׁרֵת בַּצָּפוֹן, וְדָמָן טָעוּן שְׁתֵּי מַתָּנוֹת שֶׁהֵן אַרְבַּע. וְנֶאֱכָלִין לִפְנִים מִן הַקְּלָעִים לְזִכְרֵי כְהֻנָּה, בְּכָל מַאֲכָל, לְיוֹם וָלַיְלָה, עַד חֲצוֹת.

[ו] **הַתּוֹדָה** וְאֵיל נָזִיר קָדָשִׁים קַלִּים. שְׁחִיטָתָן בְּכָל מָקוֹם בָּעֲזָרָה, וְדָמָן טָעוּן שְׁתֵּי מַתָּנוֹת שֶׁהֵן אַרְבַּע. וְנֶאֱכָלִין בְּכָל הָעִיר, לְכָל אָדָם, בְּכָל מַאֲכָל, לְיוֹם וָלַיְלָה, עַד חֲצוֹת. הַמּוּרָם מֵהֶם כַּיּוֹצֵא בָהֶם, אֶלָּא שֶׁהַמּוּרָם נֶאֱכָל לַכֹּהֲנִים, לִנְשֵׁיהֶם וְלִבְנֵיהֶם וּלְעַבְדֵּיהֶם.

he would pour onto the western base of the Outer Altar; but if he failed to apply it [the leftover blood on the base], he has not prevented [atonement].

[2] **פָּרִים** *[Regarding] the bulls that are completely burned and he-goats that are completely burned, their slaughter is in the north, and the reception of their blood in a service-vessel is in the north. Their blood requires sprinkling toward the Curtain and upon the Golden Altar. Every one of these applications is essential. The leftover blood he would pour onto the western base of the Outer Altar; but if he failed to apply it [the leftover blood on the base], he has not prevented [atonement]. Both these and those [the Yom Kippur offerings] are burned in the place where the [Altar] ashes are deposited.*

[3] **חַטָּאת** *[Regarding] sin-offerings of the community and of the individual — the communal sin-offerings are the following: the he-goats of Rosh Chodesh and festivals — their slaughter [of all sin-offerings] is in the north and the reception of their blood in a service-vessel is in the north. Their blood requires four applications, [one] on [each of] the four corners [of the Altar]. How is it done? He [the Kohen] ascended the [Altar] ramp, turned to the surrounding ledge and arrived at the southeast [corner], the northeast, the northwest, and the southwest. The leftover blood he would pour out on the southern base. They are eaten within the [Courtyard] curtains, by males of the priesthood, prepared in any manner, on the same day and that night until midnight.*

[4] **הָעוֹלָה** *The elevation-offering is among the most holy offerings. Its slaughter is in the north and the reception of its blood in a service-vessel is in the north. Its blood requires two applications that are equivalent to four. It requires flaying and dismemberment, and it is entirely consumed by the fire.*

[5] **זִבְחֵי** *[Regarding] communal peace-offerings and [personal] guilt-offerings — the guilt-offerings are as follows: the guilt-offering for thefts, the guilt-offering for misuse of sacred objects, the guilt-offering [for violating] a betrothed maidservant, the guilt-offering of a Nazirite, the guilt-offering of a metzora, and a guilt-offering in case of doubt — their slaughter is in the north and the reception of their blood in a service-vessel is in the north. Their blood requires two applications that are equivalent to four. They are eaten within the [Courtyard] curtains, by males of the priesthood, prepared in any manner, on the same day and that night until midnight.*

[6] **הַתּוֹדָה** *The thanksgiving-offering and the ram of a Nazirite are offerings of lesser holiness. Their slaughter is anywhere in the Courtyard, and their blood requires two applications that are equivalent to four. They are eaten throughout the City [of Jerusalem] by anyone, prepared in any manner, on the same day and that night until midnight. The [priestly] portion separated from them is treated like them, except that that portion may be eaten only by the Kohanim, their wives, children and slaves.*

[ז] **שְׁלָמִים** קָדָשִׁים קַלִּים. שְׁחִיטָתָן בְּכָל מָקוֹם בָּעֲזָרָה, וְדָמָן טָעוּן שְׁתֵּי מַתָּנוֹת שֶׁהֵן אַרְבַּע. וְנֶאֱכָלִין בְּכָל הָעִיר, לְכָל אָדָם, בְּכָל מַאֲכָל, לִשְׁנֵי יָמִים וְלַיְלָה אֶחָד. הַמּוּרָם מֵהֶם כַּיּוֹצֵא בָהֶם, אֶלָּא שֶׁהַמּוּרָם נֶאֱכָל לַכֹּהֲנִים, לִנְשֵׁיהֶם וְלִבְנֵיהֶם וּלְעַבְדֵיהֶם.

[ח] **הַבְּכוֹר** וְהַמַּעֲשֵׂר וְהַפֶּסַח קָדָשִׁים קַלִּים. שְׁחִיטָתָן בְּכָל מָקוֹם בָּעֲזָרָה, וְדָמָן טָעוּן מַתָּנָה אֶחָת, וּבִלְבַד שֶׁיִּתֵּן כְּנֶגֶד הַיְסוֹד. שָׁנָה בַאֲכִילָתָן: הַבְּכוֹר נֶאֱכָל לַכֹּהֲנִים, וְהַמַּעֲשֵׂר לְכָל אָדָם. וְנֶאֱכָלִין בְּכָל הָעִיר, בְּכָל מַאֲכָל, לִשְׁנֵי יָמִים וְלַיְלָה אֶחָד. הַפֶּסַח אֵינוֹ נֶאֱכָל אֶלָּא בַלַּיְלָה, וְאֵינוֹ נֶאֱכָל אֶלָּא עַד חֲצוֹת, וְאֵינוֹ נֶאֱכָל אֶלָּא לִמְנוּיָו, וְאֵינוֹ נֶאֱכָל אֶלָּא צָלִי.

בָּרַיְתָא דר' יִשְׁמָעֵאל – סִפְרָא, פְּתִיחָה

רַבִּי יִשְׁמָעֵאל אוֹמֵר: בִּשְׁלֹשׁ עֶשְׂרֵה מִדּוֹת הַתּוֹרָה נִדְרֶשֶׁת בָּהֶן. (א) מִקַּל וָחֹמֶר; (ב) וּמִגְּזֵרָה שָׁוָה; (ג) מִבִּנְיַן אָב מִכָּתוּב אֶחָד, וּמִבִּנְיַן אָב מִשְּׁנֵי כְתוּבִים; (ד) מִכְּלָל וּפְרָט; (ה) וּמִפְּרָט וּכְלָל; (ו) כְּלָל וּפְרָט וּכְלָל, אִי אַתָּה דָן אֶלָּא כְּעֵין הַפְּרָט; (ז) מִכְּלָל שֶׁהוּא צָרִיךְ לִפְרָט, וּמִפְּרָט שֶׁהוּא צָרִיךְ לִכְלָל; (ח) כָּל דָּבָר שֶׁהָיָה בִכְלָל וְיָצָא מִן הַכְּלָל לְלַמֵּד, לֹא לְלַמֵּד עַל עַצְמוֹ יָצָא, אֶלָּא לְלַמֵּד עַל הַכְּלָל כֻּלּוֹ יָצָא; (ט) כָּל דָּבָר שֶׁהָיָה בִכְלָל וְיָצָא לִטְעוֹן טוֹעַן אֶחָד שֶׁהוּא כְעִנְיָנוֹ, יָצָא לְהָקֵל וְלֹא לְהַחֲמִיר; (י) כָּל דָּבָר שֶׁהָיָה בִכְלָל וְיָצָא לִטְעוֹן טוֹעַן אַחֵר שֶׁלֹּא כְעִנְיָנוֹ, יָצָא לְהָקֵל וּלְהַחֲמִיר; (יא) כָּל דָּבָר שֶׁהָיָה בִכְלָל וְיָצָא לִדּוֹן בַּדָּבָר הֶחָדָשׁ, אִי אַתָּה יָכוֹל לְהַחֲזִירוֹ לִכְלָלוֹ, עַד שֶׁיַּחֲזִירֶנּוּ הַכָּתוּב לִכְלָלוֹ בְּפֵרוּשׁ; (יב) דָּבָר הַלָּמֵד מֵעִנְיָנוֹ, וְדָבָר הַלָּמֵד מִסּוֹפוֹ; (יג) וְכֵן שְׁנֵי כְתוּבִים הַמַּכְחִישִׁים זֶה אֶת זֶה, עַד שֶׁיָּבוֹא הַכָּתוּב הַשְּׁלִישִׁי וְיַכְרִיעַ בֵּינֵיהֶם.

יְהִי רָצוֹן מִלְּפָנֶיךָ, יהוה אֱלֹהֵינוּ וֵאלֹהֵי אֲבוֹתֵינוּ, שֶׁיִּבָּנֶה בֵּית הַמִּקְדָּשׁ בִּמְהֵרָה בְיָמֵינוּ, וְתֵן חֶלְקֵנוּ בְּתוֹרָתֶךָ. וְשָׁם נַעֲבָדְךָ בְּיִרְאָה כִּימֵי עוֹלָם וּכְשָׁנִים קַדְמוֹנִיּוֹת.

שְׁלָמִים *The peace-offerings are offerings of lesser holiness. Their slaughter is anywhere in the Courtyard, and their blood requires two applications that are equivalent to four. They are eaten throughout the City [of Jerusalem] by anyone, prepared in any manner, for two days and one night. The [priestly] portion separated from them is treated like them, except that that portion may be eaten only by the Kohanim, their wives, children and slaves.*

[8] **הַבְּכוֹר** *The firstborn and tithe of animals and the pesach-offering are offerings of lesser holiness. Their slaughter is anywhere in the Courtyard, and their blood requires a single application, provided he applies it above the base. They differ in their consumption: The firstborn is eaten by Kohanim, and the tithe by anyone. They are eaten throughout the City [of Jerusalem], prepared in any manner, for two days and one night. The pesach-offering is eaten only at night and it may be eaten only until midnight; it may be eaten only by those registered for it; and it may be eaten only if roasted.*

Introduction to *Sifra*

רַבִּי יִשְׁמָעֵאל *Rabbi Yishmael says: Through thirteen rules is the Torah elucidated: (1) Through a conclusion inferred from a lenient law to a strict one, and vice versa; (2) through tradition that similar words in different contexts are meant to clarify one another; (3) through a general principle derived from one verse, and a general principle derived from two verses; (4) through a general statement limited by a specification; (5) through a specification broadened by a general statement; (6) through a general statement followed by a specification followed, in turn, by another general statement — you may only infer whatever is similar to the specification; (7) when a general statement requires a specification or a specification requires a general statement to clarify its meaning; (8) anything that was included in a general statement, but was then singled out from the general statement in order to teach something, was not singled out to teach only about itself, but to apply its teaching to the entire generality; (9) anything that was included in a general statement, but was then singled out to discuss a provision similar to the general category, has been singled out to be more lenient rather than more severe; (10) anything that was included in a general statement, but was then singled out to discuss a provision not similar to the general category, has been singled out both to be more lenient and more severe; (11) anything that was included in a general statement, but was then singled out to be treated as a new case, cannot be returned to its general statement unless Scripture returns it explicitly to its general statement; (12) a matter elucidated from its context, or from the following passage; (13) similarly, two passages that contradict one another — until a third passage comes to reconcile them.*

יְהִי רָצוֹן *May it be Your will, HASHEM, our God and the God of our forefathers, that the Holy Temple be rebuilt, speedily in our days, and grant us our share in Your Torah, and may we serve You there with reverence as in days of old and in former years.*

קדיש דרבנן

Mourners recite קַדִּישׁ דְּרַבָּנָן. **See Laws §135-136.**

יִתְגַּדַּל וְיִתְקַדַּשׁ שְׁמֵהּ רַבָּא. (.Cong – אָמֵן.) בְּעָלְמָא דִּי בְרָא כִרְעוּתֵהּ, וְיַמְלִיךְ מַלְכוּתֵהּ, בְּחַיֵּיכוֹן וּבְיוֹמֵיכוֹן וּבְחַיֵּי דְכָל בֵּית יִשְׂרָאֵל, בַּעֲגָלָא וּבִזְמַן קָרִיב. וְאִמְרוּ: אָמֵן.

(.Cong – אָמֵן. יְהֵא שְׁמֵהּ רַבָּא מְבָרַךְ לְעָלַם וּלְעָלְמֵי עָלְמַיָּא.)

יְהֵא שְׁמֵהּ רַבָּא מְבָרַךְ לְעָלַם וּלְעָלְמֵי עָלְמַיָּא.

יִתְבָּרַךְ וְיִשְׁתַּבַּח וְיִתְפָּאַר וְיִתְרוֹמַם וְיִתְנַשֵּׂא וְיִתְהַדָּר וְיִתְעַלֶּה וְיִתְהַלָּל שְׁמֵהּ דְּקֻדְשָׁא בְּרִיךְ הוּא (.Cong – בְּרִיךְ הוּא) לְעֵלָּא מִן כָּל בִּרְכָתָא וְשִׁירָתָא תֻּשְׁבְּחָתָא וְנֶחֱמָתָא, דַּאֲמִירָן בְּעָלְמָא. וְאִמְרוּ: אָמֵן. (.Cong – אָמֵן.)

עַל יִשְׂרָאֵל וְעַל רַבָּנָן, וְעַל תַּלְמִידֵיהוֹן וְעַל כָּל תַּלְמִידֵי תַלְמִידֵיהוֹן, וְעַל כָּל מָאן דְּעָסְקִין בְּאוֹרַיְתָא, דִּי בְאַתְרָא הָדֵין וְדִי בְכָל אֲתַר וַאֲתַר. יְהֵא לְהוֹן וּלְכוֹן שְׁלָמָא רַבָּא, חִנָּא וְחִסְדָּא וְרַחֲמִין, וְחַיִּין אֲרִיכִין, וּמְזוֹנֵי רְוִיחֵי, וּפֻרְקָנָא מִן קֳדָם אֲבוּהוֹן דִּי בִשְׁמַיָּא (וְאַרְעָא). וְאִמְרוּ: אָמֵן. (.Cong – אָמֵן.)

יְהֵא שְׁלָמָא רַבָּא מִן שְׁמַיָּא, וְחַיִּים (טוֹבִים) עָלֵינוּ וְעַל כָּל יִשְׂרָאֵל. וְאִמְרוּ: אָמֵן. (.Cong – אָמֵן.)

Take three steps back. Bow left and say . . . עֹשֶׂה; bow right and say . . . הוּא; bow forward and say וְעַל כָּל . . . אָמֵן. Remain standing in place for a few moments, then take three steps forward.

עֹשֶׂה שָׁלוֹם בִּמְרוֹמָיו, הוּא בְּרַחֲמָיו יַעֲשֶׂה שָׁלוֹם עָלֵינוּ, וְעַל כָּל יִשְׂרָאֵל. וְאִמְרוּ: אָמֵן. (.Cong – אָמֵן.)

◄§ פסוקי דזמרה §►

INTRODUCTORY PSALM TO PESUKEI D'ZIMRAH

תהלים ל

מִזְמוֹר שִׁיר חֲנֻכַּת הַבַּיִת לְדָוִד. אֲרוֹמִמְךָ יהוה כִּי דִלִּיתָנִי, וְלֹא שִׂמַּחְתָּ אֹיְבַי לִי. יהוה אֱלֹהָי, שִׁוַּעְתִּי אֵלֶיךָ וַתִּרְפָּאֵנִי. יהוה הֶעֱלִיתָ מִן שְׁאוֹל נַפְשִׁי, חִיִּיתַנִי מִיָּרְדִי בוֹר. זַמְּרוּ לַיהוה חֲסִידָיו, וְהוֹדוּ לְזֵכֶר קָדְשׁוֹ. כִּי רֶגַע בְּאַפּוֹ, חַיִּים בִּרְצוֹנוֹ, בָּעֶרֶב יָלִין בֶּכִי וְלַבֹּקֶר רִנָּה. וַאֲנִי אָמַרְתִּי בְשַׁלְוִי, בַּל אֶמּוֹט לְעוֹלָם. יהוה בִּרְצוֹנְךָ הֶעֱמַדְתָּה לְהַרְרִי עֹז, הִסְתַּרְתָּ פָנֶיךָ הָיִיתִי נִבְהָל. אֵלֶיךָ יהוה אֶקְרָא, וְאֶל אֲדֹנָי אֶתְחַנָּן. מַה בֶּצַע בְּדָמִי, בְּרִדְתִּי אֶל שָׁחַת, הֲיוֹדְךָ עָפָר, הֲיַגִּיד אֲמִתֶּךָ. שְׁמַע יהוה וְחָנֵּנִי, יהוה הֱיֵה עֹזֵר לִי. ❖ הָפַכְתָּ מִסְפְּדִי לְמָחוֹל לִי, פִּתַּחְתָּ שַׂקִּי, וַתְּאַזְּרֵנִי שִׂמְחָה. לְמַעַן יְזַמֶּרְךָ כָבוֹד וְלֹא יִדֹּם, יהוה אֱלֹהַי לְעוֹלָם אוֹדֶךָּ.

THE RABBIS' KADDISH

Mourners recite the Rabbis' *Kaddish*. See *Laws* §135-136.
[A transliteration of this *Kaddish* appears on page 485.]

יִתְגַּדַּל May His great Name grow exalted and sanctified (Cong.— Amen.) in the world that He created as He willed. May He give reign to His kingship in your lifetimes and in your days, and in the lifetimes of the entire Family of Israel, swiftly and soon. Now respond: Amen.

(Cong.— Amen. May His great Name be blessed forever and ever.)
May His great Name be blessed forever and ever.

Blessed, praised, glorified, exalted, extolled, mighty, upraised, and lauded be the Name of the Holy One, Blessed is He (Cong.— Blessed is He) — beyond any blessing and song, praise and consolation that are uttered in the world. Now respond: Amen. (Cong.— Amen.)

Upon Israel, upon the teachers, their disciples and all of their disciples and upon all those who engage in the study of Torah, who are here or anywhere else; may they and you have abundant peace, grace, kindness, and mercy, long life, ample nourishment, and salvation from before their Father Who is in Heaven (and on earth). Now respond: Amen. (Cong. — Amen.)

May there be abundant peace from Heaven, and (good) life, upon us and upon all Israel. Now respond: Amen. (Cong.— Amen.)

Take three steps back. Bow left and say, 'He Who makes peace . . .';
bow right and say, 'may He . . .'; bow forward and say, 'and upon all Israel . . .'
Remain standing in place for a few moments, then take three steps forward.

He Who makes peace in His heights, may He, in His compassion, make peace upon us, and upon all Israel. Now respond: Amen. (Cong.— Amen.)

ᴥ PESUKEI D'ZIMRAH ᴥ

INTRODUCTORY PSALM TO PESUKEI D'ZIMRAH

Psalm 30

מִזְמוֹר A psalm — a song for the inauguration of the Temple— by David. I will exalt You, HASHEM, for You have drawn me up and not let my foes rejoice over me. HASHEM, my God, I cried out to You and You healed me. HASHEM, You have raised my soul from the lower world, You have preserved me from my descent to the Pit. Make music to HASHEM, His devout ones, and give thanks to His Holy Name. For His anger endures but a moment; life results from His favor. In the evening one lies down weeping, but with dawn — a cry of joy! I had said in my serenity, 'I will never falter.' But, HASHEM, all is through Your favor — You supported my greatness with might; should You but conceal Your face, I would be confounded. To You, HASHEM, I would call and to my Lord I would appeal. What gain is there in my death, when I descend to the Pit? Will the dust acknowledge You? Will it declare Your truth? Hear, HASHEM, and favor me; HASHEM, be my Helper! Chazzan— You have changed for me my lament into dancing; You undid my sackcloth and girded me with gladness. So that my soul might make music to You and not be stilled, HASHEM my God, forever will I thank You.

קדיש יתום

Mourners recite קַדִּישׁ יָתוֹם. See *Laws* §132-134.

יִתְגַּדַּל וְיִתְקַדַּשׁ שְׁמֵהּ רַבָּא. (.Cong – אָמֵן.) בְּעָלְמָא דִּי בְרָא כִרְעוּתֵהּ,
וְיַמְלִיךְ מַלְכוּתֵהּ, בְּחַיֵּיכוֹן וּבְיוֹמֵיכוֹן וּבְחַיֵּי דְכָל בֵּית יִשְׂרָאֵל,
בַּעֲגָלָא וּבִזְמַן קָרִיב. וְאִמְרוּ: אָמֵן.

(.Cong – אָמֵן. יְהֵא שְׁמֵהּ רַבָּא מְבָרַךְ לְעָלַם וּלְעָלְמֵי עָלְמַיָּא.)
יְהֵא שְׁמֵהּ רַבָּא מְבָרַךְ לְעָלַם וּלְעָלְמֵי עָלְמַיָּא.

יִתְבָּרַךְ וְיִשְׁתַּבַּח וְיִתְפָּאַר וְיִתְרוֹמַם וְיִתְנַשֵּׂא וְיִתְהַדָּר וְיִתְעַלֶּה
וְיִתְהַלָּל שְׁמֵהּ דְּקֻדְשָׁא בְּרִיךְ הוּא (.Cong – בְּרִיךְ הוּא) – לְעֵלָּא מִן כָּל
בִּרְכָתָא וְשִׁירָתָא תֻּשְׁבְּחָתָא וְנֶחֱמָתָא, דַּאֲמִירָן בְּעָלְמָא. וְאִמְרוּ: אָמֵן.
(.Cong – אָמֵן.)

יְהֵא שְׁלָמָא רַבָּא מִן שְׁמַיָּא, וְחַיִּים עָלֵינוּ וְעַל כָּל יִשְׂרָאֵל. וְאִמְרוּ:
אָמֵן. (.Cong – אָמֵן.)

Take three steps back. Bow left and say . . . עֹשֶׂה; bow right and say . . . הוּא; bow forward and say
וְעַל כָּל . . . אָמֵן. Remain standing in place for a few moments, then take three steps forward.

עֹשֶׂה שָׁלוֹם בִּמְרוֹמָיו, הוּא יַעֲשֶׂה שָׁלוֹם עָלֵינוּ, וְעַל כָּל יִשְׂרָאֵל.
וְאִמְרוּ: אָמֵן. (.Cong – אָמֵן.)

(Some recite this short Kabbalistic declaration of intent before beginning Pesukei D'zimrah:)

(הֲרֵינִי מְזַמֵּן אֶת פִּי לְהוֹדוֹת וּלְהַלֵּל וּלְשַׁבֵּחַ אֶת בּוֹרְאִי. לְשֵׁם יִחוּד
קֻדְשָׁא בְּרִיךְ הוּא וּשְׁכִינְתֵּיהּ עַל יְדֵי הַהוּא טָמִיר וְנֶעֱלָם, בְּשֵׁם כָּל יִשְׂרָאֵל.)

Pesukei D'zimrah begins with the recital of בָּרוּךְ שֶׁאָמַר, which is recited while standing.
The *tzitzis* are not held during its recitation, and are not kissed at its conclusion.

בָּרוּךְ שֶׁאָמַר וְהָיָה הָעוֹלָם, בָּרוּךְ הוּא. בָּרוּךְ עֹשֶׂה
בְרֵאשִׁית, בָּרוּךְ אוֹמֵר וְעֹשֶׂה, בָּרוּךְ גּוֹזֵר
וּמְקַיֵּם, בָּרוּךְ מְרַחֵם עַל הָאָרֶץ, בָּרוּךְ מְרַחֵם עַל הַבְּרִיּוֹת, בָּרוּךְ
מְשַׁלֵּם שָׂכָר טוֹב לִירֵאָיו, בָּרוּךְ חַי לָעַד וְקַיָּם לָנֶצַח, בָּרוּךְ פּוֹדֶה
וּמַצִּיל, בָּרוּךְ שְׁמוֹ. בָּרוּךְ אַתָּה יהוה אֱלֹהֵינוּ מֶלֶךְ הָעוֹלָם, הָאֵל
הָאָב הָרַחֲמָן הַמְהֻלָּל בְּפֶה עַמּוֹ, מְשֻׁבָּח וּמְפֹאָר בִּלְשׁוֹן חֲסִידָיו
וַעֲבָדָיו, וּבְשִׁירֵי דָוִד עַבְדֶּךָ. נְהַלֶּלְךָ יהוה אֱלֹהֵינוּ, בִּשְׁבָחוֹת
וּבִזְמִרוֹת. נְגַדֶּלְךָ וּנְשַׁבֵּחֲךָ וּנְפָאֶרְךָ וְנַזְכִּיר שִׁמְךָ וְנַמְלִיכְךָ, מַלְכֵּנוּ
אֱלֹהֵינוּ. ❖ יָחִיד, חֵי הָעוֹלָמִים, מֶלֶךְ מְשֻׁבָּח וּמְפֹאָר עֲדֵי עַד שְׁמוֹ
הַגָּדוֹל. בָּרוּךְ אַתָּה יהוה, מֶלֶךְ מְהֻלָּל בַּתִּשְׁבָּחוֹת. (.Cong – אָמֵן.)

◆§ Permitted responses during Pesukei D'zimrah

From this point until after *Shemoneh Esrei* conversation is forbidden. During *Pesukei D'zimrah* [from בָּרוּךְ שֶׁאָמַר until יִשְׁתַּבַּח, p. 272] certain congregational and individual responses

[e.g., בָּרוּךְ הוּא וּבָרוּךְ שְׁמוֹ] are omitted. The following responses, however, should be made: אָמֵן, *Amen,* after any blessing; *Kaddish; Borchu; Kedushah;* and the Rabbis' *Modim.* Additionally, one should join the congregation in reciting the first verse of the *Shema,* and may recite the אֲשֶׁר יָצַר blessing if he had to relieve himself

MOURNER'S KADDISH

Mourners recite the Mourners' *Kaddish*. *See Laws* §132-134.
[A transliteration of this *Kaddish* appears on page 486.]

יִתְגַּדַּל *May His great Name grow exalted and sanctified* (Cong.— *Amen.) in the world that He created as He willed. May He give reign to His kingship in your lifetimes and in your days, and in the lifetimes of the entire Family of Israel, swiftly and soon. Now respond: Amen.*

(Cong.— *Amen. May His great Name be blessed forever and ever.*)
May His great Name be blessed forever and ever.

Blessed, praised, glorified, exalted, extolled, mighty, upraised, and lauded be the Name of the Holy One, Blessed is He (Cong.— *Blessed is He) — beyond any blessing and song, praise and consolation that are uttered in the world. Now respond: Amen.* (Cong.— *Amen.)*

May there be abundant peace from Heaven, and life, upon us and upon all Israel. Now respond: Amen. (Cong.— *Amen.)*

Take three steps back. Bow left and say, 'He Who makes peace . . .';
bow right and say, 'may He . . .'; bow forward and say, 'and upon all Israel . . .'
Remain standing in place for a few moments, then take three steps forward.

He Who makes peace in His heights, may He make peace upon us, and upon all Israel. Now respond: Amen. (Cong.— *Amen.)*

(Some recite this short Kabbalistic declaration of intent before beginning *Pesukei D'zimrah:*)

(*I now prepare my mouth to thank, laud, and praise my Creator. For the sake of the unification of the Holy One, Blessed is He, and His Presence, through Him Who is hidden and inscrutable — [I pray] in the name of all Israel.*)

Pesukei D'zimrah begins with the recital of בָּרוּךְ שֶׁאָמַר, *Blessed is He Who spoke . . .*, which is recited while standing. The tzitzis are not held during its recitation, and are not kissed at its conclusion.

בָּרוּךְ שֶׁאָמַר *Blessed is He Who spoke, and the world came into being — blessed is He. Blessed is He Who maintains Creation; blessed is He Who speaks and does; blessed is He Who decrees and fulfills; blessed is He Who has mercy on the earth; blessed is He Who has mercy on the creatures; blessed is He Who gives goodly reward to those who fear Him; blessed is He Who lives forever and endures to eternity; blessed is He Who redeems and rescues — blessed is His Name! Blessed are You, HASHEM, our God, King of the universe, the God, the merciful Father, Who is lauded by the mouth of His people, praised and glorified by the tongue of His devout ones and His servants and through the psalms of David Your servant. We shall laud You, HASHEM, our God, with praises and songs. We shall exalt You, praise You, glorify You, mention Your Name and proclaim Your reign, our King, our God.* Chazzan— *O Unique One, Life-giver of the worlds, King Whose great Name is eternally praised and glorified. Blessed are You, HASHEM, the King Who is lauded with praises.* (Cong.— *Amen.)*

during *Pesukei D'zimrah.*

If one is in the middle of *Pesukei D'zimrah* and the congregation has already reached the Torah reading, it is preferable that he not be called to the Torah. However, if (a) one is the only *Kohen* or Levite present, or (b) the *gabbai* inadvertently called him to the Torah, then he may recite the blessings and even read the portion softly along with the Torah reader.

If after beginning *Pesukei D'zimrah* one realizes that he has forgotten to recite the morning Blessings of the Torah (p. 194), he should pause to recite them and their accompanying verses. Likewise, if he fears that he will not reach the *Shema* before the prescribed time (see *Laws* §55), he should recite all three para-

דברי הימים א טז:ח-לו

הוֹדוּ לַיהוה קִרְאוּ בִשְׁמוֹ, הוֹדִיעוּ בָעַמִּים עֲלִילֹתָיו. שִׁירוּ לוֹ,
זַמְּרוּ לוֹ, שִׂיחוּ בְּכָל נִפְלְאֹתָיו. הִתְהַלְלוּ בְּשֵׁם קָדְשׁוֹ,
יִשְׂמַח לֵב מְבַקְשֵׁי יהוה. דִּרְשׁוּ יהוה וְעֻזּוֹ, בַּקְּשׁוּ פָנָיו תָּמִיד. זִכְרוּ
נִפְלְאֹתָיו אֲשֶׁר עָשָׂה, מֹפְתָיו וּמִשְׁפְּטֵי פִיהוּ. זֶרַע יִשְׂרָאֵל עַבְדּוֹ, בְּנֵי
יַעֲקֹב בְּחִירָיו. הוּא יהוה אֱלֹהֵינוּ, בְּכָל הָאָרֶץ מִשְׁפָּטָיו. זִכְרוּ
לְעוֹלָם בְּרִיתוֹ, דָּבָר צִוָּה לְאֶלֶף דּוֹר. אֲשֶׁר כָּרַת אֶת אַבְרָהָם,
וּשְׁבוּעָתוֹ לְיִצְחָק. וַיַּעֲמִידֶהָ לְיַעֲקֹב לְחֹק, לְיִשְׂרָאֵל בְּרִית עוֹלָם.
לֵאמֹר, לְךָ אֶתֵּן אֶרֶץ כְּנָעַן, חֶבֶל נַחֲלַתְכֶם. בִּהְיוֹתְכֶם מְתֵי מִסְפָּר,
כִּמְעַט וְגָרִים בָּהּ. וַיִּתְהַלְּכוּ מִגּוֹי אֶל גּוֹי, וּמִמַּמְלָכָה אֶל עַם אַחֵר.
לֹא הִנִּיחַ לְאִישׁ לְעָשְׁקָם, וַיּוֹכַח עֲלֵיהֶם מְלָכִים. אַל תִּגְּעוּ
בִמְשִׁיחָי, וּבִנְבִיאַי אַל תָּרֵעוּ. שִׁירוּ לַיהוה כָּל הָאָרֶץ, בַּשְּׂרוּ מִיּוֹם
אֶל יוֹם יְשׁוּעָתוֹ. סַפְּרוּ בַגּוֹיִם אֶת כְּבוֹדוֹ, בְּכָל הָעַמִּים נִפְלְאֹתָיו.
כִּי גָדוֹל יהוה וּמְהֻלָּל מְאֹד, וְנוֹרָא הוּא עַל כָּל אֱלֹהִים. ❖ כִּי כָּל
אֱלֹהֵי הָעַמִּים אֱלִילִים, (pause) וַיהוה שָׁמַיִם עָשָׂה.

הוֹד וְהָדָר לְפָנָיו, עֹז וְחֶדְוָה בִּמְקֹמוֹ. הָבוּ לַיהוה מִשְׁפְּחוֹת
עַמִּים, הָבוּ לַיהוה כָּבוֹד וָעֹז. הָבוּ לַיהוה כְּבוֹד שְׁמוֹ, שְׂאוּ
מִנְחָה וּבֹאוּ לְפָנָיו, הִשְׁתַּחֲווּ לַיהוה בְּהַדְרַת קֹדֶשׁ. חִילוּ מִלְּפָנָיו
כָּל הָאָרֶץ, אַף תִּכּוֹן תֵּבֵל בַּל תִּמּוֹט. יִשְׂמְחוּ הַשָּׁמַיִם וְתָגֵל הָאָרֶץ,
וְיֹאמְרוּ בַגּוֹיִם, יהוה מָלָךְ. יִרְעַם הַיָּם וּמְלֹאוֹ, יַעֲלֹץ הַשָּׂדֶה וְכָל
אֲשֶׁר בּוֹ. אָז יְרַנְּנוּ עֲצֵי הַיָּעַר, מִלִּפְנֵי יהוה, כִּי בָא לִשְׁפּוֹט אֶת
הָאָרֶץ. הוֹדוּ לַיהוה כִּי טוֹב, כִּי לְעוֹלָם חַסְדּוֹ. וְאִמְרוּ הוֹשִׁיעֵנוּ
אֱלֹהֵי יִשְׁעֵנוּ, וְקַבְּצֵנוּ וְהַצִּילֵנוּ מִן הַגּוֹיִם, לְהֹדוֹת לְשֵׁם קָדְשֶׁךָ,
לְהִשְׁתַּבֵּחַ בִּתְהִלָּתֶךָ. בָּרוּךְ יהוה אֱלֹהֵי יִשְׂרָאֵל מִן הָעוֹלָם וְעַד
הָעֹלָם, וַיֹּאמְרוּ כָל הָעָם, אָמֵן, וְהַלֵּל לַיהוה.

❖ רוֹמְמוּ יהוה אֱלֹהֵינוּ וְהִשְׁתַּחֲווּ לַהֲדֹם רַגְלָיו, קָדוֹשׁ הוּא.[1]
רוֹמְמוּ יהוה אֱלֹהֵינוּ וְהִשְׁתַּחֲווּ לְהַר קָדְשׁוֹ, כִּי קָדוֹשׁ יהוה אֱלֹהֵינוּ.[2]

וְהוּא רַחוּם יְכַפֵּר עָוֹן וְלֹא יַשְׁחִית, וְהִרְבָּה לְהָשִׁיב אַפּוֹ, וְלֹא
יָעִיר כָּל חֲמָתוֹ.[3] אַתָּה יהוה, לֹא תִכְלָא רַחֲמֶיךָ מִמֶּנִּי, חַסְדְּךָ

---

graphs of *Shema.*

In all cases of permitted responses it is preferable to respond between psalms, whenever possible. Thus, for example, if one realizes that the congregation is approaching *Kedushah,* he should not begin a new psalm, but should wait for the congregation to recite *Kedushah,* then continue his prayers.

The responses permitted above do not apply during the 'blessing' portions of בָּרוּךְ שֶׁאָמַר

I Chronicles 16:8-36

הוֹדוּ *Give thanks to HASHEM, declare His Name, make His acts known among the peoples. Sing to Him, make music to Him, speak of all His wonders. Glory in His holy Name, be glad of heart, you who seek HASHEM. Search out HASHEM and His might, seek His Presence always. Remember His wonders that He wrought, His marvels and the judgments of His mouth. O seed of Israel, His servant, O children of Jacob, His chosen ones — He is HASHEM, our God, over all the earth are His judgments. Remember His covenant forever — the word He commanded for a thousand generations — that He made with Abraham and His vow to Isaac. Then He established it for Jacob as a statute, for Israel as an everlasting covenant; saying, 'To you I shall give the Land of Canaan, the lot of your heritage.' When you were but few in number, hardly dwelling there, and they wandered from nation to nation, from one kingdom to another people. He let no man rob them, and He rebuked kings for their sake: 'Dare not touch My anointed ones, and to My prophets do no harm.' Sing to HASHEM, everyone on earth, announce His salvation daily. Relate His glory among the nations, among all the peoples His wonders. That HASHEM is great and exceedingly lauded, and awesome is He above all heavenly powers.* Chazzan— *For all the gods of the peoples are nothings — but HASHEM made heaven!*

Glory and majesty are before Him, might and delight are in His place. Render to HASHEM, O families of the peoples, render to HASHEM honor and might. Render to HASHEM honor worthy of His Name, take an offering and come before Him, prostrate yourselves before HASHEM in His intensely holy place. Tremble before Him, everyone on earth, indeed, the world is fixed so that it cannot falter. The heavens will be glad and the earth will rejoice and say among the nations, 'HASHEM has reigned!' The sea and its fullness will roar, the field and everything in it will exult. Then the trees of the forest will sing with joy before HASHEM, for He will have arrived to judge the earth. Give thanks to HASHEM, for He is good, for His kindness endures forever. And say, 'Save us, O God of our salvation, gather us and rescue us from the nations, to thank Your Holy Name and to glory in Your praise!' Blessed is HASHEM, the God of Israel, from This World to the World to Come — and let the entire people say, 'Amen and praise to God!'

Chazzan— *Exalt HASHEM, our God, and bow at His footstool; He is holy!*[1] *Exalt HASHEM, our God, and bow at His holy mountain; for holy is HASHEM, our God.*[2]

He, the Merciful One, is forgiving of iniquity and does not destroy; frequently, He withdraws His anger, not arousing His entire rage.[3] *You, HASHEM — withhold not Your mercy from me; may Your kindness*

---

(1) *Psalms* 99:5. (2) 99:9. (3) 78:38.

and וִישְׁתַּבַּח [i.e., from the words בָּרוּךְ אַתָּה ה׳, *Blessed are You, HASHEM,* until the blessing's   conclusion] where no interruptions are permitted.

וַאֲמָתְךָ תָּמִיד יִצְּרְוּנִי.¹ זְכֹר רַחֲמֶיךָ יהוה וַחֲסָדֶיךָ, כִּי מֵעוֹלָם
הֵמָּה.² תְּנוּ עֹז לֵאלֹהִים, עַל יִשְׂרָאֵל גַּאֲוָתוֹ, וְעֻזּוֹ בַּשְּׁחָקִים. נוֹרָא
אֱלֹהִים מִמִּקְדָּשֶׁיךָ, אֵל יִשְׂרָאֵל הוּא נֹתֵן עֹז וְתַעֲצֻמוֹת לָעָם, בָּרוּךְ
אֱלֹהִים.³ אֵל נְקָמוֹת יהוה, אֵל נְקָמוֹת הוֹפִיעַ. הִנָּשֵׂא שֹׁפֵט הָאָרֶץ,
הָשֵׁב גְּמוּל עַל גֵּאִים.⁴ לַיהוה הַיְשׁוּעָה, עַל עַמְּךָ בִרְכָתֶךָ סֶּלָה.⁵
❖ יהוה צְבָאוֹת עִמָּנוּ, מִשְׂגָּב לָנוּ אֱלֹהֵי יַעֲקֹב סֶלָה.⁶ יהוה צְבָאוֹת,
אַשְׁרֵי אָדָם בֹּטֵחַ בָּךְ.⁷ יהוה הוֹשִׁיעָה, הַמֶּלֶךְ יַעֲנֵנוּ בְיוֹם קָרְאֵנוּ.⁸

הוֹשִׁיעָה אֶת עַמֶּךָ, וּבָרֵךְ אֶת נַחֲלָתֶךָ, וּרְעֵם וְנַשְּׂאֵם עַד
הָעוֹלָם.⁹ נַפְשֵׁנוּ חִכְּתָה לַיהוה, עֶזְרֵנוּ וּמָגִנֵּנוּ הוּא. כִּי בוֹ יִשְׂמַח
לִבֵּנוּ, כִּי בְשֵׁם קָדְשׁוֹ בָטָחְנוּ. יְהִי חַסְדְּךָ יהוה עָלֵינוּ, כַּאֲשֶׁר יִחַלְנוּ
לָךְ.¹⁰ הַרְאֵנוּ יהוה חַסְדֶּךָ, וְיֶשְׁעֲךָ תִּתֶּן לָנוּ.¹¹ קוּמָה עֶזְרָתָה לָּנוּ,
וּפְדֵנוּ לְמַעַן חַסְדֶּךָ.¹² אָנֹכִי יהוה אֱלֹהֶיךָ הַמַּעַלְךָ מֵאֶרֶץ מִצְרָיִם,
הַרְחֶב פִּיךָ וַאֲמַלְאֵהוּ.¹³ אַשְׁרֵי הָעָם שֶׁכָּכָה לּוֹ, אַשְׁרֵי הָעָם שֶׁיהוה
אֱלֹהָיו.¹⁴ ❖ וַאֲנִי בְּחַסְדְּךָ בָטַחְתִּי, יָגֵל לִבִּי בִּישׁוּעָתֶךָ, אָשִׁירָה
לַיהוה, כִּי גָמַל עָלָי.¹⁵

The following prayer should be recited with special intensity.

יְהִי כְבוֹד יהוה לְעוֹלָם, יִשְׂמַח יהוה בְּמַעֲשָׂיו.¹⁶ יְהִי שֵׁם יהוה
מְבֹרָךְ, מֵעַתָּה וְעַד עוֹלָם. מִמִּזְרַח שֶׁמֶשׁ עַד מְבוֹאוֹ, מְהֻלָּל
שֵׁם יהוה. רָם עַל כָּל גּוֹיִם יהוה, עַל הַשָּׁמַיִם כְּבוֹדוֹ.¹⁷ יהוה
שִׁמְךָ לְעוֹלָם, יהוה זִכְרְךָ לְדֹר וָדֹר.¹⁸ יהוה בַּשָּׁמַיִם הֵכִין כִּסְאוֹ,
וּמַלְכוּתוֹ בַּכֹּל מָשָׁלָה.¹⁹ יִשְׂמְחוּ הַשָּׁמַיִם וְתָגֵל הָאָרֶץ, וְיֹאמְרוּ
בַגּוֹיִם יהוה מָלָךְ.²⁰ יהוה מֶלֶךְ,²¹ יהוה מָלָךְ,²² יהוה יִמְלֹךְ לְעֹלָם
וָעֶד.²³ יהוה מֶלֶךְ עוֹלָם וָעֶד, אָבְדוּ גוֹיִם מֵאַרְצוֹ.²⁴ יהוה הֵפִיר עֲצַת
גּוֹיִם, הֵנִיא מַחְשְׁבוֹת עַמִּים.²⁵ רַבּוֹת מַחֲשָׁבוֹת בְּלֶב אִישׁ, וַעֲצַת
יהוה הִיא תָקוּם.²⁶ עֲצַת יהוה לְעוֹלָם תַּעֲמֹד, מַחְשְׁבוֹת לִבּוֹ לְדֹר
וָדֹר.²⁷ כִּי הוּא אָמַר וַיֶּהִי, הוּא צִוָּה וַיַּעֲמֹד.²⁸ כִּי בָחַר יהוה בְּצִיּוֹן,
אִוָּהּ לְמוֹשָׁב לוֹ.²⁹ כִּי יַעֲקֹב בָּחַר לוֹ יָהּ, יִשְׂרָאֵל לִסְגֻלָּתוֹ.³⁰ כִּי לֹא
יִטֹּשׁ יהוה עַמּוֹ, וְנַחֲלָתוֹ לֹא יַעֲזֹב.³¹ ❖ וְהוּא רַחוּם יְכַפֵּר עָוֹן וְלֹא
יַשְׁחִית, וְהִרְבָּה לְהָשִׁיב אַפּוֹ, וְלֹא יָעִיר כָּל חֲמָתוֹ.³² יהוה הוֹשִׁיעָה,
הַמֶּלֶךְ יַעֲנֵנוּ בְיוֹם קָרְאֵנוּ.³³

---

(1) Psalms 40:12. (2) 25:6. (3) 68:35-36. (4) 94:1-2. (5) 3:9. (6) 46:8. (7) 84:13. (8) 20:10.
(9) 28:9. (10) 33:20-22. (11) 85:8. (12) 44:27. (13) 81:11. (14) 144:15. (15) 13:6. (16) 104:31.
(17) 113:2-4. (18) 135:13. (19) 103:19. (20) I Chronicles 16:31. (21) Psalms 10:16.
(22) 93:1 et al. (23) Exodus 15:18. (24) Psalms 10:16. (25) 33:10. (26) Proverbs 19:21.
(27) Psalms 33:11. (28) 33:9. (29) 132:13. (30) 135:4. (31) 94:14. (32) 78:38. (33) 20:10.

and Your truth always protect me.¹ Remember Your mercies, HASHEM, and Your kindnesses, for they are from the beginning of the world.² Render might to God, Whose majesty hovers over Israel and Whose might is in the clouds. You are awesome, O God, from Your sanctuaries, O God of Israel — it is He Who grants might and power to the people, blessed is God.³ O God of vengeance, HASHEM, O God of vengeance, appear! Arise, O Judge of the earth, render recompense to the haughty.⁴ Salvation is HASHEM's, upon Your people is Your blessing, Selah.⁵ Chazzan— HASHEM, Master of Legions, is with us, a stronghold for us is the God of Jacob, Selah.⁶ HASHEM, Master of Legions, praiseworthy is the person who trusts in You.⁷ HASHEM, save! May the King answer us on the day we call.⁸

Save Your people and bless Your heritage, tend them and elevate them forever.⁹ Our soul longed for HASHEM — our help and our shield is He. For in Him will our hearts be glad, for in His Holy Name we trusted. May Your kindness, HASHEM, be upon us, just as we awaited You.¹⁰ Show us Your kindness, HASHEM, and grant us Your salvation.¹¹ Arise — assist us, and redeem us by virtue of Your kindness.¹² I am HASHEM, your God, Who raised you from the land of Egypt, open wide your mouth and I will fill it.¹³ Praiseworthy is the people for whom this is so, praiseworthy is the people whose God is HASHEM.¹⁴ Chazzan— As for me, I trust in Your kindness; my heart will rejoice in Your salvation. I will sing to HASHEM, for He dealt kindly with me.¹⁵

The following prayer should be recited with special intensity.

יְהִי May the glory of HASHEM endure forever, let HASHEM rejoice in His works.¹⁶ Blessed be the Name of HASHEM, from this time and forever. From the rising of the sun to its setting, HASHEM's Name is praised. High above all nations is HASHEM, above the heavens is His glory.¹⁷ 'HASHEM' is Your Name forever, 'HASHEM' is Your memorial throughout the generations.¹⁸ HASHEM has established His throne in the heavens, and His kingdom reigns over all.¹⁹ The heavens will be glad and the earth will rejoice, they will proclaim among the nations, 'HASHEM has reigned!'²⁰ HASHEM reigns,²¹ HASHEM has reigned,²² HASHEM shall reign for all eternity.²³ HASHEM reigns forever and ever, even when the nations will have perished from His earth.²⁴ HASHEM annuls the counsel of nations, He balks the designs of peoples.²⁵ Many designs are in man's heart, but the counsel of HASHEM — only it will prevail.²⁶ The counsel of HASHEM will endure forever, the designs of His heart throughout the generations.²⁷ For He spoke and it came to be; He commanded and it stood firm.²⁸ For God selected Zion, He desired it for His dwelling place.²⁹ For God selected Jacob as His own, Israel as His treasure.³⁰ For HASHEM will not cast off His people, nor will He forsake His heritage.³¹ Chazzan— He, the Merciful One, is forgiving of iniquity and does not destroy; frequently He withdraws His anger, not arousing His entire rage.³² HASHEM, save! May the King answer us on the day we call.³³

אַשְׁרֵי יוֹשְׁבֵי בֵיתֶךָ, עוֹד יְהַלְלוּךָ סֶּלָה.[1] אַשְׁרֵי הָעָם שֶׁכָּכָה לּוֹ,
אַשְׁרֵי הָעָם שֶׁיהוה אֱלֹהָיו.[2]

תְּהִלָּה לְדָוִד,

תהלים קמה

אֲרוֹמִמְךָ אֱלוֹהַי הַמֶּלֶךְ, וַאֲבָרְכָה שִׁמְךָ לְעוֹלָם וָעֶד.

בְּכָל יוֹם אֲבָרְכֶךָּ, וַאֲהַלְלָה שִׁמְךָ לְעוֹלָם וָעֶד.

גָּדוֹל יהוה וּמְהֻלָּל מְאֹד, וְלִגְדֻלָּתוֹ אֵין חֵקֶר.

דּוֹר לְדוֹר יְשַׁבַּח מַעֲשֶׂיךָ, וּגְבוּרֹתֶיךָ יַגִּידוּ.

הֲדַר כְּבוֹד הוֹדֶךָ, וְדִבְרֵי נִפְלְאֹתֶיךָ אָשִׂיחָה.

וֶעֱזוּז נוֹרְאוֹתֶיךָ יֹאמֵרוּ, וּגְדוּלָּתְךָ אֲסַפְּרֶנָּה.

זֵכֶר רַב טוּבְךָ יַבִּיעוּ, וְצִדְקָתְךָ יְרַנֵּנוּ.

חַנּוּן וְרַחוּם יהוה, אֶרֶךְ אַפַּיִם וּגְדָל חָסֶד.

טוֹב יהוה לַכֹּל, וְרַחֲמָיו עַל כָּל מַעֲשָׂיו.

יוֹדוּךָ יהוה כָּל מַעֲשֶׂיךָ, וַחֲסִידֶיךָ יְבָרְכוּכָה.

כְּבוֹד מַלְכוּתְךָ יֹאמֵרוּ, וּגְבוּרָתְךָ יְדַבֵּרוּ.

לְהוֹדִיעַ לִבְנֵי הָאָדָם גְּבוּרֹתָיו, וּכְבוֹד הֲדַר מַלְכוּתוֹ.

מַלְכוּתְךָ מַלְכוּת כָּל עֹלָמִים, וּמֶמְשַׁלְתְּךָ בְּכָל דּוֹר וָדֹר.

סוֹמֵךְ יהוה לְכָל הַנֹּפְלִים, וְזוֹקֵף לְכָל הַכְּפוּפִים.

עֵינֵי כֹל אֵלֶיךָ יְשַׂבֵּרוּ, וְאַתָּה נוֹתֵן לָהֶם אֶת אָכְלָם בְּעִתּוֹ.

While reciting the verse פּוֹתֵחַ,
concentrate intently on its meaning.

פּוֹתֵחַ אֶת יָדֶךָ,

וּמַשְׂבִּיעַ לְכָל חַי רָצוֹן.

צַדִּיק יהוה בְּכָל דְּרָכָיו, וְחָסִיד בְּכָל מַעֲשָׂיו.

קָרוֹב יהוה לְכָל קֹרְאָיו, לְכֹל אֲשֶׁר יִקְרָאֻהוּ בֶאֱמֶת.

רְצוֹן יְרֵאָיו יַעֲשֶׂה, וְאֶת שַׁוְעָתָם יִשְׁמַע וְיוֹשִׁיעֵם.

שׁוֹמֵר יהוה אֶת כָּל אֹהֲבָיו, וְאֵת כָּל הָרְשָׁעִים יַשְׁמִיד.

❖ תְּהִלַּת יהוה יְדַבֶּר פִּי, וִיבָרֵךְ כָּל בָּשָׂר שֵׁם קָדְשׁוֹ לְעוֹלָם וָעֶד.

וַאֲנַחְנוּ נְבָרֵךְ יָהּ, מֵעַתָּה וְעַד עוֹלָם, הַלְלוּיָהּ.[3]

תהלים קמו

הַלְלוּיָהּ, הַלְלִי נַפְשִׁי אֶת יהוה. אֲהַלְלָה יהוה בְּחַיָּי, אֲזַמְּרָה
לֵאלֹהַי בְּעוֹדִי. אַל תִּבְטְחוּ בִנְדִיבִים, בְּבֶן אָדָם
שֶׁאֵין לוֹ תְשׁוּעָה. תֵּצֵא רוּחוֹ, יָשֻׁב לְאַדְמָתוֹ, בַּיּוֹם הַהוּא

(1) *Psalms* 84:5. (2) 144:15. (3) 115:8.

אַשְׁרֵי *Praiseworthy are those who dwell in Your house; may they always praise You, Selah!*[1] *Praiseworthy is the people for whom this is so, praiseworthy is the people whose God is HASHEM.*[2]

Psalm 145   *A psalm of praise by David:*

א *I will exalt You, my God the King,*
    and I will bless Your Name forever and ever.

ב *Every day I will bless You, and I will laud Your Name forever and ever.*

ג *HASHEM is great and exceedingly lauded,*
    and His greatness is beyond investigation.

ד *Each generation will praise Your deeds to the next*
    and of Your mighty deeds they will tell.

ה *The splendrous glory of Your power*
    and Your wondrous deeds I shall discuss.

ו *And of Your awesome power they will speak,*
    and Your greatness I shall relate.

ז *A recollection of Your abundant goodness they will utter*
    and of Your righteousness they will sing exultantly.

ח *Gracious and merciful is HASHEM,*
    slow to anger, and great in [bestowing] kindness.

ט *HASHEM is good to all; His mercies are on all His works.*

י *All Your works shall thank You, HASHEM,*
    and Your devout ones will bless You.

כ *Of the glory of Your kingdom they will speak,*
    and of Your power they will tell;

ל *To inform human beings of His mighty deeds,*
    and the glorious splendor of His kingdom.

מ *Your kingdom is a kingdom spanning all eternities,*
    and Your dominion is throughout every generation.

ס *HASHEM supports all the fallen ones and straightens all the bent.*

ע *The eyes of all look to You with hope*
    and You give them their food in its proper time;

פ *You open Your hand, and satisfy*   While reciting the verse, 'You open . . .'
    the desire of every living thing.   concentrate intently on its meaning.

צ *Righteous is HASHEM in all His ways and magnanimous in all His deeds.*

ק *HASHEM is close to all who call upon Him —*
    to all who call upon Him sincerely.

ר *The will of those who fear Him He will do;*
    and their cry He will hear, and save them.

ש *HASHEM protects all who love Him; but all the wicked He will destroy.*

ת Chazzan— *May my mouth declare the praise of HASHEM*
    and may all flesh bless His Holy Name forever and ever.
We will bless God from this time and forever, Halleluyah![3]

Psalm 146

הַלְלוּיָהּ *Halleluyah! Praise HASHEM, O my Soul! I will praise HASHEM while I live, I will make music to my God while I exist. Do not rely on nobles, nor on a human being for he holds no salvation. When his spirit departs he returns to his earth, on that day*

אָבְדוּ עֶשְׁתֹּנֹתָיו. אַשְׁרֵי שֶׁאֵל יַעֲקֹב בְּעֶזְרוֹ, שִׂבְרוֹ עַל יהוה אֱלֹהָיו. עֹשֶׂה שָׁמַיִם וָאָרֶץ, אֶת הַיָּם וְאֶת כָּל אֲשֶׁר בָּם, הַשֹּׁמֵר אֱמֶת לְעוֹלָם. עֹשֶׂה מִשְׁפָּט לַעֲשׁוּקִים, נֹתֵן לֶחֶם לָרְעֵבִים, יהוה מַתִּיר אֲסוּרִים. יהוה פֹּקֵחַ עִוְרִים, יהוה זֹקֵף כְּפוּפִים, יהוה אֹהֵב צַדִּיקִים. יהוה שֹׁמֵר אֶת גֵּרִים, יָתוֹם וְאַלְמָנָה יְעוֹדֵד, וְדֶרֶךְ רְשָׁעִים יְעַוֵּת. ✧ יִמְלֹךְ יהוה לְעוֹלָם, אֱלֹהַיִךְ צִיּוֹן, לְדֹר וָדֹר, הַלְלוּיָהּ.

תהלים קמז

הַלְלוּיָהּ, כִּי טוֹב זַמְּרָה אֱלֹהֵינוּ, כִּי נָעִים נָאוָה תְהִלָּה. בּוֹנֵה יְרוּשָׁלַיִם יהוה, נִדְחֵי יִשְׂרָאֵל יְכַנֵּס. הָרֹפֵא לִשְׁבוּרֵי לֵב, וּמְחַבֵּשׁ לְעַצְּבוֹתָם. מוֹנֶה מִסְפָּר לַכּוֹכָבִים, לְכֻלָּם שֵׁמוֹת יִקְרָא. גָּדוֹל אֲדוֹנֵינוּ וְרַב כֹּחַ, לִתְבוּנָתוֹ אֵין מִסְפָּר. מְעוֹדֵד עֲנָוִים יהוה, מַשְׁפִּיל רְשָׁעִים עֲדֵי אָרֶץ. עֱנוּ לַיהוה בְּתוֹדָה, זַמְּרוּ לֵאלֹהֵינוּ בְכִנּוֹר. הַמְכַסֶּה שָׁמַיִם בְּעָבִים, הַמֵּכִין לָאָרֶץ מָטָר, הַמַּצְמִיחַ הָרִים חָצִיר. נוֹתֵן לִבְהֵמָה לַחְמָהּ, לִבְנֵי עֹרֵב אֲשֶׁר יִקְרָאוּ. לֹא בִגְבוּרַת הַסּוּס יֶחְפָּץ, לֹא בְשׁוֹקֵי הָאִישׁ יִרְצֶה. רוֹצֶה יהוה אֶת יְרֵאָיו, אֶת הַמְיַחֲלִים לְחַסְדּוֹ. שַׁבְּחִי יְרוּשָׁלַיִם אֶת יהוה, הַלְלִי אֱלֹהַיִךְ צִיּוֹן. כִּי חִזַּק בְּרִיחֵי שְׁעָרָיִךְ, בֵּרַךְ בָּנַיִךְ בְּקִרְבֵּךְ. הַשָּׂם גְּבוּלֵךְ שָׁלוֹם, חֵלֶב חִטִּים יַשְׂבִּיעֵךְ. הַשֹּׁלֵחַ אִמְרָתוֹ אָרֶץ, עַד מְהֵרָה יָרוּץ דְּבָרוֹ. הַנֹּתֵן שֶׁלֶג כַּצָּמֶר, כְּפוֹר כָּאֵפֶר יְפַזֵּר. מַשְׁלִיךְ קַרְחוֹ כְפִתִּים, לִפְנֵי קָרָתוֹ מִי יַעֲמֹד. יִשְׁלַח דְּבָרוֹ וְיַמְסֵם, יַשֵּׁב רוּחוֹ יִזְּלוּ מָיִם. ✧ מַגִּיד דְּבָרָיו לְיַעֲקֹב, חֻקָּיו וּמִשְׁפָּטָיו לְיִשְׂרָאֵל. לֹא עָשָׂה כֵן לְכָל גּוֹי, וּמִשְׁפָּטִים בַּל יְדָעוּם, הַלְלוּיָהּ.

תהלים קמח

הַלְלוּיָהּ, הַלְלוּ אֶת יהוה מִן הַשָּׁמַיִם, הַלְלוּהוּ בַּמְּרוֹמִים. הַלְלוּהוּ כָל מַלְאָכָיו, הַלְלוּהוּ כָּל צְבָאָיו. הַלְלוּהוּ שֶׁמֶשׁ וְיָרֵחַ, הַלְלוּהוּ כָּל כּוֹכְבֵי אוֹר. הַלְלוּהוּ שְׁמֵי הַשָּׁמַיִם, וְהַמַּיִם אֲשֶׁר מֵעַל הַשָּׁמַיִם. יְהַלְלוּ אֶת שֵׁם יהוה, כִּי הוּא צִוָּה וְנִבְרָאוּ. וַיַּעֲמִידֵם לָעַד לְעוֹלָם, חָק נָתַן וְלֹא יַעֲבוֹר. הַלְלוּ אֶת יהוה מִן הָאָרֶץ, תַּנִּינִים וְכָל תְּהֹמוֹת. אֵשׁ וּבָרָד, שֶׁלֶג וְקִיטוֹר, רוּחַ סְעָרָה עֹשָׂה דְבָרוֹ. הֶהָרִים וְכָל גְּבָעוֹת, עֵץ פְּרִי וְכָל אֲרָזִים. הַחַיָּה וְכָל בְּהֵמָה, רֶמֶשׂ וְצִפּוֹר כָּנָף. מַלְכֵי אֶרֶץ וְכָל לְאֻמִּים, שָׂרִים וְכָל שֹׁפְטֵי אָרֶץ. בַּחוּרִים וְגַם בְּתוּלוֹת, זְקֵנִים עִם נְעָרִים. ✧ יְהַלְלוּ אֶת

his plans all perish. Praiseworthy is one whose help is Jacob's God, whose hope is in HASHEM, his God. He is the Maker of heaven and earth, the sea and all that is in them, Who safeguards truth forever. He does justice for the exploited; He gives bread to the hungry; HASHEM releases the bound. HASHEM gives sight to the blind; HASHEM straightens the bent; HASHEM loves the righteous. HASHEM protects strangers; orphan and widow He encourages; but the way of the wicked He contorts. Chazzan— HASHEM shall reign forever — your God, O Zion — from generation to generation. Halleluyah!

Psalm 147

הַלְלוּיָהּ Halleluyah! For it is good to make music to our God, for praise is pleasant and befitting. The Builder of Jerusalem is HASHEM, the outcast of Israel He will gather in. He is the Healer of the broken-hearted, and the One Who binds up their sorrows. He counts the number of the stars, to all of them He assigns names. Great is our Lord and abundant in strength, His understanding is beyond calculation. HASHEM encourages the humble, He lowers the wicked down to the ground. Call out to HASHEM with thanks, with the harp sing to our God — Who covers the heavens with clouds, Who prepares rain for the earth, Who makes mountains sprout with grass. He gives to an animal its food, to young ravens that cry out. Not in the strength of the horse does He desire, and not in the legs of man does He favor. HASHEM favors those who fear Him, those who hope for His kindness. Praise HASHEM, O Jerusalem, laud your God, O Zion. For He has strengthened the bars of your gates, and blessed your children in your midst; He Who makes your borders peaceful, and with the cream of the wheat He sates you; He Who dispatches His utterance earthward; how swiftly His commandment runs! He Who gives snow like fleece, He scatters frost like ashes. He hurls His ice like crumbs — before His cold, who can stand? He issues His command and it melts them, He blows His wind — the waters flow. Chazzan— He relates His Word to Jacob, His statutes and judgments to Israel. He did not do so for any other nation, such judgments — they know them not. Halleluyah!

Psalm 148

הַלְלוּיָהּ Halleluyah! Praise HASHEM from the heavens; praise Him in the heights. Praise Him, all His angels; praise Him, all His legions. Praise Him, sun and moon; praise Him, all bright stars. Praise Him, the most exalted of the heavens and the waters that are above the heavens. Let them praise the Name of HASHEM, for He commanded and they were created. And He established them forever and ever, He issued a decree that will not change. Praise HASHEM from the earth, sea giants and all watery depths. Fire and hail, snow and vapor, stormy wind fulfilling His word. Mountains and all hills, fruitful trees and all cedars. Beasts and all cattle, crawling things and winged fowl. Kings of the earth and all governments, princes and all judges on earth. Young men and also maidens, old men together with youths. Chazzan— Let them praise the

שֵׁם יהוה, כִּי נִשְׂגָּב שְׁמוֹ לְבַדּוֹ, הוֹדוֹ עַל אֶרֶץ וְשָׁמָיִם. וַיָּרֶם קֶרֶן לְעַמּוֹ, תְּהִלָּה לְכָל חֲסִידָיו, לִבְנֵי יִשְׂרָאֵל עַם קְרֹבוֹ, הַלְלוּיָהּ.

תהלים קמט

הַלְלוּיָהּ, שִׁירוּ לַיהוה שִׁיר חָדָשׁ, תְּהִלָּתוֹ בִּקְהַל חֲסִידִים. יִשְׂמַח יִשְׂרָאֵל בְּעֹשָׂיו, בְּנֵי צִיּוֹן יָגִילוּ בְמַלְכָּם. יְהַלְלוּ שְׁמוֹ בְמָחוֹל, בְּתֹף וְכִנּוֹר יְזַמְּרוּ לוֹ. כִּי רוֹצֶה יהוה בְּעַמּוֹ, יְפָאֵר עֲנָוִים בִּישׁוּעָה. יַעְלְזוּ חֲסִידִים בְּכָבוֹד, יְרַנְּנוּ עַל מִשְׁכְּבוֹתָם. רוֹמְמוֹת אֵל בִּגְרוֹנָם, וְחֶרֶב פִּיפִיּוֹת בְּיָדָם. לַעֲשׂוֹת נְקָמָה בַּגּוֹיִם, תּוֹכֵחוֹת בַּלְאֻמִּים. ❖ לֶאְסֹר מַלְכֵיהֶם בְּזִקִּים, וְנִכְבְּדֵיהֶם בְּכַבְלֵי בַרְזֶל. לַעֲשׂוֹת בָּהֶם מִשְׁפָּט כָּתוּב, הָדָר הוּא לְכָל חֲסִידָיו, הַלְלוּיָהּ.

תהלים קנ

הַלְלוּיָהּ, הַלְלוּ אֵל בְּקָדְשׁוֹ, הַלְלוּהוּ בִּרְקִיעַ עֻזּוֹ. הַלְלוּהוּ בִגְבוּרֹתָיו, הַלְלוּהוּ כְּרֹב גֻּדְלוֹ. הַלְלוּהוּ בְּתֵקַע שׁוֹפָר, הַלְלוּהוּ בְּנֵבֶל וְכִנּוֹר. הַלְלוּהוּ בְּתֹף וּמָחוֹל, הַלְלוּהוּ בְּמִנִּים וְעֻגָב. הַלְלוּהוּ בְצִלְצְלֵי שָׁמַע, הַלְלוּהוּ בְּצִלְצְלֵי תְרוּעָה. ❖ כֹּל הַנְּשָׁמָה תְּהַלֵּל יָהּ, הַלְלוּיָהּ. כֹּל הַנְּשָׁמָה תְּהַלֵּל יָהּ, הַלְלוּיָהּ.

בָּרוּךְ יהוה לְעוֹלָם, אָמֵן וְאָמֵן.[1] בָּרוּךְ יהוה מִצִּיּוֹן, שֹׁכֵן יְרוּשָׁלָיִם, הַלְלוּיָהּ.[2] בָּרוּךְ יהוה אֱלֹהִים אֱלֹהֵי יִשְׂרָאֵל, עֹשֵׂה נִפְלָאוֹת לְבַדּוֹ. ❖ וּבָרוּךְ שֵׁם כְּבוֹדוֹ לְעוֹלָם, וְיִמָּלֵא כְבוֹדוֹ אֶת כָּל הָאָרֶץ, אָמֵן וְאָמֵן.[3]

One must stand from וַיְבָרֶךְ דָּוִיד, until after the phrase אַתָּה הוּא ה' הָאֱלֹהִים; however, there is a generally accepted custom to remain standing until after completing אָז יָשִׁיר (p. 112).

דברי הימים א כט:י-יג

וַיְבָרֶךְ דָּוִיד אֶת יהוה לְעֵינֵי כָּל הַקָּהָל, וַיֹּאמֶר דָּוִיד: בָּרוּךְ אַתָּה יהוה, אֱלֹהֵי יִשְׂרָאֵל אָבִינוּ, מֵעוֹלָם וְעַד עוֹלָם. לְךָ יהוה הַגְּדֻלָּה וְהַגְּבוּרָה וְהַתִּפְאֶרֶת וְהַנֵּצַח וְהַהוֹד, כִּי כֹל בַּשָּׁמַיִם וּבָאָרֶץ; לְךָ יהוה הַמַּמְלָכָה וְהַמִּתְנַשֵּׂא לְכֹל לְרֹאשׁ. וְהָעֹשֶׁר וְהַכָּבוֹד מִלְּפָנֶיךָ, וְאַתָּה מוֹשֵׁל It is customary to set aside something for charity at this point. בַּכֹּל, וּבְיָדְךָ כֹּחַ וּגְבוּרָה, וּבְיָדְךָ לְגַדֵּל וּלְחַזֵּק לַכֹּל. וְעַתָּה אֱלֹהֵינוּ מוֹדִים אֲנַחְנוּ לָךְ, וּמְהַלְלִים לְשֵׁם תִּפְאַרְתֶּךָ.

Name of HASHEM, for His Name alone will have been exalted; His glory is above earth and heaven. And He will have exalted the pride of His nation, causing praise for all His devout ones, for the Children of Israel, His intimate people. Halleluyah!

Psalm 149

הַלְלוּיָהּ Halleluyah! Sing to HASHEM a new song, let His praise be in the congregation of the devout. Let Israel exult in its Maker, let the Children of Zion rejoice in their King. Let them praise His Name with dancing, with drums and harp let them make music to Him. For HASHEM favors His nation, He adorns the humble with salvation. Let the devout exult in glory, let them sing joyously upon their beds. The lofty praises of God are in their throats, and a double-edged sword is in their hand — to execute vengeance among the nations, rebukes among the governments. Chazzan– To bind their kings with chains, and their nobles with fetters of iron. To execute upon them written judgment — that will be the splendor of all His devout ones. Halleluyah!

Psalm 150

הַלְלוּיָהּ Halleluyah! Praise God in His Sanctuary; praise Him in the firmament of His power. Praise Him for His mighty acts; praise Him as befits His abundant greatness. Praise Him with the blast of the shofar; praise Him with lyre and harp. Praise Him with drum and dance; praise Him with organ and flute. Praise Him with clanging cymbals; praise Him with resonant trumpets. Chazzan– Let all souls praise God, Halleluyah! Let all souls praise God, Halleluyah!

בָּרוּךְ Blessed is HASHEM forever, Amen and Amen.[1] Blessed is HASHEM from Zion, Who dwells in Jerusalem, Halleluyah.[2] Blessed is HASHEM, God, the God of Israel, Who alone does wonders. Chazzan– Blessed is His glorious Name forever, and may all the earth be filled with His glory, Amen and Amen.[3]

One must stand from here until after the phrase 'It is You, HASHEM the God'; however, there is a generally accepted custom to remain standing until after completing the Song at the Sea (p. 112).

I Chronicles 29:10-13

וַיְבָרֶךְ And David blessed HASHEM in the presence of the entire congregation; David said, 'Blessed are You, HASHEM, the God of Israel our forefather from This World to the World to Come. Yours, HASHEM, is the greatness, the strength, the splendor, the triumph, and the glory, even everything in heaven and earth; Yours, HASHEM, is the It is customary to set kingdom, and the sovereignty over every leader. aside something for Wealth and honor come from You and You rule charity at this point. everything — in Your hand is power and strength and it is in Your hand to make anyone great or strong. So now, our God, we thank You and praise Your splendrous Name.'

---

(1) *Psalms* 89:53. (2) 135:21. (3) 72:18-19.

נחמיה ט:ו-יא

אַתָּה הוּא יהוה לְבַדֶּךָ, אַתָּה עָשִׂיתָ אֶת הַשָּׁמַיִם, שְׁמֵי הַשָּׁמַיִם וְכָל צְבָאָם, הָאָרֶץ וְכָל אֲשֶׁר עָלֶיהָ, הַיַּמִּים וְכָל אֲשֶׁר בָּהֶם, וְאַתָּה מְחַיֶּה אֶת כֻּלָּם, וּצְבָא הַשָּׁמַיִם לְךָ מִשְׁתַּחֲוִים. ✧ אַתָּה הוּא יהוה הָאֱלֹהִים אֲשֶׁר בָּחַרְתָּ בְּאַבְרָם, וְהוֹצֵאתוֹ מֵאוּר כַּשְׂדִּים, וְשַׂמְתָּ שְּׁמוֹ אַבְרָהָם. וּמָצָאתָ אֶת לְבָבוֹ נֶאֱמָן לְפָנֶיךָ —

— וְכָרוֹת עִמּוֹ הַבְּרִית לָתֵת אֶת אֶרֶץ הַכְּנַעֲנִי הַחִתִּי הָאֱמֹרִי וְהַפְּרִזִּי וְהַיְבוּסִי וְהַגִּרְגָּשִׁי, לָתֵת לְזַרְעוֹ, וַתָּקֶם אֶת דְּבָרֶיךָ, כִּי צַדִּיק אָתָּה. וַתֵּרֶא אֶת עֳנִי אֲבֹתֵינוּ בְּמִצְרָיִם, וְאֶת זַעֲקָתָם שָׁמַעְתָּ עַל יַם סוּף. וַתִּתֵּן אֹתֹת וּמֹפְתִים בְּפַרְעֹה וּבְכָל עֲבָדָיו וּבְכָל עַם אַרְצוֹ, כִּי יָדַעְתָּ כִּי הֵזִידוּ עֲלֵיהֶם, וַתַּעַשׂ לְךָ שֵׁם כְּהַיּוֹם הַזֶּה. ✧ וְהַיָּם בָּקַעְתָּ לִפְנֵיהֶם, וַיַּעַבְרוּ בְתוֹךְ הַיָּם בַּיַּבָּשָׁה, וְאֶת רֹדְפֵיהֶם הִשְׁלַכְתָּ בִמְצוֹלֹת, כְּמוֹ אֶבֶן בְּמַיִם עַזִּים.

שירת הים

שמות יד:ל-טו:יט

וַיּוֹשַׁע יהוה בַּיּוֹם הַהוּא אֶת־יִשְׂרָאֵל מִיַּד מִצְרָיִם, וַיַּרְא יִשְׂרָאֵל אֶת־מִצְרַיִם מֵת עַל־שְׂפַת הַיָּם: ✧ וַיַּרְא יִשְׂרָאֵל אֶת־הַיָּד הַגְּדֹלָה אֲשֶׁר עָשָׂה יהוה בְּמִצְרַיִם, וַיִּירְאוּ הָעָם אֶת־יהוה, וַיַּאֲמִינוּ בַּיהוה וּבְמֹשֶׁה עַבְדּוֹ:

אָז יָשִׁיר־מֹשֶׁה וּבְנֵי יִשְׂרָאֵל אֶת־הַשִּׁירָה הַזֹּאת לַיהוה, וַיֹּאמְרוּ לֵאמֹר, אָשִׁירָה לַיהוה כִּי־גָאֹה גָּאָה, סוּס וְרֹכְבוֹ רָמָה בַיָּם: עָזִּי וְזִמְרָת יָהּ וַיְהִי־לִי לִישׁוּעָה, זֶה אֵלִי וְאַנְוֵהוּ, אֱלֹהֵי אָבִי וַאֲרֹמְמֶנְהוּ: יהוה אִישׁ מִלְחָמָה, יהוה שְׁמוֹ: מַרְכְּבֹת פַּרְעֹה וְחֵילוֹ יָרָה בַיָּם, וּמִבְחַר שָׁלִשָׁיו טֻבְּעוּ בְיַם־סוּף: תְּהֹמֹת יְכַסְיֻמוּ, יָרְדוּ בִמְצוֹלֹת כְּמוֹ־אָבֶן: יְמִינְךָ יהוה נֶאְדָּרִי בַּכֹּחַ, יְמִינְךָ יהוה תִּרְעַץ אוֹיֵב: וּבְרֹב גְּאוֹנְךָ תַּהֲרֹס קָמֶיךָ, תְּשַׁלַּח חֲרֹנְךָ יֹאכְלֵמוֹ כַּקַּשׁ: וּבְרוּחַ אַפֶּיךָ נֶעֶרְמוּ מַיִם, נִצְּבוּ כְמוֹ־נֵד

Nehemiah 9:6-11

It is You alone, HASHEM, You have made the heaven, the most exalted heaven and all their legions, the earth and everything upon it, the seas and everything in them and You give them all life; the heavenly legions bow to You. Chazzan– It is You, HASHEM the God, Who selected Abram, brought him out of Ur Kasdim and made his name Abraham. You found his heart faithful before You —

— and You established the covenant with him to give the land of the Canaanite, Hittite, Emorite, Perizzite, Jebusite, and Girgashite, to give it to his offspring; and You affirmed Your word, for You are righteous. You observed the suffering of our forefathers in Egypt, and their outcry You heard at the Sea of Reeds. You imposed signs and wonders upon Pharaoh and upon all his servants, and upon all the people of his land. For You knew that they sinned flagrantly against them, and You brought Yourself renown as [clear as] this very day. Chazzan– You split the Sea before them and they crossed in the midst of the Sea on dry land; but their pursuers You hurled into the depths, like a stone into turbulent waters.

THE SONG AT THE SEA

Exodus 14:30-15:19

וַיּוֹשַׁע HASHEM saved — on that day — Israel from the hand of Egypt, and Israel saw the Egyptians dead on the seashore. Chazzan– Israel saw the great hand that HASHEM inflicted upon Egypt and the people feared HASHEM, and they had faith in HASHEM and in Moses, His servant.

Then Moses and the Children of Israel chose to sing this song to HASHEM, and they said the following:

I shall sing to HASHEM for He is exalted above the arrogant, having hurled horse with its rider into the sea.

God is my might and my praise, and He was a salvation for me. This is my God, and I will build Him a Sanctuary; the God of my father, and I will exalt Him.

HASHEM is Master of war, through His Name HASHEM.

Pharaoh's chariots and army He threw into the sea; and the pick of his officers were mired in the Sea of Reeds.

Deep waters covered them; they descended in the depths like stone.

Your right hand, HASHEM, is adorned with strength; Your right hand, HASHEM, smashes the enemy.

In Your abundant grandeur You shatter Your opponents; You dispatch Your wrath, it consumes them like straw.

At a blast from Your nostrils the waters were heaped up; straight as

אָמַר   קָפְאוּ תְהֹמֹת בְּלֶב־יָם: נֹזְלִים,
תִּמְלָאֵמוֹ   אֲחַלֵּק שָׁלָל,   אוֹיֵב, אֶרְדֹּף אַשִּׂיג
נָשַׁפְתָּ   אָרִיק חַרְבִּי, תּוֹרִישֵׁמוֹ יָדִי: נַפְשִׁי,
צָלֲלוּ כַּעוֹפֶרֶת בְּמַיִם,   בְרוּחֲךָ כִּסָּמוֹ יָם,
מִי   מִי־כָמֹכָה בָּאֵלִם יהוה,   אַדִּירִים:
נוֹרָא תְהִלֹּת עֹשֵׂה   כָּמֹכָה נֶאְדָּר בַּקֹּדֶשׁ,
נָחִיתָ   נָטִיתָ יְמִינְךָ, תִּבְלָעֵמוֹ אָרֶץ: פֶלֶא:
נֵהַלְתָּ בְעָזְּךָ אֶל־נְוֵה   בְחַסְדְּךָ עַם־זוּ גָּאָלְתָּ,
חִיל   שָׁמְעוּ עַמִּים יִרְגָּזוּן,   קָדְשֶׁךָ:
אָז נִבְהֲלוּ אַלּוּפֵי   אָחַז יֹשְׁבֵי פְּלָשֶׁת:
נָמֹגוּ   אֵילֵי מוֹאָב יֹאחֲזֵמוֹ רָעַד,   אֱדוֹם,
תִּפֹּל עֲלֵיהֶם אֵימָתָה   כֹּל יֹשְׁבֵי כְנָעַן:
עַד־   בִּגְדֹל זְרוֹעֲךָ יִדְּמוּ כָּאָבֶן,   וָפַחַד,
עַד־יַעֲבֹר עַם־זוּ   יַעֲבֹר עַמְּךָ יהוה,
מָכוֹן   תְּבִאֵמוֹ וְתִטָּעֵמוֹ בְּהַר נַחֲלָתְךָ,   קָנִיתָ:
מִקְּדָשׁ אֲדֹנָי כּוֹנֲנוּ   לְשִׁבְתְּךָ פָּעַלְתָּ יהוה,
יָדֶיךָ:   יהוה ׀ יִמְלֹךְ לְעֹלָם וָעֶד:

יהוה יִמְלֹךְ לְעֹלָם וָעֶד. (יהוה מַלְכוּתֵהּ קָאֵם, לְעָלַם וּלְעָלְמֵי עָלְמַיָּא.) כִּי בָא סוּס פַּרְעֹה בְּרִכְבּוֹ וּבְפָרָשָׁיו בַּיָּם, וַיָּשֶׁב יהוה עֲלֵהֶם אֶת מֵי הַיָּם, וּבְנֵי יִשְׂרָאֵל הָלְכוּ בַיַּבָּשָׁה בְּתוֹךְ הַיָּם. ✧ כִּי לַיהוה הַמְּלוּכָה, וּמֹשֵׁל בַּגּוֹיִם.[1] וְעָלוּ מוֹשִׁעִים בְּהַר צִיּוֹן, לִשְׁפֹּט אֶת הַר עֵשָׂו, וְהָיְתָה לַיהוה הַמְּלוּכָה.[2] וְהָיָה יהוה לְמֶלֶךְ עַל כָּל הָאָרֶץ, בַּיּוֹם הַהוּא יִהְיֶה יהוה אֶחָד וּשְׁמוֹ אֶחָד.[3] (וּבְתוֹרָתְךָ כָּתוּב לֵאמֹר: שְׁמַע יִשְׂרָאֵל יהוה אֱלֹהֵינוּ יהוה אֶחָד.[4])

Stand while reciting יִשְׁתַּבַּח . . . The fifteen expressions of praise —
שִׁיר וּשְׁבָחָה . . . בְּרָכוֹת וְהוֹדָאוֹת — should be recited without pause, preferably in one breath.

יִשְׁתַּבַּח שִׁמְךָ לָעַד מַלְכֵּנוּ, הָאֵל הַמֶּלֶךְ הַגָּדוֹל וְהַקָּדוֹשׁ, בַּשָּׁמַיִם וּבָאָרֶץ. כִּי לְךָ נָאֶה יהוה אֱלֹהֵינוּ וֵאלֹהֵי אֲבוֹתֵינוּ, שִׁיר וּשְׁבָחָה, הַלֵּל וְזִמְרָה, עֹז וּמֶמְשָׁלָה, נֶצַח גְּדֻלָּה וּגְבוּרָה, תְּהִלָּה וְתִפְאֶרֶת, קְדֻשָּׁה וּמַלְכוּת, בְּרָכוֹת וְהוֹדָאוֹת מֵעַתָּה וְעַד עוֹלָם. ✧ בָּרוּךְ אַתָּה יהוה, אֵל מֶלֶךְ גָּדוֹל בַּתִּשְׁבָּחוֹת, אֵל הַהוֹדָאוֹת, אֲדוֹן הַנִּפְלָאוֹת, הַבּוֹחֵר בְּשִׁירֵי זִמְרָה, מֶלֶךְ אֵל חַי הָעוֹלָמִים. (Cong.– אָמֵן.)

a wall stood the running water, the deep waters congealed in the heart of the sea.

The enemy declared: 'I will pursue, I will overtake, I will divide plunder; I will satisfy my lust with them; I will unsheathe my sword, my hand will impoverish them.'

You blew with Your wind — the sea enshrouded them; the mighty ones sank like lead in the waters.

Who is like You among the heavenly powers, HASHEM! Who is like You, mighty in holiness, too awesome for praise, doing wonders!

You stretched out Your right hand — the earth swallowed them.

You guided in Your kindness this people that You redeemed; You led with Your might to Your holy abode.

Peoples heard — they were agitated; convulsive terror gripped the dwellers of Philistia.

Then the chieftains of Edom were confounded, trembling gripped the powers of Moab, all the dwellers of Canaan dissolved.

May fear and terror befall them, at the greatness of Your arm may they be still as stone; until Your people passes through, HASHEM, until this people You have acquired passes through.

You shall bring them and implant them on the mount of Your heritage, the foundation of Your dwelling-place, which You, HASHEM, have made: the Sanctuary, my Lord, that Your hands established.

HASHEM shall reign for all eternity.

HASHEM shall reign for all eternity. (HASHEM — His kingdom is established forever and ever.) When Pharaoh's cavalry came — with his chariots and horsemen — into the sea and HASHEM turned back the waters of the sea upon them, the Children of Israel walked on the dry bed amid the sea. Chazzan— For the sovereignty is HASHEM's and He rules over nations.[1] The saviors will ascend Mount Zion to judge Esau's mountain, and the kingdom will be HASHEM's.[2] Then HASHEM will be King over all the world, on that day HASHEM will be One and His Name will be One.[3] (And in Your Torah it is written: Hear O Israel: HASHEM is our God, HASHEM, the One and Only.[4])

Stand while reciting 'May Your Name be praised . . .'
The fifteen expressions of praise — 'song and praise. . .blessings and thanksgivings' —
should be recited without pause, preferably in one breath.

יִשְׁתַּבַּח May Your Name be praised forever — our King, the God, the great and holy King — in heaven and on earth. Because for You is fitting — O HASHEM, our God, and the God of our forefathers — song and praise, lauding and hymns, power and dominion, triumph, greatness and strength, praise and splendor, holiness and sovereignty, blessings and thanksgivings from this time and forever. Chazzan— Blessed are You, HASHEM, God, King exalted through praises, God of thanksgivings, Master of wonders, Who chooses musical songs of praise — King, God, Life-giver of the world.   (Cong.— Amen.)

---

(1) *Psalms* 22:29. (2) *Ovadiah* 1:21. (3) *Zechariah* 14:9. (4) *Deuteronomy* 6:4.

The *chazzan* recites חֲצִי קַדִּישׁ.

יִתְגַּדַּל וְיִתְקַדַּשׁ שְׁמֵהּ רַבָּא. (.Cong – אָמֵן.) בְּעָלְמָא דִּי בְרָא כִרְעוּתֵהּ. וְיַמְלִיךְ מַלְכוּתֵהּ, בְּחַיֵּיכוֹן וּבְיוֹמֵיכוֹן וּבְחַיֵּי דְכָל בֵּית יִשְׂרָאֵל, בַּעֲגָלָא וּבִזְמַן קָרִיב. וְאִמְרוּ: אָמֵן.

(.Cong – אָמֵן. יְהֵא שְׁמֵהּ רַבָּא מְבָרַךְ לְעָלַם וּלְעָלְמֵי עָלְמַיָּא.)

יְהֵא שְׁמֵהּ רַבָּא מְבָרַךְ לְעָלַם וּלְעָלְמֵי עָלְמַיָּא.

יִתְבָּרַךְ וְיִשְׁתַּבַּח וְיִתְפָּאַר וְיִתְרוֹמַם וְיִתְנַשֵּׂא וְיִתְהַדָּר וְיִתְעַלֶּה וְיִתְהַלָּל שְׁמֵהּ דְּקֻדְשָׁא בְּרִיךְ הוּא (.Cong – בְּרִיךְ הוּא) – לְעֵלָּא מִן כָּל בִּרְכָתָא וְשִׁירָתָא תֻּשְׁבְּחָתָא וְנֶחֱמָתָא, דַּאֲמִירָן בְּעָלְמָא, וְאִמְרוּ: אָמֵן. (.Cong – אָמֵן.)

In some congregations the *chazzan* chants a melody during his recitation of בָּרְכוּ, so that the congregation can then recite יִתְבָּרַךְ.

Chazzan bows at בָּרְכוּ and straightens up at ה'.

יִתְבָּרַךְ וְיִשְׁתַּבַּח וְיִתְפָּאַר וְיִתְרוֹמַם וְיִתְנַשֵּׂא שְׁמוֹ שֶׁל מֶלֶךְ מַלְכֵי הַמְּלָכִים, הַקָּדוֹשׁ בָּרוּךְ הוּא. שֶׁהוּא רִאשׁוֹן וְהוּא אַחֲרוֹן, וּמִבַּלְעָדָיו אֵין אֱלֹהִים.[1] סֶלָה, לָרֹכֵב

בָּרְכוּ אֶת יהוה הַמְּבֹרָךְ.

Congregation, followed by *chazzan*, responds, bowing at בָּרוּךְ and straightening up at ה'.

בָּרוּךְ יהוה הַמְּבֹרָךְ לְעוֹלָם וָעֶד.

בָּעֲרָבוֹת, בְּיָהּ שְׁמוֹ, וְעִלְזוּ לְפָנָיו.[2] וּשְׁמוֹ מְרוֹמַם עַל כָּל בְּרָכָה וּתְהִלָּה.[3] בָּרוּךְ שֵׁם כְּבוֹד מַלְכוּתוֹ לְעוֹלָם וָעֶד. יְהִי שֵׁם יהוה מְבֹרָךְ, מֵעַתָּה וְעַד עוֹלָם.[4]

ברכות קריאת שמע

It is preferable that one sit while reciting the following series of prayers — particularly the *Kedushah* verses, קָדוֹשׁ קָדוֹשׁ and בָּרוּךְ כְּבוֹד — until *Shemoneh Esrei*.

בָּרוּךְ אַתָּה יהוה אֱלֹהֵינוּ מֶלֶךְ הָעוֹלָם, יוֹצֵר אוֹר וּבוֹרֵא חֹשֶׁךְ, עֹשֶׂה שָׁלוֹם וּבוֹרֵא אֶת הַכֹּל.[5]

הַמֵּאִיר לָאָרֶץ וְלַדָּרִים עָלֶיהָ בְּרַחֲמִים, וּבְטוּבוֹ מְחַדֵּשׁ בְּכָל יוֹם תָּמִיד מַעֲשֵׂה בְרֵאשִׁית. מָה רַבּוּ מַעֲשֶׂיךָ יהוה, כֻּלָּם בְּחָכְמָה עָשִׂיתָ, מָלְאָה הָאָרֶץ קִנְיָנֶךָ.[6] הַמֶּלֶךְ הַמְרוֹמָם לְבַדּוֹ מֵאָז, הַמְשֻׁבָּח וְהַמְפֹאָר וְהַמִּתְנַשֵּׂא מִימוֹת עוֹלָם. אֱלֹהֵי עוֹלָם, בְּרַחֲמֶיךָ הָרַבִּים רַחֵם עָלֵינוּ, אֲדוֹן עֻזֵּנוּ, צוּר מִשְׂגַּבֵּנוּ, מָגֵן יִשְׁעֵנוּ, מִשְׂגָּב בַּעֲדֵנוּ. אֵל בָּרוּךְ גְּדוֹל דֵּעָה, הֵכִין וּפָעַל זָהֳרֵי חַמָּה, טוֹב יָצַר כָּבוֹד לִשְׁמוֹ, מְאוֹרוֹת נָתַן סְבִיבוֹת עֻזּוֹ, פִּנּוֹת צְבָאָיו קְדוֹשִׁים רוֹמְמֵי שַׁדַּי, תָּמִיד מְסַפְּרִים כְּבוֹד אֵל

◆§ Interruptions During the Blessings of the Shema

As a general rule, no אָמֵן or other prayer response may be recited between בָּרְכוּ and

Shemoneh Esrei, but there are exceptions. The main exception is 'between chapters' [בֵּין הַפְּרָקִים] of the *Shema* Blessings — i.e., after יוֹצֵר הַמְּאוֹרוֹת and בָּאַהֲבָה ... הַבּוֹחֵר, and between the three chapters of *Shema*. At those points, אָמֵן (but not

The *chazzan* recites Half-*Kaddish*.

יִתְגַּדַּל *May His great Name grow exalted and sanctified* (Cong.– *Amen.*) *in the world that He created as He willed. May He give reign to His kingship in your lifetimes and in your days, and in the lifetimes of the entire Family of Israel, swiftly and soon. Now respond: Amen.*

(Cong.– *Amen. May His great Name be blessed forever and ever.*)

May His great Name be blessed forever and ever.

Blessed, praised, glorified, exalted, extolled, mighty, upraised, and lauded be the Name of the Holy One, Blessed is He (Cong.– *Blessed is He*) — *beyond any blessing and song, praise and consolation that are uttered in the world. Now respond: Amen.* (Cong.– *Amen.*)

In some congregations the *chazzan* chants a melody during his recitation of *Borchu*, so that the congregation can then recite *'Blessed, praised . . .'*

Chazzan bows at 'Bless' and straightens up at 'HASHEM.'

Bless HASHEM, the blessed One.

Congregation, followed by *chazzan*, responds, bowing at *'Blessed'* and straightening up at *'HASHEM.'*

Blessed is HASHEM, the blessed One, for all eternity.

Blessed, praised, glorified, exalted and upraised is the Name of the King Who rules over kings — the Holy One, Blessed is He. For He is the First and He is the Last and aside from Him there is no god.[1] Extol Him — Who rides the highest heavens — with His Name, YAH,

and exult before Him.[2] His Name is exalted beyond every blessing and praise.[3] Blessed is the Name of His glorious kingdom for all eternity. Blessed be the Name of HASHEM from this time and forever.[4]

BLESSINGS OF THE SHEMA

It is preferable that one sit while reciting the following series of prayers — particularly the *Kedushah* verses, *'Holy, holy, holy . . .'* and *'Blessed is the glory . . .'* — until *Shemoneh Esrei.*

בָּרוּךְ *Blessed are You, HASHEM, our God, King of the universe, Who forms light and creates darkness, makes peace and creates all.[5]*

הַמֵּאִיר *He Who illuminates the earth and those who dwell upon it, with compassion; and in His goodness renews daily, perpetually, the work of Creation. How great are Your works, HASHEM, You make them all with wisdom, the world is full of Your possessions.[6] The King Who was exalted in solitude before Creation, Who is praised, glorified, and upraised since days of old. Eternal God, with Your abundant compassion be compassionate to us — O Master of our power, our rocklike stronghold, O Shield of our salvation, be a stronghold for us. The blessed God, Who is great in knowledge, prepared and worked on the rays of the sun; the Beneficent One fashioned honor for His Name, emplaced luminaries all around His power; the leaders of His legions, holy ones, exalt the Almighty, constantly relate the honor of God*

---

(1) Cf. *Isaiah* 44:6. (2) *Psalms* 68:5. (3) Cf. *Nehemiah* 9:5.
(4) *Psalms* 113:2. (5) Cf. *Isaiah* 45:7. (6) *Psalms* 104:24.

שְׁמוֹ וּבָרוּךְ הוּא (בָּרוּךְ) may be responded to any blessing. Some responses, however, are so important that they are permitted at any point in the *Shema* blessings. They are:
(a) In *Kaddish*, עָלְמַיָּא . . . שְׁמֵהּ רַבָּא יְהֵא אָמֵן and the אָמֵן after בְּעָלְמָא דַּאֲמִירָן; (b) the response to בָּרְכוּ (even of one called to the Torah); and (c) during

the *chazzan's* repetition of *Shemoneh Esrei* — 1) in *Kedushah*, the verses . . . קָדוֹשׁ קָדוֹשׁ קָדוֹשׁ; 2) בָּרוּךְ כְּבוֹד ה' מִמְּקוֹמוֹ and כְּבוֹדוֹ; 3) the three words מוֹדִים אֲנַחְנוּ לָךְ הָאֵל הַקָּדוֹשׁ.
During the recital of the two verses שְׁמַע and בָּרוּךְ שֵׁם, absolutely no interruptions are permitted.

וּקְדָשָׁתוֹ. תִּתְבָּרַךְ יהוה אֱלֹהֵינוּ עַל שֶׁבַח מַעֲשֵׂה יָדֶיךָ, וְעַל מְאוֹרֵי אוֹר שֶׁעָשִׂיתָ, יְפָאֲרוּךָ, סֶּלָה.

תִּתְבָּרַךְ צוּרֵנוּ מַלְכֵּנוּ וְגֹאֲלֵנוּ, בּוֹרֵא קְדוֹשִׁים. יִשְׁתַּבַּח שִׁמְךָ לָעַד מַלְכֵּנוּ, יוֹצֵר מְשָׁרְתִים, וַאֲשֶׁר מְשָׁרְתָיו כֻּלָּם עוֹמְדִים בְּרוּם עוֹלָם, וּמַשְׁמִיעִים בְּיִרְאָה יַחַד בְּקוֹל דִּבְרֵי אֱלֹהִים חַיִּים וּמֶלֶךְ עוֹלָם. כֻּלָּם אֲהוּבִים, כֻּלָּם בְּרוּרִים, כֻּלָּם גִּבּוֹרִים, וְכֻלָּם עֹשִׂים בְּאֵימָה וּבְיִרְאָה רְצוֹן קוֹנָם. ❖ וְכֻלָּם פּוֹתְחִים אֶת פִּיהֶם בִּקְדֻשָּׁה וּבְטָהֳרָה, בְּשִׁירָה וּבְזִמְרָה, וּמְבָרְכִים וּמְשַׁבְּחִים וּמְפָאֲרִים וּמַעֲרִיצִים וּמַקְדִּישִׁים וּמַמְלִיכִים —

אֶת שֵׁם הָאֵל הַמֶּלֶךְ הַגָּדוֹל הַגִּבּוֹר וְהַנּוֹרָא קָדוֹשׁ הוּא.[2] ❖ וְכֻלָּם מְקַבְּלִים עֲלֵיהֶם עֹל מַלְכוּת שָׁמַיִם זֶה מִזֶּה, וְנוֹתְנִים רְשׁוּת זֶה לָזֶה, לְהַקְדִּישׁ לְיוֹצְרָם, בְּנַחַת רוּחַ בְּשָׂפָה בְרוּרָה וּבִנְעִימָה. קְדֻשָּׁה כֻּלָּם כְּאֶחָד עוֹנִים וְאוֹמְרִים בְּיִרְאָה:

Congregation recites aloud:

קָדוֹשׁ קָדוֹשׁ קָדוֹשׁ יהוה צְבָאוֹת, מְלֹא כָל הָאָרֶץ כְּבוֹדוֹ.[3]

וְהָאוֹפַנִּים וְחַיּוֹת הַקֹּדֶשׁ בְּרַעַשׁ גָּדוֹל מִתְנַשְּׂאִים לְעֻמַּת שְׂרָפִים. לְעֻמָּתָם מְשַׁבְּחִים וְאוֹמְרִים:

Congregation recites aloud:

בָּרוּךְ כְּבוֹד יהוה מִמְּקוֹמוֹ.[4]

לָאֵל בָּרוּךְ נְעִימוֹת יִתֵּנוּ. לְמֶלֶךְ אֵל חַי וְקַיָּם, זְמִרוֹת יֹאמֵרוּ, וְתִשְׁבָּחוֹת יַשְׁמִיעוּ. כִּי הוּא לְבַדּוֹ פּוֹעֵל גְּבוּרוֹת, עֹשֶׂה חֲדָשׁוֹת, בַּעַל מִלְחָמוֹת, זוֹרֵעַ צְדָקוֹת, מַצְמִיחַ יְשׁוּעוֹת, בּוֹרֵא רְפוּאוֹת, נוֹרָא תְהִלּוֹת, אֲדוֹן הַנִּפְלָאוֹת. הַמְחַדֵּשׁ בְּטוּבוֹ בְּכָל יוֹם תָּמִיד מַעֲשֵׂה בְרֵאשִׁית. כָּאָמוּר: לְעֹשֵׂה אוֹרִים גְּדֹלִים, כִּי לְעוֹלָם חַסְדּוֹ.[5] ❖ אוֹר חָדָשׁ עַל צִיּוֹן תָּאִיר, וְנִזְכֶּה כֻלָּנוּ מְהֵרָה לְאוֹרוֹ. בָּרוּךְ אַתָּה יהוה, יוֹצֵר הַמְּאוֹרוֹת. (אָמֵן. —Cong.)

אַהֲבָה רַבָּה אֲהַבְתָּנוּ יהוה אֱלֹהֵינוּ, חֶמְלָה גְדוֹלָה וִיתֵרָה חָמַלְתָּ עָלֵינוּ. אָבִינוּ מַלְכֵּנוּ, בַּעֲבוּר אֲבוֹתֵינוּ שֶׁבָּטְחוּ בְךָ, וַתְּלַמְּדֵם חֻקֵּי חַיִּים, כֵּן תְּחָנֵּנוּ וּתְלַמְּדֵנוּ. אָבִינוּ הָאָב הָרַחֲמָן הַמְרַחֵם, רַחֵם עָלֵינוּ, וְתֵן בְּלִבֵּנוּ לְהָבִין וּלְהַשְׂכִּיל, לִשְׁמוֹעַ לִלְמֹד

and His sanctity. May You be blessed, HASHEM, our God, beyond the praises of Your handiwork and beyond the bright luminaries that You have made — may they glorify You — Selah!

תִּתְבָּרֵךְ *May You be blessed, our Rock, our King and our Redeemer, Creator of holy ones; may Your Name be praised forever, our King, O Fashioner of ministering angels; all of Whose ministering angels stand at the summit of the universe and proclaim — with awe, together, loudly — the words of the living God and King of the universe.[1] They are all beloved; they are all flawless; they are all mighty; they all do the will of their Maker with dread and reverence.* Chazzan— *And they all open their mouth in holiness and purity, in song and hymn — and bless, praise, glorify, revere, sanctify and declare the kingship of —*

אֶת שֵׁם *The Name of God, the great, mighty, and awesome King; holy is He.[2]* Chazzan— *Then they all accept upon themselves the yoke of heavenly sovereignty from one another, and grant permission to one another to sanctify the One Who formed them, with tranquillity, with clear articulation, and with sweetness. All of them as one proclaim His holiness and say with awe:*

Congregation recites aloud:

'Holy, holy, holy is HASHEM, Master of Legions, the whole world is filled with His glory.'[3]

וְהָאוֹפַנִּים *Then the Ofanim and the holy Chayos, with great noise, raise themselves towards the Seraphim. Facing them they give praise saying:*

Congregation recites aloud:

'Blessed is the glory of HASHEM from His place.'[4]

לְאֵל *To the blessed God they shall offer sweet melodies; to the King, the living and enduring God, they shall sing hymns and proclaim praises. For He alone effects mighty deeds, makes new things, is Master of wars, sows kindnesses, makes salvations flourish, creates cures, is too awesome for praise, is Lord of wonders. In His goodness He renews daily, perpetually, the work of creation. As it is said: '[Give thanks] to Him Who makes the great luminaries, for His kindness endures forever.'[5]* Chazzan— *May You shine a new light on Zion, and may we all speedily merit its light. Blessed are You, HASHEM, Who fashions the luminaries.*   (Cong.— *Amen.*)

אַהֲבָה *With an abundant love have You loved us, HASHEM, our God; with exceedingly great pity have You pitied us. Our Father, our King, for the sake of our forefathers who trusted in You and whom You taught the decrees of life, may You be equally gracious to us and teach us. Our Father, the merciful Father, Who acts mercifully, have mercy upon us, instill in our hearts to understand and elucidate, to listen, learn*

---

(1) Cf. *Jeremiah* 10:10. (2) Cf. *Deuteronomy* 10:17; *Psalms* 99:3.
(3) *Isaiah* 6:3. (4) *Ezekiel* 3:12. (5) *Psalms* 136:7.

וּלְלַמֵּד, לִשְׁמֹר וְלַעֲשׂוֹת וּלְקַיֵּם אֶת כָּל דִּבְרֵי תַלְמוּד תּוֹרָתְךָ בְּאַהֲבָה. וְהָאֵר עֵינֵינוּ בְּתוֹרָתֶךָ, וְדַבֵּק לִבֵּנוּ בְּמִצְוֹתֶיךָ, וְיַחֵד לְבָבֵנוּ לְאַהֲבָה וּלְיִרְאָה אֶת שְׁמֶךָ, וְלֹא נֵבוֹשׁ לְעוֹלָם וָעֶד. כִּי בְשֵׁם קָדְשְׁךָ הַגָּדוֹל וְהַנּוֹרָא בָּטָחְנוּ, נָגִילָה וְנִשְׂמְחָה בִּישׁוּעָתֶךָ.

וַהֲבִיאֵנוּ לְשָׁלוֹם מֵאַרְבַּע כַּנְפוֹת הָאָרֶץ, וְתוֹלִיכֵנוּ קוֹמְמִיּוּת לְאַרְצֵנוּ. כִּי אֵל פּוֹעֵל

The tzitzis are not gathered at this point and are not kissed during the last paragraph of the Shema.

יְשׁוּעוֹת אָתָּה, וּבָנוּ בָחַרְתָּ מִכָּל עַם וְלָשׁוֹן. ❖ וְקֵרַבְתָּנוּ לְשִׁמְךָ הַגָּדוֹל סֶלָה בֶּאֱמֶת, לְהוֹדוֹת לְךָ וּלְיַחֶדְךָ בְּאַהֲבָה. בָּרוּךְ אַתָּה יהוה, הַבּוֹחֵר בְּעַמּוֹ יִשְׂרָאֵל בְּאַהֲבָה. (אָמֵן. —Cong.)

שמע

Immediately before its recitation concentrate on fulfilling the positive commandment of reciting the Shema twice daily. It is important to enunciate each word clearly and not to run words together. For this reason, vertical lines have been placed between two words that are prone to be slurred into one and are not separated by a comma or a hyphen. See Laws §95-109.

When praying without a minyan, begin with the following three-word formula:

אֵל מֶלֶךְ נֶאֱמָן.

Recite the first verse aloud, with the right hand covering the eyes, and concentrate intently upon accepting God's absolute sovereignty.

שְׁמַע | יִשְׂרָאֵל, יהוה | אֱלֹהֵינוּ, יהוה | אֶחָד:[2]

בָּרוּךְ שֵׁם כְּבוֹד מַלְכוּתוֹ לְעוֹלָם וָעֶד. —In an undertone

While reciting the first paragraph (דברים ו:ה-ט), concentrate on accepting the commandment to love God.

וְאָהַבְתָּ אֵת | יהוה | אֱלֹהֶיךָ, בְּכָל־לְבָבְךָ, וּבְכָל־נַפְשְׁךָ, וּבְכָל־מְאֹדֶךָ: וְהָיוּ הַדְּבָרִים הָאֵלֶּה, אֲשֶׁר | אָנֹכִי מְצַוְּךָ הַיּוֹם, עַל־לְבָבֶךָ: וְשִׁנַּנְתָּם לְבָנֶיךָ, וְדִבַּרְתָּ בָּם, בְּשִׁבְתְּךָ בְּבֵיתֶךָ, וּבְלֶכְתְּךָ בַדֶּרֶךְ, וּבְשָׁכְבְּךָ וּבְקוּמֶךָ: וּקְשַׁרְתָּם לְאוֹת | עַל־יָדֶךָ, וְהָיוּ לְטֹטָפֹת בֵּין | עֵינֶיךָ: וּכְתַבְתָּם | עַל־מְזֻזוֹת בֵּיתֶךָ, וּבִשְׁעָרֶיךָ:

While reciting the second paragraph (דברים יא:יג-כא), concentrate on accepting all the commandments and the concept of reward and punishment.

וְהָיָה, אִם־שָׁמֹעַ תִּשְׁמְעוּ אֶל־מִצְוֹתַי, אֲשֶׁר | אָנֹכִי מְצַוֶּה | אֶתְכֶם הַיּוֹם, לְאַהֲבָה אֶת־יהוה | אֱלֹהֵיכֶם וּלְעָבְדוֹ, בְּכָל־לְבַבְכֶם, וּבְכָל־נַפְשְׁכֶם: וְנָתַתִּי מְטַר־אַרְצְכֶם בְּעִתּוֹ, יוֹרֶה וּמַלְקוֹשׁ, וְאָסַפְתָּ דְגָנֶךָ וְתִירֹשְׁךָ וְיִצְהָרֶךָ: וְנָתַתִּי | עֵשֶׂב | בְּשָׂדְךָ לִבְהֶמְתֶּךָ, וְאָכַלְתָּ וְשָׂבָעְתָּ: הִשָּׁמְרוּ לָכֶם, פֶּן־יִפְתֶּה לְבַבְכֶם, וְסַרְתֶּם וַעֲבַדְתֶּם | אֱלֹהִים | אֲחֵרִים, וְהִשְׁתַּחֲוִיתֶם לָהֶם: וְחָרָה אַף־יהוה בָּכֶם, וְעָצַר | אֶת־הַשָּׁמַיִם, וְלֹא־יִהְיֶה מָטָר, וְהָאֲדָמָה לֹא

teach, safeguard, perform, and fulfill all the words of Your Torah's teaching with love. Enlighten our eyes in Your Torah, attach our hearts to Your commandments, and unify our hearts to love and fear Your Name,[1] and may we not feel inner shame for all eternity. Because we have trusted in Your great and awesome holy Name, may we exult and

The *tzitzis* are not gathered at this point and are not kissed during the last paragraph of the *Shema*.

rejoice in Your salvation. Bring us in peacefulness from the four corners of the earth and lead us with upright pride to our land. For You effect salvations, O God; You have chosen us from among every people and tongue. Chazzan— *And You have brought us close to Your great Name forever in truth, to offer praiseful thanks to You, and proclaim Your Oneness with love. Blessed are You,* HASHEM, *Who chooses His people Israel with love.*   (Cong.— *Amen.*)

THE SHEMA

Immediately before its recitation concentrate on fulfilling the positive commandment of reciting the *Shema* twice daily. It is important to enunciate each word clearly and not to run words together. See *Laws* §95-109.

When praying without a *minyan*, begin with the following three-word formula:
God, trustworthy King.

Recite the first verse aloud, with the right hand covering the eyes, and concentrate intently upon accepting God's absolute sovereignty.

Hear, O Israel: HASHEM is our God, HASHEM, the One and Only.[2]

In an undertone— *Blessed is the Name of His glorious kingdom for all eternity.*

While reciting the first paragraph (*Deuteronomy* 6:5-9), concentrate on accepting the commandment to love God.

וְאָהַבְתָּ *You shall love* HASHEM, *your God, with all your heart, with all your soul and with all your resources. Let these matters that I command you today be upon your heart. Teach them thoroughly to your children and speak of them while you sit in your home, while you walk on the way, when you retire and when you arise. Bind them as a sign upon your arm and let them be tefillin between your eyes. And write them on the doorposts of your house and upon your gates.*

While reciting the second paragraph (*Deuteronomy* 11:13-21), concentrate on accepting all the commandments and the concept of reward and punishment.

וְהָיָה *And it will come to pass that if you continually hearken to My commandments that I command you today, to love* HASHEM, *your God, and to serve Him, with all your heart and with all your soul — then I will provide rain for your land in its proper time, the early and late rains, that you may gather in your grain, your wine, and your oil. I will provide grass in your field for your cattle and you will eat and be satisfied. Beware lest your heart be seduced and you turn astray and serve gods of others and bow to them. Then the wrath of* HASHEM *will blaze against you. He will restrain the heaven so there will be no rain and the ground will not*

---

(1) Cf. *Psalms* 86:11. (2) *Deuteronomy* 6:4.

תִּתֵּן אֶת־יְבוּלָהּ, וַאֲבַדְתֶּם | מְהֵרָה מֵעַל הָאָרֶץ הַטֹּבָה | אֲשֶׁר | יהוה נֹתֵן לָכֶם: וְשַׂמְתֶּם | אֶת־דְּבָרַי | אֵלֶּה, עַל־לְבַבְכֶם וְעַל־נַפְשְׁכֶם, וּקְשַׁרְתֶּם | אֹתָם לְאוֹת | עַל־יֶדְכֶם, וְהָיוּ לְטוֹטָפֹת בֵּין | עֵינֵיכֶם: וְלִמַּדְתֶּם | אֹתָם | אֶת־בְּנֵיכֶם, לְדַבֵּר בָּם, בְּשִׁבְתְּךָ בְּבֵיתֶךָ, וּבְלֶכְתְּךָ בַדֶּרֶךְ, וּבְשָׁכְבְּךָ וּבְקוּמֶךָ: וּכְתַבְתָּם | עַל־מְזוּזוֹת בֵּיתֶךָ, וּבִשְׁעָרֶיךָ: לְמַעַן | יִרְבּוּ | יְמֵיכֶם וִימֵי בְנֵיכֶם, עַל הָאֲדָמָה | אֲשֶׁר נִשְׁבַּע | יהוה לַאֲבֹתֵיכֶם לָתֵת לָהֶם, כִּימֵי הַשָּׁמַיִם | עַל־הָאָרֶץ:

במדבר טו:לז-מא

The *tzitzis* are not kissed.

וַיֹּאמֶר | יהוה | אֶל־מֹשֶׁה לֵּאמֹר: דַּבֵּר | אֶל־בְּנֵי | יִשְׂרָאֵל, וְאָמַרְתָּ אֲלֵהֶם, וְעָשׂוּ לָהֶם צִיצִת, עַל־כַּנְפֵי בִגְדֵיהֶם לְדֹרֹתָם, וְנָתְנוּ | עַל־צִיצִת הַכָּנָף, פְּתִיל תְּכֵלֶת: וְהָיָה לָכֶם לְצִיצִת, וּרְאִיתֶם | אֹתוֹ, וּזְכַרְתֶּם | אֶת־כָּל־מִצְוֹת | יהוה, וַעֲשִׂיתֶם | אֹתָם, וְלֹא תָתוּרוּ | אַחֲרֵי לְבַבְכֶם וְאַחֲרֵי | עֵינֵיכֶם, אֲשֶׁר־אַתֶּם זֹנִים | אַחֲרֵיהֶם: לְמַעַן תִּזְכְּרוּ, וַעֲשִׂיתֶם | אֶת־כָּל־מִצְוֹתָי, וִהְיִיתֶם קְדֹשִׁים לֵאלֹהֵיכֶם: אֲנִי יהוה | אֱלֹהֵיכֶם, אֲשֶׁר הוֹצֵאתִי | אֶתְכֶם | מֵאֶרֶץ מִצְרַיִם,

Concentrate on fulfilling the commandment of remembering the Exodus from Egypt.

לִהְיוֹת לָכֶם לֵאלֹהִים, אֲנִי | יהוה | אֱלֹהֵיכֶם: אֱמֶת —

Although the word אֱמֶת belongs to the next paragraph, it is appended to the conclusion of the previous one.

יהוה אֱלֹהֵיכֶם אֱמֶת. — *Chazzan repeats*

וְיַצִּיב וְנָכוֹן וְקַיָּם וְיָשָׁר וְנֶאֱמָן וְאָהוּב וְחָבִיב וְנֶחְמָד וְנָעִים וְנוֹרָא וְאַדִּיר וּמְתֻקָּן וּמְקֻבָּל וְטוֹב וְיָפֶה הַדָּבָר הַזֶּה עָלֵינוּ לְעוֹלָם וָעֶד. אֱמֶת אֱלֹהֵי עוֹלָם מַלְכֵּנוּ צוּר יַעֲקֹב, מָגֵן יִשְׁעֵנוּ, לְדֹר וָדֹר הוּא קַיָּם, וּשְׁמוֹ קַיָּם, וְכִסְאוֹ נָכוֹן, וּמַלְכוּתוֹ וֶאֱמוּנָתוֹ לָעַד קַיֶּמֶת. וּדְבָרָיו חָיִים וְקַיָּמִים, נֶאֱמָנִים וְנֶחֱמָדִים לָעַד וּלְעוֹלְמֵי עוֹלָמִים. ✧ עַל אֲבוֹתֵינוּ וְעָלֵינוּ, עַל בָּנֵינוּ וְעַל דּוֹרוֹתֵינוּ, וְעַל כָּל דּוֹרוֹת זֶרַע יִשְׂרָאֵל עֲבָדֶיךָ.

עַל הָרִאשׁוֹנִים וְעַל הָאַחֲרוֹנִים, דָּבָר טוֹב וְקַיָּם לְעוֹלָם וָעֶד, אֱמֶת וֶאֱמוּנָה חֹק וְלֹא יַעֲבֹר. אֱמֶת שָׁאַתָּה הוּא יהוה אֱלֹהֵינוּ וֵאלֹהֵי אֲבוֹתֵינוּ, ✧ מַלְכֵּנוּ מֶלֶךְ אֲבוֹתֵינוּ, גֹּאֲלֵנוּ גֹּאֵל אֲבוֹתֵינוּ, יוֹצְרֵנוּ צוּר יְשׁוּעָתֵנוּ, פּוֹדֵנוּ וּמַצִּילֵנוּ מֵעוֹלָם שְׁמֶךָ, אֵין אֱלֹהִים זוּלָתֶךָ.

yield its produce. And you will swiftly be banished from the goodly land
which HASHEM gives you. Place these words of Mine upon your heart and
upon your soul; bind them for a sign upon your arm and let them be tefillin
between your eyes. Teach them to your children, to discuss them, while
you sit in your home, while you walk on the way, when you retire and
when you arise. And write them on the doorposts of your house and upon
your gates. In order to prolong your days and the days of your children
upon the ground that HASHEM has sworn to your ancestors to give them,
like the days of the heaven on the earth.

Numbers 15:37-41
The *tzitzis* are not kissed.

וַיֹּאמֶר *And HASHEM said to Moses saying: Speak to the Children of
Israel and say to them that they are to make themselves tzitzis
on the corners of their garments, throughout their generations. And they
are to place upon the tzitzis of each corner a thread of techeiles. And it
shall constitute tzitzis for you, that you may see it and remember all the
commandments of HASHEM and perform them; and not explore after
your heart and after your eyes after which you stray. So that you may
remember and perform all My commandments; and be holy to your*

Concentrate on fulfill-   *God. I am HASHEM, your God, Who has removed you*
ing the commandment   *from the land of Egypt to be a God to You; I am*
of remembering the   *HASHEM your God — it is true —*
Exodus from Egypt.

Although the word אֱמֶת, *'it is true,'* belongs to the next paragraph,
it is appended to the conclusion of the previous one.

Chazzan repeats: **HASHEM, your God, is true.**

וְיַצִּיב *And certain, established and enduring, fair and faithful, beloved
and cherished, delightful and pleasant, awesome and powerful,
correct and accepted, good and beautiful is this affirmation to us forever
and ever. True — the God of the universe is our King; the Rock of Jacob
is the Shield of our salvation. From generation to generation He endures
and His Name endures and His throne is well established; His
sovereignty and faithfulness endure forever. His words are living and
enduring, faithful and delightful forever and to all eternity;* Chazzan— *for
our forefathers and for us, for our children and for our generations, and
for all the generations of Your servant Israel's offspring.*

עַל *Upon the earlier and upon the later generations, this affirmation is
good and enduring forever. True and faithful, it is an unbreakable
decree. It is true that You are HASHEM, our God and the God of our
forefathers,* Chazzan— *our King and the King of our forefathers, our
Redeemer, the Redeemer of our forefathers; our Molder, the Rock of our
salvation; our Liberator and our Rescuer — this has ever been Your
Name. There is no God but You.*

עֶזְרַת אֲבוֹתֵינוּ אַתָּה הוּא מֵעוֹלָם, מָגֵן וּמוֹשִׁיעַ לִבְנֵיהֶם אַחֲרֵיהֶם בְּכָל דּוֹר וָדוֹר. בְּרוּם עוֹלָם מוֹשָׁבֶךָ, וּמִשְׁפָּטֶיךָ וְצִדְקָתְךָ עַד אַפְסֵי אָרֶץ. אַשְׁרֵי אִישׁ שֶׁיִּשְׁמַע לְמִצְוֹתֶיךָ, וְתוֹרָתְךָ וּדְבָרְךָ יָשִׂים עַל לִבּוֹ. אֱמֶת אַתָּה הוּא אָדוֹן לְעַמֶּךָ וּמֶלֶךְ גִּבּוֹר לָרִיב רִיבָם. אֱמֶת אַתָּה הוּא רִאשׁוֹן וְאַתָּה הוּא אַחֲרוֹן, וּמִבַּלְעָדֶיךָ אֵין לָנוּ מֶלֶךְ¹ גּוֹאֵל וּמוֹשִׁיעַ. מִמִּצְרַיִם גְּאַלְתָּנוּ יהוה אֱלֹהֵינוּ, וּמִבֵּית עֲבָדִים פְּדִיתָנוּ. כָּל בְּכוֹרֵיהֶם הָרָגְתָּ, וּבְכוֹרְךָ גָּאָלְתָּ, וְיַם סוּף בָּקַעְתָּ, וְזֵדִים טִבַּעְתָּ, וִידִידִים הֶעֱבַרְתָּ, וַיְכַסּוּ מַיִם צָרֵיהֶם, אֶחָד מֵהֶם לֹא נוֹתָר.² עַל זֹאת שִׁבְּחוּ אֲהוּבִים וְרוֹמְמוּ אֵל, וְנָתְנוּ יְדִידִים זְמִרוֹת שִׁירוֹת וְתִשְׁבָּחוֹת, בְּרָכוֹת וְהוֹדָאוֹת, לְמֶלֶךְ אֵל חַי וְקַיָּם, רָם וְנִשָּׂא, גָּדוֹל וְנוֹרָא, מַשְׁפִּיל גֵּאִים, וּמַגְבִּיהַּ שְׁפָלִים, מוֹצִיא אֲסִירִים, וּפוֹדֶה עֲנָוִים, וְעוֹזֵר דַּלִּים, וְעוֹנֶה לְעַמּוֹ בְּעֵת שַׁוְּעָם אֵלָיו.

Rise for *Shemoneh Esrei*. Some take three steps backward here; others do so before צוּר יִשְׂרָאֵל.

٭ תְּהִלּוֹת לְאֵל עֶלְיוֹן, בָּרוּךְ הוּא וּמְבֹרָךְ. מֹשֶׁה וּבְנֵי יִשְׂרָאֵל לְךָ עָנוּ שִׁירָה בְּשִׂמְחָה רַבָּה וְאָמְרוּ כֻלָּם:

מִי כָמֹכָה בָּאֵלִם יהוה, מִי כָּמֹכָה נֶאְדָּר בַּקֹּדֶשׁ, נוֹרָא תְהִלֹּת עֹשֵׂה פֶלֶא.³ ٭ שִׁירָה חֲדָשָׁה שִׁבְּחוּ גְאוּלִים לְשִׁמְךָ עַל שְׂפַת הַיָּם, יַחַד כֻּלָּם הוֹדוּ וְהִמְלִיכוּ וְאָמְרוּ:

יהוה יִמְלֹךְ לְעֹלָם וָעֶד.⁴

It is forbidden to interrupt or pause between גָּאַל יִשְׂרָאֵל and *Shemoneh Esrei*, even for *Kaddish, Kedushah* or *Borchu*.

٭ **צוּר יִשְׂרָאֵל,** קוּמָה בְּעֶזְרַת יִשְׂרָאֵל, וּפְדֵה כִנְאֻמֶךָ יְהוּדָה וְיִשְׂרָאֵל. גֹּאֲלֵנוּ יהוה צְבָאוֹת שְׁמוֹ, קְדוֹשׁ יִשְׂרָאֵל.⁵ בָּרוּךְ אַתָּה יהוה, גָּאַל יִשְׂרָאֵל.

٭ שְׁמוֹנֶה עֶשְׂרֵה – עֲמִידָה ٭

Take three steps backward, then three steps forward. Remain standing with feet together while reciting *Shemoneh Esrei*. Recite it with quiet devotion and without interruption, verbal or otherwise. Although it should not be audible to others, one must pray loudly enough to hear himself.

אֲדֹנָי שְׂפָתַי תִּפְתָּח, וּפִי יַגִּיד תְּהִלָּתֶךָ.⁶

אבות

Bend the knees at בָּרוּךְ; bow at אַתָּה; straighten up at ה'.

בָּרוּךְ אַתָּה יהוה אֱלֹהֵינוּ וֵאלֹהֵי אֲבוֹתֵינוּ, אֱלֹהֵי אַבְרָהָם, אֱלֹהֵי יִצְחָק, וֵאלֹהֵי יַעֲקֹב, הָאֵל הַגָּדוֹל הַגִּבּוֹר

עֶזְרַת **The Helper** of our forefathers are You alone, forever, Shield and Savior for their children after them in every generation. At the zenith of the universe is Your dwelling, and Your justice and Your righteousness extend to the ends of the earth. Praiseworthy is the person who obeys Your commandments and takes to his heart Your teaching and Your word. True — You are the Master for Your people and a mighty King to take up their grievance. True — You are the First and You are the Last, and other than You we have no king,[1] redeemer, or savior. From Egypt You redeemed us, HASHEM, our God, and from the house of slavery You liberated us. All their firstborn You slew, but Your firstborn You redeemed; the Sea of Reeds You split; the wanton sinners You drowned; the dear ones You brought across; and the water covered their foes — not one of them was left.[2] For this, the beloved praised and exalted God; the dear ones offered hymns, songs, praises, blessings, and thanksgivings to the King, the living and enduring God — exalted and uplifted, great and awesome, Who humbles the haughty and lifts the lowly; withdraws the captive, liberates the humble, and helps the poor; Who responds to His people upon their outcry to Him.

Rise for *Shemoneh Esrei*. Some take three steps backward at this point;
others do so before צוּר יִשְׂרָאֵל, *'Rock of Israel.'*

Chazzan— Praises to the Supreme God, the blessed One Who is blessed. Moses and the Children of Israel exclaimed a song to You with great joy and they all said:

'Who is like You among the heavenly powers, HASHEM! Who is like You, mighty in holiness, too awesome for praise, doing wonders.'[3] Chazzan— With a new song the redeemed ones praised Your Name at the seashore, all of them in unison gave thanks, acknowledged [Your] sovereignty, and said:

'HASHEM shall reign for all eternity.'[4]

It is forbidden to interrupt or pause between 'Who redeemed Israel' and *Shemoneh Esrei*,
even for *Kaddish, Kedushah* or *Borchu*.

צוּר יִשְׂרָאֵל Chazzan— Rock of Israel, arise to the aid of Israel and liberate, as You pledged, Judah and Israel. Our Redeemer — HASHEM, Master of Legions, is His Name — the Holy One of Israel.[5] Blessed are You, HASHEM, Who redeemed Israel.

⁕ SHEMONEH ESREI — AMIDAH ⁂

Take three steps backward, then three steps forward. Remain standing with feet together while reciting *Shemoneh Esrei*. Recite it with quiet devotion and without interruption, verbal or otherwise. Although it should not be audible to others, one must pray loudly enough to hear himself.

My Lord, open my lips, that my mouth may declare Your praise.[6]

PATRIARCHS

Bend the knees at 'Blessed'; bow at 'You'; straighten up at 'HASHEM.'

בָּרוּךְ Blessed are You, HASHEM, our God and the God of our forefathers, God of Abraham, God of Isaac, and God of Jacob; the great, mighty,

---

(1) Cf. *Isaiah* 44:6. (2) *Psalms* 106:11. (3) *Exodus* 15:11. (4) 15:18. (5) *Isaiah* 47:4. (6) *Psalms* 51:17.

וְהַנּוֹרָא, אֵל עֶלְיוֹן, גּוֹמֵל חֲסָדִים טוֹבִים וְקוֹנֵה הַכֹּל, וְזוֹכֵר חַסְדֵי אָבוֹת, וּמֵבִיא גוֹאֵל לִבְנֵי בְנֵיהֶם, לְמַעַן שְׁמוֹ בְּאַהֲבָה.

Bend the knees at בָּרוּךְ; *bow at* אַתָּה; *straighten up at* ה'.

מֶלֶךְ עוֹזֵר וּמוֹשִׁיעַ וּמָגֵן. בָּרוּךְ אַתָּה יהוה, מָגֵן אַבְרָהָם.

גבורות

אַתָּה גִּבּוֹר לְעוֹלָם אֲדֹנָי, מְחַיֶּה מֵתִים אַתָּה, רַב לְהוֹשִׁיעַ. מְכַלְכֵּל חַיִּים בְּחֶסֶד, מְחַיֶּה מֵתִים בְּרַחֲמִים רַבִּים, סוֹמֵךְ נוֹפְלִים, וְרוֹפֵא חוֹלִים, וּמַתִּיר אֲסוּרִים, וּמְקַיֵּם אֱמוּנָתוֹ לִישֵׁנֵי עָפָר. מִי כָמוֹךָ בַּעַל גְּבוּרוֹת, וּמִי דּוֹמֶה לָּךְ, מֶלֶךְ מֵמִית וּמְחַיֶּה וּמַצְמִיחַ יְשׁוּעָה. וְנֶאֱמָן אַתָּה לְהַחֲיוֹת מֵתִים. בָּרוּךְ אַתָּה יהוה, מְחַיֶּה הַמֵּתִים.

During the chazzan's repetition, Kedushah (below) is recited at this point.

קדושת השם

אַתָּה קָדוֹשׁ וְשִׁמְךָ קָדוֹשׁ, וּקְדוֹשִׁים בְּכָל יוֹם יְהַלְלוּךָ סֶּלָה. בָּרוּךְ אַתָּה יהוה, הָאֵל הַקָּדוֹשׁ.

בינה

אַתָּה חוֹנֵן לְאָדָם דַּעַת, וּמְלַמֵּד לֶאֱנוֹשׁ בִּינָה. חָנֵּנוּ מֵאִתְּךָ דֵּעָה בִּינָה וְהַשְׂכֵּל. בָּרוּךְ אַתָּה יהוה, חוֹנֵן הַדָּעַת.

קדושה

When reciting *Kedushah,* one must stand with his feet together and avoid any interruptions. One should rise on his toes when saying the words קָדוֹשׁ, קָדוֹשׁ, קָדוֹשׁ; בָּרוּךְ (of בָּרוּךְ כְּבוֹד); and יִמְלֹךְ.

נְקַדֵּשׁ אֶת שִׁמְךָ בָּעוֹלָם, כְּשֵׁם שֶׁמַּקְדִּישִׁים אוֹתוֹ בִּשְׁמֵי מָרוֹם, כַּכָּתוּב עַל יַד נְבִיאֶךָ, וְקָרָא זֶה אֶל זֶה וְאָמַר: — Cong. then Chazzan

קָדוֹשׁ קָדוֹשׁ קָדוֹשׁ יהוה צְבָאוֹת, מְלֹא כָל הָאָרֶץ כְּבוֹדוֹ.[1] — All

לְעֻמָּתָם בָּרוּךְ יֹאמֵרוּ: — Chazzan

בָּרוּךְ כְּבוֹד יהוה, מִמְּקוֹמוֹ.[2] — All

וּבְדִבְרֵי קָדְשְׁךָ כָּתוּב לֵאמֹר: — Chazzan

יִמְלֹךְ יהוה לְעוֹלָם, אֱלֹהַיִךְ צִיּוֹן לְדֹר וָדֹר, הַלְלוּיָהּ.[3] — All

— Chazzan only concludes לְדוֹר וָדוֹר נַגִּיד גָּדְלֶךָ וּלְנֵצַח נְצָחִים קְדֻשָּׁתְךָ נַקְדִּישׁ, וְשִׁבְחֲךָ אֱלֹהֵינוּ מִפִּינוּ לֹא יָמוּשׁ לְעוֹלָם וָעֶד, כִּי אֵל מֶלֶךְ גָּדוֹל וְקָדוֹשׁ אָתָּה. בָּרוּךְ אַתָּה יהוה, הָאֵל הַקָּדוֹשׁ.

Chazzan continues . . . אַתָּה חוֹנֵן *(above).*

and awesome God, the supreme God, Who bestows beneficial kind-
nesses and creates everything, Who recalls the kindnesses of the
Patriarchs and brings a Redeemer to their children's children, for His
Name's sake, with love. O King, Helper, Savior, and Shield.

Bend the knees at 'Blessed'; bow at 'You'; straighten up at 'HASHEM.'

Blessed are You, HASHEM, Shield of Abraham.

GOD'S MIGHT

אַתָּה You are eternally mighty, my Lord, the Resuscitator of the
dead are You; abundantly able to save. He sustains the living
with kindness, resuscitates the dead with abundant mercy, supports the
fallen, heals the sick, releases the confined, and maintains His faith to
those asleep in the dust. Who is like You, O Master of mighty deeds, and
who is comparable to You, O King Who causes death and restores life
and makes salvation sprout! And You are faithful to resuscitate the
dead. Blessed are You, HASHEM, Who resuscitates the dead.

During the chazzan's repetition, Kedushah (below) is recited at this point.

HOLINESS OF GOD'S NAME

אַתָּה You are holy and Your Name is holy, and holy ones praise
You every day, forever. Blessed are You, HASHEM, the holy
God.

INSIGHT

אַתָּה You graciously endow man with wisdom and teach insight to a
frail mortal. Endow us graciously from Yourself with wisdom,
insight, and discernment. Blessed are You, HASHEM, gracious Giver of
wisdom.

KEDUSHAH

When reciting Kedushah, one must stand with his feet together and avoid any interruptions. One
should rise on his toes when saying the words *Holy, holy, holy; Blessed is;* and *HASHEM shall reign.*

Cong. —נְקַדֵּשׁ *We shall sanctify Your Name in this world, just as they*
then *sanctify it in heaven above, as it is written by Your prophet,*
Chazzan *"And one [angel] will call another and say:*

All—'Holy, holy, holy is HASHEM, Master of Legions, the whole world
is filled with His glory.' "[1]

Chazzan—*Those facing them say 'Blessed':*

All—'Blessed is the glory of HASHEM from His place.'[2]

Chazzan—*And in Your holy Writings the following is written:*

All—'HASHEM shall reign forever — your God, O Zion — from generation
to generation, Halleluyah!'[3]

Chazzan only concludes— *From generation to generation we shall relate Your
greatness and for infinite eternities we shall proclaim Your holiness. Your praise,
our God, shall not leave our mouth forever and ever, for You, O God, are a great
and holy King. Blessed are You, HASHEM, the holy God.*

Chazzan continues אַתָּה חוֹנֵן, *You graciously endow . . .* (above).

---

(1) *Isaiah* 6:3. (2) *Ezekiel* 3:12. (3) *Psalms* 146:10.

תשובה

הֲשִׁיבֵנוּ אָבִינוּ לְתוֹרָתֶךָ, וְקָרְבֵנוּ מַלְכֵּנוּ לַעֲבוֹדָתֶךָ, וְהַחֲזִירֵנוּ בִּתְשׁוּבָה שְׁלֵמָה לְפָנֶיךָ. בָּרוּךְ אַתָּה יהוה, הָרוֹצֶה בִּתְשׁוּבָה.

סליחה

Strike the left side of the chest with the right fist while reciting the words חָטָאנוּ and פָּשָׁעְנוּ.

סְלַח לָנוּ אָבִינוּ כִּי חָטָאנוּ, מְחַל לָנוּ מַלְכֵּנוּ כִּי פָשָׁעְנוּ, כִּי מוֹחֵל וְסוֹלֵחַ אָתָּה. בָּרוּךְ אַתָּה יהוה, חַנּוּן הַמַּרְבֶּה לִסְלוֹחַ.

גאולה

רְאֵה בְעָנְיֵנוּ, וְרִיבָה רִיבֵנוּ, וּגְאָלֵנוּ¹ מְהֵרָה לְמַעַן שְׁמֶךָ, כִּי גּוֹאֵל חָזָק אָתָּה. בָּרוּךְ אַתָּה יהוה, גּוֹאֵל יִשְׂרָאֵל.

During his repetition the *chazzan* recites עֲנֵנוּ at this point. See *Laws* §61-63.
[If he forgot to recite it at this point, he may insert it in שְׁמַע קוֹלֵנוּ, p. 128].

עֲנֵנוּ יהוה עֲנֵנוּ, בְּיוֹם צוֹם תַּעֲנִיתֵנוּ, כִּי בְצָרָה גְדוֹלָה אֲנָחְנוּ. אַל תֵּפֶן אֶל רִשְׁעֵנוּ, וְאַל תַּסְתֵּר פָּנֶיךָ מִמֶּנּוּ, וְאַל תִּתְעַלַּם מִתְּחִנָּתֵנוּ. הֱיֵה נָא קָרוֹב לְשַׁוְעָתֵנוּ, יְהִי נָא חַסְדְּךָ לְנַחֲמֵנוּ, טֶרֶם נִקְרָא אֵלֶיךָ עֲנֵנוּ, כַּדָּבָר שֶׁנֶּאֱמַר: וְהָיָה טֶרֶם יִקְרָאוּ וַאֲנִי אֶעֱנֶה, עוֹד הֵם מְדַבְּרִים וַאֲנִי אֶשְׁמָע.² כִּי אַתָּה יהוה הָעוֹנֶה בְּעֵת צָרָה, פּוֹדֶה וּמַצִּיל בְּכָל עֵת צָרָה וְצוּקָה. בָּרוּךְ אַתָּה יהוה, הָעוֹנֶה בְּעֵת צָרָה.

רפואה

רְפָאֵנוּ יהוה וְנֵרָפֵא, הוֹשִׁיעֵנוּ וְנִוָּשֵׁעָה, כִּי תְהִלָּתֵנוּ אָתָּה,³ וְהַעֲלֵה רְפוּאָה שְׁלֵמָה לְכָל מַכּוֹתֵינוּ, °°כִּי אֵל מֶלֶךְ רוֹפֵא נֶאֱמָן וְרַחֲמָן אָתָּה. בָּרוּךְ אַתָּה יהוה, רוֹפֵא חוֹלֵי עַמּוֹ יִשְׂרָאֵל.

ברכת השנים

בָּרֵךְ עָלֵינוּ יהוה אֱלֹהֵינוּ אֶת הַשָּׁנָה הַזֹּאת וְאֶת כָּל מִינֵי תְבוּאָתָהּ לְטוֹבָה, וְתֵן בְּרָכָה עַל פְּנֵי הָאֲדָמָה, וְשַׂבְּעֵנוּ מִטּוּבֶךָ, וּבָרֵךְ שְׁנָתֵנוּ כַּשָּׁנִים הַטּוֹבוֹת. בָּרוּךְ אַתָּה יהוה, מְבָרֵךְ הַשָּׁנִים.

°°At this point one may interject a prayer for one who is ill:

יְהִי רָצוֹן מִלְּפָנֶיךָ יהוה אֱלֹהַי וֵאלֹהֵי אֲבוֹתַי, שֶׁתִּשְׁלַח מְהֵרָה רְפוּאָה שְׁלֵמָה מִן הַשָּׁמַיִם, רְפוּאַת הַנֶּפֶשׁ וּרְפוּאַת הַגּוּף

for a male—לַחוֹלֶה (patient's name) בֶּן (mother's name) בְּתוֹךְ שְׁאָר חוֹלֵי יִשְׂרָאֵל.

for a female—לַחוֹלָה (patient's name) בַּת (mother's name) בְּתוֹךְ שְׁאָר חוֹלֵי יִשְׂרָאֵל.

Continue—כִּי אֵל ...

REPENTANCE

הֲשִׁיבֵנוּ *Bring us back, our Father, to Your Torah, and bring us near, our King, to Your service, and influence us to return in perfect repentance before You. Blessed are You, HASHEM, Who desires repentance.*

FORGIVENESS

Strike the left side of the chest with the right fist while reciting the words 'erred' and 'sinned.'

סְלַח *Forgive us, our Father, for we have erred; pardon us, our King, for we have willfully sinned; for You pardon and forgive. Blessed are You, HASHEM, the gracious One Who pardons abundantly.*

REDEMPTION

רְאֵה *Behold our affliction, take up our grievance, and redeem us[1] speedily for Your Name's sake, for You are a powerful Redeemer. Blessed are You, HASHEM, Redeemer of Israel.*

During his repetition the chazzan recites עֲנֵנוּ, 'Answer us,' at this point. See Laws §61-63. [If he forgot to recite it at this point, he may insert it in שְׁמַע קוֹלֵנוּ, 'Hear our voice' (p. 128).]

עֲנֵנוּ *Answer us, HASHEM, answer us, on this day of our fast, for we are in great distress. Do not pay attention to our wickedness; do not hide Your Face from us; and do not ignore our supplication. Please be near to our outcry; please let Your kindness comfort us — before we call to You answer us, as it is said: 'And it will be that before they call, I will answer; while they yet speak, I will hear.'[2] For You, HASHEM, are the One Who responds in time of distress, Who redeems and rescues in every time of distress and woe. Blessed are You, HASHEM, Who responds in time of distress.*

HEALTH AND HEALING

רְפָאֵנוּ *Heal us, HASHEM — then we will be healed; save us — then we will be saved, for You are our praise.[3] Bring complete recovery for all our ailments, °°for You are God, King, the faithful and compassionate Healer. Blessed are You, HASHEM, Who heals the sick of His people Israel.*

YEAR OF PROSPERITY

בָּרֵךְ *Bless on our behalf — O HASHEM, our God — this year and all its kinds of crops for the best, and give a blessing on the face of the earth, and satisfy us from Your bounty, and bless our year like the best years. Blessed are You, HASHEM, Who blesses the years.*

°°At this point one may interject a prayer for one who is ill:

May it be Your will, HASHEM, my God, and the God of my forefathers, that You quickly send a complete recovery from heaven, spiritual healing and physical healing to the patient (name) *son/daughter of* (mother's name) *among the other patients of Israel.*   Continue: *For You are God . . .*

---

(1) Cf. Psalms 119:153-154. (2) Isaiah 65:24. (3) Cf. Jeremiah 17:14.

קיבוץ גליות

תְּקַע בְּשׁוֹפָר גָּדוֹל לְחֵרוּתֵנוּ, וְשָׂא נֵס לְקַבֵּץ גָּלֻיּוֹתֵינוּ, וְקַבְּצֵנוּ יַחַד מֵאַרְבַּע כַּנְפוֹת הָאָרֶץ.¹ בָּרוּךְ אַתָּה יהוה, מְקַבֵּץ נִדְחֵי עַמּוֹ יִשְׂרָאֵל.

דין

הָשִׁיבָה שׁוֹפְטֵינוּ כְּבָרִאשׁוֹנָה, וְיוֹעֲצֵינוּ כְּבַתְּחִלָּה², וְהָסֵר מִמֶּנּוּ יָגוֹן וַאֲנָחָה, וּמְלוֹךְ עָלֵינוּ אַתָּה יהוה לְבַדְּךָ בְּחֶסֶד וּבְרַחֲמִים, וְצַדְּקֵנוּ בַּמִּשְׁפָּט. בָּרוּךְ אַתָּה יהוה, מֶלֶךְ אוֹהֵב צְדָקָה וּמִשְׁפָּט.

ברכת המינים

וְלַמַּלְשִׁינִים אַל תְּהִי תִקְוָה, וְכָל הָרִשְׁעָה כְּרֶגַע תֹּאבֵד, וְכָל אֹיְבֶיךָ מְהֵרָה יִכָּרֵתוּ, וְהַזֵּדִים מְהֵרָה תְעַקֵּר וּתְשַׁבֵּר וּתְמַגֵּר וְתַכְנִיעַ בִּמְהֵרָה בְיָמֵינוּ. בָּרוּךְ אַתָּה יהוה, שׁוֹבֵר אֹיְבִים וּמַכְנִיעַ זֵדִים.

צדיקים

עַל הַצַּדִּיקִים וְעַל הַחֲסִידִים, וְעַל זִקְנֵי עַמְּךָ בֵּית יִשְׂרָאֵל, וְעַל פְּלֵיטַת סוֹפְרֵיהֶם, וְעַל גֵּרֵי הַצֶּדֶק וְעָלֵינוּ, יֶהֱמוּ רַחֲמֶיךָ יהוה אֱלֹהֵינוּ, וְתֵן שָׂכָר טוֹב לְכָל הַבּוֹטְחִים בְּשִׁמְךָ בֶּאֱמֶת, וְשִׂים חֶלְקֵנוּ עִמָּהֶם לְעוֹלָם, וְלֹא נֵבוֹשׁ כִּי בְךָ בָּטָחְנוּ. בָּרוּךְ אַתָּה יהוה, מִשְׁעָן וּמִבְטָח לַצַּדִּיקִים.

בנין ירושלים

וְלִירוּשָׁלַיִם עִירְךָ בְּרַחֲמִים תָּשׁוּב, וְתִשְׁכּוֹן בְּתוֹכָהּ כַּאֲשֶׁר דִּבַּרְתָּ, וּבְנֵה אוֹתָהּ בְּקָרוֹב בְּיָמֵינוּ בִּנְיַן עוֹלָם, וְכִסֵּא דָוִד מְהֵרָה לְתוֹכָהּ תָּכִין. בָּרוּךְ אַתָּה יהוה, בּוֹנֵה יְרוּשָׁלָיִם.

מלכות בית דוד

אֶת צֶמַח דָּוִד עַבְדְּךָ מְהֵרָה תַצְמִיחַ, וְקַרְנוֹ תָּרוּם בִּישׁוּעָתֶךָ, כִּי לִישׁוּעָתְךָ קִוִּינוּ כָּל הַיּוֹם. בָּרוּךְ אַתָּה יהוה, מַצְמִיחַ קֶרֶן יְשׁוּעָה.

קבלת תפלה

שְׁמַע קוֹלֵנוּ יהוה אֱלֹהֵינוּ, חוּס וְרַחֵם עָלֵינוּ, וְקַבֵּל בְּרַחֲמִים וּבְרָצוֹן אֶת תְּפִלָּתֵנוּ, כִּי אֵל שׁוֹמֵעַ תְּפִלּוֹת וְתַחֲנוּנִים אָתָּה. וּמִלְּפָנֶיךָ מַלְכֵּנוּ רֵיקָם אַל תְּשִׁיבֵנוּ,

If *chazzan* forgot to say עֲנֵנוּ before, he says it at this point but omits the concluding blessing (בָּרוּךְ ... צָרָה).

INGATHERING OF EXILES

תְּקַע Sound the great shofar for our freedom, raise the banner to gather our exiles and gather us together from the four corners of the earth.[1] Blessed are You, HASHEM, Who gathers in the dispersed of His people Israel.

RESTORATION OF JUSTICE

הָשִׁיבָה Restore our judges as in earliest times and our counselors as at first;[2] remove from us sorrow and groan; and reign over us — You, HASHEM, alone — with kindness and compassion, and justify us through judgment. Blessed are You, HASHEM, the King Who loves righteousness and judgment.

AGAINST HERETICS

וְלַמַּלְשִׁינִים And for slanderers let there be no hope; and may all wickedness perish in an instant; and may all Your enemies be cut down speedily. May You speedily uproot, smash, cast down, and humble the wanton sinners — speedily in our days. Blessed are You, HASHEM, Who breaks enemies and humbles wanton sinners.

THE RIGHTEOUS

עַל הַצַּדִּיקִים On the righteous, on the devout, on the elders of Your people the Family of Israel, on the remnant of their scholars, on the righteous converts and on ourselves — may Your compassion be aroused, HASHEM, our God, and give goodly reward to all who sincerely believe in Your Name. Put our lot with them forever, and we will not feel ashamed, for we trust in You. Blessed are You, HASHEM, Mainstay and Assurance of the righteous.

REBUILDING JERUSALEM

וְלִירוּשָׁלַיִם And to Jerusalem, Your city, may You return in compassion, and may You rest within it, as You have spoken. May You rebuild it soon in our days as an eternal structure, and may You speedily establish the throne of David within it. Blessed are You, HASHEM, the Builder of Jerusalem.

DAVIDIC REIGN

אֶת צֶמַח The offspring of Your servant David may You speedily cause to flourish, and enhance his pride through Your salvation, for we hope for Your salvation all day long. Blessed are You, HASHEM, Who causes the pride of salvation to flourish.

ACCEPTANCE OF PRAYER

שְׁמַע Hear our voice, HASHEM our God, pity and be compassionate to us, and accept — with compassion and favor — our prayer, for God Who hears prayers and supplications are You. From before Yourself, our King, turn us not away empty-handed,

---

(1) Cf. *Isaiah* 11:12. (2) Cf. 1:26.

°° כִּי אַתָּה שׁוֹמֵעַ תְּפִלַּת עַמְּךָ יִשְׂרָאֵל בְּרַחֲמִים. בָּרוּךְ אַתָּה יהוה, שׁוֹמֵעַ תְּפִלָּה.

עבודה

רְצֵה יהוה אֱלֹהֵינוּ בְּעַמְּךָ יִשְׂרָאֵל וּבִתְפִלָּתָם, וְהָשֵׁב אֶת הָעֲבוֹדָה לִדְבִיר בֵּיתֶךָ. וְאִשֵּׁי יִשְׂרָאֵל וּתְפִלָּתָם בְּאַהֲבָה תְקַבֵּל בְּרָצוֹן, וּתְהִי לְרָצוֹן תָּמִיד עֲבוֹדַת יִשְׂרָאֵל עַמֶּךָ.

וְתֶחֱזֶינָה עֵינֵינוּ בְּשׁוּבְךָ לְצִיּוֹן בְּרַחֲמִים. בָּרוּךְ אַתָּה יהוה, הַמַּחֲזִיר שְׁכִינָתוֹ לְצִיּוֹן.

הודאה

Bow at מוֹדִים; straighten up at 'ה. In his repetition the *chazzan* should recite the entire מוֹדִים aloud, while the congregation recites מוֹדִים דְּרַבָּנָן softly.

מוֹדִים אֲנַחְנוּ לָךְ, שָׁאַתָּה הוּא יהוה אֱלֹהֵינוּ וֵאלֹהֵי אֲבוֹתֵינוּ לְעוֹלָם וָעֶד. צוּר חַיֵּינוּ, מָגֵן יִשְׁעֵנוּ אַתָּה הוּא לְדוֹר וָדוֹר. נוֹדֶה לְּךָ וּנְסַפֵּר תְּהִלָּתֶךָ עַל חַיֵּינוּ הַמְּסוּרִים בְּיָדֶךָ, וְעַל נִשְׁמוֹתֵינוּ הַפְּקוּדוֹת לָךְ, וְעַל נִסֶּיךָ שֶׁבְּכָל יוֹם עִמָּנוּ, וְעַל נִפְלְאוֹתֶיךָ וְטוֹבוֹתֶיךָ שֶׁבְּכָל עֵת, עֶרֶב וָבֹקֶר וְצָהֳרָיִם. הַטוֹב כִּי לֹא כָלוּ רַחֲמֶיךָ, וְהַמְרַחֵם כִּי לֹא תַמּוּ חֲסָדֶיךָ,² מֵעוֹלָם קִוִּינוּ לָךְ.

מוֹדִים דְּרַבָּנָן

מוֹדִים אֲנַחְנוּ לָךְ, שָׁאַתָּה הוּא יהוה אֱלֹהֵינוּ וֵאלֹהֵי אֲבוֹתֵינוּ, אֱלֹהֵי כָל בָּשָׂר, יוֹצְרֵנוּ, יוֹצֵר בְּרֵאשִׁית. בְּרָכוֹת וְהוֹדָאוֹת לְשִׁמְךָ הַגָּדוֹל וְהַקָּדוֹשׁ, עַל שֶׁהֶחֱיִיתָנוּ וְקִיַּמְתָּנוּ. כֵּן תְּחַיֵּנוּ וּתְקַיְּמֵנוּ, וְתֶאֱסוֹף גָּלֻיּוֹתֵינוּ לְחַצְרוֹת קָדְשֶׁךָ, לִשְׁמוֹר חֻקֶּיךָ וְלַעֲשׂוֹת רְצוֹנֶךָ, וּלְעָבְדְּךָ בְּלֵבָב שָׁלֵם, עַל שֶׁאֲנַחְנוּ מוֹדִים לָךְ. בָּרוּךְ אֵל הַהוֹדָאוֹת.

°°During the silent *Shemoneh Esrei* one may insert either or both of these personal prayers.

For livelihood:

אַתָּה הוּא יהוה הָאֱלֹהִים, הַזָּן וּמְפַרְנֵס וּמְכַלְכֵּל מִקַּרְנֵי רְאֵמִים עַד בֵּיצֵי כִנִּים. הַטְרִיפֵנִי לֶחֶם חֻקִּי, וְהַמְצֵא לִי וּלְכָל בְּנֵי בֵיתִי מְזוֹנוֹתַי קֹדֶם שֶׁאֶצְטָרֵךְ לָהֶם, בְּנַחַת וְלֹא בְצַעַר, בְּהֶתֵּר וְלֹא בְאִסּוּר, בְּכָבוֹד וְלֹא בְבִזָּיוֹן, לְחַיִּים וּלְשָׁלוֹם, מִשֶּׁפַע בְּרָכָה וְהַצְלָחָה, וּמִשֶּׁפַע בְּרָכָה עֶלְיוֹנָה, כְּדֵי שֶׁאוּכַל לַעֲשׂוֹת רְצוֹנֶךָ וְלַעֲסוֹק בְּתוֹרָתֶךָ וּלְקַיֵּם מִצְוֹתֶיךָ. וְאַל תַּצְרִיכֵנִי לִידֵי מַתְּנַת בָּשָׂר וָדָם. וִיקֻיַּם בִּי מִקְרָא שֶׁכָּתוּב: פּוֹתֵחַ אֶת יָדֶךָ, וּמַשְׂבִּיעַ לְכָל חַי רָצוֹן.³ וְכָתוּב: הַשְׁלֵךְ עַל יהוה יְהָבְךָ וְהוּא יְכַלְכְּלֶךָ.⁴

For forgiveness:

אָנָּא יהוה, חָטָאתִי עָוִיתִי וּפָשַׁעְתִּי לְפָנֶיךָ, מִיּוֹם הֱיוֹתִי עַל הָאֲדָמָה עַד הַיּוֹם הַזֶּה (וּבִפְרָט בַּחֵטְא ....). אָנָּא יהוה, עֲשֵׂה לְמַעַן שִׁמְךָ הַגָּדוֹל, וּתְכַפֶּר לִי עַל עֲוֹנִי וַחֲטָאַי וּפְשָׁעַי שֶׁחָטָאתִי וְשֶׁעָוִיתִי וְשֶׁפָּשַׁעְתִּי לְפָנֶיךָ, מִנְּעוּרַי עַד הַיּוֹם הַזֶּה. וּתְמַלֵּא כָּל הַשֵּׁמוֹת שֶׁפָּגַמְתִּי בְּשִׁמְךָ הַגָּדוֹל.

Continue — כִּי אַתָּה ...

°° *for You hear the prayer of Your people Israel with compassion. Blessed are You, HASHEM, Who hears prayer.*

TEMPLE SERVICE

רְצֵה *Be favorable, HASHEM, our God, toward Your people Israel and their prayer and restore the service to the Holy of Holies of Your Temple. The fire-offerings of Israel and their prayer accept with love and favor, and may the service of Your people Israel always be favorable to You.*

וְתֶחֱזֶינָה *May our eyes behold Your return to Zion in compassion. Blessed are You, HASHEM, Who restores His Presence to Zion.*

THANKSGIVING [MODIM]

Bow at 'We gratefully thank You'; straighten up at 'HASHEM.' In his repetition the *chazzan* should recite the entire *Modim* aloud, while the congregation recites *Modim of the Rabbis* softly.

מוֹדִים *We gratefully thank You, for it is You Who are HASHEM, our God and the God of our forefathers for all eternity; Rock of our lives, Shield of our salvation are You from generation to generation. We shall thank You and relate Your praise*[1] *— for our lives, which are committed to Your power and for our souls that are entrusted to You; for Your miracles that are with us every day; and for Your wonders and favors in every season — evening, morning, and afternoon. The Beneficent One, for Your compassions were never exhausted, and the Compassionate One, for Your kindnesses never ended*[2] *— always have we put our hope in You.*

MODIM OF THE RABBIS

מוֹדִים *We gratefully thank You, for it is You Who are HASHEM, our God and the God of our forefathers, the God of all flesh, our Molder, the Molder of the universe. Blessings and thanks are due Your great and holy Name for You have given us life and sustained us. So may You continue to give us life and sustain us and gather our exiles to the Courtyards of Your Sanctuary, to observe Your decrees, to do Your will and to serve You wholeheartedly. [We thank You] for inspiring us to thank You. Blessed is the God of thanksgivings.*

°°During the silent *Shemoneh Esrei* one may insert either or both of these personal prayers.

For forgiveness:

אָנָּא *Please, O HASHEM, I have erred, been iniquitous, and willfully sinned before You, from the day I have existed on earth until this very day (and especially with the sin of . . .). Please, HASHEM, act for the sake of Your Great Name and grant me atonement for my iniquities, my errors, and my willful sins through which I have erred, been iniquitous, and willfully sinned before You, from my youth until this day. And make whole all the Names that I have blemished in Your Great Name.*

For livelihood:

אַתָּה *It is You, HASHEM the God, Who nourishes, sustains, and supports, from the horns of re'eimim to the eggs of lice. Provide me with my allotment of bread; and bring forth for me and all members of my household, my food, before I have need for it; in contentment but not in pain, in a permissible but not a forbidden manner, in honor but not in disgrace, for life and for peace; from the flow of blessing and success and from the flow of the Heavenly spring, so that I be enabled to do Your will and engage in Your Torah and fulfill Your commandments. Make me not needful of people's largesse; and may there be fulfilled in me the verse that states, 'You open Your hand and satisfy the desire of every living thing'*[3] *and that states, 'Cast Your burden upon HASHEM and He will support you.'*[4]

Continue: *For You hear the prayer . . .*

---

(1) Cf. *Psalms* 79:13. (2) Cf. *Lamentations* 3:22. (3) *Psalms* 145:16. (4) 55:23.

וְעַל כֻּלָּם יִתְבָּרַךְ וְיִתְרוֹמַם שִׁמְךָ מַלְכֵּנוּ תָּמִיד לְעוֹלָם וָעֶד.

Bend the knees at בָּרוּךְ; bow at אַתָּה; straighten up at 'ה.

וְכֹל הַחַיִּים יוֹדוּךָ סֶּלָה, וִיהַלְלוּ אֶת שִׁמְךָ בֶּאֱמֶת, הָאֵל יְשׁוּעָתֵנוּ וְעֶזְרָתֵנוּ סֶלָה. בָּרוּךְ אַתָּה יהוה, הַטּוֹב שִׁמְךָ וּלְךָ נָאֶה לְהוֹדוֹת.

THE CHAZZAN DOES NOT RECITE THE PRIESTLY BLESSING

שלום

שִׂים שָׁלוֹם, טוֹבָה, וּבְרָכָה, חֵן, וָחֶסֶד וְרַחֲמִים עָלֵינוּ וְעַל כָּל יִשְׂרָאֵל עַמֶּךָ. בָּרְכֵנוּ אָבִינוּ, כֻּלָּנוּ כְּאֶחָד בְּאוֹר פָּנֶיךָ, כִּי בְאוֹר פָּנֶיךָ נָתַתָּ לָּנוּ, יהוה אֱלֹהֵינוּ, תּוֹרַת חַיִּים וְאַהֲבַת חֶסֶד, וּצְדָקָה, וּבְרָכָה, וְרַחֲמִים, וְחַיִּים, וְשָׁלוֹם. וְטוֹב בְּעֵינֶיךָ לְבָרֵךְ אֶת עַמְּךָ יִשְׂרָאֵל, בְּכָל עֵת וּבְכָל שָׁעָה בִּשְׁלוֹמֶךָ. בָּרוּךְ אַתָּה יהוה, הַמְבָרֵךְ אֶת עַמּוֹ יִשְׂרָאֵל בַּשָּׁלוֹם.

יִהְיוּ לְרָצוֹן אִמְרֵי פִי וְהֶגְיוֹן לִבִּי לְפָנֶיךָ, יהוה צוּרִי וְגֹאֲלִי.[1]

Chazzan's repetition of Shemoneh Esrei ends here. Individuals continue below:

אֱלֹהַי, נְצוֹר לְשׁוֹנִי מֵרָע, וּשְׂפָתַי מִדַּבֵּר מִרְמָה,[2] וְלִמְקַלְלַי נַפְשִׁי תִדּוֹם, וְנַפְשִׁי כֶּעָפָר לַכֹּל תִּהְיֶה. פְּתַח לִבִּי בְּתוֹרָתֶךָ, וּבְמִצְוֹתֶיךָ תִּרְדּוֹף נַפְשִׁי. וְכָל הַחוֹשְׁבִים עָלַי רָעָה, מְהֵרָה הָפֵר עֲצָתָם וְקַלְקֵל מַחֲשַׁבְתָּם. עֲשֵׂה לְמַעַן שְׁמֶךָ, עֲשֵׂה לְמַעַן יְמִינֶךָ, עֲשֵׂה לְמַעַן קְדֻשָּׁתֶךָ, עֲשֵׂה לְמַעַן תּוֹרָתֶךָ. לְמַעַן יֵחָלְצוּן יְדִידֶיךָ, הוֹשִׁיעָה יְמִינְךָ וַעֲנֵנִי.[3]

Some recite verses pertaining to their names here. See page 482.

יִהְיוּ לְרָצוֹן אִמְרֵי פִי וְהֶגְיוֹן לִבִּי לְפָנֶיךָ, יהוה צוּרִי וְגֹאֲלִי.

עֹשֶׂה שָׁלוֹם בִּמְרוֹמָיו, הוּא יַעֲשֶׂה שָׁלוֹם עָלֵינוּ, וְעַל כָּל יִשְׂרָאֵל. וְאִמְרוּ: אָמֵן.

Bow and take three steps back. Bow left and say . . . עֹשֶׂה; bow right and say . . . הוּא יַעֲשֶׂה; bow forward and say . . . וְעַל כָּל . . . אָמֵן.

יְהִי רָצוֹן מִלְּפָנֶיךָ יהוה אֱלֹהֵינוּ וֵאלֹהֵי אֲבוֹתֵינוּ, שֶׁיִּבָּנֶה בֵּית הַמִּקְדָּשׁ בִּמְהֵרָה בְיָמֵינוּ, וְתֵן חֶלְקֵנוּ בְּתוֹרָתֶךָ. וְשָׁם נַעֲבָדְךָ בְּיִרְאָה, כִּימֵי עוֹלָם וּכְשָׁנִים קַדְמוֹנִיּוֹת. וְעָרְבָה לַיהוה מִנְחַת יְהוּדָה וִירוּשָׁלָיִם, כִּימֵי עוֹלָם וּכְשָׁנִים קַדְמוֹנִיּוֹת.[4]

THE INDIVIDUAL'S RECITATION OF SHEMONEH ESREI ENDS HERE.

The individual remains standing in place until the chazzan reaches Kedushah — or at least until the chazzan begins his repetition — then he takes three steps forward. The chazzan himself, or one who is praying alone, should remain in place for a few moments before taking three steps forward.

For all these, may Your Name be blessed and exalted, our King, continually forever and ever.

Bend the knees at 'Blessed'; bow at 'You'; straighten up at 'HASHEM.'

Everything alive will gratefully acknowledge You, Selah! and praise Your Name sincerely, O God of our salvation and help, Selah! Blessed are You, HASHEM, Your Name is 'The Beneficent One' and to You it is fitting to give thanks.

THE CHAZZAN DOES NOT RECITE THE PRIESTLY BLESSING

PEACE

שִׂים שָׁלוֹם *Establish peace, goodness, blessing, graciousness, kindness, and compassion upon us and upon all of Your people Israel. Bless us, our Father, all of us as one, with the light of Your countenance, for with the light of Your countenance You gave us, HASHEM, our God, the Torah of life and a love of kindness, righteousness, blessing, compassion, life, and peace. And may it be good in Your eyes to bless Your people Israel at every time and every hour with Your peace. Blessed are You, HASHEM, Who blesses His people Israel with peace.*

May the expressions of my mouth and the thoughts of my heart find favor before You, HASHEM, my Rock and my Redeemer.[1]

Chazzan's repetition of Shemoneh Esrei ends here. Individuals continue below:

אֱלֹהַי *My God, guard my tongue from evil and my lips from speaking deceitfully.*[2] *To those who curse me, let my soul be silent; and let my soul be like dust to everyone. Open my heart to Your Torah, then my soul will pursue Your commandments. As for all those who design evil against me, speedily nullify their counsel and disrupt their design. Act for Your Name's sake; act for Your right hand's sake; act for Your sanctity's sake; act for Your Torah's sake. That Your beloved ones may be given rest; let Your right hand save, and respond to me.*[3]

Some recite verses pertaining to their names at this point. See page 482.

May the expressions of my mouth and the thoughts of my heart find favor before You, HASHEM, my Rock and my Redeemer.[1] *°°He Who makes peace in*

Bow and take three steps back. Bow left and say, 'He Who makes peace ...'; bow right and say, 'may He make peace ...'; bow forward and say, 'and upon ... Amen.'

His heights, may He make peace upon us, and upon all Israel. Now respond: Amen.

יְהִי רָצוֹן *May it be Your will, HASHEM, our God and the God of our forefathers, that the Holy Temple be rebuilt, speedily in our days. Grant us our share in Your Torah, and may we serve You there with reverence, as in days of old and in former years. Then the offering of Judah and Jerusalem will be pleasing to HASHEM, as in days of old and in former years.*[4]

THE INDIVIDUAL'S RECITATION OF *SHEMONEH ESREI* ENDS HERE.

The individual remains standing in place until the chazzan reaches Kedushah — or at least until the chazzan begins his repetition — then he takes three steps forward. The chazzan himself, or one who is praying alone, should remain in place for a few moments before taking three steps forward.

---

(1) *Psalms* 19:15. (2) Cf. 34:14. (3) 60:7; 108:7. (4) *Malachi* 3:4.

The *chazzan* recites Half-*Kaddish*:

יִתְגַּדַּל וְיִתְקַדַּשׁ שְׁמֵהּ רַבָּא. (.Cong – אָמֵן.) בְּעָלְמָא דִּי בְרָא כִרְעוּתֵהּ. וְיַמְלִיךְ מַלְכוּתֵהּ, בְּחַיֵּיכוֹן וּבְיוֹמֵיכוֹן וּבְחַיֵּי דְכָל בֵּית יִשְׂרָאֵל, בַּעֲגָלָא וּבִזְמַן קָרִיב. וְאִמְרוּ: אָמֵן.

(.Cong – אָמֵן. יְהֵא שְׁמֵהּ רַבָּא מְבָרַךְ לְעָלַם וּלְעָלְמֵי עָלְמַיָּא.)

יְהֵא שְׁמֵהּ רַבָּא מְבָרַךְ לְעָלַם וּלְעָלְמֵי עָלְמַיָּא.

יִתְבָּרַךְ וְיִשְׁתַּבַּח וְיִתְפָּאַר וְיִתְרוֹמַם וְיִתְנַשֵּׂא וְיִתְהַדָּר וְיִתְעַלֶּה וְיִתְהַלָּל שְׁמֵהּ דְּקֻדְשָׁא בְּרִיךְ הוּא (.Cong – בְּרִיךְ הוּא) – לְעֵלָּא מִן כָּל בִּרְכָתָא וְשִׁירָתָא תֻּשְׁבְּחָתָא וְנֶחֱמָתָא, דַּאֲמִירָן בְּעָלְמָא. וְאִמְרוּ: אָמֵן.

(.Cong – אָמֵן.)

❧ הוצאת ספר תורה ❧

From the moment the Ark is opened until the Torah is returned to it, one must conduct himself with the utmost respect, and avoid unnecessary conversation. It is commendable to kiss the Torah as it is carried to the *bimah* [reading table] and back to the Ark.

All rise and remain standing until the Torah is placed on the *bimah*.
The Ark is opened. Before the Torah is removed the congregation recites:

וַיְהִי בִּנְסֹעַ הָאָרֹן וַיֹּאמֶר מֹשֶׁה, קוּמָה יהוה וְיָפֻצוּ אֹיְבֶיךָ וְיָנֻסוּ מְשַׂנְאֶיךָ מִפָּנֶיךָ.' כִּי מִצִּיּוֹן תֵּצֵא תוֹרָה, וּדְבַר יהוה מִירוּשָׁלָיִם.² בָּרוּךְ שֶׁנָּתַן תּוֹרָה לְעַמּוֹ יִשְׂרָאֵל בִּקְדֻשָּׁתוֹ.

זוהר ויקהל שסט:א

בְּרִיךְ שְׁמֵהּ דְּמָרֵא עָלְמָא, בְּרִיךְ כִּתְרָךְ וְאַתְרָךְ. יְהֵא רְעוּתָךְ עִם עַמָּךְ יִשְׂרָאֵל לְעָלַם, וּפֻרְקַן יְמִינָךְ אַחֲזֵי לְעַמָּךְ בְּבֵית מַקְדְּשָׁךְ, וּלְאַמְטוּיֵי לָנָא מִטּוּב נְהוֹרָךְ, וּלְקַבֵּל צְלוֹתָנָא בְּרַחֲמִין. יְהֵא רַעֲוָא קֳדָמָךְ, דְּתוֹרִיךְ לָן חַיִּין בְּטִיבוּתָא, וְלֶהֱוֵי אֲנָא פְקִידָא בְּגוֹ צַדִּיקַיָּא, לְמִרְחַם עָלַי וּלְמִנְטַר יָתִי וְיַת כָּל דִּי לִי, וְדִי לְעַמָּךְ יִשְׂרָאֵל. אַנְתְּ הוּא זָן לְכֹלָּא, וּמְפַרְנֵס לְכֹלָּא, אַנְתְּ הוּא שַׁלִּיט עַל כֹּלָּא. אַנְתְּ הוּא דְּשַׁלִּיט עַל מַלְכַיָּא, וּמַלְכוּתָא דִּילָךְ הִיא. אֲנָא עַבְדָּא דְקֻדְשָׁא בְּרִיךְ הוּא, דְּסָגִידְנָא קַמֵּהּ וּמִקַּמָּא דִּיקַר אוֹרַיְתֵהּ בְּכָל עִדָּן וְעִדָּן. לָא עַל אֱנָשׁ רָחִיצְנָא, וְלָא עַל בַּר אֱלָהִין סָמִיכְנָא, אֶלָּא בֵּאֱלָהָא דִשְׁמַיָּא, דְּהוּא אֱלָהָא קְשׁוֹט, וְאוֹרַיְתֵהּ קְשׁוֹט, וּנְבִיאְוֹהִי קְשׁוֹט, וּמַסְגֵּא לְמֶעְבַּד טַבְוָן וּקְשׁוֹט. בֵּהּ אֲנָא רָחִיץ, וְלִשְׁמֵהּ קַדִּישָׁא יַקִּירָא אֲנָא אֵמַר תֻּשְׁבְּחָן. יְהֵא רַעֲוָא קֳדָמָךְ, דְּתִפְתַּח לִבָּאִי בְּאוֹרַיְתָא, וְתַשְׁלִים מִשְׁאֲלִין דְּלִבָּאִי, וְלִבָּא דְכָל עַמָּךְ יִשְׂרָאֵל, לְטַב וּלְחַיִּין וְלִשְׁלָם. (אָמֵן.)

The Torah is removed from the Ark and presented to the *chazzan*, who accepts it in his right arm. He then turns to the Ark, bows while raising the Torah, and recites:

גַּדְּלוּ לַיהוה אִתִּי וּנְרוֹמְמָה שְׁמוֹ יַחְדָּו.³

The chazzan recites Half-Kaddish:

יִתְגַּדַּל *May His great Name grow exalted and sanctified* (Cong.— *Amen.*) *in the world that He created as He willed. May He give reign to His kingship in your lifetimes and in your days, and in the lifetimes of the entire Family of Israel, swiftly and soon. Now respond: Amen.*

(Cong.— *Amen. May His great Name be blessed forever and ever.*)
May His great Name be blessed forever and ever.

Blessed, praised, glorified, exalted, extolled, mighty, upraised, and lauded be the Name of the Holy One, Blessed is He (Cong.— *Blessed is He*) — *beyond any blessing and song, praise and consolation that are uttered in the world. Now respond: Amen.* (Cong.— *Amen.*)

❧ REMOVAL OF THE TORAH FROM THE ARK ❧

From the moment the Ark is opened until the Torah is returned to it, one must conduct himself with the utmost respect, and avoid unnecessary conversation. It is commendable to kiss the Torah as it is carried to the *bimah* [reading table] and back to the Ark.
All rise and remain standing until the Torah is placed on the *bimah*.
The Ark is opened. Before the Torah is removed the congregation recites:

וַיְהִי בִּנְסֹעַ *When the Ark would travel, Moses would say, 'Arise, HASHEM, and let Your foes be scattered, let those who hate You flee from You.'[1] For from Zion the Torah will come forth and the word of HASHEM from Jerusalem.[2] Blessed is He Who gave the Torah to His people Israel in His holiness.*

Zohar, Vayakhel 369a

בְּרִיךְ שְׁמֵהּ *Blessed is the Name of the Master of the universe, blessed is Your crown and Your place. May Your favor remain with Your people Israel forever; may You display the salvation of Your right hand to Your people in Your Holy Temple, to benefit us with the goodness of Your luminescence and to accept our prayers with mercy. May it be Your will that You extend our lives with goodness and that I be numbered among the righteous; that You have mercy on me and protect me, all that is mine and that is Your people Israel's. It is You Who nourishes all and sustains all; You control everything. It is You Who controls kings, and kingship is Yours. I am a servant of the Holy One, Blessed is He, and I prostrate myself before Him and before the glory of His Torah at all times. Not in any man do I put trust, nor on any angel do I rely — only on the God of heaven Who is the God of truth, Whose Torah is truth and Whose prophets are true and Who acts liberally with kindness and truth. In Him do I trust, and to His glorious and holy Name do I declare praises. May it be Your will that You open my heart to the Torah and that You fulfill the wishes of my heart and the heart of Your entire people Israel for good, for life, and for peace. (Amen.)*

The Torah is removed from the Ark and presented to the *chazzan*, who accepts it in his right arm. He turns to the Ark, bows while raising the Torah, and recites:

Declare the greatness of HASHEM with me, and let us exalt His Name together.[3]

(1) *Numbers* 10:35. (2) *Isaiah* 2:3. (3) *Psalms* 34:4.

The *chazzan* turns to his right and carries the Torah to the *bimah*, as the congregation responds:

לְךָ יהוה הַגְּדֻלָּה וְהַגְּבוּרָה וְהַתִּפְאֶרֶת וְהַנֵּצַח וְהַהוֹד כִּי כֹל בַּשָּׁמַיִם וּבָאָרֶץ, לְךָ יהוה הַמַּמְלָכָה וְהַמִּתְנַשֵּׂא לְכֹל לְרֹאשׁ.

רוֹמְמוּ יהוה אֱלֹהֵינוּ, וְהִשְׁתַּחֲווּ לַהֲדֹם רַגְלָיו, קָדוֹשׁ הוּא. רוֹמְמוּ יהוה אֱלֹהֵינוּ, וְהִשְׁתַּחֲווּ לְהַר קָדְשׁוֹ, כִּי קָדוֹשׁ יהוה אֱלֹהֵינוּ.

אַב הָרַחֲמִים הוּא יְרַחֵם עַם עֲמוּסִים, וְיִזְכֹּר בְּרִית אֵיתָנִים, וְיַצִּיל נַפְשׁוֹתֵינוּ מִן הַשָּׁעוֹת הָרָעוֹת, וְיִגְעַר בְּיֵצֶר הָרַע מִן הַנְּשׂוּאִים, וְיָחֹן אוֹתָנוּ לִפְלֵיטַת עוֹלָמִים, וִימַלֵּא מִשְׁאֲלוֹתֵינוּ בְּמִדָּה טוֹבָה יְשׁוּעָה וְרַחֲמִים.

The Torah is placed on the *bimah* and prepared for reading.
The *gabbai* uses the following formula to call a *Kohen* to the Torah:

וְתִגָּלֶה וְתֵרָאֶה מַלְכוּתוֹ עָלֵינוּ בִּזְמַן קָרוֹב, וְיָחֹן פְּלֵיטָתֵנוּ וּפְלֵיטַת עַמּוֹ בֵּית יִשְׂרָאֵל לְחֵן וּלְחֶסֶד וּלְרַחֲמִים וּלְרָצוֹן. וְנֹאמַר אָמֵן. הַכֹּל הָבוּ גֹדֶל לֵאלֹהֵינוּ וּתְנוּ כָבוֹד לַתּוֹרָה. כֹּהֵן° קְרַב, יַעֲמֹד (insert name) הַכֹּהֵן.

°If no *Kohen* is present, the *gabbai* says: "אִם אֵין כָּאן כֹּהֵן, יַעֲמֹד (name) יִשְׂרָאֵל (לֵוִי) בִּמְקוֹם כֹּהֵן."

בָּרוּךְ שֶׁנָּתַן תּוֹרָה לְעַמּוֹ יִשְׂרָאֵל בִּקְדֻשָּׁתוֹ. (תּוֹרַת יהוה תְּמִימָה מְשִׁיבַת נָפֶשׁ, עֵדוּת יהוה נֶאֱמָנָה מַחְכִּימַת פֶּתִי. פִּקּוּדֵי יהוה יְשָׁרִים מְשַׂמְּחֵי לֵב, מִצְוַת יהוה בָּרָה מְאִירַת עֵינָיִם. יהוה עֹז לְעַמּוֹ יִתֵּן, יהוה יְבָרֵךְ אֶת עַמּוֹ בַשָּׁלוֹם. הָאֵל תָּמִים דַּרְכּוֹ, אִמְרַת יהוה צְרוּפָה, מָגֵן הוּא לְכֹל הַחוֹסִים בּוֹ.)

Congregation, then *gabbai*:

וְאַתֶּם הַדְּבֵקִים בַּיהוה אֱלֹהֵיכֶם, חַיִּים כֻּלְּכֶם הַיּוֹם.

The reader shows the *oleh* (person called to the Torah) the place in the Torah. The *oleh* touches the Torah with a corner of his *tallis,* or the belt or mantle of the Torah, and kisses it.
He then begins the blessing, bowing at בָּרְכוּ, and straightening up at 'ה.

בָּרְכוּ אֶת יהוה הַמְבֹרָךְ.

Congregation, followed by *oleh*, responds, bowing at בָּרוּךְ, and straightening up at 'ה.

בָּרוּךְ יהוה הַמְבֹרָךְ לְעוֹלָם וָעֶד.

Oleh continues:

בָּרוּךְ אַתָּה יהוה אֱלֹהֵינוּ מֶלֶךְ הָעוֹלָם, אֲשֶׁר בָּחַר בָּנוּ מִכָּל הָעַמִּים, וְנָתַן לָנוּ אֶת תּוֹרָתוֹ. בָּרוּךְ אַתָּה יהוה, נוֹתֵן הַתּוֹרָה. (Cong.— אָמֵן.)

After his Torah portion has been read, the *oleh* recites:

בָּרוּךְ אַתָּה יהוה אֱלֹהֵינוּ מֶלֶךְ הָעוֹלָם, אֲשֶׁר נָתַן לָנוּ תּוֹרַת אֱמֶת, וְחַיֵּי עוֹלָם נָטַע בְּתוֹכֵנוּ. בָּרוּךְ אַתָּה יהוה, נוֹתֵן הַתּוֹרָה. (Cong.— אָמֵן.)

THE *MI SHEBEIRACH* PRAYER FOR A SICK PERSON APPEARS ON PAGE 140.

The *chazzan* turns to his right and carries the Torah to the *bimah,* as the congregation responds:

לְךָ Yours, HASHEM, is the greatness, the strength, the splendor, the triumph, and the glory; even everything in heaven and earth; Yours, HASHEM, is the kingdom, and the sovereignty over every leader.[1] Exalt HASHEM, our God, and bow at His footstool; He is Holy! Exalt HASHEM, our God, and bow to His holy mountain; for holy is HASHEM, our God.[2]

אַב הָרַחֲמִים May the Father of compassion have mercy on the nation that is borne by Him, and may He remember the covenant of the spiritually mighty. May He rescue our souls from the bad times, and upbraid the evil inclination to leave those borne by Him, graciously make us an eternal remnant, and fulfill our requests in good measure, for salvation and mercy.

The Torah is placed on the *bimah* and prepared for reading.
The *gabbai* uses the following formula to call a *Kohen* to the Torah:

וְתִגָּלֶה And may His kingship over us be revealed and become visible soon, and may He be gracious to our remnant and the remnant of His people the Family of Israel, for graciousness, kindness, mercy, and favor. And let us respond, Amen. All of you ascribe greatness to our God and give honor to the Torah. Kohen,° approach. Stand (name) son of (father's name) the Kohen.

°If no *Kohen* is present, the *gabbai* says: 'There is no Kohen present,
stand (name) son of (father's name) an Israelite (Levite) in place of the Kohen.'

Blessed is He Who gave the Torah to His people Israel in His holiness. (The Torah of HASHEM is perfect, restoring the soul; the testimony of HASHEM is trustworthy, making the simple one wise. The orders of HASHEM are upright, gladdening the heart; the command of HASHEM is clear, enlightening the eyes.[3] HASHEM will give might to His nation; HASHEM will bless His nation with peace.[4] The God Whose way is perfect, the promise of HASHEM is flawless, He is a shield for all who take refuge in Him.[5])

Congregation, then *gabbai:*

You who cling to HASHEM, your God, you are all alive today.[6]

The reader shows the *oleh* (person called to the Torah) the place in the Torah. The *oleh* touches the Torah with a corner of his *tallis,* or the belt or mantle of the Torah, and kisses it. He then begins the blessing, bowing at 'Bless,' and straightening up at 'HASHEM.'

Bless HASHEM, the blessed One.

Congregation, followed by *oleh,* responds, bowing at 'Blessed,' and straightening up at 'HASHEM.'

Blessed is HASHEM, the blessed One, for all eternity.

Oleh continues:

בָּרוּךְ Blessed are You, HASHEM, our God, King of the universe, Who selected us from all the peoples and gave us His Torah. Blessed are You, HASHEM, Giver of the Torah.   (Cong.— Amen.)

After his Torah portion has been read, the *oleh* recites:

בָּרוּךְ Blessed are You, HASHEM, our God, King of the universe, Who gave us the Torah of truth and implanted eternal life within us. Blessed are You, HASHEM, Giver of the Torah.   (Cong.— Amen.)

THE *MI SHEBEIRACH* PRAYER FOR A SICK PERSON APPEARS ON PAGE 140.

---

(1) *I Chronicles* 29:11. (2) *Psalms* 99:5,9. (3) 19:8-9. (4) 29:11. (5) 18:31. (6) *Deuteronomy* 4:4.

﴾ קריאת התורה ﴿

דברים ד:כה-מ

כה – כִּי־תוֹלִיד בָּנִים וּבְנֵי בָנִים וְנוֹשַׁנְתֶּם בָּאָרֶץ וְהִשְׁחַתֶּם וַעֲשִׂיתֶם פֶּסֶל תְּמוּנַת כֹּל וַעֲשִׂיתֶם הָרַע בְּעֵינֵי־יְהֹוָה אֱלֹהֶיךָ לְהַכְעִיסוֹ: הַעִידֹתִי בָכֶם הַיּוֹם אֶת־הַשָּׁמַיִם וְאֶת־הָאָרֶץ כִּי־אָבֹד תֹּאבֵדוּן מַהֵר מֵעַל הָאָרֶץ אֲשֶׁר אַתֶּם עֹבְרִים אֶת־הַיַּרְדֵּן שָׁמָּה לְרִשְׁתָּהּ לֹא־תַאֲרִיכֻן יָמִים עָלֶיהָ כִּי הִשָּׁמֵד תִּשָּׁמֵדוּן: וְהֵפִיץ יְהֹוָה אֶתְכֶם בָּעַמִּים וְנִשְׁאַרְתֶּם מְתֵי מִסְפָּר בַּגּוֹיִם אֲשֶׁר יְנַהֵג יְהֹוָה אֶתְכֶם שָׁמָּה: וַעֲבַדְתֶּם־שָׁם אֱלֹהִים מַעֲשֵׂה יְדֵי אָדָם עֵץ וָאֶבֶן אֲשֶׁר לֹא־יִרְאוּן וְלֹא יִשְׁמְעוּן וְלֹא יֹאכְלוּן וְלֹא יְרִיחֻן: וּבִקַּשְׁתֶּם מִשָּׁם אֶת־יְהֹוָה אֱלֹהֶיךָ וּמָצָאתָ כִּי תִדְרְשֶׁנּוּ בְּכָל־לְבָבְךָ וּבְכָל־נַפְשֶׁךָ: לוי – בַּצַּר לְךָ וּמְצָאוּךָ כֹּל הַדְּבָרִים הָאֵלֶּה בְּאַחֲרִית הַיָּמִים וְשַׁבְתָּ עַד־יְהֹוָה אֱלֹהֶיךָ וְשָׁמַעְתָּ בְּקֹלוֹ: כִּי אֵל רַחוּם יְהֹוָה אֱלֹהֶיךָ לֹא יַרְפְּךָ וְלֹא יַשְׁחִיתֶךָ וְלֹא יִשְׁכַּח אֶת־בְּרִית אֲבֹתֶיךָ אֲשֶׁר נִשְׁבַּע לָהֶם: כִּי שְׁאַל־נָא לְיָמִים רִאשֹׁנִים אֲשֶׁר־הָיוּ לְפָנֶיךָ לְמִן־הַיּוֹם אֲשֶׁר בָּרָא אֱלֹהִים | אָדָם עַל־הָאָרֶץ וּלְמִקְצֵה הַשָּׁמַיִם וְעַד־קְצֵה הַשָּׁמָיִם הֲנִהְיָה כַּדָּבָר הַגָּדוֹל הַזֶּה אוֹ הֲנִשְׁמַע כָּמֹהוּ: הֲשָׁמַע עָם קוֹל אֱלֹהִים מְדַבֵּר מִתּוֹךְ־הָאֵשׁ כַּאֲשֶׁר־שָׁמַעְתָּ אַתָּה וַיֶּחִי: אוֹ | הֲנִסָּה אֱלֹהִים לָבוֹא לָקַחַת לוֹ גוֹי מִקֶּרֶב גּוֹי בְּמַסֹּת בְּאֹתֹת וּבְמוֹפְתִים וּבְמִלְחָמָה וּבְיָד חֲזָקָה וּבִזְרוֹעַ נְטוּיָה וּבְמוֹרָאִים גְּדֹלִים כְּכֹל אֲשֶׁר־עָשָׂה לָכֶם יְהֹוָה אֱלֹהֵיכֶם בְּמִצְרַיִם לְעֵינֶיךָ: אַתָּה הָרְאֵתָ לָדַעַת כִּי יְהֹוָה הוּא הָאֱלֹהִים אֵין עוֹד מִלְבַדּוֹ: ישראל (מפטיר) – מִן־הַשָּׁמַיִם הִשְׁמִיעֲךָ אֶת־קֹלוֹ לְיַסְּרֶךָ וְעַל־הָאָרֶץ הֶרְאֲךָ אֶת־אִשּׁוֹ הַגְּדוֹלָה וּדְבָרָיו שָׁמַעְתָּ מִתּוֹךְ הָאֵשׁ: וְתַחַת כִּי אָהַב אֶת־אֲבֹתֶיךָ וַיִּבְחַר בְּזַרְעוֹ אַחֲרָיו וַיּוֹצִאֲךָ בְּפָנָיו בְּכֹחוֹ הַגָּדֹל מִמִּצְרָיִם: לְהוֹרִישׁ גּוֹיִם גְּדֹלִים וַעֲצֻמִים מִמְּךָ מִפָּנֶיךָ לַהֲבִיאֲךָ לָתֶת־לְךָ אֶת־אַרְצָם נַחֲלָה כַּיּוֹם הַזֶּה: וְיָדַעְתָּ הַיּוֹם וַהֲשֵׁבֹתָ

⌇ৡ Torah Reading

The Torah reading of Tishah B'Av encapsules Jewish history: the spiritual sloth that leads to idolatry and exile, the encouragement that it is in our power to arouse God's mercy — and that it is surely in His power to bring about the final redemption. In his warning that exile may be impending, Moses says that the main source of

tragedy is that *you will have been long in the land.* For all its imperfections, the generation that experienced the Exodus and the miracles of the Wilderness and the conquest of the Land would not be quick to sin so grievously. But as the years and generations go by, people tend to grow stale, to take their advantages for granted, to forget the sense of freshness and spiritual

❧ **TORAH READING** ❧

Deuteronomy 4:25-40

Kohen — *When you beget children and grandchildren and will have been long in the land, you will grow corrupt and make a graven image of anything, and you will do evil in the eyes of HASHEM, your God, to anger Him. I appoint heaven and earth this day to bear witness that you will surely perish quickly from the land that you are crossing the Jordan to possess; you will not have lengthy days upon it, for you will be utterly destroyed. HASHEM will scatter you among the peoples, and you will be left few in number among the nations where HASHEM will lead you. There you will worship gods, the handiwork of man, of wood and stone, which do not see, do not hear, do not eat, and do not smell. From there you will seek HASHEM, your God, and you will find Him — if you search for Him with all your heart and all your soul.*

Levi — *When you are in distress and all these things have befallen you — at the end of days — you shall return unto HASHEM, your God, and hearken to His voice. For HASHEM, your God, is a merciful God, He shall not abandon you nor destroy you, and He shall not forget the covenant of your forefathers that He swore to them. For inquire now regarding the early days that were before you, from the day when HASHEM created man on the earth, and from one end of heaven to the other end of heaven, has there been anything like this great thing or has anything like it been heard? Has a people ever heard the voice of God speaking from amid the fire, as you heard, and survived? Or has any god ever miraculously come to take for himself one nation from the midst of another, with challenges, with signs, with wonders, with war, with a strong hand, with an outstretched arm, and with greatly awesome deeds, like everything that HASHEM, your God, did for you in Egypt before your eyes? You have been shown to know that HASHEM — He is the God! — there is none beside Him.*

Third (Maftir) — *From heaven He caused you to hear His voice in order to discipline you, and on earth He showed you His great fire, and you heard His words from amid the fire. Because He loved your forefathers He chose their offspring after them, and took it out before Him with His great strength from Egypt; to drive away before you nations that are greater and mightier than you, to bring you, to give you their land as an inheritance, as on this day. You are to know this day and take*

striving that brought them to their high plateau of success. Once that happens and they begin to look for new stimuli, they will begin to explore the lifestyle of their neighbors and experiment with it. In ancient times, this meant idolatry. Today, it can mean any of the numerous isms and beliefs that have led Jews astray once they have grown weary of their eternal tradition and sought more fashionable ways of life and belief.

But the Torah assures us that even after the exile takes place, there is always hope. From its place of distress, Israel will seek God and find Him, and the nation will repent and return to God. The Torah exhorts us to remember that God redeemed us in an unprecedented display of mercy and love. His love for us stems from the covenant with the Patriarchs, a phenomenon that is eternal and can never be diminished by sin or exile. Therefore we must always be aware that redemption *will* come again, and that it is in

אֶל־לְבָבֶךָ כִּי יהוה הוּא הָאֱלֹהִים בַּשָּׁמַיִם מִמַּעַל וְעַל־הָאָרֶץ
מִתָּחַת אֵין עוֹד: וְשָׁמַרְתָּ אֶת־חֻקָּיו וְאֶת־מִצְוֹתָיו אֲשֶׁר אָנֹכִי
מְצַוְּךָ הַיּוֹם אֲשֶׁר יִיטַב לְךָ וּלְבָנֶיךָ אַחֲרֶיךָ וּלְמַעַן תַּאֲרִיךְ יָמִים
עַל־הָאֲדָמָה אֲשֶׁר יהוה אֱלֹהֶיךָ נֹתֵן לְךָ כָּל־הַיָּמִים:

מִי שֶׁבֵּרַךְ לְחוֹלֶה / PRAYER FOR A SICK PERSON

מִי שֶׁבֵּרַךְ אֲבוֹתֵינוּ אַבְרָהָם יִצְחָק וְיַעֲקֹב, מֹשֶׁה אַהֲרֹן דָּוִד וּשְׁלֹמֹה,

for a woman	for a man
הוּא יְבָרֵךְ וִירַפֵּא אֶת הַחוֹלָה	הוּא יְבָרֵךְ וִירַפֵּא אֶת הַחוֹלֶה
(mother's name) בַּת (patient's name)	(mother's name) בֶּן (patient's name)
יִתֵּן (supplicant's name)שֶׁ בַּעֲבוּר	יִתֵּן (supplicant's name)שֶׁ בַּעֲבוּרוֹ.°°
לִצְדָקָה בַּעֲבוּרָהּ.°° בִּשְׂכַר זֶה,	לִצְדָקָה בַּעֲבוּרוֹ. בִּשְׂכַר זֶה,
הַקָּדוֹשׁ בָּרוּךְ הוּא יִמָּלֵא רַחֲמִים	הַקָּדוֹשׁ בָּרוּךְ הוּא יִמָּלֵא רַחֲמִים
עָלֶיהָ, לְהַחֲלִימָהּ וּלְרַפֹּאתָהּ	עָלָיו, לְהַחֲלִימוֹ וּלְרַפֹּאתוֹ
וּלְהַחֲזִיקָהּ וּלְהַחֲיוֹתָהּ, וְיִשְׁלַח לָהּ	לְהַחֲזִיקוֹ וּלְהַחֲיוֹתוֹ, וְיִשְׁלַח לוֹ
מְהֵרָה רְפוּאָה שְׁלֵמָה מִן הַשָּׁמַיִם,	מְהֵרָה רְפוּאָה שְׁלֵמָה מִן הַשָּׁמַיִם,
לִרְמַ״ח אֵבָרֶיהָ, וּלְכָל גִּידֶיהָ, בְּתוֹךְ	לְכָל אֵבָרָיו, וְשַׁסָּ״ה גִּידָיו, בְּתוֹךְ
שְׁאָר חוֹלֵי יִשְׂרָאֵל, רְפוּאַת הַנֶּפֶשׁ, וּרְפוּאַת הַגּוּף, הַשְׁתָּא, בַּעֲגָלָא וּבִזְמַן
קָרִיב. וְנֹאמַר: אָמֵן. (.Cong— אָמֵן)

°°Many congregations substitute:

בַּעֲבוּר שֶׁכָּל הַקָּהָל מִתְפַּלְּלִים בַּעֲבוּרוֹ (בַּעֲבוּרָהּ)

חֲצִי קַדִּישׁ

After the last *oleh* has completed his closing blessing, the reader recites Half-Kaddish.

יִתְגַּדַּל וְיִתְקַדַּשׁ שְׁמֵהּ רַבָּא. (.Cong— אָמֵן) בְּעָלְמָא דִּי בְרָא כִרְעוּתֵהּ.
וְיַמְלִיךְ מַלְכוּתֵהּ, בְּחַיֵּיכוֹן וּבְיוֹמֵיכוֹן וּבְחַיֵּי דְכָל בֵּית יִשְׂרָאֵל,
בַּעֲגָלָא וּבִזְמַן קָרִיב. וְאִמְרוּ: אָמֵן.
(.Cong— אָמֵן. יְהֵא שְׁמֵהּ רַבָּא מְבָרַךְ לְעָלַם וּלְעָלְמֵי עָלְמַיָּא.)
יְהֵא שְׁמֵהּ רַבָּא מְבָרַךְ לְעָלַם וּלְעָלְמֵי עָלְמַיָּא.
יִתְבָּרַךְ וְיִשְׁתַּבַּח וְיִתְפָּאַר וְיִתְרוֹמַם וְיִתְנַשֵּׂא וְיִתְהַדָּר וְיִתְעַלֶּה וְיִתְהַלָּל
שְׁמֵהּ דְּקֻדְשָׁא בְּרִיךְ הוּא (.Cong— בְּרִיךְ הוּא) — לְעֵלָּא מִן כָּל בִּרְכָתָא
וְשִׁירָתָא תֻּשְׁבְּחָתָא וְנֶחֱמָתָא, דַּאֲמִירָן בְּעָלְמָא. וְאִמְרוּ: אָמֵן. (.Cong— אָמֵן)

הַגְבָּהָה וּגְלִילָה

The Torah Scroll is raised and each person looks at the Torah and recites aloud:

וְזֹאת הַתּוֹרָה אֲשֶׁר שָׂם מֹשֶׁה לִפְנֵי בְּנֵי יִשְׂרָאֵל,¹
עַל פִּי יהוה בְּיַד מֹשֶׁה.²

to your heart that HASHEM is the only God — in heaven above and on the earth below — there is none other. You shall observe His decrees and His commandments that I command you this day, so that He will do good to you and to your children after you, and so that you will long remain on the land that HASHEM, your God, gives you, for all the years.

PRAYER FOR A SICK PERSON

מִי שֶׁבֵּרַךְ He Who blessed our forefathers Abraham, Isaac and Jacob, Moses and Aaron, David and Solomon — may He bless and heal the sick person (patient's Hebrew name) son/daughter of (patient's mother's Hebrew name) because (name of supplicant) will contribute to charity on his/her behalf.°° In reward for this, may the Holy One, Blessed is He, be filled with

for a man	for a woman
compassion for him to restore his health, to heal him, to strengthen him, and to revivify him. And may He send him speedily a complete recovery from heaven for his two hundred forty-eight organs and three hundred sixty-five blood vessels, among the other	compassion for her to restore her health, to heal her, to strengthen her, and to revivify her. And may He send her speedily a complete recovery from heaven for all her organs and all her blood vessels, among the other

sick people of Israel, a recovery of the body and a recovery of the spirit, may a recovery come speedily, swiftly and soon. Now let us respond: Amen.

(Cong.—Amen.)

°°Many congregations substitute:
because the entire congregation prays for him (her)

HALF KADDISH

After the last *oleh* has completed his closing blessing, the reader recites Half-*Kaddish*.

יִתְגַּדַּל May His great Name grow exalted and sanctified (Cong.— Amen.) in the world that He created as He willed. May He give reign to His kingship in your lifetimes and in your days, and in the lifetimes of the entire Family of Israel, swiftly and soon. Now respond: Amen.

(Cong.— Amen. May His great Name be blessed forever and ever.)
May His great Name be blessed forever and ever.

Blessed, praised, glorified, exalted, extolled, mighty, upraised, and lauded be the Name of the Holy One, Blessed is He (Cong.— Blessed is He) — beyond any blessing and song, praise and consolation that are uttered in the world. Now respond: Amen. (Cong.— Amen.)

HAGBAHAH AND GELILAH

The Torah Scroll is raised and each person looks at the Torah and recites aloud:

This is the Torah that Moses placed before the Children of Israel,[1] upon the command of HASHEM, through Moses' hand.[2]

(1) *Deuteronomy* 4:44. (2) *Numbers* 9:23.

our hands to hasten it through repentance.

Thus, the Torah reading is a ray of hope amid the gloom and tragedy of Tishah B'Av. The Destruction of the Temple and the resultant exile are still with us, and this is the day that does not let us forget that. But exile is not more a part of our history than is redemption. The difference is that exile, long though it may be, is a temporary condition; the coming of Messiah is the permanent and natural state of Jewry, may it happen speedily in our days.

Some add:

עֵץ חַיִּים הִיא לַמַּחֲזִיקִים בָּהּ, וְתֹמְכֶיהָ מְאֻשָּׁר.[1] דְּרָכֶיהָ דַרְכֵי נֹעַם, וְכָל נְתִיבוֹתֶיהָ שָׁלוֹם.[2] אֹרֶךְ יָמִים בִּימִינָהּ, בִּשְׂמֹאולָהּ עֹשֶׁר וְכָבוֹד.[3] יהוה חָפֵץ לְמַעַן צִדְקוֹ, יַגְדִּיל תּוֹרָה וְיַאְדִּיר.[4]

After the Torah Scroll has been wound, tied and covered,
the *maftir* recites the *Haftarah* blessings.

ברכה קודם ההפטרה

בָּרוּךְ אַתָּה יהוה אֱלֹהֵינוּ מֶלֶךְ הָעוֹלָם, אֲשֶׁר בָּחַר בִּנְבִיאִים טוֹבִים, וְרָצָה בְדִבְרֵיהֶם הַנֶּאֱמָרִים בֶּאֱמֶת, בָּרוּךְ אַתָּה יהוה, הַבּוֹחֵר בַּתּוֹרָה וּבְמֹשֶׁה עַבְדּוֹ, וּבְיִשְׂרָאֵל עַמּוֹ, וּבִנְבִיאֵי הָאֱמֶת וָצֶדֶק: (אָמֵן. –Cong.)

הפטרה

ירמיה ח:יג-ט:כג

אָסֹף אֲסִיפֵם נְאֻם־יהוה אֵין עֲנָבִים בַּגֶּפֶן וְאֵין תְּאֵנִים בַּתְּאֵנָה וְהֶעָלֶה נָבֵל וָאֶתֵּן לָהֶם יַעַבְרוּם: עַל־מָה אֲנַחְנוּ יֹשְׁבִים הֵאָסְפוּ וְנָבוֹא אֶל־עָרֵי הַמִּבְצָר וְנִדְּמָה־שָּׁם כִּי יהוה אֱלֹהֵינוּ הֲדִמָּנוּ וַיַּשְׁקֵנוּ מֵי־רֹאשׁ כִּי חָטָאנוּ לַיהוה: קַוֵּה לְשָׁלוֹם וְאֵין טוֹב לְעֵת מַרְפֵּה וְהִנֵּה בְעָתָה: מִדָּן נִשְׁמַע נַחְרַת סוּסָיו מִקּוֹל מִצְהֲלוֹת אַבִּירָיו רָעֲשָׁה כָּל־הָאָרֶץ וַיָּבוֹאוּ וַיֹּאכְלוּ אֶרֶץ וּמְלוֹאָהּ עִיר וְיֹשְׁבֵי בָהּ: כִּי הִנְנִי מְשַׁלֵּחַ בָּכֶם נְחָשִׁים צִפְעֹנִים אֲשֶׁר אֵין־לָהֶם לָחַשׁ וְנִשְּׁכוּ אֶתְכֶם נְאֻם־יהוה: מַבְלִיגִיתִי עֲלֵי יָגוֹן עָלַי לִבִּי דַוָּי: הִנֵּה־קוֹל שַׁוְעַת בַּת־עַמִּי מֵאֶרֶץ מַרְחַקִּים הַיהוה אֵין בְּצִיּוֹן אִם־מַלְכָּהּ אֵין בָּהּ מַדּוּעַ הִכְעִסוּנִי בִּפְסִלֵיהֶם בְּהַבְלֵי נֵכָר: עָבַר קָצִיר כָּלָה קָיִץ וַאֲנַחְנוּ לוֹא נוֹשָׁעְנוּ: עַל־שֶׁבֶר בַּת־עַמִּי הָשְׁבָּרְתִּי קָדַרְתִּי שַׁמָּה הֶחֱזִקָתְנִי: הַצֳרִי אֵין בְּגִלְעָד אִם־רֹפֵא אֵין שָׁם כִּי מַדּוּעַ לֹא עָלְתָה אֲרֻכַת בַּת־עַמִּי: מִי־יִתֵּן רֹאשִׁי מַיִם וְעֵינִי מְקוֹר דִּמְעָה וְאֶבְכֶּה יוֹמָם וָלַיְלָה אֵת חַלְלֵי בַת־עַמִּי: מִי־יִתְּנֵנִי בַמִּדְבָּר מְלוֹן

---

(1) *Proverbs* 3:18. (2) 3:17. (3) 3:16. (4) *Isaiah* 42:21.

◆§ The Haftarah

Unlike the Torah reading, which is primarily hopeful, the *Haftarah* is an almost unrelieved dirge. Indeed, it is read with the sad cantillation of Eichah until the last two verses, which, with their brief depiction of what is worthwhile and praiseworthy in human beings, points the way

toward ultimate salvation. Jeremiah, the prophet of the Destruction and the author of *Eichah*, directed this harsh prophecy at his wayward brethren, in the vain hope that it would stir them to repent.

The *Haftarah* begins with a picture of the terror that the people felt. Their towns and farms

Some add:

עֵץ *It is a tree of life for those who grasp it, and its supporters are praiseworthy.[1] Its ways are ways of pleasantness and all its paths are peace.[2]
Lengthy days are at its right; at its left are wealth and honor.[3] HASHEM desired,
for the sake of its [Israel's] righteousness, that the Torah be made great and
glorious.[4]*

After the Torah Scroll has been wound, tied and covered,
the *maftir* recites the *Haftarah* blessings.

BLESSING BEFORE THE HAFTARAH

בָּרוּךְ *Blessed are You, HASHEM, our God, King of the universe, Who
has chosen good prophets and was pleased with their words
that were uttered with truth. Blessed are You, HASHEM, Who chooses the
Torah; Moses, His servant; Israel, His nation; and the prophets of truth
and righteousness.* (Cong.— Amen.)

ᵃ{ **HAFTARAH** }ᵃ

Jeremiah 8:13-9:23

I shall utterly destroy them, the words of HASHEM, there will be no
grapes on the grapevine and no dates on the date palm, the leaf will
wither, and what I have given them will pass away. 'Why do we remain
here? Let us gather and come to fortified cities, there to be silent; for
HASHEM, our God, has silenced us and given us poisonous water, for we
have sinned to HASHEM. We are hoping for peace, but there is no good;
for a time of healing, but behold! there is terror.'

From Dan was heard the snorting of his steeds, at the sound of his
mighty ones' footsteps the whole land quaked; they came and devoured
the land and its fullness, the city and its inhabitants. For behold! — I
shall incite against you snakes, serpents, that cannot be charmed, and
they shall bite you — the words of HASHEM. I seek strength against
sorrow, but my heart is sick within me. Behold! the voice of My people's
daughter from distant lands: 'Is HASHEM not in Zion, is its king not
within it?' Why have they angered Me with their graven idols, with
their alien vanities?

'The harvest has passed, the summer has ended, but we were not
saved.'

Over the collapse of my people's daughter have I been shattered; I
am blackened, desolation has gripped me. Is there no balm in Gilead, is
there no healer there? Why has no recovery come to my people's
daughter? If only someone would turn my head to water and my eye to
a spring of tears, then I would cry all day and night for the slain of my
daughter's people!

If only someone would make for me in the desert an inn for

---

were desolate and they fled to the cities, but
there, too, they found no refuge. Foolishly and
vainly they asked, Is HASHEM not in Zion, is its

king not within it?; as if the God Whom they
had spurned and the king who had been shorn
of his power could help them.

אָרְחִים וְאֶעֶזְבָה אֶת־עַמִּי וְאֵלְכָה מֵאִתָּם כִּי כֻלָּם מְנָאֲפִים
עֲצֶרֶת בֹּגְדִים: וַיַּדְרְכוּ אֶת־לְשׁוֹנָם קַשְׁתָּם שֶׁקֶר וְלֹא לֶאֱמוּנָה
גָבְרוּ בָאָרֶץ כִּי מֵרָעָה אֶל־רָעָה | יָצָאוּ וְאֹתִי לֹא־יָדָעוּ
נְאֻם־יְהוָֹה: אִישׁ מֵרֵעֵהוּ הִשָּׁמֵרוּ וְעַל־כָּל־אָח אַל־תִּבְטָחוּ כִּי
כָל־אָח עָקוֹב יַעְקֹב וְכָל־רֵעַ רָכִיל יַהֲלֹךְ: וְאִישׁ בְּרֵעֵהוּ יְהָתֵלּוּ
וֶאֱמֶת לֹא יְדַבֵּרוּ לִמְּדוּ לְשׁוֹנָם דַּבֶּר־שֶׁקֶר הַעֲוֵה נִלְאוּ: שִׁבְתְּךָ
בְּתוֹךְ מִרְמָה בְּמִרְמָה מֵאֲנוּ דַעַת־אוֹתִי נְאֻם־יְהוָֹה: לָכֵן כֹּה אָמַר
יְהוָֹה צְבָאוֹת הִנְנִי צוֹרְפָם וּבְחַנְתִּים כִּי־אֵיךְ אֶעֱשֶׂה מִפְּנֵי
בַּת־עַמִּי: חֵץ °שָׁחוּט לְשׁוֹנָם מִרְמָה דִבֵּר בְּפִיו שָׁלוֹם אֶת־רֵעֵהוּ
יְדַבֵּר וּבְקִרְבּוֹ יָשִׂים אָרְבּוֹ: הַעַל־אֵלֶּה לֹא־אֶפְקָד־בָּם נְאֻם־יְהוָֹה
אִם בְּגוֹי אֲשֶׁר־כָּזֶה לֹא תִתְנַקֵּם נַפְשִׁי: עַל־הֶהָרִים אֶשָּׂא בְכִי
וָנֶהִי וְעַל־נְאוֹת מִדְבָּר קִינָה כִּי נִצְּתוּ מִבְּלִי־אִישׁ עֹבֵר וְלֹא
שָׁמְעוּ קוֹל מִקְנֶה מֵעוֹף הַשָּׁמַיִם וְעַד־בְּהֵמָה נָדְדוּ הָלָכוּ: וְנָתַתִּי
אֶת־יְרוּשָׁלַ‍ִם לְגַלִּים מְעוֹן תַּנִּים וְאֶת־עָרֵי יְהוּדָה אֶתֵּן שְׁמָמָה
מִבְּלִי יוֹשֵׁב: מִי־הָאִישׁ הֶחָכָם וְיָבֵן אֶת־זֹאת וַאֲשֶׁר דִּבֶּר פִּי־יְהוָֹה
אֵלָיו וְיַגִּדָהּ עַל־מָה אָבְדָה הָאָרֶץ נִצְּתָה כַמִּדְבָּר מִבְּלִי עֹבֵר:
וַיֹּאמֶר יְהוָֹה עַל־עָזְבָם אֶת־תּוֹרָתִי אֲשֶׁר נָתַתִּי לִפְנֵיהֶם וְלֹא־
שָׁמְעוּ בְקוֹלִי וְלֹא־הָלְכוּ בָהּ: וַיֵּלְכוּ אַחֲרֵי שְׁרִרוּת לִבָּם וְאַחֲרֵי
הַבְּעָלִים אֲשֶׁר לִמְּדוּם אֲבוֹתָם: לָכֵן כֹּה־אָמַר יְהוָֹה צְבָאוֹת
אֱלֹהֵי יִשְׂרָאֵל הִנְנִי מַאֲכִילָם אֶת־הָעָם הַזֶּה לַעֲנָה וְהִשְׁקִיתִים
מֵי־רֹאשׁ: וַהֲפִצוֹתִים בַּגּוֹיִם אֲשֶׁר לֹא יָדְעוּ הֵמָּה וַאֲבוֹתָם
וְשִׁלַּחְתִּי אַחֲרֵיהֶם אֶת־הַחֶרֶב עַד כַּלּוֹתִי אוֹתָם: כֹּה אָמַר יְהוָֹה
צְבָאוֹת הִתְבּוֹנְנוּ וְקִרְאוּ לַמְקוֹנְנוֹת וּתְבוֹאֶינָה וְאֶל־הַחֲכָמוֹת
שִׁלְחוּ וְתָבוֹאנָה: וּתְמַהֵרְנָה וְתִשֶּׂנָה עָלֵינוּ נֶהִי וְתֵרַדְנָה עֵינֵינוּ

° שׁוֹחֵט כ'

Then Jeremiah speaks of his personal despair at the degradation of his people. He is
blackened. There is no balm to soothe his
hurt. He wishes his eyes had enough tears for
him to express his heartbreak. On the other
hand, when he views their grievous sins, he
wishes there were an inn in an isolated desert
where he could escape from them. They are
immoral and traitorous to God. Their tongues
are like bows shooting arrows of falsehood and

slander. Consequently, God must smelt them
and test them, in the hope that through punishment and suffering they will repent. So the
punishment comes, and it is harsh indeed — but
the behavior of the nation leaves God no
alternative.

'Why did it happen?' the prophet asks. Because they forsook the Torah, upon which the
Sages comment that God declares, 'I wish they
had forsaken Me, but not forsaken My Torah,

guests, then I would forsake my people and leave them; for they are all adulterers, a band of traitors. 'They bend their tongue with falsehood like a bow, not for good faith have they grown strong in the land, for they progress from evil to evil, but Me they did not know' — the words of HASHEM. 'Every man beware of his fellow, and do not trust any kin; for every kinsman acts perversely, and every fellow mongers slander. Every man mocks his fellow and they do not speak the truth; they train their tongue in speaking falsehood, striving to be iniquitous. Your dwelling is amid deceit, through deceit they refuse to know Me' — the words of HASHEM.

Therefore, so says HASHEM, Master of Legions, 'Behold! I shall smelt them and test them — for what then can I do for My people's daughter? Their tongue is a drawn arrow, speaking deceit; with his tongue one speaks peace, but in his heart he lays his ambush. Shall I not punish them for these?' — the words of HASHEM — 'For a nation like this, shall My soul not take vengeance?'

'For the mountains I shall raise a wailing and lament, and for the pasture of the wilderness a dirge, for they will have become desolate without a passerby and they will not have heard the sound of flocks; from the bird of heaven to cattle they have wandered off and gone. I shall make Jerusalem heaps of rubble, a lair of snakes; and the cities of Judah I shall turn to desolation, without inhabitant.'

Who is the wise man who will understand this, to whom the mouth of HASHEM speaks — let him relate it: 'For what reason did the land perish, become parched like a desert, without passerby?'

And HASHEM said, 'Because they forsook My Torah that I put before them, and did not heed My voice nor follow it. They followed the wantonness of their heart, and after the baal-idols, as their fathers taught them!'

Therefore, so says HASHEM, Master of Legions, the God of Israel, 'Behold! — I feed this people wormwood and give them poisonous water to drink. I shall scatter them among the nations whom they did not know, neither they nor their fathers; I shall send the sword after them until I destroy them!'

So said HASHEM, Master of Legions, 'Contemplate, summon the dirge-women and let them come, and send for the wise women and let them come.'

Let them hurry and raise up a lament for us, let our eyes run with

---

because its spiritual glow would have turned them back to the good.' This has remained a lesson for all time: The Torah is Israel's ultimate hope of restoration to its former position of glory.

The *Haftarah* concludes with another timeless guide to the road map of life. Let people never seek their glory in transient and inconsequential matters such as ordinary wisdom, strength and wealth. Only knowledge of God is

דִּמְעָה וְעַפְעַפֵּינוּ יִזְּלוּ־מָיִם: כִּי קוֹל נְהִי נִשְׁמַע מִצִּיּוֹן אֵיךְ שֻׁדָּדְנוּ בֹּשְׁנוּ מְאֹד כִּי־עָזַבְנוּ אָרֶץ כִּי הִשְׁלִיכוּ מִשְׁכְּנוֹתֵינוּ: כִּי־שְׁמַעְנָה נָשִׁים דְּבַר־יהוה וְתִקַּח אָזְנְכֶם דְּבַר־פִּיו וְלַמֵּדְנָה בְנוֹתֵיכֶם נֶהִי וְאִשָּׁה רְעוּתָהּ קִינָה: כִּי־עָלָה מָוֶת בְּחַלּוֹנֵינוּ בָּא בְּאַרְמְנוֹתֵינוּ לְהַכְרִית עוֹלָל מִחוּץ בַּחוּרִים מֵרְחֹבוֹת: דַּבֵּר כֹּה נְאֻם־יהוה וְנָפְלָה נִבְלַת הָאָדָם כְּדֹמֶן עַל־פְּנֵי הַשָּׂדֶה וּכְעָמִיר מֵאַחֲרֵי הַקּוֹצֵר וְאֵין מְאַסֵּף: כֹּה ן אָמַר יהוה אַל־יִתְהַלֵּל חָכָם בְּחָכְמָתוֹ וְאַל־יִתְהַלֵּל הַגִּבּוֹר בִּגְבוּרָתוֹ אַל־יִתְהַלֵּל עָשִׁיר בְּעָשְׁרוֹ: כִּי אִם־בְּזֹאת יִתְהַלֵּל הַמִּתְהַלֵּל הַשְׂכֵּל וְיָדֹעַ אוֹתִי כִּי אֲנִי יהוה עֹשֶׂה חֶסֶד מִשְׁפָּט וּצְדָקָה בָּאָרֶץ כִּי־בְאֵלֶּה חָפַצְתִּי נְאֻם־יהוה:

ברכות לאחר ההפטרה

After the *Haftarah* is read, the *oleh* recites the following blessings.

בָּרוּךְ אַתָּה יהוה אֱלֹהֵינוּ מֶלֶךְ הָעוֹלָם, צוּר כָּל הָעוֹלָמִים, צַדִּיק בְּכָל הַדּוֹרוֹת, הָאֵל הַנֶּאֱמָן הָאוֹמֵר וְעֹשֶׂה, הַמְדַבֵּר וּמְקַיֵּם, שֶׁכָּל דְּבָרָיו אֱמֶת וָצֶדֶק. נֶאֱמָן אַתָּה הוּא יהוה אֱלֹהֵינוּ, וְנֶאֱמָנִים דְּבָרֶיךָ, וְדָבָר אֶחָד מִדְּבָרֶיךָ אָחוֹר לֹא יָשׁוּב רֵיקָם, כִּי אֵל מֶלֶךְ נֶאֱמָן (וְרַחֲמָן) אָתָּה. בָּרוּךְ אַתָּה יהוה, הָאֵל הַנֶּאֱמָן בְּכָל דְּבָרָיו. (אָמֵן.) –Cong.

רַחֵם עַל צִיּוֹן כִּי הִיא בֵּית חַיֵּינוּ, וְלַעֲלוּבַת נֶפֶשׁ תּוֹשִׁיעַ בִּמְהֵרָה בְיָמֵינוּ. בָּרוּךְ אַתָּה יהוה, מְשַׂמֵּחַ צִיּוֹן בְּבָנֶיהָ. (אָמֵן.) –Cong.

שַׂמְּחֵנוּ יהוה אֱלֹהֵינוּ בְּאֵלִיָּהוּ הַנָּבִיא עַבְדֶּךָ, וּבְמַלְכוּת בֵּית דָּוִד מְשִׁיחֶךָ, בִּמְהֵרָה יָבֹא וְיָגֵל לִבֵּנוּ, עַל כִּסְאוֹ לֹא יֵשֵׁב זָר וְלֹא יִנְחֲלוּ עוֹד אֲחֵרִים אֶת כְּבוֹדוֹ, כִּי בְשֵׁם קָדְשְׁךָ נִשְׁבַּעְתָּ לּוֹ, שֶׁלֹּא יִכְבֶּה נֵרוֹ לְעוֹלָם וָעֶד. בָּרוּךְ אַתָּה יהוה, מָגֵן דָּוִד. (אָמֵן.) –Cong.

---

worthwhile — and if that is someone's priority, then even his wisdom, strength, and wealth are praiseworthy, because they have become his tools in the service of God.

tears and our pupils flow with water. For the sound of lament would be
heard in Zion: 'How we have been plundered, how greatly we are
shamed, for we have left the land, for our dwellings have cast us out!
Hearken, O women, to the word of HASHEM and let your ears absorb the
word of his mouth, and teach a lament to your daughters, and each
woman a dirge to her friend. For death has ascended through our
windows, it has come into our palaces to cut down infants from the
marketplace, young men from the streets.'

Speak thus — the words of HASHEM — 'Human corpses will fall like
dung on the open field and like a sheaf behind the harvester, but none
shall gather them up.'

So says HASHEM, 'Let not the wise man laud himself with his wisdom,
and let not the strong man laud himself with his strength, and let not the
rich man laud himself with his wealth. Only with this may one laud
himself — discernment in knowing Me, for I am HASHEM Who does
kindness, justice, and righteousness in the land, for in these is My
desire,' the words of HASHEM.

BLESSINGS AFTER THE HAFTARAH

After the *Haftarah* is read, the *oleh* recites the following blessings.

בָּרוּךְ Blessed are You, HASHEM, King of the universe, Rock of all
eternities, Righteous in all generations, the trustworthy God,
Who says and does, Who speaks and fulfills, all of Whose words are true
and righteous. Trustworthy are You, HASHEM, our God, and trustworthy are Your words, not one of Your words is turned back to its
origin unfulfilled, for You are God, trustworthy (and compassionate)
King. Blessed are You, HASHEM, the God Who is trustworthy in all His
words.   (Cong.— Amen.)

רַחֵם Have mercy on Zion for it is the source of our life; to the one who
is deeply humiliated bring salvation speedily, in our days.
Blessed are You, HASHEM, Who gladdens Zion through her children.
                                                          (Cong.— Amen.)

שַׂמְּחֵנוּ Gladden us, HASHEM, our God, with Elijah the prophet, Your
servant, and with the kingdom of the House of David, Your
anointed, may he come speedily and cause our heart to exult. On his
throne let no stranger sit nor let others continue to inherit his honor,
for by Your holy Name You swore to him that his heir will not be
extinguished forever and ever. Blessed are You, HASHEM, Shield of
David.   (Cong.— Amen.)

הכנסת ספר תורה

Chazzan takes the Torah in his right arm and recites:

יְהַלְלוּ אֶת שֵׁם יהוה, כִּי נִשְׂגָּב שְׁמוֹ לְבַדּוֹ –

Congregation responds:

– הוֹדוֹ עַל אֶרֶץ וְשָׁמָיִם. וַיָּרֶם קֶרֶן לְעַמּוֹ, תְּהִלָּה לְכָל חֲסִידָיו, לִבְנֵי יִשְׂרָאֵל עַם קְרֹבוֹ, הַלְלוּיָהּ.[1]

As the Torah is carried to the Ark, the congregation recites Psalm 24, לְדָוִד מִזְמוֹר.

לְדָוִד מִזְמוֹר, לַיהוה הָאָרֶץ וּמְלוֹאָהּ, תֵּבֵל וְיֹשְׁבֵי בָהּ. כִּי הוּא עַל יַמִּים יְסָדָהּ, וְעַל נְהָרוֹת יְכוֹנְנֶהָ. מִי יַעֲלֶה בְהַר יהוה, וּמִי יָקוּם בִּמְקוֹם קָדְשׁוֹ. נְקִי כַפַּיִם וּבַר לֵבָב, אֲשֶׁר לֹא נָשָׂא לַשָּׁוְא נַפְשִׁי וְלֹא נִשְׁבַּע לְמִרְמָה. יִשָּׂא בְרָכָה מֵאֵת יהוה, וּצְדָקָה מֵאֱלֹהֵי יִשְׁעוֹ. זֶה דּוֹר דֹּרְשָׁיו, מְבַקְשֵׁי פָנֶיךָ, יַעֲקֹב, סֶלָה. שְׂאוּ שְׁעָרִים רָאשֵׁיכֶם, וְהִנָּשְׂאוּ פִּתְחֵי עוֹלָם, וְיָבוֹא מֶלֶךְ הַכָּבוֹד. מִי זֶה מֶלֶךְ הַכָּבוֹד, יהוה עִזּוּז וְגִבּוֹר, יהוה גִּבּוֹר מִלְחָמָה. שְׂאוּ שְׁעָרִים רָאשֵׁיכֶם, וּשְׂאוּ פִּתְחֵי עוֹלָם, וְיָבֹא מֶלֶךְ הַכָּבוֹד. מִי הוּא זֶה מֶלֶךְ הַכָּבוֹד, יהוה צְבָאוֹת הוּא מֶלֶךְ הַכָּבוֹד, סֶלָה.

As the Torah is placed into the Ark,
the congregation recites the following verses:

וּבְנֻחֹה יֹאמַר, שׁוּבָה יהוה רִבְבוֹת אַלְפֵי יִשְׂרָאֵל.[2] קוּמָה יהוה לִמְנוּחָתֶךָ, אַתָּה וַאֲרוֹן עֻזֶּךָ. כֹּהֲנֶיךָ יִלְבְּשׁוּ צֶדֶק, וַחֲסִידֶיךָ יְרַנֵּנוּ. בַּעֲבוּר דָּוִד עַבְדֶּךָ אַל תָּשֵׁב פְּנֵי מְשִׁיחֶךָ.[3] כִּי לֶקַח טוֹב נָתַתִּי לָכֶם, תּוֹרָתִי אַל תַּעֲזֹבוּ. ❖ עֵץ חַיִּים הִיא לַמַּחֲזִיקִים בָּהּ, וְתֹמְכֶיהָ מְאֻשָּׁר.[5] דְּרָכֶיהָ דַרְכֵי נֹעַם, וְכָל נְתִיבֹתֶיהָ שָׁלוֹם.[6] הֲשִׁיבֵנוּ יהוה אֵלֶיךָ וְנָשׁוּבָה, חַדֵּשׁ יָמֵינוּ כְּקֶדֶם.[7]

---

(1) *Psalms* 148:13-14. (2) *Numbers* 10:36. (3) *Psalms* 132:8-10.
(4) *Proverbs* 4:2. (5) 3:18. (6) 3:17. (7) *Lamentations* 5:21.

RETURNING THE TORAH

Chazzan takes the Torah in his right arm and recites:

Let them praise the Name of HASHEM, for His Name alone will have been exalted —

Congregation responds:

— *His glory is above earth and heaven. And He will have exalted the pride of His people, causing praise for all His devout ones, for the Children of Israel, His intimate nation. Halleluyah!*[1]

As the Torah is carried to the Ark, the congregation
recites Psalm 24, 'Of David a psalm.'

לְדָוִד *Of David a psalm. HASHEM's is the earth and its fullness, the inhabited land and those who dwell in it. For He founded it upon seas, and established it upon rivers. Who may ascend the mountain of HASHEM, and who may stand in the place of His sanctity? One with clean hands and pure heart, who has not sworn in vain by My soul and has not sworn deceitfully. He will receive a blessing from HASHEM and just kindness from the God of his salvation. This is the generation of those who seek Him, those who strive for Your Presence — Jacob, Selah. Raise up your heads, O gates, and be uplifted, you everlasting entrances, so that the King of Glory may enter. Who is this King of Glory? — HASHEM, the mighty and strong, HASHEM, the strong in battle. Raise up your heads, O gates, and raise up, you everlasting entrances, so that the King of Glory may enter. Who then is the King of Glory? HASHEM, Master of Legions, He is the King of Glory. Selah!*

As the Torah is placed into the Ark,
the congregation recites the following verses:

וּבְנֻחֹה *And when it rested he would say, 'Return, HASHEM, to the myriad thousands of Israel.'*[2] *Arise, HASHEM, to Your resting place, You and the Ark of Your strength. Let Your priests be clothed in righteousness, and Your devout ones will sing joyously. For the sake of David, Your servant, turn not away the face of Your anointed.*[3] *For I have given you a good teaching, do not forsake My Torah.*[4] Chazzan— *It is a tree of life for those who grasp it, and its supporters are praiseworthy.*[5] *Its ways are ways of pleasantness and all its paths are peace.*[6] *Bring us back to You, HASHEM, and we shall return, renew our days as of old.*[7]

﴾ קינות ﴿

ו.

שָׁבַת[1] סוֹרוּ[2] מְנִי שִׁמְּעוּנִי עוֹבְרַי,[3]

סְחִי וּמָאוֹס הֱשִׂימוּנִי[4] בְּעֶדְרֵי חֲבֵרַי,[5]

סֻכּוֹתָה[6] מִשְׁכַּן מִסְכּוֹת דְּבִירַי,

סֻכּוֹת[7] וְהָבְלְגוּ גְבוּרַי,

סָפְקוּ כַף[8] וּמָעֲדוּ אֲבָרַי,

כָּסְלָה כָל אַבִּירַי.[9]

נָפְלָה[10] עוֹדֵינוּ[11] בְּצוּל דְּכוּיָה,

עֵינִי[12] חֻבְּתָה לַחֲזוֹן בֶּן בֶּרֶכְיָה,*

עַד[13] פִּלְאֵי גַלְגַּל* חֲבוּיָה,[14]

עֵינִי[15] מְעוֹלֶלֶת בֵּינָנִית נְכוּיָה,*

עָשָׂה[16] וְנִחַם וַיִּקְרָא לִבְכִיָּה,

וְנָם עַל אֵלֶּה אֲנִי בוֹכִיָּה.[17]

עָל[18] פָּנַי[19] פָּרַת נִפְּצוּ חֲסִידֶיהָ,*

פְּלַגֵּי[20] סוּף זָכְרָה כְּעָרוּ יְסוֹדֶיהָ,[21]

---

(1) *Eichah* 5:15. (2) 4:15. (3) Some editions read עוֹכְרַי, *those who besmirched me.* (4) Cf. *Eichah* 3:45. (5) Cf. *Song of Songs* 1:7. (6) *Eichah* 3:44. (7) Cf. 3:43. (8) 2:15. (9) Cf. 1:15. (10) 5:16. (11) Cf. 4:17. (12) 3:51. (13) 3:50. (14) Some editions read חֲכוּיָה, *awaited.* (15) *Eichah* 3:49. (16) 2:17. (17) 1:16. (18) 5:17. (19) 4:16. (20) 3:48. (21) Cf. *Psalms* 137:7.

◆§ שָׁבַת — *Everything came to a standstill!* R' Elazar HaKalir, one of the earliest *paytanim* (composers of liturgical poems), was a master at weaving seemingly diverse elements into a well-constructed, albeit difficult to understand, whole. In this first *kinnah* of the morning service, he has linked the verses of the respective chapters of *Eichah* into an intricate chain according to the following formula:

(a) each stanza contains six lines that correspond to the six alphabets of *Eichah* (chapters one, two and four contain 22 verses each, and are arranged according to an *aleph-beis* acrostic; chapter three comprises three verses beginning with א, three with ב, and so on);

(b) the first line of each sextet begins with the opening word or phrase of the corresponding verse in chapter six of *Eichah* (these do not follow an *aleph-beis* format), and is followed by the opening word or phrase of the corresponding verse in chapter five;

(c) the second line of each sextet begins with the opening word or phrase of the corresponding verse in chapter four;

(d) the next three lines correspond to the respective triad of verses in chapter three, each set in the reverse order of its appearance in *Eichah*;

(e) the fifth line of each stanza corresponds to the verses in chapter two; and

(f) the final line is taken in its entirety from chapter one, and determines the stanza's rhyme syllable. [All of the words and phrases taken from *Eichah* appear in dark type in the Hebrew text.]

The concluding stanza deviates from the established pattern. Its first five lines contain an acrostic of the author's name אֶלְעָזָר, *Elazar,* and it closes with the refrain of the following *kinnah,* thus serving as a connective between the two.

Interestingly, the *kinnah* includes only eight stanzas taken from the last eight verses (or, in chapter three, the last eight triads) of the chapter

⅍ **KINNOS** ⅏

6.

ס   *Everything came to a standstill!*[1]*
  'Turn away[2] *from me!' those who exiled me*[3] *made me hear.*
  They made me a filth and refuse[4]
  amidst the flocks of my fellow [nations].[5]
  You have enveloped[6] *Your [heavenly] Tabernacle,*
    that it not see my [earthly] Temple.
  You have enveloped Yourself,[7] *so my warriors are overpowered.*
  They [my enemies] clapped their hands [in derision][8]
    and my limbs faltered
  as they trampled all my heroes.[9]

ע   *[Jerusalem] has fallen,*[10] *it remains*[11] *sunk in the watery depths.*
  My eye[12] *still longs for the vision of [Zechariah]*
    the son of Berechiah,＊
  but until[13] *[we are shown] miracles [like those] of Gilgal,*＊
    [that prophecy] has been hidden.[14]
  My eye[15] *brings forth tears, because we are crippled by quicksand.*＊
  He [God] caused[16] *[the Destruction], then regretted it,*
    summoning [Israel] to cry,
  saying, 'Over these things I weep.'[17]

פ   *On*[18] *the surface*[19] *of the Euphrates her pious ones were mutilated;*＊
  yet she remembered the splitting[20] *of the Sea of Reeds,*
    even while her foundation was being destroyed.[21]

---

of *Eichah.* Many commentators therefore regard this *kinnah* as the conclusion of a 14-stanza *kerovah* (*piyut* recited at various points during the *chazzan's* repetition of the *Shemoneh Esrei*) written by R' Elazar HaKalir, and recited by some congregations. That *kerovah* is based on the first 14 verses of *Eichah's* chapters.

לַחֲזוֹן בֶּן בְּרֶכְיָה — *For the vision of [Zechariah] the son of Berechiah.* Zechariah's prophecies are full of hope and optimism. The Talmud points especially to his proclamation: *Thus says HASHEM, Master of Legions, 'Elderly men and women will yet sit in the streets of Jerusalem, each with his staff in hand due to old age. And the streets of the city will be filled with boys and girls; they will be playing in the streets'* (Zechariah 8:4-5; see *Makkos* 24b).

פִּלְאֵי גִלְגָּל — *Miracles [like those of] Gilgal.* While the Israelites were encamped at Gilgal, they won many battles in miraculous fashion. For example, at Gibeon, God caused the sun to remain in the skies long after it should have set. Thus, Joshua and his forces were able to annihilate the enemy, before they had a chance to retreat under cover of

night. Additionally, God caused a heavy hailstorm to rain upon the five armies allied against Israel so that *more had died by the hailstones than had been put to the sword by the Children of Israel* (Joshua 10:11).

בִּינָנִית נְכוּיָה — *Crippled by quicksand.* The word בִּינָנִית is derived from יָוֵן, *thick mud* (as in *Psalms* 40:3 and 69:3). Thus, the phrase means that we are lost in a quagmire of troubles.

Alternatively, the word is derived from יָוָן, *Greece,* and is an allusion to חָכְמַת יְוָנִית, *Greek* wisdom, a form of sign-language code instrumental (to a degree) in sowing the seeds that led to the Destruction of the Second Temple (see *Menachos* 64b; see also *Bava Kamma* 83a).

עַל פְּנֵי פְרָת נִפְּצוּ חֲסִידֶיהָ — *On the surface of the Euphrates her pious ones were mutilated.* The Midrash teaches that when Nebuchadnezzar saw the renowned Levite singers who once sang in the Temple, he demanded that they serenade him as he feasted merrily over his victory, *'Sing for us from Zion's song!'* (Psalms 137:3). Without any hesitation, the Levites hung their precious musical instruments on the trees and deliberately

פָּחַד¹ חֲטָא שִׁילֹה* תָּכַף סוֹדְיָה,

פָּצוּ² חֲזִירֵי יַעַר³ אַיֵּה חֲסִידֶיהָ,

פָּצוּ⁴ מַעֲשֵׂה עָרְיָה לְנִדְיָה,

פָּרְשָׂה צִיּוֹן בְּיָדֶיהָ.⁵

עַל הַר צִיּוֹן⁶ צָדוּ⁷ שְׁאוֹנֵי מְדָנַי,

צָפוּ עַל רָאשֵׁי⁸ צִיּוֹן זְדוֹנַי,

צָמְתוּ⁹ בְּנֹב לַעֲמוֹד¹⁰* זְדוֹנַי,

צוֹד¹¹ נָצַרְתָּ לְעוֹרֵר מְדָנַי,

צָעַק¹² עַמִּי בִּימֵי בֶן דִּינַי,*

צַדִּיק הוּא יהוה.¹³

אַתָּה¹⁴ קַלִּים¹⁵ הִכְבַּדְתָּ וּמֶעֳדַּי עַרְמוֹנִי,

קֵרַבְתָּ¹⁶ בֹּא אֵלַי וַיַּחֲרִימוֹנִי,

קָרָאתִי¹⁷ לְיוֹשְׁבֵי גִבְעוֹן עוֹד הֵם זְרְמוֹנִי,

קוֹלִי לְהַשְׁמִיעַ¹⁸ בָּעֶרֶב* הִגְרִימוֹנִי,

קוּמִי¹⁹ עֲבוּרִי בְּהָתֵל הֶעֱרִימוֹנִי,

קָרָאתִי לַמְאַהֲבַי* הֵמָּה רִמּוֹנִי.²⁰

לָמָה²¹ רוּחַ אַפֵּינוּ²² לַטֶּבַח שְׁמָרוּ,²³

רָאִיתָ²⁴ כִּי כְתַנּוּר עוֹרָם²⁵ כָּמָרוּ,²⁶

רָאִיתָ²⁷ כִּי עָמָל וָכַעַס בְּאַוֶּיךָ גָּמָרוּ,

רִבְתָּ²⁸ בְּיַד יְחֶזְקֵאל לִנְקֹם כְּמוֹ מָרוּ,

(1) Eichah 3:47. (2) 3:46. (3) Cf. Psalms 80:14. (4) Eichah 2:16. (5) 1:17. (6) 5:18. (7) 4:18. (8) Cf. 3:54. (9) 3:53. (10) See Isaiah 10:32. (11) Eichah 3:52; some editions read צור, but that is erroneous since the corresponding verse in Eichah reads צוד (Beis Levi). (12) 2:18. (13) 1:18. (14) 5:19. (15) 4:19. (16) Cf. 3:57. (17) 3:55. (18) Cf. 3:56. (19) 2:19. (20) 1:19. (21) 5:20. (22) 4:20. (23) See prefatory comments to kinnah 11. (24) Cf. Eichah 3:60. (25) Some editions read עוֹרִי, my skin; some read עוֹרֵנוּ, our skin. (26) Cf. Eichah 5:10. (27) Cf. 3:59. (28) 3:58.

mutilated their fingers, making it impossible for them to play the stringed instruments. Thus they did flatly refuse to play for Nebuchadnezzar but declared, 'How can we sing the song of HASHEM?' (ibid. 137:4). We cannot make any more music with these crippled hands!' (Pesikta Rabasi 31).

פָּחַד חֲטָא שִׁילֹה — *The dread of the sins of Shiloh.* Jeremiah had warned the nation that just as the

Tabernacle at Shiloh had come to destruction because of the sins of the sons of Eli the *Kohen Gadol,* so would the *Beis HaMikdash* be destroyed because of the people's sinfulness (see *Jeremiah* 7:12 and 26:6). And now that his message had been ignored, his dread prophecy came true.

בְּנֹב לַעֲמוֹד — *To stand [against me] at Nob.* King Saul, in his mistaken belief that the *Kohanim* of

The dread[1] of the sins of Shiloh* was swiftly fulfilled
   by the conspirators against her.
They jeered,[2] those wild boars of the forest,[3]
   'Where are her pious ones?'
They uncovered[4] shameful acts in order to disgrace her.
And Zion spread her hands [in despair].[5]

צ On Mt. Zion[6] an ambush was laid[7] by the enemy hordes.
My vicious enemies surged over the heads[8] of Zion.
My vicious enemies gathered[9]
   to stand [against me] at Nob.[10]*
You preserved [the memory of][11]
   that sin in order to incite my foes.
My nation cried out[12] in the days of the son of Dinai,*
   'He, HASHEM, is righteous!'[13]

ק You[14] elevated the lowly[15]
   and they denuded me of my jewelry.
You caused them to close in[16]
   on me and they devastated me.
I called[17] to the citizens of Gibeon [for help],
   but they too drowned me.
I cried out loud[18] [for relief] in Arabia,* but they crushed me.
'Arise![19] Travel through [safely]!' is how they mocked me.
   I called for my lovers,* but they deceived me.[20]

ר Why[21] did they anticipate butchering [King Josiah,][22]
   the very life breath of our nostrils?[23]
You have seen[24] how they scorched their skin[25] like a furnace.[26]
You have seen[27] how they consummated
   offensive and outrageous acts within Your desirous [Temple].
You admonished[28] [Israel] through Ezekiel,
   warning that Your revenge would match their rebelliousness.

---

the Tabernacle at Nob were conspiring with
David against him, had eighty-five Kohanim
slain, along with their wives, children, neighbors
and cattle (I Samuel 22:12-19). The Talmud
reports that on the day of that slaughter, God
ordained that retribution for that act will take
place (in a later year) on the ninth of Av
(Sanhedrin 95a).

בֶּן דִּינַי — The son of Dinai. Eliezer ben Dinai was
an infamous murderer (Sotah 47a; Kesubos 27a).
His unsuccessful revolt against Roman domination brought swift retribution and heavy blood-
shed (see Shir HaShirim Rabbah 2:7). Josephus
(Antiquities XX, 8) describes how he was captured and brought to Rome for trial.

בַּעֲרָב — In Arabia. When the captive Israelites
were led through the Ishmaelite lands of Arabia,
the local populace met them and appeared
interested in helping them. The Arabs pretended
friendship and sympathy, and offered food
and drink. However, the bread they offered had
been oversalted in order to cause the Jews
great and painful thirst. Then the Ishmaelites
proferred leather canteens filled, not with water,
but with air. When the captives raised the
containers to their mouths, the hot, stagnant air
entered their bodies and they died (Tanchuma,
Yisro 5).

לַמְאַהֲבַי — To my lovers. The prophet compares
alliance with foreign nations (rather than a
return of God and reliance on His salvation) to
an illicit affair with a pseudo-lover.

רְאֵה¹ וְנִכְחִידֵם מִגּוֹי² אָמְרוּ,

רְאֵה יהוה כִּי צַר לִי מֵעַי חֳמַרְמָרוּ.³

הֲשִׁיבֵנוּ⁴ שִׁישִׁי⁵ שְׁמַע לְגוֹי צֹאנִי,

שַׁבְתָּם⁶ רְמֹס חֲצֵרַי⁷ לְהַדְכִּיאָנִי,

שְׂפָתַי⁸ מְשׁוֹרְרֵי דְּבִיר דָּמְמוּ לְהַדְאִיבֵנִי,

שָׁמַעְתָּ⁹ זְמוֹרוֹת¹⁰ אַף הֵכִין לְטַאטְאָנִי,

שָׁכְבוּ¹¹ וְנָדוּ חָצָץ לְהַבְרִיאָנִי,*¹²

שָׁמְעוּ כִּי נֶאֱנָחָה אָנִי.¹³

כִּי¹⁴ תָם¹⁵ חָקַתָ בְּכֶס אוֹפַנֶּיךָ,

תָּשִׁיב לָהֶם גְּמוּל¹⁶ כְּאָז חֲזוֹת פָּנֶיךָ,

תִּרְדּוֹף¹⁷ לְצַלְמוֹן יוֹעֲצֵי¹⁸ עַל צְפוּנֶיךָ,¹⁹

תִּתֵּן²⁰ לְהַבְהֵב נוֹתְצֵי פְּנִינֶיךָ,

תִּקְרָא²¹ לְשַׁבְּרָם כּוֹס כָּמוּס בְּפָנֶיךָ,²²

תָּבֹא כָל רָעָתָם לְפָנֶיךָ.²³

תָּבֹא אֶל צָר אֲשֶׁר כֻּלָּנוּ,

לִמְבוֹא חֲמָת²⁴ בְּחֵמָה נֶהֱלָנוּ,

עַד לַחְלַח וְחָבוֹר הֻגְלָנוּ,²⁵

זָקֵן וּבָחוּר וּבְתוּלָה כְּבָלָנוּ,²⁶

רָם הַבֵּט נָא עַמְּךָ כֻּלָּנוּ,²⁷

זְכֹר יהוה מֶה הָיָה לָנוּ.²⁸

---

(1) *Eichah* 2:20. (2) *Psalms* 83:5. (3) *Eichah* 1:20. (4) 5:21. (5) 4:21.
(6) 3:63. (7) *Isaiah* 1:12. (8) *Eichah* 3:62. (9) 3:61.
(10) Cf. *Ezekiel* 8:17; see the commentaries there. (11) *Eichah* 2:21. (12) Cf. 3:17.
(13) 1:21. (14) 5:22. (15) 4:22; see Rashi to *Ezekiel* 1:5. (16) *Eichah* 3:64. (17) 3:66.
(18) Some editions read רֵעַ יוֹעֲצֵי, *those who plot evil.* (19) Cf. *Psalms* 83:4.
(20) *Eichah* 3:65. (21) 2:22. (22) Some editions read בְּפָנֶיךָ, *before You.* (23) 1:22.
(24) Cf. *Amos* 6:14. (25) *II Kings* 17:6. (26) Cf. *Jeremiah* 51:22. (27) *Isaiah* 64:8. (28) *Eichah* 5:1.

חָצָץ לְהַבְרִיאָנִי — *They [my captors] fed me pebbles.* God had told the prophet (*Ezekiel* 12:3) to prepare easily portable cooking utensils for use during the trip into exile. The purpose of the command was that others might follow his example and thus be prepared to cope with the

See[1] how [our enemies] have said,
'Let us obliterate them from nationhood!'[2]
Observe, HASHEM, how distressed I am;
my insides churn![3]

ש Bring us back to You;[4] [and fulfill the threat You made]
to the nation which exiled us, 'Rejoice [and exult,
O daughter of Edom. . .to you too will the cup
(of punishment) pass].'[5]
[Crush] their dwelling places,[6]
just as they trampled my courtyards[7] to crush me.
They stilled the lips[8] of the Temple singers,
and made me miserable.
You heard[9] their derisive songs[10]
of how they would sweep me away.
When they [my nation] rested[11] after they had traveled,
they [my captors] fed me pebbles.[12]*
They heard how I sighed.[13]

ת For[14] You engraved the likeness of the perfect one [Jacob][15]
on the throne of Your angelic Ofanim.
[Therefore] mete out their punishment[16] as on the day
[Israel] beheld Your countenance [at the Sea of Reeds];
chase[17] into the dark shadows of Hell all those who plot[18]
against [Israel,] the ones You shelter;[19]
consign[20] into the flame those who smashed
Your precious gem[like Temples].
Designate[21] [a date on which they will be forced] to drink
the intoxicating cup [of retribution] hidden in Your corners.[22]
Let all their wickedness come before You.[23]

א May [retribution] come upon the tormentor
who tried to destroy us completely.
ל In fury he led us to the entrance of Hamath.[24]
ע Unto Halah and Habor he exiled us.[25]
ז Old man, youth and maiden — he shackled us [all].[26]
ר O Supreme One, please look down,
for we are all Your nation.[27]
Remember, HASHEM, what has befallen us![28]

---

rigors of the journey. But the people jeered at
him and did not obey. Therefore, the exiles had
to knead their dough in pits dug into the ground
and their bread became mixed with grit (*Rashi*
to *Eichah* 3:16).

ז.

אֵיכָה אָצְתָּ בְּאַפְּךָ,* לְאַבֵּד בְּיַד אֲדוֹמִים אֲמוּנֶיךָ,
וְלֹא זָכַרְתָּ בְּרִית בֵּין הַבְּתָרִים¹ אֲשֶׁר בֵּרַרְתָּ לִבְחוּנֶיךָ,
וּבְכֵן בְּטִינוּ, זְכֹר יהוה מֶה הָיָה לָנוּ.²

אֵיכָה גָּעַרְתָּ בִּגְעָרָתֶךָ, לְגָלוֹת בְּיַד גֵּאִים גְּאוּלֶיךָ,
וְלֹא זָכַרְתָּ דְּלִיגַת דִּלּוּג דֶּרֶךְ* אֲשֶׁר דָּלַגְתָּ לְדִגְלֶיךָ,
וּבְכֵן דִּבַּרְנוּ, זְכֹר יהוה מֶה הָיָה לָנוּ.

אֵיכָה הָגִתָ בְּהֶגְיוֹנֶךָ, לַהֲדוֹף בְּיַד הוֹלְלִים הֲמוֹנֶיךָ,
וְלֹא זָכַרְתָּ וְעוּד וָתֵק וְסֵת* אֲשֶׁר וְעַדְתָּ לְוֹעֵדֶיךָ,
וּבְכֵן וְקוֹנַנּוּ, זְכֹר יהוה מֶה הָיָה לָנוּ.

אֵיכָה זָנַחְתָּ בְּזַעְמֶךָ לְזַלְזֵל בְּיַד זָרִים זְבוּלֶךָ,
וְלֹא זָכַרְתָּ חִתּוּן חֻקֵּי חוֹרֵב אֲשֶׁר חָקַקְתָּ לַחֲמוּלֶיךָ,
וּבְכֵן חֻוִּינוּ, זְכֹר יהוה מֶה הָיָה לָנוּ.

אֵיכָה טָרַחְתָּ בְּטָרְחֶךָ,* לִטְרוֹף בְּיַד טוֹרְפִים³ טְלָאֶיךָ,
וְלֹא זָכַרְתָּ יְקַר יְדִידוּת יֹשֶׁר אֲשֶׁר יִחַדְתָּ לְיוֹדְעֶיךָ,
וּבְכֵן יָלַלְנוּ, זְכֹר יהוה מֶה הָיָה לָנוּ.

אֵיכָה כּוֹנַנְתָּ בְּכַעְסֶךָ, לְכַלּוֹת בְּיַד כְּפִירִים כַּרְמֶךָ,
וְלֹא זָכַרְתָּ לֹא לִזְנוֹחַ לְעוֹלָם⁴ אֲשֶׁר לָמַדְתָּ לִלְקוּחֶיךָ,
וּבְכֵן לָהַגְנוּ, זְכֹר יהוה מֶה הָיָה לָנוּ.

---

(1) *Genesis* ch. 15. (2) *Eichah* 5:1.
(3) Some editions read טְמֵאִים, *the unclean.* (4) Cf. *Eichah* 3:31.

אֵיכָה אַצְתָּ בְּאַפֶּךְ ◆◆ — *How did You rush in Your
fury.* This *kinnah,* by R' Elazar HaKalir — who
signed his name, אֶלְעָזָר, in the acrostic of the final
stanza — follows a complex alphabetical form.
Each of the first eleven stanzas is constructed in
the following manner:

אֵיכָה א . . תָ בָא . . ךְ, לְא . . בְּיַד א . . יִם א . . ךְ,
וְלֹא זָכַרְתָּ ב . . ב . . ב . . אֲשֶׁר ב . . תָ לְב . . ךְ,
וּבְכֵן ב . . נוּ זְכֹר ה' מֶה הָיָה לָנוּ.
אֵיכָה ג . . תָ בְּג . . ךְ, לְג . . בְּיַד ג . . יִם ג . . ךְ,
וְלֹא זָכַרְתָּ ד . . ד . . ד . . אֲשֶׁר ד . . תָ לְד . . ךְ,
וּבְכֵן ד . . נוּ זְכֹר ה' מֶה הָיָה לָנוּ.

The alphabet is repeated five times for odd-
numbered letters (. . . ה,ג,א) and six times for
even-numbered letters (. . . ו,ד,ב). This repetition
alludes to the Five Books of the Torah and the Six

Orders of the Mishnah. Even the merit of Torah
study was ineffective in protecting Israel when its
actions became degenerate (*Kol BeRamah*).

דְּלִיגַת דִּלּוּג דֶּרֶךְ — *The contraction of the road.*
When the Israelites left Sinai, they traveled three
days and arrived at Kadosh Barnea — an eleven-
day journey under usual circumstances! (See
Rashi to *Deut.* 1:2.) Alternatively, this refers to the
four-hundred-year period of slavery prophesied
in the Covenant Between the Parts (*Genesis* 15:13)
that was condensed to two hundred and ten
years, from Jacob's arrival in Egypt until the
Exodus (see *Targum* to *Song of Songs* 2:8).

וְעוּד וָתֵק וְסֵת — *The Assembly Hall, the seasonal
stronghold.* This alludes to the *Beis HaMikdash,*

7.

א O How did You rush in Your fury to exterminate
　　Your faithful ones at the hand of the Edomites,
ב and not recall the Covenant Between the Parts[1]
　　by which You selected those whom You tested?
Therefore we have proclaimed,
'Remember, HASHEM, what has befallen us!'[2]

ג How did You reproach with Your rebuke,
　　to exile at the hand of the haughty those You had once redeemed,
ד and not recall the contraction of the road
　　You had shortened for Your flag-bearing tribes?
Therefore we have spoken,
'Remember, HASHEM, what has befallen us!'

ה How did You plan in Your thoughts
　　to push Your multitudes into the hand of the raucous,
ו and not recall the Assembly Hall, the seasonal stronghold*
　　You had designated for Your meeting partners?
Therefore, we have lamented,
'Remember, HASHEM, what has befallen us!'

ז How did You abandon Your Temples in Your rage,
　　to suffer indignity at the hands of aliens,
ח and not recall the betrothal of [Israel to the] Laws of Sinai
　　that You have carved for the recipients of Your compassion?
Therefore we have related,
'Remember, HASHEM, what has befallen us!'

ט How did You take pains in exerting Yourself* to cause
　　Your sheep to be torn asunder by the hand of the predators,[3]
י and not recall the [merit of the] precious, beloved upright [Torah]
　　that You designated for those who know You?
Therefore we have wailed,
'Remember, HASHEM, what has befallen us!'

כ How did You concentrate in Your anger, to devastate
　　Your vineyard [Israel] at the hand of the vandalizing villain,
ל and not recall that You taught Your acquired people that
　　[You would] not abandon [them] forever?[4]
Therefore we have cried,
'Remember, HASHEM, what has befallen us!'

---

the spiritual stronghold at which all of Israel would assemble during three seasons (Pesach, Shavuos, Succos) each year.

אֵיכָה טָרַחְתָּ בְּטָרְדֶּךָ — *How did You take pains in exerting Yourself.* For eighteen years a heavenly voice resounded through the halls of Nebuchad-

אֵיכָה מֻלֵּאת בְּמוֹאֲסֵךְ, לִמְחוֹת בְּיַד מוֹנִים מְנַשְּׁאָיִךְ,
וְלֹא זָכַרְתָּ נְשִׂיאַת נוֹצַת נֶשֶׁר אֲשֶׁר נָשָׂאתָ לִנְשׂוּאָיִךְ,
וּבְכֵן נָהִינוּ, זְכוֹר יהוה מֶה הָיָה לָנוּ.

אֵיכָה שָׁחַתָּ בְּסַעֲרֵךְ, לְסַגֵּר בְּיַד סֵעֲפִים סַהֲדֶיךָ,
וְלֹא זָכַרְתָּ עֹז עֲדִי עֲדָיִים* אֲשֶׁר עִטַּרְתָּ לַעֲבָדֶיךָ,
וּבְכֵן עָנִינוּ, זְכוֹר יהוה מֶה הָיָה לָנוּ.

אֵיכָה פָּצְתָּ בְּפַחְדֵּךְ, לְפַגֵּר בְּיַד פָּרִיצִים פְּלִיאָיִךְ,
וְלֹא זָכַרְתָּ צַהֲלַת צְבִי צַדִּיק² אֲשֶׁר צָפַנְתָּ לִצְבָאָיִךְ,
וּבְכֵן צָעַקְנוּ, זְכוֹר יהוה מֶה הָיָה לָנוּ.

אֵיכָה קָרָאתָ בְּקִרְיָאתֶךְ, לִקְנוֹת בְּיַד קָמִים קְרוּאָיִךְ,
וְלֹא זָכַרְתָּ רֶגֶשׁ רֶכֶב רִבּוֹתַיִם³ אֲשֶׁר רָצִיתָ לְרֵעֶיךָ,
וּבְכֵן רָגַנּוּ, זְכוֹר יהוה מֶה הָיָה לָנוּ.

אֵיכָה שָׁאַפְתָּ בְּשַׁאֲפֵךְ, לְשַׁלּוֹת בְּיַד שׁוֹדְדִים שְׁלָמֶיךָ,
וְלֹא זָכַרְתָּ תֹּקֶף תַּלְתַּלֵּי תְאַר אֲשֶׁר תִּכַּנְתָּ לִתְמִימֶיךָ,
וּבְכֵן תָּאַנּוּ, זְכוֹר יהוה מֶה הָיָה לָנוּ.

תָּאַנּוּ לִשְׁפּוֹךְ דְּמָעוֹת כַּמָּיִם,
עַל מֶה בְּיוֹם זֶה נִשְׁבִּינוּ פַעֲמָיִם,
זָכְרִי בִּהְיוֹתִי בְּשַׁלְוָה יוֹשֶׁבֶת בִּירוּשָׁלָיִם,
רָגַנְתִּי וְעַתָּה אֶאֱדֶה עַד חוּג שָׁמָיִם.

---

(1) Cf. *Ezekiel 16:7.* (2) Cf. *Isaiah 24:16;* some editions read, צַהֲלַת צְבִי צֶדֶק, *the joyous song of the desirable [Land (cf. Ezekiel 20:15) of] righteousness (cf. Isaiah 1:16).* (3) Cf. *Psalms 68:18.*

---

nezzar's palace. It cried: 'O perpetrator of evil! Go destroy your Master's Temple, for His children do not listen to Him' (*Midrash Eichah,* intro. 23).

עֲדִי עֲדָיִים — *Twin Torah-crowns.* When Israel was asked to accept the Torah, the nation cried out, נַעֲשֶׂה וְנִשְׁמָע, '*We will do and we will hear'* (*Exodus 24:7*), placing נַעֲשֶׂה, *we will do,* before נִשְׁמָע, *we will hear.* Thus they undertook to fulfill all of God's commandments, even before they knew what was expected of them. This devotion was rewarded when 600,000 ministering angels approached Israel and placed two crowns upon each Jew's head — one for נַעֲשֶׂה, and one for נִשְׁמָע (*Shabbos* 88a).

רֶגֶשׁ רֶכֶב רִבּוֹתַיִם — *The assembly [You attended with an] entourage of [more than] twice ten thousand.* The translation and interpolation are based on a midrashic account of God's descent upon Mount Sinai. The psalmist states: *The chariot of God is twice ten thousand, thousands*

מ How did You speak in Your contempt, to eradicate
 at the hand of tormentors those who had exalted You,
נ and not recall the flight on eagle's feathers
 when You carried aloft those whom You had exalted?

      Therefore we have moaned,
     'Remember, HASHEM, what has befallen us!'

ס How did You speak out in Your stormy rage,
 to confine Your witnesses by the hand of free thinkers,
ע and not recall the mighty twin Torah-crowns[1]*
 with which You crowned Your servants?

      Therefore we have cried out,
     'Remember HASHEM, what has befallen us!'

פ How did You utter in Your awesomeness,
 to murder Your wondrous people by the hand of law breakers,
צ and not recall the joyous song of the desirable righteous[2]
 that You have concealed for Your legions?

      Therefore we have shouted,
     'Remember HASHEM, what has befallen us!'

ק How did You proclaim in Your proclamation, to give over those
 You had once summoned to the hand of those who oppose You,
ר and not recall the assembly [You attended with an] entourage
 of [more than] twice ten thousand,[3]*
 at which You favored your friends?

      Therefore we have protested,
     'Remember HASHEM, what has befallen us!'

ש How You aspire with Your aspiration,
 to disperse Your perfect ones at the hand of pillagers,
ת and not recall the strength of the Temple Mount's stature
 which You prepared for Your wholesome ones?

      Therefore we have groaned,
     Remember HASHEM, what has befallen us!'

אל We have groaned; pouring out [our hearts] like water,
ע because on this day we were taken captive twice.
ז I recall how I dwelt serenely in Jerusalem.
ד I have complained, but now, I shall raise aloft [my laments]
 to the sphere of heaven.

---

of angels, my Lord is among them, at Sinai in
holiness (Psalms 68:18). R' Avudimi of Haifa
explained that twenty-two thousand ['twice ten
thousand' plus two thousand, the minimum that

can be called 'thousands'] ministering angels
accompanied God when He descended upon
Mount Sinai to give the Torah to Israel (see
Rashi to Psalms 68:18).

ח

אַאֲדֶה* עַד חוּג שָׁמַיִם,

אֵלֶּה אִתִּי שָׁמַיִם,

אֶתְאוֹנֵן מִי יִתֵּן רֹאשִׁי מַיִם.¹   אָאוֹר יוֹם מַחֲרִיבֵי פְעָמִים,

אַבְחִין בְּבִכְיַי לֵיל מִדְבָּר,²

אַבְחֶנָּה לֵיל מֵלִיל* וּמִדְבָּר מִמִּדְבָּר,*

אֶשְׁאַג מִי יִתְּנֵנִי בַמִּדְבָּר.³   אַבְכֶּה אִתִּי עוֹלַת מִדְבָּר,

אֶגְדַּע וְאֶנָּשֵׁל כְּנֹקֶף זַיִת,

אֶגְרֶה אִתִּי כָּל בְּנֵי בַיִת,

אֲרַשֶּׁה מִי יִתְּנֵנִי שָׁמִיר וָשָׁיִת.⁴   אֶגְרוֹם שֶׁיֹּאמַר בַּעַל הַבַּיִת,

אֶדְוֶה בְּכָל לֵב לְהַמְצִיאֵהוּ,

אֵדְעָה מִלִּין בָּם לְאִמְצֵהוּ.

אֶדְאַג אַיֵּה רוֹעֶה וְלֹא אֶמְצָאֵהוּ,   אֲקוֹנֵן מִי יִתֵּן יָדַעְתִּי וְאֶמְצָאֵהוּ.⁵

אֶהְפְּכָה וְאֶתְהַפְּכָה כְּאוֹפָן בְּמִלַּי,

אֶהְגֶּה פָנִים בְּפָנִים לְתַנּוֹת עֲמָלִי,

אֲצְרַח מִי יִתֵּן אֵפוֹא וְיִכָּתְבוּן מִלָּי.⁶   אָהֵהוּ חֶרֶס וְסָהַר מִלְּהַגִּיהַּ לְמוֹלִי,

אוֹרַח מִשְׁפְּטֵי גוֹנְבֵי עֲלֵי,*

אוֹדִיעַ בְּבִצְעִי וּמַעֲלִי,

אֶפְעֶה מִי יִתֵּן שׁוֹמֵעַ לִי.⁷   אוֹמְלְלוּ מַזָּלוֹת בְּקָרְעֵי מְעִילִי,

אָזְדָה כְּהוּפְרָה הָאֶבְיוֹנָה,*⁸

אֶזְכְּרָה כִּי הָיִיתִי מֵחַתְנָה,

אֶגּוֹר מִי יִתֵּן לִי אֵבֶר כַּיּוֹנָה.⁷   אָזִיל פְּלָגִים כְּבִרְכַּת הָעֶלְיוֹנָה,⁶

אֶאֱדֶה — *Would that I could soar.* The translation of this rare word is based on הִנֵּה כַנֶּשֶׁר יִדְאֶה, *Behold! It shall fly as an eagle* (Jeremiah 48:40). Alternatively the word is related to אִיד which *Targum* (Job 21:30) renders תְּבִירָא, *destruction,* and Ibn Ezra explains as a *dark cloud.*

אַבְחֶנָּה לֵיל מֵלִיל — *I would differentiate between night and night.* On that first tragic night of Tishah B'Av in the wilderness, the nation heard the Spies' slanderous reports regarding the Land of Canaan, and they wept. But that was a בְּכִיָּה שֶׁל חִנָּם, *an uncalled for* (or, *needless*) *weeping.* The tragic events that occurred on later Tishah B'Avs, however, were the source of true weeping. Thus we distinguish between tonight's weeping and that first night's weeping.

וּמִדְבָּר מִמִּדְבָּר — *And between wilderness and wilderness,* i.e., between the Wilderness of Sinai where we ate the heavenly manna, drank from the Well of Miriam and were protected by the Clouds of Glory, and the wilderness of exile where we were starving, thirsty and at the mercy of the elements and both four-legged and two-legged predators.

Once, the foreign overlords of *Eretz Yisrael* forbade the bringing of *bikkurim* (first-fruit offerings) to Jerusalem and stationed sentries on the roads to prevent the Jews from doing so. Pious men of that generation arose and placed baskets of *bikkurim*, covered with dried figs, into large wooden vessels shaped like a pestle, which was used for pressing dried figs into cakes, and carried them on their shoulders to Jerusalem. When the sentries inquired about the contents, the Jews would say that they were taking the dried figs to

8.

א *Would that I could soar* to the sphere of heaven;*
   I would make the heavens lament with me!
   I would curse the day on which I was twice destroyed.

ת *I would lament, 'Would that my head were [a stream of] water.'[1]*

ב *I would contemplate the crying of that night in the wilderness;[2]*
   I would differentiate between night and night*
      and between wilderness and wilderness.*
   I would inspire all who emerged from the wilderness to cry with me,

ש *as I would roar, 'Would that I were [once again]*
      in the Wilderness [of Sinai].'[3]

ג *[I would cry,] 'My limbs are amputated, my fruits are fallen,*
      like a beaten olive.'
   I would provoke the entire household* [to cry] with me;
   I would cause the Master of the Household Himself to say,

ר *'Would that I allowed Myself [to tread upon Israel's enemies,*
      as if they were] thorns and thistles!''[4]

ד *I would cause my whole heart to grow faint*
      as I [would struggle to have Him make Himself available [to me].
   Would that I knew the appropriate words
      to encourage Him to forgive me].
   I would worry, 'Where is the Shepherd?' — but not be able to find Him,

ק *I would lament, 'Would that I be permitted to know,*
      so that I might find him.'[5]

ה *I would turn round and round with my words*
      like an [ever-spinning] wheel,
   I would speak with Him face to face to bemoan my woes.
   The sun and moon would howl together and refuse to shine upon me,

צ *I would shriek, 'Would that my words [of lamentation]*
      be recorded [for posterity].'[6]

ו *The just ways of the pestle-thieves*
   I would reveal by [contrasting them with] my greed and treachery.
   Even the constellations were distraught when
      I ripped my [priestly] vestments [at the Temple's destruction],

פ *I would scream, 'Would that He give heed to me!'[7]*

ז *We were exiled when the desirous [Temple]* was ruined,[8]*
   I would remember that I was once wed [to the holy Torah],
   I would shed tears that stream forth as from a mountaintop cistern;[9]

ע *I would exclaim, 'Would that I had wings like a dove.'[10]*

---

(1) *Jeremiah* 8:23, see *Targum*. (2) Some editions read יְלֵל מִדְבָּר, *the wailing of the wilderness*. (3) *Jeremiah* 9:1. (4) Cf. *Isaiah* 27:4. (5) *Job* 23:3. (6) 19:23. (7) Cf. 31:35. (8) Cf. *Ecclesiates* 12:5. (9) Cf. *Isaiah* 7:3. (10) *Psalms* 55:7.

---

a mortar where they would press them with their pestle. Therefore, they were given the appellation *pestle-thieves* because they would *steal the hearts*, i.e., deceive the sentries with the pretext of the pestle (*Taanis* 28a).

הָאֲבִיוֹנָה — *The desirous [Temple].* The translation follows *Rashi* and *Ibn Ezra* (*Ecclesiastes* 12:5) who render 'lust for conjugal pleasures.' Some regarded this as a compound word from אָב, *father* or *patriarch*, and יוֹנָה, *dove*, i.e., Abraham, Isaac

אָח נִפְשָׁע מִקִּרְיַת עֹזּ אֶל צוּר,

אָחוּ בְּלִי מָיִם² בְּאַף לַעֲצוֹר,

אָחַז קָמוֹת לִקְצוֹר וְעוֹלֵלוֹת לִבְצוֹר,

אָשִׂיחָה **מִי** יוֹבִילֵנִי עִיר מָצוֹר.³

אֶטַּע אָהֳלֵי אַפַּדְנִי⁴ בְּצַלְמָוֶת,

אָטוּסָה וְאֶשְׁכְּוֹנָה⁵ עַד חֲצַר מָוֶת,

אֶטְפֹּל אֶת הַמְחַכִּים לַמָּוֶת,*

אֶנְהֶה **מִי** גֶבֶר יִחְיֶה וְלֹא יִרְאֶה מָוֶת.⁶

אֵילוּתִי לְעֶזְרָתִי⁷ תַּרְתִּי חֲזוֹת,

אֵימָתִי בְּכָל שָׁנָה אוֹמֶרֶת הִיא הַשָּׁנָה הַזֹּאת,

אֵדַע לַכֹּל כִּי מוּדַעַת זֹאת,⁸ **אִם** לֹא כִּי יַד יהוה עָשְׂתָה זֹּאת.⁹

אָכוֹף לְךָ רֹאשׁ יהוה חֵילִי,

אֶכְרַע לְךָ בֶּרֶךְ לְחַתֵּל מַחֲלִי,

אֶכְתִּירְךָ בְּשִׁיר מִשִׁירֵי מְחוֹלִי,*   אַכֵּן **מִי** יִתֶּנְךָ כְּאָח לִי.¹⁰

אַל תִּשְׁכַּח צַעֲקַת אֲרִיאֵל,¹¹

אֵלָיו לֶאֱגוֹר יְהוּדָה וְיִשְׂרָאֵל,

אַלְפֵי שִׁנְאָן¹² אֲשֶׁר מָסַר אֵל,

לֵאמֹר **מִי** יִתֵּן מִצִּיּוֹן יְשׁוּעַת יִשְׂרָאֵל.¹³

יִשְׂרָאֵל מֵעַט בִּדְרָכַי לֹא הָלָכוּ,

עֲזָבְוּנִי וַעֲזָבְתִּים וּפָנַי מֵהֶם נֶהְפָּכוּ,

רָגַנְתִּי וְהֶלַלְתִּי* וּמֵעַי וְלִבִּי נִשְׁפָּכוּ,

אֵיכָה תִפְאַרְתִּי מֵרֹאשׁוֹתַי הִשְׁלִיכוּ.

(1) Proverbs 18:19; see Nazir 23a. (2) Job 8:11. (3) Psalms 60:11. (4) Cf. Daniel 11:45.
(5) Cf. Psalms 55:7. (6) 89:49. (7) 22:20. (8) Isaiah 12:5. (9) Job 12:9.
(10) Song of Songs 8:1. (11) See commentary to kinnah 37. (12) Psalms 68:18. (13) 53:7.

and Jacob, the Patriarchs of Israel, the nation compared to a dove (see e.g., *Song of Songs* 2:14). The verse then alludes to the Talmudic teaching, תַּמּוּ זְכוּת אָבוֹת, *the merits of the Patriarchs have ended* (*Shabbos* 55a), and means that since we no longer had the merits of the אָבוֹת to protect us, the Temple was destroyed (*Matteh Levi*).

חֲצַר מָוֶת ... הַמְחַכִּים לַמָּוֶת — *Death's Courtyard ... those who wait for death.* חֲצַרְמָוֶת, *Hazarmaveth*, was a seventh-generation descendant of Noah. According to the Midrash, he was the progenitor of a tribe of impoverished people who ate animal fodder, dressed in papyrus reed garments, and eagerly anticipated death

(*Bereishis Rabbah* 37:8). The *paytan* compares the plight of exiled Israel to the lives of those unfortunates.

מְחוֹלִי — *My machalas.* The מַחֲלַת, *machalas*, is a musical instrument used by the Levite orchestra in the Temple (see *Psalms* 53:1 and 88:1). The word מְחוֹלִי [and מַחֲלַת] can also be cognate with מַחֲלָה, *sickness*, and refer to Israel's heartache over the Destruction of the two Temples (*Rashi* to *Psalms* ibid.). Alternatively, the word may be related to מָחוֹל, *a circle dance.* Accordingly the stitch is based on the verse, *You have changed for me my lament into dancing ...* (*Psalms* 30:12), and means that when redemption comes

ח Brother [Israel] separated by sinfulness from [Jerusalem]
     the mighty city[1] and exiled to Tyre;
  like a meadow without water,[2]
     because God withheld [rain] in [His] wrath.
  He held [Jerusalem] in His grasp like grain standing to be reaped
     and grapes ready to be harvested;

ס I would speak, 'Would that I be brought to the fortified city!'[3]

ט I would pitch my palatial tents[4] in the very shadow of death
     [for life is worthless in exile];
  I would fly off and find rest[5] in Death's Courtyard,
     [where] I would associate with those who wait for death.*

נ I would whimper, '[Would that I die, for] which man lives on
     [through interminable tragedy] and will never see death?'[6]

י I seek to witness [the fulfillment of my plea],
     'O my Strength [God], come to my assistance!'[7]
  My awe-inspiring nation proclaims every year,
     'This is the year [of redemption]!'
  [When that time comes I shall announce to everyone,
     so that it will be universally known,[8]

מ that had the hand of God not wrought all this
     [it could not have happened]![9]

כ I shall bow my head to You [in penitence], HASHEM,
     my source of strength;
  I shall bend my knee [in supplication] to You,
     to bandage my exile-wounds.
  I shall crown You with song, with the melodies of my machalas.*
  I will concentrate [my prayer] to request,
     'Would that You were as a brother to me!'[10]

ל Do not forget the scream of Ariel [the Beis HaMikdash],[11]
  to assemble to him Judah and Israel.
  The thousands of protective angels[12]
     whom God designated [to guard Jerusalem],
  saying, 'Would that out of Zion shall emerge Israel's salvations!'[13]

אל [To this request God responds:] 'From the moment Israel ceased
     to follow My ways;

עז they abandoned Me, so I abandoned them and
     turned My countenance away from them!'

ר I grumbled and I groaned,* my innards and my heart
     were spilled out [in grief];
  O how they have thrown my splendor from my head!

You will have changed מֶחֱלִי, my exile-wounds,
into מָחוֹלִי, my dancing.

רָגַנְתִּי וְהֶלֶלְתִּי — I grumbled and I groaned. The
speaker here may be God continuing His lament
from the previous two lines, i.e. Israel abandoned
Me ... and threw My splendor [Divine crowns

from the prayers of the righteous (see *Chagigah*
13b with *Tosafos*)] from My head. Alternatively,
the lament may revert to Israel's words: From the
time God abandoned me ... the enemy nations
have thrown my splendor [the *Beis HaMikdash*]
from my head [Jerusalem].

ט.

אֵיכָה תִפְאַרְתִּי מֵרֹאשׁוֹתַי הִשְׁלִיכוּ,*
וּכְנֶגֶד כִּסֵּא הַכָּבוֹד* צֶלֶם הִמְלִיכוּ,
בְּחַלְּלָם* תְּנָאי אֲשֶׁר חוֹזֵי נִמְלְכוּ,
וְנָם אִם בְּחֻקֹּתַי תֵּלֵכוּ.[1]

לָמָה[2] תָרִיבוּ אֵלַי כֻּלְּכֶם,[3] חָזְקוּ עָלַי דִּבְרֵיכֶם,[4]
מִיֶּדְכֶם הָיְתָה זֹּאת לָכֶם.[5]

בֶּלַע שׁוֹפְטַי בְּמוֹעֲצוֹת עֻוְּתָם,
וּפָנִים הִסְתִּיר מֵהֶם כְּשָׁר עַוָּתָם,
וַיֹּאמֶר לְאָבָק מִטְרָם[6] לְהַבְעִיתָם,
חָלֶף וְנָתַתִּי גִשְׁמֵיכֶם בְּעִתָּם.[7]

סָחִי וּמָאוֹס שָׂמָנִי,[8] כָּלָה בְאַפּוֹ וַיִּשְׂטְמֵנִי,[9]
נִחוּמָיו מְהֵרָה יְשַׁעְשְׁעוּנִי.[10]

גָּדַע רוּם קַרְנָם[11] וְעֲלוּמָם הִקְצִיר,[12]
וּבְאַבְחַת חֶרֶב שַׁעֲרֵיהֶם הֵצִיר,[13]
מִזֵּי רָעָב עָשׁ בַּקָּצִיר,
תָּמוּר וְהִשִּׂיג לָכֶם דַּיִשׁ אֶת בָּצִיר.[14]

דָּרַךְ קַשְׁתּוֹ וְכִלָּה בְחֶרֶץ,
וְכַבַּרְזֶל עָפַל עָפֵל שְׁמֵי אֶרֶץ,[15]
פְּרָצֵנִי שְׁלֹשׁ עֶשְׂרֵה פֶרֶץ,*
תַּחַת וְנָתַתִּי שָׁלוֹם בָּאָרֶץ.[16]

איכה תִפְאַרְתִּי מֵרֹאשׁוֹתַי הִשְׁלִיכוּ — *O how they have thrown My splendor from My head.* Parashas Bechukosai (*Leviticus* chapters 26-27) begins with the idyllic blessings that await the Jewish people if they prove themselves worthy of God's esteem. The portion proceeds to the תּוֹכָחָה, *Admonition*, a terrifying prediction of the curses and plagues which will inevitably befall the Jewish people if they betray their solemn covenant with God. This composition [by R' Elazar HaKalir] vividly depicts how Israel did indeed turn away from God and progressively forfeited, one by one, the blessings which God had in store for them and ultimately their evil ways forced God to fulfill the harsh prophecies of the admonition.

Appropriately, the acrostic of this *kinnah* is arranged according to the א״ת ב״ש order of the alphabet. In this arrangement, the first letter of the *aleph-beis* is paired with the last, the second letter is exchanged for the second to last, and so on. This pattern alludes to Israel who foolishly exchanged the first and best, God, for the last and worst, the idols.

The first word of each quatrain is taken from the respective verse of the second chapter of *Eichah*, thus forming an *aleph-beis* acrostic. The second word begins with the complementary letter in the א״ת ב״ש formation. The last stitch of each stanza is the opening of the corresponding verse in *Leviticus* 26:3-24.

Throughout this *kinnah*, the *paytan* shifts back and forth between first, second and third person. This indicates a continuously changing narrator. In some stanzas, God (as it were) mourns His splendor, the *Beis HaMikdash*, that 'they' [a reference to either the wicked king Manasseh (see *II Kings* 21:4-7) during the First Temple era; or the

9.

א־ת O *how they have thrown My splendor from My head,*
   when they enthroned an idol [in the Temple that is]
      correspondent to [My] Throne of Glory.

When they [Israel] defiled *the condition My prophets had advised,*
   and said, 'If you will follow My decrees.' [1]

   Why [2] *do you all quarrel with Me?* [3]
   Your words have come strongly against Me. [4]
   From your own hand has this befallen you. [5]

ב־ש *He swallowed up my judges because of their perverted advice;*
   and He concealed His countenance from them
      when He saw their perverseness.

He turned their rain to dust [6] *to frighten them,*
   instead of [fulfilling the blessing]:

   I will give you your rains in their proper season. [7]
   He made me as filth and refuse [among the nations]. [8]
   He annihilated me with His wrath and despised me. [9]
   May His comforting swiftly cheer me. [10]

ג־ר *He cut down the pinnacle of their pride* [11]
   and cut short their youth; [12]
with the butchery of the sword he laid siege to their gates. [13]

He caused them to be swollen from starvation
   during the [abundant] harvest;
instead of the blessing:

   And your threshing shall reach for you, until the vintage. [14]

ד־ק *He bent His bow and cut down completely,*
   and as with iron He solidified the heavens [15]
      [to prevent them from giving rain].

He breached me with thirteen breaches, *
   instead of [the blessing], And I will make peace in the land. [16]

---

(1) *Leviticus* 26:3. (2) Some early editions omit this stanza. (3) *Jeremiah* 2:29. (4) *Malachi* 3:13.
(5) Cf. 1:9. (6) Cf. *Deuteronomy* 28:24. (7) *Leviticus* 26:4. (8) Cf. *Eichah* 3:45. (9) Cf. *Job* 16:9.
(10) *Psalms* 94:19. (11) Cf. *Eichah* 2:3. (12) Cf. *Psalms* 89:46. (13) Cf. *Ezekiel* 21:20.
(14) *Leviticus* 26:5. (15) Cf. 26:19. (16) 26:6.

---

pagan conquerors of the Second Temple] turned into a sanctuary for idolatry. In other stanzas, Israel ruefully laments its forsaking תִּפְאַרְתִּי מְרַאֲשׁוֹתַי, *the splendor of my head,* i.e., the Torah's laws (see commentary to בְּחַלְּלָם, below). And in some stanzas the gentile nations taunt Israel in its degradation.

Alternatively, the entire *kinnah* represents the words of one speaker, so distraught in his mourning that he variously refers to himself introspectively in the first person, admonishes himself as an outsider using the second person, and hangs his guilt on a third party, but realizes that he means himself.

וּכְנֶגֶד כִּסֵּא הַכָּבוֹד — *Correspondent to [My] Throne of Glory.* The Midrash teaches that the celestial

Throne of Glory rests directly above the *Beis HaMikdash* on earth (*Mechilta* cited by *Rashi* to *Exodus* 15:17; *Targum* to *Jeremiah* 17:12).

בְּחַלְּלָם — *When they defiled.* This reference to Israel in the third person indicates that God is the speaker. However, some editions read בְּחַלְּלִי, *when I defiled,* implying that Israel is the speaker. (See commentary above.)

שְׁלֹשׁ עֶשְׂרֵה פֶּרֶץ — *Thirteen breaches.* A lattice-work fence, ten handbreadths high, stood within the walls surrounding the Temple Mount. This fence, called the סוֹרֵג, *soreig,* served as a boundary, past which neither a Jew contaminated by contact with a corpse nor a gentile was permitted to enter. When the Greeks conquered the Land

הָיָה צוּרְכֶם וּמָעֻזְּכֶם וּמִשְׂגַּבְּכֶם,

הָפַךְ לְאַכְזָר וְנִלְחַם בָּכֶם,

הַנּוֹצָרְכֶם רַחֲקָכֶם, חוֹשְׁקָכֶם תְּעַבְכֶם,

וְאַיֵּה הַבְּטָחַת וּרְדַפְתֶּם אֶת אוֹיְבֵיכֶם.[1]

וַיַּחֲמֹס פִּנַּת צֶדֶק מְלֵאָה,

כִּי בְּמַשְׂכִּיּוֹתֶהָ מָצָא כָּל טֻמְאָה,

וּמְכַבְּדֶיהָ הִזִּילוּהָ כְּדָוָה מִטַּמְּאָה,[2]

בְּשִׂנּוּי וְרָדְפוּ מִכֶּם חֲמִשָּׁה מֵאָה.[3]

זָנַח עֶלְיוֹן קִרְיַת מוֹעֲדֵיכֶם,

וְהֶאֱבִיל שַׁעֲרֵי חֵיל עֲמִידַת רַגְלֵיכֶם,

מִי בִקֵּשׁ זֹאת[4] פָּץ וְהִגְלָכֶם,

וְגָמַר אָמַר וּפָנִיתִי אֲלֵיכֶם.[5]

חָשַׁב שְׂנוֹא אוֹם לֶקֶט כַּשּׁוֹשָׁן[6]

וּמְחֵלֶב עוֹלָלֶיהָ אוֹתָהּ דִּשַּׁן,*

קִיטוֹר חֶפְתָּהּ הוֹעֲלָה כַּכִּבְשָׁן,

וְשָׁאֲלוּ אַיֵּה דָגָן תְּמוּר וַאֲכַלְתֶּם יָשָׁן נוֹשָׁן.[7]

טָבְעוּ נִכְסֵי רוֹבְדֵי דוּכָנִי,*

בְּגַיְא חֲמַת כְּנִקְטַל מְכַהֲנִי,*

הֲרֵי כַּמָּה שָׁנִים גֻּלָּה יְסוֹד מְכוֹנִי,

וְסַע מִתּוֹכִי אָמַר וְנָתַתִּי מִשְׁכָּנִי.[8]

יָשְׁבוּ מְבַכִּים מִנַּאַק מְתֵיכֶם,*[9]

בְּאַרְבַּע מִיתוֹת הִפִּיל מְתֵיכֶם,

חֶרֶב וְרָעָב וְחַיָּה וְדֶבֶר* שִׁחֵתְכֶם,[10]

---

(1) *Leviticus* 26:7. (2) Cf. *Eichah* 1:8. (3) *Leviticus* 26:8. (4) *Isaiah* 1:12. (5) *Leviticus* 26:9. (6) Cf. *Song of Songs* 2:2. (7) *Leviticus* 26:10. (8) *Leviticus* 26:11. (9) Cf. *Job* 24:12. (10) Cf. *Ezekiel* 14:21.

during the Second Temple era, they angrily broke through the *soreig* in thirteen places to register their indignation at being denied entrance. In subsequent years, the Hasmonean kings repaired these breaches (see *Middos* 2:3 with *Tos. Yom Tov*; *Shekalim* 6:8).

וּמְחֵלֶב עוֹלָלֶיהָ אוֹתָהּ דִּשַּׁן — *And [the enemy's soil] was enriched with the fat of her [slaughtered] infants.* The heathen farmers fertilized their vineyards for seven years with the blood of the slaughtered Jews (*Gittin* 57a).

דוּכָנִי — *My [Temple] platform.* The *Kohanim* would ascend a platform to bless the nation with the Priestly Blessing, and the Levite orchestra to accompany the daily Altar service.

בְּנִקְטַל מְכַהֲנִי — *When . . . my priests were murdered.* This refers to the tragic events following immediately after the destruction of the First Temple. Nebuzaradan, the chief executioner for the Babylonian king, captured Seraiah the *Kohen Gadol* and his deputy Zefaniah, along with seventy other officials, and transported them to Babylonia. There he delivered them into the hands of King Nebuchadnezzar who executed them at Rivlah in the land of Hamath

ה-צ He had been your Rock, your Fortification and your Stronghold,
  but now He has become ruthless and wages war against you.
  He Who once watched you closely has set you afar;
    He Who once yearned for you has come to despise you.
  And where is the pledge: And you shall chase after your enemies?[1]

ו-פ He despoiled [Jerusalem,] the cornerstone [of the world,
    that had been] filled with righteousness,
  because beneath her mosaic floors
    He found every manner of impurity.
  Those who had once respected her
    disparage her like a woman unclean.[2]
  Thus was perverted [the blessing]:
    And five of you shall chase after one hundred [of the enemy].[3]

ז-ע The Exalted One has rejected the metropolis
    of your festival [assemblies],
  and brought mourning to the gates of the rampart
    upon which you were stationed.
  'Who asked you for this [to trample My courtyards]?'[4]
    cried He, as He sent you into exile,
  and He nullified His statement,
    'And I will turn [My attention] towards you!'[5]

ח-ס He made His plans [to show how] He despised the nation
    that He had once picked [from among the others]
    like a rose [from the thorns],[6]
  and [the enemy's soil] was enriched*
    with the fat of her [slaughtered] infants.
  The smoke from her [burning Temple] canopy
    arose as from a furnace,
  and the [starving] people asked, 'Where is the grain?' in place of
    [the blessing]: And you shall eat your old, well-preserved foods.[7]

ט-נ They drowned and slaughtered [Kohanim and Leviim]
    who once mounted the tiers of my [Temple] platform.*
  When, in the valley of Hamath, my priests were murdered.*
  Behold, many years have passed since
    my Temple's foundation has been laid bare,
  and gone from my midst is He Who said:
    'I shall make My dwelling place [among you].'[8]

י-מ They sat down to weep because of the cry of
    those dying among you.[9]*
  He struck down your people with four forms of death:
    He destroyed you with the sword, starvation,
    wild beast and the plague.[10]*

(see *II Kings* 25:18-21).

מִנַּאֲקַת מֵתֵיכֶם — *Because of the cry of those dying among you* [lit., *the cry of your dead*]. Since the dead cannot cry, the phrase must refer to the cry of those in the throes of death. Alternative-

ly, it means the screams of the relatives of the dead.

וְדֶבֶר — *And the plague.* This indicates that הִפִּיל, *He struck down,* refers to God, as germ warfare was unknown at that time.

כְּסֶר צֶלֶם פָּץ' וְהִתְהַלַּכְתִּי בְּתוֹכְכֶם.²

כָּלוּ לְשׁוֹד כְּרֶגַע אָהֳלֵיכֶם,
וּבָכֶם נִשְׁבָּעוּ* מְהוֹלְלֵיכֶם,³
לְחֵיקְכֶם נִשְׁפְּכוּ נַפְשׁוֹת עוֹלְלֵיכֶם,⁴
בְּמָאׇסְכֶם שִׂיחַ אֲנִי יהוה אֱלֹהֵיכֶם.⁵

לְאִמּוֹתָם בַּלְכּוֹל אָנָה שֹׁוֵעוּ,
וְצוּר לְמַלְאָכָיו שָׁח מֶנִּי שְׁעוּ,⁶
אֶרֶץ הַכַּרְמֶל⁷ הֲבֵאתִים וְשָׁעֲשֵׁעוּ,
וְשֹׂנְאוּ מוֹכִיחַ וְאִם לֹא תִשְׁמָעוּ.⁸

מָה אֲעִידֵךְ* יְשִׁישַׁיִךְ עִם גּוּרַיִךְ⁹ בֹּסָּסוּ,
אוֹמְרִים עַל סוּס נָנוּס* עַל כֵּן נָסוּ,¹⁰
נִלְאֵיתִי נְשׂוֹא¹¹ עֲוֹנֹתֵיכֶם כְּהוֹעֲמָסוּ,
וַאֲיַסֶּרְכֶם כְּנָמַתִּי אִם בְּחֻקֹּתַי תִּמְאָסוּ.¹²

נְבִיאַיִךְ תָּעוּ* תַּרְמִית שָׁוְא חָזוּת,¹³
וְאֶדְרוֹשׁ לִסְלֹחַ וּפִצְתִּי אֵי לָזֹאת,¹⁴
פִּתִּיתִים וּכְנֶגְדִּי הֵשִׁיבוּ עַזּוּת,
וְאָנַפְתִּי וְשָׁחַתִּי אַף אֲנִי אֶעֱשֶׂה זֹּאת.¹⁵

סָפְקוּ חָרְקוּ שָׁרְקוּ מוֹנַי,¹⁶
מִבִּפְנִים וּמִבַּחוּץ לְהַצְמִית אֱמוּנַי,¹⁷
כִּי בְנֵי זֵדִים חֻלְּלוּ צְפוּנַי,
לְרָעָה וְלֹא לְטוֹבָה נָם וְנָתַתִּי פָנַי.¹⁸

פָּצוּ זֵדִים לְפָנַי מִי תְחַלֶּה,
עִם כֶּבֶד עָוֹן פָּקַד וַיִּלְאֶה,
לֹא תְחַכּוּ עוֹד לְמוֹפֵת וָפֶלֶא,
אָנַף וְנָסַע וְנָם וְאִם עַד אֵלֶּה.¹⁹

(1) Cf. Numbers 14:9. (2) Leviticus 26:12. (3) Cf. Psalms 102:9. (4) Cf. Eichah 2:12. (5) Leviticus 26:13. (6) Cf. Isaiah 22:4; see Rashi there. (7) Cf. Jeremiah 2:7. (8) Leviticus 26:14. (9) Cf. II Chronicles 36:16-17. (10) Cf. Isaiah 30:16. (11) 1:14. (12) Cf. Leviticus 26:15. (13) Cf. Eichah 2:14; Micah 3:5-7; Ezekiel 13:8-10. (14) Jeremiah 5:7. (15) Leviticus 26:16. (16) Cf. Eichah 2:15. (17) Cf. 1:20; Deuteronomy 32:25. (18) Leviticus 26:17. (19) 26:18.

וּבָכֶם נִשְׁבָּעוּ — Would use you as a curse. If one of the enemy took an oath and wished to reinforce it, he would say, 'If I am not telling the truth may I be cursed in the worst possible way, in the manner which the conquered Jews suffer!' (Rashi to Psalms 12:9).

מָה אֲעִידֵךְ — How can I admonish you ...? The word אֲעִידֵךְ is derived from the root עוד which can mean either warn, admonish, or testify. The translation here follows Midrash Eichah (2:13).

And as [God] their protective shadow departed[1]
    [so did His pledge], 'And I shall walk in your midst.'[2]

כ-ל In but one moment all of your tents were totally destroyed by pillage,
    and your taunters would use you as a curse.[3]*
    The blood of your infants was spilled into your bosom,[4]
    because you abominated the utterance, 'I am HASHEM, your God.'[5]

ל-ב To their mothers they cried out, 'The food — where is it?'
    But the Rock [God] said to His angels
    [when they took up the children's cause], 'Turn away from Me![6]
    For I brought them into a fertile land[7] where they found all delights,
    but they despised the admonition, "If you will not give heed . . ."'[8]

מ-י How can I admonish you,* [when because of your obstinacy]
    they have trampled both your dignified elders and your cubs?[9]
    They would say [to those who rebuked them],*
    'We will flee on horseback!'* So they [were caused to] flee
    [but never returned]!'[10]
    I am utterly exhausted from carrying[11] your sins,
    for they are a burden [upon Me].
    Therefore, I have disciplined you as I said,
    'If you will abominate My decrees . . .'[12]

נ-ט Your prophets led you astray* with deceit and vain visions.[13]
    I sought to forgive you [but you refused to repent] so I cried out,
    'How shall I [pardon you] for this?'[14]
    I tried to persuade them [to repent],
    but they answered Me with brazenness.
    I was infuriated and declared, 'I will even do this to you . . .'[15]

ס-ח My tormentors clapped, gnashed (their teeth) and hissed[16]
    [as they prepared] to decimate my faithful ones
    from inside and out,[17]
    because the sons of the wanton desecrated my hidden treasures.
    To inflict harm and not help, He said, 'I will set My face . . .'[18]

פ-ז The wanton ones jeered at us, 'Before Whom do you pray?
    [You are] a nation heavy with iniquity;
    He has abandoned you and is wearied [by your sins].
    Therefore, wait no longer for sign and wonder.'
    He is angered and has departed, saying,
    'If despite all this [you refuse to obey].'[19]

According to others, the phrase means, *Whom can I bring to testify to you* that their suffering equals yours? (*Zohar; Targum; Rashi*), for צָרַת רַבִּים חֲצִי נֶחָמָה, *general suffering is half of assuagement*, i.e., grieving and troubles are easier to bear when one knows that there are others in the same dire circumstances (*Ibn Kaspi*).

עַל סוּס נָנוּס — *We will flee on horseback!* When warned by the prophets that the only way to avert impending disaster is a combination of repentance and quiet confidence in God's salva-

tion, the nation proudly refused to pay heed. Instead they replied, 'We will flee on horseback!' They meant, 'We will ally ourselves with Egypt who will supply us with mighty steeds. Thus shall we escape the threat of annihilation. Then, when the enemy leaves our land, we will return home safe and sound!' For this, God caused them to flee, but did not allow them to return (*Isaiah* 30:15-16 with *Rashi*).

תָּעוּ — *Led you astray* [or, *strayed*]. Since this *kinnah* follows an א"ת ב"ש pattern (see above), a word beginning with ט (the letter corresponding

עָשָׂה וַיָּרֶם קָדְקֹד בְּנֵי שָׁאוֹן,
וְדָמִי שִׁכְּרֵנִי בְּגֵיא צִמָּאוֹן,
וּבְכָל שָׁנָה וְשָׁנָה הוֹסִיף יָגוֹן עַל אוֹן,
מֵעַט כָּעַס וְנָם **וְשָׁבַרְתִּי אֶת גְּאוֹן.**[1]

צָעַק הוֹי הוֹי וְאַשְׁפַּתּוֹ הֵרִיק,
מִפֹּה וּמִפֹּה הֵבִיא עָלַי מַעֲרִיק,
וּבְלַעֲגֵי מָעוֹג שִׁנֵּי צָר הֶחֱרִיק,[2]
וְכָלָה כֹּחִי בְּנֻאָם **וְתַם לָרִיק.**[3]

קוּמִי דָפְקִי שַׁוְּעִי אַל דֳּמִי,[4]
וּתְנִי כְאוֹב מֵאֶרֶץ קוֹלֵךְ וָדְמִי,
מִי רֹאשׁ הִשְׁקַנִי וְהִדְמִי,
וְחָשַׁךְ הַלּוּכִי בְּנֻאָם **וְאִם תֵּלְכוּ עִמִּי.**[6]

רְאֵה גּוֹרָל אִוִּיתָ הוּשַׂם לָרוֹעִים לְעָיַת,[7]
וְלִקְאַת מִדְבָּר הָיִיתִי דְמוּיַת,
גּוֹלָה כְנוּיַת וְסוּרָה גְנוּיַת,[8]
בְּשָׁמְעִי **וְהִשְׁלַחְתִּי בָכֶם אֶת חַיַּת.**[9]

שָׁכְבוּ בְּעָלוּף כְּתוֹא מִכְמָר וְאֵין דּוֹלֶה,[10]
הַמְּלֵאִים גְּעַר וְאֵין מַרְפֵּא עוֹלֶה,
הֲרֵי כַּמֶּה שָׁנִים הֶמְמַנִּי לְהִתְכַּלֶּה,
אֱנוֹשִׁים בְּוִכּוּחַ **וְאִם בְּאֵלֶּה.**[11]

תִּקְרָא אֵיד עוֹלֶלֶת עַל אַדְמוֹנִי,
לְסַחֲפוֹ וּלְשַׁסְּפוֹ שִׁבְעָתַיִם כְּאוֹנִי,
תְּהוֹם צָרַי בְּצֵאת קוֹל מֵאַרְמוֹנִי,
כְּנֶהֱמַמְתִּי בְרִיב **וְהָלַכְתִּי אַף אָנִי.**[12]

אַף אֲנִי לָכוּד* בְּיוֹקֵשׁ שִׁכָּרוֹן,
עָרְבָה שִׂמְחָה וְהִשְׁבִּית חָרוֹן,
לָאָרֶץ אֵשֵׁב וְאֶהְגֶּה בְגָרוֹן,
אֵיכָה יָשְׁבָה חֲבַצֶּלֶת הַשָּׁרוֹן.[13]

---

to נ in (א״ת ב״ש) is expected here. Perhaps the
proper reading here is טָעוּ, *caused to err* or *erred*,
which is homophonous with תָּעוּ and similar in
meaning. Moreover, the only appearance of the

root טעה in Scriptures (*Ezekiel* 13:10) speaks of
the 'prophets' whose vain visions lulled the
nation into a false sense of security. Indeed, the
wording of the *kinnah* seems to be based on that

ע-י   *He proceeded to raise the heads of the tempestuous sons,*
     and He made me drunk on my own blood in the waterless valley;
   year after year He added anguish to [my] mourning,
   since the moment He was angered and said,
     'And I will shatter the pride [of your strength].'[1]

צ-ה   *He cried out, 'Woe! Woe!'*
     even though He emptied His quiver [against me].
   From here and from there He brought pursuers against me.
   They mock me for the sake of a breadloaf
     and cause the oppressor to gnash his teeth [at me].[2]
   He drained my strength with the statement,
     'And [your strength] will be used up in vain.'[3]

ק-ד   *Arise and pound [on the gates of heaven],*
     cry out, 'Do not be silent!'[4]
   Set your voice [in prayer] as the [muffled sound of]
     necromancy [arising] from the earth,[5] *then remain still.*
   He silenced me by making me drink bitter waters.
   He darkened my path, when He stated,
     'But if you will go against Me.'[6]

ר-ג   *Behold, the lot You had once desired*
     has been made into rubble heaps,[7]
   and I have come to resemble the [wandering] desert bird.
   They nickname me 'Exile,' and humiliate me as 'Displaced,'[8]
   so I have heard [the fulfillment of],
     'And I will send forth wild beasts against you.'[9]

ש-ב   *They lie in a swoon like a wild ox in a snare with none to release it.*[10]
   [They are] steeped in rebuke, yet no healing has emerged.
   Lo, [these] many years has He completely crushed me.
   We are pained by the admonition, 'And if despite this . . .'[11]

ת-א   *Designate a day of doom for the red one [Edom],*
     as You did [when you afflicted me],
   to eradicate him and to slash him seven times more than my pain.
   Confound my tormentors when the cry goes forth from my palace,
   as I was shocked by the rebuke, 'And I will also go [against you]'[12]

     I have also been trapped* in the snare of drunkenness.
     [Only after my] joy was confounded
       [by the Temple's destruction] did [His] anger subside.
     I will sink down to the earth and murmur in my throat,
     'O how the Rose of Sharon[13] *sits!'*

---

(1) *Leviticus* 26:19. (2) Cf. *Psalms* 35:16. (3) *Leviticus* 26:20. (4) Cf. *Psalms* 83:2.
(5) Cf. *Isaiah* 29:4. (6) *Leviticus* 26:21. (7) Cf. *Psalms* 79:1. (8) Cf. *Isaiah* 49:21.
(9) *Leviticus* 26:22. (10) Cf. *Isaiah* 51:20. (11) *Leviticus* 26:23. (12) 26:24. (13) *Song of Songs* 2:1.

passage (ibid. 13:9-10). Nevertheless, we have retained the word תָעוּ because in similar passages (e.g., *Michah* 3:5-7) the root תעה is used in Scriptures, and because that is how it appears in virtually all editions.

אַף אֲנִי לָכוּד — *I have also been trapped.* Many a *kinnah* of the series attributed to R' Elazar HaKalir ends with a stanza that links it with the following *kinnah*, i.e., the closing word or stich of one is identical with the opening word or stich of

י.

אֵיכָה יָשְׁבָה חֲבַצֶּלֶת הַשָּׁרוֹן,*
וְדָמַם רוֹן מִפִּי נוֹשְׂאֵי אָרוֹן,*
וְנָעוּ מִמִּשְׁמְרוֹתָם כֹּהֲנִים בְּנֵי אַהֲרֹן,
כְּנִמְסַר הַבַּיִת בְּמִסָרְבֵי **מָרוֹן.***

בָּכָה תִבְכֶּה מְחֻמֶּשֶׁת סְפָרִים,*
כְּנֶהֱרַג כֹּהֵן וְנָבִיא בְּיוֹם הַכִּפּוּרִים,
וְעַל דָּמוֹ נִשְׁחֲטוּ פְרָחִים כִּצְפִירִים,
וְנָדוּ כִצְפָרִים, כֹּהֲנֵי **צִפּוֹרִים.***

גָּלְתָה מֵאַרְצָהּ כַּלָּה מְקֻשָּׁטָה,
בַּעֲוֹן מַעְשְׂרוֹת וּשְׁמִטָּה,
וּבְאַרְבַּעַת שְׁפָטִים* הֻשְׁפָּטָה,
וּמֶעְדָּיָה הֻפְשָׁטָה, מִשְׁמֶרֶת **מִפְשָׁטָה.**

דַּרְכֵי הֵיכָל שָׁמְמוּ כְּנִפְרַץ כָּתְלוֹ,
וְהַמְּעִיל כְּנִקְרַע פְּתִילוֹ,
הוּרַד וְהֻשְׁפַּל מִתְּלוֹ,
וְנָע מִשְׁתִּילוֹ, כֹּהֵן עַיְתָה **לוֹ.***

---

the next. Such a linking stanza is evident between *kinnos* 7-8, 8-9, 11-12 and 19-20, and such is the nature of this stanza. However, many early editions do not contain this stanza, which leads to the contention that it is not the work of R' Elazar, but was inserted by some later *paytan* in order to connect this and the following *kinnah*. Indeed, *Maharil* argues that *kinnah* 15 was originally juxtaposed with this *kinnah* and he would recite that *kinnah* at this point (see commentary there for his reasoning). If so, this stanza could not have been part of the original *kinnah*, as it would be entirely out of place.

◆§ אֵיכָה יָשְׁבָה חֲבַצֶּלֶת הַשָּׁרוֹן — *O how the Rose of Sharon sits.* The Talmud (*Taanis* 26a-27a) teaches that the early prophets, David and Samuel, established twenty-four מִשְׁמָרוֹת כְּהֻנָּה, *priestly watches*, to scrupulously perform the Temple services. Each *mishmar* (watch) served for one week, on a rotation basis. The names of the watches in the First Temple are enumerated in *I Chronicles*, chapter 24. This *kinnah* describes the watches of the Second Temple which were then known under different names. According to many commentators, these new names were the names of each *mishmar's* home city. This is the

approach followed in the translation and commentary. Some commentators explain the new names as pejoratives and expound on the particular offense by which each *mishmar* earned its nickname. The commentary includes only those pejorative interpretations found in the Talmud.

In composing this *kinnah*, R' Elazar HaKalir used the opening word or phrase of the respective verses in the first chapter of *Eichah* to begin each stanza. Thus, the stanzas contain an alphabetical acrostic. The second word of each stanza begins with the corresponding letter of the א״ת ב״ש arrangement of the *aleph-beis*. The name of the corresponding *mishmar* appears in the last line.

חֲבַצֶּלֶת הַשָּׁרוֹן — *The Rose of Sharon.* The *Beis HaMikdash* was affectionately called חֲבַצֶּלֶת, *Rose.* The Midrash teaches that חֲבַצֶּלֶת is a contraction of the words חֲבוּיָה בְּצֵל, *sheltered in the shade*, i.e., in good times God loved Israel and their Temple so much that he hovered over them and provided them with the most intense protection under the shade of His Divine Presence, the *Shechinah* (*Shir HaShirim Rabbah* 2).

וְדָמַם רוֹן מִפִּי נוֹשְׂאֵי אָרוֹן — *And joy has been silenced from the mouths of those who carried the*

10.

א O how the Rose of Sharon[1]* sits* [alone]
and joy has been silenced from the mouths
   of those who carried the Ark;*
And the Kohanim, the sons of Aaron
   were removed from their watches,
When the Temple was given over to the rebels of Maron.*

ב The [people endowed with the] Five Books* wept and wept,
when the priest and prophet [Zechariah] was slain on Yom Kippur,
   when in vengeance for his blood,
   blossoming children were butchered like goats,
And the Kohanim of Sepphoris* wandered like birds.

ג The bejewelled bride was exiled from her land
because of the iniquity of the tithes and the Sabbatical year.
She was condemned to suffer four types of affliction,*
And the watch of Mifshatah was stripped of her ornaments.

ד The roads to the Sanctuary were silenced
   when its wall was breached;
and the [bells on the High Priest's] tunic [were silenced]
   when its threads were ripped apart.
[The Temple] was pulled down and lowered from its Mount,
And the Kohen from Aysah-Lo was uprooted from his planting.

---

(1) Song of Songs 2:1.

Ark. According to Rambam (Sefer HaMitzvos, aseh 34 and shoresh 3), the Kohanim were the bearers of the Ark throughout the generations. Only during the early years in the Wilderness, when there were very few Kohanim, did the Leviim carry the Ark. Ramban (ibid.) disagrees and states that the Leviim were charged with carrying the Ark whenever this would become necessary throughout the generations. Most commentators to kinnos follow Ramban's view. Thus, רוֹן refers to the joyous song the Levite bearers of the Ark sang on the platform in the Temple courtyard. Indeed, the Talmud relates that the Levite choir was interrupted in mid-verse when the enemy conquered the Beis HaMikdash (Taanis 29a). However, the translation of רוֹן as joy [see Psalms 30:6 where רְנָה, synonymous with רוֹן, is used as the opposite of בְּכִי, weeping], rather than joyous song, allows the kinnah to be understood even according to Rambam's view that the Kohanim bore the Ark.

בְּמִסְרְבֵי מָרוֹן — The rebels of Maron. The town of Maron was situated on a mountain and only could be reached by a narrow road (see Rosh Hashanah 18a and Eruvin 22b). It was the home of the first mishmar, יְהוֹיָרִיב, Jehoiarib. The Talmud states that it was during this mishmar's tour of duty that Jerusalem was captured (Taanis 29a), and expounds on the name Jehoiarib: יָ־הּ הֵרִיב עִם בָּנָיו עַל שֶׁמָּרוּ וְסָרְבוּ בּוֹ, God contended

with His children because they were rebellious and defiant against Him (Yerushalmi Taanis 4:5).

מֵחֲמֵשֶׁת סְפָרִים — The [people endowed with the] Five Books. This refers either to Israel, the Torah nation (as indicated by the interpolation), or to the Torah itself which metaphorically wept bitterly when Zechariah was assassinated (see kinnah 34).

כֹּהֲנֵי צִיפּוֹרִים — The Kohanim of Sepphoris. The city of קִיטְרוֹן, Kitron (see Judges 1:30), was also called צִיפּוֹרִי or צִיפּוֹרִים, Sepphoris, because it sat on a mountaintop like a high-soaring צִיפּוֹר, bird (Megillah 6a). It was the home town of the second watch, יְדַעְיָה, Jedaiah, whose name the Talmud explains as יָדַע יָ־הּ, God knew, what evil was in the depths of their hearts and so He exiled them 'לְצִיפּוֹרִין, to Sepphoris,' or, in a variant reading, 'כְּצִיפּוֹרִים, like birds' (Yerushalmi Taanis 4:5). The paytan merges both readings.

וּבְאַרְבַּעַת שְׁפָטִים — Four types of affliction: sword, starvations, wild beast and plague (see Ezekiel 14:21; see also kinnah 9).

עַיָּתָה לוֹ — Aysah-Lo. This was the city of the fourth watch, שְׂעוֹרִים, Seorim. Perhaps it is identical with עַיַּת, Aiath, the first city taken by Sennacherib when he moved against Jerusalem (Isaiah 10:28 with Rashi). The Vilna Gaon identifies that place with Gilgal.

הָיוּ אוֹיְבִים מַלְעִיבִים בְּלוֹחֲמֵי לֶחֶם,[1]
כְּבֻטְּלוּ הֲלֹא פָרֹס לָרָעֵב לֶחֶם,[2]
וְהִרְעִיבוּ וְהִצְמָאוּ מִמַּיִם וּמִלֶּחֶם,
כְּבֻטְּלוּ שְׁתֵּי הַלֶּחֶם, מִבֵּית לֶחֶם.*

וַיֵּצֵא הֲדַר אוֹם בַּכֶּסֶף נֶחְפָּת,[3]
וּתְמוּרוֹ אֵפֶר עַל רֹאשָׁהּ חָפַת,
וְנֵרוֹת נִכְבּוּ וּמְנוֹרָה נִכְפָּת,
כְּפָשְׁעוּ בְלֶחֶם וּפַת, נִלְכְּדָה יוֹדְפַת.*[4]

זָכְרָה זְמַן אֲשֶׁר נַעֲשֶׂה וְנִשְׁמָע[5] הֵשִׁיבוּ,
וְעַתָּה עֲנוֹת אָמֵן לֹא אָבוּ,
לַעֲנָה וָרֹאשׁ[6] שָׂבְעוּ וְרָווּ,
וְהִקְצוּ וְהִלְעִבוּ, כֹּהֲנֵי עֵילְבוּ.

חֵטְא חָטְאָה וְאָמְרָה לֶאֱלִיל זֶה אֵל,
וְהִלְעִיגָה וְתִעְתְּעָה בְּחוֹזֵי אֵל,
עֲבוּר כֵּן הִקְנָאָה בְּמַרְגִּיזֵי אֵל,
וַיֵּצֵא מִמְּעוֹן אֵל, כְּפַר עֻזִּיאֵל.

טֻמְאָתָהּ הֶחֱנִיפָה תֵבֵל,
וְנַעֲלָה רַב הַחוֹבֵל,
וְעָנָן אֲבַק רַגְלָיו כְּאָבֵל,
וְאֵין מִתְכַּרְבֵּל, בְּכֹהֲנֵי אַרְבֵּל.

יָדוֹ פָּרַשׂ צָר בְּבֵית זְבוּל,
כִּי כָלְיָה חִיַּבְתִּי כְּדוֹר הַמַּבּוּל,
כִּסְאוֹ הֵשִׁית לַחֲבוּל וּנְבוּל,
וַיֵּצֵא בְּכֶבֶל כָּבוּל, כֹּהֵן כָּבוּל.*[7]

כָּל עַמָּה קוֹנְנוּ קִינָה,
כִּי הִכְעִיסוּ לְאֵל קַנָּא,
בְּגוֹיֵי נָבָל אוֹתָם קִנֵּא,
וְנָדְדָה מִקְנֶה, מִשְׁמֶרֶת אֶלְקָנָה.

בֵּית לֶחֶם — *Bethlehem.* The fifth watch, מַלְכִּיָּה, *Malciah,* was headquartered in Bethlehem. Additionally, בֵּית לֶחֶם, literally, *House of Bread,* alludes to the *Beis HaMikdash.* For as the

Midrash teaches, as long as the Show Bread was placed on the שֻׁלְחָן, *Table,* each Sabbath, and the Two Loaves were brought every Shavuos in the Temple, the nation's flour and bread would

ה　*They ridiculed those who fought in the battle [for Torah observance],*[1]
　when they ignored [the verse],
　　'Shall you not break bread with the hungry?'[2]
　Thus, they hungered and thirsted for water and for bread,
　when the offering of the two loaves
　　was discontinued, from Bethlehem.*

ו　*Beauty has left the nation once sheltered by the silver[like Torah],*[3]
　in its place ashes cover her head.
　The candles have been extinguished
　　and the Menorah has been bent [to the ground].
　When they willfully sinned with [their failure
　　to give the poor] portions of bread,
　the [fortress] of Yodpath[4] *was captured.*

ז　*Remember the moment when they replied,*
　'We shall do and we shall listen!'[5]
　But now [when they are admonished] they do not confirm [their sins].
　They were sated and filled with wormwood and bitter gall;[6]
　The Kohanim of Aylevu were shunned and shamed.

ח　*She sinned greatly when she addressed the idol*
　　and said, 'This is God!'
　She mocked and ridiculed God's seers,
　therefore He took revenge through those who infuriated God,
　and [Kohanim from] the village of Uziel
　　had to depart from God's dwelling.

ט　*Her contamination has defiled the inhabited world,*
　and the Captain of the ship has ascended [to his heavenly dwelling].
　Clouds are on His feet like dust on [the bare feet of the] mourner,
　and there is none among the Kohanim of Arbel
　　who clads himself in the [priestly] vestments.

י　*The enemy spread out his hand against the [Divine] dwelling,*
　for I was culpable to extinction like the generation of the Flood.
　The enemy subjected God's throne to mutilation and degradation,
　And the Kohanim of Cabul[7]* *went out [into exile] chained in leg irons.*

כ　*Her entire nation chanted a lamentation,*
　because they angered the zealous God;
　He took revenge against them through a degenerate nation,
　And the watch of Elkanah wandered [into exile] from its nest.

---

(1) Cf. *Proverbs* 9:5; *Chagigah* 14a. (2) *Isaiah* 58:7. (3) Cf. *Psalms* 68:14 with *Rashi*. (4) Some editions read יוֹרְפָת, *Yurfath*. (5) *Exodus* 24:7. (6) Cf. *Eichah* 3:15. (7) See *Joshua* 19:27 and *I Kings* 9:13.

be blessed. But since these were stopped, blessing no longer lies in the bread. Nonetheless, in the future they will be restored (*Yalkut Shimoni* II:565).

יוֹדְפָת — *Yodpath*. A Galilean fortress, mentioned in *Arachin* (32a) as a city that was walled from the time Joshua entered the land.

כָּבוּל — *Cabul*. In return for supplying many of the materials for the *Beis HaMikdash* and Solomon's Palace, King Hiram of Tyre was presented with twenty cities in the land of Cabul, but he was not satisfied (*I Kings* 9:10-13). The Talmud explains that the inhabitants of this area of the Galilee were so wealthy that they would attire themselves in silver and gold. If so,

לֹא לַמָּרוֹם עֵין צָפַת,
וְכֶסֶף עַל חֶרֶשׁ חִפַּת,
וּבְחִזּוּק מוּסָר הִרְפַּת,
וְנֶהֱרַס וְנִלְפַּת, כֹּהֵן **צָפַת**.

מִמָּרוֹם הִשְׁמִיעַ נִלְאֵיתִי טְעוֹן,[1]
וְהִכְנִי בְּעִנָּרוֹן וּבְשִׁגָּעוֹן,
וּפָקַד עָלַי עֲוֹן נוֹב וְגִבְעוֹן,[2]
וְנַעֲשָׂה מִמָּעוֹן, מִשְׁמֶרֶת **בֵּית** כֹּהֵן **מָעוֹן**.

נִשְׁקַד עוֹל עָוֹן וְנִכְאָב,
כְּהוֹשַׁבְתִּי אֲנוּנָה מִבְּלִי אָב,
וְנִמְנַעְתִּי מִלְּצַפְצֵף בְּמִנִּים וְעֻגָב,
וְנָשְׂאָה עָלַי קִינָה, מִשְׁמֶרֶת **יֶשֶׁבְאָב.**∗

סֶלָה אַבִּירֵי מוֹרֵי הוֹרָיָה,
וְלֹא נִזְכַּר לִי עֲקֵדַת מוֹרִיָּה,
וּמֶרֶב מֶרֶד וּמְרִיָּה,
הוּצַגָּה עֵרוֹם וְעֶרְיָה,[4] מִשְׁמֶרֶת **מַעֲדְיָה.**[3]

עַל גַּבִּי חָרְשׁוּ חוֹרְשִׁים וְהֶאֱרִיכוּ מַעֲנִית,[5]
וְהֵרִיקוּ עָלַי חֶרֶב וַחֲנִית,[6]
וְהִרְבֵּיתִי צוֹמוֹת וְתַעֲנִית,
וּמִצּוֹרַת תָּכְנִית,[7] יָצְאָה **יָוְנִית.**

פֶּרְשָׂה וְאֵין יָד שׁוֹלֵחַ,
כִּי לֹא הֶאֱמִינָה בְּהַשְׁכֵּם וְשָׁלוֹחַ,[8]
וְהָשְׁבַּתָּה בְּרִית מֶלַח,[9]
וְאֵין שֶׁמֶן מִמְלָח, בְּרֹאשׁ **מַמְלָח.**

צַדִּיק הוּא יהוה כִּי פִיהוּ מָרַת,[10]
וְעָרוּ עָרוּ עַד הַיְסוֹד בָּהּ[11] הוֹעֲרַת,
וּתְמוּר עֻזִּי וְזִמְרָת,[12]
קִינִים עָלֶיהָ נֶחֱרַת, וּבְקַצְוֵי אֶרֶץ נִזְרַת **נִצְרַת.**

---

(1) Cf. *Isaiah* 1:14. (2) See *I Samuel* 22:19. (3) Some editions read מַעֲרְיָה, *Maariah*. (4) Cf. *Hosea* 2:5.
(5) Cf. *Psalms* 129:3. (6) Cf. *Ezekiel* 28:7. (7) 43:11. (8) Cf. *Jeremiah* 25:4; 29:19. (9) Cf. *Leviticus* 2:13.
(10) Cf. *Eichah* 1:18. (11) Cf. *Psalms* 137:7. (12) *Exodus* 15:2.

ל *Not heavenward did [their] eye peer;*
[Their external piety was like] silverplate overlaid on earthenware.
And as [God's] admonition intensified, [their strength] waned.
The Kohanim of Safed were knocked down and captured.

מ *From on high He sounded [the cry],*
   'I am exhausted from carrying [the burden of your sins].'[1]
Then He afflicted me with blindness and madness.
He visited upon me the iniquity
   of [the massacre] of Nob and Gibeon,[2]
and the watch from Beis Ma'on departed from the Temple.

נ *The burden of my iniquities has accumulated and causes me pain.*
When I was forced to sit like a mourning daughter,
   without [my] Father,
and I was silenced from playing the organ and flute,
the watch of Jeshebeab* raised a lament for me.

ס *He has trampled all of my heroes, the teachers of God's Law,*
And the [merit of Abraham's] binding [Isaac as an offering]
   on Mount Moriah was not recalled on my behalf;
Because of the enormity of my rebellion and insurrection,
the watch of Maadiah[3] *has been put on display, naked and bare.*[4]

ע *On my back the plowers plowed, they lengthened the furrow,*[5]
they bared sword and spear against me;[6]
so I have increased fasts and afflictions;
and the [watch of] Yevanis departed from
   the perfectly formed design [of the Temple].[7]

פ *She [Israel] spread [her hands in prayer],*
   but no [helping hand] was sent.
Because she did not believe [in God's prophets]
   who arose early and were sent [to admonish her].[8]
The [sacrificial service's] Covenant of Salt was discontinued,[9]
and the well-blended oil of anointment is no longer
   on the head [of the Kohen Gadol] from Mamlah.

צ *It is HASHEM Who is righteous for His utterance was disobeyed.*[10]
[Therefore the enemy cried,] 'Destroy! Destroy!
   Bare it to its very foundation!'[11]
Instead of singing, 'God is my might and my praise,'[12]
   laments were engraved for her,
and the watch of Nitzrath was scattered to the ends of the earth.

---

why was Hiram displeased? Because such wealthy people would not serve him properly (*Shabbos* 54a). According to the Talmud, Cabul was destroyed because there was strife among its citizens (*Yerushalmi Taanis* 4:5).

יְשָׁבְאָב — *Jeshebeab.* Although the *paytan* does not refer to any of the other watches by their Scriptural names as recorded in *I Chronicles* (24:7-18), in this case he makes an exception.

According to those who interpret the names used by the *paytan* as geographical locations (see the opening comment to this *kinnah*), it is not unreasonable to assume that this *mishmar* lived in a town that bore its name. Following the opinion that these names are allusions to the sins of the *Kohanim* (see ibid.), *Beis Levi* surmises that this *mishmar* was righteous in all its deeds. Thus, it was not given a pejorative nickname.

קָרָאתִי לְצוּרִי וְקוֹלִי לֹא עָרַב,

וְקוֹנַנְתִּי בַיַּעַר בַּעֶרֶב,

וְכָבָה נֵר הַדּוֹלֵק בְּמַעֲרָב,

וְרֵיחוֹ לֹא עָרַב, **מַאֲכָלָה עָרָב.**

רְאֵה כִּי הִסְעַרְתִּי כָאֳנִיָּה,

בְּתַאֲנִיָּה וַאֲנִיָּה,[1]

וּקְהָלִי כַצֹּאן לַטֶּבַח[2] מְנוּיָה,

וְנָעָה מֵחֲנוּיָה, **מִגְדַּל נוּנְיָה.**

שִׁמְעוּ כִּי נִזְהַמְתִּי בְּצַחֲנָה,

וְנִשְׂרְפָה דָּת מָרוֹם שְׁבוּיָה,[3]*

וְהוּשַׁתִּי לְשַׁמָּה וְעַרְבּוּבְיָה,

וּמֵהֶסְתֵּר חֲבוּיָה, נָדָה בֵּית **חוֹבְיָה.**

שִׁמְעוּ כִּי נִזְהַמְתִּי בְּצַחֲנָה,

וְסָתַם מֶנִּי תְחִנָּה,

וְלֹא נָתַן לִי רַחֲמִים וַחֲנִינָה,

וּמִקִּרְיַת חָנָה,[4] נָעָה **כְּפַר יוֹחֲנָה.**

תָּבֹא רָעַת שָׂמוּנִי הַדָּמִין,

וְשָׁתוּ שְׁעָרֵי שׁוֹמֵמִין,[5]

וְהֵשִׁיב אָחוֹר יָמִין,[6]

וּבַעֲוֹן פְּסִילִים נָעָה גִּנְּתוֹן **צַלְמִין.**

תָּבֹא תַמְרִיחַ, וְחָשְׁכִּי תַּזְרִיחַ,

וְכַדְּשָׁא עַצְמוֹתֵינוּ תַּפְרִיחַ,[7]

וְרֵיחַ נִיחוֹחֵינוּ כְּקֶדֶם תָּרִיחַ,

וּמִשֻּׁלְחָנָךְ תַּאֲרִיחַ, שׁוּלֵי **חֲמַת אָרִיחַ.**

(וַיְקוֹנֵן יִרְמְיָהוּ עַל יֹאשִׁיָּהוּ.)*

This view is borne out by the Talmud's statement (*Succah* 56b) that Bilgah, the *mishmar* following Jeshebeab, would arrive late (or not at all) when it was their week to serve in the Temple. At those times, the *Kohanim* of Jeshebeab would dutifully remain at their posts. For this, Bilgah's watch was punished (see ibid.) and Jeshebeab was rewarded.

דָּת מָרוֹם שְׁבוּיָה — *The Law captured from heaven.* During the forty-day period that Moses was atop Mount Sinai, he ascended to heaven to receive the Torah to bring it down to Israel. When the ministering angels complained to God that a mortal did not belong among them, He replied, 'He has ascended to take the Torah.'

The angels argued, 'This precious treasure, which was hidden away for the equivalent of 974 generations before the world was created, should not be given to mortal man.'

ק I called out to my Rock [of salvation], but my voice was not pleasing.
   I lamented in the Arabian forest,
      for the Western Lamp [which burnt wondrously
         in the Temple] was extinguished,
      and the fragrance [of the incense offered in the Temple
         by the watch] from Achalah Arav was not pleasing.

ר Behold, I am storm tossed like a [floundering] ship,
   moaning and mourning;[1]
   my congregation resembles a flock of sheep prepared for slaughter,[2]
   [the watch from] the Tower of Nuniyah was made
      to wander from Chanuyah [in Jerusalem].

ש [When] they heard that I went forth into captivity,
   the Law captured from heaven[3]* was burnt.
   I was placed in abandonment and chaos,
      and [the watch] from Hoviah was exiled from [the Temple]
         where God's concealed Presence was once hidden.

ש They heard that I was befouled by the stench [of my sins],
   and that [God] had sealed [the gates of prayer] to my supplication,
   and bestowed upon me neither compassion nor grace.
   So [the watch] from the village of Yohanah was made to wander
      from [Jerusalem,] the City of [David's] encampment.[4]

ת May evil befall those who cut my limbs to pieces,
   and desolated my gateways;[5]
   [God] has now withdrawn His right hand,[6]
   and for the iniquity of idols, [the watch from]
      Ginthon-tzalmin was made to wander.

ת O come and spread soothing balm [on my wounds]
      and illuminate my darkness,
   and let our [dry] bones blossom forth as verdure.[7]
   Accept graciously the fragrance of our pleasing offerings
      as in days of yore;
   and offer [the] final [watch] from Hamath-Ariach
      hospitality at your Altar-table.
(And Jeremiah lamented over Josiah.)*

---

(1) Eichah 2:5. (2) Cf. Jeremiah 12:3. (3) Cf. Psalms 68:19. (4) Cf. Isaiah 29:1.
(5) Cf. Eichah 1:4. (6) Cf. 2:3. (7) Cf. Isaiah 66:14.

God then summoned Moses to counter the arguments of the angels. Moses reasoned with them, 'Angels do not need the Torah. You have no parents to honor, no possibility of conforming to the requirements of kashrus, and no Egyptian bondage to remember.'

The holy angels admitted the truth of Moses' words and consented to allow the Torah out of the heavenly domain, for they realized that its precepts apply only to man and to his world (Shabbos 88b).

Since the angels sought to keep the Torah captive in the heavens until Moses captured it for mankind by his convincing arguments, the paytan describes the Torah as 'captured from heaven.'

וַיְקוֹנֵן ... יֹאשִׁיָּהוּ — And Jeremiah lamented over Josiah. Although this verse is printed at the end of this kinnah in many editions, the consensus of the commentators considers it a mistake. It is really the opening verse of the next kinnah, and that is how it appears in most early editions.

יא.

וַיְקוֹנֵן יִרְמְיָהוּ עַל יֹאשִׁיָהוּ.*¹

אֵיכָה אֵלִי* קוֹנֵנוּ מֵאֵלָיו,
בֶּן שְׁמוֹנֶה שָׁנָה הֵחֵל לִדְרֹשׁ מֵאֱלֹהָיו,*²
בְּנֵי חָם* בְּעָבְרָם חָנוּ עָלָיו,
וְלֹא הִזְכַּר לוֹ שְׁגוּיֵי מִפְעָלָיו.

גַּם בְּכָל מַלְכֵי יִשְׂרָאֵל אֲשֶׁר קָמוּ לְגָדוֹר,
לֹא קָם כָּמוֹהוּ מִימוֹת אֲבִיגָדוֹר,*³
דָּבַק בּוֹ חֵטְא לֵיצָנֵי הַדּוֹר,
אֲשֶׁר קָמוּ אַחַר הַדֶּלֶת לִסְדּוֹר.⁴

וַיְקוֹנֵן יִרְמְיָהוּ עַל יֹאשִׁיָהוּ — *And Jeremiah lamented over Josiah.* This *kinnah* is the most important and authentic lament we recite on Tishah B'Av (except for the Book of *Eichah*) because its recitation was ordained by the prophet Jeremiah [Yirmeyahu] himself following the tragic death of King Josiah [Yoshiyahu]: *...And all of Judah and Jerusalem mourned over Yoshiyahu. And Yirmeyahu lamented over Yoshiyahu; and all of the male singers and the female singers have mentioned Yoshiyahu in their laments to this day and made them a statute in Israel, and behold, they are written in the Book of Lamentations* (II Chronicles 35:24,25).

Why was the death of Yoshiyahu considered a tragedy of such proportion that it must be remembered by *all* of Israel for *all* time? Because *never* in all of Jewish history was there a leader as great as this king who sparked a massive nationwide wave of *teshuvah*, repentance, which had such a positive effect on Israel that the First Temple was almost saved from doom and preserved for future generations — as Scripture states: *And like him there was no king before him who returned to HASHEM with all his heart and all his soul and with all his resources in accordance with all the Torah teachings of Moses, nor did anyone equal to him ever arise afterwards* (II Kings 23:25).

Yoshiyahu's grandfather, the notorious King Menashe, had fanatically dedicated the early years of his reign to a campaign of utterly stripping the Jewish people of every vestige of true faith in God. With single-minded devotion, Menashe planted idols in every corner of his kingdom, even in the Holy of Holies itself! Although Menashe repented in his later years, it was beyond his ability to rip out the bitter root of idolatry he had planted so deeply within the heart of the Jewish people.

Amon, Menashe's son, was an idolater who corrupted Judah for twenty-two years until he

was assassinated by his palace guards. His son Yoshiyahu was eight years old when he began his reign and he reigned thirty-one years in Jerusalem (II Kings 22:1).

So thoroughly had Yoshiyahu's predecessors eradicated the Torah's influence from the Jewish people that it appears that the king of the Jewish people *never saw a Sefer Torah* for the first eighteen years of his reign. In the eighteenth year, the *Kohen Gadol*, Hilkiah [Chilkiyahu, father of the prophet Yirmeyahu], began to make long overdue repairs on the Temple structure. In the course of this work, he discovered a Torah Scroll which had been hidden for generations — since the time of the wicked King Ahaz, father of Hezekiah [Chizkiyahu] and grandfather of Menashe (*Metzudas David*). Chilkiyahu was shocked when he opened the Scroll to the תוֹכֵחָה, *Admonition,* recorded in *Deuteronomy* (chs. 27 and 28), *HASHEM will carry off [to captivity] both you and the king whom you shall raise over yourself, to a nation which neither you nor your fathers have known* (*Deut.* 28:36); and, אָרוּר אֲשֶׁר לֹא-יָקִים אֶת דִּבְרֵי הַתּוֹרָה-הַזֹּאת לַעֲשׂוֹת אוֹתָם, *Cursed be he who does not uphold all the words of this Torah, to fulfill them* (*Deut.* 27:26). When King Yoshiyahu heard this, he was so shaken that he ripped his clothing (II *Chron.* 34:19) in anguish over all the years he had neglected the Torah out of sheer ignorance. Then he cried out, עָלֵינוּ לְהָקִים, *It is incumbent upon us to uphold [the Torah]!* (*Yerushalmi Sotah* 5:4; *Midrash HaGadol, Devarim* 27:26).

Yoshiyahu swiftly convened a massive assembly of all the leaders and elders of Judah and Jerusalem and read to them from this new-found treasure, the Torah Scroll. Together, they entered a solemn covenant to keep all the teachings of the Torah with all their heart and soul. Yoshiyahu appointed agents to search out and destroy every vestige of idolatry in the land. They were successful in eradicating every *apparent* heathen

11.

'And Jeremiah lamented over Josiah.' [1]*

א *Arouse the lament of 'Eichah'* for one of the mightiest [kings],*
   who after eight years began to search for His God. [2]*

ב *Yet when the sons of Ham* passed through and encamped against him,*
   none of his meritorious deeds were recalled [to stand] in his favor.

ג *Also, of all the kings who arose to defend [against idolatry],*
   no one like him arose since the days of Avigdor [Moses]. [3]*

ד *The sin of that generation's scorners clung to him —*
   those who stood [idols] behind the door. [4]

---

(1) *II Chronicles* 35:25. (2) Cf. 34:3. (3) Cf. *II Kings* 23:25. (4) Cf. *Isaiah* 57:8.

image and the vast majority of people did join in Yoshiyahu's penitence, but a stubborn minority persisted in the pagan beliefs that had taken such firm root over the generations. They invented an ingenious method for concealing their idols. They split their doors in two and they split their idols in two, down the middle. They attached one half of the idol to each half door in such a way that when the doors were closed the two idol halves came together to be whole, but when the doors were opened the idol was split in half and each piece was concealed behind the open door. When Yoshiyahu's detectives came to search for idols they opened the doors and found nothing (*Eichah Rabbah* 1:18). This *kinnah* laments that these surreptitious idolaters undermined all of Yoshiyahu's efforts to purify Israel.

In the last year of Yoshiyahu's reign, Pharaoh Necho, the king of Egypt, which is southwest of Israel, decided to wage war against Assyria which lies northeast of Israel. He asked Yoshiyahu for permission to march his troops through his land as this was the fastest and shortest route to Assyria. However, Yoshiyahu refused because God promised that when the Jewish people do His will, '... a sword will not pass through your land' (*Leviticus* 26:6). This means that the blessing of peace will be so pervasive that (a) foreign armies will not even attempt to use *Eretz Yisrael* en route to battle with a different country (*Sifra* and *Rashi* ibid.), and (b) the Jews will be so strong and meritorious that no army would be able to force its way through (see *Taanis* 22a,b).

Yirmeyahu the prophet sent word to Yoshiyahu to allow Pharaoh to pass through. He warned Yoshiyahu that his generation was not as righteous as he imagined and that there were still significant groups of secret idolaters. Tragically, Yoshiyahu, in his righteous zeal, refused to face reality and continued to entertain illusions of total perfection for the Jewish people. He ignored the prophet's harsh warning and instead sought advice from the prophetess Huldah whom he felt would see things in a more sympathetic light. This was a fatal mistake — to ignore the advice of the leading prophet of God and to accuse him of excessive harshness.

This *kinnah* describes King Yoshiyahu's tragic and untimely death when he went out to battle Pharaoh Necho to prevent him from crossing his territory. With his last breath, Yoshiyahu repented his sin against Yirmeyahu but it was too late. Not only was Yoshiyahu personally doomed, but the entire kingdom of Judah was now set on a course of irrevocable, ultimate destruction. Hence, the enormous tragedy of Yoshiyahu's death, because with him died the very last hope and opportunity to save the Temple and the Jewish people.

אֵיכָה אֶלִי — *The lament of 'Eichah.'* Specifically, this refers to the fourth chapter of the Book of *Eichah* which also begins with the word אֵיכָה. That elegy was originally pronounced over Yoshiyahu's death and is the *kinnah* referred to in the verse from *II Chronicles* that introduces this *kinnah* (*Rashi* to *Eichah* 4:1). For this reason the *paytan* begins each line of this *kinnah* with the first word of the corresponding verse in *Eichah* 4.

בֶּן שְׁמוֹנֶה שָׁנָה הֵחֵל לִדְרוֹשׁ מֵאֱלֹהָיו — *Who after eight years* [lit., *at eight years old*] *began to search for His God.* Actually, it was Yoshiyahu's reign that began when he was eight years old. And it was in the eighth year of his reign (when he was sixteen years old) that Yoshiyahu felt the first stirrings of *teshuvah* in his heart and *began to search for the God of David*, his ancestor (*II Chronicles* 34:3, see *Malbim*). Nevertheless, since a newly crowned king is considered like a new-born baby (see *Yoma* 22b), the *paytan* refers to Yoshiyahu in the eighth year of his reign as an eight-year-old.

בְּנֵי חָם — *The sons of Ham.* This refers to Pharaoh Necho (see above) of Egypt. מִצְרַיִם, *Mitzrayim*, the progenitor of Egypt was a son of חָם, *Ham*, the son of Noah (see *Genesis* 10:6).

אֲבִיגְדוֹר — *Avigdor [Moses].* The Talmud (*Megillah* 13a) and Midrash (*Vayikra Rabbah* 1:3) record ten names by which Moses was known: Moshe, Toviah, Yered, Avi Gedor (or Avigdor), Chaver, Avi Socho, Yekusiel, Avi Zanoach, Shemayah and Nesanel (see *I Chronicles* 4:18, 24:6).

הָאוֹכְלִים זֶרַע שִׁיחוֹר,

כִּתְּמוּ הַטּוֹב פְּחֲמוֹ מִשָּׁחוֹר,

וַיִּגְדַּל עָוֹן וְהֵשִׁיב יָמִין אָחוֹר,[1]

וְעוֹד לֹא שָׁלַח יָדוֹ מִן הֶחָוֹר.[2]

זַכּוּ אֲמָרָיו כְּנָם דַּת לְהָקִים,

בְּצַע אִמְרָתוֹ[3] בְּאָרוּר אֲשֶׁר לֹא יָקִים,[4]

חָשַׁךְ תָּאֳרוֹ כְּנֶאֶצוּ רְחוֹקִים,

בְּבֶצַע מוֹאֲסֵי דַת וְחֻקִים.

טוֹבִים רָעִים[5] נִקְרְאוּ בְּשָׁלְחוֹ מַלְאָךְ,

מַה לִּי וָלָךְ הַיּוֹם לְתַלְאָךְ,[6]

יָדֵי עַם הָאָרֶץ דָּמִים בְּמַלְאָךְ,

תֵּעָנֵשׁ בְּבִצְעִי אֶת פְּנֵי פְלָאָךְ.

כָּלָה הֲמוֹנִי לֶכֶת אֲרַם נַהֲרַיִם,

לְמַעַן לֹא תַעֲבוֹר חֶרֶב[7] כָּל שֶׁהוּא בְּאֶפְרַיִם,

וְלֹא שָׁמַע לַחוֹזֶה לָשׁוּב אֲחוֹרַיִם,

כִּי גְזֵרָה נִגְזְרָה לְסַכְסֵךְ מִצְרַיִם בְּמִצְרָיִם.[8]*

מְחַטֵּאת סְתִירַת מְזוּזוֹת,

חֲזוֹן עֲנָתוֹתִי[9] הֶחֱלוּ לְבַזּוֹת,

נָעוּ עֲנָמִים לֵחוֹמוֹ לְהַבְזוֹת.

וְלֹא חֲסַב פָּנָיו[10] וְסָפְדוּ עַל זֹאת.*

סוּרוּ הֵעִידוּ עַד לֹא שְׁאִיָּה,

וַיְמָאֲנוּ סוּר וּמָט יְסוֹד* נְשִׁיָּה,

פְּנֵי קְרָב כְּקָרֵב וְלֹא עָלְתָה לּוֹ רְטִיָּה,[11]

וַיּוֹרוּ הַמּוֹרִים לַמֶּלֶךְ יֹאשִׁיָּה.[12]

עוֹדֶנּוּ עוֹצֶם עֵינָיו בְּגֵוָיו נוֹחֲצִים,

חֵץ אַחַר חֵץ מוֹרִים וְלוֹחֲצִים,

מִצְרַיִם בְּמִצְרָיִם — *Egyptian . . . against Egyptian.* According to the prophecy of Isaiah (19:2), Egypt would be destroyed through internal strife as *I will cause Egyptian to contend against Egyptian; each man to wage battle against his*

brother and against his friend; city against city and kingdom against kingdom.

עַל זֹאת — 'For this . . .' Yirmeyahu bemoaned the death of Yoshiyahu with the words: עַל זֹאת . . ., *For this shall you all gird yourselves in*

ה   [Thus] those who ate the produce of the Nile
        darkened [Josiah's] handsome,
            glowing countenance blacker than charcoal.

ו   [As] iniquity increased, He withdrew His right hand;[1]
        and He has not yet returned His hand through the opening.[2]

ז   Pure were his words when he spoke of upholding the Law;
        and he carried out His decree,[3]
            'Cursed be he who upholds not [the Torah].'[4]

ח   His features darkened [in anger] when the estranged [Jews]
        were defiant [of God]; through the corruption
            of those who despised the Law and the statutes.

ט   The bad ones were called good[5] when he [Pharaoh Necho]
        sent a messenger [saying],
            'Why should you and I do battle today?'[6]

י   'You will be filling the hands of your countrymen with blood;
        and you will be punished [for preventing me] from
            fulfilling the desire of your miracle worker [God].'

כ   [But] he [Josiah] stopped his [Pharaoh's] hordes
        from marching to Mesopotamia, so that
            not even one sword would pass through[7] Ephraim.

ל   He failed to heed the seer [Jeremiah] who said to turn back,
        for it was [divinely] decreed that Egyptian should
            contend against Egyptian.[8]*

מ   This resulted from the sin of concealing [idols behind] the doorposts,
        when they began to scoff at [the prophecies of Jeremiah,]
            the seer from Anathoth.[9]

נ   The Anamite [Egyptians] moved onward to mutilate
        his [Josiah's] flesh; yet he did not turn his face [in retreat][10]
            and they eulogized him with, 'For this . . .'*

ס   'Turn back!' they warned him before the disaster would strike,
        but he refused to turn back, and [Josiah]
            the righteous foundation* of the world collapsed.

פ   When the vanguard of the battle lines approached,
        healing [salvation][11] was not available to him,
            when the archers shot at King Josiah.[12]

ע   While he was yet closing his eyes, they continued,
        swiftly shooting and driving arrow after arrow into his body.

---

(1) Cf. *Eichah* 2:3. (2) Cf. *Song of Songs* 5:4. (3) *Eichah* 2:17. (4) *Deuteronomy* 27:26. (5) Some editions read טוֹבִים רֵעִים נִקְרָאוּ, *They were called good friends.* (6) Cf. *II Chronicles* 35:21. (7) Cf. *Leviticus* 26:6. (8) Cf. *Isaiah* 19:2. (9) See *Jeremiah* 1:1. (10) Cf. *II Chronicles* 35:22. (11) Some editions read שְׁעִיָה which can mean either *salvation* or *prayer.* (12) Cf. *II Chronicles* 35:23; some editions read הַיֹּרִים (as in the Scriptural verse), rather than הַמּוֹרִים, but the meaning is the same.

sackloth, lament and wail, for HASHEM'*s burning anger has not turned from us* (*Jeremiah* 4:8).

יְסוֹד — *[Josiah] the [righteous] foundation.* The interpolations are based on the verse: וְצַדִּיק יְסוֹד

צָדְדוּהוּ וְשָׂמְוּהוּ כַּמַּטָּרָה לַחִצִּים,
וַיִּזְרְקוּ בוֹ שְׁלֹשׁ מֵאוֹת חִצִּים.[1]

קַלִּים[2] הָטּוּ אַחֲרָיו אֱזוֹן מוֹצָא פִּיהוּ,
וְעַד מִצְוֵי נֶפֶשׁ מַעֲשָׂיו הֵפִיהוּ,
רִוּחַ שְׂפָתָיו הִפְצָה מִפִּיהוּ,
צַדִּיק הוּא יהוה* כִּי מָרִיתִי פִיהוּ.[3]

שִׁישִׁי נוֹף* כִּי קִנֵּא זַעַם,
לְשַׁלֵּם שְׁאוֹנָם בַּעֲוֹן בִּצְעָם,[4]
תַּם כֶּתֶם הַטּוֹב עִם זוּ* בְּפִשְׁעָם,
וַיְקוֹנֵן עָלָיו כָּל אֵיכָה יוֹעַם.[5]

תָּם בְּמִקְרֶה אֶחָד* כּוֹס מְגִדוֹ לִשְׁתּוֹת,
בְּמוֹעֵד שְׁנַת הַשְּׁמִטָּה[6] כְּנֶגַע הַקָּהֵל לֵאתוֹת,
תָּלָה בְּעֶשְׂרִים וּשְׁתַּיִם* מֵהֲרוֹס שָׁתוֹת,
כִּי סָפְדוּ לוֹ אֵיכָה בְּעֶשְׂרִים וּשְׁתַּיִם אוֹתִיּוֹת.

אוֹתוֹת קִינוֹת* לְבָטֵה מְחוֹלִי,
עֵת כִּי שָׁכַחְתִּי מְחוֹלְלִי,[7]
זַמּוֹתִי כִּי לָעַד יַאֲהִילִי,
רָשַׁעְתִּי וְנָסַעְתִּי וְנָטַשׁ אָהֳלִי.

---

(1) Eichah Rabbah 1:53; cf. Sanhedrin 48b. (2) Cf. Isaiah 18:2. (3) Cf. Eichah 1:18; Eichah Rabbah 1:53. (4) Alternatively: Because God's fury has avenged, repaying [Israel's] multitudes for the sin of their corruption. (5) Eichah ch. 4. (6) Deuteronomy 31:10; see Sotah 41a. (7) Cf. Deuteronomy 32:18.

עוֹלָם, a righteous person is the foundation of the world (Proverbs 10:25; see Chagigah 12b).

צַדִּיק הוּא ה' . . . — 'It is HASHEM Who is righteous . . .' With three hundred well-aimed arrows, the Egyptians pierced Yoshiyahu's body like a sieve. As the king breathed his last, Yirmeyahu swiftly ran over to his side to catch the dying words of this great tzaddik. Yoshiyahu completely accepted the punishment that God had

meted out to him and realized that he deserved it. 'It is HASHEM Who is righteous, for I disobeyed His utterance — and I disobeyed the utterances of His representative, the prophet Yirmeyahu!' (Midrash Eichah 1:53).

נוֹף — Nof, an Egyptian city mentioned in Isaiah (19:13), Jeremiah (2:16 et al.) and Ezekiel (30:13,16) and usually identified with Memphis.

צ *They trapped him, made him a target for [their] arrows,*
   and shot three hundred arrows into him.[1]

ק *The swift-footed [emissary Jeremiah][2] inclined behind him,*
   to hear his [final] words;
   and until his soul was forced out of him,
   his deeds adorned him.

ר *The breath of his lips burst forth from his mouth,*
   'It is HASHEM Who is righteous,*
   for I have disobeyed His utterance.'[3]

ש *Rejoice [while you can], O Nof,**
   because [God's] fury shall avenge,
   repaying [your] hordes for the sin of their corruption.[4]

ת *The good, golden one [Joshiah] has died*
   because of this nation's* guilt,
   and [Jeremiah] lamented him: 'Alas, the gold is dimmed . . .'[5]

   [The righteous Josiah] died under the same circumstances
   [as the wicked Ahab],* when he drank the cup [of retribution]
   at Megiddo;
   it was the Festival [of Succos in a year following a] Sabbatical year[6]
   when the time of national assembly arrived.
   For twenty-two [years,* God] suspended
   the utter destruction of the Temple
   because they eulogized [Josiah with the lament of] 'Eichah,'
   [composed] in the order of the twenty-two letters
   [of the aleph-beis].

א-ל *My dance degenerated into signs of lament,**

ע *at the time I forgot my Creator;[7]*

ז *I expected that He would eternally shelter me,*

ר *but I was wicked and was forced to depart,*
   for my Tent was abandoned [by God].

עם זו — *This nation.* In the Song of the Sea, Israel is called עַם זוּ גָּאָלְתָּ, *'this nation' that You redeemed* (Exodus 15:13), and עַם זוּ קָנִיתָ, *'this nation' that You have acquired* (ibid. 15:16). Moreover, Isaiah (43:21) calls Israel, עַם זוּ יָצַרְתִּי לִי, *'this nation' which I have fashioned for Myself.* Based on these passages, the *paytanim* often refer to Israel as עַם זוּ, *this nation.*

בְּמִקְרֶה אֶחָד — *Under the same circumstances [as the wicked Ahab],* who also succumbed to an enemy archer's arrow on the battlefield (see I King 22:34-35).

בְּעֶשְׂרִים וּשְׁתַּיִם — *For twenty-two [years].* The calculation of these years is as follows: After the death of Yoshiyahu, his son Jehoahaz [Yehoachaz] reigned for three months, Jehoiakim [Yehoyakim] for eleven years, Jehoiachim [Yehoyachin] for three months and ten days, and the last king of Judah, Zedekiah [Zidkiyahu], for eleven years, for a total of twenty-two years, six months and ten days (Beis Levi).

אוֹתוֹת קִינוֹת — *Signs of lament.* The singular noun אוֹת can mean either *letter of the alphabet* or *sign.* Usually the plural אוֹתוֹת is used for *signs* and the plural אוֹתִיּוֹת for *letters.* But sometimes they are interchanged. Thus, some render this phrase *alphabetically arranged lamentations.*

יב.

אָהֳלִי אֲשֶׁר תָּאַבְתָּ עַד לֹא בְרֵאשִׁית*

עִם כִּסֵּא כָבוֹד לְצָרְפוֹ,*

לָמָּה לָנֶצַח¹ שֻׁדַּד בְּיַד שׁוֹדְדִים,

וְנִהְיֵיתָ כְּרוֹעָה בְּעֶטְיָה² וְרָעַשְׁתְּ וְרָגַנְתְּ,

וְעַתָּה מַה לִּי פֹה.³

אָהֳלִי אֲשֶׁר קוֹמַמְתָּ לְאֵיתָנֵי אָרֶץ,⁴

בְּחֶרְדַּת מִי אֵיפֹא,*⁵

לָמָּה לָנֶצַח צֻמַּת בְּיַד צָרִים,

וְנִהְיֵיתָ כְּצִפּוֹר בּוֹדֵד עַל גַּגּ⁶ מַר צוֹרֵחַ, מַה לִּידִידִי פֹה.⁷

אָהֳלִי אֲשֶׁר פַּצְתָּ לְמַעֲנוּ לְצִיר,

וְאַתָּה עֲמוֹד עֶמְדִי פֹה,⁸

לָמָּה לָנֶצַח עִרְעַר בְּיַד עֲרֵלִים,⁹

וְנִהְיֵיתָ כְּשׂוֹנֵא וְצָר,¹⁰ וְאַיֵּה אֲוַוי מוֹשַׁב פֹה.¹¹

אָהֳלִי אֲשֶׁר נָחִיתָ בְּעַנְנֵי הוֹד,

לְזֹאת אֲשֶׁר יֶשְׁנוֹ פֹה וְאֵינֶנּוּ פֹה,¹²

לָמָּה לָנֶצַח מוֹאָס בְּיַד מוֹרְדִים,

וְנִהְיֵיתָ כְּגִבּוֹר לֹא יוּכַל לְהוֹשִׁיעַ,¹³

מַה לְּךָ פֹה וּמִי לְךָ פֹה.¹⁴

אָהֳלִי אֲשֶׁר כֻּנַּנְתָּ מוּל מָכוֹן לְשִׁבְתֶּךָ*¹⁵

לַחוֹפֵף לְחַפּוֹ,

---

§§ אָהֳלִי — **My Tent.** Each stanza begins אָהֳלִי, *My Tent,* which variously alludes to either the *Mishkan* (Tabernacle) that accompanied Israel through the Wilderness for forty years, or to one or the other of the two Temples. According to Ibn Ezra (Eichah 2:4), the *Beis HaMikdash* is referred to as a tent, because just as when fire touches a tent, it begins to burn instantly, so did the *Beis HaMikdash* catch fire in an instant.

The *kinnah* is a series of triplets, each of which follows the same pattern: (a) The first line begins אָהֳלִי אֲשֶׁר, *My Tent that,* followed by a letter of the reverse alphabetical arrangement known as תַשְׁרַ"ק; and ends with the syllable פוֹ or פֹּה. (b) the second line begins לָמָּה לָנֶצַח, *why*

is it forever ..., followed by the next letter of תַשְׁרַ"ק; and ends with the syllable יָם-; (c) the third line begins וְנִהְיֵיתָ כְּ-, *And why have You become ...,* followed by a תַשְׁרַ"ק letter; (d) the second part of the line is a Scriptural passage that ends with the word פֹה or פֹּה.

The final stanza contains an acrostic of the author's name אֶלְעָזָר, *Elazar.*

עַד לֹא בְרֵאשִׁית — *Even before Creation* [lit., when there was no beginning]. The Talmud states that the *Beis HaMikdash* is one of seven things (or concepts) created before the world. The other six are: תּוֹרָה, *Torah;* תְּשׁוּבָה, *repentance;* גַּן עֵדֶן, *the Garden of Eden;* גֵּיהִנֹּם, *Hell;*

12.

ת My Tent,* that You yearned, even before Creation,*
    to align with Your [celestial] Throne of Glory,*
ש why is it forever[1] plundered by the hand of plunderers?
ר And why have You become like a shepherd veiled
    [in mourning over his lost flocks],[2]
  as You stormed and grumbled,   'And now, what have I here?'[3]

ק My Tent that You erected for the powerful [Patriarchs] of the Land,[4]
    with [Isaac's] shudder [when he wondered],
    'Who is this then [that will dare to destroy the Temple]?'[5]*
צ why is it forever slashed to pieces by tormentors?
  And why have You become like a lonely bird on a rooftop,[6]
  screeching bitterly,   'What is My beloved doing here?'[7]

פ My Tent that You spoke about to the emissary [Moses], saying,
    'You stand with me here [so I may teach you
    about the Tabernacle],'[8]
ע why is it forever stripped bare by the hand of the uncircumcised?[9]
ס And why have You become like an enemy and tormentor?[10]
                  What has become of [Your] desire
              that Your habitation be here [in Zion]?[11]

נ My Tent that You guided with clouds of splendor,
    for the sake of those who are here and for those who are not here,[12]
מ why is it forever made contemptuous by the hand of rebels?
ל And why have You become like a warrior unable to save,[13]
                    [while the enemy mocks,]
   'What have You here and whom have You here?'[14]

כ My Tent that You positioned as a foundation
    for Your [celestial] dwelling[15]* that hovers over it like a canopy,

---

(1) *Eichah* 5:20. (2) Cf. *Song of Songs* 1:7. (3) *Isaiah* 52:5. (4) Some editions read לְאֵיתָנֵי עוֹלָם,
the powerful of the world, or, *the powerful of yore*. (5) Cf. *Genesis* 27:33. (6) *Psalms* 102:8.
(7) Cf. *Jeremiah* 11:15. (8) Cf. *Deuteronomy* 5:28. (9) Some editions read עוֹבְדֵי כּוֹכָבִים, *star
worshipers*, some read נָכְרִים, *strangers*, and some read אוֹיְבִים, *enemies*. Obviously, the hand of
the censor has been at work here, and the whims of the various censors had to be adhered to
by the printing shops. (10) Cf. *Eichah* 2:5. (11) Cf. *Psalms* 132:13. (12) Cf. *Deuteronomy* 29:14.
(13) *Jeremiah* 14:9. (14) *Isaiah* 22:16. (15) Cf. *Exodus* 15:17.

כֵּסֵא הַכָּבוֹד, *God's Throne of Glory*; and שְׁמוֹ שֶׁל
מָשִׁיחַ, *the name of the Messiah* (*Pesachim* 54a;
Nedarim 39b).

עִם כִּסֵּא כָבוֹד לְצָרְפוֹ — *To align with Your
[celestial] Throne of Glory*. According to the
Midrash, the *Throne of Glory* in heaven is
directly above the *Beis HaMikdash* on earth
(*Mechilta* cited by *Rashi* to *Exodus* 15:17;
Targum to *Jeremiah* 17:12).

בְּחֶרְדַּת מִי אֵיפֹא — *With [Isaac's] shudder [when*

he wondered], 'Who is this then [that will dare
to destroy the Temple]?' According to the
paytan, Isaac did not tremble because Jacob had
pre-empted Esau's blessing. Rather, Isaac saw in
a prophetic vision that descendants of the one
standing before him would someday destroy the
Beis HaMikdash.

כּוֹנַנְתָּ מוּל מָכוֹן לְשִׁבְתֶּךָ — *That You positioned as a
foundation for Your [celestial] dwelling.* The
Midrash teaches that the celestial *Beis HaMikdash* is aligned with the terrestrial *Beis HaMik-*

לָמָה לָנֶצַח יוֹעָה בְּיַד יְהִירִים,

וְנִהְיֵיתָ כְּטָס בֶּחָלָל וְאֵין עוֹד נָבִיא,   וְנִמְתַּ הַאֵין פֹּה.[1]

אָהֳלִי אֲשֶׁר חָנִיתָ מֵאָז

בְּתָאָיו מִפֹּה וּמִפֹּה,[2]

לָמָה לָנֶצַח זֻנַּח בְּיַד זָרִים,

וְנִהְיֵיתָ כְּוָתִיק יוֹצֵא חוּצָה,   וְלֹא עָבַר פֹּה.

אָהֳלִי אֲשֶׁר הֵכַנְתָּ לְהַשְׁלִיךְ בּוֹ לְפָנֶיךָ

גּוֹרָל* פֹּה,[3]

לָמָה לָנֶצַח דּוּחָה בְּיַד דָּמִים,[4]

וְנִהְיֵיתָ כְּגֵר בָּאָרֶץ, וְנִמְתָּ   כִּי לֹא נָסוֹב עַד בּוֹאוּ פֹּה.[5]

אָהֳלִי אֲשֶׁר בַּעֲוֹן בִּצְעִי,

חָשְׁכוּ כּוֹכְבֵי נִשְׁפּוֹ,*[6]

לָמָּה לָנֶצַח אָפֵל בְּיַד אֵמוֹת,

וְנִהְיֵיתָ כְּאֹרֵחַ בַּמָּלוֹן,   וְעוֹד מִי לְךָ פֹּה.[7]

אָחוֹר וָקֶדֶם[8] מִפֹּה וּמִפֹּה,*

לְכָל דּוֹר וָדוֹר נוֹדַע קִצְפּוֹ וְחֶפּוֹ,

עַל מֶה מִכָּל אוֹם שָׁת עָלַי כַּפּוֹ,

זֹאת בַּעֲלִיל כִּי פִיד חָקוּק בְּכַפּוֹ,

רְפוּאָתִי בְּטוּחָה כִּי רֶגַע בְּאַפּוֹ,[9]

וְעַד עַתָּה אֵיכָה יָעִיב יָעֵיב בְּאַפּוֹ.[10]

---

(1) I Kings 22:7. (2) Cf. Ezekiel 40:21. (3) Cf. Joshua 18:6. (4) Some editions read either דּוֹמִים (see Rashi to Isaiah 21:11) or דּוֹמִים (a contraction of אֲדוֹמִים), both of which mean Edomites; some editions read אֲחֵרִים, others. Once again, the censors have left their stamp on this kinnah. (5) I Samuel 16:11. (6) Cf. Job 3:8. (7) Genesis 19:12. (8) Cf. Psalms 139:5. (9) 30:6. (10) Eichah 2:1.

---

dash (Tanchuma, Mishpatim 18, cited by Rashi to Exodus 28:17).

גּוֹרָל — Lots. Four times each day the Kohanim would assemble in the Beis HaMikdash. At those times lots would be drawn to determine who would perform the various aspects of the Altar service. The method by which the selec-

tions were made and the particular tasks assigned at each lottery are discussed in chapter two of tractate Yoma.

כּוֹכְבֵי נִשְׁפּוֹ — [Evening-]star-like luster. The word נֶשֶׁף alludes to brightness shining through the dark, and can mean both morning and evening (Pesachim 2b). The interpolation of

י   *why is it forever shoveled aside by the hand of the arrogant?*
ט   *And why have You become like [a bird] flying in an empty void?*
    And why is there no longer any prophet, as You have said,
                      'Is there no [prophet] here?' [1]

ח   *My Tent where You encamped since yore in the chambers*
    flanking this side and that, [2]
ז   *why is it forsaken forever [and left] in the hand of aliens?*
ו   *And why have You become like a brave veteran*
    who [suddenly] runs out [in terror],
                unable to return [to his place] here?

ה   *My Tent where You established the casting of lots**
    in Your Presence, [3]
ד   *why is it forever pushed into the hand of the bloodthirsty?* [4]
ג   *And why have You become like a foreigner in the land,*
    and announced
        that You would not return [to Your celestial Temple]
        until [Israel] returns here [to terrestrial Jerusalem]? [5]

ב   *My Tent that, because of the sin of my avarice,*
    has had its [evening-]star-like luster* darkened, [6]
א   *why is it forever blackened at the hand of the nations?*
    And why have You become like a transient at an inn [begging],
        'Do you have anyplace else here [for me to rest]?' [7]

א   *After and before* [8] *[the Temple's destruction],*
    both this time and that,*
ל   *in each and every generation God's anger*
    and protective shelter are made known.
ע   *So why, of all nations,*
    has He pressed His [punishing] hand upon me?
ז   *This is evident, although my destruction is engraved on His Palm,*
ר   *nevertheless, my healing is certain,*
    for His anger is but for a moment. [9]
           Still, [I wonder,] how has He clouded me
           until now in His anger? [10]

'evening' into the translation is thus arbitrary and could just as well read 'morning.' The meaning remains unchanged.

אָחוֹר וָקֶדֶם מִפֹּה וּמִפֹּה — *After and before . . . both this time and that.* The translation of this phrase in a temporal sense follows *Matteh Levi* who understands it as an allusion to the generations following and preceding the Destruction. Alternatively, the phrase is spatial in meaning and is translated, *West and east, from here and from there* (see *Targum* to Isaiah 9:11 and Job 23:8).

יג.

אֵי **כֹּה** אָמֶר כּוֹרֵת לְאָב בְּפֶצַח,

בִּבְרִית בֵּין הַבְּתָרִים **כֹּה** יִהְיֶה' לָנֶצַח,

וְהֵן עַתָּה בִּלְעוּ עֲצָמַי בְּרֶצַח,

לָמָה אֱלֹהִים זָנַחְתָּ לָנֶצַח.‏²

אֵי **כֹּה** גָּשׁ כְּשֶׂה לְעוֹלָה לִרְצוֹתֶךָ,

נֵלְכָה עַד **כֹּה**³ פִּתּוּ בְּעֵדוֹתֶיךָ,

וְהֵן עַתָּה דָּקְרוּ כְּפֶלַח רַעְיָתֶךָ,

יֶעְשַׁן אַפְּךָ בְּצֹאן מַרְעִיתֶךָ.‏²

אֵי **כֹּה** הַבְטָחַת עֲקֻדִים נְקֻדִּים⁴ בְּמַשּׂוּאוֹת,

אִם **כֹּה** יֹאמַר⁵ כֹּה יוֹחַשׁ אוֹת,

וְהֵן עַתָּה וְכֵחְתָּ עִיר מָלֵאָה תְּשׁוּאוֹת,⁶

הָרִימָה פְעָמֶיךָ לְמַשֻּׁאוֹת.‏⁷

אֵי **כֹּה** זָם וְהָרַג מִצְרִי בְּגַן נָעוּל⁸ בַּקְּדֶשׁ,

וַיִּפֶן **כֹּה** וָכֹה⁹ חָתַם בַּעֲדַת קֹדֶשׁ,

וְהֵן עַתָּה חֶלְקָם אָכַל חָדָשׁ,¹⁰

כָּל הֵרַע אוֹיֵב בַּקֹּדֶשׁ.‏⁷

---

(1) *Genesis* 15:5. (2) *Psalms* 74:1. (3) *Genesis* 22:5. (4) 31:11-13. (5) 31:8.
(6) Cf. *Isaiah* 22:2. (7) *Psalms* 74:3. (8) Cf. *Song of Songs* 4:12; see *Shemos Rabbah* 1:29.
(9) *Exodus* 2:12. (10) Cf. *Hosea* 5:7, see Rashi there.

‏אֵי כֹּה ... ‏ — *Where is [the merit of the word]* '*so.*' The Midrash teaches that the *mitzvah* of *Bircas Kohanim* (the Priestly Blessing), which is introduced with the word כֹּה, '*so*' *shall you bless the Children of Israel,* was given in the merit of the three Patriarchs, about each of whom Scripture uses the word כֹּה, so. Regarding Abraham it is written, כֹּה, *so shall your offspring be* (*Genesis* 15:5); about Isaac it is said, *I and the lad* [i.e., Isaac] *will go* כֹּה, *so far* [i.e., yonder] (ibid. 22:5); and of Jacob the Torah states, כֹּה, *so shall you say to the House of Jacob* (*Exodus* 19:3; *Bereishis Rabbah* 43:8).

When God utilizes the term כֹּה, He demonstrates an intense degree of הַשְׁגָּחָה פְּרָטִית, *Divine Providence,* and reveals manifest love for His Chosen People. This *kinnah* laments that all the merits of the Patriarchs, the *Kohanim,* and various other personages and events that Scripture describes with the word כֹּה, *so,* could not

prevent the Temple's destruction when Israel turned away from God's service, and God concealed His Presence from the nation.

The events recalled are: בְּרִית בֵּין הַבְּתָרִים, *the Covenant Between the Parts* (*Genesis* ch. 15); עֲקֵדַת יִצְחָק, *the offering of Isaac* (ibid., ch. 22); the dream in which Jacob was promised prosperity despite Laban's dishonesty in paying Jacob's wages (ibid. 31:1-16); Moses' killing an Egyptian taskmaster who had been beating a Jew (*Exodus* 2:11-12); Moses' encounter with God at the Burning Bush, where he was charged with redeeming the Israelite slaves from Egypt (ibid. 3:1-4:17); the Covenant of Circumcision and the *pesach* offering (ibid. 12:43-50); the Giving of the Torah at Mount Sinai (ibid. chs. 19-20); the Priestly Blessing (*Numbers* 6:22-27); Balaam's attempted curses that were transformed into blessings (ibid. chs. 22-24); the selection of the Tribe of Levi to minister in the

13.

א   *Where is [the merit of the word] 'so,'*[*]
     promised with a proclamation to [our] father [Abraham]
     at the Covenant Between the Parts,
     'So shall [your offspring] always be [as numerous as the stars]?'[1]
ב   *Behold now, how my bones are swallowed up murderously.*
     Why, O God, have you abandoned us
     [for what seems like an] eternity?[2]

ג   *Where is [the merit of the word] 'so,' [mentioned*
     when Abraham] approached [with his son] as with a sheep
     for a burnt offering to please You?
     They persuaded [the others to stay behind, saying],
     'We shall go so far,'[3] *[in order to fulfill] Your testimonies.*
ד   *Behold now, how Your beloved ones are speared like a piece of fruit.*
     Why does Your wrath smolder against the sheep of Your pasture?[2]

ה   *Where is [the merit of the word] 'so,' in the promise [to Jacob]*
     in the dark of night [when you promised him an abundance of]
     striped and spotted [sheep]?[4]
     When [Laban] would say,
     '[With sheep marked] so [I will reward you],'[5]
     so was the sign swiftly fulfilled.
ו   *Behold now, how You admonished [Jerusalem,]*
     the city once filled with a chorus of jubilation.[6]
     Lift Your footsteps to wreak [eternal] ruin[7]
     [upon the enemy who destroyed this holy city].

ז   *Where is [the merit of the word] 'so,' when [Moses]*
     intentionally killed an Egyptian [who was beating a Jew]
     in [view of the Israelites, who are like] a garden locked in[8]
     with holiness? He turned like so and like so,[9] *and the matter*
     [of the Egyptian's death] was kept sealed
     within the holy congregation [of Israel].
ח   *Behold now, how their portion was devoured in the month*
     [of tragedy, Av],[10] *when all of the enemy's wickedness*
     was wreaked in the Sanctuary.[7]

Sanctuary (ibid. 8:5-22); the conquest of Jericho (*Joshua* ch. 6); and the more than four hundred prophecies recorded in Scriptures that begin with the words כה אָמַר ה', *so said HASHEM.*

  The first line of each stanza begins אֵי כֹה, *Where is [the merit of the word] 'so,'* followed by the respective letter of the *aleph-beis.* The third line begins וְהֵן עַתָּה, *Behold now, how*

. . .,followed by the next letter of the alphabet. The last stitch of each stanza is taken from the first ten verses of psalm 74. The author of this *kinnah,* R' Elazar HaKalir (whose name, atypically, does not appear), draws upon the verses of this psalm to express Israel's bewilderment and confusion over the drastic change in their relationship with God, that brought about their ruination.

אִי כֹּה טוֹב* כְּשַׁלַּח גְּאוֹל עֲבָדֶיךָ,

כֹּה תֹאמַר¹ לְשַׁלַּח עַם לְעָבְדֶךָ,

וְהֵן עַתָּה יָשְׁבוּ בוֹגְדִים בְּבֵית וְעֵדֶיךָ,

שָׁאֲגוּ צוֹרְרֶיךָ בְּקֶרֶב מוֹעֲדֶיךָ.²

אִי כֹּה בְּרִיתוֹת חֲדָשׁוֹת בְּרִיתוֹת,*

בְּכֹה אָמַר כַּחֲצוֹת לַיְלָה בְּמוֹפְתֵי אוֹתוֹת,³

וְהֵן עַתָּה לְהָקוּ בְּנַעֲלֵיהֶם לְאֹתוֹת,

שָׂמוּ אוֹתוֹתָם אוֹתוֹת.*²

אִי כֹּה מִשְׁמַע וּמֹשֶׁה עָלָה,

כֹּה תֹאמַר⁴ לְנָוַת בַּיִת מֶעְלָה,

וְהֵן עַתָּה נַאֲסוּהָ בְּנֵי עַוְלָה,

יֻנַּע כְּמֵבִיא לְמֶעְלָה.⁵

אִי כֹּה שִׂיחַ שִׁשִּׁים אוֹתִיּוֹת הַקְּדוּמוֹת,*

כֹּה תְבָרְכוּ⁶ לְשִׁשִּׁים גִּבּוֹרִים⁷ דוֹמוֹת,

וְהֵן עַתָּה עָתְקוּ רְדוּמוֹת,

בְּסֻכָּךְ עֵץ קַרְדֻּמּוֹת.*⁵

---

(1) *Exodus* 3:14. (2) *Psalms* 74:4. (3) *Exodus* 11:4. (4) 19:3. (5) *Psalms* 74:5; some editions read, וְהֵן עַד עַתָּה לֹא שָׁבוּ בְּנֵי גוֹלָה, *Behold how, until now, the exiles have not returned*, but this fits neither the alphabetic nor the repetitive aspects of the *kinnah*. It may be the result of a censor's whim. (6) *Numbers* 6:23. (7) Cf. *Song of Songs* 3:7.

טוב — *Tov[iah, Moses]*. Expounding on the verse that describes the birth of Moses, *And she [Yocheved] saw that he [her newborn son] was* טוֹב, *good* (*Exodus* 2:2), the Talmud explains that she named him טוּבִיָּה, which means *God is good* (*Sotah* 12a). Pharaoh's daughter named him מֹשֶׁה, *Moses*, three months later when she drew him out of the waters of the Nile (*Exodus* 2:10).

[Although popularly pronounced as if it were spelled טוּבְיָה, *Tuvyah*, lit., *goodness of God*, the proper vowelization of this name is טוּבִיָּה (see for example, *Zechariah* 6:10 and *Ezra* 2:60).]

בְּרִיתוֹת חֲדָשׁוֹת בְּרִיתוֹת — *When new [blood-] covenants were sealed*. When the Israelites were to be set free from Egyptian slavery, they had no merits by which to be redeemed. So God gave them the *mitzvah* of the *pesach* offering, but forbade the uncircumcised from partaking of it (*Exodus* 12:44,48). Since most of them had not been circumcised in Egypt, they had to submit to the covenant of *milah* before they could offer the *pesach*. Then the blood of the *milah* and the blood of the offerings mingled. And it was in the merit of these two blood-related *mitzvos* that the nation was redeemed (*Shemos Rabbah* 19:5). The *paytan* refers to these *mitzvos* as 'new covenants,' since one, the *pesach*, was indeed new, and the other, *milah*, had fallen into disuse and was then renewed.

שָׂמוּ אוֹתוֹתָם אוֹתוֹת — *They have made their signs for signs*. These words refer to the destruction of the First *Beis HaMikdash* at the hands of Nebuchadnezzar. He received heavenly signs which were meant to encourage his assault on Jerusalem and he was wise enough to pay heed to those messages. Thus *they* [the attackers] *made their* [Heaven-sent] *signs for* [meaningful] *signs*.

Nebuchadnezzar had not been sure whether to attack Israel or Ammon, so he had consulted seers, who foretold victory over Israel. He then shot arrows into the air, aimed in all directions. He observed that all of the arrows flew towards the south, in the direction of the Holy Land

ט *Where is [the merit of the word] 'so,' when Tov[iah, Moses]**
   was sent to redeem Your servants?
   [When You said,] 'So shall you say
   [unto the Children of Israel] [1]
   this nation must be sent out to serve You.

י *Behold now, how traitors occupy Your House of Meeting,*
   [as it is written,] Your enemies have roared
   amidst Your meeting place. [2]

כ *Where is [the merit of the word] 'so,' when new*
   [blood-]covenants were sealed*
   [when the Jews were redeemed from Egypt]?
   [Moses said,] 'So says [HASHEM]:
   About midnight [I shall go out among the Egyptians]
   with miraculous signs!' [3]

ל *Behold, now, how they have gathered to come into [the Temple]*
   in their shoes; They have made their signs for signs! [2]*

מ *Where is [the merit of the word] 'so,' which was heard*
   when Moses ascended [Mount Sinai
   and God told him to tell Israel],
   'So shall you say unto [the women,] [4]
   the distinguished homemakers?'

נ *Behold, now, how the sons of iniquity blaspheme Him*
   and it is regarded as an attack on [God] above. [5]

ס *Where is [the merit of the the word] 'so,' mentioned at*
   [the beginning of] the sixty-letter premier [benediction],*
   'So shall you bless' [6] *which is like sixty mighty warriors?'* [7]

ע *But, now, behold, the once slumbering [Babylonian Empire]*
   has reawakened [and ascended] to power
   and its axes are in the wooden thicket. [5]*

(Babylon is in the north). Thus assured, he confidently marched to Jerusalem (*Midrash Shocher Tov* 74:4).

Others interpret the passage as an allusion to the Destruction of the Second *Beis HaMikdash.* The Talmud describes how Titus entered the Temple, unsheathed his sword and stabbed the holy פָּרוֹכֶת, *curtain*, for he imagined that he could thereby cut God away from Israel. Blood began to flow from the curtain. Titus interpreted this as an אוֹת, *sign*, that he had slain God Himself (*Gittin* 56b). The blood was actually a Divine sign to Israel that God was 'suffering' over their tragic plight. Thus, *they* [the Romans] made אוֹתוֹתָם, *their signs* [the ones intended for encouraging Israel], for אוֹתוֹת, *signs* [for themselves and in their own favor] (*Sforno*).

שָׁשִׁים אוֹתִיּוֹת הַקְּרוּמוֹת — *The sixty-letter pre-*

mier [benediction]. בִּרְכַּת כֹּהֲנִים, *the Priestly Blessing*, contains exactly sixty letters. These are alluded to in the verse, *Behold the couch of the King of Peace, sixty of Israel's mightiest warriors surround it* (*Song of Songs* 3:7). Since all the blessings promised in the Torah are contingent upon Israel's fulfillment of the *mitzvos* (see, e.g., *Leviticus* 22:3-13 and *Deuteronomy* 28:1-14), while the Priestly Blessing is given with no conditions attached, it is called 'the premier benediction' (*Beis Levi*).

בְּסָבְךָ עֵץ קַרְדֻּמּוֹת — *Its axes are in the wooden thicket.* The Talmud (*Sanhedrin* 96b) relates that when the Babylonian multitudes laid siege to Jerusalem, King Nebuchadnezzar sent to his general Nebuzaradan three hundred mules laden with axes made of specially hardened iron which could smash through barriers of iron. At

אֵי כֹּה פָּץ לָקֹוב עָם וּבֵרַךְ עַם קְדוֹשֶׁיךָ,

בְּשׁוּב וְכֹה תְדַבֵּר' הוּמַר לִקְדוֹשֶׁיךָ,

וְהֵן עַתָּה צָרוּ עַל עִיר קָדְשֶׁךָ,

שִׁלְחוּ בָאֵשׁ מִקְדָּשֶׁיךָ.²

אֵי כֹּה קִיחַת לֵוִיִּם שְׁלֵמֶיךָ,

כֹּה תַעֲשֶׂה לָהֶם לְטַהֲרָם' לְבֵית עוֹלָמֶיךָ,

וְהֵן עַתָּה רָעֲשׁוּ וְהִרְעִישׁוּ שָׁמֶיךָ,

לָאָרֶץ חִלְּלוּ מִשְׁכַּן שְׁמֶךָ.²

אֵי כֹּה שִׁבְעַת שׁוֹפְרוֹת עָרֶץ,

כֹּה תַעֲשֶׂה שֵׁשֶׁת יָמִים' לְהַפִּיל חוֹמָה לָאָרֶץ,

וְהֵן עַתָּה שְׁעָרִים טָבְעוּ בָאָרֶץ,⁵

שָׂרְפוּ כָל מוֹעֲדֵי אֵל בָּאָרֶץ.⁶

אֵי כֹּה תְּשׁוּעוֹת אֲסָמֵי אוֹצָר,

בְּכֹה אָמַר אֲשֶׁר לַחוֹזִים נָצָר,⁷

וְהֵן עַתָּה תִּפְּחוּ פְרָחַי בַּחָצָר,

עַד מָתַי אֱלֹהִים יְחָרֶף צָר.⁸

---

(1) *Numbers* 23:5. (2) *Psalms* 74:7. (3) Cf. *Numbers* 8:7. (4) *Joshua* 6:3. (5) Cf. *Eichah* 2:9. (6) *Psalms* 74:8. (7) Some editions read אֲשֶׁר לַדּוֹרוֹת נָצָר, *designated for the generations.* (8) *Psalms* 74:10.

first the Babylonians were entirely unsuccessful and they wasted this entire stock of unique weapons on an assault on just one of Jerusalem's many gates, all to no avail; the axes shattered while the gate held firm. Nebuzaradan was completely demoralized and he wished to lift the siege and retreat, for he feared that he would meet the disastrous fate of Sennacherib whose vast army perished to a man when he besieged the Holy City. But a קוֹל בַּת, *heavenly voice,* resounded and said to Nebuzaradan: 'Don't be hasty. The moment has just arrived for the Temple to be destroyed and the Sanctuary to be consumed in fire.' Nebuzaradan had but one axe left in his arsenal. He threw it at the gate and it didn't even strike it with its metal head, but with its dull wooden handle, yet it smashed the iron gate wide open! This fulfilled King David's prophetic lamentation, '*It is regarded as an attack on [God] above, its axes are in the wooden*

פ *Where is [the merit of the word]* 'so,' *when*
  [the wicked Balaam] opened his mouth to curse —
  but instead blessed — Your holy nation?
  [You commanded Balaam,] 'Return
  [to Balak, the king who hired you]
  and **so** *shall you say,'*[1] *[that the curses were]*
  transformed [into blessings] for Your holy ones.

צ *Behold, now, how they have set upon Your holy city;*
  they have sent Your Sanctuary up in flames.[2]

ק *Where is [the merit of the word]* 'so,' *when the Levites,*
  Your perfect [attendants], were taken
  [into Your service with the words],
  *'***So** *you shall do unto them, to purify them'*[3]
  for your Eternal Temple?

ר *Behold, now, how they have stormed [the earthly Temple]*
  and thereby caused Your heaven[ly Temple] to tremble;
  to the ground have they desecrated the Abode of Your Name.[2]

ש *Where is [the merit of the word)* 'so,' *[when the Jews circled*
  the walls of Jericho and seven priests sounded]
  seven powerful ram's horns? [For You had said,]
  *'***So** *shall you do for six days,*[4] *to topple the wall to the ground.'*

ש *Behold, now, how the gates [of our Holy Temple]*
  have sunk into the ground;[5] *[and] they have burned*
  all of God's meeting places on earth.[6]

ת *Where is [the merit of the word]* 'so,'
  [which assured] salvation emanating from
  [the Holy Temple described as]
  the storehouse brimming with abundance.
  [The prophecies of future redemption which God]
  designated for His visionaries[7] *[all began with the words],*
  *'***So** *says [HASHEM].'*

ת *Behold, now, how my flower[-like children]*
  lie bloated [from starvation] in each courtyard.
  How long, O God, will the tormentor revile?[8]

---

thicket' (Psalms 74:5), i.e., this wondrous assault   tantamount to an attack on the celestial Temple
on the gates of the earthly Temple below was   Above (Rashi ibid.).

יד.

אֵיכָה* אֶת אֲשֶׁר כְּבָר עָשׂוּהוּ,¹
תָּבַע מֶנִּי לִגְבוֹת נְשִׁיֵּהוּ,
אֲשֶׁר עַד לֹא שְׁחָקִים נִמְתָּחוּ,
בְּשֶׁלִּי רָמַז הֱיוֹת אֶרֶץ תֹּהוּ.²

בֶּלַע בְּאוֹת עַרְבִית וְשַׁחֲרִית,³
גֵּאֶה מַגִּיד מֵרֵאשִׁית אַחֲרִית,⁴
בָּנוּי וְחָרֵב וּבָנוּי בְּאַחֲרִית,
וּמְחוֹבִי קַלְקָלָתוֹ הֶחֱרִית.

הֶחֱרִית אִישׁוֹן חֹשֶׁךְ מִידַּע,
וְקַדְמוֹנִים חָזֵהוּ מִגְדָּע,
אָז לְרָאשֵׁי דוֹרוֹת נְתוּצוֹ נוֹדַע,
עַד לֹא עֲשׂוּי קַרְנוֹתָיו גֻּדַּע.⁵

גֻּדַּע גֹּבַהּ קוֹמַת יְצִיר צָר,*
זֶה סֶפְרִי⁶ לְפָנָיו הוּבְצָר,
גָּלְמִי רָאוּ עֵינֶיךָ⁷ הֻפְצָר,
כְּהַעֲבִיר לְפָנָיו כָּל נֶעֱצָר.*

דֶּרֶךְ דֹּחַף מִבֵּית הָאוֹצָר,
וְהֶרְאָהוּ כִּי הַמַּצָּע קָצָר,*⁸

---

(1) *Ecclesiastes* 2:12. (2) *Genesis* 1:2. (3) Cf. 1:5. (4) *Isaiah* 46:10.
(5) *Eichah* 2:3. (6) *Genesis* 5:1. (7) *Psalms* 139:16. (8) Cf. *Isaiah* 28:20.

איכה ⊱— *Alas.* From the very beginning of Creation, God foresaw that the *Beis HaMikdash* would be built, destroyed, and rebuilt. Thus, the Torah states: בְּרֵאשִׁית בָּרָא אֱלֹהִים, *In the beginning God created* (*Genesis* 1:1), an allusion to building . . .; then, וְהָאָרֶץ הָיְתָה תֹהוּ וָבֹהוּ, *the earth was astonishingly empty* (1:2), a hint of destruction . . .; finally, וַיֹּאמֶר אֱלֹהִים יְהִי אוֹר, *God said, 'Let there be light'* (1:3), indicating a rebuilding (*Midrash Bereishis Rabbah* 2:5). This *kinnah* describes how all the Patriarchs and forebears of the Jewish people were privy to foreknowledge regarding the first two phases, but were not permitted to learn the secret of the third phase — the time of the End — when the Temple will be rebuilt.

R' Moshe Chaim Luzzatto explains in *Daas Tevunos* that God created the forces of evil in this world — and allows them to temporarily overpower the good — to provide the good with an opportunity to summon forth all of its latent inner strength and to ultimately obliterate evil. The triumph of the dark forces over those of light is always temporary, because the light is destined to burst out with hitherto untapped brilliance to ultimately wash away the stain of darkness. The Midrash (ibid.) concludes that the prophet Isaiah also had this idea in mind when he proclaimed: *Arise and shine, for your light has arrived, and the glory of* HASHEM *has dawned upon you. For, behold, darkness shall shroud the earth and deep gloom the nations, but* HASHEM *will dawn over you and His glory will be visible over you. And the nations shall walk by your shining light and kings by the brightness of your rising!* (*Isaiah* 60:1-3).

In the intricate tapestry of this *kinnah*, R' Elazar HaKalir wove together a triple *aleph-beis* and his signature (for the most part doubled). Each group of three stanzas is arranged in the following format: The first words of stanzas one and two are taken from the respective verses in

14.

א *Alas** — *that it has already been done;*[1]
   He [God] demanded payment of His debt from me.

א *For before the heavens had been spread out,*
   He alluded to my [Temple's Destruction in the verse],
   'And the earth was astonishingly empty.'[2]

ב *He intimated an omen [symbolizing the Destruction as]*
   evening and [the future rebuilding as] morning;[3]
   thus did the Glorious One announce the final outcome
   at the very beginning.[4]

ב *It would be built and destroyed and then rebuilt in the end,*
   yet it was because of my guilt that its ruination was inscribed.

   א *God inscribed [in the Torah] the blackness and dark*
      so that it would be known, and the ancient
      [Patriarchs and prophets] had visions of it
      having been cut down.

   א *From early times the leaders of the generations knew*
      that it would be shattered. Even before [the Temple]
      was completed, its dignity was already cut down
      [in the Divine design].[5]

ג *He cut down the towering stature of [Adam,]*
   the creature He had fashioned [with His own hands];*
   this very book [of generations of mankind][6]
   was revealed before him;

ג *additional proof [of this revelation is in the verse],*
   Your eyes saw my as yet unshaped future
   [and in your book all were recorded],'[7]
   as You passed before him all [the souls]
   stored [in heaven until their time to be born].*

ד *He had just stepped into the treasure house [of Eden]*
   when he was evicted. Thus God demonstrated to him
   that the couch is too short.[8]*

---

chapter two of *Eichah*; the next word and the
first word of line three begin with the same letter
as that word; the third stanzas of the respective
group contain a double acrostic of the author's
name, אֶלְעָזָר בִּירַבִּי קַלִּיר, *Elazar son of R' Kalir*;
the last word of the second stanza is repeated as
the first word of the third, and the last word of
the third is repeated as the first word of the
following stanza.

גָּרַע גֹּבַהּ קוֹמַת יְצִיר צָר — *He cut down the towering
stature of [Adam,] the creature He had fashioned
[with His own hands].* Before Adam sinned by
eating the forbidden fruit, He stood from the
earth to heaven (see *Chagigah* 12a). His spiritual
capacity was virtually limitless. There was no
facet of creation, from the most mundane to the
most sublime, that Adam did not encompass.
Nothing was hidden from him. More — no
one ever comprehended better than he how

each of his actions could determine the course of
creation. However, after Adam sinned, God
laid His hand upon him and diminished his
stature until he was able to hide *among the trees
of the Garden* (Genesis 3:8; *Bereishis Rabbah*
19:9).

כְּהַעֲבִיר לְפָנָיו כָּל נֶעֱצָר — *As You passed before
him all [the souls] stored [in heaven until their
time to be born].* Adam foresaw the fate of all
future generations, as Scripture relates: זֶה סֵפֶר
תּוֹלְדֹת אָדָם, *This is the account* [lit., *book*] *of the
descendants of Adam* (Genesis 5:1). The Talmud
(*Avodah Zarah* 5a) explains that this verse
implies that God showed Adam every generation
with its expositors, sages and leaders.

כִּי הַמַּצָּע קָצַר — *That the couch is too short,* i.e.,
when man arrogantly defies God there is no room
for both of them to dwell together, and man must

דָּוֶה לִבּוֹ כְּבָט בִּיאַת צָר,
וַיְקוֹנֵן עָלָיו אֵיכָה בְּאַיֶּכָּה* בְּעֵת צָר.

צוּר הֶרְאָה לוֹ מַה שֶּׁהָיָה,
נִתַּץ קִיר נָטוּי וְגֶדֶר הַדְּחוּיָה,²
לְדוֹרוֹת לְמֵד נְהוֹת נְהִי נִהְיָה,
עַל שֶׁבֶר אֲשֶׁר הָיָה.

הָיָה הַנּוֹעַר מִמִּזְרָח,³
בֵּין בְּתָרִים⁴ אוֹרוֹ כְּזָרַח,
וְהֶרְאָהוּ אַרְבַּע מַלְכִיּוֹת בְּרֶדֶם וְצָרַח,
כִּי טָבַע שַׁעַר הַמִּזְרָח.⁵

וַיַּחֲמוֹס וַיְנַצֵּל זֵרָה,
וַיַּרְא הַשְׁלָכַת נִזְרָה,*
וְאֵימָה נוֹפֶלֶת עָלָיו כְּבִדְזָרָה,⁶
וְצִדֵּק מִדַּת הַדִּין כְּאָז רָאָה.

רָאָה עֵרֹם וְעֶרְיָה⁷ וְנֶאֱנַח,
וְלַעֲקוּדוֹ סוֹד זֶה פִּעֲנַח,
עֲשָׂשָׂה מִכַּעַס עֵינוֹ⁸ וְלֹא נָח,
מֵרְאוֹת גְּזוֹעַ טוֹב זָנַח.⁹

זָנַח זֹהַר תָּם בַּמַּחֲזֶה,
כִּי לֹא הֶאֱמִין בִּנְאָם זֶה,
זָן עֵינוֹ בַּמָּקוֹם הַזֶּה,
וְשֵׁר שְׁמוּמוֹ וַיְקוֹנֵן אֵין זֶה.¹⁰

(1) Genesis 3:9. (2) Cf. Psalms 62:4. (3) Cf. Isaiah 41:2. (4) See Genesis 15. (5) Cf. Eichah 2:9. (6) Cf. Genesis 15:12. (7) Cf. Ezekiel 16:7. (8) Cf. Psalms 6:8. (9) Cf. Hosea 8:3. (10) Genesis 28:17.

be dismissed. Interestingly, this verse also alludes to the Destruction of the *Beis HaMikdash.* The Talmud (*Sanhedrin* 103b; *Yoma* 9b) relates that when the sinful King Menashe placed an idol in the Sanctuary, God said, 'The couch is too short to support a man and his two wives,' i.e., the *Beis HaMikdash,* in which God made His Presence rest, could not tolerate the rival, idolatrous worship. And so it was to be destroyed.

אֵיכָה בְּאַיֶּכָּה — *'Eichah! Alas!' [as alluded to] in . . . 'Where are you?'* When Adam and Eve tried to hide their nakedness after eating the forbidden fruit, God approached to admonish them with the word, 'אַיֶּכָּה, *Where are you?'* The *paytan* plays on the similarity between that word and the word, אֵיכָה, *alas.* Both words are spelled with the same letters and differ only in vowelization. Thus, they are taken as an allusion that the ultimate cause of the Destruction was Adam's initial sin. The commentators disagree regarding the speaker of the word אֵיכָה in this comparison. Either it was said by God after the actual Destruction, or it was spoken by Adam when he was shown the vision of the Destruction.

ד His [Adam's] heart ached upon foreseeing the entry
of the enemy [into the Temple]; and he lamented
in time of distress over [the destroyed Temple]
with the word, 'Eichah! Alas!' [as alluded to]
in [God's call to him], 'Where are you?'¹*

> ל [Similarly,] God showed [the enemy that
> the Destruction of the Temple was] an accomplished fact;
> thus, he [merely] smashed an already crumbled wall
> and an already toppled fence;²
>
> ל nevertheless, God taught all future generations
> to mourn the actual destruction with doleful lament
> over the Destruction when it actually happened.

ה [The Patriarch Abraham] was inspired to arise
from [Ur-kasdim in] the East,³ until his light shone forth
[in the Holy Land] at the Covenant Between the Parts.⁴

ה In his sleep, [God] showed [Abraham a vision of] the Four Kingdoms
[which would subjugate his descendants in exile], and he screamed
when the Eastern [Temple] Gate sank [into the earth].⁵

ו He ripped apart [the Temple] and confiscated her tiara.
[Abraham] saw the throwing-away of her crown;*

ו and he was seized with terror when [he saw his children] scattered.⁶
Nevertheless, he affirmed the righteousness of
the Divine Attribute of Strict Justice, despite all that he foresaw.

> ע He foresaw [his children exiled] bare and naked⁷
> and he groaned, and to his sacrificially bound [son Isaac]
> he revealed this secret [of the future exile];
>
> ע his eye dimmed with anguish⁸ and he could not rest, because
> he saw his offspring abandoned by the One Who is Good.⁹

ז The illustrious perfect [Patriarch Jacob] abandoned
what he saw in the vision [of Israel's future descent]
and would not believe this pronouncement;

ז but when his eyes totally absorbed [all that was destined
to transpire on] this place, he foresaw its desolation
and lamented, 'This cannot be!'¹⁰

זְרָה ... נוְרָה — *Her tiara ... her crown.* Some
commentators understand this as an allusion to
the three crowns spoken of in *Avos* (4:17). They
are the crowns of Torah scholarship, priesthood, and kingship. When the *Beis HaMikdash* was destroyed, Israel had to forfeit these
three crowns. This interpretation is difficult
because only two crowns are mentioned in the
kinnah.

Perhaps the *paytan* means to teach that although the crown of priesthood was lost with the

Destruction, and the crown of kingship was lost
with the Exile, the crown of Torah can never be
removed from the Jewish people, despite their
centuries-long homeless wandering through the
Diaspora.

Alternatively, this refers to the three 'crowned'
vessels in the Sanctuary: הָאָרוֹן, *the Ark,* in which
the Tablets of the Ten Commandments rested
(see *Exodus* 25:11); הַשֻּׁלְחָן, *the Table,* for the
Panim Loaves (ibid. 25:24); and הַמִּזְבֵּחַ, *the
Golden Altar,* upon which the Incense was

חָשַׁב חֲשׁוֹשׁ בְּעוֹלִים וְיוֹרְדִים,

וַיָּבֶן כִּי בוֹ יְהוּ רוֹדִים,

חֲנִיכָיו עַל מֶה בְּדִינוֹ חֲרֵדִים,

וּמֵהֶם תָּבַע זְבוּל מוֹרְדִים.

מוֹרְדִים זְבוּל וּמַצְפּוֹנָיו נִבְעוּ,[1]

וּמַסְמְרוֹת נְעָלֵימוֹ* בְּקַרְקָעִיתוֹ קָבְעוּ,

זִיו שְׁעָרָיו מֶנִּי מַה נִתְבָּעוּ,

וְהִנָּם טְמוּנִים בָּאָרֶץ כִּי טָבְעוּ.[2]

טָבְעוּ טוֹרְדִים לֵידַע זְמָן,

כִּי לְגַלּוֹת קֵץ אָב זְמָן,[3]

טוֹב מִשֶּׁגִּלָּה לוֹ קֵץ מְזֻמָּן,

הָשַׁע וְהִבְלִיג[4] וְקֵץ כָּמָן.

יָשְׁבוּ וְשָׁאֲלוּ לְאָב לֵידַע,

זְמַן קֵץ הַפְּלָאוֹת מָתַי יִתְוַדַּע,[5]

יָקַן לְיוֹם יְשׁוּעָה וְלֹא נוֹדַע,

עַד כִּי בְּעִתּוֹ יוּחַשׁ[6] וְיִתְוַדַּע.

יִתְוַדַּע רָז לְבָם נִסְתַּכְּלוּ,

וְנִכְסְתָה מֵהֶם וְלֹא יוּכְלוּ,

רֵעֶיךָ מִקִּנְאַת בֵּיתְךָ נֶאֱכָלוּ,[7]

וּבְיָגוֹן חַיֵּימוֹ כָּלוּ.[8]

כָּלוּ בְּסִלֵּי צִיר כְּשָׁלַח,

וְנָם שְׁלַח נָא בְּיַד תִּשְׁלָח,[9]

כִּי מַה בֶּצַע לִי לְהִשְׁתַּתְּלַח,

וְאַחֲרֵי גִלְעָדִי יִשְׁלַח.

לְאֻמּוֹתָם לִבָּם עוֹלְלֵי סוֹף,

אֵיזֶה יוֹם הַכָּסוּף,

offered (ibid. 30:3). The Talmud correlates: (a) the Altar's crown with the crown of priesthood that Aaron merited and took for his descendants; (b) the Table's crown with the crown of kingship (as in the expression, שֻׁלְחָן שֶׁל מְלָכִים, *a royal table*) that David merited and took for his offspring; and (c) the Ark's crown with the crown of Torah scholarship, but that crown is still available and whoever desires to wear it can attain it [through diligent study] (*Yoma* 72b).

ח He pondered and grew apprehensive about
[the angels] who ascended and descended [the celestial ladder],
for he understood [that the heathen nations would ascend to power
and then come down] to oppress [Israel].

ח O why does He [God] terrify His disciples [Israel]
with such retribution, then exact punishment from them
[for the Destruction of] the Temple by [the heathen] rebels?

י [Heathen] rebels stripped bare Your Temple
and its hidden [treasures],[1] they riddled the [Temple] floor
with their hob-nailed shoes.*

י Why were its shining gates demanded
[as punishment for my sins]? Behold them,
hidden in the earth for they have sunk.[2]

ט [Jacob's sons] probed deeply and exerted themselves
to discover the time [appointed for the final redemption],
and their father was on the verge of disclosing the End of Days].[3]

ט But He Who is Good after revealing the End [to Jacob],
turned it away [from him] and reinforced [this removal],[4]
thus He hid [knowledge of] the End.

י They sat and beseeched their father to inform [them]
when the inscrutable End would be disclosed;[5]

י they waited hopefully for the day of salvation,
but it will not be made known until its designated time,
or it will be made known earlier [if Israel has special merits].[6]

ר Their hearts sought to discover the secret [of the End],
but they were unable to for it was
absolutely concealed from them.

ר Your beloved ones [Israel] are consumed with vengeance
for [the Destruction of] Your House,[7]
and their lives are spent in sorrow.[8]

כ Spent were the hopes of the emissary [Moses] when he was sent forth
[and foresaw that the Jews would again be exiled], so he said,
'Send, please, through the agency of another messenger;[9]

כ for what is there for me to gain by being sent
[since the Jews will be exiled again anyway],
and after me [Elijah] the Gileadite will have to be sent
out [to announce the final redemption]?

ל The infants at the [Sea of] Reeds asked their mothers
with heartfelt sincerity, 'Which is that yearned-for day?'

---

(1) Cf. *Obadiah* 1:6. (2) Cf. *Eichah* 2:9. (3) See *Rashi* to *Genesis* 49:1. (4) Cf. *Psalms* 39:14.
(5) Cf. *Daniel* 12:6. (6) Cf. *Isaiah* 60:22. (7) Cf. *Psalms* 69:10. (8) Cf. 31:11. (9) *Exodus* 4:13.

וּמַסְמְרוֹת נַעֲלֵימוֹ — *With their hob-nailed shoes*. In   prohibited from wearing shoes while per-
the place so holy that the *Kohanim* were   forming the Temple Service, these brazen hea-

לָבָּם הֵכִין לְשׁוֹרֵר מְסוֹף,¹
יהוה יִמְלוֹךְ בִּזְרוֹעַ חָשׂוּף.²

חָשׂוּף זְרוֹעוֹ **בְּיַד** רָמָה,
וְנִגְלָה בִּימִין רוֹמֵמָה,³
בָּנִים כְּשָׂרוּ חֵמָה זְרוּמָה,
קָצְרָה נַפְשָׁם בְּגֵיא אֱדוֹם* לָדַעַת עַל מָה.

מַה מָּצָאתָ עַוְלָתָה בִּי,
כִּי בָגוֹד בָּגַדְתָּ בִּי,⁴
מִמִּדְבָּר הֲמַרְתָּ בִּי,⁵
וְעַד עַתָּה לֹא הֶאֱמַנְתָּ בִּי.

נְבִיאַיִךְ נָטְעֵי אֲבִיגְדוֹר,⁶
נִשְׁתַּבְּרוּ פְּרָצוֹת לִגְדוֹר,
נִגְלֵיתִי בְּיוֹם נָקָם⁷ לִסְדוֹר,
וְלֹא קִדְּשׁוּ פְּרִיצֵי הַדוֹר.

הַדּוֹר יָזְמוּ דְעַת סוֹד וְדָפְקוּ,
הִשְׁבַּעְתִּי אֶתְכֶם* שָׁמְעוּ וּפָקְקוּ,⁸
יַחַד כְּשָׁמְעָם כֵּן נִתְמַקְמְקוּ,
וְעַל כַּפַּיִם סָפְקוּ.

סָפְקוּ שָׂשׂוּ בָּאֵי הָאָרֶץ,
כְּנָפְלוּ בְּיָדָם מַלְכֵי אָרֶץ,
סָבְרוּ כִּי יִשְׁעָם יָרֶץ,
וְעַל יָדָם יִתְכּוֹנֵן מְשׂוֹשׂ כָּל הָאָרֶץ.⁹

פָּצוּ פִיהֶם חַג לַיָי בְּשִׁילֹה,¹⁰
דָּמוּ כִּי לָעַד יִהְיֶה שָׁם מוֹשָׁלוֹ,
פָּעֲלוּ שֶׁקֶר וְהֵשִׁילוֹ,
עַד כִּי יָבֹא שִׁילֹה.*¹¹

thens came tramping in with their nail-studded shoes.

הִשְׁבַּעְתִּי אֶתְכֶם — *I adjure you.* This phrase appears four times in *Song of Songs* (2:7, 3:5, 5:8, 8:4). According to the Midrash, God made Israel take four oaths: That it would not rebel against the sovereign governments; that it would not seek to hasten the End; that it would not reveal the Torah's mysteries to other nations; and that it would not attempt to ascend from the Diaspora by force (*Shir Rabbah* 2:7). When these

ל So He prepared their hearts to sing at the Sea of Reeds,[1]
'HASHEM shall reign, through [the power of] His uncovered arm!'[2]

ב His arm is uncovered and His hand is lifted on high,
and [His strength] is revealed through
[His] upraised right hand.[3]

ב When [His] sons witnessed [His] wrath streaming down,
their spirits were anxious, in the [exile of the] valley
of Edom, to know why [they were so severely punished].

מ [God responded,] 'What wrong did you find in Me
that caused you to defy Me?[4]

מ Since the Wilderness you have rebelled against Me[5]
and to this very day you still do not believe in Me!'

נ Your prophets, the plantings of Avigdor [Moses],[6]
[were sent,] but they were broken by the many breaches
[in Torah observance] that they had to mend.

נ I revealed Myself [to them and told them] to arrange
[prophecy regarding] a day of retribution,[7]
but the unbridled sinners of the generation
[did not heed their warnings and]
did not sanctify themselves [with repentance].

י [The Sages of every] generation desired to know the secret
[time of Messiah's advent] and pushed [to hasten] it,
but then they heard [God cry out], 'I adjure you,*
[O Israel, not to attempt to force the Messiah's arrival,]'[8]
and they sealed [their mouths].

י When they all heard this together, their [hearts] melted,
and they clapped their hands [in anguish].

ס But those who entered the Land [with Joshua] clapped for joy
when the kings of the land [of Canaan] fell into their hands;

ס because they hoped their Savior would show them favor,
and, that by their hand, [Jerusalem] the joy of all the earth[9]
would be established.

פ They opened their mouths and announced,
'A festival for HASHEM in Shiloh!'[10]
They imagined that His reign would continue there forever;

פ but they acted deceitfully, so they were thrown out
until the advent of Shiloh [the Messiah].[11]*

---

(1) See *Sotah* 30b. (2) Cf. *Isaiah* 52:10. (3) Cf. *Psalms* 118:16. (4) Cf. *Jeremiah* 5:11. (5) Cf. 2:11.
(6) See commentary to *kinnah* 11. (7) Cf. *Isaiah* 63:4. (8) *Song of Songs* 2:7; 3:5; 5:8; 8:4.
(9) *Psalms* 48:3. (10) Cf. *Judges* 21:19. (11) *Genesis* 49:10.

---

oaths were demanded of them, the people's
hearts melted in anguish.

שילה — *Shiloh [the Messiah.]* The Talmud states
four opinions regarding the Messiah's given

שִׁילֹה רָצָה כַּחַלָּה מֵעִסָּה,*

וְנִמְאַס כַּאֲשֶׁר בּוֹ נַעֲשָׂה,[1]

רְאוּ מַה עֶבְרָה עוֹשָׂה,

לְכֹל אֲשֶׁר חָפֵץ עָשָׂה.[2]

עָשָׂה עַמִּי אוֹת[3] בְּצִבְיוֹן,

וּלְעֻתּוֹ חָשׁ עֲלֵי קִשָּׁיוֹן,

עֻלַּפְתִּי כְּחָרֵב בְּצִיּוֹן,[4]

עַד אֲשֶׁר יוֹפִיעַ אֱלֹהִים מִצִּיּוֹן.[5]

צָעַק צִיּוֹן אֵיךְ נָתָן,

לָשׂוּם עָלַי גּוֹי אֵיתָן,[6]

צָהַל וְרָקַע עַל הַמִּפְתָּן,

וּבַחֲמָתוֹ חִתִּיתוֹ נָתָן.[7]

נָתָן בְּעִתּוֹתוֹ עֵת הוֹבִילַנִי רוֹקְמִי,

תַּרְתִּי לַעַד בָּהּ לְקוֹמְמִי,

בָּשְׁתִּי וְגַם נִכְלַמְתִּי[8] בֵּל בַּהֲקִימִי,

וּבָחֲרִי אַף נָם לִי קוּמִי.

קוּמִי קַשַׁבְתִּי בְּהַזְנָחָה,

קוּמִי וּלְכִי כִּי לֹא זֹאת הַמְּנוּחָה,[9]

קַצְתִּי בְחַיַּי[10] מֵאֲנָחָה,

וְהִגַּשְׁתִּי וְלֹא עָרְבָה מִנְחָה.[11]

רְאֵה רַע נַפְשִׁי זְנוּחָה,

מִשָּׁלוֹם וּמִשַׁלְוָה וּמֵהֲנָחָה,

רְטוּשָׁה בְּהֶרֶי נֶשֶׁף[12] זְנוּחָה,

גַּם שָׁם לֹא נָחָה.

נָחָה יָדוֹ בָּם וּבָהּ נִכְווּ,

אֲנוּשִׁים* עַל רֹאשָׁם כְּרָכְבוּ,[13]

---

name: מְנַחֵם, Menachem; שִׁילֹה, Shiloh; יִנּוֹן, Yinon; and חֲנִינָה, Chaninah (Sanhedrin 98b). It is noteworthy that the initial letters of these four names spell מָשִׁיחַ, Messiah.

שִׁילֹה רָצָה כְּחַלָּה מֵעִסָּה — He [God] showed favor to Shiloh, as if it were challah from the dough. Shiloh was the site of the first permanent Tabernacle. The paytan compares this to chal-

ר He [God] showed favor to Shiloh, as if it were challah
    from the dough,* but [later] abominated it
    because of what was committed there
    [by the officiating priests].[1]

ר Observe what sin accomplishes,
    with the One Who does Whatever He pleases.[2]

ע He offered me a sign [of hope][3] when He was pleased;
    but when the time called for it, He hastened [retribution]
    for [our] stubborn defiance.

ע I fell faint, as if from the dry heat of a parched land,[4]
    [not to be revived] until God appears from Zion.[5]

צ Zion cried out, 'How did [God] permit me
    to be dominated by a powerful nation[6]

צ that gleefully trampled on the [Temple's] threshold,
    and sowed terror in its fury?'[7]

    ב He Who fashioned me cast His awe
        [upon the heathen nations] when He brought me
        [into the land of Canaan] and I imagined that
        I would be established within it for eternity.

    ב But I was shamed and humiliated[8] when the idol of Bel
        was erected [inside the Temple]; and with angry fury
        He told me, 'Arise [and leave this land]!'

ק 'Arise!' is what I heard in abandonment,
    'Arise, and go forth! For this is not the resting place!'[9]

ק I have become disgusted with my life,[10]
    because of [my incessant] groaning,
    I approached [God with offerings]
    but my gift proved undesirable.[11]

ר Behold the sorry state of my forlorn spirit,
    bereft of peace, serenity and composure,

ר torn apart and forsaken in [Exile's] mountains of darkness,[12]
    and there too finding no rest.

    י [God] laid His hand [heavily] upon them [Israel]
        and they were burnt by it, as weaklings*
        rode over their heads.[13]

---

(1) See *I Samuel* 2:11 ff. (2) Cf. *Psalms* 115:3. (3) Cf. 86:17. (4) *Isaiah* 25:5.
(5) Cf. *Psalms* 50:2. (6) Cf. *Jeremiah* 5:15. (7) Cf. *Ezekiel* 32:26.
(8) *Jeremiah* 31:18. (9) Cf. *Micah* 2:10. (10) *Genesis* 27:46.
(11) Cf. *Malachi* 3:3-4. (12) Cf. *Jeremiah* 13:16. (13) Cf. *Psalms* 66:12.

---

lah, the first portion of dough separated from
each batch and presented to a *Kohen*.

אֲנוּשִׁים — *Weaklings*. The translation follows

Rashi (*Jeremiah* 17:9) who renders אָנֻשׁ as *sickly*.
According to *Targum* (ibid.) the word means
powerful. Some editions of *Kinnos* read אֱנוֹשִׁים,
frail mortals.

יָגְעוּ עַל נַהֲרוֹת בָּבֶל¹ כְּנִתְעַבְּבוּ,*
וּכְעוֹלְלוּ עוֹלְלֵי חוּצָה שָׁבְבוּ.²

שָׁבְבוּ שׁוֹבִים גּוֹיִם מַדְקִירִים,³
מִתְעוֹלְלִים בָּמוֹ כְּמוֹ בְקָרִים,
שֶׁהֵם יָזְבוּ מְדְקָרִים,⁴
וּמֵי פְרָת קְרָבֵימוֹ דּוֹקְרִים.*

תִּקְרָא תֶקֶף טֶבַח וּמֶסֶךְ לְמַבְקִירִים,
קִיר עֶרָה מְקַרְקְרִים,
וְכָל עַם וְלָשׁוֹן בָּם סוֹקְרִים,
וַעֲלֵיהֶם מְקוֹנְנִים בְּנֵי צִיּוֹן הַיְקָרִים.⁵

הַיְקָרִים קוֹל בְּרָמָה הִשְׁמִיעוּ לִבְכֹּה,⁶
לָמָה זֶה וְעַל מַה זֶה הֻקְרַנוּ כֹּה,
יַחַד זֶה אוֹמֵר בְּכֹה וְזֶה אוֹמֵר בְּכֹה,
רָגְנוּ לְהָמִיר לְשׁוֹן אֵיכָה בִּלְשׁוֹן אִי כֹה.⁷

יָגְעוּ עַל נַהֲרוֹת בָּבֶל כְּנִתְעַבְּבוּ — *They were worn
down when detained along the rivers of Babylon.*
When the Jewish captives arrived at the Euphrates River, Nebuchadnezzar and his retinue
were sailing leisurely on the river while being
entertained by musicians. The nobles of Israel
trudged by the river bank, naked and chained
together with heavy iron shackles. Nebuchadnezzar noticed them and asked of his attendants,

'Why are these captives allowed to walk with
noble, upright bearing? Is there no burden we
can place on them to bend them over?' The cruel
overseers filled huge casks with sand and placed
them on the captives' backs until they doubled
over from the weight. At that moment all the
Jews burst out in tears and their anguished cries
arose to the highest heavens (*Midrash Tehillim*
137).

 י *They were worn down when detained*
along the rivers of Babylon;[1]*
for they were repaid in kind for their deeds,
lying [asleep] out in the open.[2]

שׁ *The captors slept [peacefully], having stabbed*
their [Jewish captives'] bodies,[3]
treating them as if they were cattle.

שׁ *Now they pine away, stricken,*[4]
*while the waters of the Euphrates ulcerate their innards.**

ת *Summon forth, O Powerful One,*
the [day of] slaughter and the cup [of agony]
for those who repudiate You,
those who shattered the ruined wall,
while all nations and tongues [stood by and] watched;
for [only] the precious sons of Zion[5]
lamented over these [Jewish tragedies].

ק *The precious [Patriarchs] let a voice of weeping be heard on high,*[6]

ל *[crying,] 'Why is this? And why did it happen so?'*

י *In unison, one said, 'This is the reason,'*
and the other said, 'That is the reason.'

ר *but all lamented that they had been made*
to transform the expression, 'How?' into the expression,
'Where is [the Divine promise], "So [says HASHEM]'?'[7]

---

(1) *Psalms* 137:1. (2) Cf. *Eichah* 2:21. (3) Some editions read גְּוְיָם מַבְקִירִים, *having left their bodies to the elements.* (4) *Eichah* 4:9. (5) 4:2. (6) Cf. *Jeremiah* 31:14. (7) See commentary to *kinnah* 13.

Many editions read גָּעוּ, *they cried*, in place of יָגְעוּ, *they were worn down.* Both versions allude to the same Midrash. However, the format of the *kinnah* indicates that this verse should begin with the letter י.

וּמֵי פְרָת קָרְבִּימוֹ דוֹקְרִים — *While the waters of the Euphrates ulcerate their innards.* Why did the

Jews weep so bitterly by the river of Babylon? R' Yochanan taught that the Jews were entirely unaccustomed to the harsh, sharp nature of the waters of the Euphrates River, so it had a lethal effect on them. Far more Jews died as a result of drinking these foreign waters than fell to the sword of Nebuchadnezzar! (*Midrash Tehillim* 137).

טו.

אֵיכָה אַשְׁפָּתוֹ פָּתוּחַ כְּקֶבֶר,[1]
וְלִרְוֹדִי בְּאַף הוֹסִיף אָבֶר,
אֲנִי הַגֶּבֶר.

אֵיכָה אֶשָּׂא עֲוֹן הָג,
וְחָסַם פִּי מְפַלֵּל לַהַג,
אוֹתִי נָהַג.

אֵיכָה אֵץ זַעֲמוֹ לִשְׁפּוֹךְ,
הָכֵיל נִלְאֵיתִי וְנָם שְׁפוֹךְ,[2]
אַךְ בִּי יָשׁוּב יַהֲפוֹךְ.

זְכוֹר אֲפִיפָתִי בְּשָׁרָב,
וְנָם כִּי יִנָּטוּ צִלְלֵי עָרֶב,[3]
וְהֵבֵאתִי עֲלֵיכֶם חָרֶב.

בָּכֹה תִבְכֶּה בְּעֵת כֹּל חֲסָרַי,
וּכְעָזְבִי אֹרַח יִסָּרַי,[4]
בִּלָּה בְשָׂרִי וְעוֹרִי.

בִּלַּע בַּיִת לָרוֹם מְזַקֵּף,
וְכַבַּרְזֶל סְבִכַי נִקַּף,[5]
בָּנָה עָלַי וַיַּקַּף.

בְּנֵי בִטְנִי לֶאֱכוֹל[6] הִקְשִׁיבָנִי,
מִנִּי צָר אָחוֹר הֱשִׁיבָנִי,[7]
בְּמַחֲשַׁכִּים הוֹשִׁיבָנִי.

נַחֲלוֹתֵינוּ כְּנֻטְּשׁוּ בְּיַד לוֹחֵם,
נָם לֹא אָחוּס וְלֹא אֲרַחֵם,
בְּשִׁבְרִי לָכֶם מַטֵּה לָחֶם.

גֻּלְּתָה גְהוּצָה לַעֲטוֹת עֶדְיִי,
מֻחְפָּה לְגָלוּת בְּהִתְעַתְּדִי,
גָּדַר בַּעֲדִי.

אֵיכָה אַשְׁפָּתוֹ ‎‎§ — *Alas! For His arrow case.* The longest and most intricate of our Tishah B'Av recitations, this *kinnah* was composed by R' Elazar HaKalir, based on two Scriptural sources.

As explained in the Overview, the longest and the most sorrowful section of Jeremiah's *Eichah* is the third chapter which he composed after King Yehoyakim brazenly burnt the original

15.

א Alas! For His arrow case is open like a grave[1] [waiting for death],
and He has added a wing to my furious attacker.
I am the man [who has seen affliction by the rod of His anger].

א [God] said, 'Alas! How can I bear sin?'
Thus, my mouth was sealed from uttering prayer.
He has driven me [into unrelieved darkness].

א Alas! For He has rushed to pour out His wrath,
[saying,] 'I have tired of [exercising restraint]!'
And He said, 'Pour forth!'[2]
But only against me did He turn [His hand].

Remembering [how I sinned with the Golden Calf]
during my wandering in the parched Wilderness,
He said, 'The shadows of [Exiles's] evening shall be drawn out,[3]
and I will bring a sword against you [to avenge My covenant]!'

ב She [Zion] weeps and weeps, 'At the time I lost all,
and when I abandoned the [righteous] path of my admonition,[4]
He wore away my flesh and skin.'

ב He consumed the Temple which rose to lofty heights,
and with iron have my branches been pruned.[5]
He besieged and encircled me [with bitterness and travail].

ב He [Moses] informed me that [a time would come when]
I would be forced to eat the children of my womb.[6]
[And this occurred when] He caused us
to retreat before the oppressor,[7]
[and] He placed me in darkness [like the eternally dead].

When our heritage [the Temple] was abandoned
into the hand of the [enemy] soldier,
He said, 'I will neither pity nor show compassion [for you],
When I break the staff of bread for you!'

ג Exiled is she who cleansed herself [of sin in order]
to adorn herself with [spiritual] crowns [at Sinai].
From the bridal canopy she was destined to be exiled
[for serving the Golden Calf].
[She cries,] 'He has made a wall for me
[so that I cannot return to my land].'

---

(1) Cf. *Jeremiah* 5:16. (2) Cf. 6:11. (3) 6:4. (4) Cf. *Proverbs* 15:10.
(5) Cf. *Isaiah* 10:34. (6) Cf. *Deuteronomy* 28:53. (7) Cf. *Psalms* 44:11.

---

version of *Eichah*. That chapter vividly foretells the impending *Churban* in alphabetic sequence, using three verses for every letter of the Hebrew alphabet. Essential segments of all those verses are cited in this *kinnah*. The second major component of this lament is the *Tochachah* /

Admonition recorded in *Leviticus* (ch. 26), in which Moses graphically predicted the Destruction of the First Temple which came to pass in Jeremiah's day some nine hundred years later. *Ramban* in his commentary on the Torah (ibid.) demonstrates how each and every one of Moses'

גָּדַע גְּאוֹן נָדִיב וָשׁוֹעַ,
וְהֵשִׁיב יָמִין אָחוֹר מִלְּהוֹשִׁיעַ,
גַּם כִּי אֶזְעַק וַאֲשַׁוֵּעַ.

גַּם גָּבַר עָלַי פּוֹרְכִי,
וּבְנַאֲקִי סָתַם חֲרַכִּי,
גָּדַר דְּרָכַי.

יְתוֹמִים גְּרוּשִׁים מֵאֲחֻזּוֹת,
וְלֹא שָׁב אַפּוֹ בְּכָל זֹאת,[2]
וַאֲמַר אִם בְּזֹאת.

דַּרְכֵי דִין סָךְ לְהַאֲבִילִי,
וּלְגָלוֹת שֶׁשַׁךְ הוֹבִילִי,
דֹּב אֹרֵב הוּא לִי.

דֶּרֶךְ דּוֹחֵק עַל בָּמוֹתַי לְהִשְׁתָּרֵר,
שְׁעוּ מִנִּי בִּבְכִי אֲמָרֵר,[3]
דְּרָכַי סוֹרֵר.

דָּבַק דּוֹלְקִי וְצָדַנִי בְּרִשְׁתּוֹ,
עָלַי לִלְטוֹשׁ מַחֲרַשְׁתּוֹ,[4]
דָּרַךְ קַשְׁתּוֹ.

מֵימֵינוּ דָּלַח[5] וְנָם אֲשִׁימְכֶם,
גֵּיא גָלוּת אֲטִילְכֶם לְהַכְלִימְכֶם,
וְהָלַכְתִּי עִמָּכֶם.

הָיוּ הָה לְיוֹם בְּכִיּוֹתַי,
וְצָרֶבֶת אֵשׁ כְּוִיּוֹתַי,
הֵבִיא בְּכִלְיוֹתָי.

הָיָה הוֹלֵךְ לְפָנַי מַזְעִימִי,
וְכַעֲסִיס דָּמִי הִטְעִימִי,[6]
הָיִיתִי שְׂחוֹק לְכָל עַמִּי.

הָאוֹכְלִים הַקְדֵּשׁ פֶּסַח בְּלֵיל שִׁמּוּרִים,
הֶאֱכִילָם בְּכָפָן רָאשֵׁי חֲמוּרִים,[7]
הִשְׂבִּיעַנִי בַמְּרוֹרִים.

ג He cut down the pride of noble and chief,
  and turned His right hand back,[1] not to save,
  even as I would cry out and plead.

ג Even [when] those who broke my back overpowered me,
  and when I screamed [in prayer], He sealed
    the windows [of heaven to my pleas];
  He walled up my roads.

> [We were] like orphans banished from ancestral estates,
> yet, despite all this [suffering], His anger has not subsided,[2]
> rather He said, 'If in spite of this [you fail to hearken to Me
> . . .I will chastise you seven-fold for your sins]!'

ד He has filled with thorns the roads once jubilant [with pilgrims],
    to cause me to mourn. And He led me into
    the Babylonian exile [on these very same roads].
  He is [like] a lurking bear to me.

ד The attacker trampled on my neck to display his sovereignty.
  [Please] turn from me, that I may express
    [my] bitterness with weeping.[3]
  He has strewn my paths with thorns.

ד My pursuer caught up to me and snared me in his net,
  he honed his plow blade [as a weapon] against me;[4]
  he bent his bow [and set me as a target for his arrow].

> He muddied our waters[5] and said, 'I will devastate you!
> I will cast you into the valley of exile
>   to utterly degrade you.
> I will behave toward you [with a fury of indifference].'

ה There were [cries of] 'Ho' on the day of my weeping,
  [and the hot tears] scalded [my face] with a fiery blister.
  He shot [His arrows] into my vitals.

ה He who enraged me stood [arrogantly] in front of me,
  and he forced me to taste my own blood
    as if it were sweet nectar.[6]
  [Thus] have I become a laughingstock to all my people.

ה Those who would eat the sacred flesh of
    the Pesach offering on the guarded night,
  He fed donkey heads during famine.[7]
  He filled me with bitterness.

---

(1) Cf. *Eichah* 2:3. (2) Cf. *Isaiah* 5:25. (3) Cf. *Isaiah* 22:4. (4) *I Samuel* 13:20.
(5) *Ezekiel* 32:2. (6) Cf. *Isaiah* 49:26. (7) Cf. *II Kings* 6:25.

---

warnings came true when Israel's sins finally forced God to unleash His anger against them. Thus, after every three verses from the Book of *Eichah*, the kinnah cites the corresponding verse from the *Tochachah*.

In the complex format of this *kinnah*, each letter of the *aleph-beis* appears ten times in the following manner: The respective letter is represented by four three-line stanzas. The first word in stanza one of each four-stanza group is the

עַל צַוָּארֵנוּ הַשָּׁרִיג וְחָלָל שְׁכֶם,
וְנָם אֶפְקוֹד עַל עֲווֹנוֹתֵיכֶם,
וַאֲכַלְתֶּם בְּשַׂר בְּנֵיכֶם.

וַיֵּצֵא וְקַדְקֹד סָפַח[1] וְרָצַץ,
וְחִזַּק מוֹסְרַי בִּי וָאֶתְלוֹצֵץ,[2]
וַיִּגְרַס בֶּחָצָץ.

וַיַּחְמֹס וַיְנַצֵּל מֵעֶדְיִי[3] לְהַכְפִּישִׁי,
וּמִגְּבַהּ לִתְהוֹם הִרְפִּישִׁי,
וַתִּזְנַח מִשָּׁלוֹם נַפְשִׁי.

וַיִּגְדַּל וְכָבֵד נְאַק רְצָחַי,
וּבְקָדְקֳדִי עָלָה צְנָחַי,
וָאֹמַר אָבַד נִצְחִי.

מִצְרַיִם וְכוּשׁ שָׂח אֲשִׁיבְכֶם,[4]
וְאֶשְׁפּוֹטְכֶם כְּזִמּוֹתֵיכֶם,
וְהִשְׁמַדְתִּי אֶת בָּמוֹתֵיכֶם.

זָכְרָה זֹאת כִּי נִבְאַשׁ נִרְדִּי,
וּלְכַלֵּה פָץ מִכְּבוֹד רֵדִי,
זְכָר עָנְיִי וּמְרוּדִי.

זָנַח זְבוּל וְלֵב הִקְשִׁיחַ,
וּבְהִתְעַבְּרוֹ עִם מָשִׁיחַ,[5]
זָכוֹר תִּזְכּוֹר וְתָשִׁיחַ.[6]

זְכוּת זְקֵנַי וּפָעֳלָם אָבִיא,
כִּי בְכֵן פֶּרֶץ נְתִיבִי,
זֹאת אָשִׁיב אֶל לִבִּי.

אֲבוֹתֵינוּ זָעֲקוּ וְכָלוּ מִדְּבָה,
וְשָׂח עַל רָעָתֵנוּ כִּי רַבָּה,
וְנָתַתִּי אֶת עָרֵיכֶם חָרְבָּה.

חֵטְא חָז כִּי בְעָוֹן נִכְתַּמְנוּ,[7]
תְּמוּר כִּי בְּצִדְיוֹן נִזְהַמְנוּ,
חַסְדֵי יהוה כִּי לֹא תָמְנוּ.

He braided ropes [of our sins] upon our necks
and crippled our shoulder[-like Temple], for He said,
'I shall visit [upon you] retribution for your iniquities!
And you shall eat the flesh of your sons.'

ו *And He went forth afflicting and smashing heads with leprosy,[1]*
and it was smashed and He tightened my bonds,
because I scorned [the admonitions of His prophets],[2]
He ground my teeth on gravel.

ו *He pillaged [the Holy Temple] and stripped me of*
my [spiritual] adornments,[3] covering me with dust,
[He lowered me] from the loftiest heights to
[muddy me in] the depths.
My soul despaired of having peace.

ו *The cry of my murdered one grew louder and stronger,*
until my scream reverberated in my skull
And I said, 'Gone is my strength!'

'To Egypt and to Kush,' said God, 'shall I return you;[4]
and I shall judge you in accordance with your scheming;
And I shall destroy your high altars.'

ו *He [God] remembered when [my sin with*
the Golden Calf] purified my nard.
Therefore He told the bride, "Descend from [your place of] honor!'
O remember my afflictions and my sorrow.

ו *He abandoned His Temple and stiffened His heart,*
[because] of His anger with the anointed one [King Josiah].[5]
[My soul] remembers well, and makes me despondent.[6]

ו *I shall bring My ancestors' merit and*
their achievement [to God's attention],
because my path was justly breached [due to my iniquity].
This I bear in mind [therefore I still hope].

Our forefathers cried and were annihilated
because of the [spies'] slander;
and when our wickedness multiplied, [He proclaimed,]
'I shall lay waste to your cities.'

ח *He saw sin [within me], for I was stained by iniquity;[7]*
for we filthied ourselves in the Wilderness,
exchanging [God for the Golden Calf].
[Yet,] HASHEM's kindness surely has not ended.

---

(1) Cf. *Isaiah* 3:17. (2) Cf. 28:22. (3) Cf. *Exodus* 33:6. (4) Cf. *Deuteronomy* 28:68.
(5) See commentary to *kinnah* 11. (6) *Eichah* 3:20; as evidenced by the rhyme scheme,
the *paytan* used the כְּתִיב, *Masoretic spelling*, in place of the קְרִי, *Masoretic pronunciation*
(וְתָשִׁיחַ instead of וְתָשׂוֹחַ or וְתָשׁוּחַ); nevertheless, most editions read וְתָשׂוּחַ. (7) Cf. *Jeremiah* 2:22.

---

first word of the corresponding verse in chapter   same letter of the alphabet. Stanza two follows
one of *Eichah*; the next word begins with the   the same format but the first word is from

חָשַׁב חוֹרְשֵׁי לְקַרְקֵר (קִיר)¹ יְקָרִים,

וְמַר יְבְכָּיוּן² מַכְתֵי סוֹקְרִים,

חֲרָשִׁים לַבְּקָרִים.

חָשַׁךְ חֶזְוֹן מַגִּישֵׁי אִשָּׁי,

קִיר כְּעוּר לְגַשְּׁשִׁי,³

חֶלְקִי יהוה אָמְרָה נַפְשִׁי.

עֲבָדִים חַסְּמוּנִי מִלְּגְדּוֹר פֶּרֶץ,

וְתוֹכְחוֹת קָשׁוֹת פָּץ בְּחֶרֶץ,

וַהֲשִׁמּוֹתִי אֲנִי אֶת הָאָרֶץ.

טֻמְאָתָהּ טָפְלָה וְנָטָה קָו,⁴

וְלֹא נָסוֹג אָחוֹר מִקְוָיו,

טוֹב יהוה לְקוָיו.

טָבְעוּ טִירוֹתַי וּפִי צַר דָּמָם,⁵

וְכָל עוֹבֵר עָלַי שָׁרַק וְשָׁמָם,⁶

טוֹב וְיָחִיל וְדוּמָם.

טוֹבִים טַפִּים נִכְּלוּ בְּהוֹסִיפִי לִמְעוֹל,

וּכְמַעֲלָלַי חָרָה בִי לִפְעוֹל,

טוֹב לַגֶּבֶר כִּי יִשָּׂא עוֹל.

בְּנַפְשֵׁנוּ נָבִיא טֶרֶף נִכְרֶה,⁷

כִּי כְּמוֹ בָּרַחַת וּבַמִּזְרֶה,⁸

נָם וְאֶתְכֶם אֱזָרֶה.

יָדוֹ יָרָה בִּי אוֹר כִּסְדוֹם,

וְעַל כָּל אֵלֶּה הוֹנָאַתְנִי בַת אֱדוֹם,

יֵשֵׁב בָּדָד וְיִדֹּם.

יֵשְׁבוּ יְגוֹנִים בָּנַי עָלַי חוֹפֵיהוּ,

כִּי כָבֵד עָלַי אַכְפֵּהוּ,⁹

יִתֵּן בֶּעָפָר פִּיהוּ.

---

chapter two of *Eichah*. And in stanza three the first word is from chapter four. The third stich of each of these three stanzas is the opening phrase from the respective verses of chapter three (which has three verses for each letter). Thus, the group's *aleph-beis* letter appears three times in each of these stanzas: the first two words of line one and the first word of line three, for a total of nine times. The fourth stanza of each group begins with the first word of the respective verse in chapter five of *Eichah*. This is followed by a word beginning with the group's code letter (its

ח *The one who plowed over me planned*
    to tear down [the wall of]¹ the precious ones,
    and [the angels] who perceive my wounds cry bitterly,²
    [the angels] who are renewed every morning.

ח *He deprived [the priests] who bring*
    [offerings to] my [Altar] fire of their prophetic vision,
    like the sightless, I must grope for the wall.³
    [Nevertheless,] 'HASHEM is my portion,' says my soul.
        [The Babylonian soldier-]slaves prevented us
            from repairing the breach,
            because He had spoken sharply with harsh admonition,
            And I Myself shall bring the land to desolation.

ט *She [Zion] attached her [idolatrous] impurity [to the Temple],*
    so [God] stretched out the measuring line [of retribution].⁴
    Yet He did not turn away from those who sincerely hope to Him;
    [for] HASHEM is good to those who trust in Him.

ט *My turrets sank into the earth, and*
    my mouth became silenced with tribulation.⁵
    and whoever passed me whistled [in amazement]
    and wondered [what I did to deserve such punishment].⁶
    [Still, I declare,] 'It is good to hope submissively
    [for HASHEM's salvation].'

ט *The finest infants were exterminated*
    when I continued to sin even more,
    and in proportion to my misdeeds, [God's anger]
    flared against me, to act.
    It is good for a man that he bear the yoke [of discipline in his youth,
    so that he not stray when he is older].
        With [danger to] our lives is our food purchased,⁷
        and [we are tossed about] as if with
            a winnowing shovel or a pitchfork,⁸
        [thus fulfilling the curse,] 'And [like grain in the field]
        shall I scatter you [among the nations].'

י *His hand shot fire at me as [He did] against Sodom,*
    and in addition to all that, He caused the [Roman]
        daughter of Edom to torment me.
    Let one sit in solitude and be submissive [for it is God
        Who has laid His hand upon him].

י *My children sit in anguish over His sheltering canopy,*
    because His [God's] burden weighs heavily upon them.⁹
    [Therefore] let him put his mouth to the dust
        [in absolute submission to God, as there may yet be hope].

---

(1) Many editions omit the word in parentheses; if included, it refers to the walls of the *Beis HaMikdash*. (2) Isaiah 33:7. (3) Cf. 59:10. (4) *Eichah* 2:8. (5) Alternatively: *the tormentor's mouth was silent.* (6) Cf. *Jeremiah* 18:16, 19:8. (7) Some editions read טֶרֶף נִבְרָה, *our food is supplied.* (8) Isaiah 30:24. (9) Cf. *Job* 33:7; some editions read אַפָּהוּ, *His [God's] anger.*

יְדֵי יוֹסְרִי שָׁתוּ בִּי מֶחִי,
וְקַשַּׁבְתִּי מִפִּי צַר שְׁחִי,
יִתֵּן לְמַכֵּהוּ לֶחִי.

עוֹרֵנוּ יוּעַם כְּחֶרֶשׂ בַּקֶּרֶץ,
וּגְוִיּוֹתֵינוּ שָׂמְנוּ כָּאָרֶץ,[1]
אָז תִּרְצֶה הָאָרֶץ.

כָּל כְּבוֹד תַּאֲרֵנוּ הֻכְלָם,
וְצוּר אוֹרְחוֹתָיו חֶסֶד[2] כֻּלָּם,
כִּי לֹא יִזְנַח לְעוֹלָם.

כָּלוּ[3] כִמְעַט כִּי בִי נִלְחַם,
וְעַל הָרָעָה הוּא נִחַם,[4]
כִּי אִם הוֹגָה וְרִחַם.

כָּלָה כַעֲסוֹ וְהִצִּית לְהָבוֹ,
וּבְתַכְלִית שָׁשָׂה מְאוֹרֵי אוֹר* כִּבּוֹ,
כִּי לֹא עִנָּה מִלִּבּוֹ.

נָשִׁים כִּפְרוּעוֹת יוֹשְׁבוֹת שָׁמָּה,
בְּכָל שָׁנָה וְשָׁנָה מַזְכִּירוֹת אַשְׁמָה,
כָּל יְמֵי הַשַּׁמָּה.

לֹא אֲלֵיכֶם לוֹחֲצֵי גִילָיו,
וְעַל בָּנָיו הֶעֱבִיר גַּלָּיו,[5]
לְדַכֵּא תַּחַת רַגְלָיו.

לְאִמּוֹתָם עֵת כָּמֹהוּ מִשְׁבֵּר,
יַעַן כִּי גָרוֹן פָּתְחוּ כְּקֶבֶר,[6]
לְהַטּוֹת מִשְׁפַּט גָּבֶר.

לֹא לִמְחוֹת[7] פָּץ לְעַם קְרוֹבוֹ,
וְאֵיךְ מִתַּעַר הוֹצִיא חַרְבּוֹ,[8]
לְעַוֵּת אָדָם בְּרִיבוֹ.

שָׂרִים לְכוּדִים הוֹצִיא מִשְּׁעָרִים,
תֵּת כַּתְּאֵנִים הַשּׁוֹעָרִים,[9]
לְעוֹלֵל אֶת הַנִּשְׁאָרִים.[10]

א The hands of those who punish me shower me with blows,
  and I have heard from the mouth of the tormentor, Bend low,
  offer a cheek to his smiter.'
        Our skin has become dark like earthenware
            because of pogroms,
        and we [submissively] made our bodies like the ground.[1]
        Thus, may land will be appeased.

ב [Although] all the splendor of our features has been humiliated,
  [we have faith that] all of the Creator's paths reflect total kindness;[2]
  For [the Lord] does not reject forever.

ב [We] were almost annihilated,[3] He Himself waged war against us,
  but then He reconsidered the evil[4] [with which He afflicted us].
  [For,] even if He afflicts [at first], He [later] pities.

ב He spent His anger when He lit his flame,
  which had been cooling for six [annual cycles of the] luminaries,*
  for He does not torment capriciously.
        Women sat devastated with their hair unkempt,
            and each and every year [on Tishah B'Av] they recall
            [and confess] the sins [that brought about the Destruction].
        As long as it lies desolate.

ל [God did] not [bring suffering] upon you
      who tyrannize those who emulate [God's ways]!
  Rather, upon his own sons did God cause
      His [destructive] waves to roll.[5]
  To crush [them] under His feet.

ל [Children cried out] to their mothers when they were pining for food,
  [The children were punished] because
      their [parents'] throats had gaped like an open grave,[6]
  to deny another man justice.

ל He did not declare that His intimate people be eradicated.[7]
  How then did He draw His sword from its sheath,[8]
  to wrong a man in his conflict?
            The captive noblemen were removed
                from the gateways [of Jerusalem],
            and they were ill-treated like rotten figs,[9]
            to be harvested to their very remainder.[10]

---

(1) Cf. *Isaiah* 51:23; some editions read בָּאָרֶץ, *(we placed our bodies) on the ground.* (2) Cf. *Psalms* 25:10. (3) Some editions read כָּלִינוּ, which includes the interpolated 'we' of the translation; however, since this stich corresponds to *Eichah* 2:11, it should begin כָּלוּ. (4) Cf. *Joel* 2:13. (5) Cf. *Psalms* 42:8. (6) Cf. 5:10. (7) Cf. *II Kings* 14:27. (8) Cf. *Ezekiel* 21:8. (9) *Jeremiah* 29:17. (10) Cf. 6:9.

---

tenth appearance). The final stich of this stanza is the opening phrase of the corresponding verse from *Leviticus* 26:25-46. [Some commentators assume that this *kinnah* is a companion to *kinnah* 9, in which the stanzas end with the first phrases of the verses from *Leviticus* 26:3-24.]

שִׁשָּׁה מְאוֹרֵי אוֹר — *Six [annual cycles of the] luminaries.* When the nation's sinfulness reached the maximum that God would overlook, He commanded the angel Gabriel to throw two coals from the celestial fires upon the city of Jerusalem (see *Ezekiel* 10:2). For six years, Gabriel allowed

מִמָּרוֹם מְגִלָּה כָתַב וַנֶּהִי,
קִינִים וָהֶגֶה וָהִי,[1]
מִי זֶה אָמַר וַתֶּהִי.

מָה אֲעִידֵךְ מְאוּמָה מִלְּהֵרָצָה,[2]
נְתוּנָה בְּיַד מֵרִיב וּמִתְנַצָּה,[3]
מִפִּי עֶלְיוֹן לֹא תֵצֵא.

מֵחַטְּאת מַדִּיחֵי שָׁוְא[4] אֱקוֹנֵן,
מְנַחֲמַי כְּמַיִן מִתְרוֹנֵן,[5]
מַה יִּתְאוֹנֵן.

בַּחוּרִים מוֹטְטוּ כְּשֵׁל בִּי לְהָרֶב,
וּשְׁכִינָה הוֹעֲלָה מִקֶּרֶב,
וְכָשְׁלוּ אִישׁ בְּאָחִיו כְּמִפְּנֵי חָרֶב.

נִשְׁקַד נִטַּל עוֹל פּוֹרְכֵינוּ,
וַיִּתְעֵב שַׁי עוֹרְכֵינוּ,
נַחְפְּשָׂה דְרָכֵינוּ.

נְבִיאַיִךְ נָאֲצוּ לִקְרוֹץ עַפְעַפַּיִם,[6]
וְאַכְזְרוּ עָלֵינוּ אֶרֶךְ אַפַּיִם,
נִשָּׂא לְבָבֵנוּ אֶל כַּפָּיִם.

נָעוּ וְנָדוּ רֹאשׁ[7] בְּמַהֲמוֹרֵינוּ,
רְשָׁעִים מַפִּילִים בְּמִכְמוֹרֵינוּ,[8]
נַחְנוּ פָשַׁעְנוּ וּמָרִינוּ.

זְקֵנִים וְנִינָם לָרֹב סְגוּגִים,
אֲכָלוּם וְהֵשִׁיתוֹם מָשָׁל בַּגּוֹיִם,[9]
כֵּנָם וַאֲבַדְתֶּם בַּגּוֹיִם.

סִלָּה שָׁמַי קְטוֹרָה בְּאַף,[10]*
וְאֶפְעַר פִּי וָאֶשְׁאַף,[11]
סַכּוֹתָה בְּאַף.

---

the coals to cool in his hands before he actually threw them. He was certain that Israel's repentance would soon be forthcoming. When he realized that the people were steadfast in their evil ways, he decided to cast the fire upon them in a way that would wipe them out without a trace remaining. But God intervened, 'Gabriel, Gabriel, take your time; take your time, for among them there are some who treat one another righteously.'

But then an accusing angel appeared before the Throne of Glory and said, 'Master of the universe, will this wicked man be permitted to say haughtily, "I have destroyed God's Home,

מ   *From Above He wrote a scroll while moaning,*
      lament, murmuring and woe.[1]
      [For] who [other than the Lord] can say something,
        and it will be fulfilled?

מ   *What slightest example can I adduce for you*
      [of another nation's suffering] to bring consolation?[2]
      [Has any other nation] been delivered into
        the hand of antagonist and foe?[3]
      Has it not issued from the mouth of the Most High?

מ   *I shall lament over the sins of the worthless,[4]*
      deceptive [soothsayers].
      Yet my Comforter [has not forsake me; rather,]
      He is as one arousing Himself from wine.[5]
      So what is there to complain about?
          Youths crumbled, they increasingly stumbled within me,
          while the Divine Presence ascended
            [and departed] from our midst.
          And they stumble over one another
            as if [running] before the sword.

נ   *Heavy upon us is the yoke of those who crush us,*
      for He has rejected our well-ordered prayers.
      [Therefore,] let us search [and examine] our ways
      [to see where we erred].

נ   *Your [false] prophets with winking eyelids caused abomination,[6]*
      therefore, He Who is slow to anger treated us harshly.
      Let us lift our hearts to [the One Who dwells above] the clouds!

נ   *Everyone shook and wagged their heads[7]*
      [in disbelief] at the deep pits [of our woes];
      even the wicked who made us fall into our nets
      [were amazed by the enormity of our tragedy].[8]
      [All because] we have transgressed and rebelled
      [but God has not yet forgiven].
          Grandparents and their offspring increased abundantly,
          [the conquerors] devoured them and made them
            into a simile [for misfortune] amongst the nations.[9]
          As He had said, 'You will become lost among the nations.'

ס   *[The Kohanim] who offered incense were trampled in fury,[10]**
      while my mouth opened wide and I gasped [in bewilderment][11]
      [for] You have enveloped Yourself in anger.

---

(1) Cf. *Ezekiel* 2:9. (2) See commentary to *kinnah* 9. (3) Cf. *Eichah* 2:14. (4) Cf. *Eichah* 2:14.
(5) Cf. *Psalms* 78:65. (6) Cf. *Proverbs* 10:10. (7) Cf. *Jeremiah* 18:16. (8) Cf. *Psalms* 141:10.
(9) 44:15. (10) Cf. *Deuteronomy* 33:10. (11) Cf. *Psalms* 119:131.

---

and burned His Sanctuary?'''

    Immediately, God replied, 'If so, let fire descend from above and burn it!' (*Midrash Eichah* 1:41).

שָׁמֵי קְטוֹרָה בָּאַף — *[The Kohanim] who offered incense . . . in fury.* The *paytan* plays on the dual meaning of the word אַף. The Torah verse that this stich paraphrases reads, יָשִׂימוּ קְטוֹרָה בְּאַפֶּךָ,

סָפְקוּ שׁוֹטְנַי כַּף וָאֶשְׁתּוֹנָן,
וְאֶזְעַק חָמָס וְאֶתְאוֹנָן,
סַכּוֹתָה בֶעָנָן.

סוֹרוּ טָמֵא סָחוּ מַאֲשִׁימֵינוּ,
בְּהִנָּתֵן כַּבַּרְזֶל שָׁמֵינוּ,
סְחִי וּמָאוֹס תְּשִׂימֵנוּ.

שָׁבַת מְשׂוֹשׂ שִׂמְחַת מְשׁוֹרְרִים,
וְרוֹדְפַי קַלּוּ מִנְּשָׁרִים,
לְאַבֵּד הַנִּשְׁאָרִים.

עַל אֵלֶּה עֲשָׁקוּנוּ בְּחֵרוּפֵיהֶם,
וְהִגְדִּילוּ שָׁאוֹן גְּדוּפֵיהֶם,
פָּצוּ עָלַי פִּיהֶם.

פָּצוּ פָּעֲרוּ פֶה מִבְּאֵר שַׁחַת,
וְאִטְּרוּ עָלַי בְּתוֹכַחַת,
פַּחַד וָפָחַת.

פְּנֵי פָאֵר חֻפַּת מְעוֹנִי,
הִקְמִיל וְהֵקִים מְעַנִּי,
פַּלְגֵי מַיִם תֵּרַד עֵינִי.

נָפְלָה עֲטֶרֶת עֹז מִשְׁעָנָם,
וְצָרֵי בְּשִׁבְעָה דִינִים דָּנָם,[3]
וְהִתְוַדּוּ אֶת עֲוֹנָם.

פֶּרְשָׂה פּוֹצְצָה אוֹי כִּי סָגְרָה,
תְּמוּר עֹז מַתְנֶיהָ בְּשַׂק חָגְרָה,
עֵינִי נִגְּרָה.

עָשָׂה עֶבְרָתוֹ וַיֶּחֱרָה,
וְעָרַף אֶת מָדוֹן מִגְרֶה,[4]
עַד יַשְׁקִיף וְיֵרֶא.

עוֹדֶנּוּ עָף כָּבוֹד וְעָלָה,
וְעֹשֶׁר מַסָּעוֹת הוֹעֲלָה,
עֵינִי עוֹלְלָה.

ס My accusers clapped hands [with glee over my sorrows]
        and caused me sharp pain,
     and I would scream out over the corruption
        [perpetrated against me]¹ and I mourned,
     [because] You wrapped Yourself in a cloud
        [that no prayer can pierce].

ע 'Away, unclean one,' our persecutors said,
        when our skies were rendered as hard as iron [allowing no rainfall].
     [Thus,] You made us as filth and refuse [among the nations].

        The joyous jubilation of the singers has ceased,
        for those who chased me were swifter than eagles
        to destroy the remnant.

ע Because of these [sins] they abused us with their curses,
     and they intensified the din of their blasphemies,
        [when] they opened their mouths against us.

פ They opened their mouth wider than the Well of Destruction
     they closed me in with rebuke,
     panic and pitfall [were ours].

פ The majestic appearance of my canopied Temple
     he cut down. He stood my oppressor erect.
     [Therefore,] my eye sheds streams of water.

        Fallen is their crown of strength, their [pillar of] support;
        for God² afflicted them with seven harsh punishments.³
        [This would bring them] to confess their sin.

פ [Zion] spread [her arms in distress], she cried,
        'Woe!' for she was locked [into captivity]!
     Instead of [girding] her loins with power,
        she now girds herself with sackcloth.
     My eye will flow [with endless tears].

צ [God] smote with His fury and it continued to burn,
     and He beheaded those [evildoers] who instigated
        the strife [that alienated God from Israel].⁴
     [Yet, how long must we wait] until [HASHEM] looks down
        and takes notice [of our shame].

צ [Divine] Glory soared continually heavenward,
        [away from the Temple] it ascended in ten stages
        [to provide Israel with ten opportunities to repent].
     [Over this] my eyes have brought me grief.

---

(1) *Job* 19:7. (2) See *Eichah* 2:4. (3) See *Leviticus* 26:18, 24, 28. (4) Cf. *Proverbs* 15:18.

They shall place incense before You. The literal   *You.* The word אף can also mean *anger* or *fury,*
meaning of בְּאַפֶּךָ is *in Your nose,* hence *before*   for flaring nostrils are a sign of anger (see *Rashi*

עַל זֶה פָּסַק גּוֹי נָעֲמָם,
וְשָׂח לֹא אֶעֱזְבֵם בְּכַף זוֹעֲמָם,
אַף אֲנִי אֵלֵךְ עִמָּם.

צַדִּיק צַר צְעָדַי לִסְפּוֹר,[1]
וּכְעַקַּלָּתִי יָשָׁר וָאֶכְפּוֹר,
צוֹד צָדוּנִי כַּצִּפּוֹר.

צָעַק צוּרִי וְסָכֵךְ מֵעֲבוֹר,
וּבְחַלְלֵי עָרֵךְ לִשְׁבּוֹר,
צָמְתוּ בַבּוֹר.

צָדוּ צְעָדַי וְסָע דּוֹרְשִׁי,
וְכַעֲלוֹתָם עָלַי לְדוֹרְשִׁי,[2]
צָפוּ מַיִם עַל רֹאשִׁי.

עַל הַר צִיּוֹן צָבְאוּ לְהַכְרִיתִי,
וְצוּר שָׂח אֶחְמוֹל עַל שְׁאֵרִיתִי,
וְזָכַרְתִּי אֶת בְּרִיתִי.

קָרָאתִי קְשׁוֹב חֶרְפַּת מוֹנַי,
עַל הַלֶּחִי מַכִּים בָּנַי,
קָרָאתִי שִׁמְךָ יהוה.

קוּמִי קְרָאַי כִּי לֹא יִכָּלֵם,
עַל יֶתֶר לְמַקְנִיאַי יְשַׁלֵּם,[3]
קוֹלִי שָׁמָעְתָּ אַל תַּעְלֵם.

קַלִּים קְדָחוּנִי וְעַלְמָתָ מַרְאֵךְ,
הָשֵׁב בַּגּוֹיִם מוֹרָאֵךְ,[4]
קָרַבְתָּ בְּיוֹם אֶקְרָאֵךְ.

אַתָּה יהוה קֵץ אַל תְּכַזֵּב,[5]
עַד מָתַי כְּחֹרֶשׁ אֶעֱזֹב,[6]
וְהָאָרֶץ תֵּעָזֵב.

רְאֵה רְגַז מַכַּת אֱנוּשִׁי,
וָאוֹמַר בְּהִנָּטְשִׁי בַּגֶּשִׁי,
רַבְתָּ אֲדֹנָי רִיבֵי נַפְשִׁי.

רְאֵה רֹב בְּעַתּוּתִי,

For this the beauty of their pleasant [Temple shrine] has ended,
  although the Creator stated, 'I shall never abandon them
    into the hands of [the enemies] who frustrate them,
  [nevertheless,] even I shall behave towards them
    [in a punitive manner].'

צ The Righteous One once [lovingly] observed
    my footsteps and counted them,[1]
  but ever since I corrupted the straight and denied
    [God's sovereignty],
  I have been ensnared like a bird.

צ My Rock shouted [a command] and sealed [the heavens]
    [to prevent my entreaties] from passing through;
  and when I profaned [God's sanctity], He prepared to break [me].
  So they cut off [my life] in a pit.

צ [The enemy hounded] my footsteps, but the One
    Who had sought my welfare departed;[2]
  and when [the enemy] overpowered me and sought [my downfall],
  waters flowed over my head.

On Mount Zion [the enemy legions] assembled to cut me down,
  but the Creator said, 'I will take pity on My [people's] remnant
  and I will remember My covenant [with them].'

ק I called out, 'Listen carefully [O God] to my detractors' insults!'
    [See how] they smack my sons on the cheek!
  I called Your Name, HASHEM.'

ק Arise! Call out [O Israel to your God], for He will not shame you!
  He will surely repay the haughtiness of those who disturbed me.[3]
  You have heard my voice; do not shut [Your ear from my prayer].

ק Vulgar barbarians burnt me,
    but You were oblivious to what You saw,
  re-establish Your fear over the nations[4]
  You would always draw near on the day I would call You.

O You, HASHEM, do not misrepresent the [time of the] End,[5]
  O how long shall I be abandoned like a [lonely] forest?[6]
  [As You stated,] 'The land will be bereft.'
  Behold the turmoil caused by my mortal wound,
    yet [even though] I seem to be forsaken and forgotten,
      I shall [still] say,
  'You always championed my cause, O my Lord.'

ר Behold my extraordinary terror,

---

(1) Cf. Job 31:4. (2) Some editions read כְּיָם לְנָרְשִׁי, to drive me away like the [rolling] sea.
(3) Some editions read וְיִתְעַנְגוּ לְרֹב שָׁלוֹם, and may they delight in abundant peace,
cf. Psalms 37:11. (4) Cf. 9:21. (5) Cf. Habakkuk 2:3. (6) Cf. Isaiah 17:9.

---

to Exodus 15:8). Thus, Malbim expounds regard-   enter through the nose, one to torment the soul,
ing the Scriptural verse: Both anger and incense   the other to restore it.

הֶשָׁמּוֹת כָּל עֲדָתִי,

רָאִיתָה יהוה עַוָּתָתִי.

רוּחַ רָפָתָה בִּי מֵאֵימָתָם,

לְבַלְעִי הֶעֱלוּ חֲמָתָם,

רָאִיתָה כָּל נִקְמָתָם.

לָמָּה בְּרָחוֹק תַּעֲמוֹד[2] בִּדְבָרִם עַזּוֹת,[3]

נָמַת הַנְּשָׁמָה אוֹשִׁיב פְּרָזוֹת,[4]

וְאַף גַּם זֹאת.

שִׁמְעוּ שֶׁנּוּקַשְׁתִּי בִּדְחִיפָתָם,

וּכְיֵלֶךְ עָלָה עֵיפָתָם,

שָׁמַעְתָּ חֶרְפָּתָם.

שָׁכְבוּ שׁוֹחֲחִים בְּנֵי מִיגוֹנָם,

וְשׁוֹבֵיהֶם גָּאָה מְאֹד גְּאוֹנָם,

שִׂפְתֵי קָמַי וְהֶגְיוֹנָם.

שִׁישִׁי שׁוֹסֵתִי כִּי בִּי יַד מֵטָה,

מְשֻׁפֶּלֶת עַד[5] שְׁאוֹל מָטָה,

שַׁבְתָּם וְקִימָתָם הַבִּיטָה.

הֲשִׁיבֵינוּ שָׁלֵם שְׁלוּם שָׁנִים,

וְתֹאמַר אֶפְדֵּם מִשָּׁאוֹנִים,

וְזָכַרְתִּי לָהֶם בְּרִית רִאשׁוֹנִים.

תָּבֹא תְּשׁוּר מֵעַנִּי לָמוֹל,

הֵם שֶׁגָּבוּ חַיִל וְאוֹוְיֶךְ אָמוֹל,

תָּשִׁיב לָהֶם גְּמוּל.

תִּקְרָא תְּגַלֶּה יוֹם כָּמוּס בְּלֵב,

וּמְחַפְּשֵׂי עוֹלוֹת לִפְעוֹל מִלֵּב,[6]

תִּתֵּן לָהֶם מִגְנַּת לֵב.

תַּם תַּכְלִית תָּקְפָּם לְלָכְדֵם,

יִפְּלוּ בְּלִי לְהַעֲמִידָם,[7]

תִּרְדּוֹף בְּאַף וְתַשְׁמִידֵם.

כִּי תָמִיד דּוֹקְרִים וְשׂוֹחֲקִים,

וּמִתּוֹרָתְךָ אָנוּ לֹא רוֹחֲקִים,

הֲשִׁיבֵנוּ וְהוֹרֵנוּ אֵלֶּה הַחֻקִּים.

because You have ruined my entire flock,
    You have seen, HASHEM, the injustices I suffer.

ר   My spirit sagged[1] within me because of their intimidation,
    for they stirred up their wrath in order to swallow me.
    You have seen all their vengeance.

> Why do You stand aloof[2] when they speak brazenness?[3]
> Have You not said, I shall restore the desolate [city of Jerusalem
>   and it will be secure] without walls?[4]
> For despite all this [that they have done,
>   I shall not annul My covenant with them].

ש   They [the enemy] heard that I was battered from their shoving,
    so they rose against me like a locust plague.
    Haven't You heard their insults [regarding me]?

ש   My sons lay bent and cringing from their agony,
    while their captors' haughtiness grew ever more powerful,
    the speech and thoughts of my enemies.

ש   Rejoice, O You who plundered me,
        for the [punishing] hand of [God] has fallen upon me,
    and I have been dragged down to the grave.[5]
    Observe their sitting down [to plot against me]
        and their rising up [to take action].

> Return us to [Jeru]salem and repay [us for the]
>   years [we suffered in exile].
> And say, 'I shall release them from the roaring masses!
>   I shall remember for their sake the covenant of the ancients.'

ת   Come and observe those who torment me in order to cut me down,
    they performed mighty military feats
        in order to destroy Your desirous [Temple].
    Pay them back their due.

ת   Divulge and publicize the date [of redemption] sealed in [Your] heart.
    But as for those who search their hearts[6] to work evil,
    give them a broken heart.

ת   Let the gist of their power cease,
    let them be humbled, never to be permitted to rise,[7]
    pursue them in anger and destroy them.

> Because [our enemies] stab and scorn us continuously,
>   yet we are not alienated from Your Torah,
> O bring us back and guide us [on the path of] these decrees
>   [that HASHEM gave at Mount Sinai, through Moses].

---

(1) Cf. *Judges* 8:3. (2) Cf. *Psalms* 10:1. (3) Cf. *Proverbs* 18:23. (4) Cf. *Zechariah* 2:8. (5) Cf. *Isaiah* 57:9. (6) Some editions read וְהֵטִיבָה לָנוּ לְהָסִיר מֶנּוּ מְגִינַת לֵב, *be good to us, to remove from us a broken heart.* (7) Some editions read תַּצִילֵנִי ממוקְשֵׁי בְּנֵי אָדָם, *save me from the snares of humankind,* / שׁוֹטְנִים לְהַפִּיל בְּלִי לְהַעֲמִידָם, *to humble accusers that they never be permitted to arise;* some editions read תִּשְׁלַח חִישׁ עֶזְרָךְ, *swiftly dispatch Your assistance,* / וְרַחֵם עַל בָּנֶיךָ, *and have mercy on Your sons,* / הַמְצַפִּים לִישׁוּעָתֶךָ, *who long for Your salvation.*

טז.

זָכוֹר* אֲשֶׁר עָשָׂה צַר בִּפְנִים,*[1]
שָׁלַף חַרְבּוֹ וּבָא לִפְנַי וְלִפְנִים,
נַחֲלָתֵנוּ בְּעֵת כְּטַמֵּא לֶחֶם הַפָּנִים,
וְגִדֵּר פָּרְכֶת בַּעֲלַת שְׁתֵּי פָנִים.*[2]

יְתוֹמִים גֹּעַל בְּמָגֵן מְאָדָּם,*[3]
וַיְמַדֵּד קָו* כְּמַרְאֵה אֲדַמְדָּם,
מֵימֵינוּ דָלַח וְהִשְׁכִּיר חִצָּיו מִדָּם,[5]
כְּיָצָא מִן הַבַּיִת וְחַרְבּוֹ מְלֵאָה דָם.

עַל הֲגוֹתוֹ הֲוֹות גֶּבֶר,
וְנָטָה אֶל אֵל יָדוֹ לְמוּלוֹ לְגַבֵּר,[6]
מִצְרַיִם וְכָל לְאוֹם אִם בָּם גָּבֵר,
אֲנִי בְּתוֹךְ אַוִּיו אָרוּץ אֵלָיו בְּצַנָּאר.*[7]

אֲבוֹתֵינוּ זָרָה כְּהַכְנִיסוֹ[9] בַּחוֹרָיו אָכְלָה אֵשׁ,[8]

זָכוֹר ✦—*Remember.* The Roman general Titus — whose words and actions represent the unique arrogance and ruthlessness of the entire Roman nation, the seed of the proud and bloodthirsty Esau — destroyed the Second Temple. The Talmud (*Gittin* 56b) relates that he began his assault on Jerusalem with an insolent declaration of war — not merely against the Jews — but against the Almighty, God of Israel, Himself! Titus shouted out the verse from Scripture: אֵי אֱלֹהֵימוֹ צוּר חָסָיוּ בוֹ, *Where is their God, the Rock in Whom they have trusted?* (*Deuteronomy* 32:37).

Avos d'Rabbi Nosson (1:6) states that King David had Titus in mind when he supplicated before God: אַל תְּבוֹאֵנִי רֶגֶל גַּאֲוָה, *Let not the foot of the arrogant overtake me* (*Psalms* 36:12), because Titus' insufferable arrogance against God was unsurpassed. When he entered the Temple sanctuary he banged on the altar and taunted: "O Wolf! O Wolf! You are a monarch and I am a monarch! Come, let us do battle with one another!'

Nor was Titus alone in this defiance. He was merely continuing the attitude of his father Vespasian, who had begun the siege against Jerusalem and had continued it until he was elected Emperor of Rome. Then he appointed his son Titus to complete the destruction of the city. Therefore many Midrashim which describe the destruction refer to one or the other of these wicked men, or to both.

God allowed the brutal Roman legions to vanquish their Jewish victims. Jerusalem was reduced to rubble; the Temple was destroyed. The human toll was staggering: 'The number of captives was 97,000. The number of those who perished (from starvation or pestilence) or were slaughtered by the sword was one million and one hundred thousand' (Josephus, *Wars of the Jews* VI, 9:3). Even after Jerusalem fell, the Romans relentlessly hunted down every Jew they could find. Thus, they supplied victims for cruel torture for the amusement of Titus and his cohorts in sensational celebrations throughout the Roman Empire.

To emphasize how important this victory over the Jews was, a special coin was minted and issued to commemorate this event. On one side appears the head of Vespasian garlanded by a victory wreath, the reverse side depicts a Roman legionnaire leaning on his spear, while a forlorn figure representing the Jews weeps pitifully under a palm tree. The inscription reads, *Judea Capta* — Judah is a captive! Moreover, Titus had a huge monument erected to mark this great triumph, an arch upon which are engraved scenes of the sacred vessels being plundered from the *Beis HaMikdash*. This Arch of Titus, which has endured for almost 2000 years, is one of the most dramatic structures of the Imperial Capital, and is a constant reminder to us that we have not yet fully repented the sins that vouchsafed to Titus the power to destroy our *Beis HaMikdash*.

This *kinnah*, by R' Elazar HaKalir, depicts

16.

א Remember* what the tormentor [Titus]
    perpetrated in the Temple;[1]*
  he unsheathed his sword and entered
    the innermost chamber [the Holy of Holies].

ב He struck terror throughout [the land of] our heritage
    when he desecrated the show bread,
  and he impaled the two-sided[2] Curtain.*

ג He besmirched the orphaned [nation] with a red [bloody] shield;[3]*
  and measured them [for death][4] along a blood-red line.

ד He muddied our waters, and inebriated his arrows with blood,[5]
  as he emerged from the Temple with his blood-soaked sword.

ה [We mourn] because of the evil plans and words of the man
    who stretched his hand out against God,
  attempting to vanquish Him.[6]

ו [He bragged,] '[Despite the downfall of] Egypt and the other nations,
    that He conquered, I shall rush with [haughty] neck[7]*
  within His own desirable Temple.'

ז [In the times of] our ancestors, fire consumed His young men[8]
    [Aaron's sons Nadab and Abihu] when they brought
  an alien [fire into the Tabernacle],[9]

---

(1) Cf. *Zechariah* 14:10; some editions read בִּפְנִים, *within.* (2) Some editions read בְּבַעֲלַת שְׁתֵּי פָנִים, *with a double-edged [blade].* (3) Cf. *Nahum* 2:4. (4) Cf. *II Samuel* 8:2. (5) Cf. *Deuteronomy* 32:42. (6) Cf. *Job* 15:25. (7) 15:26. (8) *Psalms* 78:63. (9) See *Leviticus* 10:1-2.

Titus' wicked acts when he entered and destroyed the Temple. The first and third line of each quatrain begin with the opening words of the corresponding verses in chapter five of *Eichah.* The second words of those lines form an *aleph-beis* acrostic.

זְכוֹר אֲשֶׁר עָשָׂה צַר בִּפְנִים — *Remember what the tormentor perpetrated in the Temple.* The Talmud (*Gittin* 56b) relates that when Titus entered the Holy Temple he cursed and blasphemed the God of Israel. He dragged a prostitute into the Holy of Holies and unrolled a holy Torah scroll and committed unspeakably lewd acts upon it. He then unsheathed his sword (already bloodied with the blood of countless Jewish victims) and slashed the פָּרֹכֶת, *Curtain* (that separated the Sanctuary from the Holy of Holies), to shreds. A miracle occurred and blood began to flow from the curtain. Thus Titus imagined that he had actually pierced and slain God Himself!

פָּרֹכֶת בַּעֲלַת שְׁתֵּי פָנִים — *The two-sided Curtain.* The *Paroches* was woven in an intricate manner with various designs depicted on each of its sides. Two views are stated in the Talmud: (a) 'A lion on one side, and a lion on the other,' i.e., the same picture was visible from either side (or, as some explain, the front view of the lion on the front of the curtain, and the back view of the same lion on

the reverse); or, (b) 'a lion on one side and an eagle on the other,' i.e., totally different scenes on each side (*Yerushalmi Shekalim* 8:2).

יְתוֹמִים גְעַל בְּמָגֵן מֵאָדָם — *He besmirched the orphaned [nation] with a red [bloody] shield.* Josephus (*Wars of the Jews* VI, 5:1) described the misery and destruction brought about by Titus:

'There was a shout of the Roman legions as they marched together, and a sad clamor of the people, now surrounded by fire and sword ... Many who were worn away by starvation so that their mouths were almost closed, when they saw the Holy House on fire they exerted their last strength and broke out in groans and outcry. The mountains around the city returned the echo and increased the noise... The Temple Mount was seething with fire in every part, and the blood was even more than the fire...for the ground was not visible because of the dead bodies that covered it; the soldiers went over heaps of those bodies in pursuit of the fleeing.'

בְּצַוָּאר — *With [haughty] neck.* The translation is based upon *Rashi's* interpretation of this phrase in *Job* 15:26 (see also *Psalms* 75:6). Alternatively, it is an allusion to the Temple and Altar both of which are compared to the straight neck of stately stature (see commentaries to *Song of Songs* 4:4 and 7:5).

וְזֶה זוֹנָה צוֹעָה הִכְנִיס' וְלֹא נִכְוָה בָאֵשׁ,*

עֲבָדִים חָתוּ בְּתוֹכוֹ לַבַּת אֵשׁ,

וְעַל מָה בְּבֵית אֵשׁ,² מִמָּרוֹם שָׁלַח אֵשׁ.*³

בְּנַפְשֵׁנוּ טָבַעְנוּ כְּהוֹצִיא כְּלֵי שָׁרֵת,

וְשָׂמָם בָּאֳנִי שַׁיִט בָּם לְהַשְׁרֵת,

עוֹרֵנוּ נָמַק כְּהִשְׁכִּים מְשָׁרֵת,

וְלֹא מָצָא תִּשְׁעִים וּשְׁלֹשָׁה כְּלֵי שָׁרֵת.*

נָשִׁים בִּשָּׂרוּ כִּי בָא עָרִיץ,

בְּקַרְקַע הַבַּיִת נֶעֱלָיו הֶחֱרִיץ,⁴

שָׂרִים* לְפָתוּ כְּבוֹא פָרִיץ,

בְּבֵית קֹדֶשׁ הַקֳּדָשִׁים צַחֲנָתוֹ הִשְׁרִיץ.

בַּחוּרִים מִבַּחוּץ צָגוּ מְחֻזָּקִים,

וְתָרוּ כִּי יוּזַק בְּשִׁשִּׁים רִבּוֹא מַזִּיקִים,*

זְקֵנִים נִבְעָתוּ כְּהֶרְשׁוּהוּ מִשְׂחָקִים⁵

עֲשׂוֹת רְצוֹנוֹ וְהוּא אָסוּר בַּזִּקִים.⁶

שָׁבַת סוֹטֵן וַיָּבֹא אַדְמוֹן,

וַיִּסֹּב חוֹמָה וַיְעַוֵּת הָמוֹן,

נָפְלָה עֶבְרָה עַל נִינֵי פֶצֶל לַח וְלוּז וְעַרְמוֹן,⁷

עַד כִּי נָטַשׁ מָדוֹק אַרְמוֹן.

בָּחוּרָיו אָכְלָה אֵשׁ ... וְלֹא נִכְוָה בָאֵשׁ — *Fire consumed His young men [Aaron's sons Nadab and Abihu]...yet he [Titus] was not burnt by the fire.* These two eldest sons of Aaron were pious and holy but they erred in their service on the very day of the Tabernacle's inauguration, Rosh Chodesh Nissan 2449. Bolts of fire burst forth from the Holy of Holies, entered their nostrils and consumed their innards, yet their outer flesh and garments remained perfectly intact. The fact that they were punished so severely for their error, while Titus who intentionally committed every form of atrocity and sacrilege was left unscathed, demonstrates that they entered the House of God when it was at the height of its sanctity, and God's Presence permeated its environs with unsurpassed intimacy and intensity. Therefore, the slightest deviation caused a serious flaw in the awesome level of sanctity maintained at that moment. Titus, however, entered the Temple only after God's Presence departed in anger over the sins of Israel. Therefore, his victory was truly a hollow one, because he destroyed an empty shell, a meaningless facade. Although Titus' intentions were entirely evil, God left him unharmed. This demonstrated that Titus was unwittingly a tool of the Divine will to destroy the Temple from which the sins of Israel had chased the protective *Shechinah.*

בְּבֵית אֵשׁ — *In the House of [God, the All-consuming] Fire.* Alternatively, the *Beis HaMikdash* is the House of the Altar and Menorah fires, both of which had miraculous elements: The Altar fire was never extinguished, even though it stood in the open air (see *Avos* 5:7); the נֵר מַעֲרָבִי, *western lamp,* of the Menorah would still be burning, long after the other lamps (with the same amount of oil and same size wicks) had gone out (see *Shabbos* 22b).

וְעַל מָה...מִמָּרוֹם שָׁלַח אֵשׁ — *Why...did He send a fire from on high?* The translation treats the

> *while this man [Titus] brought a reclining harlot[1]*
>> *inside [the Holy of Holies], yet he was not burnt by the fire.**

ח *[A lowly] slave-nation stoked the flames within it;*
> *Why upon this House of [God, the All-consuming] Fire,[2]*
>> *did He send a fire from on high?[3]**

ט *Our souls sank, when he removed the service vessels,*
> *and placed them on oared ships,*
>> *that he might be served with them.*
> *Our very skin seemed to melt away [in agony]*
> *when the ministering priest arose early*
> *and didn't find the [full complement of] ninety-three service vessels.**

כ *The women were terrified when they saw the ruthless one enter*
> *and riddle the Temple floor with his [hob-nailed] boots.[4]*

ל *Princes* cringed in [helpless] fear when the wanton one entered,*
> *he splattered the Holy of Holies with his foul stench.*

מ *Outside, young men [Jewish defenders] stood firm,*
> *they thought he [Titus] would be harmed by the*
>> *six hundred thousand demons [they saw entering with him].**

נ *Elders panicked when he [Titus] was given free reign by heaven[5]*
> *to do as he pleased, while He [God] appeared*
>> *to be shackled in chains.[6]*

ס *When the Satanic one [Babylon] withdrew,*
> *the ruddy one [Rome] arrived;*
>> *he surrounded the wall and shocked the populace.*

ע *The wrath [of God] fell upon the descendants of he [Jacob]*
> *who had peeled fresh [branches of] almond and chestnut,[7]*
>> *to the point where the palace was abandoned by heaven.*

---

(1) Cf. *Jeremiah* 2:20. (2) Cf. *Deuteronomy* 4:24. (3) *Eichah* 1:13. (4) See *kinnah* 13. (5) Some editions read מְחָזָקִים, *from the powerful [heavens]*. (6) *Jeremiah* 40:1. (7) See *Genesis* 30:37.

---

entire line as a rhetorical question. Alternatively, it comprises a question and answer: *How could this happen to the House of Fire? — He sent a fire from on high!*

תִּשְׁעִים וּשְׁלֹשָׁה כְּלֵי שָׁרֵת — *Ninety-three service vessels.* Each morning, the *Kohanim* of the day's watch would remove exactly ninety-three vessels needed for the Temple service (*Tamid* 3:4). On the morning of the day on which the *Beis HaMikdash* was to fall, the *Kohanim* could not find all ninety-three vessels — something that had never happened before.

שָׂרִים — *Princes.* This refers either to the nobility of Jerusalem, or to the heavenly angels who are called שָׂרִים. When the sinful were admonished that Jerusalem would be destroyed unless they would mend their ways, they replied, 'We know the Divine Names that are the lifeblood of the various angels appointed over the elements. Should we be attacked, we will call upon the

angels to surround us with walls of water, or fire, or iron.' But God confounded them by exchanging each angel's role with another's. Thus, when the people called upon the angels that formerly protected them, the answer was always the same, 'That is no longer within my realm.' These angels now cringed because they were unable to help Israel (*Yalkut Shimoni* II:1023).

וְתָרוּ כִּי יוּזַק בְּשִׁשִּׁים רִבּוֹא מַזִּיקִים — *They thought he [Titus] would be harmed by the six hundred thousand demons.* When the Roman enemies came to destroy Jerusalem, six hundred thousand demons waited at the gateway of the Temple to attack and harm them. However, the demons realized that God Himself witnessed the atrocities the Romans perpetrated, yet remained silent, as it is written: *He withdrew His right hand in the presence of the enemy.* Therefore the demons said, 'If God does not interfere, we too will not interfere!' (*Devarim Rabbah* 1:17).

עַל פֶּתַח הַר הַבַּיִת הֵחֵל לָבֹא,

בְּיַד אַרְבָּעָה רָאשֵׁי טַפְסָרָיו לְהַחֲרִיבוֹ,

עַל צַד מַעֲרָבִי לְזֵכֶר הִשְׂרִיד בּוֹ,*

וְצָג אַחַר כְּתָלֵנוּ וְלֹא רָב רִיבוֹ.

אַתָּה קָצַפְתָּ וְהִרְשֵׁיתָ לְפַנּוֹת,

יְלָדִים אֲשֶׁר אֵין בָּהֶם כָּל מְאוּם מִשָּׁם לְהַפְנוֹת,[1]

לָמָּה רָגְשׁוּ גוֹיִם[2] וְלֹא שָׁעְתָּ אֶל הַמִּנְחָה פְנוֹת,[3]

וְשִׁלְּחוּם בְּאֶרֶץ עוּץ בְּשָׁלֹשׁ סְפִינוֹת.*

הֱשִׁיבֵנוּ שַׁוְּעוּ כְּבָאוּ בְּנִבְכֵי יָם,[4]

וְשִׁתְּפוּ עַצְמָם יַחַד לִנְפּוֹל בַּיָּם,

שִׁיר וְתִשְׁבָּחוֹת שׁוֹרְרוּ כְּעַל יָם,

כִּי עָלֶיךָ הוֹרַגְנוּ[5] בִּמְצוּלוֹת יָם.

כִּי תְהוֹמוֹת בָּאוּ עַד נַפְשָׁם,

כָּל זֹאת בָּאַתְנוּ וְלֹא שְׁכַחֲנוּךָ חִלּוּ לְמַמָּשָׁן,[6]

תִּקְוָתָם נָתְנוּ לְמֵשִׁיב מִבָּשָׁן,[7]

וּבַת קוֹל נִשְׁמְעָה עוּרָה לָמָּה תִישָׁן.[8]

---

(1) Daniel 1:4. (2) Psalms 2:1. (3) Cf. Malachi 2:13. (4) Cf. Job 38:16.
(5) Psalms 44:23. (6) Cf. 44:21. (7) Cf. 68:23. (8) 44:24.

עַל צַד מַעֲרָבִי לְזֵכֶר הִשְׂרִיד בּוֹ — *On the Western Side, as a memorial, they left over a remnant of it.* The Midrash states: When Vespasian besieged Jerusalem, he assigned four different generals to raze the four sections of the city. The western sector fell to the lot of a general named Pangar. In heaven it was decreed that the Western Wall of the Temple Mount should not be destroyed and, indeed, while the other three generals destroyed their sectors, Pangar allowed the Western Wall to stand intact. Vespasian summoned him and demanded an explanation, to which Pangar responded, 'I swear that my intention is only to glorify your reputation, O royal master! Had I obliterated every last vestige of this metropolis of Jerusalem, later generations would have no idea of the scope of your victory, for they might think that Jerusalem was no more than a tiny town. But now that I have left over this massive Western Wall as a memorial, it will be known for all time that your majesty conquered a major city of colossal proportions!'

The Emperor said to him, 'You have defended yourself very well, nevertheless, since you failed to follow my command you must climb to the top of a tower and throw yourself off. If you survive, I will let you live; but if you die, then indeed you will have received the death penalty you deserve!' Pangar threw himself off the top of a tower and was killed, for Rabban Yochanan ben Zakkai had uttered a curse against him saying, 'Your own heart knows what your real intentions are! You claim to have preserved the Western Wall for the glory of Vespasian, but in your heart you know full well that you desire a memorial to commemorate the utter defeat and destruction of the Jewish people!' (*Midrash Eichah* 1:32).

וְשִׁלְּחוּם בְּאֶרֶץ עוּץ בְּשָׁלֹשׁ סְפִינוֹת — *They sent them [the children] away to the land of Uz in three ships.* This is based on the narrative related in the Talmud (*Gittin* 57b) and the Midrash (*Midrash Eichah*) and presented here in composite form: Vespasian (or Titus) filled three galleys with four hundred of the finest youths of Jerusalem, boys and girls, and sent

פ *Upon the entrance of the Temple Mount*
       he [Titus] began to advance,
   to destroy it through the hand of his four chief commanders.

צ *On the Western side, as a memorial,*
       they left over a remnant of it,*
   and He [God] stood behind our wall,
       but did not fight on its behalf.

ק *You [God] were so enraged that You allowed them to empty*
       [the Temple of its contents],
   and to remove from there [Jerusalem]
       the unblemished children.[1]

ר *Why do You allow the nations to gather [against me]?*
       while You ignore my offering, paying it no attention?[3]
   They sent them [the children] away
       to the land of Uz in three ships.*

ש *'Bring us back!' [to life in the Hereafter] they cried out*
       as they sunk into the sea's depths,[4]
   as they united themselves with a solemn pact
       to cast themselves into the sea as one.
   They sang song and praises as [Israel did] at the Sea of Reeds,
       chanting, 'Because for Your sake we are killed[5]
       in the depths of the Sea!'

ת *Even as the depths were about to take their souls,*
       they prayed to the Real One, saying,
       'All this has befallen us, yet we have not forgotten You!'[6]
   They placed their hope in the One [Who promised]
       to bring them back from Bashan,[7]
   and a heavenly voice was heard, 'Awaken!
       Why do You seem to sleep?'[8]

---

them off to Rome for immoral purposes. The children realized this and preferred taking their own lives to living in sin, yet they were uncertain whether suicide is permissible under such circumstances. They feared they might forfeit their share in the World to Come. God inspired them with a holy spirit to expound a verse from Scripture which gave them guidance and comfort: My Lord promised, 'I will bring back from Bashan (i.e. those threatened by בּוּשָׁה, immoral disgrace), I will bring back from the depths of the sea' (i.e. God will resurrect and reward those who drown themselves in the sea in order to preserve their purity and to sanctify God's name) (Psalms 68:23). Upon hearing this, all the maidens leaped into the sea without any hesitation. The youths immediately followed their inspiring example.

As they performed this ultimate act of *Kiddush Hashem*, Sanctification of God's Holy Name, those on the first ship cried out, *'Have we forgotten the Name of our God and extended our hands to a strange god?'* (ibid. 44:21). Those on the second ship cried out, *'Is it not so that God can examine this? For He knows the secrets of the heart!'* (44:22). Those on the third ship cried out, *'Because for Your sake we are killed all the time, we are considered as sheep for slaughter'* (44:23).

Concerning these young and innocent martyrs Jeremiah laments: *'Over these people I weep; my eyes run with water ... My children have been destroyed, because the enemy has prevailed'* (Lamentations 1:16). And about them does the remainder of this *kinnah* speak.

יז.

אִם* תֹּאכַלְנָה נָשִׁים פִּרְיָם עוֹלְלֵי טִפּוּחִים,[1] אַלְלַי לִי.[2]

אִם תְּבַשֵּׁלְנָה נָשִׁים רַחְמָנִיּוֹת יְלָדִים[3]

הַמְּדֻדִּים טְפָחִים טְפָחִים,* אַלְלַי לִי.

אִם תָּגֹזְנָה פְּאַת רֹאשָׁם וְתִקְשְׁרֶנָּה לְסוּסִים פּוֹרְחִים,* אַלְלַי לִי. אַלְלַי לִי.

אִם תִּדְבַּק לְשׁוֹן יוֹנֵק לְחִכּוֹ[4] בְּצִמְאוֹן צְחִיחִים, אַלְלַי לִי.

אִם תְּהֻמֶּינָה זוֹ לְעֻמַּת זוֹ

בּוֹאִי וּנְבַשֵּׁל אֶת בָּנֵינוּ צוֹרְחִים, אַלְלַי לִי.

אִם תְּעֻדֶּנָה זוֹ לָזוֹ

תְּנִי בְנֵךְ וְהוּא חָבוּי מִנְתָּח נְתָחִים,[5] אַלְלַי לִי.

אִם תְּזַמֵּינָה בְּשַׂר אָבוֹת לַבָּנִים* בִּמְעָרוֹת וְשִׂיחִים, אַלְלַי לִי. אַלְלַי לִי.

אִם תְּחַיֵּבְנָה בָּנוֹת אֶל חֵיק אִמּוֹתָם נִתְפָּחִים,[6] אַלְלַי לִי.

אִם תָּטֹסְנָה רוּחוֹת עוֹלְלִים

בִּרְחוֹבוֹת קִרְיָה תְּפוּחִים,[7] אַלְלַי לִי.

אִם תְּיַקְּרֶנָה בְּשִׁכּוּל רֶחֶם וְצֹמֶק שָׁדַיִם[8]

וְאֵם עַל בָּנִים שַׁחִים, אַלְלַי לִי.

אִם תְּבַשֵּׁלְנָה שְׁמוֹנֶה מֵאוֹת מָגִנִּים בַּעֲרָב אֱלוֹחִים, אַלְלַי לִי.

---

(1) *Eichah* 2:20. (2) *Job* 10:15. (3) Cf. *Eichah* 4:10. (4) Cf. 4:4; *Psalms* 137:6.
(5) See *II Kings* 6:28-29. (6) Cf. *Eichah* 2:12. (7) Cf. 2:11. (8) Cf. *Hosea* 9:14.

◆§ אם — *If [it could happen that.]* This *kinnah* describes in horrible detail how the scope of the Destruction was not merely confined to material objects. Rather, this event ripped out the very moral fiber of the people and utterly distorted their essential personality traits. The Talmud teaches that the Jewish nation is identified by three basic qualities, they are רַחְמָנִים, בַּיְשָׁנִים, וְגוֹמְלֵי חֲסָדִים, *compassionate, modest, and performers of kindness* (*Yevamos* 79a). The intense suffering of the Destruction crazed the Jewish People and stripped them of the most elementary, normal human feelings and emotions, to the point where mothers relished the opportunity to cook the flesh of their own babes in order to still their hunger, and children were not revolted to consume the remains of their dead parents.

Concurrently, the heathen conquerors, already barbaric, were roused to an unprecedented level of cruelty and depravity and perpetrated every form of unspeakable atrocity against their Jewish victims.

In the closing stanza of this *kinnah*, the author, R' Elazar HaKalir, reveals the true reason for this atmosphere of utter inhumanity. It all stemmed from the astonishing crime which the Jewish nation committed as a whole. Two hundred and fifty years before the destruction of the Temple, in the reign of King Joash, the prophet and priest Zechariah ben Jehoiada admonished the nation in the Temple courtyard on Yom Kippur. So perverted were the people that instead of heeding the rebuke of their spiritual leader, they cold-bloodedly stoned and murdered their holiest leader, on the holiest day of the year, in the holiest location on earth. It was this crime which totally corrupted the Jewish people and distorted their nature and for this God exacted terrible vengeance at the time of the Temple's Destruction.

Each line of the *kinnah* begins with . . . אִם, *if*, followed by the third person feminine prefix. The second letters of the second words of each line form the *aleph-beis*. The letters א מ ת spell the word אֱמֶת, *truth* or *it is true*. Perhaps this is an allusion to that which the *paytan* writes in the closing stanza, namely, that God was in full accord with the punishments described in the first twenty-two verses of the *kinnah*. Similarly, we find that when the Sages wished to eradicate the overpowering *yetzer hara* of idolatry from Israel, a note fell from heaven on which was written אֱמֶת, *it is true*. This proved that God

17.

א　If [it could happen that]* women ate the fruit
　　of their own [womb], the babes of their care —[1]　　alas unto me![2]

ב　If [it could happen that] compassionate women cooked [their own]
　　children[3] whom they had so carefully measured
　　　　handbreadth by handbreadth* —　　　　　　　alas unto me!

ג　If [it could happen that] the locks of their hair were torn from
　　their heads when they were tied [by their hair] to fleet horses* —
　　　　　　　　　　　　　　　　　　　　　　　alas unto me!

ד　If [it could happen that] the tongue of the nursing babe would
　　adhere to its palate[4] through unmitigated thirst — alas unto me!

ה　If [it could happen that] one [mother] cried out to another,
　　'Come, let us cook our screeching children!' —　　alas unto me!

ו　If [it could happen that after devouring one of their babies,]
　　the two met [and the mother of the eaten child said],
　　'Give your son!' But he was already cut to pieces
　　and hidden away [for his mother to enjoy alone] —[5] alas unto me!

ז　If [it could happen that] fathers' flesh was waiting for
　　[their] sons* [to eat] in caves and ditches —　　alas unto me!

ח　If [it could happen that] daughters were condemned to die
　　in their mother's bosom, swollen [with hunger] —[6] alas unto me!

ט　If [it could happen that] the spirits of infants soared [heavenward]
　　from their swollen corpses
　　[which were lying] in the city's streets —[7]　　　alas unto me!

י　If [it could happen that] women were weighed down
　　by miscarriage of womb and dryness of breast,[8]
　　and that mother [lamented] over dying sons —　　alas unto me!

כ　If [it could happen that] eight hundred [young Kohanim
　　who bore decorative gold] shields were trapped;
　　in Arabia [they fell to] foul decay —　　　　　　alas unto me!

---

agreed to their plan, for אֱמֶת is the signet of God (*Yoma* 69b; *Sanhedrin* 63a).

The significance of these letters is that they come at the beginning, middle and end of the *aleph-beis*. Thus they allude to the fact that God is the First, the Last and has no equal or partner (*Yerushalmi Sanhedrin* 1:1). Accordingly, with this scheme, as with the alphabetical arrangement, the *paytan* intimates that the sins of the generation ran the gamut from א to ת.

טְפָחִים טְפָחִים — *Handbreadth by handbreadth.* The Talmud relates that when Doeg ben Yosef died, his widow was left with a young son. Each year, she would measure his growth by handbreadths and donate an equivalent amount of gold coins to the Temple treasury in honor of her son. But when the siege intensified against Jerusalem, she was caught in the throes of starvation until she slaughtered and ate her precious son (*Yoma* 38b).

וְתִקְשָׁרְנָה לְסוּסִים פּוֹרְחִים — *When they were tied*

[by their hair] to fleet horses. The Midrash recounts how, after the Destruction, Miriam bas Baisos, wife of the *Kohen Gadol* Yehoshua ben Gamla, was tied by her hair to the tails of Arabian steeds and was dragged from Jerusalem to Lud (*Midrash Eichah* 1:47).

בְּשַׂר אֲבוֹת לַבָּנִים — *Fathers' flesh ... for [their] sons.* When the siege was at its peak and the hunger most intense, one man of a group went out to find a corpse they could scavenge. When he chanced upon his own father's body, he buried it in a shallow grave and made a sign to enable him to recognize the spot. Then he returned empty-handed to his comrades. They sent out a second man to seek food. He returned with a corpse which they proceeded to eat. Later the first scout asked, 'I was unable to find anything to eat. Where did you find this body?' The second described how he had exhumed it from a freshly dug grave which was marked in such and such a manner. And the first screamed, 'Woe is me! For

אִם תְּלַהֲטֶנָה רוּחָם בְּמִינֵי מְלוּחִים וְנוֹדוֹת נְפוּחִים,*   אַלְלַי לִי.

אִם תְּמַעֲטֶנָה מֵאֶלֶף מֵאָה

וּמִמֵּאָה עֲשָׂרָה עַד אֶחָד לְמַפָּחִים,   אַלְלַי לִי.

אִם תָּנְסֶנָה לְמָסַךְ הֵיכָל שְׁמוֹנִים אֶלֶף כֹּהֲנִים פְּרָחִים,   אַלְלַי לִי.

אִם תִּשָּׂרַפְנָה שָׁם כָּל אוֹתָם הַנְּפָשׁוֹת

כְּקוֹצִים כְּסוּחִים,   אַלְלַי לִי.

אִם תֵּעָרַפְנָה עַל דָּם נָקִי

שְׁמוֹנִים אֶלֶף כֹּהֲנִים מְשׁוּחִים,²   אַלְלַי לִי.

אִם תִּפָּחְנָה נְפָשׁוֹת מְדֻקָּרִים מֵרֵיחַ תְּנוּבוֹת שִׂיחִים,³   אַלְלַי לִי.

אִם תִּצָּבַרְנָה עַל אֶבֶן אַחַת

תִּשְׁעָה קַבִּין מוֹחֵי יְלָדִים מֻנָּחִים,   אַלְלַי לִי.

אִם תּוּקַעֲנָה שְׁלֹשׁ מֵאוֹת יוֹנְקִים

עַל שׂוֹכָה אַחַת מְתוּחִים,   אַלְלַי לִי.

אִם תֵּרָאֶינָה רַכּוֹת וַעֲנֻגּוֹת⁴ כְּבוּלוֹת

עַל יַד רַב טַבָּחִים,   אַלְלַי לִי.

אִם תִּשְׁכַּבְנָה בֵּין שְׁפַתָּיִם⁵* בְּנוֹת נְדִיבִים מְשֻׁבָּחִים,   אַלְלַי לִי.

אִם תִּתְעַלַּפְנָה הַבְּתוּלוֹת וְהַבַּחוּרִים

בְּצִמָּאוֹן צְחִיחִים,   אַלְלַי לִי.

וְרוּחַ הַקֹּדֶשׁ לְמוּלָם מַרְעִים,

הוֹי עַל כָּל שְׁכֵנַי הָרָעִים,

מַה שֶּׁהִקְרָאָם מוֹדִיעִים,

וְאֵת אֲשֶׁר עָשׂוּ לֹא מוֹדִיעִים,

אִם תֹּאכַלְנָה נָשִׁים פִּרְיָם מַשְׁמִיעִים,

וְאִם יֵהָרֵג בְּמִקְדַּשׁ יהוה כֹּהֵן וְנָבִיא לֹא מַשְׁמִיעִים.

---

(1) Cf. *Amos* 5:3. (2) See *kinnah* 34. (3) Cf. *Eichah* 4:9.
(4) Cf. *Deuteronomy* 28:56. (5) Cf. *Psalms* 68:14; *Genesis* 49:14.

I have eaten my father's flesh!' (*Midrash Eichah* 1:45).

וְנוֹדוֹת נְפוּחִים — *Wineskins [deviously] inflated with [hot, stale] air.* Various Midrashim describe how, when the captives were led through the lands of Arabia, the Ishmaelites met them on the way and appeared to be friendly and sympathetic. They offered bread and other foods all of which had been oversalted. Soon the Jews asked for something to drink. The Ishmaelites offered them leather canteens that they had filled with air and left hanging in the sun. Thinking they were full of refreshing liquid, the unfortunate captives — whose hands were tied behind their back — bit off the plugs with their teeth. The hot, stagnant air in the bags filled their lungs and killed them (*Tanchuma Yisro* 5; *Midrash Eichah; Yerushalmi Taanis* 4:5).

בֵּין שְׁפַתָּיִם — *On the open roadsides* [lit., *between the borders*]. The translation and interpretation follow *Rashi* (*Genesis* 49:14 and *Psalms* 68:14). The captive women were not permitted to sleep

ל If [it could happen that] their breath was set on fire
   with a variety of salty foods and [they died while trying to drink
   from] wineskins [deviously] inflated with [hot, stale] air* —
                                       alas unto me!

מ If [it could happen that] they were decimated
   from one thousand to one hundred, from one hundred to ten,
   until but one [remained][1] — a source of terrible sorrow —
                                       alas unto me!

נ If [it could happen that] eighty thousand fledgling priests
   fled to the sheltering Sanctuary —   *alas unto me!*

ס If [it could happen that] all those souls
   were burned there like dry thorn cuttings —   *alas unto me!*

ע If [it could happen that] eighty thousand anointed priests
   were beheaded over the innocent blood [of Zechariah] — [2]
                                       alas unto me!

פ If [it could happen that] the souls [of the starving defenders] were
   swollen and stricken by the [tantalizing] aroma of the fruits
   of the field [that they could not attain] — [3]   *alas unto me!*

צ If [it could happen that] heaped on one stone
   were nine kab-measures of children's brains — *alas unto me!*

ק If [it could happen that] three hundred suckling babes
   were hung [to die], stretched out on a single branch —
                                       alas unto me!

ר If [it could happen that] delicate, pampered women[4]
   were seen in iron chains, under the hand of the chief butcher —
                                       alas unto me!

ש If [it could happen that] the daughters of distinguished royalty
   took their rest on the open roadsides — [5]*   *alas unto me!*

ת If [it could happen that] young maidens and young men
   fainted from the dehydrating thirst —   *alas unto me!*
But the Holy Spirit raged back at them:
'Woe unto all my wicked neighbors!
Those [tragedies] which befell them, they publicize,
   but that [evil] which they perpetrated, they do not publicize.
If [it happened that] women ate the fruit of their own [womb],
   they let it be heard,
but if [it happened that] they murdered a Prophet-Priest
   in God's Sanctuary,
   they did not let that be heard!'

---

in the cities they passed on their way to Babylon, but had to sleep out in the open, exposed to the elements. Some interpret that these women were publicly violated when they were made to lie on the roadsides.

Various other interpretations of this phrase are possible: The noble daughters were forced to work as kitchen slaves and had to sleep among the racks of pots (see *Ibn Ezra* to *Psalms* 68:14); they were forced to till the soil and sleep between the furrows (see *Rashbam* to *Genesis* 49:14); they were forced to carry heavy double burdens and collapsed under their weight (see *Sforno* ibid.). None of these views are mutually exclusive, for all of these atrocities may have been perpetrated against the captives.

יח.

וְאַתָּה אָמַרְתָּ* הֵיטֵב אֵיטִיב עִמָּךְ,[1]
וְנִפְלִינוּ אֲנִי וְעַמָּךְ,[2]
וְלָמָּה בְּנֵי בְלִיַּעַל חִלְּלוּ שְׁמָךְ,
וְלֹא שָׁפַכְתָּ עֲלֵיהֶם זַעְמָךְ.

אַתָּה גִדַּלְתָּ וְרוֹמַמְתָּ בָּנִים[3] לְהָנֵק,
כַּאֲשֶׁר יִשָּׂא הָאוֹמֵן אֶת הַיּוֹנֵק,[4]
וְלָמָּה דּוֹדָנִים דָּרְצוּ לְנַק,
וְאַרְיֵה גוֹרוֹתָיו לַחֲנֵק.[5]

אַתָּה הֵינַקְתָּ דְּבַשׁ מִסֶּלַע,[6]
וַתּוֹצִיא נוֹזְלִים מִסָּלַע,[7]
וְלָמָּה שׁוֹפְטֵיהֶם נִשְׁמְטוּ בִּידֵי סֶלַע,[8]
וְעוֹלְלֵיהֶם נֻפְּצוּ אֶל הַסָּלַע.[9]

אַתָּה זָנַחְתָּ וַתִּמְאַס[10] כָּל גּוֹי,
לָקַחַת גּוֹי מִקֶּרֶב גּוֹי,[11]
וְלָמָּה חָשׁ וְעָלָה עַל אַרְצִי גּוֹי,
וְאָמְרוּ לְכוּ וְנַכְחִידֵם מִגּוֹי.[12]

אַתָּה טֵאטֵאת שִׁשִּׁים וּשְׁמוֹנִים,
לְהָבִיא גּוֹי שׁוֹמֵר אֱמוּנִים,
וְלָמָּה יָזְמוּ מוֹאָבִים וְעַמּוֹנִים,
לְעַם זוּ[13] בַּקְּרוּבִים מוֹנִים.*

אַתָּה כּוּנַנְתָּ לְשֶׁבֶת הוֹדֶךָ,[14]
הַר זֶה קָנְתָה יְמִינְךָ וְיָדֶךָ,[15]

◀§ **וְאַתָּה אָמַרְתָּ** — *And You have said.* The stark
contrast between God's extremely close relationship with the Jewish people in early times and
His aloofness at the time of the Destruction is
highlighted in this *kinnah*, by R' Elazar HaKalir.
Each odd-numbered line begins with the word
אַתָּה, *You,* and describes some aspect of the
closeness that permeated the relationship in the
past. Each even-numbered line begins with וְלָמָּה, *so
why* have You, O God, permitted such drastic
change? The second words of the respective lines
form an alphabetical acrostic. The final stanza
acknowledges that God is righteous in all His
deeds, and we must accept responsibility for the
bitter tragedies that are the consequences of our

misguided action.

It is not clear why the first stanza begins with
a connective ו, *and,* while the remaining stanzas
do not. If anything, the opposite would be
expected. Indeed, many old editions omit the
opening ו.

שִׁשִּׁים וּשְׁמוֹנִים — *The sixty and the eighty.* This is
based on the verse: שִׁשִּׁים הֵמָּה מְלָכוֹת וּשְׁמֹנִים
פִּילַגְשִׁים, *There are sixty queens and eighty
concubines* (Song of Songs 6:8). Rashi (ibid.),
based on the Midrash, explains that *sixty queens*
refers to the offspring of Abraham who were
noble people, when compared to the rest of the
world. The family heads directly descended from

18.

א And You have said,* 'I will surely do good with you!'[1]
   [And You acquiesced when Moses requested,]
   'Let us be differentiated [from all the nations], I and Your people.'[2]

ב So, why, when worthless men desecrated Your Name,
   did you fail to pour out Your fury upon them?

ג You have reared and raised children,[3]
   nurturing [with the milk and honey of the Holy Land],
   as a nurse who carries the suckling babe.[4]

ד So, why did You allow [their Ishmaelite] cousins to prance with joy
   as the leonine [Nebuchadnezzar of Babylon]
   strangled their young cubs?[5]

ה You have caused [Israel] to suck honey from the rock,[6]
   and You brought forth flowing waters from the rock.[7]

ו So, why did their judges go astray through [their hearts] of stone[8]
   and cause their infants to be smashed against the rock?[9]

ז You have abandoned and rejected[10] every nation,
   but have taken one nation from the midst of another nation.[11]

ח So, why did [You allow] a [heathen] nation
   to arise speedily against my land, saying,
   'Come let us cut them off from nationhood.'[12]

ט You have swept away the sixty and the eighty*
   in order to bring forth the one nation which guards the faith.

י So, why did You allow the Moabites and Ammonites
   to conspire against this nation,[13] to denounce them
   because of the Cherubim?*

כ You aligned [Your earthly Temple] with Your majestic Throne,[14]
   on the mountain You acquired with Your right hand.[15]

---

(1) *Genesis* 32:13. (2) Cf. *Exodus* 33:16. (3) Cf. *Isaiah* 1:2. (4) *Numbers* 11:12. (5) Cf. *Nahum* 2:13.
(6) Cf. *Deuteronomy* 32:13. (7) Cf. *Psalms* 78:16. (8) Cf. 141:6. (9) Cf. 137:9. (10) Cf. 89:39.
(11) Cf. *Deuteronomy* 4:34. (12) *Psalms* 83:5. (13) See commentary to *kinnah* 11.
(14) See commentary to *kinnah* 5. (15) Cf. *Psalms* 78:54.

---

him were: the sixteen of Keturah; Isaac and his two children; Ishmael and his twelve family heads; the twelve sons of Jacob; and the sixteen family heads of Esau; a total of sixty. The vast majority of these nations were rejected by God in favor of Israel. *Eighty concubines* refers to Noah and his descendants until Abraham. The family heads descending from those leaving the Ark to rebuild and repopulate the earth add up to eighty. And just as queens are superior to concubines, so are Abraham and his descendants more esteemed than all others.

בְּכְרוּבִים מוֹנִים — *To denounce them because of the Cherubim.* The Midrash relates that when the Babylonian hordes entered into the Holy Temple the troops of Ammon and Moab joined them.

However, whereas all the marauders greedily looted silver, gold and precious treasures, the Ammonites and Moabites turned their attention exclusively towards destroying the Torah which states: *No Ammonite or Moabite shall enter into the congregation of* HASHEM (*Deuteronomy* 23:4). Furthermore, they burst into the Holy of Holies and seized the two golden Cherubs which were atop the Ark-cover. They placed them on display in an open cage and paraded them all around Jerusalem. They mocked the Jews with derision and scorn, saying, 'Didn't you all think that the Jews were special because they spurned idolatry? Look what we found in their holiest inner sanctum! Graven images! They are no better than the rest of us!' (*Midrash Eichah* intro. 9; 1:4).

וְלָמָּה לְאָחוֹר הֵשַׁבְתָּ יְמִין יָדֶךָ,[1]
וַתְּנַבֵּל כִּסֵּא כְבוֹדֶךָ.[2]

אַתָּה מָרוֹם לְעוֹלָם יהוה[3] וְרִאשׁוֹן,
כּוֹנַנְתָּ מָרוֹם מֵרִאשׁוֹן,[4]
וְלָמָּה נֹאֵץ רָשָׁע[5] בְּפֶה וְלָשׁוֹן,
עַד כִּי נָגַע צָר בְּאִישׁוֹן.

אַתָּה שַׁשְׁתָּ לְטוֹב עָלֵימוֹ,
בְּשִׂיחַ תְּבִאֵמוֹ וְתִטָּעֵמוֹ,[6]
וְלָמָּה עָרִיץ* חֵרֵף וְאָמַר אֵי אֱלֹהֵימוֹ,[7]
אֲשֶׁר יֹאכַל חֵלֶב זְבָחֵימוֹ.

אַתָּה פוֹרַרְתָּ בְעָזְּךָ יָם,[8]*
וַתָּסֶךְ בִּדְלָתַיִם יָם,[9]
וְלָמָּה צָלַלְתִּי עַד נִבְכֵי יָם,[10]
וַיִּגְדַּל שִׁבְרִי כַּיָּם.[11]

וְאַתָּה קָדוֹשׁ יוֹשֵׁב תְּהִלּוֹת קְדוֹשִׁים,[12]
בְּקֶרֶב יְשִׁישִׁים הַמְּקֻדָּשִׁים,
וְלָמָּה רָגְשׁוּ גוֹיִם עַם קְדֵשִׁים,[13]
וְהֵשִׁמּוּ בֵּית קֹדֶשׁ הַקֳּדָשִׁים.

וְאַתָּה שְׁמַע אֱלֹהֵינוּ כִּי הָיִינוּ חֶרְפָּה,
וְסֻכָּתְךָ בָּאֵשׁ נִשְׂרָפָה,
וְלָמָּה תְבַלַּע נַחֲלַת[14] חֵפָה,
תַּצְמִיחַ תְּרוּפָה וְעָלֵינוּ חוֹפְפָה.

וְאַתָּה צַדִּיק עַל כָּל הַבָּא,[15]
לְךָ אֲדֹנָי הַצְּדָקָה וְנַצְדִּיקָךְ בְּחִבָּה,
וְלָמָּה נָהִינוּ וְלָנוּ הַדִּבָּה,
כִּי כָל זֹאת בָּאַתְנוּ בְּחוֹבָה.

עָרִיץ — *The ruthless oppressor.* According to the Talmud (*Gittin* 56b), the wicked Titus shouted, *'Where is their God?'* as he desecrated the inner sanctum of the Temple (see commentary to *kinnah* 16).

Beis Levi says that afterwards, Titus and his soldiers offered animal sacrifices to their pagan gods in the ruins of our Holy Temple. All the while they mocked the God of Israel, saying, *'Since He allows us to worship other gods in His Temple, He must venerate our gods too. Why, then, does He not come to partake of the fattest*

ל Why, then, did You withdraw Your majestic right hand[1]
   and allow Your Throne of Glory to be derogated?[2]

מ You remain exalted forever, HASHEM![3] and You are the very first.
   Indeed, you established the exalted [Temple]
      from the first [even before Creation].[4]

נ So, why did You allow the wicked to revile You[5]
      with his mouth and tongue,
   until the tormentor attacked [the Temple,] the apple of Your eye?

ס You rejoiced to bestow goodness upon them,
      as the statement 'You shall bring them,
      and implant them (on the mount of Your heritage).'[6]

ע So, why did You allow the ruthless oppressor*
      to blaspheme and taunt, 'Where is their God[7]
   Who would eat the fats of their slaughter?'

פ 'You shattered the sea with Your might,'[8]*
      then You held back the seawaters with double doors.[9]

צ So, why am I now drowning [in tragedy]
      unto the very depths of the sea,[10]
   and my ruination has grown as huge as the ocean?[11]

ק You are the Holy One, enthroned upon the praises of the holy ones[12]
      You dwell in the counsel of the sacred elders
      (the seventy sages of the Sanhedrin).

ר So, why do the profligate nations gather[13]
      to lay waste to the Temple's Holy of Holies?

ש And You, our God, hear how we have been disgraced
      while Your Tabernacle was burnt in fire.

ת So, why do You swallow up the heritage[14] You once sheltered?
      Cause a healing balm to blossom forth
      and hover protectively over us!

But You are righteous in all that happens;[15]
   Yours, My Lord, is the righteousness,
      and we shall proclaim Your righteousness with love.
So, why do we moan, when the [evil] words are ours?
For all this has befallen us as a result of [our] guilt!

---

(1) Cf. *Eichah* 2:3. (2) Cf. *Jeremiah* 14:21. (3) Cf. *Psalms* 92:9. (4) Cf. *Jeremiah* 17:12.
(5) Cf. *Psalms* 10:13. (6) *Exodus* 15:17. (7) *Deuteronomy* 32:37. (8) *Psalms* 74:13.
(9) Cf. *Job* 38:8. (10) 38:16. (11) Cf. *Eichah* 2:13. (12) Cf. *Psalms* 22:4; some editions
omit the prefix ו from this and the next two verses that begin וְאַתָּה. (13) Cf. 2:1.
(14) Cf. *II Samuel* 20:19. (15) *Nehemiah* 9:33.

---

of our sacrifices?'

אַתָּה פוֹרַרְתָּ בְעָזְּךָ יָם — *You shattered the sea
with Your might.* You split the Sea of Reeds so
Israel could cross on dry land. When the

Egyptians entered, You returned the waters to
their natural condition to drown them, yet You
kept Israel safe from the raging, flooding waters, by holding them back as if with a dike of
double doors.

יט.

לְךָ אֲדֹנָי הַצְּדָקָה* בְּאוֹתוֹת אֲשֶׁר הִפְלֵאתָ מֵאָז וְעַד עָתָּה,

וְלָנוּ בֹּשֶׁת הַפָּנִים בִּבְחִינָה אֲשֶׁר נִצְרַפְנוּ¹ וְאוֹתָנוּ תִּעַבְתָּ,

לְךָ אֲדֹנָי הַצְּדָקָה בְּגוֹי מִקֶּרֶב גּוֹי לָקַחַת בְּמַסּוֹת,²

וְלָנוּ בֹּשֶׁת הַפָּנִים בְּדֹפִי אֲשֶׁר נִמְצָא בָנוּ כְּמַעֲשֵׂיהֶם עָשׂוֹת.

לְךָ אֲדֹנָי הַצְּדָקָה בְּהָלְכוּ אֱלֹהִים לִפְדּוֹת לוֹ לְעָם,³

וְלָנוּ בֹּשֶׁת הַפָּנִים בְּוַיַּמְרוּ עַל יָם בְּיַם סוּף⁴ גּוֹי בֵּאלֹהָיו בְּפִשְׁעָם,

לְךָ אֲדֹנָי הַצְּדָקָה בְּזָכֹר וְאַתֶּם עֵדַי וַאֲנִי אֱלֹהִים,⁵

וְלָנוּ בֹּשֶׁת הַפָּנִים בְּחָרְפֵנוּ יהוה בְּסִין קוּם עֲשֵׂה לָנוּ אֱלֹהִים.⁶

לְךָ אֲדֹנָי הַצְּדָקָה בְּטַעַם שֶׁהִטְעַמְתָּנוּ כְּצַפִּיחִית בִּדְבָשׁ,⁷

וְלָנוּ בֹּשֶׁת הַפָּנִים בְּיוֹם הִקְרַבְנוּ לְפָנָיו סֹלֶת וְשֶׁמֶן וּדְבָשׁ.*⁸

לְךָ אֲדֹנָי הַצְּדָקָה בְּכָלְכּוֹל מָן וּבְאֵר וְעַמּוּד עָנָן,

וְלָנוּ בֹּשֶׁת הַפָּנִים בְּלֶחֶם הַקְּלוֹקֵל*⁹ אֲבוֹתֵינוּ בְּאָהֳלֵיהֶם בְּרָגְנָן,¹⁰

לְךָ אֲדֹנָי הַצְּדָקָה בַּמִּדְבָּר לֹא חָסַרְנוּ דָבָר,¹¹

וְלָנוּ בֹּשֶׁת הַפָּנִים בְּנָאֲצוֹת לָבָן וַחֲצֵרוֹת וְדִי זָהָב*¹² כְּמִדְבָּר.

לְךָ אֲדֹנָי הַצְּדָקָה בְּסִיחוֹן וְעוֹג¹³ וְכָל מַמְלְכוֹת כְּנַעַן,¹⁴

---

(1) Cf. *Jeremiah* 9:6. (2) *Deuteronomy* 4:34. (3) *II Samuel* 7:23. (4) *Psalms* 106:7.
(5) Cf. *Isaiah* 43:12. (6) *Exodus* 32:1. (7) 16:31. (8) Cf. *Ezekiel* 16:19. (9) *Numbers* 21:5.
(10) Cf. *Deuteronomy* 1:27. (11) Cf. 2:7. (12) 1:1. (13) See *Numbers* 21:21-35. (14) See *Joshua* ch. 12.

לְךָ ה' הַצְּדָקָה ❧ — *Yours, my Lord, is the righteousness.* R' Elazar HaKalir based this *kinnah* on the Midrash (*Tanchuma, Re'eh* 16) which expounds on the verse continuing the theme expressed in the preceding *kinnah's* conclusion — *Yours, my Lord, is the righteousness* (*Daniel* 9:7). R' Elazar HaKalir illustrates a number of applications of this verse. Each odd-numbered line begins with the opening phrase of the Scriptural verse לְךָ ה' הַצְּדָקָה, *Yours, my Lord, is the righteousness,* and each even-numbered line begins with the phrase וְלָנוּ בֹּשֶׁת הַפָּנִים, *and ours is the shamefacedness.* The next word of each line begins with the respective letter of the *aleph-beis* after the prefix בְּ, *because of* or *in regard to.*

הִקְרַבְנוּ לְפָנָיו סֹלֶת וְשֶׁמֶן וּדְבָשׁ — *We brought it an offering of fine flour with oil and honey.* Regarding Israel's sinfulness with idolatry, the prophet Ezekiel admonishes that their betrayal is all the more shocking because God's own special gifts to Israel were used as offerings to idols. *My bread which I gave you — fine flour, oil and honey did I feed you — you placed it before them . . .* (*Ezekiel* 16:19). Rashi cites a Midrash that this refers to the *manna* that was placed in worship before the Golden Calf. Rashi there cites the verses from *Nehemiah* (9:18-19) that state: *Although they had made themselves a molten calf . . . You, in Your great compassion, did not forsake them in the Wilderness . . .*

בְּלֶחֶם הַקְּלוֹקֵל — *About . . . the destructive bread.* The word קְלוֹקֵל means either *destructive* (see *Metzudos* to *Jeremiah* 4:24) or *extremely light* (see *Ibn Ezra* to *Numbers* 21:5). Rashi (*Numbers* 21:5 and *Avodah Zarah* 5b) explains that since the *manna* is perfect food, it is digested in its entirety, producing no waste material. After a period of eating nothing but *manna*, the people no longer had the need to defecate. Instead of showing thankfulness for this miraculous food, they complained, 'This bread will destroy us. It enters our bodies but does not leave. Eventually we will be bloated and become sick and die.' The Talmud (*Avodah Zarah* 5a-b) cites this as an example of כְּפוּי טוֹבָה, *ingratitude.*

לָבָן נַחֲצֵרוֹת וְדִי זָהָב — *Laban, Hazeroth and Di-zahab.* Moses began his reprimand to the nation before his death with a seemingly inno-

19.

א Yours, my Lord, is the righteousness,* because of
    the wondrous signs You have displayed from then until now;

ב and ours is the shamefacedness, because of the trials
    with which You sought to refine us,[1]
    [but as a result of our failure] You despised us.

ג Yours, my Lord, is the righteousness,
    because You have taken [our] nation
    from amidst another nation, with miracles;[2]

ד and ours is the shamefacedness, because of the hypocrisy
    to be found within us as we emulated [Egypt's abominable] deeds.

ה Yours, my Lord is the righteousness, because God went out
    to redeem us as a people unto Himself;[3]

ו and ours is the shamefacedness,
    because they [our forefathers] rebelled
    on the shore of the Sea of Reeds,[4]
    the nation sinning against its God!

ז Yours, my Lord, is the righteousness,
    when we recall the proclamation,
    'You are witnesses, and I am God!'[5]

ח and, ours is the shamefacedness,
    because we blasphemed HASHEM in
    [the Wilderness of] Sin [when we demanded of Aaron],
    'Arise and create a god for us!'[6]

ט Yours, my Lord, is the righteousness,
    because You fed us [the manna]
    that tasted like dough fried in honey;[7]

י and ours is the shamefacedness,
    because on the day [we made the Golden Calf],
    we brought it an offering of fine flour with oil and honey.[8]*

כ Yours, my Lord, is the righteousness,
    because You provided us with the manna,
    the well and the pillar of clouds;

ל and ours is the shamefacedness,
    because our forefathers grumbled in their tents[10]
    about [the manna and called it] the destructive bread.[9]*

מ Yours, my Lord, is the righteousness,
    because in the wilderness we lacked for nothing;[11]

נ and ours is the shamefacedness, because we defied You
    at Laban, Hazeroth and Di-zahab[12]* as related [by Moses].

ס Yours, my Lord, is the righteousness, because of
    [how You waged war for us with] Sihon and Og[13]
    and all the kings of Canaan;[14]

וְלָנוּ בְּשֶׁת הַפָּנִים בְּעָכָן אֲשֶׁר מָעַל בְּחֵרֶם בְּלִי מָצָא מַעַן.[1]

לְךָ אֲדֹנָי הַצְּדָקָה בְּפֹעַל אֲשֶׁר פָּעַלְתָּ בְּאַרְבָּעָה עָשָׂר מוֹשִׁיעִים,*

וְלָנוּ בְּשֶׁת הַפָּנִים בְּצֶלֶם מִיכָה כִּי בוֹ אֲנַחְנוּ פוֹשְׁעִים.[2]

לְךָ אֲדֹנָי הַצְּדָקָה בְּקִימַת שִׁילֹה וְנֹב וְגִבְעוֹן* וּבֵית עוֹלָמִים,

וְלָנוּ בְּשֶׁת הַפָּנִים בְּרֶשַׁע שֶׁנִּמְצָא בָּנוּ שֶׁחָרְבוּ וּבָם אָנוּ נִכְלָמִים.

לְךָ אֲדֹנָי הַצְּדָקָה בִּשְׁנֵי חָרְבָּנוֹת שֶׁחָרְבוּ בְּבִצְעֵנוּ
וַאֲנַחְנוּ קַיָּמִים,

וְלָנוּ בְּשֶׁת הַפָּנִים בְּשׁוּבֵנוּ אֵלֶיךָ בְּכָל לֵב שֶׁתָּשׁוּב אֵלֵינוּ
בְּרַחֲמִים.

לְךָ אֲדֹנָי הַצְּדָקָה בִּתְשַׁע מֵאוֹת שָׁנָה* שֶׁהָיְתָה
שִׂנְאָה כְּבוּשָׁה מִלְּהִשָּׁמַע,

וְלָנוּ בְּשֶׁת הַפָּנִים כְּטֶבַע אִישׁ חֲמוּדוֹת,
הַטֵּה אֱלֹהַי אָזְנְךָ וּשְׁמָע.[3]

---

(1) See *Joshua* 7:10-26. (2) See *Judges* chs. 17-18. (3) *Daniel* 9:18.

---

cent recollection of their itinerary through the Wilderness. Close inspection reveals a deeper meaning to Moses' words. Firstly, not all the place names enumerated by Moses appear elsewhere in the Torah. This raises the question of why they were omitted from the list of encampments given in *Numbers* (ch. 33). Secondly, at each of the places mentioned by Moses that does appear earlier, the nation struck a rebellious pose. Three of the names on Moses' litany are לָבָן, *Laban*, חֲצֵרוֹת, *Hazeroth*, and דִּי זָהָב, *Di-za-*

hab (*Deuteronomy* 1:1). *Rashi* cites a Midrash that לָבָן is not a place name but means *white* and refers to the *manna* which the Torah describes as white (*Exodus* 16:31). Thus, Laban alludes to the Israelites' ingratitude when they grumbled about the *manna*.

חֲצֵרוֹת is mentioned elsewhere and was the site of both Korah's uprising and Miriam's *tzaraas* punishment when she spoke slanderously about her brother Moses (see *Numbers* 12:14-16).

ע and ours is the shamefacedness, because of Achan
who appropriated for himself from the forbidden booty
[of Jericho] and found no excuse [for his crime].[1]

פ Yours, my Lord, is the righteousness,
because of all that You accomplished through
the fourteen savior[—Judges];*

צ and ours is the shamefacedness, because of
Micah's idol through which we transgressed.[2]

ק Yours, my Lord, is the righteousness,
because You erected [Tabernacles] at Shiloh, Nob, Gibeon*
and the Eternal Temple [in Jerusalem];

ר and ours is the shamefacedness,
because the evil in our midst
caused each one's destruction,
and in their loss we have been humiliated.

ש Yours, my Lord, is the righteousness,
because although the Destructions of the two Temples
were caused by our corruption, we ourselves were spared;

ש and ours is the shamefacedness,
because we should have repented to You wholeheartedly,
so that You would return to us with compassion.

ת Yours, my Lord, is the righteousness
because of the [almost] nine centuries*
throughout which You withheld Your anger
[over our sins] and didn't broadcast it;

ת and ours is the shamefacedness,
because [Daniel] the man of delights pleaded with You
[to end the Babylonian Exile after a mere seventy years,
even though we were not worthy,] saying,
'Incline Your ear, O my God, and hear!'[3]

דִי זָהָב, literally, *sufficient gold*, is also not a place name. Rather, it alludes to the Golden Calf made by the nation because God had endowed them with abundant gold (see also *Hosea* 2:10).

בְּאַרְבָּעָה עָשָׂר מוֹשִׁיעִים — *The fourteen savior[-Judges]*. These are the fourteen leaders of Israel from the death of Moses until the era of the prophets which began with Samuel. They were called שׁוֹפְטִים, *Judges*, and their tenures are the subject of the Scriptural Book of that name.

שִׁילֹה וְנוֹב וְגִבְעוֹן — *Shiloh, Nob, Gibeon*. These were the successive sites of the Tabernacle before the בֵּית עוֹלָמִים, *Eternal Temple*, was erected by King Solomon.

בְּתֵשַׁע מֵאוֹת שָׁנָה — *Because of the [almost] nine centuries*. When Israel left Egypt, some of the nation carried out idols with them. For close to nine hundred years, God remained silent. But when idolatry became rampant in the days of Ezekiel, God revived the memory of that treachery and admonished the nation for it (*Vayikra Rabbah* 7:1; cited by *Rashi* to *Ezekiel* 20:5).

ב.

הַטֵּה אֱלֹהַי אָזְנֶֽךָ,*¹

לְתִפְלֶצֶת מְנַאֲצֵת מִי לִי בַשָּׁמָֽיִם,*²

וּשְׁמָע

שַׁאֲגַת צוֹרְרֶֽיךָ הָאוֹמְרִים עָֽרוּ עָֽרוּ עַד הַיְסוֹד³ שַֽׁעַר הַשָּׁמָֽיִם.*⁴

הַטֵּה אֱלֹהַי אָזְנֶֽךָ,

לְרִגְשַׁת הַדּוֹבֶֽרֶת עַל צַדִּיק עָתָק,*⁵

וּשְׁמָע

קוֹל שָׁאוֹן מֵעִיר⁶ בְּחֵמָה שְׁפוּכָה לְשַׁתֵּק.

הַטֵּה אֱלֹהַי אָזְנֶֽךָ,

לְצִיר שֻׁלַּח וְנָם קֽוּמוּ וְנָקֽוּמָה עָלֶֽיהָ לַמִּלְחָמָה,⁷

וּשְׁמָע

פְּלָצוּת הוֹמִים בָּא הָעֵת אִתּוֹ בְּבֵיתוֹ לְהִלָּחֲמָה.

הַטֵּה אֱלֹהַי אָזְנֶֽךָ,

לְעָצוּ עֵצָה וְחָשְׁבוּ מְזִמָּה בַּל יוּכָֽלוּ,

וּשְׁמָע

שִׂיחַת נוֹעֲצוּ לֵב יַחְדָּו עָלֶֽיךָ⁸ עָלוֹת נִסְתַּכָּֽלוּ.

הַטֵּה אֱלֹהַי אָזְנֶֽךָ,

לְנִאֲצוּ וְשִׁלְּחוּ בָאֵשׁ מִקְדַּשׁ מוֹרָא,⁹

וּשְׁמָע

מְחָרְפֶֽיךָ מַדְמִימֵי תוֹדָה וְקוֹל זִמְרָה.¹⁰

הַטֵּה אֱלֹהַי אָזְנֶֽךָ,

לְלֵצִים לָצוֹן חָמְדוּ לָהֶם,¹¹

וּשְׁמָע

כָּל חֶרְפָּתָם אֲשֶׁר חֵרְפֽוּךָ¹² וְהַפֵּל אֵימָתְךָ עֲלֵיהֶם.

הַטֵּה אֱלֹהַי אָזְנֶךָ — *Incline Your ear, my God.* As in the preceding *kinnah*, R' Elazar HaKalir based this composition on a verse from the Book of *Daniel, Incline Your ear, my God, and hear* (9:18). The contention of this lament is that the gentile marauders, who are supposedly God's agents to punish Israel and to destroy the Temple, are not merely enemies of the Jewish people; rather, they are the enemies of God

Himself. This is vividly and unquestionably evident by the way in which they curse, blaspheme and taunt God. Therefore Israel argues with God, 'How can You, O God, allow these heathens to continue unchecked? They claim that since the Temple site remains desolate it proves that God was destroyed together with His Abode! You, O God, must stop them because they are far greater enemies of heaven than we

20.

ת *Incline Your ear, my God,[1]* to the licentious ones who*
    blaspheme saying, 'Whom do I have [to fear] in heaven?'[2]*

ש *And hear the roaring of Your enemies who declare,*
    'Destroy! Destroy! unto the very foundation[3] of
    [the Temple which is] the gateway to heaven.'[4]*

ר *Incline Your ear, my God, to the gathering of those*
    who speak falsehood against* the Righteous One;[5]

ק *and hear the sound of tumult [arising]*
    from the [conqueror's capital] city,[6]
    silence it with an outpouring of rage.

צ *Incline Your ear, my God, to the emissary [Obadiah*
    who was] sent [to rally the gentile nations] and proclaim,
    'Arise! Let us arise against her [the Roman Empire] in war!'[7]

פ *And hear the horrifying sound of those who scream,*
    'The time has come to wage war
    [against God] in His own Temple!'

ע *Incline Your ear, my God, to those who conspired and*
    concocted an evil scheme that was impossible to carry out;

ס *and hear the uttering of those*
    who singleheartedly take counsel [against You],[8]
    and foolishly rise up against You.

נ *Incline Your ear, my God, to those who blasphemed*
    and set fire to the awe-inspiring Temple;[9]

מ *and hear [the curses] of those who deride You,*
    who silence the sound of thanksgiving and song.[10]

ל *Incline Your ear, my God, to the scorners who relish ridicule,[11]*

כ *and hear all the disgrace with which they disgrace You,[12]*
    and make Your fear befall them.

---

(1) *Daniel* 9:18. (2) *Psalms* 73:25. (3) *137:3.* (4) *Genesis* 28:17.
(5) Cf. *Psalms* 31:19. (6) *Isaiah* 66:6. (7) *Obadiah* 1:1. (8) *Psalms* 83:6.
(9) Cf. *74:7.* (10) *Isaiah* 51:3. (11) Cf. *Proverbs* 1:22. (12) *Psalms* 79:12.

---

are, despite our sins. Therefore we beseech You, O God, to return, rebuild the Temple and demonstrate how mistaken they are!'

In each stanza the first line begins הַטֵּה אֱלֹהַי ... ל אָזְנְךָ, *Incline Your ear, my God, to . . .*, and the second line begins וּשְׁמַע, *and hear.* These phrases are followed by a word beginning with the respective letter of the reverse-alphabetical formulation known as תַשְׁרַ״ק.

מִי לִי בַשָּׁמַיִם — *'Whom do I have [to fear] in heaven?'* According to the translation, these words were spoken by the Roman soldier in direct defiance of God, as if to say, 'I need fear none in heaven.' Alternatively, these are Israel's words: The heathens ask *whom I have in heaven*

to protect me. They claim that even God has forsaken me.

שַׁעַר הַשָּׁמַיִם — *The gateway to heaven.* When Jacob awoke from his prophetic vision of the angels ascending and descending a ladder stretching from earth to heaven, he declared, *'How awesome is this place! This is none other than the House of God and this is the gateway to heaven!'* (Genesis 28:17).

עָתָק — *Falsehood.* The translation follows *Rashi's* first interpretation of this word (*Psalms* 31:19). In an alternate explanation, *Rashi* has *harsh*; thus, in this *kinnah*, 'those who speak harshly about the Righteous One.'

הַטֵּה אֱלֹהַי אָזְנֶךָ,
לְיָהֲרוּ וְהוֹצִיאוּ כְרוּבִים בִּרְחוֹבוֹת מְחַזְּרִים,
וּשְׁמַע
טָרְחֹת טְנוּפָם* כְּהֶעֱלוּ עַל מִזְבַּחֲךָ חֲזִירִים.

הַטֵּה אֱלֹהַי אָזְנֶךָ,
לְחִלְּלוּ וְטִנְּפוּ בֵּית קֹדֶשׁ הַקֳּדָשִׁים,
וּשְׁמַע
זֵדִים מְזַרְקִים לְמוּלְךָ מִילוֹת קְדוֹשִׁים.*

הַטֵּה אֱלֹהַי אָזְנֶךָ,
לְלוֹעֲזִים מְעִיזִים מֵצַח לְכוּ וְנִלָּחֲמָה אִתּוֹ בְּבֵיתוֹ,
וּשְׁמַע
הַוּוֹת הוֹלְלִים מְהַלְּלִים כִּי אֵין הָאִישׁ בְּבֵיתוֹ.[1]

הַטֵּה אֱלֹהַי אָזְנֶךָ,
לְדוֹבֶרֶת אֲנִי וְאַפְסִי עוֹד,[2]
וּשְׁמַע
גְדוּפֶיהָ וְחֵרוּפֶיהָ מִשְׁתַּחֲצֶת עַד כִּסְאֲךָ עוֹד.

הַטֵּה אֱלֹהַי אָזְנֶךָ,
לְבוֹזָה וּמַלְעֶגֶת[3] מַה תּוֹחִילִי וְאֵינוּ נִבְנֶה,
וּשְׁמַע
בְּכִית מַסְפִּידִים וְקוֹרְאִים[4] וּמְחַכִּים מָתַי יִבָּנֶה.

הַטֵּה אֱלֹהַי אָזְנֶךָ,
לְאוֹמְרִים עֲזַב וְשָׁכַח וְנָטַשׁ וְלָעַד שׁוֹמֵם,
וּשְׁמַע
אָנְקָתֵנוּ, וְקַנֵּא קִנְאָתֵנוּ,
וְהָאֵר פָּנֶיךָ עַל מִקְדָּשְׁךָ הַשָּׁמֵם.[5]

טְנוּפָם — *Their filth.* Idolatrous offerings are considered nothing more than filth, as the prophet (*Isaiah* 28:8) declares: *For all the tables [i.e., altars] are full of vomit and excrement, without the Omnipresent* (See *Avos* 3:4). Moreover, the idols themselves are so considered, as it

is written: צֵא תֹּאמֶר לוֹ, *Say unto him [the idol], 'You are excrement!'* (ibid. 30:22; see *Radak* there, and *Maharshal* to *Shabbos* 82a).

מִילוֹת קְדוֹשִׁים — *The circumcised organs ... from the holy ones.* The Amalekites would

י Incline Your, ear, my God, to those
   who haughtily removed the Cherubim
   [from the Ark Cover in the Holy of Holies]
   and paraded them around the streets;

ט and hear how they burdened You with their filth*
   when they offered up swine on Your Altar.

ח Incline Your ear, my God, to those who desecrated
   and filthied the chamber of the Holy of Holies;

ז and hear how the wanton ones
   flung at You the circumcised organs
   [they cruelly severed] from the holy ones.*

ו Incline Your ear, my God, to the
   brazen-browed foreigners [who declare],
   'Let us go forth and wage war with Him in His own House';

ה and hear the treacherous mockery of the scorners,
   'The Man is not in His House!'[1]

ד Incline Your ear, my God, to those who boast,
   'I am [everything] and anything else is nothing!'[2]

ג And hear the curses and disgraces [of the nation]
   whose arrogance reaches up to Your very Throne.

ב Incline Your ear, my God,
   to the disparagement and ridicule,[3]
   'Where is your hope? Your Temple will never be rebuilt!'

ב And hear the weeping of those who mourn and cry out[4]
   and yearn, 'When will it be built [again]?'

א Incline Your ear, my God, to those who claim
   that [the Temple] is abandoned, forgotten and cast aside,
   forever will it be desolate.

א And hear our anguished cry and zealously take up our cause;
   and let Your countenance shine upon
   Your desolate Sanctuary.[5]

---

(1) *Proverbs* 7:19. (2) *Isaiah* 47:8. (3) Cf. *Nehemiah* 2:19.
(4) Some editions read וְקוֹרְעִים, *and rend [their garments]*,
in place of וְקוֹרְאִים, *and cry out*. (5) *Daniel* 9:17.

---

mutilate their Jewish victims, then throw their
organs skyward while calling out blas-
phemously to God, 'Here, this is what You have
chosen! Take what is Yours!' (*Midrash
Tanchuma, Ki Seitzei* 10).

כא.

אַרְזֵי הַלְּבָנוֹן* אַדִּירֵי הַתּוֹרָה,

בַּעֲלֵי תְרֵיסִין* בְּמִשְׁנָה וּבִגְמָרָא,

גִּבּוֹרֵי כְחַ* עֲמֵלֶיהָ בְּטָהֳרָה,

דָּמָם נִשְׁפַּךְ וְנָשְׁתָה גְבוּרָה,

הֵנָם קְדוֹשֵׁי הַרוּגֵי מַלְכוּת עֲשָׂרָה,

וְעַל אֵלֶּה אֲנִי בוֹכִיָּה וְעֵינִי נִגְּרָה.

זֹאת בְּזָכְרִי אֶזְעַק בְּמָרָה,

חֶמְדַּת יִשְׂרָאֵל כְּלֵי הַקֹּדֶשׁ נֵזֶר וַעֲטָרָה,

טְהוֹרֵי לֵב קְדוֹשִׁים מֵתוּ בְּמִיתָה חֲמוּרָה,

יָדוּ גוֹרָל* מִי רִאשׁוֹן לַחֶרֶב בְּרוּרָה,

כִּנְפוֹל גּוֹרָל עַל רַבָּן שִׁמְעוֹן* פָּשַׁט צַוָּארוֹ וּבָכָה כְּנִגְזְרָה גְזֵרָה,*

לְרַבָּן שִׁמְעוֹן² חָזַר הַהֶגְמוֹן לְהָרְגוֹ בְּנֶפֶשׁ נְצוּרָה,

מִזֶּרַע אַהֲרֹן* שָׁאַל בְּבַקָּשָׁה לִבְכּוֹת עַל בֶּן הַגְּבִירָה,

---

אַרְזֵי הַלְּבָנוֹן — *Cedars of Lebanon*. This *kinnah*, whose author is unknown [although some ascribe it to יְחִיאֵל בֶּן מָאִיר, whose name may appear in the acrostic], is a dramatic highlight of the Tishah B'Av service. It depicts the tragic execution of the עֲשָׂרָה הֲרוּגֵי מַלְכוּת, *Ten Martyrs*.

Numerous *piyutim, kinnos* and *selichos* have been written about the Ten Martyrs, all of which seemingly place them as contemporaneous. It should be noted, however, that while all ten of these righteous men were murdered by the Romans during the Mishnaic period, their executions did not take place at the same time, nor could they have, since two of the ten did not even live in the same generation as the other eight. Namely, Rabban Shimon ben Gamliel and Rabbi Yishmael the *Kohen Gadol* lived before the Destruction of the Second Temple, and were murdered shortly thereafter, while the others were all killed after the Bar Kochba revolt, more than sixty years later. The liturgical accounts of the martyrdom were not meant as historical records, but as dramatic accounts of the story, in order to evoke feelings of loss and repentance on the part of the congregation.

The Talmud teaches: 'The death of the righteous is a tragedy equal to the burning of the Temple of our God' (*Rosh Hashanah* 18a). Thus, it is appropriate to mourn the loss of these righteous sages on Tishah B'Av, the day our Temple was destroyed in fire.

In the *chazzan's* repetition of the *Amidah* during *Mussaf* on Yom Kippur, the Day of Atonement, we read another *piyut* describing the death of the Ten Martyrs titled אֵלֶּה אֶזְכְּרָה, *These shall I recall.* It is included in the Yom Kippur

service because the Talmud (*Moed Katan* 28a) states: 'The death of the righteous atones for the sins of Israel,' and it is on Yom Kippur that we seek to arouse the merit of the martyrs. The Yom Kippur version of this story is lengthier and explains that the death of the Ten Martyrs was an atonement for the sin of the ten sons of Jacob who were involved in the sale of Joseph into slavery (see *Genesis* ch. 37). That heartless deed sowed the seeds of future dissension and senseless hatred in Israel. But it was not until the Second Temple was destroyed due to שִׂנְאַת חִנָּם, *baseless hatred*, that Israel reaped the bitter fruits of that deed (*Yoma* 9b). Then, after the Temple's destruction, God brought about the death of ten holy martyrs who sanctified His Name in atonement for the sin of the ten brothers. For it was the still-present influence of their act that continued to prevent their offspring from living in brotherhood and harmony.

This *kinnah* lists only eight of the Ten Martyrs. In the Yom Kippur liturgy and other sources the other two are given as Rabbi Chanina ben Chachinai, one of Rabbi Akiva's earlier disciples and Rabbi Yehudah (or Elazar) ben Dama. Some versions add the name of Rabbi Yehudah HaNachtom in place of ben Dama.

אַרְזֵי הַלְּבָנוֹן — *Cedars of Lebanon*. The righteous are thus described by the psalmist: *A righteous man will flourish like a date palm*, כְּאֶרֶז בַּלְּבָנוֹן יִשְׂגֶּה, *like a cedar in Lebanon he will grow tall* (*Psalms* 92:13).

בַּעֲלֵי תְרֵיסִין — *Shield-carriers* [lit., *masters of the shields*]. The Talmud uses this when referring to the sages in the academy of Rabban Gamliel,

21.

א *Cedars of Lebanon,* giants of Torah,*

ב *shield-carriers* of Mishnah and Gemara,*

ג *powerful warriors,* exerting themselves over it in purity,*

ד *their blood was spilt and [their] greatness removed [from us].*

ה *Behold, they are the holy Ten Martyrs*
   executed by the [Roman] government,

ו *and for these do I weep and my eye overflows.[1]*

ז *When I remember this I scream in bitterness.*

ח *The most desirable in Israel, the holy vessels, crown and tiara,*

ט *pure of heart and consecrated, they suffered a harsh death.*

י *They cast lots* to determine whom to put to the sword first.*

כ *When the lot fell on Rabban Shimon [ben Gamliel],**
   he stretched out his neck and wept as the decree was issued.*

ל *The overlord, with soul steeped in evil,*
   turned to slay Rabban Shimon.[2]

מ *[Rabbi Yishmael, the Kohen Gadol,] the scion of Aaron**
   asked permission to cry over this son of royalty.

---

(1) Cf. *Eichah* 1:16; 3:49. (2) Some editions read רַבִּי יִשְׁמָעֵאל, *Rabbi Yishmael.*

nassi of Israel and son of Rabban Shimon, the first of the Ten Martyrs. Among those described with this title was Rabbi Chutzpis the Interpreter, ninth of the Martyrs (*Berachos* 27b). They are called shield-carriers either because they metaphorically do battle with each other in debating the fine points of Torah law, or because of their role in enforcing the law as interpreted by the *nassi* and his academy (*Aruch*).

גְּבוֹרֵי כֹחַ — *Powerful warriors.* Perhaps this is an even greater accolade than earlier ones, for the psalmist depicts the angels with this term (see *Psalms* 103:20).

יַדּוּ גוֹרָל — *They cast lots.* Rabban Shimon ben Gamliel and Rabbi Yishmael the *Kohen Gadol* were seized by the Romans at the time of the Temple's destruction. When they were about to be killed, each begged the executioner, 'Please kill me first, so that I will not be forced to witness the death of my beloved colleague!' The executioner was amazed by the pure love for one another and said, 'In that case we will cast lots to decide who should die first!'

רַבָּן שִׁמְעוֹן — *Rabban Shimon [ben Gamliel],* נָשִׂיא, *Prince,* of Israel, a great grandson of Hillel and a direct descendant of the royal family of King David. He was the first of the Ten Martyrs to die. *Mishnah Berurah* (53:35) quotes *Sefer Chassidim* who relates that when Rabban Shimon ben Gamliel was about to die he asked Rabbi Yishmael, 'My dear brother, why am I being subjected to die such an ignominious death [like a common criminal]?'

Rabbi Yishmael replied, 'Perhaps when you preached in public before the masses you were filled with too much personal pleasure and you thereby benefited personally from words of Torah?' Rabban Shimon responded, 'My brother, you have comforted and consoled me!'

וּבָכָה כְּנִגְזְרָה גְזֵרָה — *And wept as the decree was issued.* The much more detailed version in the *piyut* אֵלֶה אֶזְכְּרָה (see above) relates that the Roman ruler informed the martyrs that they would be executed as retribution for the sale of Joseph by his brothers. They asked for a three-day period during which they would determine whether their deaths had been decreed by the Heavenly Tribunal. Rabbi Yishmael the Kohen Gadol uttered God's secret Name by which miracles can be performed, and ascended to heaven. There he met the angel Gabriel who told him, 'Accept it upon yourselves . . . for I have heard . . . that you have been destined for this.'

The *kinnah* informs us that Rabban Shimon wept as he heard Rabbi Yishmael report that their deaths had been decreed in heaven.

מִזֶּרַע אַהֲרֹן — *The scion of Aaron.* Although his name is not mentioned in this *kinnah*, other sources identify him as Rabbi Yishmael ben Elisha the *Kohen Gadol* (see *kinnah* 23). According to those sources, the Roman governor who condemned Rabbi Yishmael to death had a daughter who was impressed with the Rabbi's appearance, for he was as handsome as Joseph in his prime. She begged her father to spare the Rabbi for her personal gratification. Her father replied, 'If it is his face that impresses you, we can preserve it.' In an incredible display of cruelty, the governor gave orders that Rabbi Yishmael be skinned alive and the skin on his face be mounted like a trophy and preserved in fragrant balsam. They flayed the flesh off his face until they reached the top of his head where *tefillin* were

נָטַל רֹאשׁוֹ וּנְתָנוֹ עַל אַרְכְּבוֹתָיו מְנוֹרָה הַטְּהוֹרָה,*

שָׂם עֵינָיו עַל עֵינָיו וּפִיו עַל פִּיו בְּאַהֲבָה גְמוּרָה,

עָנָה וְאָמַר פֶּה הַמִּתְגַּבֵּר בַּתּוֹרָה,

פִּתְאוֹם נִקְנְסָה עָלָיו מִיתָה מִשְׁנָה וַחֲמוּרָה,

צִוָּה לְהַפְשִׁיט אֶת רֹאשׁוֹ בְּתַעַר הַשְּׂכִירָה,

קַיָּם בְּעוֹרוֹ אָמְרוּ לְנַפְשֵׁךְ שְׁחִי וְנַעֲבֹרָה,¹

רָשָׁע הַפּוֹשֵׁט עֵת הִגִּיעַ לִמְקוֹם תְּפִלִּין מִצְוַת בָּרָה,

צָעַק צְעָקָה* וְנִזְדַּעְזְעָה עוֹלָם וְאֶרֶץ הִתְפּוֹרֲרָה.

מֵאַחֲרָיו הֵבִיאוּ אֶת רַבִּי עֲקִיבָא*

עוֹקֵר הָרִים וְטוֹחֲנָן זוּ בָזוּ בִּסְבָרָה,

וְסָרְקוּ אֶת בְּשָׂרוֹ בְּמַסְרֵק שֶׁל בַּרְזֶל לְהִשְׁתַּבְּרָה,

יָצְתָה נִשְׁמָתוֹ בְּאֶחָד וּבַת קוֹל אָמְרָה,

אַשְׁרֶיךָ רַבִּי עֲקִיבָא גוּפָךְ טַהוֹר בְּכָל מִינֵי טָהֳרָה.

בֶּן בָּבָא רַבִּי יְהוּדָה* אַחֲרָיו, הֵבִיאוּ בְּשִׁבָּרוֹן לֵב וְאַזְהָרָה,

נֶהֱרַג בֶּן שִׁבְעִים שָׁנָה בִּידֵי אֲרוּרָה,

יוֹשֵׁב בְּתַעֲנִית הָיָה נָקִי וְחָסִיד בִּמְלַאכְתּוֹ לְמַהֲרָה.

רַבִּי חֲנִינָא² בֶּן תְּרַדְיוֹן* אַחֲרָיו מַקְהִיל קְהִלּוֹת בְּצִיּוֹן שָׁעֲרָה,

---

positioned. Until that point Rabbi Yishmael bore the excruciating physical pain in silence, but when they stripped him of this precious spiritual possession he let out a terrifying scream.

The Talmud relates that once every seventy years the Romans would reenact the following scene: A healthy man (representing Esau) would ride on the back of a cripple (symbolic of Jacob, who had a temporary limp after doing battle with the angel — see *Genesis* 32:24-32). 'Esau' would be wearing the garments once worn by Adam and later the property of Esau and would hold aloft the preserved head of Rabbi Yishmael. All this, to prove Esau's continued supremacy over Jacob, i.e., Israel (*Avodah Zarah* 11b with *Rashi*).

מְנוֹרָה הַטְּהוֹרָה — *'O pure Menorah!'* Torah scholars are beacons of light that guide people along the paths that lead to heaven. Or, in the words of King Solomon: נֵר מִצְוָה וְתוֹרָה אוֹר, *A mitzvah is a lamp and the Torah is light* (*Proverbs* 6:23).

צָעַק צְעָקָה — *He ... let such a scream.* For some reason the alphabetical acrostic is discontinued after the first twenty letters and omits the letter ש and ת. Perhaps some lines of the original composition have been lost or removed by the censors.

רַבִּי עֲקִיבָא — *Rabbi Akiva.* Rabbi Akiva's death at the age of one hundred and twenty took place about sixty years after the destruction of the Temple (circa 135 C.E.). After Bar Kochba's

unsuccessful uprising against the Romans, they enacted extremely harsh decrees proscribing the practice of Judaism in general and prohibiting the study and teaching of Torah in particular. Rabbi Akiva believed that without Torah study the Jewish people suffer a demise worse than death, so he ignored the Roman decree and taught Torah at massive public gatherings. The Romans imprisoned him and finally executed him on Yom Kippur.

Rabbi Akiva was tortured to death in this barbaric manner:

It was the time of the morning *Shema* reading when R' Akiva was taken out to be murdered publicly. During his frightful ordeal he accepted God's sovereignty upon himself by reciting the *Shema* joyously, oblivious to the pain. Turnus Rufus, the Roman commander who ordered the barbarous execution, was flabbergasted. 'Have you no feeling of pain that you can laugh in the face of such intense suffering!' he exclaimed. Even R' Akiva's own students wondered, 'Our teacher, even to this extent?'

The dying sage explained, 'All my life I was concerned over a phrase of the Torah. We are taught in the *Shema* to accept God's sovereignty and decrees upon ourselves, בְּכָל נַפְשֶׁךָ, *with all your soul* (*Deuteronomy* 6:5) — this implies that we must serve God even if it means forfeiting our life. I used to wonder if I would ever have the

נ He took [Rabban Shimon's severed] head and placed it
   on his lap [and lamented], 'O pure Menorah!'*

ס He placed his eyes upon his eyes, and his mouth
   upon his mouth in absolute love.

ע He cried out and said, 'O mouth that strengthened itself in Torah,

פ how suddenly a violent and cruel death has been inflicted upon you!'

צ He [the overlord] ordered them to strip the skin off
   [Rabbi Yishmael's] head with a sharp razor.

ק With his skin he fulfilled the prophecy: 'They [the enemy]
   said to your soul, "Prostrate yourself that we may walk over you!"'[1]

ר When the wicked one who flayed him
   reached the place of the tefillin, the brilliant mitzvah,

He [Rabbi Yishmael] let out such a scream* that
   the whole world quaked and the earth crumbled into little pieces.

After him they brought forth Rabbi Akiva*
   who uprooted mountains [of halachic problems]
   and ground them one against the other by thorough analysis.

They combed his flesh with an iron comb in order to break him.
   His soul departed while he declared,
   '[God is] One' and a heavenly voice proclaimed,

'Fortunate are you, Rabbi Akiva;
   your body has been purified with every type of purity!'

After him they brought forth Rabbi Yehudah ben Bava,*
   a man of humble heart, and scrupulous [in avoiding sin],
   he was killed at age seventy by the hands of the cursed [nation].

He was immersed in fasting; clean and pious,
   alacritous in his service.

Rabbi Chanina[2] ben Teradyon* came after him, [condemned because]
   he assembled crowds [to study Torah] within the gates of Zion.

---

(1) *Isaiah* 51:23. (2) Some editions read חֲנַנְיָא or חֲנַנְיָה, *Chananiah.*

privilege of serving God to such a degree. Now that the chance has come to me, shall I not grasp it with joy?'

He repeated the first verse of *Shema* — Hear, O Israel, HASHEM is our God, HASHEM is One — and as he drew out the word אֶחָד, One, his soul left him.

A heavenly voice was heard saying, 'You are praiseworthy, Rabbi Akiva, for your soul left you as you proclaimed God's Oneness! ... You are praiseworthy, Rabbi Akiva, for you are ready to enter the life of the World to Come' (*Berachos* 61b; *Yerushalmi Berachos* 9:5).

רַבִּי יְהוּדָה בֶּן בָּבָא — *Rabbi Yehudah ben Bava.* Moses ordained his disciple Joshua, thus investing him with the God-given authority to render halachic judgments and to impose certain fines. The chain of *Semichah* ordination remained unbroken, handed down from teacher to disciple, for almost fifteen centuries until the Romans issued a decree prohibiting Rabbis (under pain of death) from ordaining their students. Rabbi

Yehudah ben Bava was determined to guarantee the perpetuation of the chain of *Semichah*. He secretly ordained five of his greatest disciples near a mountain pass in a secluded area between the cities of Usha and Shefaram. These illustrious students were: Rabbi Meir, Rabbi Yehudah bar Illai, Rabbi Shimon bar Yochai, Rabbi Yossi ben Chalafta and Rabbi Elazar ben Shamua, the tenth martyr (other opinions add a sixth disciple, Rabbi Nechemiah, see *Sanhedrin* 13b-14a).

Unfortunately, the Romans heard about this convocation and sent troops to execute the master and his disciples. Seventy-year-old Rabbi Yehudah ben Bava commanded his students, 'Run away, my sons, and I will stand firm before them like an immovable boulder.' Rabbi Yehudah blocked the narrow mountain path with his body and the Romans could not budge him. Only after they pierced his body with three hundred iron spears and made him like a sieve did he fall dead.

רַבִּי חֲנִינָא בֶּן תְּרַדְיוֹן — *Rabbi Chanina ben Teradyon.* The Talmud (*Avodah Zarah* 18a)

יוֹשֵׁב וְדוֹרֵשׁ וְסֵפֶר תּוֹרָה עִמּוֹ, וְהִקִּיפוּהוּ בְּחַבְלֵי זְמוֹרָה,

אֶת הָאוֹר הִצִּיתוּ בָהֶם וּכְרָכְוּהוּ בְּסֵפֶר תּוֹרָה,

סְפוֹגִין שֶׁל צֶמֶר הִנִּיחוּ עַל לִבּוֹ שֶׁלֹּא יָמוּת מְהֵרָה.

חָסִיד רַבִּי יֶשֵׁבָב הַסּוֹפֵר* הֲרָגְוּהוּ עִם עֲמוֹרָה,

זְרָקְוּהוּ וְהִשְׁלִיכְוּהוּ לַכְּלָבִים וְלֹא הֻקְבַּר בִּקְבוּרָה,

יָצְאָה בַּת קוֹל עָלָיו שֶׁלֹּא הִנִּיחַ כְּלוּם מִתּוֹרַת מֹשֶׁה לְשָׁמְרָה,

וְאַחֲרָיו רַבִּי חוּצְפִּית* בְּיוֹם עֶבְרָה,

עוֹף הַפּוֹרֵחַ נִשְׂרַף בַּהֶבֶל פִּיו כְּבַמְּדוּרָה.

צַדִּיק רַבִּי אֶלְעָזָר בֶּן שַׁמְּוּעַ* בָּאַחֲרוֹנָה נֶהֱרַג בְּמַדְקִירָה,

יוֹם עֶרֶב שַׁבָּת הָיָה זְמַן קִדּוּשׁ וַיְקַדֵּשׁ וַיִּקְרָא,

חֶרֶב שָׁלְפוּ עָלָיו וְלֹא הִנִּיחְוּהוּ בַּחַיִּים לְגָמְרָה,

יָצְאָה נִשְׁמָתוֹ בְּבָרָא אֱלֹהִים' יוֹצֵר וְצָר צוּרָה.

כָּהֲנָה וְכָהֲנָה הוֹסִיפוּ בְּנֵי עַוְלָה לַעֲנוֹת בְּגֶעְרָה,

בִּסְקִילָה שְׂרֵפָה הֶרֶג וְחֶנֶק מִי יוּכַל לְשַׁעֲרָה,

נוֹתֶרֶת מִמֶּנָּה יֹאכְלוּ אֲרָיוֹת שֶׂה פְזוּרָה,²

חֵזֶה הַתְּנוּפָה וְשׁוֹק הַתְּרוּמָה*³ טָרְפוּ אַרְיֵה וְהַבְּפִירָה,

יֵיטִיב יהוה וְלֹא יוֹסִיף עוֹד לְיַסְּרָה,⁴

אַמֵּץ בִּרְכַּיִם כּוֹשְׁלוֹת⁵ חֵלֶק יַעֲקֹב⁶ וּמוֹשִׁיעַ בְּעֵת צָרָה,⁷

לְצֶדֶק יִמְלָךְ מֶלֶךְ,⁸ יֵאָמֵר שַׁלְּמוּ יְמֵי אֶבְלֵךְ,⁹ לְאוֹרוֹ נִסַּע וְנֵלֵךְ.

---

(1) Genesis 2:3. (2) Cf. Jeremiah 50:17. (3) Cf. Leviticus 7:34. (4) Cf. 26:18. (5) Cf. Isaiah 35:3. (6) Jeremiah 10:16. (7) Cf. 14:8. (8) Isaiah 32:1. (9) 60:20.

teaches that the pretext to execute Rabbi Chanina was that he violated the Roman edict against teaching the Torah publicly. The Romans wrapped him in the Torah Scroll that he always kept with him and set it afire. To prolong his agony, they packed his chest with water-soaked wool. To his horrified daughter and student, Rabbi Chanina said, 'The parchment is consumed, but the letters fly up in the air.' The Roman executioner was deeply moved by Rabbi Chanina's holiness and asked, 'If I remove the wool from your heart, will I have a share in the World to Come?' Rabbi Chanina promised that he would, whereupon the Roman removed the wet wool and put more wood on the fire, so that the agony would end quickly. Then, the Roman threw himself into the fire and died. A heavenly voice proclaimed, 'Rabbi Chanina and his executioner are about to enter the World to Come.'

רַבִּי יֶשֵׁבָב הַסּוֹפֵר — *Rabbi Yeshevav the Scribe.* Rabbi Yeshevav was Rabbi Akiva's colleague. It was said of him that he was as great as Moses in every respect other than prophecy. The Romans

murdered him while he was reciting the *Shema*, as he was reading the portion dealing with the *mitzvah* of the *tzitzis* fringes. He died on a high level of purity for he had been fasting all that day, but the Romans were determined to subject his remains to degradation. They refused to allow him to be buried; instead, they had wild dogs drag his pure and holy body through the streets.

רַבִּי חוּצְפִּית — *Rabbi Chutzpis.* In Talmudic times, a מְתוּרְגְּמָן, literally, *interpreter*, would repeat and explain the lecture of the *rosh yeshivah.* Rabbi Chutzpis was one day short of his 130th birthday and his last wish was for one more day of life in order to recite the *Shema* for another evening and morning. But his wish was not granted.

The Romans devised a particularly sadistic barbarism for Rabbi Chutzpis. Since he was renowned for his rhetorical skill and his golden tongue, before they killed him they cut out his tongue and tossed it into the trash heap. This was a particularly disturbing torture, for Rabbi Chutzpis never used his tongue to speak anything other than words of Torah. The Talmud

While he sat with a Torah Scroll and taught,
  they surrounded him with bundles of vines.
They set them on fire, and wrapped him in the Torah Scroll
  [from which he taught].
They placed tufts of [water-soaked] wool on his heart,
  so that he would not die quickly.
The pious one, Rabbi Yeshevav the Scribe,* was killed
  by the descendants of [Sodom and] Amorah.
They threw him down and flung him to the dogs,
  so he was not buried in a proper grave.
A heavenly voice went forth [and said] that he did not fail
  to observe any detail of the Torah of Moses.
And after him on the day of wrath, they [killed] Rabbi Chutzpis,*
  [who taught Torah with such fiery zeal that a] bird
  flying [above him] would be burnt
  by the breath of his mouth as if on the Altar pyre.
The righteous Rabbi Elazar ben Shamua* was the last;
  he was killed by stabbing.
It was on a Friday as the day turned to the holy Sabbath,
  so he began the Kiddush and recited [the opening passage].
They unsheathed a sword over him,
  and did not allow him to live to finish it.
His soul departed with [the words] 'which God created,'[1]
  [thereby acknowledging Him as] the Creator
  Who fashioned every creature's form.
Again and again in this manner, the sons of iniquity
  continued to torture [us] with rebuke.
With stoning, burning, beheading and strangling —
  who can calculate [the enormity of the tragedy]?
What remained of it, the scattered flock, the lions consumed.[2]
The breast of the waving and the thigh of the raising-up[3]*
  the lion and his daughter tore to pieces.
May HASHEM show [His] benevolence [to us]
  and never again make us suffer.[4]
Strengthen the faltering knees,[5] O You Who are Jacob's portion,[6]
  and his savior in times of distress.[7]
For the sake of righteousness He [God] shall reign as king.[8]
He will say [to Israel], 'The days of your mourning have come to
  an end!'[9] Then we shall venture forth and walk in His light!

---

relates that when Elisha ben Avuyah, a well-known Sage of Mishnaic times, saw Rabbi Chutzpis' tongue being chewed up by a swine in the trash heap, he could not fathom that a just God would allow such 'injustice,' and he turned heretic. The Talmud, however, explains Rabbi Chutzpis' degradation as proof that שְׂכַר מִצְוָה בְּהַאי עָלְמָא לֵיכָּא, *reward for mitzvah observance is not forthcoming in this world,* but in the World to Come (*Kiddushin* 39b).

רַבִּי אֶלְעָזָר בֶּן שַׁמּוּעַ — *Rabbi Elazar ben Shamua.* One of the five great disciples ordained by Rabbi Yehudah ben Bava (see above), he was the last of the Ten Martyrs. He was killed at the age of one hundred and five.

חֲזֵה הַתְּנוּפָה וְשׁוֹק הַתְּרוּמָה — *The breast of the waving and the thigh of the raising-up.* The flesh of these innocent victims was regarded by God as the choicest and finest of Altar offerings.

כב.

הַחֲרִישׁוּ מִמֶּנִּי* וַאֲדַבֵּרָה, וְיַעֲבֹר עָלַי מָה,[1]

חָמָס אֶזְעַק וְשֹׁד[2] לְךָ שׁוֹכֵן שָׁמַיְמָה,

הֲצִיקַתְנִי רוּחִי וְלֹא אוּכַל אֶדֹּמָה,

כַּיּוֹלֵדָה אֶפְעֶה אֶשְׁאַף וְאֶשְׁאָמָה,[3]

מִסְפֵּד מַר אֶעֱשֶׂה וַאֲקוֹנֵן בִּנְהִימָה,

דִּבְרֵי שַׁאֲגוֹתַי יֻתְּכוּ כְּיָמָּה,[4]

סִפְרִי עַל עֲדָתִי אֲשֶׁר נִתְּנָה לְשַׁמָּה,

אָרִיד בְּשִׂיחִי וְאָהִימָה,[5] וְקוֹל נְהִי אָרִימָה.

אֵיךְ שָׁבַת מָשׂוֹשׂ וְעָרְבָה שִׂמְחָה,

כָּל פָּנִים פָּארוּר[6] וְכָל רֹאשׁ קָרְחָה,

וְכָל זָקָן גְּדוּעָה[7] וְעַל כָּל לֵב אֲנָחָה,

מֵאָז נִתְעוֹרֵר גּוֹי עַז דּוֹרֵשׁ שׂוּחָה,[8]

סָלָה אַבִּירַי[9] הוֹגֵי עֹז מִבְטַחָה,

בְּתוּלוֹתַי וּבַחוּרַי נָסַח בִּנְסִיחָה,

בְּרֹאשׁ כָּל חוּצוֹת[10] נִבְלָתָן כַּסּוּחָה,[11]

עוֹלָלַי וְטַפַּי[12] נֶחְשְׁבוּ כְּצֹאן טִבְחָה,[12]

אֵילִילָה עַל זֹאת[13] וְדִמְעָתִי עַל לֶחָה,[14]

הֵאָסְפוּ אֵלַי דְּוּוּיֵי צֹאן נִדָּחָה,

לְהַרְבּוֹת הַבְּכִי וּלְהָרִים צְוָחָה,

הֵילִילוּ שָׁמַיִם וְזַעֲקִי אֲדָמָה.

אָרִיד בְּשִׂיחִי וְאָהִימָה, וְקוֹל נְהִי אָרִימָה.

אֶרְאֶלִּים* צְאוּ וְצַעֲקוּ[15] מָרָה,

סְפוֹד תַּמְרוּר הֶאָגְדוּ בַּחֲבוּרָה,[16]

קוֹל כַּחוֹלָה צָרָה כְּמַבְכִּירָה,[17]

הִתְאוֹנְנוּ עַל עֲדַת שֶׂה פְזוּרָה,

עֲלֵימוֹ כִּי נִגְזְרָה גְזֵרָה, בָּחֳרִי אַף וָזַעַם וְעֶבְרָה,[18]

וְנִתְוַעֲדוּ בִּפְרִישׁוּת וּבְטָהֳרָה, לְקַדֵּשׁ שֵׁם הַגָּדוֹל וְהַנּוֹרָא,

---

◆§ הַחֲרִישׁוּ מִמֶּנִּי — *Be silent and leave me be.* In vivid prose and sharp detail this *kinnah,* of unknown authorship, captures the anguish of a survivor of an unknown massacred community whose emotions are still storming and seething and whose tears are not yet dry. It describes the untenable tragedy of loving parents forced to slaughter their cherished children by their own hand, to save them from excruciating torture and mutilation at the hand of the enemy. All this was

22.

Be silent and leave me be* so that I may speak out;
  let whatever may befall me,[1]
I shall scream to You, Who dwells in the Heavens,
  over the violence and pillage.[2]
My spirit presses me and I cannot remain still,
I shall cry like a woman in birth travail, I shall pant and gasp.[3]
I shall compose a bitter dirge and I shall lament as I moan.
The words of my roars shall roll out like [the waves of] the sea.[4]
I eulogize my community which has been given over to desolation.
     I shall lament as I speak and I shall moan,[5]
       and I shall raise the sound of lament.
O how joy is halted and gladness darkened;
every face is blackened[6] and every head is bald,
every beard is clipped[7] and on every heart a sigh,
ever since the powerful nation aroused itself to seek
     [the means to cast us into] the pit,[8]
He trampled my heroes,[9] those who study
  our secure stronghold [the Torah].
My maidens and my youths, he uprooted with devastation;
on every street corner[10] their corpses lay like refuse.[11]
My infants and my babes were treated like sheep for the slaughter.[12]
About this shall I wail,[13] my tears on [my] cheek.[14]
Gather around me, O suffering lost sheep,
to intensify [your] weeping and to scream even louder.
Howl, O Heaven, and shout out, O Earth.
     I shall lament as I speak and I shall moan, and I shall raise the sound of lament.
O Erelim,* go forth and shout[15] bitterly,
assemble in groups for most bitter eulogy,[16]
cry like a woman in travail, with the pain
  of one undergoing her first childbirth.[17]
Mourn for the flock of scattered sheep,
for the decree was issued against them
with blazing anger, rage and wrath.[18]
They gathered themselves in abstinence and purity
to sanctify the Great and Awesome Name,

---

(1) Cf. *Job* 13:13. (2) Cf. *Habakkuk* 1:2-3. (3) *Isaiah* 42:14. (4) Cf. *Job* 3:24. (5) *Psalms* 55:3.
(6) Cf. *Joel* 2:6. (7) Cf. *Jeremiah* 48:37; some editions read גְּרוּעָה, *diminished,* which is the
word used in Scriptures. (8) Some editions read כּוֹרָה שׁוּחָה, *to dig a pit;* cf. *Jeremiah* 18:22.
(9) Cf. *Eichah* 1:15. (10) 2:19. (11) Cf. *Isaiah* 5:25. (12) Cf. *Psalms* 44:23. (13) Cf. *Micah* 1:8.
(14) Cf. *Eichah* 1:2. (15) Cf. *Isaiah* 33:7. (16) Cf. *Jeremiah* 6:26. (17) Cf. 4:31. (18) Cf. *Psalms* 78:49.

---

performed in a spirit of utmost piety and purity
to sanctify the Name of God. Furthermore, it
describes how the greatest Torah scholars were
murdered and how their books and manuscripts
were mercilessly consigned to the flames.

It concludes with a question and a challenge to
God, 'How long will You continue to witness this
indifferently? ... Will You not seek revenge for

the blood spilled like gushing streams?'

The particular tragedy about which this *kinnah* was written is unknown. It very aptly describes any one of many massacres and pogroms
that have formed a large part of Jewish history.

אֶרְאֵלִים — *Erelim.* We lack the vocabulary to
distinguish between the varieties of angels.

וְאִישׁ אֶת אָחִיו חִזְּקוּ בְּעֶזְרָה,[1]
לְהִדָּבֵק בְּיִרְאָה טְהוֹרָה, בְּלִי כְּרוֹעַ לַעֲבוֹדָה זָרָה,
וְלֹא חָסוּ גֶּבֶר וּגְבִירָה,
עַל בָּנִים צְפִירַת תִּפְאָרָה,
אֲבָל אָזְרוּ גְּבוּרָה יְתֵרָה,
לַהֲלוֹם רֹאשׁ וְלִקְרוֹץ שִׁדְרָה,
וְאֵלֵימוֹ דִּבְּרוּ בַּאֲמִירָה,
לֹא זָכִינוּ לְגַדֶּלְכֶם לַתּוֹרָה,
נַקְרִיבְכֶם כְּעוֹלָה וְהַקְטָרָה,
וְנִזְכֶּה עִמָּכֶם לְאוֹרָה, הַצְּפוּנָה מֵעֵין כֹּל וַעֲלוּמָה.
אָרִיד בְּשִׂיחִי וְאָהִימָה, וְקוֹל נְהִי אָרִימָה.

אָז הִסְכִּימוּ גְּדוֹלִים וּקְטַנִּים,
לְקַבֵּל בְּאַהֲבָה דִּין שׁוֹכֵן מְעוֹנִים,
וּזְקֵנִים דְּשֵׁנִים וְרַעֲנַנִּים,[2] הֵם הָיוּ תְּחִלָּה נִדּוֹנִים,
וְיָצְאוּ לִקְרַאתָם עַזֵּי פָנִים, וְנֶהֶרְגוּ הַמּוֹנִים הַמּוֹנִים,
וְנִתְעָרְבוּ פְדָרִים עִם פַּרְשְׁדוֹנִים,
וְהָאָבוֹת אֲשֶׁר הָיוּ רַחֲמָנִים,
נֶהְפְּכוּ לְאַכְזָר כַּיְּעֵנִים,[3]
וְהֵפִיסוּ עַל אָבוֹת וְעַל בָּנִים,
וּמִי שֶׁגּוֹרָל עָלָה לוֹ רִאשׁוֹנִים,
הוּא נִשְׁחָט בַּחֲלָפוֹת וְסַכִּינִים,
וּבַחוּרִים עֲלֵי תוֹלָע אֱמוּנִים,[4]
הֵם לָחֲכוּ עָפָר כַּתַּנִּינִים,[5]
וְהַכַּלּוֹת לְבוּשׁוֹת שָׁנִים, מְעֻלָּפוֹת בִּזְרוֹעוֹת חֲתָנִים,
מְנֻתָּחוֹת בְּחֶרֶב וְכִידוֹנִים,
זִכְרוּ זֹאת קָהָל עֲדַת נְבוֹנִים,
וְאַל תֶּחֱשׁוּ מֵהַרְבּוֹת קִינִים,
וְהַסְפִּידוּ עַל חֲסִידִים וַהֲגוּנִים,
אֲשֶׁר צָלְלוּ בַּמַּיִם הַזֵּידוֹנִים,
לְזֵכֶר זֹאת נַפְשִׁי עֲגוּמָה.
אָרִיד בְּשִׂיחִי וְאָהִימָה, וְקוֹל נְהִי אָרִימָה.

and each man encouraged the other with succor,[1]
[enabling him] to embrace [God] with pure awe,
and not to kneel to strange gods.
Neither a man nor a woman showed weakening pity
for the [children whose] faces were like a splendid tiara.
Instead, they girded themselves with abnormal courage
to smash the head and sever the spine.
Then they addressed them with these words,
'We merited not to raise you in the Torah['s ways],
let us then bring you nearer [to God],
    like burnt-offering and incense.
May we merit sharing with you the light
that is is concealed and hidden from the eyes of all.
    I shall lament as I speak and I shall moan, and I shall raise the sound of lament.

Then young and old agreed
to accept lovingly the decision
    of the One Who Dwells in the heavens.
The aged who were nevertheless still vigorous and fresh,[2]
it was they who were judged the first [to be executed].
The insolent [enemy] went forth against them
and slaughtered multitudes upon multitudes,
until there was a [gruesome heap] of
    intermingled fats and intestinal wastes.
Then the Fathers who were once compassionate
turned cruel as ostriches,[3]
and they cast lots over parents and children
and whomever the lot came upon first,
he was slaughtered with blades and knives.
Youths brought up in scarlet clothing[4]
now licked the dust like serpents;[5]
and brides dressed in scarlet
swooned into the arms of their husbands,
[where they were] butchered by sword and spears.
Remember this, assembled congregation of the wise,
and dare not be silenced from abundant lamentations!
Eulogize the pious and proper ones
who sank in the treacherous waters.
At the memory of this, my soul is grieved.
    I shall lament as I speak and I shall moan, and I shall raise the sound of lament.

(1) Cf. *Isaiah* 41:6. (2) Cf. *Psalms* 92:15. (3) Cf. *Eichah* 4:3. (4) Cf. 4:5. (5) Cf. *Micah* 7:17.

Rambam (*Yesodei HaTorah* 2:7) enumerates ten levels: *Chayos, Ofanim, Erelim, Chashmalim, Seraphim, Malachim, Elohim, Bnei Elohim, Cheruvim,* and *Ishim*.

תּוֹרָה תּוֹרָה חִגְרִי שַׂק וְהִתְפַּלְּשִׁי בָּאֵפָרִים,

אֵבֶל יָחִיד עֲשִׂי לָךְ וּמִסְפַּד תַּמְרוּרִים,¹

עַל תּוֹפְשֵׂי מְשׁוֹטַיִךְ וּפוֹרְשֵׂי מַכְמוֹרִים,

מַלָּחַיִךְ וְחוֹבְלַיִךְ בְּמַיִם אַדִּירִים,²

עוֹרְכֵי מַעֲרָכֵךְ, מְיַשְּׁרֵי הֲדוּרִים,³

מְפַעֲנְחֵי צְפוּנַיִךְ וּמְגַלֵּי מִסְתּוֹרִים,

מִי יְקַצֶּה בִּגְבָעוֹת וּמִי יְסַתֵּת בֶּהָרִים,

וּמִי יְפָרֵק הֲוָיוֹת וּמִי יְתָרֵץ שְׁבָרִים,

מִי יַפְלִיא נְזִירוֹת וּמִי יַעֲרוֹךְ נְדָרִים,

מִי יְשַׁדֵּד מַעֲמַקַּיִךְ וְחָתוּ אִכָּרִים,

וּמִי יִלְחוֹם מִלְחַמְתֵּךְ וְיָשׁוּב לַשְּׁעָרִים,

כְּלֵי מִלְחָמָה אָבְדוּ וְנָפְלוּ גִבּוֹרִים.⁴

אַשְׁרֵיהֶם מַשְׂכִּילִים כָּרְקִיעַ זוֹהֲרִים,⁵

בִּמְנוּחוֹת שָׁלוֹם נָחוּ יְשָׁרִים, אוֹי וַאֲבוֹי שׁוֹד וָשֶׁבֶר לְנוֹתָרִים,

לִמְדִיבַת נֶפֶשׁ⁷ וַחֲבָלִים וְצִירִים,

לְכִלְיוֹן עֵינַיִם⁷ צַלְמָוֶת וְלֹא סְדָרִים,

עֶרֶב אֹמְרִים מִי יִתֵּן צְפָרִים, וּבֹקֶר מְצַפִּים מִי יְגַלֶּה אוֹרִים,*

מִמַּרְאֵה עֵינֵימוֹ אֲשֶׁר הֵמָּה שָׁרִים,⁸

מִחוּץ שִׁכְּלָה חֶרֶב וְאֵימָה מֵחֲדָרִים,⁹*

עַד מָתַי תַּבִּיט רוֹאֶה כָּל סְתָרִים,

קַנֵּא לְתוֹרָתְךָ אֲשֶׁר שְׂרָפוּהָ זָרִים,

קְלָאוּהָ פְּרָעוּהָ קְרָעוּהָ לִגְזָרִים,

כְּסִירִים סְבוּכִים הִגְדִּילוּ הַמְּדוּרִים,

הַעַל אֵלֶּה תִתְאַפֵּק¹⁰ אֲדוֹן כָּל יְצוּרִים,

תִּנְקוֹם דָּם הַנִּשְׁפָּךְ כַּמַּיִם הַמֻּגָּרִים,

מִשּׁוֹד עֲנִיִּים מֵאַנְקַת סְעוּרִים,¹¹

עִם שָׁבֵי פֶשַׁע לַעֲוֹנִים וּמְרוֹרִים רַחֲמָה,

אוֹתָם בַּל תַּחֲרִימָה, קַרְנָם הַגְבִּיהַּ וְהָרִימָה.

אָרִיד בְּשִׂיחִי וְאָהִימָה וְקוֹל נְהִי נְהִי אָרִימָה.

מִי יְגַלֶּה אוֹרִים — *O who will remove the daylight [and bring on evening]?* The root גלה has two diametrically opposite meanings. It can mean *to exile, to remove,* or *to uncover, to reveal.* The translation uses the first meaning. Alternatively, the phrase may be translated according to the second meaning, *O who will reveal the night-time luminaries?*

Torah, O Torah, gird yourself in sackcloth and roll yourself in ashes,
make yourself mourn for your only son; [recite the] most bitter eulogy¹
over those who hold the oars and spread the nets,
your sailors and those who man the ropes through
      the mighty waters² [of the sea of Talmud],
[They are the ones] who organize [Torah themes according to]
      logical arrangements that clarify complicated issues.³
who explain Your hidden [wisdom] and uncover its secrets.
Who will [now] cut through the heights,
      and who will [now] carve through the mountains?
Who will [now] clarify the issues, and who will [now]
      answer the [earth-]shattering [questions]?
Who will [now] interpret the [intricacies of] Nazirite vows, and who will
      [now] arrange [the complex laws of] oaths [and their annulment]?
Who will plow through your depths when
      the farmers have been cut down?
And who will wage your battles and return [Israel]
      to the gates [of the House of Torah Study],
[now that] the weapons are lost, and the heroes have fallen?⁴
Fortunate are those wise [martyrs] who are radiant as the firmament,⁵
these upright ones rest in peaceful repositories.
Woe and wailing, plunder and devastation; for the survivors,
for those miserable of spirit,⁶ travail and torment;
for those of failing eyes,⁷ the shadow of death and anarchy.
Eveningtime they say, 'O who will make it morning!'
And morning they anxiously say, 'O who will remove the daylight
      [and bring on evening]?'*
[This,] because of the [frightful] sights their eyes behold.⁸
Outside the sword cuts down while terror reigns within;⁹*
O how long will You watch [indifferently],
      You Who sees everything hidden?
Avenge Your Torah, which strangers have burnt;
they scorched it, they vandalized it, they ripped it to pieces.
They enlarged the pyre [with stacks of Torah volumes]
      like piles of tangled thornbrush.
Shall You restrain Yourself¹⁰ over such deeds,
      O Master of everything created?
Seek revenge for the blood spilled like falling waters,
for the plundering of the poor, for the cry of the storm-tossed.¹¹
Upon the people who repent transgression,
      who are sated with wormwood and bitterness,
take pity; do not allow them to be annihilated.
Elevate and exalt their honor.

   I shall lament as I speak and I shall moan, and I shall raise the sound of lament.

---

(1) Cf. *Jeremiah* 6:26. (2) Cf. *Ezekiel* 27:27-29. (3) Cf. *Isaiah* 45:2. (4) Cf. *II Samuel* 1:27. (5) Cf. *Daniel* 12:3. (7) Cf. *Deuteronomy* 28:65. (8) Cf. 28:67. (9) Cf. 32: 25. (10) *Isaiah* 64:11. (11) Cf. *Psalms* 12:6.

מֵחֲדָרִים . . . מחוץ — *Outside . . . within* [lit., *from the chambers*]. The translation follows one of the interpretations given by *Rashi* (*Deuteronomy* 32:25). According to *Rashi's* other interpre-

כג.

וְאֶת נָוִי חַטָּאתִי הַשָּׁמַיְמָה,*
וְדִמְעָתִי עַל לֶחְיִי אַזְרִימָה.
וּבַיּוֹם זֶה נְהִי נִהְיָה אָרִימָה,
וְאָהִימָה מִיָּמִים יָמִימָה.

אֲבָל לֵב וְנִחוּם חָדַל חָדוֹל,
וּמִכָּל כְּאֵב צִירִי נִבְדַּל בָּדוֹל,
עַל בֵּן וּבַת רַבִּי יִשְׁמָעֵאל כֹּהֵן גָּדוֹל,
זִכְרָם יְקוֹד בְּלִבָּבִי אָשִׂימָה.
וְאָהִימָה מִיָּמִים יָמִימָה.

עֵת נִשְׁבּוּ וְנָפְלוּ לִשְׁנֵי אֲדוֹנִים,
וְהֵם שְׁכֵנִים זֶה לְעֻמַּת זֶה חוֹנִים,
וַיְסַפְּרוּ זֶה לָזֶה עִנְיָנִים,
זֶה אָמַר מַשְׁבִּיַת צִיּוֹנִים,
שָׁבִיתִי שִׁפְחָה לְבוּשַׁת שָׁנִים,
כַּלְּבָנָה בְּזִיו וּקְלַסְתֵּר פָּנִים,
וּבְתֹאַר כִּקְצִיעָה וְיָמִימָה.*
וְאָהִימָה מִיָּמִים יָמִימָה.

רֵעֵהוּ סִפֵּר לוֹ בְּכִפְלַיִם,
הֵן אֲנִי מַשְׁבִּי יְרוּשָׁלַיִם,
שָׁבִיתִי עֶבֶד יְפֵה עֵינַיִם,
כַּשֶּׁמֶשׁ בְּתָקְפּוֹ עֵת צָהֳרַיִם,
בָּא וּנְזַוְּגֵם וּנְחַלְּקָה בִּנְתַּיִם,
בּוֹלְדוֹת כְּמוֹ כּוֹכְבֵי שָׁמַיִם,
לִשְׁמֹעַ זֹאת תִּצַּלְנָה אָזְנַיִם,
לִזְכֹּר זֹאת אֶת מַדַּי אַפְרִימָה.
וְאָהִימָה מִיָּמִים יָמִימָה.

כְּהִסְכִּימוּ עַל זֹאת שְׁנֵיהֶם יַחַד,
לָעֶרֶב זוּגוֹם בְּחֶדֶר אֶחָד,
וְהָאֲדוֹנִים מִבַּחוּץ לִבָּם כְּאֶחָד,

23.

My sin caused the destruction of my Temple,*
so I shall cause my tears to run down my cheeks;
and on this day I shall raise a doleful lament.
>   And I shall moan [about this] each year on this day.

The heart mourns, yet refuses consolation,
and from all other pain is my pain set apart,
upon [the fate of] the son and daughter of Rabbi Yishmael
>   the Kohen Gadol;
>   I shall set their memory as a fire in my heart.
>   And I shall moan [about this] each year on this day.

When they were captured, they fell to two different masters,
who were neighbors dwelling across from one another;
they discussed their affairs between themselves.
One said, 'From the captivity of Zion
I have captured a maid-servant dressed in scarlet-wool,
[her] features as bright as the moon,
>   as beautiful as Keziah and Jemimah!'*
>   And I shall moan [about this] each year on this day.

His neighbor responded with double [those praises],
'I [too] have come from the captivity of Jerusalem,
where I captured a man-servant with eyes so beautiful,
as the sun in its full splendor at high noon!
Come, let us pair them and divide between us
their children who will be abundant as the stars of the heavens!'
At these tidings all ears will ring;
>   to commemorate this, I shall rend my robe!
>   And I shall moan [about this] each year on this day.

Once the two of them had approved this [plan],
they paired [brother and sister] together that evening in one room.
The masters waited outside, their hearts as one,

---

tations: *Outside* refers to the battlefield outside the city, and *chambers* refers to the fugitives from the battlefield who succumbed to the terror throbbing in the chamber of their hearts; or *outside* alludes to overt idolatry (see, e.g., Jeremiah 11:13) and *chambers* to covert idolatry (see, e.g., Ezekiel 8:12).

וְאֵת נְוֵי חַטָּאתִי הַשְּׁמִימָה § — *My sin caused the destruction of my Temple.* The story of the son and daughter of R' Yishmael ben Elisha, the Kohen Gadol, (see kinnah 21) is related in the Talmud (Gittin 58a). It is interesting to note that the Midrash contains a very similar, though more complicated, narrative about the son and

daughter of Tzaddok HaKohen (*Midrash Eichah* 1:46). In each case, the young pair's moral purity set an example of chastity and righteousness that became an example for future generations. Neither youth nor maiden complained about the personal tragedy each underwent. Rather, it was the *chillul Hashem*, the desecration of God's Holy Name, that was the point of their plaints. And it was for this reason that Jeremiah prophetically wailed and lamented for this brother and sister so many centuries earlier.

וּבְתֹאַר כְּקְצִיעָה וְיָמִימָה — *As beautiful as Keziah and Jemimah.* Job had three daughters:

וְהֵם בּוֹכִים בְּמַר נֶפֶשׁ וָפַחַד,
עַד בְּקֶר בְּכִיתָם לֹא הִדְמִימָה.
וְאָהִימָה מִיָּמִים יָמִימָה.

זֶה יִסְפּוֹד בְּחִיל וּבְקִיר לֵב יִמְסֶה,
נִין אַהֲרֹן אֵיךְ לְשִׁפְחָה יְהִי נוֹשֵׂא,
וְהִיא גַם הִיא תְּיַלֵּל בְּתִגְרַת שׁוֹסֶה,
בַּת יוֹכֶבֶד אֵיךְ לְעֶבֶד תִּנָּשֵׂא,
אוֹי כִּי זֹאת גָּזַר אוֹמֵר וְעֹשֶׂה,
לָזֹאת יִבְכּוּ עָשׁ וּכְסִיל וְכִימָה.[1]
וְאָהִימָה מִיָּמִים יָמִימָה.

אוֹר בְּקֶר זֶה אֶת זֶה כְּהַכִּירוּ,
הוֹי אָחִי וְהוֹי אָחוֹת הִגְבִּירוּ.
וְנִתְדַּבְּקוּ יַחַד וְנִתְחַבָּרוּ,
עַד יָצְתָה נִשְׁמָתָם בִּנְשִׁימָה.
וְאָהִימָה מִיָּמִים יָמִימָה.

לָזֹאת יְקוֹנֵן יִרְמְיָהוּ בְּשָׁאיָה,
גְּזֵרָה זֹאת תָּמִיד אֲנִי בוֹכִיָּה,
וּבִלְבָבִי יְקַד יְקוֹד וּכְוִיָּה,
עַל בֵּן וּבַת מִסְפֵּד רַב אַרְעִימָה.[2]
אָרִיד בְּשִׂיחִי וְאָהִימָה,
וְקוֹל נְהִי אָרִימָה.

Jemimah, Keziah and Keren-happuch. *And there were not to be found in all the land,* women as beautiful as the daughter of Job (Job 42:15).

but [the young couple] wept with bitter soul and fear,
> their weeping was not stilled until the morning.
>> And I shall moan [about this] each year on this day.

He mourned all atremble; inside, his heart was melting,
'A scion of Aaron, can he be wed to a maid-servant?'
While she also bemoaned her captor's deal,
'A daughter of Yocheved, can she be wed to a slave?'
Woe! For this is the decree of [God],
Who says [something] and does [it].
> Upon this [tragedy], even [the constellations] Ursa,
> Orion and Pleiades[1] weep!
>> And I shall moan [about this] each year on this day.

At the light of dawn, they recognized one another,
they intensified [their cries], 'Woe! Brother!' and 'Woe! Sister!'
They embraced each other and were cleaved together,
> until both their souls left them, in the very same breath.
>> And I shall moan [about this] each year on this day.

For this Jeremiah lamented amidst the Destruction,
'I shall weep continually,
and in my heart is kindled a flame and a burn,
for this son and daughter I will thunder forth a great lament.[2]
> I shall lament as I speak, and I shall moan,
> and I shall raise the sound of lament.'

---

(1) *Job* 9:9; see commentary to *kinnah* 5.
(2) Some editions read אֲצִימָה, but the meaning is the same.

כד.

עַל חֻרְבַּן בֵּית הַמִּקְדָּשׁ,

כִּי הוּרַס וְכִי הוּדָשׁ,

אֶסְפּוֹד בְּכָל שָׁנָה וְשָׁנָה מִסְפֵּד חָדָשׁ,

עַל הַקְּדֶשׁ וְעַל הַמִּקְדָּשׁ.

תִּסָּתֵר לְאַלֵּם תַּרְשִׁישִׁים* מֵרוֹן,

כְּזִעְזַעְתָּ עוֹלָם מִפְּנֵי חָרוֹן,

כְּלַהֲטָה הָאֵשׁ בֵּין שְׁנֵי בַּדֵּי אָרוֹן.

שְׁנֵי מִקְדָּשִׁים אֲשֶׁר בְּמַעְלָה וּבְמַטָּה,

זֶה עַל גַּב זֶה הוּאָפְלוּ בַּעֲלָטָה,

וְנִחַמְתָּ אַחֲרִישׁ וְאֶתְאַפַּק¹ וְאַבִּיטָה.

רָאשֵׁי הַבַּדִּים כְּנִגְנְזוּ* מִבֵּין הַפָּרוֹכוֹת,*

וְאַרְבַּע גְּחָלִים* בִּדְבִיר מְהַלְּכוֹת,

וְאַרְבָּעִים יְסוֹד עַד תְּהוֹם מְלַחֲכוֹת.

קֹדֶשׁ הַקֳּדָשִׁים מִבֵּית קֹדֶשׁ כְּנִבְדַּד,

שָׁחַתָּ וְהֵילַלְתָּ אָהֳלֵי שַׁדָּד,³

וְנִחַמְתָּ אַכֶּה כַף עַל כַּף⁴ וְאֶשְׁאַג הֵידָד.⁵

צְפִירַת תִּפְאַרְתֵּךְ כְּנִתְּנָה בְּיַד צָר,

וְכָל כְּלֵי חֶמְדָּה אִוּוּי בֵּית הָאוֹצָר,⁶

וּלְךָ הַכֹּחַ וְהַגְּבוּרָה⁷ וְנָמוּ עָצֵר.

---

the terrestrial and celestial Temples. Here we grieve over the diminution of benefits derived from the phenomena of nature.

The *kinnah* follows a reverse-alphabetical format, beginning with the second stanza.

לְאַלֵּם תַּרְשִׁישִׁים — *To silence the celestial angels.* On three occasions when the angels in their heavenly array were about to begin their daily songs of God's praises, He stopped them: during the flood in Noah's time; when the Egyptians were drowning in the Sea of Reeds; and at the Destruction of the *Beis HaMikdash* (*Midrash Eichah*, intro. 24, as interpreted by *Yefeh Anaf*). The *paytan* alludes to the flood and the drowning with the words, *when You made the world shudder before Your fiery anger,* and to the Destruction with, *when the*

24.

Over the Destruction of the Temple,
that was torn down and trampled upon,
I shall lament with a new elegy every year,
for the holy [vessels] and for the Sanctuary.

ת   You hid Yourself in order to silence
    the celestial angels* from their songs,
When You made the world shudder before Your fiery anger,
[and] when the flames flared between the two poles of the Ark.

ש   When these two Temples, the one above and the one below —
    one directly over the other — were[1] both enshrouded in darkness,
You said, 'I will be silent, I will hold myself back,[2] I will observe.'

ר   When the heads of the poles were [removed
    from] behind the Curtains,* and hidden,*
four [flaming] coals* blazed in the Holy of Holies
and the forty foundation pillars were burnt to the depths.

ק   When the Holy of Holies was desolated
    and ceased to be a holy habitation,
You proclaimed and wailed, 'My Tent is plundered!'[3]
And you said, 'I shall clap My hands,
    one on the other,[4] and I shall roar, "O woe!"'[5]

צ   When the crown of Your glory [the Temple]
    was delivered into the hands of Your tormentors,
with all the precious vessels,
    the most desirable of the treasure house;[6]
You to Whom belongs the strength and the power[7]
    allowed them to exult, 'He has been restrained!'

---

(1) See kinnah 5. (2) Isaiah 42:14. (3) Jeremiah 10:20. (4) Cf. Ezekiel 21:22. (5) See Jeremiah 48:33 with Rashi. (6) Cf. Hosea 13:15. (7) Cf. I Chronicles 29:11.

---

flames flared between the two poles of the Ark (Beis Levi).

מִבֵּין הַפָּרוֹכוֹת — *Behind the Curtains.* Although the Torah speaks of only one *Paroches*-Curtain in the Tabernacle, there were two in the Second Temple (see Yoma 47a).

כְּנִגְנְזוּ — *When the ...were [removed ...] and hidden.* The Talmudic Sages discuss the fate of the Ark. Some maintain that it was taken by Nebuchadnezzar when he conquered the First Temple. Others hold, and this is the opinion of the *paytan*, that when King Josiah was informed by the prophets of the impending Destruction, he had the Ark removed from its place in the Holy of Holies and hidden in one of the underground passageways that Solomon had built beneath the *Beis HaMikdash* (Yoma 54b; Shekalim 6:2).

וְאַרְבַּע גֶּחָלִים — *Four [flaming] coals.* While the enemy was debating how to set fire to the *Beis HaMikdash*, the angels were debating with God (as it were) whether to permit the Destruction to take place. Finally, the Divine Attribute of Strict Justice came to the fore and said, 'Master of the world, do You want this wicked man to be able to boast, "I have destroyed God's Temple! I have burnt His Sanctuary!" No! It is better that a heavenly fire be sent down upon it ... Then, if the Babylonians claim supremacy because of their victory, Jerusalem will be able to retort, "You have slain an already dying lion! You have ground already milled flour! You have kindled an already burned city!"' (Midrash Eichah 1:41). Suddenly the conquerors looked up and saw four flaming coals descend from heaven upon the four corners of the Temple and set it afire (Pesikta Rabbah 27:6).

פְּנֵי הַכִּסֵּא אָז אָפֵלוּ,

וְגָבְהֵי שָׁמַיִם לְקַדְרוּת הוּשְׁפֵּלוּ,

יָכִין וּבוֹעֵז לְהִשְׁתַּבֵּר כְּנָפֵלוּ,

עֲשָׂרָה שֻׁלְחָנוֹת* אָז שֻׁלָּלוּ,

וּלְעוֹרְכֵיהֶם נָמוּ אַיֵּה אֲדוֹן אֵלּוּ,

לְאוֹצְרוֹת שִׁנְעָר לַקֳּדָשִׁים כְּהוּנְחָלוּ.

שְׂרָפִים עוֹמְדִים³ נָעוּ מִמַּעֲמָד,

כְּנֶהֶרְסוּ מְכוֹנוֹת⁴ מִתּוֹךְ מַחֲמָד,

וְזֵדִים קָרְאוּ יְמֵי הַשָּׁמַד.

נְחֹשֶׁת יָם⁵ וַעֲשָׂרָה כִּיּוֹרוֹת,⁶

כְּנִמְסְרוּ לַבֵּל וְהִנָּם שְׁבוּרוֹת,*

וּשְׁנֵי הַמְּאוֹרוֹת מֵאָז קְדוּרוֹת.⁷

מַעֲשֵׂה הָאוֹפַנִּים אֲשֶׁר בַּמֶּרְכָּבָה,⁸

כְּהוּרְדוּ לָאָרֶץ זָהַר הָרָקִיעַ כָּבָה,

חוֹלֵשׁ עַל גּוֹיִם⁹* לִפְנֵי כְרוּבִים בָּא.

לִוְיוֹת הַמּוֹרָד¹⁰ מֵעֵת הוֹרְדוּ,

וְהַטְּלָלִים לִבְרָכָה לֹא יָרְדוּ,

אֲנָשִׁים רָעִים עַל בָּמֳתֵי עָב דָּדוּ.¹¹

כָּל כְּלֵי כֶסֶף וּכְלֵי הַזָּהָב,

קֳצָצוּ וְשֻׁסּוּ מִבֵּית הַלַּהַב,

בְּצֵאת הֶהָדָר שָׁחֲחוּ עוֹזְרֵי רָהַב.¹²

יוֹם אֲשֶׁר נִקְרָא מְהוּמָה וּמְבוּכָה,¹³

לַהֲקַת מַלְאָכִים כְּאִשָּׁה מְצֵרָה נְבוֹכָה,

דִּבּוּר פָּתַח וְעָנוּ אַחֲרָיו אֵיכָה.

---

(1) See *I Kings* 7:21. (2) See *II Chronicles* 4:8. (3) See commentary to *kinnah* 22, s.v. אֶרְאֵלִים, *Erelim*. (4) See *I Kings* 7:27ff. (5) See 7:23 ff. (6) See 7:38. (7) Cf. *Joel* 2:10. (8) Cf. *I Kings* 7:33. (9) *Isaiah* 14:12. (10) See *I Kings* 7:29. (11) Cf. *Isaiah* 14:14. (12) Cf. *Eichah* 1:6; *Job* 9:13. (13) Cf. *Isaiah* 22:5.

עֲשָׂרָה שֻׁלְחָנוֹת — *Ten Tables.* The Torah ordains that a Golden Table be placed in the Sanctuary, upon which the *Panim*-breads are arranged. When King Solomon built the *Beis HaMikdash*, he enhanced that Table by placing five more to its right and five to its left (see *Rashi* to *II Chronicles* 4:8). These should not be confused with the thirteen tables of the Second Temple (see *Shekalim* 6:4) which served an entirely different purpose.

וְהִנָּם שְׁבוּרוֹת — *And behold, they were broken.* When these sturdy copper vessels were brought to Babylon for idolatrous purposes, they suddenly broke apart of their own accord (*Arugas HaBosem*).

פ   Then [the heavens] facing the Throne [of Glory] were darkened,
and the celestial heights were plunged into blackness,
when [the two Temple pillars called] Yachin and Boaz[1]
     fell and were smashed.

ע   Ten Tables[2]* were then taken as booty;
and to [the priests] who once set them, [the enemy] said,
     'Where is the Master of these [tables]?'
when [they were taken] to the treasure houses
     of Shinar [Babylon], and bequeathed to harlots.

ס   The stationary Seraphim[3] were removed from their positions,
when the bases [of the washstands][4]
     were demolished within the [Temple of God's] delight,
while strangers proclaimed [that period as]
     'The Days of Destruction'.

נ   When the copper [pool known as 'the] Sea [of Solomon'][5]
     and the ten washbasins[6]
were given over to the [worshipers of the idol]
     Bel, and, behold, they were broken —*
and ever since then the two luminaries
     [the sun and the moon] have darkened.[7]

מ   When [the copper bases] designed in the shape of
     the wheels of the [Celestial] Chariot,[8]
were lowered to the ground, the brilliance
     of the firmament was dimmed,
because [Nebuchadnezzar] who cast lots over the nations[9]*
     entered into the presence of the Cherubim [in the Holy of Holies].

ל   When the engravings of the entwined [cherubs][10]
     were taken down [from the Temple walls],
the dew ceased descending from the skies for a blessing,
while the vicious dogs [Nebuchadnezzar's hordes]
     ascended above the cloud-wreathed heights.[11]

כ   All the silver and golden vessels
were hacked to pieces and pillaged
     from the abode of the Eternal Flame.
and when the splendor departed,
     the ministering angels were demoted.[12]

י   On the day which was called 'Chaos and Confusion,'[13]
bands of angels were left perplexed like a woman in birth travail,
until [the Almighty Himself] began to speak
     [in lament and the angels] answered 'Eichah' after Him.

חוֹלֵשׁ עַל גּוֹיִם — [Nebuchadnezzar] who cast lots
over the nations. Nebuchadnezzar would de-
grade the kings of the lands he had captured, by

making them his personal servants. Daily lots
would be cast to determine which king would
serve him each day. According to the Sages, he

טָסוּ עֲמוֹנִים וּמוֹאָבִים, וְהוֹצִיאוּ הַכְּרוּבִים,
וּבִכְלִיבָה הָיוּ אוֹתָם מְסַבְּבִים,
הִנֵּה כְּכָל הַגּוֹיִם בֵּית יְהוּדָה חֲשׁוּבִים.[1]

חֵיל שַׂרְפֵי הַקֹּדֶשׁ[2] חָלַף מִגְדַּלְתּוֹ,
וְאֵל אַדִּיר שְׁמוֹ לֹא אָבָה תְהִלָּתוֹ,[3]
לַגַּלִּים הוּשַׂם בֵּית תְּפִלָּתוֹ.

זַמָּרֵי שַׁחַק הֶחֱשׁוּ מִנְּעַם,
וְנָם מַה לָּכֶם פֹּה אֵין הַיּוֹם טַעַם,
מַה תְּקַלְּסוּן לַמֶּלֶךְ בִּשְׁעַת הַזַּעַם.

וְהַכֹּהֲנִים וְהַלְוִיִּם עַל מִשְׁמְרוֹתָם נִשְׁחָטִים,
וְעַל מַחְלְקוֹתָם שַׁעֲטַת אִסְטַרְדְּיוֹטִים,
וְנָמוּ אַיֵּה מֶלֶךְ אָסוּר בָּרְהָטִים.[4]

הַכֵּלִים וְהַמְּשַׁמְּשִׁים בַּשְּׁבִי הוֹלְכִים,
וְהַשָּׂרִים וְהַסְּגָנִים בַּכֶּבֶל מְשׁוּכִּים,
וּתְמוּר בַּדִּים שַׂק חָגְרוּ מַלְאָכִים.

דָּץ לָבִיא וּפָקַח עֵינָיו,
וְהִנֵּה מִיכָאֵל מְהַלֵּךְ לְפָנָיו,
וְשָׂרִים* הוֹלְכִים כַּעֲבָדִים חָזוּ הֲמוֹנָיו.

גַּאֲוָה עֻטָּה וְכִבָּה הַמְּנוֹרָה,
וְנָטָה יָדוֹ אֶל אֵלֵי[5] הַמּוֹרָא,
וַיַּחְשִׁיךְ אוֹר עוֹטֶה אוֹרָה.[6]

בְּשַׁאֲגוֹ כָּאֲרִי בִּדְבִיר בֵּל,
בָּרַח דּוֹדִי וּכְעַל מֵת מִתְאַבֵּל,
פִּקְדוֹן הָרוּחוֹת בּוֹ בַּלַּיְלָה לֹא קִבֵּל.

אָמַר לַמַּשְׁחִיתִים חֲמָתִי הֲתִכֹּתִי,[7]
אֶת יְדִידוּת נַפְשִׁי בְּכַף אוֹיְבֶיהָ נָתַתִּי,
עָזַבְתִּי אֶת בֵּיתִי וְאֶת נַחֲלָתִי נָטַשְׁתִּי.[8]

---

also used them for immoral purposes (Rashi to
Isaiah 14:12).

וְשָׂרִים — And ... [Jewish] nobles. Alternatively,
this alludes to the Midrash that tells how, when

Nebuchadnezzar ordered crushing burdens
placed on the captives' backs to break their noble
stature, armies of angels descended to help the
Jews bear their loads (Midrash Tehillim 137).
Thus, the שָׂרִים are the celestial princes.

ט The Ammonites and Moabites swept in and took out the Cherubim,
    and paraded them around [Jerusalem] in a cage,
  saying, 'Behold, the House of Judah is to be considered
    [idolatrous] like all the nations.'[1]

ח The legions of holy Seraphim[2] were removed from their prominence,
    and God Whose Name is Mighty had no desire to be praised,[3]
  when His House of Splendor was turned into piles of ruins.

ז The angelic singers were silent from their pleasant [singing],
    because He said, 'What are you doing here? Today,
    permission [to sing] has not been given!
  How can you offer praise to the King at the time of fury?'

ו The Kohanim and the Levites were slaughtered at their watches;
    they manned their posts despite the clamor
    of the [Roman] commanders,
  who asked, 'Where is the King who is bound under the roofbeams?'[4]

ה The vessels and the ministers have gone into captivity,
    the nobles and the assistants were dragged away in shackles,
    and instead of fine linen, the angels girded themselves in sackcloth.

ד Lion[-like Nebuchadnezzar] rejoiced and opened up his eyes,
    and behold, [the archangel] Michael was going before him;
    and [Nebuchadnezzar's] hordes witnessed [Jewish] nobles*
    going [into exile] like slaves.

ג [Nebuchadnezzar] wrapped himself in arrogance
    and extinguished the Menorah,
  then he stretched out his hand against God[5] so Awesome,
    and darkened the light of God Who is enveloped in light.[6]

ב When [Nebuchadnezzar who worshiped the idol]
    roared like a lion in the Holy of Holies,
  my Beloved fled and mourned as for the dead;
    on that night He did not accept the deposited souls.*

א To the destructive angels, [God] said,
    'I have poured out My fury [over Jerusalem],[7]
  I have placed the beloved of My soul [Israel]
    into the hand of her enemies;
  I have abandoned My Temple and forsaken My estate.'[8]

---

(1) Cf. *Ezekiel* 25:8. (2) Some editions read שַׂרְפֵי מַעְלָה, *celestial* or *exalted Seraphim*.
(3) See commentary above. (4) *Song of Songs* 7:6. (5) Cf. *Job* 15:25.
(6) Cf. *Psalms* 104:2. (7) Cf. *II Chronicles* 34:25. (8) Cf. *Jeremiah* 12:7.

פִּקְדוֹן הָרוּחוֹת בּוֹ בַּלַּיְלָה לֹא קִבֵּל — *On that night He
did not accept the deposited souls.* Every night,
when a person retires, his soul ascends to the
heavens where it is held in safekeeping until
morning (see *Psalms* 31:6). Moreover, it is
invigorated and returned to its body in a fresh

and renewed state — as it is stated: *They are new
every morning; great is Your faithfulness* (*Eichah*
3:23). The *paytan* teaches us that on the night of
the Destruction, God accepted no souls, for no one
was able to sleep. Or, perhaps, no one could fall
asleep, because God would not accept the souls.

כה.

מִי יִתֵּן רֹאשִׁי מַיִם* וְעֵינִי מְקוֹר נוֹזְלַי,

וְאֶבְכֶּה כָל יְמוֹתַי וְלֵילַי,¹

אֶת חַלְלֵי טַפַּי וְעוֹלָלַי, וִישִׁישֵׁי קְהָלַי,

וְאַתֶּם עֲנוּ אֲבוֹי אוֹי² וְאַלְלַי,

וּבְכֵן בָּכֹה בְכֶה³ רַב וְהֶרֶב,

עַל בֵּית יִשְׂרָאֵל וְעַל עַם יהוה כִּי נָפְלוּ בֶחָרֶב.⁴

וְדָמוֹעַ תִּדְמַע⁵ עֵינִי וְאֵלְכָה לִי שְׂדֵה בוֹכִים,

וַאֲבַכֶּה עַמִּי מָרֵי לֵבָב הַנְּבוֹכִים,

עַל בְּתוּלוֹת הַיָּפוֹת וִילָדִים הָרַכִּים,

בְּסִפְרֵיהֶם נִכְרָכִים וְלַטֶּבַח נִמְשָׁכִים,

אָדְמוּ עֶצֶם⁶ מִפְּנִינִים סַפִּירִים וְנוֹפְכִים,

כְּמוֹ טִיט חוּצוֹת⁷ נִדָּשִׁים וְנִשְׁלָכִים,

סוּרוּ טָמֵא קָרְאוּ לָמוֹ⁸ מִלְּקָרֶב,

עַל בֵּית יִשְׂרָאֵל וְעַל עַם יהוה כִּי נָפְלוּ בֶחָרֶב.

‎מִי יִתֵּן רֹאשִׁי מַיִם — *Would that my head were water.* Significantly, this is the first *kinnah* recited on the Ninth of Av that is apparently unrelated to the destruction of the two Temples. Indeed, this elegy mourns the calamity that befell the Jewish communities of the Rhineland — Worms, Speyer and Mainz (Mayence) — in the year 1096, during the First Crusade, over one thousand years after the destruction of the Second Temple. The inclusion of this lament in the Tishah B'Av ritual serves to demonstrate that the source and cause of all Jewish tragedies in exile can and must be traced back to the Destruction of our Temple. The following incident illustrates this concept vividly.

When the Jewish people became aware of the awesome devastation that befell our nation at the hands of the murderous Nazis in World War II, many sought to establish a new day of national mourning to commemorate *Churban Europa*. The contemporary Torah leaders were consulted. Among the responses was that of the *Brisker Rav, R' Yitzchak Zev Soloveitchik,* who said that the reply to this question lies in the *kinnah* before us. Why didn't the great Rabbis and Sages of that generation — among them the greatest of the *Rishonim*, including Rashi — establish a *new* day of national mourning to commemorate that *new* tragedy? The author of this *kinnah* addresses this question and provides this insight:

Please take to your hearts to compose a bitter eulogy, / because their massacre is deservant of mourning and rolling in dust / as was the burning of the House of our God, its Hall and its Palace. / However, we cannot add a (new) day (of mourning) over ruin and conflagration, / nor may we mourn any earlier — only later. / Instead, today (on Tishah B'Av), I will arouse my sorrowful wailing, / and I will eulogize and wail and weep with a bitter soul, / and my groans are heavy from morning until evening.

Thus, the essential purpose of this *kinnah* is to drive home this lesson: There are really no *new* tragedies befalling Israel. All of our woes stem from one tragic source — the Destruction of the Temple on Tishah B'Av. To establish a new day of mourning would detract from the significance of Tishah B'Av and obscure its lesson and message. (See Rashi to *II Chronicles* 35:25.)

This *kinnah* also answers another major question. Why does the exile continue? Why does God visit fresh calamities upon His people? Where have we gone astray?

One of the main reasons for the continuation of our exile is because Jews are often quite content and comfortable in their adopted, alien homelands and have all but lost their desire to return to the poverty and hardships of *Eretz Yisrael*. Slowly the Jew ceases to identify with his true home, the Holy Land, and begins to feel intense pride in his citizenship in his new country.

The destruction of the Jewish community of Worms in the German Rhineland was the work of the crusaders. How ironic! The crusaders were willing to leave everything behind — homes,

25.

Would that my head were water,*
  and my eye a fount of flowing tears,
that I might spend all my days and nights weeping,[1]
for my slaughtered children and infants,
and for the venerable oldsters of my congregation.
I call upon all of you to respond [to my cry], 'Vay! Ay![2] Woe!'
  And cry profusely[3] and intensify your weeping!
  Over the House of Israel and over the nation of HASHEM,
  because they have fallen by the sword![4]

My eye shall be filled with copious tears,[5]
  and I shall get me to the weeper's field.
I shall arouse the bitter of heart,
  the confounded ones, to weep with me,
over the beautiful maidens and the tender lads,
wrapped in their scrolls and dragged to the slaughter.
Their appearance was ruddier[6] than rubies,
  [more dazzling] than sapphires and gems,
yet they were trampled and discarded like the mud in the streets.[7]
  'Turn away from the unclean [Jew]!'
  they called to each other,[8] lest they come too close.
  Over the House of Israel and over the nation of HASHEM,
  because they have fallen by the sword!

---

(1) Cf. *Jeremiah* 8:23. (2) Cf. *Proverbs* 23:29. (3) Cf. *Ezra* 10:1. (4) Cf. *II Samuel* 1:12. (5) *Jeremiah* 13:17. (6) *Eichah* 4:7. (7) *II Samuel* 22:43. (8) *Eichah* 4:15.

---

families, occupations — in order to conquer the Holy Land they called Palestine, while the Jews themselves were filled with no such zeal to regain their own homeland! In heaven, this irony did not go unnoticed, but aroused a terrible denunciation against the Jewish people, and especially against the Jews of Worms and her neighboring communities.

The classic work on Jewish history, *Seder HaDoros*, by R' Yechiel Halperin, records the following observation in his entry for the year 5380 (1620):

> The author of the commentary *Sefer Meiras Eynayim (SMA)* on the *Shulchan Aruch* explained why the Jewish community of Worms suffered far more persecution, pogroms and evil decrees than other congregations. That *kehillah* was founded by Jewish exiles who made their way to Germany following the Destruction of the First Temple. After seventy years of exile, many Jews returned from Babylon to *Eretz Yisrael* and Jerusalem, but none returned from Worms. The community in Jerusalem wrote to the *kehillah* in Worms and urged them to join their new settlement in Jerusalem . . . but the complacent Jews of Worms dismissed this invitation out of hand. Instead, they responded, 'You stay where you are in the great Jerusalem, and we will continue to stay where we are in our little Jerusalem!' This arrogant response was due to the prosperity and prestige the Jews of Worms enjoyed in the eyes of the local gentiles and their princes.

The success of Worms was its undoing! The prosperity of the Jew in exile is nothing more than a Divine test to see whether it will cause the Jew to forget his homeland and his heritage. Worms and the Rhineland failed and suffered bitterly. In our own times, the vast majority of the German *kehillah* failed, because, as *Meshech Chochmah (Bechukosai)* observes, 'They began to call Berlin, Jerusalem!'

◄§ The Calamity of the First Crusade

On November 27, 1096, in Clermont (southeastern France) Pope Urban II called upon faithful Christians to join in arms to liberate the city of Jerusalem and its holy sites from the hands of the Moslem infidels who occupied it. Those who answered the call affixed crosses to their garments, and the campaign became known as *le Croisade* (from *croix*, French for cross), or the Crusade. At first, the Crusade seemed to pose no threat to the Jews who resided in peace with their Christian neighbors, but soon enough it became clear that the crusaders did not wish to wait until they reached far-off Palestine to 'avenge the

וְתֵרַד עֵינִי דִּמְעָה וְאֵילִילָה וְאָנוּדָה,

וְלִבְכִּי וְלַחֲגוֹר שַׂק אֶקְרָא לְהַסְפִּידָה,

מִפַּז יְקָרָה וְזָהָב חֲמוּדָה,

פְּנִימָה כְּבוּדָה[2] כְּבוֹד כָּל כְּלִי חֶמְדָּה,

רְאִיתִיהָ קְרוּעָה שְׁכוּלָה וְגַלְמוּדָה,[3]

הַתּוֹרָה וְהַמִּקְרָא וְהַמִּשְׁנָה וְאַגָּדָה,

עֲנוּ וְקוֹנְנוּ זֹאת לְהַגִּידָה,

אֵי תוֹרָה תַּלְמִיד וְהַלּוֹמְדָהּ,

הֲלֹא הַמָּקוֹם מֵאֵין יוֹשֵׁב חָרֵב,[4]

עַל בֵּית יִשְׂרָאֵל וְעַל עַם יהוה כִּי נָפְלוּ בְּחָרֶב.

וְעַפְעַפַּי יִזְּלוּ מַיִם דְּמַע[5] לְהַגִּירָה,

וְאֲקוֹנֵן מַר עֲלֵי הֲרוּגֵי אַשְׁפִּירָה,*

בַּשֵּׁנִי בִּשְׁמוֹנָה בּוֹ בְּיוֹם מַרְגּוֹעַ הַקְּרָה,

מַרְגּוֹעַ נֶחְלְפוּ לְהַבְעִירָה,

נֶהֶרְגוּ בַּחוּרֵי חֶמֶד[6] וְיִשִׁישֵׁי הֲדָרָה,

נֶאֶסְפוּ יָחַד נַפְשָׁם הִשְׁלִימוּ בְּמָרָא.

עַל יִחוּד שֵׁם הַמְּיֻחָד יִחֲדוּ שֵׁם בִּגְבוּרָה,

גִּבּוֹרֵי כֹחַ עוֹשֵׂי[7] דְבָרוֹ לְמַהֲרָה,

וְכֹהֲנַי וְעָלָמַי נִגְוְעוּ כֻּלְּהֶם עֲשָׂרָה.

וּבְמַר יְגוֹנִי וְעָצְבִּי יְלֵל אַחְבִּירָה,

קְהִלּוֹת הַקֹּדֶשׁ הֲרִיגָתָם הַיּוֹם בְּזִכְרָה,

קָהָל וַרְמַיְזָא* בְּחוֹנָה וּבְחוֹרָה,

גְּאוֹנֵי אֶרֶץ וּנְקִיֵּי טָהֳרָה,

---

blood of their savior.' In truth, it was their envy of the prosperous Jewish communities that incited the vulgar rabble and the greedy nobility to punish 'the murderers of their lord' wherever they passed. It was rumored that the French leader of the Crusades, Godfrey of Bouillon, had taken a solemn vow that he would avenge the blood of the crucifixion with the blood of the Jews and that he would not tolerate even one Jewish soul remaining alive.

Early in the year 1096, the French communities, threatened with extinction if they did not submit to baptism, called upon the great Jewish communities on the Rhine to ordain a day of public fasting and prayer. The Rhenish Jews complied and prayed fervently for the welfare of their French brethren. However, they themselves felt perfectly secure, enjoying as they did the special favor of the Emperor and the local nobility.

But all too soon, the frenzied mobs of crusaders poured into Germany, thirsty for Jewish blood, and hungry for Jewish riches.

In the early spring, in the weeks between Pesach and Shavuos, violence broke out and atrocities escalated. The three Jewish communities of Speyer, Worms and Mainz felt the main brunt of the carnage, and their calamity is described in this *kinnah* (see commentary below).

הֲרוּגֵי אַשְׁפִּירָה — *The slain victims of Speyer.* On the Sabbath, the eighth of Iyar [May 3, 1096], the crusaders surrounded the synagogue in Speyer. They were unable to breach its fortifications, and

My eyes will shed tears[1] and I will wail
  and thus bestirring [friends to comfort me],
and I will call them to cry, to don sackcloth and to eulogize
that which is more precious than fine gold, more desirable than gold,
whose glory is concealed within,[2]
  honored as the most cherished vessel,
and now I see it ripped, desolate, forlorn[3] —
[namely,] the Torah, the Scriptures, the Mishnah and the Aggadah.
Raise your voice and moan and make this pronouncement,
'Where is the Torah and the student who studied it?'
  Behold, the place is desolate and no one dwells therein![4]
  Over the House of Israel and over the nation of HASHEM,
  because they have fallen by the sword!

Water will stream from my eyelids, running over with tears,[5]
as I bitterly bemoan the slain victims of Speyer.*
It happened on the eighth day of the second month [Iyar],
  on the day of tranquility [the Sabbath].
My calm was transformed into a destructive tempest.
Pleasant young men[6] were murdered
  with splendid, venerable oldsters.
They assembled together and [decided]
  to surrender their souls in reverence,
for the unification of the One and Only Name,
  they declared the unity of God with fortitude.
Strong warriors, swift to fulfill His word.[7]
And my ministers and my youths expired
  — altogether they numbered ten.

In my bitter agony and sadness, I compose elegies,
as I remember today the murder of the holy congregations;
the community of Worms,* proven and chosen.
Talmudic masters of the land, their purity unsullied.

---

(1) *Jeremiah* 13:17. (2) *Psalms* 45:14. (3) *Isaiah* 49:21. (4) Cf. *Jeremiah* 26:9.
(5) Cf. 9:17. (6) *Ezekiel* 23:12. (7) *Psalms* 103:20.

---

the assembled worshipers were able to repel their attack. Frustrated, the frenzied mob threw itself upon any Jew it could find outside the synagogue. Altogether they murdered ten men. In addition they attacked one woman who was given the choice of death or conversion. She gladly chose the former and died a martyr's death and proved to be an example for many other Jews who preferred to sanctify God's Name in death, rather than to abandon Him in life.

קְהַל וַרְמַיזָא — *The community of Worms.* On the twenty-third of Iyar [Sunday, May 18, 1096] a large force of crusaders, led by Count Emicho, mercilessly attacked the Jews of Worms who had remained confidently in their homes. There they felt safe, relying on the promises of protection offered by their Christian neighbors. Many were

slain by the crusaders and their small children were seized for forced baptism. Jewish homes were pillaged and destroyed. The greedy mob even stripped the clothing from their victims' corpses, leaving them naked. Eventually, some Jews who had found refuge in the bishop's palace managed to send clothes to cover their shame.

But for the Jews of Worms the suffering was not over. God had singled them out for double tragedy. On the following Sunday, Rosh Chodesh Sivan [May 25,] the crusaders and local rabble attacked the bishop's palace to kill the many Jews who had taken refuge there. After fierce combat the crusaders prevailed and slew every Jew they could find. When the attack came, the victims were in the midst of reciting *Hallel* (*Psalms* 113-118); with God's praises on

פְּעָמִים קִדְּשׁוּ שֵׁם הַמְּיֻחָד בְּמוֹרָא.

בְּעֶשְׂרִים וּשְׁלֹשָׁה בְּחֹדֶשׁ זִיו לְטַהֲרָה,

וּבַחֹדֶשׁ הַשְּׁלִישִׁי בִּקְרִיאַת הַלֵּל לְשׁוֹרְרָה,

הִשְׁלִימוּ נַפְשָׁם בְּאַהֲבָה קְשׁוּרָה,

אֲהִימָה עֲלֵיהֶם בִּבְכִי יְלֵל לְחַשְׁרָה,

כְּלוּלֵי כֶתֶר עַל רֹאשָׁם לְעַטְּרָה.

וְעַל אַדִּירֵי קְהַל מַגֶּנְצָא* הַהֲדוּרָה,

מִנְּשָׁרִים קַלּוּ מֵאֲרָיוֹת לְהִתְגַּבְּרָה,²

הִשְׁלִימוּ נַפְשָׁם עַל יִחוּד שֵׁם הַנּוֹרָא,

וַעֲלֵיהֶם זַעֲקַת שֶׁבֶר אֶשְׁעָרָה,

עַל שְׁנֵי מִקְדָּשֵׁי יְסוֹדָם כְּהַיּוֹם עֲרְעָרָה,

וְעַל חָרְבוֹת מְעַט מִקְדָּשֵׁי³ וּמִדְרְשֵׁי הַתּוֹרָה.

בַּחֹדֶשׁ הַשְּׁלִישִׁי בַּשְּׁלִישִׁי נוֹסַף לְדַאֲבוֹן וּמְאֵרָה,

הַחֹדֶשׁ אֲשֶׁר נֶהְפַּךְ לְיָגוֹן וְצָרָה,

בְּיוֹם מַתַּן דָּת שִׁבַּרְתִּי לְהִתְאַשְּׁרָה,

וּבְיוֹם נְתִינָתָהּ כְּמוֹ כֵן אָז חָזָרָה,

עָלְתָה לָּהּ לַמָּרוֹם לִמְקוֹם מְדוֹרָה,

עִם תִּיקָהּ וְנַרְתֵּקָהּ וְהַדּוֹרְשָׁהּ וְחוֹקְרָהּ,

לוֹמְדֶיהָ וְשׁוֹנֶיהָ בְּאִישׁוֹן כְּמוֹ בְאוֹרָה,

שִׂימוּ נָא עַל לְבַבְכֶם⁴ מִסְפֵּד מַר לְקַשְׁרָה,

כִּי שְׁקוּלָה הֲרִיגָתָם לְהִתְאַבֵּל וּלְהִתְעַפְּרָה,

כְּשׂרֵפַת בֵּית אֱלֹהֵינוּ הָאוּלָם וְהַבִּירָה,

וְכִי אֵין לְהוֹסִיף מוֹעֵד שֶׁבֶר וְתַבְעֵרָה,

וְאֵין לְהַקְדִּים זוּלָתִי לְאַחֲרָה,

תַּחַת כֵּן הַיּוֹם לְוִיָּתִי אֲעוֹרְרָה,

וְאֶסְפְּדָה וְאֵילִילָה וְאֶבְכֶּה בְּנֶפֶשׁ מָרָה,

וְאַנְחָתִי כָּבְדָה מִבֹּקֶר וְעַד עֶרֶב,

עַל בֵּית יִשְׂרָאֵל וְעַל עַם יהוה כִּי נָפְלוּ בֶחָרֶב.

---

their lips they sanctified His Name. A youth named Simchah Cohen planned to avenge his father and seven brothers who had been murdered by the crusaders. He pretended that he would accept baptism, and was taken to the church. At the moment he was to receive the sacrament, he whipped out a concealed knife and lashed out at those around him, stabbing the bishop's nephew in the act. Needless to say, the brave youth was torn to pieces by the infuriated bystanders.

All told, eight hundred Jews fell victim to the

Twice they sanctified the One and Only Name in reverence.
On the twenty-third day of the month of Ziv [Iyar],[1]
  they were purified,
and in the third month [Sivan],
  while reciting the Hallel [on Rosh Chodesh] in song,
they surrendered their soul, bound up with love.
I moan over them with a wailing cry. Saturated [with tears]
those adorned with a perfect crown upon their heads.

For the towering personalities of
  the distinguished community of Mainz;[*]
quicker than eagles, stronger than lions,[2]
they surrendered their souls while declaring
  [God's] unity and His awesome Name.
For them, I will scream out a shattering cry,
over my two Temples whose foundation were destroyed on this day,
and for the ruins of my miniature sanctuaries[3]
  and houses of Torah study.

In the third month [Sivan], on the third day,
  more misery and misfortune were added,
in this month which was turned into agony and grief.
I had hoped that on the day the Law was given [Shavuos]
  I would renew my fortune [in the merit of the Torah],
but on the very day it was given it was returned.
It arose on high, [back to] its dwelling place,
together with its cover and its case, its expounder and its examiner,
those who study it and reviewed it in the darkness [of night]
as by the light [of day].

Please take to your hearts[4] to compose a bitter eulogy,
because their massacre is deserving of mourning and rolling in dust
as was the burning of the House of our God, its Hall and its Palace.
However, [we] cannot add a [new] day
  [of mourning] over ruin and conflagration,
nor may [we] mourn any earlier — only later.
Instead, today [on Tishah B'Av], I will arouse my sorrowful wailing,
and I will eulogize and wail and weep with a bitter soul,
and my groans are heavy from morning until evening.
  Over the House of Israel and over the nation of HASHEM,
    because they have fallen by the sword!

---

(1) *I Kings* 6:1. (2) Cf. *II Samuel* 1:23. (3) Cf. *Ezekiel* 11:16. (4) Cf. *Chaggai* 2:18.

---

crusaders on those two Sundays in Worms.

קְהַל מַגֶּנְצָא — *The ... community of Mainz.*
Terribly alarmed by the massacre at Speyer and
Worms, the Jews of Mainz petitioned for the
bishop's protection and paid him 400 pieces of
silver for his promise. However, on the third of
Sivan [May 27, 1096], when Count Emicho and

his multitudes arrived at the gates of the city, the
burghers were only too happy to welcome the
crusaders and join in their attack on the Jews. The
populace led the crusaders to all the Jewish
hiding places. The Jews, led by R' Klonimos ben
R' Meshullam, valiantly resisted, but were outnumbered and weakened by their penitential
fasting. After a brief struggle, a general massacre

וְעַל אֵלֶּה אֲנִי בוֹכִיָּה וְלִבִּי נוֹהֵם נְהִימוֹת,

וְאֶקְרָא לַמְקוֹנְנוֹת וְאֶל הַחֲכָמוֹת,[2]

אֵלַי וַאֲלֵיהֶ כֻּלָּם הוֹמוֹת,

הֲיֵשׁ מַכְאוֹב לְמַכְאוֹבִי[3] לְדַמּוֹת,

מִחוּץ תְּשַׁכֶּל חֶרֶב וּמֵחֲדָרִים אֵמוֹת,[4]

חֲלָלַי חַלְלֵי חֶרֶב מוּטָלִים עֲרֵמִים וַעֲרֵמוֹת,

נִבְלָתָם כְּסוּחָה[5] לְחַיַּת אֶרֶץ וְלַבְּהֵמוֹת,

יוֹנֵק עִם אִישׁ שֵׂיבָה[6] עֲלָמִים וַעֲלָמוֹת.

מִתְעַתְּעִים בָּמוֹ מוֹנַי וּמַרְבִּים כְּלִמּוֹת,

אֵי אֱלֹהֵימוֹ אָמְרוּ צוּר חָסָיוּ בוֹ[7] עַד מוֹת,

יָבֹא וְיוֹשִׁיעַ וְיַחֲזִיר נְשָׁמוֹת,

חֲסִין יָהּ מִי כָמוֹךָ[8] נוֹשֵׂא אֲלֻמּוֹת,[9]

תֶּחֱשֶׁה וְתִתְאַפַּק[10] וְלֹא תַחְגֹּר חֵמוֹת,[11]

בֶּאֱמוֹר אֵלַי מַלְעִיגַי אִם אֱלֹהִים הוּא יָרֵב,[12]

עַל בֵּית יִשְׂרָאֵל וְעַל עַם יהוה כִּי נָפְלוּ בֶחָרֶב.

עֵינַי עֵינַי יֹרְדָה מַּיִם[13] כִּי נֶהְפַּךְ לְאֵבֶל[14] מְשׁוֹרֵר,

וְעֻגָּבִי לְקוֹל בּוֹכִים[15] מִלְהָפִיג וּלְקָרֵר,

מִי יָנוּד לִי[16] וּמִי מַחֲזִיק לְהִתְעוֹרֵר,[17]

חֵמָה בִּי יָצְאָה וְסַעַר מִתְגּוֹרֵר,[18]

אֲכָלָנִי הֲמָמַנִי[19] הַצַּר הַצּוֹרֵר,[20]

שִׁבַּר עַצְמוֹתַי[21] זוֹרֵר וּמְפָרֵר,

סִלָּה כָל אַבִּירַי[22] הַטַּבּוּר וְהַשָּׁרֵר,

רְטִיָּה וּמָזוֹר אֵין לְבָרֵר,

מַכָּתִי אֲנוּשָׁה[23] בְּאֵין מַתְעִיל וּמְזוֹרֵר,

עַל כֵּן אָמַרְתִּי שְׁעוּ מֶנִּי אֲמָרֵר,

בִּבְכִי[24] דִּמְעָתִי עַל לְחָיַי[25] לְצָרֵב,

עַל בֵּית יִשְׂרָאֵל וְעַל עַם יהוה כִּי נָפְלוּ בֶחָרֶב.

---

ensued. The victims, more than one thousand pure Jewish souls, were ignominiously thrown into nine large ditches for mass burial.

Throughout the spring and early summer, the crusaders continued to maraud and sack once proud and venerable Jewish communities, many of which had stood for over a thousand years. They brought death and destruction to Cologne,

Trier, Regensburg, Metz and Prague. In all, it is estimated that over 5,000 Jews lost their lives during the First Crusade. But worse than that, the Crusades introduced the idea of organized, massive, widespread terror against the Jews on a vast, sweeping scale — an idea that would continue, and find its ultimate, horrible expression in the awesome Nazi Holocaust.

Over these I do cry[1] and my heart moans deeply,
and I summon the wailing-women and the skilled ones.[2]
'Ay li', 'Ay lay,' they all cry with intense feeling.
Is there any pain which compares with my pain?[3]
Outside the [avenging] sword renders parents childless,
  while terror stalks the inner chambers.[4]
My dead bodies, corpses of the sword,
  are strewn about naked, both male and female.
Their cadavers rotting[5] for the wild beasts of the land
  and for the animals —
suckling baby with hoary old man,[6] young men and young maidens.

My tormentors ridicule them and humiliate them intensely.
'Where is their God,' taunt they,
  'the Rock in Whom they sought refuge[7] until death?
  Let Him come and save and restore souls!'
Who is like You, O strong One, God,[8]
  Who patiently bears the bundles[9] [of their iniquities]?
Will You remain silent and hold back,[10]
  not to gird Yourself in burning wrath,[11]
      when those who mock me say, 'If indeed there is a God,
      let Him fight[12] [on your behalf]!'
      Over the House of Israel and over the nation of HASHEM,
      because they have fallen by the sword!

My eyes, my eyes, run with water![13]
  For our singer has turned to mourning,[14]
my flute has changed over to the sound of weeping,[15]
  without relief or composure.
Who will bestir himself to console me?[16]
  And is there none to revive me with a strong embrace?[17]
[God's] wrath went forth against me,
  while a storm [of anger] gathered[18] [to harm me].
The cruel enemy[20] consumed and mutilated me.[19]
My bones he shattered,[21] strew and pulverized.
He trampled all my heroes,[22] [who were my] navel and umbilicus.
There is no bandage or medicine from which to choose.
[because] my wound is mortal,[23] beyond remedy or cure.
Therefore I said, 'Leave me alone with my bitterness,
      so that with the weeping[24] of my tears, I will blister my cheeks.[25]
      Over the House of Israel and over the nation of HASHEM,
      because they have fallen by the sword!

(1) *Eichah* 1:16. (2) Cf. *Jeremiah* 9:16. (3) Cf. *Eichah* 1:12. (4) Cf. *Deuteronomy* 32:25. (5) *Isaiah* 5:25.
(6) *Deuteronomy* 32:25. (7) Cf. 32:37. (8) Cf. *Psalms* 89:9. (9) Cf. 126:6. (10) Cf. *Isaiah* 42:14.
(11) Cf. *Psalms* 76:11. (12) *Judges* 6:31. (13) *Eichah* 1:16. (14) 5:15. (15) *Job* 30:31. (16) Cf. *Isaiah* 51:19.
(17) Cf. 64:6. (18) *Jeremiah* 30:23. (19) Cf. 51:34. (20) *Numbers* 10:9. (21) *Eichah* 3:4.
(22) 1:15. (23) *Jeremiah* 15:18. (24) *Isaiah* 22:4. (25) *Eichah* 1:2.

כו.

אָז* בַּהֲלוֹךְ יִרְמְיָהוּ עַל* קִבְרֵי אָבוֹת,

וְנָם עֲצָמוֹת חֲבִיבוֹת, מָה אַתֶּם שׁוֹכְבוֹת,

בְּנֵיכֶם גָּלוּ וּבָתֵּיהֶם חֲרֵבוֹת,

וְאַיֵּה זְכוּת אָבוֹת בְּאֶרֶץ תַּלְאוּבוֹת.*

גָּעוּ כֻּלָּם בְּקִינִים עַל חֶסְרוֹן בָּנִים,

דּוֹבְבוּ בְּקוֹל תַּחֲנוּנִים פְּנֵי שׁוֹכֵן מְעוֹנִים,

וְאַיֵּה הַבְטָחַת וְזָכַרְתִּי לָהֶם בְּרִית רִאשׁוֹנִים.[1]

הֵם הֵמִירוּ כְבוֹדוֹ בַּתֹּהוּ,[2] וְלֹא פָחֲדוּ וְלֹא רָהוּ,[3]

וָאַעֲלִים עֵינַי מֵהֶם[4] וְלֹא שָׁבוּ וְלֹא נָהוּ,

וְאֵיךְ אֶתְאַפֵּק עַל אֲמִירַת לֹא הוּא.[5]

זָעַק אַב הֶמוֹן[6] בַּעֲבוּרָם, וְחִנֵּן פְּנֵי אֵל רָם,

חִנָּם נִסִּיתִי עֶשֶׂר בְּחִינוֹת עֲבוּרָם, וְהֵן חָזִיתִי שִׁבְרָם,

וְאַיֵּה הַבְטָחַת אַל תִּירָא אַבְרָם.[7]

טָעוּ לְהוֹרוֹת[8] בַּעֲבוֹדוֹת זָרוֹת,

יָעֲצוּ לַחְצוֹב בֹּארוֹת בֹּארוֹת נִשְׁבָּרוֹת,[9]

וְאֵיךְ אֶתְאַפֵּק עַל בִּטּוּל עֲשֶׂרֶת הַדִּבְּרוֹת.

כֹּה צָוַח יִצְחָק פְּנֵי שׁוֹכֵן שַׁחַק,

לַשָּׁוְא בִּי טֶבַח הוּחַק, וְהֵן זַרְעִי נִשְׁחַק וְנִמְחַק,

וְאַיֵּה הַבְטָחַת וְאֶת בְּרִיתִי אָקִים אֶת יִצְחָק.[10]

מָרוּ בְּיִרְמְיָה, וְטִמְּאוּ הַר הַמּוֹרִיָּה,

---

(1) *Leviticus* 26:45. (2) Cf. *Jeremiah* 2:11. (3) Cf. *Isaiah* 44:8. (4) Cf. 1:15.
(5) *Jeremiah* 5:12. (6) Cf. *Genesis* 17:4. (7) 15:1. (8) Some editions read לְהוֹרוֹת,
to become estranged. (9) Cf. *Jeremiah* 2:13. (10) *Genesis* 17:21.

---

§ אָז — *Then.* In this work, R' Elazar HaKalir retells the Midrashic account (Midrash *Eichah* intro. 24) of God's reaction to the Destruction. When He saw the ruins of the burnt Sanctuary, God cried to Jeremiah, 'I feel like a father whose only son died on his wedding day! Go, summon Abraham, Isaac, Jacob, and Moses from their graves. They know how to weep (and perhaps they will arouse My mercy to return Israel to their land).' Jeremiah went to the Cave of Machpelah in Hebron to arouse the Patriarchs and to the banks of the Jordan river to awaken Moses. They all went to visit the ruins of the Temple. As they

passed from gate to desolate gate, they wailed and cried and rent their garments in mourning. Yet, all their tears and pleas failed to arouse God's mercy, that He pledge to guarantee Israel's final redemption and return, for Israel had sinned terribly and God's fury was aroused.

God relented only after the Matriarchs led by Rachel joined in with their impassioned plea and God's response is recorded by the Prophet Jeremiah:

Thus says HASHEM, 'A voice is heard in Ramah, lamentation and bitter weeping, Rachel is weeping for her children, she refuses to be comforted

26.

א *Then* when Jeremiah approached* the graves of the Patriarchs*
and said, 'O cherished bones, how can you lie still?

ב *Your sons have been exiled and their homes destroyed;*
where is the merit of their ancestors in a parched wasteland?'*

ג *They all cried out in lamentations*
over the loss of their children;

ד *they spoke in a voice of supplication before [God]*
Who dwells in the high heavens,
"Where is the assurance, 'And I shall remember for their sake
the covenant of the ancients'?"[1]

ה *[God replied,] "They exchanged My honor for utter nothingness,*[2]
and they were neither awed nor afraid [of Me].[3]

ו *Then I averted My eyes from them*[4]*, yet they did not repent*
nor did they lament;
and how can I restrain [My anger] from the statement,
'He is not [the Lord]'?"[5]

ז *Then [Abraham] the father of the multitude*[6] *cried out*
on their behalf and pleaded before God, the Most High,

ח *"For nothing was I tried with ten tests for their sake,*
for behold, how I must witness their ruination!
Where is the assurance 'Fear not, O Abram!'?"[7]

ט *[God responded,] 'They erred by permitting*[8] *idolatrous worship.*

י *They devised plans to dig [for themselves] cisterns, broken cisterns,*[9]
and how can I restrain [My anger]
over the nullification of the Ten Commandments?'

כ *Then Isaac screamed before [God] Who dwells in heaven,*

ל *"Was it for nothing that I was inscribed [in the Torah]*
as being prepared for slaughter?
For behold how my seed is crushed and obliterated.
Where is the assurance,
'And I shall fulfill My covenant with Isaac'?"[10]

מ *[God responded,] 'They have defied Jeremiah*
and defiled Mount Moriah.

---

over her children for they are not here.' Thus says
HASHEM, *'Restrain your voice from weeping and*
hold back your eyes from tears, for your efforts
will be rewarded,' says HASHEM, *'and they will*
return from the land of the enemy. And there is
hope for your future,' says HASHEM, *'for your*
children shall be restored to their own borders!'
(Jeremiah 31:14-16).

אָז בַּהֲלוֹךְ יִרְמְיָהוּ עַל — *Then when Jeremiah*
approached [lit., *walked upon*]. Since Jeremiah
was a *Kohen* (see Jeremiah 1:1), he was forbidden

from contaminating himself to the dead. There-
fore, he could not have entered the Cave of
Machpelah (see *Rashi* to Ezekiel 37:2, where
Ezekiel, also a *Kohen*, was led around a valley
filled with bones to prophesy regarding those
bones, but was not permitted to enter the valley).
Thus, עַל, *upon*, has been translated according to
its alternate meaning, *near* (see *Targum* and
Rashi to Numbers 2:20) and the phrase . . . הֲלוֹךְ
עַל is rendered *approached.*

בְּאֶרֶץ תַּלְאוּבוֹת — *In a parched wasteland,* an

נִלְאֵיתִי נְשׂוֹא¹ גְּעָיָה, עוֹלָה לִי מִנְּשִׁיָּה,
וְאֵיךְ אֶתְאַפַּק עַל הֲרִיגַת זְכַרְיָה.²

סָח יֶלֶד בְּתֶלֶף, דְּמָעוֹת כְּתַנִּין זוֹלֵף,
עוֹלָלַי אֲשֶׁר טִפַּחְתִּי³ בְּעֶלֶף,
וְאֵיךְ גֻּזּוּ מֶנִּי בְּחֶלֶף
וְאֵיךְ הֻפְרַע מֶנִּי דָמִים בְּדָמִים כַּמָּה אֶלֶף.

פָּץ רוֹעֶה נֶאֱמָן, כָּפוּשׁ בְּאֵפֶר וּמִדְמָן,
צֹאן אֲשֶׁר בְּחֵיקִי הָאֱמָן,⁴ אֵיךְ גֻּזּוּ בְּלֹא זְמָן,
וְאַיֵּה הַבְטָחַת כִּי לֹא אַלְמָן.⁵

קוֹל בְּכִי לֵאָה מְתוֹפֶפֶת עַל לְבָבֶיהָ,⁶
רָחֵל אֲחוֹתָהּ מְבַכָּה עַל בָּנֶיהָ,⁷
וְזִלְפָּה מַכָּה פָנֶיהָ, בִּלְהָה מְקוֹנֶנֶת בִּשְׁתֵּי יָדֶיהָ.

שׁוּבוּ תְמִימִים לִמְנוּחַתְכֶם,
מַלֵּא אֲמַלֵּא כָּל מִשְׁאֲלוֹתֵיכֶם,
שָׁלַחְתִּי בְּבֶלָה לְמַעַנְכֶם,⁸
הִנְנִי מְשׁוֹבֵב גָּלוּת בְּנֵיכֶם.

allusion to the Wilderness of Sinai where their ancestors accepted the Torah. As the prophet (Jeremiah 2:2) states: *So said* HASHEM, *'I shall remember for your sake the kindness of your younger days ... how you followed Me in the Wilderness in an unsown land.'*

ג I have become exhausted from bearing[1]
   the cry that rises from the land of oblivion;
and how can I restrain [My anger from avenging]
   the murder of Zechariah?'[2]

ס [Then Jacob] who was born to learning
   spoke with tears flowing [to the ground] like a [slithering] serpent,

ע 'My babes whom I have dandled [and reared][3]
   to the point of exhaustion,
how they have been torn from me, to disappear!
How there has been exacted from me, for [Zechariah's] blood,
   the blood of so many thousands!'

פ The faithful shepherd [Moses] burst forth,
   while sunk in ashes and sullied in filth,

צ 'The lambs, who were nursed at my bosom,[4]
   O how were they cut off before their time!
Where is the assurance, "It [Israel] shall not be widowed"?'[5]

ק The sound of Leah's weeping, as she pounds on her heart;[6]

ר Rachel, her sister, weeping for her sons;[7]
   Zilpah slapping her face;
      and Bilhah lamenting with her two hands [outstretched].

ש-ת [God responds,] 'Return, O wholesome ones, to your place of rest,
   I shall surely fulfill all your requests.
I was sent to Babylon, for your sake.[8]
   Behold, I shall return your children from exile!'

---

(1) Isaiah 1:14. (2) See kinnah 34. (3) Cf. Eichah 2:22. (4) Cf. Numbers 11:12. (5) Jeremiah 51:5.
(6) Cf. Nahum 2:8. (7) Cf. Jeremiah 31:14. (8) See Minchas Shai to Isaiah 43:14.

כז.

אָז בִּמְלֹאת סֵפֶק יָפָה כְּתִרְצָה,*

הֵן אֶרְאֶלָּם צָעֲקוּ חוּצָה,[2]

בֵּן חִלְּקֵיהוּ מֵאַרְמוֹן כִּיָּצָא,

אִשָּׁה יְפַת תֹּאַר מְנֻוֶּלֶת מָצָא.

גּוֹזַרְנִי עָלֶיךָ בְּשֵׁם אֱלֹהִים וְאָדָם,

אִם שֵׁד לַשֵּׁדִים אַתְּ אוֹ לִבְנֵי אָדָם,

דְּמוּת יָפְיֵךְ כִּבְשָׂר וָדָם,

פַּחְדֵּךְ וְיִרְאָתֵךְ כְּמַלְאָכִים לְבַדָּם.

הֵן לֹא שֵׁד אֲנִי וְלֹא גֹלֶם פַּחַת,

יְדוּעָה הָיִיתִי בְּשׁוּבָה וָנַחַת,

הֵן לְאֶחָד אֲנִי וְלִשְׁלֹשָׁה וְשִׁשִּׁים וְאַחַת,

וְלִשְׁנַיִם עָשָׂר וּלְשִׁבְעִים וְאַחַת.

זֶה הָאֶחָד אַבְרָהָם הָיָה,

וּבֵין הַשְּׁלֹשָׁה אָבוֹת שְׁלִישִׁיָּה,

חֹק שְׁנַיִם עָשָׂר הֵן הֵן שִׁבְטֵי יָהּ,

וְשִׁשִּׁים רִבּוֹא וְשִׁבְעִים וְאֶחָד סַנְהֶדְרֵי יָהּ.

טַעֲמִי הַקְשִׁיבִי וַעֲשִׂי תְשׁוּבָה,

יַעַן הֱיוֹתֵךְ כָּל כַּךְ חֲשׁוּבָה,

יָפָה לָךְ בְּעֶלֶץ וְלִשְׂמוֹחַ בְּטוֹבָה,

וְלֹא לְקָרֵא עוֹד בַּת הַשּׁוֹבֵבָה.

כִּי אֵיךְ אֶשְׂמַח וְקוֹלִי מָה אָרִים,

הֵן עוֹלָלַי נִתְּנוּ בְּיַד צָרִים,

לֻקְּחוּ נְבִיאַי וְדָמָם מְגֹרִים,

גָּלוּ מְלָכַי וְשָׂרַי וְכֹהֲנַי וַהֲרֵי הֵם בְּקוֹלָרִים.

מְלוֹן מִקְדָּשַׁי בַּעֲוֹנִי נָדַד,

דּוֹדִי מֵאָז נָדַד וַיִּדַּד,

Cave of Machpelah and thus serves as an appropriate introduction to *kinnah* 26 which narrates the pleas of the Patriarchs after they were aroused. According to our sequence, this *kinnah* comes later because its main theme is an

27.

א *Then, when the measure [of sin] was filled by [Israel]*
who is as beautiful as Tirtzah,* the Erelim[1] cried out in public.[2]

ב *As [Jeremiah] the son of Hilkiyah departed from the Temple,*
he met a woman of beautiful features who was filthy.

ג *[He said:] 'I command you, in the name of God and man,*
[to reveal] whether you are one of the demons or of humankind.

ד *Your graceful appearance resembles flesh and blood, but the*
terror and awe [etched on your features] is unique to the angels!'

ה *'Behold', [she replied] 'I am neither demon,*
nor worthless lump [of clay].
Rather, I was once renowned for tranquility and serenity.
I am [the representative spirit of the Jewish people, the daughter]
of one and of three,
[my offspring number] sixty with one [leader, Moses, over them];
[they stem]

ו *from twelve and [are ruled by] seventy-one!*

ז *This one [that I mentioned] was Abraham,*
and the three refers to the Patriarchs, a trio dedicated to God.

ח *The number twelve represents the tribes of God, who numbered*
sixty myriad. And the seventy-one are God's Sanhedrin.'

ט *[Jeremiah responded,] 'Harken to my advice and repent,*
considering that you are truly so distinguished.

י *It is proper for you to celebrate and to rejoice in goodness,*
no longer to be referred to as the rebellious daughter!'

כ *'But how can I rejoice? How can I raise my voice [in song]?*
Behold, my babes are delivered into the hands of my tormentors!

ל *My prophets were beaten and their blood flowed. My kings,*
my princes and my priests were exiled and behold,
they are now in shackles.

מ *My Holy Dwelling was uprooted because of my iniquity,*
since then my Beloved has fled and withered.

---

(1) See commentary to *kinnah* 22. (2) *Isaiah* 33:7.

event that occurred after the Destruction, as related in *Pesikta Rabbosi* (27): When Jeremiah returned to Jerusalem he met a woman sitting on a mountaintop, clothed in black, her hair disheveled. 'Who will console me?' she cried out.

Jeremiah responded sternly, 'If you are a real woman, speak to me, but if you are a spirit, depart!'

'I am your mother, Zion!' the woman responded.

Jeremiah said to her, 'God, Himself, will console you! Mortal men built you and mortal men destroyed you. But in the future, God Himself will rebuild you as Scripture states: *The Builder of Jerusalem is* HASHEM (*Psalms* 147:2).

The *kinnah* follows an alphabetical format, and is a conversation between Jeremiah, Israel, God, and the Patriarchs.

יָפָה כְּתִרְצָה — *Beautiful as Tirtzah.* Israel is described with this phrase in *Song of Songs* (6:4).

נְעַם אָהֳלִי בְּעַל כָּרְחִי שָׁדַד,

רַבָּתִי עָם אֵיכָה יָשְׁבָה בָדָד.[1]

שָׁחָה הָאִשָּׁה לַנָּבִיא יִרְמְיָה,

סַח לֵאלֹהֶיךָ בְּעַד מַכַּת סוֹעֲרָה עֲנִיָּה,

עַד יַעֲנֶה אֵל וְיֹאמַר דַּיָּה,

וְיַצִּילֵנִי מֵחֶרֶב וְשִׁבְיָה.

פַּלֵּל תְּחִנָּה לִפְנֵי קוֹנוֹ,

מָלֵא רַחֲמִים רַחֵם כְּאָב עַל בְּנוֹ,

צָעַק מַה לְּאָב שֶׁהֻגְלָה בְּנוֹ,

וְגַם אוֹי לַבֵּן שֶׁעַל שֻׁלְחַן אָב אֵינוֹ.

קוּם לְךָ יִרְמְיָה לָמָּה תֶחֱשֶׁה,

לֵךְ קְרָא לְאָבוֹת וְאַהֲרֹן וּמֹשֶׁה,

רוֹעִים יָבֹאוּ קִינָה לְהִנָּשֵׂא,

כִּי זְאֵבֵי עֶרֶב טָרְפוּ אֶת הַשֶּׂה.

שׁוֹאֵג הָיָה יִרְמְיָהוּ הַנָּבִיא,

עַל מַכְפֵּלָה נוֹהֵם כְּלָבִיא,

תְּנוּ קוֹל בִּבְכִי אֲבוֹת הַצְּבִי,

תְּעוּ בְנֵיכֶם וַהֲרֵי הֵם בַּשֶּׁבִי.

וְאִם כְּאָדָם עָבְרוּ בְרִית,

אַיֵּה זְכוּת כְּרוּתֵי בְרִית.

מָה אֶעֱשֶׂה לָכֶם בָּנַי,

גְּזֵרָה הִיא מִלְּפָנַי.

שָׁמֵם מִקְדָּשׁ מִבְּלִי בָאֵי מוֹעֵד,[2]

עַל כִּי יְדִידִים נִתְּנוּ לְהִמָּעֵד,

תְּשִׁיבֵם* כְּמֵאָז סוֹמֵךְ וְסוֹעֵד,

תְּרַחֵם צִיּוֹן כִּי בָא מוֹעֵד.[3]

The translation follows *Ibn Ezra* there, who explains that Tirtzah refers to the province of that name mentioned elsewhere in Scriptures (see, e.g., *I Kings* chs. 14-16). *Rashi*, however, translates homiletically, and understands כְּתִרְצָה as a contraction of כְּשֵׁאת רְצוּיָה, *when you find*

נ *My pleasant Tent was forcefully plundered.*
The city once great with people,
   alas, she now sits in solitude!'[1]

ס *The woman spoke [further] to Jeremiah,*
"Pray to your God concerning the blows
   inflicted upon the suffering, storm-tossed [people of Israel],

ע *Until God responds and says, 'Enough!'*
and saves me from sword and captivity."

פ *[Jeremiah] prayed in supplication before his Creator,*
'[O You Who are] full of compassion,
   pity [us] as a father would [pity] his son!'

צ *[God] cried, 'How does a Father feel*
   when he has exiled his son?
And woe unto the son,
   who is absent from the father's table!

ק *Arise, Jeremiah! Why should you be silent?*
Go summon the Patriarchs, and Aaron and Moses!

ר *Let these shepherds come and arouse lamentation,*
because the wolves of the night have torn the lamb to pieces.'

ש *Jeremiah the prophet roared;*
   at the [Cave of] Machpelah he growled like a lion,

ת *'Give forth [your] voice in weeping,*
   O Patriarchs of the splendid [nation]!
Your children have strayed, and behold, they are in captivity!'

[The Patriarchs replied,]
'And if, indeed, like mortals they violated the Covenant,
where is the merit of [our deeds, for we are] the ones
   with whom the covenant was signed?'
[God answered,]
'What can I do for you, My sons?
This is My irrevocable decree!
The Temple has been laid waste for lack of Festival pilgrims,[2]
because [My] beloved ones have faltered!'
'Return them* as in days of yore,
O Supporter and Sustainer, have mercy on Zion,
   for the appointed time [of redemption] has come!'[3]

---

(1) Cf. *Eichah* 1:1. (2) 1:4. (3) Cf. *Psalms* 102:14.

---

favor; in other words, Israel is beautiful when it   תְּשִׁיבֵם — *Return them.* It is unclear whether this
follows God's will and thereby finds favor in His   last verse is spoken by Jeremiah, the Patriarchs,
eyes.   or the *paytan.*

כח.

אֵיךְ תְּנַחֲמוּנִי* הֶבֶל,[1] וְכִנּוֹרִי נֶהְפַּךְ לְאֵבֶל,[2]

בְּנַחֲלַת חֶבֶל,[3] כָּבֵד עָלַי עוֹל סֵבֶל, וְאֵיךְ אֲנַחֵם.

בְּזֶה יוֹם בְּכָל שָׁנָה, עֶדֶן עָלַי שָׁנָה,

וְהִנְנִי עֲגוּמָה וַעֲגוּנָה, יוֹתֵר מֵאֶלֶף שָׁנָה,* וְאֵיךְ אֲנַחֵם.

גָּבַר חָרוֹן, וְנִגְנַז אָרוֹן,[4]

בְּמִשְׁנֶה שִׁבָּרוֹן,[5] בְּמִסְדְּרֵי מָרוֹן,[6] וְאֵיךְ אֲנַחֵם.

דִּירָתִי חָרֵבָה, וְעֶדְרִי נִשְׁבָּה,

וְרַבַּת אֳהָלִיבָה,[7] בָּדָד יָשְׁבָה,[8] וְאֵיךְ אֲנַחֵם.

הוּעַל אַרְיֵה* מִסֻּבְּכוֹ,[9] עַל אֲרִיאֵל וְהִסְבִּיכוֹ,

וְהֻגְלָה מִסְכּוֹ, מִנְחָתוֹ וְנִסְכּוֹ, וְאֵיךְ אֲנַחֵם.

וְהָרַג הֲמוֹנִים, מְשׁוּחֵי שְׁמָנִים,

בְּאַוּוּי נִמְנִים, פִּרְחֵי כֹהֲנִים, אֲלָפִים שְׁמוֹנִים, וְאֵיךְ אֲנַחֵם.

זִנְּבָם כְּחִוּוּי[10] וְהִדְבִּיא, בְּעֶזְרַת הַמַּלְבִּיא,[11]

אֲרִיוֹךְ* כְּמוֹ לָבִיא, עַל דַּם כֹּהֵן וְנָבִיא,[12] וְאֵיךְ אֲנַחֵם.

---

(1) *Job* 21:34. (2) Cf. 30:31. (3) Cf. *Deuteronomy* 32:9.
(4) See commentary to *kinnah* 24. (5) Cf. *Jeremiah* 17:18.
(6) See commentary to *kinnah* 10. (7) *kinnah* 4. (8) Cf. *Eichah* 1:1.
(9) Cf. *Jeremiah* 4:7. (10) Some editions read בְּאַוּוּי, *in the desirable [Temple]*.
(11) Some editions read בְּעֶזְרַת, but the meaning is unchanged. (12) See *kinnah* 34.

אֵיךְ תְּנַחֲמוּנִי — *How can you console me?* This alphabetical composition by R' Elazar HaKalir highlights the futility of our attempts to find consolation for the tragedy of Israel's destruction. The calamity was so enormous that it is absolutely unforgettable. Its harsh effects are still felt today, even though many centuries have elapsed. Indeed, the opening words of this *kinnah* declare that any attempt at comfort is futile. The burden of witnessing the desolation of *Eretz Yisrael* and the suffering of the Jewish people is beyond endurance. The *kinnah* ends with a proclamation that even though there can be no consolation as long as the nation remains in exile, there is always hope for redemption and ultimate consolation.

It is not clear from the context whether the speaker of this *kinnah* is God, the nation or the individual lamenter.

יוֹתֵר מֵאֶלֶף שָׁנָה — *For more than a thousand years.* This *kinnah* is usually ascribed to R' Elazar HaKalir, who lived, according to various opinions, somewhere between the second and seventh centuries C.E. In any case, he did not live a thousand years after the Destruction. Assumedly, this line originally read something like כַּמָּה מֵאוֹת שָׁנָה, *many hundreds of years,* but was changed by a later copyist who updated the *kinnah.* Alternatively, if he was (as *Tosafos* and the *Rosh* record) a second-century Tanna, then he may have had in mind the original Tishah B'Av of the Spies' slanderous report about *Eretz Yisrael.* That event would have preceded him by some fourteen centuries, a period of 'more than a thousand years.'

אַרְיֵה — *The lion [Nebuchadnezzar].* Throughout the Talmud and Midrash, and based on the Book of *Daniel* (ch. 8), Israel's long series of exiles and persecutions are always treated as four main periods of subjugation to foreign oppressors — either in *Eretz Yisrael* or in the Diaspora. These periods are known collectively as אַרְבַּע מַלְכֻיּוֹת, *the Four Kingdoms* (*Daniel* 8:22), and each is called by the name of the

28.

א *How can you console me* in vain,[1]*
when my harp has turned to mourning?[2]
Indeed, because of [the sins of Israel] the lot of [my] heritage,[3]
the yoke of the burden is heavy upon me!

So how can I be consoled?

ב *On this day, every year, times for me [are the worst],*
and behold I have been anguished and abandoned
for more than a thousand years.*   *So how can I be consoled?*

ג *Fury intensified and the Holy Ark was concealed;[4]*
disaster struck twice[5] because of those
who defiantly rebelled [against God].[6]   *So how can I be consoled?*

ד *My dwelling is in ruins and my flock is captured,*
and once-teeming Oholivah [Jerusalem][7] now sits in solitude![8]

So how can I be consoled?

ה *The lion [Nebuchadnezzar]* arose from his dense brush,[9]*
to attack God's leonine Temple;
and banished from His Tabernacle, His meal-offering and His libation.

So how can I be consoled?

ו *And he killed multitudes of blossoming Priests*
[who had been] anointed with oils.
[Their corpses] in the desirable [Temple]
were counted at eighty thousand.   *So how can I be consoled?*

ז *He attacked from behind like a snake[10] and caused [their blood]*
to flow in the leonine [Temple's] Courtyard.[11]
Arioch [General Nebuzaradan]* and the lion [King Nebuchadnezzar]
both stood over the blood of the priest and prophet [Zechariah].[12]

So how can I be consoled?

---

empire dominant in the world at that particular time. The first, called גָּלוּת בָּבֶל, *the Babylonian Exile*, began when Nebuchadnezzar king of Babylon conquered the Land of Israel and destroyed the First Temple. The second, called גָּלוּת מָדַי וּפָרַס, *the Median-Persian Exile* (ibid. 8:20), began when that empire captured the Babylonians and became the leading world power. Although the Medes permitted the Jewish return to *Eretz Yisrael* and the building of the Second Temple, the early years of that *Beis HaMikdash* were still considered a part of the exile, because Israel was not sovereign in its Land. During the entire third period, גָּלוּת יָוָן, *the Greek Exile* (ibid. 8:21), paradoxically, Israel lived on its Land and the Temple stood. Nevertheless, it was a very turbulent era marked with civil strife, foreign domination, vicious anti-religious campaigns, and the rejection of Torah

values by a large number of Jews who adopted Greek culture with all its abominations. The downfall of the Greek Empire and the rise of Rome marked the beginning of גָּלוּת אֱדוֹם, *the Edomite* or *Roman Exile*. It is this millennia-long exile that we are still in today. The *kinnah* now speaks of these Four Kingdoms and their respective atrocities.

אֲרִיוֹךְ — *Arioch [General Nebuzaradan].* In *II Kings* (ch. 25) and in *Jeremiah* (chs. 39, 52, et al.), Nebuchadnezzar's general is called נְבוּזַרְאֲדָן רַב טַבָּחִים, *Nebuzaradan the chief executioner*. In *Daniel* (2:14), he is called אַרְיוֹךְ רַב טַבָּחַיָּא, *Arioch the chief executioner*. According to the Midrash, his name was Nebuzaradan, but he was called Arioch (a diminutive of *Ari*, lion) because he roared at the Jewish captives, giving them no rest until they reached the banks of the Euphrates (*Midrash Eichah* 5:5).

חָרַשׁ לַמַּשּׁוּאוֹת, עִיר מְלֵאָה תְּשׁוּאוֹת,[1]

וּבָתֵּי סוֹפְרִים וּמִשְׁנָיוֹת, יוֹתֵר מֵאַרְבַּע מֵאוֹת,   וְאֵיךְ אֲנַחֵם.

טָסָה מָדַי, לְאַבֵּד חֲמוּדַי,

וּמָשְׁלָה בְּמַחְמַדַּי, בְּקַרְעֵי מַדַי,   וְאֵיךְ אֲנַחֵם.

יָעֲצָה לְחַנֵּק, בְּנֵי גוּר מְזַנֵּק,[2]

בְּפֶה אֶחָד לְשַׁנֵּק, זָקֵן וְיָשִׁישׁ עוֹלֵל וְיוֹנֵק,   וְאֵיךְ אֲנַחֵם.

כָּבְדָה שְׁלִישִׁית, עַל קֹדֶשׁ רֵאשִׁית,[3]

בְּשֶׁצֶף חֲרִישִׁית, בָּתָה לְהָשִׁית,   וְאֵיךְ אֲנַחֵם.

לָחֲצָה לְחַלֵּק, בְּנֵי חָלָק וְחוֹלֵק,

שֶׁאֵין לָכֶם חֵלֶק, בְּשֵׁם אֵשׁ דּוֹלֵק,[4]   וְאֵיךְ אֲנַחֵם.

מָרְדָה אֱדוֹם, עֲדוּשַׁת אָדוֹם,

וְאָצָה בְזָדוֹן, לְאַבֵּד כֵּס וַהֲדוֹם,[5]   וְאֵיךְ אֲנַחֵם.

נוֹעֲדוּ עִם אַדְמוֹן, מוֹאָב וְעַמּוֹן,

לְהַשְׁבִּית אָמוֹן,* וּלְהַחֲרִיב אַרְמוֹן,   וְאֵיךְ אֲנַחֵם.

סָלָה כָל אַבִּירַי,[6] וְעֶדְרֵי חֲבֵרַי,

וְהִבְלִיגוּ גְבוּרַי, לְעֵין כָּל עוֹבְרַי,   וְאֵיךְ אֲנַחֵם.

עָיְפָה נַפְשִׁי לְהוֹרְגִים,[7] לְמִסְפַּר הַהֲרוּגִים,

כְּאַיָּל עוֹרְגִים,[8] וְעָלֶיךָ נֶהֱרָגִים,[9]   וְאֵיךְ אֲנַחֵם.

פָּלְצוּ בְיוֹם קְרָב, בְּמִזְרָח וּבְמַעֲרָב,

עַל דָּמָם מְעֹרָב, קָהָל וְעַם רָב,*[10]   וְאֵיךְ אֲנַחֵם.

צָרוֹת עַל צָרוֹת, זוּ מִזּוֹ מְצִירוֹת,

גְּדוֹלוֹת וּבְצוּרוֹת[11] אֲרֻכּוֹת וְלֹא קְצָרוֹת,   וְאֵיךְ אֲנַחֵם.

---

(1) Cf. *Isaiah* 22:2. (2) Cf. *Deuteronomy* 33:22. (3) Cf. *Jeremiah* 2:3. (4) Some editions read
אֵל דּוֹלֵק, *the fiery God.* (5) Cf. *Isaiah* 66:1; see also *Ezekiel* 43:7. (6) *Eichah* 1:15.
(7) *Jeremiah* 4:31. (8) Cf. *Psalms* 42:2. (9) Cf. 44:23. (10) *Ezekiel* 26:7. (11) Cf. *Jeremiah* 33:3.

לְהַשְׁבִּית אָמוֹן — *To eradicate the nurturing
Torah.* The Talmud relates that when the
enemies entered the Temple, Ammonites and
Moabites entered among them. While the others
ran to plunder the silver and gold, the Ammonites and Moabites ran to plunder the Torah
itself to erase the verse (*Deuteronomy* 23:4, לֹא
יָבֹא עַמּוֹנִי וּמוֹאָבִי בִּקְהַל ה׳ , *An Ammonite or*

Moabite shall not enter the Assembly of HASHEM
(*Yevamos* 13b). The intention of Ammon and
Moab in performing this brazen act was not
merely to expunge the verse. There were many
other Torah Scrolls in the land which still
contained that verse — tearing it from the
Temple scroll would not have changed their
forbidden status. Rather, their sole aim was to

ח *[The wicked Turnus Rufus] plowed [Jerusalem] to devastation;*
   the city [once] filled with multitudes,[1]
   and more than four hundred schools studying Scripture and Mishnah.
                                                    So how can I be consoled?

ט *Media flew swiftly to annihilate my cherished ones;*
   and ruled over my precious [Temple], when I rent my robes [in sorrow].
                                                    So how can I be consoled?

י *She took counsel [from Haman] to strangle the prancing lion cub,[2]*
   with one bite to tear asunder the elderly, the aged,
      the infant and the nursing babe.   *So how can I be consoled?*

כ *The third kingdom was even more oppressive,*
   [they came] upon the premier holy [nation][3]
      like a deafening tempest, to devastate it. *So how can I be consoled?*

ל *She [Greece] pressured to separate the sons of the smooth-skinned*
      [Jacob] and [God] the One Who apportions [to each man his lot];
   [she coerced them, saying, 'Declare that you have no portion
      in the Name of [the God you call] the Flaming Fire!'[4]
                                                    So how can I be consoled?

מ *Edom, [who took his name from] the red lentils, rebelled [against God],*
   and they defiantly hastened to obliterate God's [celestial] throne
      and His [earthly] footstool.[5]   *So how can I be consoled?*

נ *Allied with Edom were Moab and Ammon,*
   [who came] to eradicate the nurturing Torah,*
      and to destroy the palatial Temple.   *So how can I be consoled?*

ס *He trampled all my heroes[6] and all the flocks of my comrades;*
   all my warriors were vanquished in full view
      of all who passed me by.   *So how can I be consoled?*

ע *My spirit is exhausted by the killers,[7]*
      by the number of the murder victims
   who call longingly like a deer,[8]
      and are slaughtered for Your sake.[9]   *So how can I be consoled?*

פ *They were horrified on the day of battle,*
      in the East and in the West,
   [when] the [flowing] blood of congregation
      and great nation[10]* intermingled.   *So how can I be consoled?*

צ *Calamities upon calamities, each more tragic than the other,*
   overwhelming and powerful,[11] enduring and not short lived.
                                                    So how can I be consoled?

---

defy God and His Torah with impunity   קָהָל וְעַם רָב — *Congregation and great nation.*
(*Lechem Dimah*).   Ironically, this phrase, used by the *paytan* to

קָשְׁרוּ צִנָּתָם, וְחָגְרוּ חֲנִיתָם וְאָסְפוּ מַחֲנוֹתָם,

וְהֶאֱרִיכוּ לְמַעֲנִיתָם,[1]*   וְאֵיךְ אֲנַחֵם.

רַבּוֹת אַנְחוֹתַי וַעֲצוּמוֹת קִינוֹתַי,

רַבּוּ נַהֲמוֹתַי, וְאַתָּה יהוה עַד מָתַי,[2]   וְאֵיךְ אֲנַחֵם.

שָׁמַעְתָּ חֶרְפָּתָם, חֵרְפְוּנִי בִּשְׂפָתָם,

שִׁבְתָּם וְקִימָתָם, אֲנִי מַנְגִּינָתָם,[3]   וְאֵיךְ אֲנַחֵם.

תִּקְוָתְכֶם אֵיפוֹא, מַה לָּכֶם פֹּה,

חָרָה אַפּוֹ, וְאֵין עוֹד לִרְפֹּא,   וְאֵיךְ אֲנַחֵם.

תְּשׁוּבוֹתֵיכֶם נִשְׁאֲרָה מֵעַל , הוֹנוּנִי עוֹבְדֵי הַבַּעַל,

עַד יַשְׁקוּף¹ מִמַּעַל, מוֹרִיד שְׁאוֹל וַיָּעַל,[5]   **וְאָז אֲנַחֵם.**

---

(1) Cf. *Psalms* 129:3. (2) 6:4. (3) Cf. *Eichah* 3:61-63. (4) Cf. 3:50. (5) *I Samuel* 2:6.

describe the masses murdered by Nebuchadnez-zar's hordes, is used by the prophet to describe those very hordes (see *Ezekiel* 26:7). וְהֶאֱרִיכוּ לְמַעֲנִיתָם — *And lengthened their fur-*	*row.* The plowman never pauses while he is in the middle of a furrow, but waits until he reaches the end of the line. Thus, the longer the furrow, the longer the oxen must toil, without any respite. This alludes to Israel in exile who

ק They tied on their armor and belted their spears;
    they gathered their camps
and lengthened their furrow.[1*]   So how can I be consoled?

ר My groans are many and my laments are powerful;
    my moanings are abundant,
      so [I ask] You, HASHEM, 'Until when?'[2]   So how can I be consoled?

ש You have heard their insults [as] they defamed me with their lips;
    when they sit and when they stand,
      I am the theme of their derisive songs.[3]   So how can I be consoled?

ת 'Where is your hope? What are you doing here?
    His fury has been aroused [against you],
      and there is no longer any cure [for you]!' So how can I be consoled?

ת 'All your answers remain lies!'
    the worshipers of the Baal taunt me.
[And this will last] until He looks down and takes notice[4]
    from above,
[until] He lowers [our enemies] to the grave,
    and raises [us out of exile].[5*]   And then I will be consoled!

---

suffered over a lengthy period, without relief (*Radak* to *Psalms* 129:3).

מוֹרִיד שָׁאוּל וַיָּעַל — *[Until] He lowers [our enemies] to the grave, and raises [us out of exile].* Alternatively, this is a descriptive phrase: *He*

Who lowers to the grave, then raises. Accordingly the paytan means: Just as God causes people to die and will eventually resurrect them, so has He caused us to sink to the depths of exile and will eventually redeem us.

כט.

אָמַרְתִּי* שְׁעוּ מִנִּי בִּבְכִי אֲמָרֵר,¹
מַר נַפְשִׁי וְרוּחִי אֲקָרֵר,
עִם לִוְיָתָן* הָעֲתִידִים לְעוֹרֵר,²

בְּבְכִי יַעֲזֹר*³ עֲלֵי יְגוֹנֵךְ,
בַּת עַמִּי הִתְאַבְּכִי בְּגִינֵךְ,
אַל תִּתְּנִי פוּגַת לָךְ, וְאַל תִּדֹּם בַּת עֵינֵךְ.⁴

גֵּעִי בִּבְכִיָּה מְעֻטֶּרֶת בַּעֲלִיזוֹת,
הָיִית מִקֶּדֶם וְהִנָּךְ לְבִזּוֹת,
אֵיכָה נִהְיָתָה הָרָעָה הַזֹּאת.⁵

דֹּמִי אַל תִּתְּנִי* פְּלֵטָה הַנִּשְׁאָרָה,
הָרִימִי קוֹל וְזַעֲקִי מָרָה,
כִּי שֶׁבֶר עַל שֶׁבֶר נִקְרָא.⁷

הֵן לְאֻמִּים עֵת נִקְבָּצוּ,
חַי עָלֶיךָ כְּרוֹת בְּרִית⁸ כְּחָפָצוּ,
עַל עַמְּךָ יַעֲרִימוּ סוֹד וְיִתְיָעָצוּ.⁹

וְנִבְּלוּ מְזִמּוֹת נְטוֹת אֲשׁוּרַי לִמְעוֹד,
מִדְּאָגָה וּמִפַּחַד לִרְעוֹד,
אָמְרוּ לְכוּ וְנַכְחִידֵם מִגּוֹי וְלֹא יִזָּכֵר שֵׁם יִשְׂרָאֵל עוֹד.¹¹

זֹאת הִשְׁמִיעוּ בְּנֵי מִקְרָאָיו,
לוּ נִחַל אִם יִקְטְלֵנוּ¹² נַעֲרִיץ לְמוֹרָאָיו,
הֵכִין יהוה זֶבַח הִקְדִּישׁ קְרוּאָיו.¹³

חֲלָלַי אָז הִרְבּוּ וְהָרְגוּ טוֹבַי,
יִסְּרוּנִי קְשׁוֹת צָרַי וְאוֹיְבַי,
הַמַּכּוֹת הָאֵלֶּה הֻכֵּיתִי בֵּית מְאַהֲבָי.¹⁴

אָמַרְתִּי *— I said.* This *kinnah* is a bitter narrative that recounts the brave martyrdom and slaughter of innocent Jews at the hand of their enemy. It laments children being butchered cruelly for the sanctification of God's name while their fathers are forced to witness this scene, reciting the *Shema* to proclaim that despite these unspeakable tragedies their faith was not shaken. The author cries out to God to avenge the blood of Israel and to speedily bring the redemption.

Each stanza comprises three lines. The third line is a Scriptural verse fragment and determines the rhyme. The initial letters of the respective stanzas form the *aleph-beis*, followed by the composer's signature, קְלוֹנִימוֹס הַקָּטָן, *Klonimos the lesser*. Perhaps he is Klonimos Yehudah who composed *kinnah* 25. If so, the events described here occurred during the First Crusade, in 1096. It

29.

א   *I said,* 'Turn away from me,*
    while I express my bitterness with weeping.'[1]
  I will soothe the bitterness of my soul and spirit [by crying]
  with those who are prepared to arouse their lament.[2]*

ב   *Assist in weeping[3]* over your agony,*
    O daughter of my nation, weep over yourself!
  Give yourself no rest, let not your eyes be silenced [from crying].[4]

ג   *Burst out weeping, O you who had been crowned with joy,*
    but now have been shamed.
  Alas! How did this evil happen?[5]

ד   *Do not hold yourself silent,[6] O you fugitive remnant,*
  call out in loud voice and cry out bitterly,
  because catastrophe occurs on [the heels] of catastrophe.[7]

ה   *Behold, when all the nations gathered together*
    at the designated time,
  O Lifegiver, they entered into a covenant against You,[8]
    as was their desire.
  Against Your nation they plot deviously and take counsel.[9]

ו   *They wove treacherous schemes, turning my steps to cause a fall;*
  to make me tremble from anxiety and fear.[10]
  They said, 'Come, let us cut them off from nationhood,
    so Israel's name will not be remembered any more!'[11]

ז   *The sons of His summoned ones proclaimed,*
  'We place our trust in Him, even if He should slay us,[12]
    we will revere His awesomeness,
  for HASHEM *has prepared a sacrifice,*
    He has consecrated His guests.'[13]

ח   *They then multiplied my corpses and slaughtered my finest;*
  my tormentors and my enemies tortured me intensively,
  these are the wounds inflicted upon me
    in the house of my [treacherous] lovers.[14]

---

(1) Cf. *Isaiah* 22:4. (2) Cf. *Job* 3:8 [7]. (3) Cf. *Isaiah* 16:9. (4) *Eichah* 2:18. (5) *Judges* 20:3.
(6) Cf. *Isaiah* 62:7. (7) *Jeremiah* 4:20. (8) Cf. *Psalms* 83:6. (9) 83:4. (10) Some editions read
אַחֲרֵי הַהֶבֶל לְהַהְבִּיל וּמִפָּנָיו לַרְעוֹד, *to misguide me after the futile [idolatry], and to tremble before it.*
(11) *Psalms* 83:5. (12) Cf. *Job* 13:15. (13) *Zephaniah* 1:7. (14) Cf. *Zechariah* 13:6.

---

is not surprising, therefore, that the medieval
censors laid a heavy hand on this *kinnah*, as is
obvious from the number and order of the
variant readings for some of the stanzas.

לְוָיָתָן — *Their lament.* The translation follows *Ibn
Ezra* (to *Job* 3:8 [7]) in his first explanation.
Accordingly, the word is third person feminine
plural possessive, a contraction of לְוָיָה שֶׁלָהֶן.
Alternatively, the word is a proper noun and
refers to the huge sea creature *Leviathan*, as if the

sailors on an about-to-capsize ship were bemoan-
ing their fate to become food for the Leviathan
(*Ibn Ezra* ibid.). *Rashi* (ibid.) understands the
word as *their conjugality,* i.e., as bereaved
partners mourning over the spouse of their
youth. In the *kinnah* this alludes to Israel
lamenting her wayward infidelity in worshiping
idols and in forsaking her first Husband, God,
Who, in return, banished her from His House.

בְּבְכִי יַעֲזֹר — *Assist in weeping.* In the verses from

טוֹב וּמֵטִיב הַבֵּט בְּצָרוֹתֵינוּ,

הִשְׁמִידוּ גִבּוֹרֵי בְּחֶתֶף מֵאַרְצֵנוּ,

כָּל נֵתַח טוֹב יָרֵךְ וְכָתֵף וְכָל מַשְׂמַגֵּינוּ.²

יַחַד לַטֶּבַח הוּבְלוּ כִּטְלָאִים וּגְדָיִים,³

בָּנוֹת מְחֻטָּבוֹת מְשֻׁבָּצוֹת עֲדִי עֲדָיִים,

גְּמוּלֵי מֵחָלָב עַתִּיקֵי מִשָּׁדָיִם.⁴

כָּבַשׁ הָאָב רַחֲמָיו* לְזֶבַח,

יְלָדָיו הִשְׁלִים כְּכָרִים לְטֶבַח,

הֵכִין לְבָנָיו מַטְבֵּחַ.⁵

לְאִמּוֹתָם נוֹאָמִים הִנְנוּ נִשְׁחָטִים וְנִטְבָּחִים,

כְּהִקְדִּישׁוּם לַטֶּבַח וְהִתִּיקוּם לַאֲבָחִים,⁶

נָשִׁים פִּרְיָם עוֹלְלֵי טִפּוּחִים.⁷

מִי יִשְׁמַע וְלֹא יִדְמַע,

הַבֵּן נִשְׁחַט וְהָאָב קוֹרֵא אֶת שְׁמַע,

מִי רָאָה כָזֹאת וּמִי שָׁמַע.⁸

נְוַת בֵּית הַיָּפָה בְּתוּלַת בַּת יְהוּדָה,

צַוָּארָהּ פָּשְׁטָה וּמַאֲכֶלֶת הִשְׁחִיזָה וְחִדְּדָה,

עַיִן רָאֲתָה וַתְּעִידָהּ.⁹

סְגֻפָה הָאֵם וּפָרְחָה רוּחָהּ,

וְנַפְשָׁהּ הַשְּׁלֵימָה לַטֶּבַח אֲרוּחָהּ כְּאָרְחָהּ,

אֵם הַבָּנִים שְׂמֵחָה.¹⁰

עָלְצוּ הַבָּנוֹת כְּנוּסוֹת וַאֲרוּסוֹת,

לְאִבְחַת חֶרֶב לְקַדֵּם דָּצוֹת וְשָׂשׂוֹת,

דָּמָם עַל צְחִיחַ סֶלַע לְבִלְתִּי הִכָּסוֹת.¹¹*

פּוֹנֶה הָאָב בִּבְכִי וִילָלָה,

עַצְמוֹ עַל חַרְבּוֹ לִדְקוֹר וּלְהַפִּילָה,

וְהוּא מִתְגּוֹלֵל בַּדָּם בְּתוֹךְ הַמְּסִלָּה.¹²

---

(1) *Ezekiel* 24:4. (2) Some editions have a variant reading of this entire stanza. מֵאֲנְתִּי בָּם לְהִשְׁתַּתֵּף צְנַף צַחֲנָתָם, *I refused to become a partner to the smelly filth [of their idols],*/ הִשְׁמִידוּ גִבּוֹרֵי כֻלָּם בְּחֶתֶף, *in one fell swoop all our warriors were obliterated,*/ כָּל נֵתַח טוֹב יָרֵךְ וְכָתֵף, *[they were like] all the best cuts [of meat], thigh and shoulder.*
(3) Cf. *Isaiah* 53:7. (4) 28:9. (5) Cf. 14:21. (6) Cf. *Jeremiah* 12:3. (7) *Eichah* 2:20.
(8) *Isaiah* 66:8. (9) Cf. *Job* 29:11. (10) *Psalms* 113:9. (11) Cf. *Ezekiel* 24:8. (12) *II Samuel* 20:12.

ט [O God] Who is good and does good, observe our misfortunes,
   for in one fell swoop our warriors were obliterated from our land,
   [they were like] all the best cuts [of meat], thigh and shoulder,[1]
      and all of our choicest [leaders].[2]

י They were led to the slaughter together, like lambs and kids;[3]
   daughters perfectly formed, adorned with jewels and ornaments,
   [and] just-weaned babies torn from the breast.[4]

כ The father suppressed his compassion*
      [to allow himself] to sacrifice.
   He surrendered his children like fatted sheep to the slaughter.
   He prepared the butchering block for his own sons.[5]

ל To their mothers they said,
      'Behold we are slaughtered and butchered!'
   when they prepared them for the slaughter
      and dragged them from their place.[6]
   Women [did this to] their own offspring,
      the babes they carefully pampered.[7]

מ Who can hear this and not shed tears?
   The son is slaughtered, and the father recites the Shema!
   Who ever saw the likes of this, who ever heard of it?[8]

נ The beautiful one who dwells within,
      the maiden daughter of Judah,
   stretched her neck [for the slaughter] and honed
      and sharpened the knife;
   [God's] Eye saw and testified [to this unsurpassed devotion].[9]

ס Tormented was the mother and her spirit flew off,
   she submitted her soul to the slaughter, [with the same love]
      as if she were preparing a meal [for her family].
   [And yet,] the mother of children rejoices.[10]

ע The daughters exulted, those wed and those betrothed,
   they rushed joyfully and gladly to the whetted sword,
   their blood [shed] on a smooth rock, never to be covered over.[11]*

פ The father turns away with weeping and wailing,
   throwing himself on his sword to be stabbed.
   He wallows in his own blood on the roadway.[12]

---

which this phrase is borrowed (Isaiah 16:9 and
Jeremiah 48:32), the word יַעְזֵר is a proper noun,
the name of a Moabite city. Nevertheless, the
translation treats it as a derivative of the root
עזר, to help or assist, because that interpretation
seems more apt. Although the word's vowelization seems to contradict this view, it is not
uncommon for paytanim to speak in wordplay
and conundrum.

כָּבַשׁ הָאָב רַחֲמָיו — The father suppressed his

compassion. The next series of stanzas describes
how parents made the supreme sacrifice in
sanctification of God's Name by offering their
children to the crusader's sword, rather than to
his baptismal font. And all the while affirming
their faith in the One True God by reciting the
Shema.

דָּמָם עַל צְחִיחַ סֶלַע לְבִלְתִּי הִכָּסוֹת — Their blood
[shed] on a smooth rock, never to be covered
over. The Scriptural verse from which this

צִדְקָה דִינָה פוֹרִיָה כְּהַקְרִיבָה עֲנָפֶיהָ,

וְתַמּוּר מִזְרָק דָּם קַבָּלָה בִּכְנָפֶיהָ,

תִּתְיַפַּח תְּפָרֵשׂ כַּפֶּיהָ.[1]

קוֹרוֹתַי מִי יָנוּד שׁוֹד וָשֶׁבֶר[2] יִשְׁתָּרֵג,

מַחֲמַד עֵינִי כְּנִמְסַר לְחֶרֶב וּלְהֶרֶג,

אִם כְּהֶרֶג הֲרוּגָיו הֹרָג.[3]

רַעְיוֹנַי נִבְהֲלוּ וַאֲחָזַתְנִי פַּלָּצוּת וָשֶׁבֶר,

בְּאַחַת* נִמְצָא הַכָּתוּב בּוֹ תִּקְוָה וָשֶׁבֶר,

כִּי זֶה לְבַדּוֹ יָבֹא לְיָרָבְעָם אֶל קָבֶר.[4]

שָׁלֵם נִמְצָא בְּכָל פָּעֳלוֹ,

נַפְשׁוֹ לָטֶבַח הַשָּׁלִים מִפַּחַד חֵילוֹ,

וְגַם קְבוּרָה לֹא הָיְתָה לּוֹ.[5]

תַּתִּי לִבִּי מָצֹא תֹכֶן עִנְיָנָיו,

יָדַעְתִּי אֲנִי צֶדֶק וְיֹשֶׁר דִּינָיו,

וְטוֹב הוּא לִירֵאֵי הָאֱלֹהִים שֶׁיִּרְאוּ מִלְּפָנָיו.[6]

קְדוֹשָׁיו לֹא יַאֲמִין[7]* הַשְׁלֵם עֲוֹנוֹתָם לְשַׁעֲרָה,[8]

סִמָּן טוֹב לְאָדָם* שֶׁלֹּא נִסְפַּד וְנִקְבַּר כְּשׁוּרָה,

בְּיוֹן עֶבְרָה לֹא יִירָא.

לְזֹאת יֶחֱרַד לִבִּי יֶתֶר בְּחַלְחָלָה,

גִּבּוֹרַי נִרְעֲצוּ וְנִכְנְעוּ לְהַשְׁפִּילָה,

כִּנְפוֹל לִפְנֵי בְּנֵי עַוְלָה.[9]

---

fragment is borrowed reads in full: *In order to arouse fury, to incite vengeance, have I placed her blood on a smooth rock, never to be covered* (Ezekiel 24:8). *Rashi* explains that since the smooth rock will not absorb the blood as the soil would, the blood will remain a visible reminder that the murderer has not received his just desserts.

בְּאַחַת — *Because of one [good deed].* In *I Kings* (ch. 14), the prophet אֲחִיָּה, *Ahijah*, tells the wicked Jeroboam's wife that God would utterly cut off every male child from the House of Jeroboam, '...and will sweep them away as one sweeps away dung... The dead of Jeroboam in the city, the dogs shall eat, and the dead in the field, the birds of the heaven shall eat.' The only

exception to this curse was Jeroboam's son אֲבִיָּה, *Abijah*, who merited a proper burial because he defied his father on one point. Jeroboam had stationed armed sentries on all the roads leading to Jerusalem to prevent any member of the Ten Tribes of Israel from making the pilgrimage to Jerusalem on the three Festivals. According to the Talmud (*Moed Kattan* 28b), Prince Abijah was on sentry duty, but deserted his post and went up to Jerusalem himself. Another opinion says that Abijah entirely abolished the sentry system his father had established.

קְדוֹשָׁיו לֹא יַאֲמִין — *He trusts not His holy ones.* When R' Yochanan would reach this verse (*Job* 15:15), he would weep. 'If He does not trust His holy ones, whom does He trust?' One day, he

צ The fruitful [mother] proclaimed the righteousness of her judgment
   as she offered her scions.
And instead of the [usual] consecrated basin [in which the sacrificial
   blood is caught], she caught [her children's blood]
   in the hem of her garments,
sobbing and spreading out her arms [in anguish].[1]

ק Who will be stirred by my tragedies wherein ruination
   and destruction[2] knitted together,
when my eye's delight was delivered
   to the sword and to the slaughter.
Was there ever a slaughter to compare with
   the murder of his victims?[3]

ר My thoughts are confounded for I am seized
   by confusion and heartbreak;
because of one [good deed]* found in him,
   Scripture gives [Abijah] hope and confidence,
for he alone of [the House of] Jeroboam
   shall come to the grave.[4]

ש [Yet,] one found perfect in his every deed,
   who gave up his life to the slaughter in awe
of God's domain, for him there was no proper burial![5]

ת I have set my heart to finding the inner meaning of His dealings.
For this I do know: His judgments are righteous and just,
   and it will be good for the God-fearing, that they
   may be awed in His Presence.[6]

ק He trusts not His holy ones,[7]*
   rather He punishes their sins even to a hair.[8]
Indeed, it is an auspicious omen for a man*
   if he is not eulogized or buried properly.
Therefore, let him not fear the day of wrath.

ל Over this my heart shudders, it palpitates with convulsion,
for my heroes are shattered and subdued, humbled
   as they fall before the iniquitous.[9]

---

(1) Jeremiah 4:31. (2) Cf. Isaiah 51:19. (3) 27:7. (4) I Kings 14:13. (5) Ecclesiates 6:3.
(6) 8:12. (7) Cf. Job 15:11. (8) Tractate Bava Kamma 50a. (9) II Samuel 3:34.

---

came upon a man picking not-yet-completely-ripe figs while leaving the ripe figs on the tree. He explained to R' Yochanan that he was going on a long journey. the not-yet-ripe fruits could be expected to last; but the already ripe could not. Said R' Yochanan, 'That must be the meaning of the verse!' Just as this man is apprehensive of how the ripe figs will fare later on, so is God apprehensive lest a young tzaddik spoil as he ages. Thus, He will sometimes take His holy ones from this world while they are still young, and not trust them to the vicissitudes that might break them of their righteousness (Chagigah 5a with Rashi).

סִמָּן טוֹב לְאָדָם — It is an auspicious omen for a man ... The Talmud teaches that God will sometimes cause a righteous person anguish after his death, in order to fully purge him of any stain on his soul caused by sin. Thus, one who does not receive proper burial, or is not eulogized in accordance with his stature, or

וְעַד מָתַי תִּהְיֶה כְּגִבּוֹר לֹא יוּכַל לְהוֹשִׁיעַ,[1]

נִקְמַת דַּם עֲבָדֶיךָ תּוֹדִיעַ,[2]

אֵל נְקָמוֹת יהוה אֵל נְקָמוֹת הוֹפִיעַ.[3]

נְקֹם נִקְמָתִי מֵאֵת מְעַנַּי,

עֵת נְקָמָה הִיא לָדוּן דִּינַי,

אֵל קַנָּא וְנוֹקֵם יהוה.[5]

יהוה כְּגִבּוֹר צֵא יְדֵי חוֹבָךְ פְּרַע,

שׁוֹבֵר כְּתוֹב שְׁטַר חוֹב תִּקְרַע,

שְׁבוֹר גְּזַר דִּינֵנוּ הָרָע.[7]

מִמָּרוֹם כְּהִסִּיק אֵשׁ בְּמַעֲזִיבָה וְתִקְרָה,

חוֹמַת אֵשׁ סָבִיב שׁוֹמֵירָה וּבֵית דִּירָה,

שַׁלֵּם יְשַׁלֵּם הַמַּבְעִיר אֶת הַבְּעֵרָה.[10]

וּכְגָמוּל גְּמוּלוֹת נָא שַׁלֵּם,[11]

(אוֹיְבַי תַּפִּיל מְהֵרָה וּתְכַלֵּם,)[12]

כִּי אֵל גְּמוּלוֹת יהוה שַׁלֵּם יְשַׁלֵּם.[13]

(שׂוֹנְאֶיךָ תַּצְמִית סַף רַעַל תַּשְׁקֵם,[14]

הֵמֵת תַּחַת יָדוֹ נָקֹם יִנָּקֵם,[15]

אִם בְּכָזֶה לֹא תִתְנַקֵּם.)[12]

הַעַל כֵּן נִקְרֵאתָ אִישׁ מִלְחָמָה,[17]

צָרֶיךָ לְכַלּוֹת וּבָהֶם לְהִנָּקְמָה,

נֹקֵם יהוה וּבַעַל חֵמָה.[18]

קַנָּא לְשִׁמְךָ עֲבוּרְךָ הָאֵל,

וּלְדַם עֲבָדֶיךָ הַשָּׁפוּךְ[19] וּלְחָרְבוֹת אֲרִיאֵל,

וּנְקוֹם נִקְמַת בְּנֵי יִשְׂרָאֵל.[20]

טְפֵי דָמָם אַחַת לְאַחַת מְנוּיוֹת,

וְיֵז נִצְחָם[21] עַל בְּגָדֶיךָ וּבְפוּרְפְּרָךְ הָיוֹת,

יָדִין בַּגּוֹיִם מָלֵא גְוִיּוֹת.[22]

נִלְאֵיתִי נְשׂא אֶת כָּל הַתְּלָאָה,

מַהֵר גְּאָלְתִּי וְתָחִישׁ הַמַּרְאָה,

כִּי יוֹם נָקָם בְּלִבִּי וּשְׁנַת גְּאוּלַי בָּאָה.[23]

---

whose unburied body is attacked by a wild beast, attains atonement through this degradation. Such a person will be spared the punish-ments of the next world (*Sanhedrin* 47a with *Rashi* and *Tosafos* [46b]).

ו *Until when will You continue to be like a warrior*
   who is unable to save?[1]
Let [Your] vengeance for the blood of Your servants become known
   [before our eyes and among the nations];[2]
O God of vengeance, HASHEM, O God of vengeance, appear![3]

ג *Take my revenge from those who tormented me,*
   [for] it is a time of vengeance,[4] to take up my grievance.
A zealous and avenging God is HASHEM.[5]

י *HASHEM, go forth like mighty warrior[6] and pay Your obligation*
   [to avenge the slaughtered];
write [Yourself] a receipt [acknowledging this action],
   and rip up the note of [Israel's] indebtedness [for their iniquities].
Break the power of the wicked and the evil one.[7]

מ *From on high [God] kindled a fire[8] on the plaster and the beam,*
a wall of fire engulfed[9] [everything from] the sentry box
   to the [Divine] Dwelling,
He who kindled the fire must surely make full restitution.[10]

ו *According to their [wicked] deeds, please do repay [them];[11]*
(humble my enemies speedily, and destroy them,)[12]
for HASHEM is a God of retribution, He will surely repay [them].[13]

ס *(Cut down Your enemies, give them to drink the cup of poison;[14]*
[as Scripture states,] 'If one dies under his hand, he shall
   surely be avenged.'[15] Will You not avenge such as these?[16])[12]

ה *Is this why You are called the Man of War,[17] because*
You destroy Your enemies as You wreak vengeance upon them?
HASHEM avenges and is Master of His fury.[18]

ק *Be zealous for Your Name, for Your sake, O God!*
And for the spilt blood of Your servants[19]
   and for the ruins of the leonine Temple.
O avenge the vengeance of the Children of Israel.[20]

ט *The drops of my blood, counted one by one,*
drippings of their lifeblood[21] on Your [royal] purple,
let Him judge the nations [on a battlefield] filled with corpses.[22]

נ *I am tired from carrying all travail,*
hasten my redemption and speedily fulfill the vision:
For the day of vengeance is in my heart,
   and the year of my redemption has arrived![23]

---

(1) Cf. *Jeremiah* 14:9. (2) Cf. *Psalms* 79:10; some editions include a longer segment of the verse and read . . . . . . נקמת בגוים לעינינו; the translation includes this phrase in the interpolation. (3) 94:1. (4) *Jeremiah* 51:6. (5) *Nahum* 1:2. (6) Cf. *Isaiah* 42:13. (7) Cf. *Psalms* 10:15; some editions read שבור גזר דיננו הרע, *Break the evil decree of our verdict.* (8) Cf. *Eichah* 1:13. (9) *Zechariah* 2:9. (10) *Exodus* 22:5. (11) *Isaiah* 59:18. (12) Some editions omit the passages in parentheses. (13) *Jeremiah* 51:56. (14) Cf. *Zechariah* 12:2. (15) Cf. *Exodus* 21:20. (16) Cf. *Jeremiah* 5:9, 29; 9:8. (17) *Exodus* 15:3. (18) *Nahum* 1:2. (19) Cf. *Psalms* 79:10. (20) Cf. *Numbers* 31:2. (21) Cf. *Isaiah* 63:3. (22) *Psalms* 110:6; some editions do not contain this stanza, but instead read: טוב ומטיב קנא לשמך, *O God One Who does good for others be zealous for Your Name,*/למען יחלצון ידידיך, *so that Your beloved ones may be released*/הושיעה ימינך, *save us with Your right hand* (*Psalms* 60:7). (23) *Isaiah* 63:4.

ל.

מְעוֹנֵי שָׁמַיִם,* שְׁחָקִים יְזַבְּלוּךְ, מְלֵאִים מֵהוֹדְךָ,
וְאַף כִּי הַבָּיִת.[1]

מַה טּוֹב וּמַה נָּעִים,[2] שִׁבְתְּךָ עִם רֵעִים, בְּכַנְפֵי צַעְצוּעִים,[3]
יַעַן הָיָה עִם לְבָבְךָ[4]   לִבְנוֹת הַבָּיִת.

נָאוֹר, אַהֲבָתְךָ הֶרְאֵיתָ לְעַמֶּךָ, כִּי הֵם נַחֲלָתֶךָ,
וְלֵידַע כִּי שְׁמֶךָ   נִקְרָא עַל הַבָּיִת.[5]

נָכְרִים שָׁם בָּאוּ, וְעַמִּים הַר יִקְרָאוּ, וְאוֹתוֹתָיו רָאוּ,
לְמַעַן יִרְאוּ כְּבוֹד יהוה   עַל הַבָּיִת.[6]

חָטָאי כִּי עָצְמוּ, אֲכָלַתְנִי קִנְאָה,[7] וְעָרָה צַר הַיְסוֹד,[8]
שָׂמְנִי שׁוֹאָה,   וְנָתַץ אֶת הַבָּיִת.[9]

חֲמוּדֵי אוֹצְרֵיהֶם, הֵבִיאוּ בְּהֵיכְלֵיהֶם, מִלְאוּ כְרֵסֵיהֶם,[10]
וְצִוָּה הַכֹּהֵן   וּפִנּוּ אֶת הַבָּיִת.[11]

מַדּוּעַ נִתְּכָה, וְחֵמָה לֹא שָׁכָכָה, עַל מַה זֶּה עָשָׂה צוּרֵנוּ כָּכָה,
לָאָרֶץ הַזֹּאת   וְלַבָּיִת.[12]

מְקוֹם כֹּהֲנַי נִגָּשׁוּ, וְשָׁם יִתְקַדְּשׁוּ, וְהֵן כָּעֵת רָפָסוּ,
הֲמוֹן גּוֹיִם רָגָשׁוּ,[13]   נָסַבּוּ עַל הַבָּיִת.[14]

בַּת קוֹל הִיא עוֹנָה, מַה תִּתְמְהוּ פֶּגַע,
סֵמֶל הַקִּנְאָה[15] הֲבֵאתֶם,   וּכְנֶגַע נִרְאָה לִי בַּבָּיִת.[16]

רְבִיצַת עוֹלָם מָלֵא, שׁוֹכֵן בְּהֵיכָלוֹ, הֲתַעֲשׂוּ צָרָה* לוֹ,

---

(1) I Kings 8:27. (2) Psalms 133:1. (3) II Chronicles 3:10. (4) Cf. 6:8. (5) Cf. I Kings 8:43.
(6) II Chronicles 7:3. (7) Cf. Psalms 69:10. (8) Cf. 137:7. (9) Leviticus 14:45.
(10) Cf. Jeremiah 51:34. (11) Leviticus 14:36. (12) II Chronicles 7:21. (13) Cf. Psalms 2:1.
(14) Genesis 19:4. (15) Ezekiel 8:3. (16) Leviticus 14:35.

---

§ מְעוֹנֵי שָׁמַיִם — *The celestial palaces.* There was a time when God was so eager to dwell in the midst of His beloved Jewish people that He contained His unlimited Being within the limited confines of the Temple's walls. His *Shechinah*-Presence was so manifest in the Temple that even a non-Jew who came to pray there could feel God's Presence. But later, Israel ignored God's Presence. They desecrated His earthly abode with abominable idolatry. To purify the Temple, God purged it with fiery flames that consumed it.

Today, Israel eagerly awaits God's return when He will surround the rebuilt Temple with a wall of protective fire so that it will never again be defiled or destroyed.

The acrostic of the stanzas spells the composer's name, מְנַחֵם בַּר יַעֲקֹב חֲזַק, *Menachem son of Yaakov, may he be strong.* (R' Menachem flourished in Worms, Germany, during the last decades of the 12th century.) The fourth, final stich of each stanza is a Scriptural fragment ending with the word בַּיִת, *house* or *Temple.*

30.

מ *The celestial palaces,* the heavens that house You,*
are filled with Your splendor, yet they cannot contain You.
How much less so the Temple?[1]

מ *How good and how pleasant[2] was Your dwelling amongst friends*
between the wings of the cherished Cherubim[3]
because it was Your heart's desire[4] to [have us] build the Temple.

נ *O Awesome One, You have displayed Your love to Your nation,*
for they are Your heritage, and You let it be known
that Your Name is identified with the Temple.[5]

נ *Gentiles [also] came there, and foreign nations*
summoned one another to the [Temple] mountain,
they saw its wondrous signs, in order that they
should see the glory of HASHEM upon the Temple.[6]

ח *However, when my sins became massive,*
jealous zeal consumed me,[7]* and the tormentor
[razed the Temple until he] laid bare its foundation,[8]
left me desolate, and smashed the Temple.[9]

ח *They [the heathens] brought into their palaces*
[Israel's] precious treasures,
they filled their bellies[10] [with spoils].
For the [supreme] Kohen [God] commanded
that they empty out the Temple.[11]

מ *Why was [God's] unrelenting fury*
poured out like molten metal?
Why did our Creator do such a thing
to this land and to the Temple?[12]

מ *The place where my priests would approach,*
there to sanctify themselves, behold,
it is now overrun [by] gentile hordes
who have gathered,[13] surrounding the Temple.[14]

ב *A [heavenly] echo replies, 'Why are you so bewildered*
by this visitation? [Have] you [not] brought
the image of jealousy[15] in[to the Sanctuary],
which seemed to me like a plague in the Temple?'[16]

ר *He whose resting place is the entire universe,*
yet dwelled in His palatial Temple,
how could you manufacture a rival* to Him

אֲכָלַתְנִי קִנְאָה — *Jealous zeal consumed me.*
Various interpretations are given for this line. It
refers to either: God's zealous anger at 'my sins'
of the preceding line; or the sin of idolatry as
represented by the סֵמֶל הַקִּנְאָה, *image of jeal-*
ousy, mentioned below; or the jealousy borne by

the heathen nations against the *Beis HaMikdash*
and which, because of my sins, they were
permitted to vent by destroying the Temple.

צָרָה — *Rival.* A polygamous man's wives are
called צָרוֹת, *rivals*, literally, *troubles*, to each
other (see, e.g., *I Samuel* 1:6 and *Yevamos* 2a).

עֵוֵּר וּפִסֵּחַ   לֹא יָבֹא אֶל הַבָּיִת.[1]

יַעַן הֻשְׁחַתֶּם מְצָאוּנְכֶם רָעוֹת, חֻלַּל הַמִּקְדָּשׁ וְהִנֵּה מִגְרָעוֹת
נָתַן לַבָּיִת.[2]

קָדוֹשׁ יִתְעַשֵּׁת, אֱמֶת לָנוּ בְּשֵׁת,[3] יְשַׁלַּח תַּחְבֻּשֶׁת,
וְחֵטְא אַל יָשֵׁת,[4]   וְחִטֵּא אֶת הַבָּיִת.[5]

בְּמָקוֹר הַנִּפְתָּח[6] וּמַעֲלֵה עַל שָׂפָה,[7] מְבַכֵּר לָחֳדָשָׁיו,
וְעָלֵהוּ לִתְרוּפָה,   מִתַּחַת מִפְתַּן הַבָּיִת.

חֲמוֹל עִיר הַחֲרֵבָה, תְּמוּר מוֹקֵשׁ שְׁבִיבָה, חוֹמַת אֵשׁ סוֹבְבָה,
לְכָבוֹד תִּהְיֶה בָהּ,[8]   אֶל דְּבִיר הַבָּיִת.[9]

זְרֵה וְהַעֲבֵר טֻמְאָה מִבֵּיתְךָ מַלְכִּי, אֱלִיל כָּלִיל תַּחֲלוֹף,[10]
וְתִקְרָא   אָנֹכִי פִּנִּיתִי הַבָּיִת.[11]

קַדֵּשׁ בֵּית מְעוֹנִי,* וְתָשׁוּב לִמְלוֹנִי, וְנִקְבְּצוּ לְגִיוֹנִי,
וְהִנֵּה כְּבוֹד יהוה,   בָּא אֶל הַבָּיִת.[12]

---

(1) *II Samuel* 5:8. (2) *I Kings* 6:6. (3) *Daniel* 9:7. (4) Cf. *Numbers* 12:11.
(5) *Leviticus* 14:52. (6) *Zechariah* 13:1. (7) Cf. *Ezekiel* 47:12. (8) Cf. *Zechariah* 2:9.
(9) *I Kings* 8:6. (10) Cf. *Isaiah* 2:18. (11) *Genesis* 24:31. (12) *Ezekiel* 43:4.

קַדֵּשׁ בֵּית מְעוֹנִי — *Sanctify the House of My Dwelling.* The translation assumes that God is still speaking. Accordingly, God says, 'I have done My part by cleansing the Sanctuary of idolatrous defilement. Now you do your part by sanctifying yourself and your environs, and by

[especially in the place of which it is written],
'A blind man or a cripple shall not enter into the Temple.'[1]

ע Because you grew immoral, evil has found you!
The Sanctuary was defiled and [God] Himself
diminished [the stature of] the Temple.[2]

ק May the Holy One reflect that shame is truly ours;[3]
May He send a cure [for our wounds] and not hold sin[4]
[against us]. May He purge the Temple.[5]

ב With the [newly] opened water source[6]
    [He will purify the Temple];
and on the bank [of this stream] will grow[7]
    fruit trees that ripen each month
and whose leaves will have curative powers,
    [because they are nurtured by the holy water]
flowing from under the threshold of the Temple.

ח Have mercy on the devastated city!
Instead of the flaming pyre [that destroyed it,
let] a [protective] wall of fire surround it,
and You shall be glorious within it,[8]
[when Your Presence returns] to the Holy of Holies of the Temple.[9]

ז Cast out and throw away all impurity from your House,
O my King! Let the idols utterly vanish,[10] and cry out,
'I alone have cleared out [the idols from] the Temple!'[11]

ק So sanctify the House of My Dwelling,* and return to My Lodging;
let My legions be gathered there [and let them proclaim],
'Behold the glory of HASHEM has entered the Temple!'[12]

---

returning your thoughts to My Lodging, so that
I may return to My Dwelling.' Alternatively, this

stanza contains Israel's plaint that God return to
'the House that I built for Your dwelling.'

לא.

אֵשׁ תּוּקַד בְּקִרְבִּי,* בְּהַעֲלוֹתִי עַל לִבִּי,   בְּצֵאתִי מִמִּצְרָיִם.

קִינִים אָעִירָה, לְמַעַן אַזְכִּירָה,   בְּצֵאתִי מִירוּשָׁלָיִם.

אָז יָשִׁיר מֹשֶׁה,¹ שִׁיר לֹא יִנָּשֶׁה,   בְּצֵאתִי מִמִּצְרָיִם.

וַיְקוֹנֵן יִרְמְיָה,* וְנָהָה נְהִי נִהְיָה,²   בְּצֵאתִי מִירוּשָׁלָיִם.

בֵּיתִי הִתְכּוֹנָן, וְשָׁכַן הֶעָנָן,³   בְּצֵאתִי מִמִּצְרָיִם.

וַחֲמַת אֵל שָׁכְנָה, עָלַי כַּעֲנָנָה,   בְּצֵאתִי מִירוּשָׁלָיִם.

גַּלֵּי יָם רָמוּ, וְכַחוֹמָה קָמוּ,⁴   בְּצֵאתִי מִמִּצְרָיִם.

זְדוֹנִים שָׁטָפוּ, וְעַל רֹאשִׁי צָפוּ,⁵   בְּצֵאתִי מִירוּשָׁלָיִם.

דְּגַן שָׁמַיִם, וּמִצּוּר יָזוּבוּ מָיִם,⁶   בְּצֵאתִי מִמִּצְרָיִם.

לַעֲנָה וּמְרוֹרִים, וּמֵי הַמָּרִים,   בְּצֵאתִי מִירוּשָׁלָיִם.

הַשְׁכֵּם וְהַעֲרֵב, סְבִיבוֹת הַר חוֹרֵב,*   בְּצֵאתִי מִמִּצְרָיִם.

קוֹרֵא אֵל אֵבֶל, עַל נַהֲרוֹת בָּבֶל,⁷   בְּצֵאתִי מִירוּשָׁלָיִם.

וּמַרְאֵה כְּבוֹד יהוה, כְּאֵשׁ אוֹכֶלֶת⁸ לְפָנַי,   בְּצֵאתִי מִמִּצְרָיִם.

וְחֶרֶב לְטוּשָׁה, וּלְטֶבַח נְטוּשָׁה,   בְּצֵאתִי מִירוּשָׁלָיִם.

זֶבַח וּמִנְחָה, וְשֶׁמֶן הַמִּשְׁחָה,   בְּצֵאתִי מִמִּצְרָיִם.

סֻגַּלְתְּ אֵל לְקוּחָה, כְּצֹאן לְטִבְחָה,   בְּצֵאתִי מִירוּשָׁלָיִם.

חַגִּים וְשַׁבָּתוֹת, וּמוֹפְתִים וְאוֹתוֹת,   בְּצֵאתִי מִמִּצְרָיִם.

תַּעֲנִית וְאֵבֶל, וּרְדוֹף הַהֶבֶל,   בְּצֵאתִי מִירוּשָׁלָיִם.

---

(1) Exodus 15:1. (2) Micah 2:4. (3) See Numbers 9:15,22. (4) Cf. Exodus 15:8. (5) Cf. Eichah 3:54. (6) Cf. Psalms 78:24,20. (7) 137:1. (8) Exodus 24:17.

◆§ אֵשׁ תּוּקַד בְּקִרְבִּי — A fire ... burns within me. The Midrash cites numerous examples of the startling contrast between our triumphant Exodus from Egypt and our tragic exit from conquered Jerusalem (Eichah Zuta 19). When Israel left Egypt their hearts were aflame with a fire of love for God and an unquenchable desire to receive the Torah at Sinai. But as the defeated Jews trudged out of Jerusalem's ruins into captivity, their hearts were shrouded in gloom and lamentations were on their lips.

Another tragedy which occurred on Tishah B'Av was the expulsion of the Jews from Spain in 1492. At that time the Spanish rabbis allowed orchestras to play before them (even on Tishah B'Av itself), in order to strengthen the spirits of the unfortunate exiles and to thank God for giving them the courage and strength not to

succumb to the pressure to convert. It was also the aim of these rabbis to teach the people that we never weep over departing from a country in exile. No matter how we prospered in that land, we weep only over our forced departure from Jerusalem (see Sefer HaTodaah).

The kinnah, of unknown authorship, follows an aleph-beis arrangement as the initial letters of the respective stanzas.

הַר חוֹרֵב — Mount Horeb. According to the Midrash (Tanchuma, Bamidbar 7), Scripture records six names for Mount Sinai: (a) הַר הָ[אֱ]לֹהִים], the Mountain of Elokim (Exodus 18:5; Psalms 68:16); (b) הַר בָּשָׁן, Mount Bashan (Psalms 68:16); (c) הַר גַּבְנֻנִּים, Mount Gavnunim (ibid.); (d) הָהָר חָמַד, the Desired Mountain (ibid. v. 17); (e) הַר חוֹרֵב, Mount Horeb (Exodus 3:1;

31.

א *A fire [of elation] burns within me,**
    when I recall in my heart [what happened],
                    when I went forth from Egypt;
    but I shall arouse lamentations,
      so that I'll remember [what occurred],
                 when I went forth from Jerusalem.

א *Then Moses chose to sing¹ a song not to be forgotten,*
                    when I went forth from Egypt;
    but Jeremiah lamented* a doleful lament,²
                 when I went forth from Jerusalem.

ב *My House [the Tabernacle] was*
    established, and the cloud rested upon it,³
                    when I went forth from Egypt;
    but God's fury rested like a heavy cloud upon me,
                 when I went forth from Jerusalem.

ג *The waves of the Sea piled high, and stood up like a wall,⁴*
                    when I went forth from Egypt;
    but the wanton enemy drowned me and poured over my head,⁵
                 when I went forth from Jerusalem.

ד *Heavenly grain and a rock from which flowed water,⁶*
                    when I went forth from Egypt;
    wormwood and bitterness and the bitter waters,
                 when I went forth from Jerusalem.

ה *From dawn to dusk, encircling Mount Horeb,**
                    when I went forth from Egypt;
    but a call to mourning by the rivers of Babylon,⁷
                 when I went forth from Jerusalem.

ו *And the appearance of the glory of HASHEM*
    was like a fire consuming⁸ before me,
                    when I went forth from Egypt;
    but abandoned to the slaughter of the sharpened sword,
                 when I went forth from Jerusalem.

ז *Sacrifices and flour offerings, and the oil of anointment,*
                    when I went forth from Egypt;
    but God's treasure was taken like sheep to the slaughter,
                 when I went forth from Jerusalem.

ח *Festivals and Sabbaths, and miracles and signs,*
                    when I went forth from Egypt;
    but fasting and mourning and the pursuit of futility,
                 when I went forth from Jerusalem.

33:6; *I Kings* 19:8); and (f) הַר סִינַי, *Mount Sinai*   וַיְקוֹנֵן יִרְמְיָה — *But Jeremiah lamented.* This
(*Exodus* 19:18).   refers to the Book of *Eichah* that *Jeremiah*

טְבוּ אֹהָלִים, לְאַרְבָּעָה דְגָלִים,*   בְּצֵאתִי מִמִּצְרָיִם.
וְאָהֳלֵי יִשְׁמְעֵאלִים, וּמַחֲנוֹת עֲרֵלִים,   בְּצֵאתִי מִירוּשָׁלָיִם.

יוֹבֵל וּשְׁמִטָּה,[1] וְאֶרֶץ שׁוֹקְטָה,   בְּצֵאתִי מִמִּצְרָיִם.
מָכוּר לַצְּמִיתוּת, וְכָרוֹת וְכָתוֹת,   בְּצֵאתִי מִירוּשָׁלָיִם.

כַּפְּרֶת וְאָרוֹן,[2] וְאַבְנֵי זִכָּרוֹן,[3]   בְּצֵאתִי מִמִּצְרָיִם.
וְאַבְנֵי הַקֶּלַע, וּכְלֵי הַבֶּלַע,   בְּצֵאתִי מִירוּשָׁלָיִם.

לְוִיִּם וְאַהֲרֹנִים, וְשִׁבְעִים זְקֵנִים,[4]   בְּצֵאתִי מִמִּצְרָיִם.
נוֹגְשִׂים וּמוֹנִים, וּמוֹכְרִים וְקוֹנִים,   בְּצֵאתִי מִירוּשָׁלָיִם.

מֹשֶׁה יִרְעֵנוּ, וְאַהֲרֹן יַנְחֵנוּ,   בְּצֵאתִי מִמִּצְרָיִם.
נְבוּכַדְנֶצַּר, וְאַנְדְּרִינוּס* קֵיסַר,   בְּצֵאתִי מִירוּשָׁלָיִם.

נַעֲרוֹךְ מִלְחָמָה, וַיהוה שָׁמָּה,[5]   בְּצֵאתִי מִמִּצְרָיִם.
רָחַק מִמֶּנּוּ, וְהִנֵּה אֵינֶנּוּ,   בְּצֵאתִי מִירוּשָׁלָיִם.

סִתְרֵי פָרֹכֶת,[6] וְסִדְרֵי מַעֲרֶכֶת,[7]   בְּצֵאתִי מִמִּצְרָיִם.
חֵמָה נִתֶּכֶת, וְעָלַי סוֹכֶכֶת,   בְּצֵאתִי מִירוּשָׁלָיִם.

עוֹלָה וּזְבָחִים, וְאִשֵּׁי נִיחוֹחִים,   בְּצֵאתִי מִמִּצְרָיִם.
בְּחֶרֶב מְדֻקָּרִים, בְּנֵי צִיּוֹן הַיְקָרִים,[8]   בְּצֵאתִי מִירוּשָׁלָיִם.

פַּאֲרֵי מִגְבָּעוֹת, לְכָבוֹד נִקְבָּעוֹת,[9]   בְּצֵאתִי מִמִּצְרָיִם.
שְׁרִיקוֹת וּתְרוּעוֹת, וְקוֹלוֹת וּזְוָעוֹת,   בְּצֵאתִי מִירוּשָׁלָיִם.

צִיץ הַזָּהָב,[10] וְהַמְשֵׁל וָרַהַב,   בְּצֵאתִי מִמִּצְרָיִם.
הֻשְׁלַךְ הַנֵּזֶר, וְאָפֵס הָעֵזֶר,   בְּצֵאתִי מִירוּשָׁלָיִם.

---

(1) See *Leviticus* 25:1-24. (2) See *Exodus* 25:10-22. (3) See 28:9-12.
(4) See *Numbers* 11:16-17,24-25. (5) Cf. *Exodus* 14:13. (6) See 26:31-33.
(7) See *Leviticus* 24:5-9. (8) *Eichah* 4:2. (9) Cf. *Exodus* 39:28. (10) See 28:36-38.

composed as a lament over the Destruction.

לְאַרְבָּעָה דְגָלִים — *[Encamped] under four flags.* The Israelite camp in the Wilderness was in the shape of a square with three tribes on each side. The Torah ordained four tribes as the head of their respective sides. Thus, for example, the tribes of Judah, Issachar and Zebulun camped on the Eastern side under the דֶּגֶל מַחֲנֵה יְהוּדָה, *flag of Judah's camp.* With a similar arrangement on each side, the nation camped under four flags (see Numbers ch. 2).

נְבוּכַדְנֶצַּר וְאַנְדְּרִינוּס — *Nebuchadnezzar and Hadrian.* The *kinnah* bewails the Destruction of both the First Temple by Nebuchadnezzar of

ט Goodly tents [encamped] under four flags,*
                              when I went forth from Egypt;
      but tents of the Ishmaelites
        and camps of the uncircumcised,
                              when I went forth from Jerusalem.

י Jubilee and Sabbatical year,¹ and the land was tranquil,
                              when I went forth from Egypt;
      but I was sold for posterity; torn apart and cut to pieces,
                              when I went forth from Jerusalem.

כ The Ark and [its] cover,² and the stones of remembrance
        [on the High Priest's shoulder],³
                              when I went forth from Egypt;
      but stones from the catapult and weapons that devour,
                              when I went forth from Jerusalem.

ל Levites and sons of Aaron and the seventy elders,⁴
                              when I went forth from Egypt;
      but tyrants and tormentors, [slave-]traders and buyers,
                              when I went forth from Jerusalem.

מ Moses provided for us, and Aaron guided us,
                              when I went forth from Egypt;
      but Nebuchadnezzar and Hadrian* the Emperor,
                              when I went forth from Jerusalem.

נ We arrayed for battle, and HASHEM was [with us] there,⁵
                              when I went forth from Egypt;
      but He was distant from us and indeed,
        He seemed not to be present,
                              when I went forth from Jerusalem.

ס The [Ark] concealed behind the Curtain,⁶
        and the [Tables's] Panim-bread arrangement,⁷
                              when I went forth from Egypt;
      but fury poured out upon me, and hovered over me,
                              when I went forth from Jerusalem.

ע Burnt offerings and sacrifices, and pleasing fire offerings,
                              when I went forth from Egypt;
      but stabbed with the sword were precious children of Zion,⁸
                              when I went forth from Jerusalem.

פ Glorious turbans, designated for [the priests'] honor,⁹
                              when I went forth from Egypt;
      but whistle calls and trumpet blasts, fearsome cries and shuddering,
                              when I went forth from Jerusalem.

צ [The High Priest's] golden Head Plate,¹⁰ monarchy and sovereignty,
                              when I went forth from Egypt;
      but the tiara was thrown down and [Divine] help vanished,
                              when I went forth from Jerusalem.

קְדֻשָּׁה וּנְבוּאָה, וּכְבוֹד יהוה נִרְאָה,¹   בְּצֵאתִי מִמִּצְרָיִם.

נִגְאָלָה וּמוֹרָאָה,² וְרוּחַ הַטֻּמְאָה,   בְּצֵאתִי מִירוּשָׁלָיִם.

רִנָּה וִישׁוּעָה, וַחֲצוֹצְרוֹת הַתְּרוּעָה,   בְּצֵאתִי מִמִּצְרָיִם.

זַעֲקַת עוֹלָל, וְנַאֲקַת חָלָל,   בְּצֵאתִי מִירוּשָׁלָיִם.

שֻׁלְחָן³ וּמְנוֹרָה,⁴ וְכָלִיל וּקְטוֹרָה,   בְּצֵאתִי מִמִּצְרָיִם.

אֱלִיל וְתוֹעֵבָה, וּפֶסֶל וּמַצֵּבָה,   בְּצֵאתִי מִירוּשָׁלָיִם.

תּוֹרָה וּתְעוּדָה, וּכְלֵי הַחֶמְדָּה,   בְּצֵאתִי מִמִּצְרָיִם.

שָׂשׂוֹן וְשִׂמְחָה, וְנָס יָגוֹן וַאֲנָחָה,⁵   בְּשׁוּבִי לִירוּשָׁלָיִם.

Babylon, and the Second Temple by the Romans, here represented by Hadrian, the emperor who crushed the Bar Kochba revolution some sixty years later.

ק Sanctity and prophecy,
   and the glory of HASHEM was manifest,[1]
                       when I went forth from Egypt;
   but abomination and filth[2] and impure spirit,
                       when I went forth from Jerusalem.

ר Joyous song and salvation, and the [triumphant] trumpet blasts,
                       when I went forth from Egypt;
   but the infant's wailing and the mortally wounded's groaning,
                       when I went forth from Jerusalem.

ש [The Tabernacle's] Table[3] and Menorah,[4]
   burnt offering and incense,
                       when I went forth from Egypt;
   but idol and abomination, graven image and [pagan] stele,
                       when I went forth from Jerusalem.

ת Torah and Testimony, and the cherished vessels,
                       when I went forth from Egypt;
   gladness and joy, while anguish and sighing will flee,[5]
                       when I return to Jerusalem!

---

(1) Cf. *Exodus* 16:10. (2) Cf. *Zephaniah* 3:1. (3) See *Exodus* 25:23-30.
(4) See 25:31-40. (5) Cf. *Isaiah* 51:11.

לב.

אֶצְבְּעוֹתַי שָׁפֵלוּ,* וְאִשְׁיוֹתַי נָפֵלוּ,¹   אוֹיָה.

בְּנֵי צִיּוֹן גָּלוּ, וְכָל אוֹיְבַי שָׁלוּ,²   אוֹי מֶה הָיָה לָנוּ.

בַּיִת וַעֲזָרוֹת, בְּיוֹם אַף נִגְרָרוֹת,³   אוֹיָה.

פְּנֵי שָׂרִים וְשָׂרוֹת, כְּמוֹ שׁוּלֵי קְדֵרוֹת,   אוֹי מֶה הָיָה לָנוּ.

גֻּלַּת הַכּוֹתֶרֶת,⁴ כְּנֵבֶל נִשְׁבֶּרֶת,⁵   אוֹיָה.

עֲטֶרֶת תִּפְאֶרֶת, לָאָרֶץ נִגְרֶרֶת,   אוֹי מֶה הָיָה לָנוּ.

דַּרְכֵי עִיר אֲבֵלוֹת,⁶ וַיֶּחְדְּלוּ הַקּוֹלוֹת⁷   אוֹיָה.

אֳרָחוֹת הַסְּלוּלוֹת, חֲשֵׁכוֹת וַאֲפֵלוֹת,   אוֹי מֶה הָיָה לָנוּ.

הֵיכָל וּכְתָלָיו, מֵעַי הָמוּ עָלָיו,⁸   אוֹיָה.

וְעַל שֻׁלְחָן וְכֵלָיו, וּמְעִיל עַל שׁוּלָיו,   אוֹי מֶה הָיָה לָנוּ.

וָוֵי הָעַמּוּדִים,⁹ בְּיַד בְּנֵי הָעֲבָדִים,   אוֹיָה.

וְהֶקֵּף רוֹבְדִים, רַבִּים וְנִכְבָּדִים,   אוֹי מֶה הָיָה לָנוּ.

זְבָחִים וּמְנָחוֹת, לַמַּשּׁוּאוֹת¹⁰ וּמַדְּחוֹת,¹¹   אוֹיָה.

הֲדַר מִזְבְּחוֹת, בְּיָגוֹן וַאֲנָחוֹת,   אוֹי מֶה הָיָה לָנוּ.

חַיִל וְהַסּוֹרֵג, לְחֶרֶב וְלַהֶרֶג,   אוֹיָה.

בִּנְיָן הַנֶּאֱרָג, נִדַּשׁ בְּמוֹרַג,   אוֹי מֶה הָיָה לָנוּ.

טְלָאִים מְבֻקָּרִים,* מֶנּוּ נֶעֱדָרִים,   אוֹיָה.

וְטַבָּעוֹת סְדוּרִים, וְנַסִּין הַהֲדוּרִים,   אוֹי מֶה הָיָה לָנוּ.

יָפְיִי נִבְרֶכֶת, אֵיכָה נֶהְפָּכֶת,   אוֹיָה.

וְגֶפֶן וּפָרֶכֶת, וּמִנְחַת מַרְבֶּכֶת,¹²   אוֹי מֶה הָיָה לָנוּ.

כִּיּוֹר עִם כַּנּוֹ, הֲתָעִיף בּוֹ וְאֵינוֹ,¹³   אוֹיָה.

הַנֵּר עִם שַׁמְנוֹ, לֻקַּח מִמְּעוֹנוֹ,   אוֹי מֶה הָיָה לָנוּ.

לֶחֶם הַפָּנִים, שָׂאוּ עָלָיו קִינִים,   אוֹיָה.

וְטוּרֵי רִמּוֹנִים, לְמִרְמָס נְתוּנִים,   אוֹי מֶה הָיָה לָנוּ.

מְנוֹרָה הַטְּהוֹרָה, אוֹרָהּ נֶעֱדָרָה,   אוֹיָה.

וּמַגְרֵפָה יְקָרָה, נְטוּלָה וַחֲסֵרָה,   אוֹי מֶה הָיָה לָנוּ.

---

(1) Cf. *Jeremiah* 50:15. (2) *Eichah* 1:5. (3) Cf. *Job* 20:28. (4) *I Kings* 7:41.
(5) Cf. *Isaiah* 30:14. (6) Cf. *Eichah* 1:4. (7) *Exodus* 9:33. (8) *Song of Songs* 5:4. (9) *Exodus* 27:10.
(10) *Psalms* 73:18. (11) Cf. *Eichah* 2:14. (12) Cf. *Leviticus* 6:14. (13) Cf. *Proverbs* 23:5.

אֶצְבְּעוֹתַי שָׁפֵלוּ — *My fingers are humbled.*
Many beautiful aspects of Jerusalem and its
crowning glory, the Temple, are described and
their disappearance is mourned in this *kinnah*.

The greatest misfortune of all is that we once
had so many opportunities to show our devotion
to God and to be close to Him in the Temple, but
now we are distant and alienated.

32.

א My fingers are humbled* and my foundations are crumbled[1] —
O woe!

The children of Zion are exiled while all my enemies are serene[2] —
woe, what has befallen us!

ב The Holy Temple and its courtyards are dragged
under on the day of wrath[3] —   O woe!
The faces of princes and princesses are [blackened]
like the bottoms of pots —   woe, what has befallen us!

ג The crown atop the colonnades[4] is shattered like a clay jug[5] — O woe!
the majestic tiara is pulled to the ground — woe, what has befallen us!

ד The city's roads mourn,[6] and the voices [of her inhabitants]
ceased[7] —   O woe!
Her smoothly paved highways are darkened and gloomy —
woe, what has befallen us!

ה The Sanctuary with its walls, O how my stomach longs for them[8] —
O woe!

And for the Table and its vessels and for the [Kohen Gadol's]
tunic [with bells] on its hem —   woe, what has befallen us!

ו The hooks of the [Tabernacle's] posts[9]
are in the hand of the [Babylonian] slave-nation —   O woe!
As are the many stately rows of flooring stone.
— woe, what has befallen us!

ז Sacrificial slaughterings and flour offerings
are destroyed[10] and pushed away[11] —   O woe!
The glorious altars are in agony and groaning —
woe, what has befallen us!

ח The cheil promenade and the [surrounding] fence
[fell] to sword and to murder —   O Woe!
The edifice decorated with woven tapestries lies crushed under
the threshing boards —   woe, what has befallen us!

ט The lambs that were examined [before being slaughtered]
have been concealed from us —   O woe!
Along with the orderly rows of [animal] shackles
and the flaying pillars —   woe, what has befallen us!

י The water pool, so lovely! O how it has been turned to ruin — O woe!
[Together with] the [golden] grapevine, the Paroches curtain
and the hot-water flour-offering[12] —   woe, what has befallen us!

כ The washbasin on its stand was gone in a blink[13] —   O woe!
The lamp with its oil has been taken from its dwelling place —
woe, what has befallen us!

ל For the Panim Bread, arouse lamentations   — O woe!
And for the rows of pomegranates [on the High Priest's tunic]
given over to be stepped upon —   woe, what has befallen us!

מ The pure Menorah, its light has vanished —   O woe!
The [Altar's] heavy coal rake was carried off and is missing —
woe, what has befallen us!

אֲוֹיָה.   **נוֹי** יָם הַנְּחֹשֶׁת,[1] לְעוֹבְדִים לַבֹּשֶׁת,
אוֹי מֶה הָיָה לָנוּ.   וּמַעֲשֵׂה הָרֶשֶׁת, וְחַלּוֹת מַרְחֶשֶׁת,[2]

אֲוֹיָה.   **סָלָתוֹת** וּנְסָכִים, מְנּוּ נֶחְשָׁכִים,
אוֹי מֶה הָיָה לָנוּ.   וּבֹעַז וְגַם יָכִין,[3] לָאָרֶץ נִשְׁלָכִים,

אֲוֹיָה.   **עַל** מַחְתָּה וּמִזְרָק, אוֹיֵב שֵׁן חָרַק,[4]
אוֹי מֶה הָיָה לָנוּ.   טְנִי גַם כּוֹז זָרַק, וְאֶת חַרְבּוֹ הַבְרָק,

אֲוֹיָה.   **פִּשְׁפְּשִׁים** וּשְׁעָרִים, אַרְצָה נִגְרָרִים,
אוֹי מֶה הָיָה לָנוּ.   הַתָּמִים וְהָאוּרִים, אֵיכָה נִסְתָּרִים,

אֲוֹיָה.   **צְפִירַת** מַעֲטָפוֹת, בְּאֵיבָה נֶהְדָּפוֹת,
אוֹי מֶה הָיָה לָנוּ.   לִשְׁכוֹת הַיָּפוֹת, וּבֵית הַחֲלָפוֹת,

אֲוֹיָה.   **קִיר** מָגֵן עֻרָה,[5] וְקִרְקֵר הֶהָרָה,[6]
אוֹי מֶה הָיָה לָנוּ.   וְזָרְקוּ הַמָּרָה, וְשָׂרְפוּ הַבִּירָה,

אֲוֹיָה.   **רָאשֵׁי** מִשְׁמָרוֹת, סְבוּכִים בְּצָרוֹת,
אוֹי מֶה הָיָה לָנוּ.   וְשָׂרֵי הָעֲשָׂרוֹת, בְּיַד בַּעֲלֵי חֲטוֹטָרוֹת,

אֲוֹיָה.   **שַׁעַר** בַּת רַבִּים,[7] לְזָאֲבֵי עֲרָבִים,[8]
אוֹי מֶה הָיָה לָנוּ.   לָקְחוּ הַכְּרוּבִים, תֻּפִּים וְאַבּוּבִים,

אֲוֹיָה.   **תָּאִים** הַנָּאִים, לַבָּנִים הַשְּׂנוּאִים,
אוֹי מֶה הָיָה לָנוּ.   בַּפָּז מְסֻלָּאִים,[9] לְחֻלְדּוֹת הַסָּנָאִים,

אֲוֹיָה.   **בָּנִים** הַיְקָרִים, בַּחֲרָבוֹת נִדְקָרִים,
אוֹי מֶה הָיָה לָנוּ.   לְוִים הַמְשׁוֹרְרִים, וְכֹהֲנִים מַקְטִירִים,

אֲוֹיָה.   **רוּבִים** וּפְרָחִים, לְחָצִים וּשְׁלָחִים,
אוֹי מֶה הָיָה לָנוּ.   בְּכוֹרוֹת וְטַפּוּחִים, בְּיָגוֹן נֶאֱנָחִים,

אֲוֹיָה.   וּמַפְתְּחוֹת זָרְקוּ, בְּשׁוֹרָם כִּי לָקוּ,
אוֹי מֶה הָיָה לָנוּ.   בְּעָוֹן נִמְקוּ,[10] וְכַפַּיִם סָפְקוּ,[11]

---

(1) *II Kings* 25:13. (2) *Leviticus* 2:7. (3) *See I Kings* 7:21. (4) *Eichah* 2:17. (5) *Cf. Isaiah* 22:6. (6) *Cf.* 22:5.
(7) *Song of Songs* 7:5. (8) *Jeremiah* 5:6. (9) *Cf. Eichah* 4:2. (10) *Cf. Leviticus* 26:39. (11) *Cf. Eichah* 2:15.

    The stanzas of this *kinnah* bear an alpha-betical acrostic, followed by the author's signature, בָּרוּךְ חֲזַק, *Baruch, may he be strong.* The first line of each stanza contains two stiches, and ends with the plaintive cry, אֲוֹיָה, *O woe!* The second line's two stiches are followed by, אוֹי מֶה הָיָה לָנוּ, *Woe, what has*

befallen us!
    The author, R' Baruch [probably R' Baruch ben Shmuel (died, Mainz, Germany, 1221)], was one of the Tosafists (*Ba'alei HaTosafos*) and served on the Mainz *beis din.* He wrote commentary to various tractates of the Talmud. His work *Sefer HaChochmah* is no longer extant.

ב   The beautiful copper pool[1] [known as King Solomon's sea]
        [is in the hands] of those who worship ignominious idols — O woe!
    Along with the [Altar's] network and the deep-fried
        loaves offering[2] —   woe, what has befallen us!

ס   Fine meal offerings and wine libations have been removed from us —
                                                                    O woe!
    And [the twin Temple columns called] Boaz and Yachin[3]
        are thrown down to the ground —   woe, what has befallen us!

ע   Over the fire pan and the blood basin, the enemy gnashed his
        teeth[4] —   O woe!
    Also, he threw down basket and jug, while he flashed his sword—
                                                        woe, what has befallen us!

פ   Small doors and large gates are dragged along the ground— O woe!
    The Urim V'Tumim, O where are they now hidden? —
                                                        woe, what has befallen us!

צ   The crown-like turbans were knocked off with malice —   O woe!
    The beautiful chambers and the repository of the slaughtering
        knives —   woe, what has befallen us!

ק   [The citizenry of] Kir [in Assyria] uncovered its battle shield[5]
        [against Jerusalem], [and the Jerusalemites]
        ran screaming into the mountains[6] —   O woe!
    They injected bitterness [into the people] and burnt down
        the palatial Temple —   woe, what has befallen us!

ר   The leaders of the [Temple] watches were entangled in troubles —
                                                                    O woe!
    And the captains of ten suffer at the hand of whippers —
                                                        woe, what has befallen us!

ש   The gate of the many-peopled city[7]
        [is abandoned to] the wolves of the wilderness[8] —   O woe!
    The Cherubim have been taken away, with the [Levites']
        drums and flutes —   woe, what has befallen us!

ת   The lovely chambers [of the Temple have been given over]
        to the despised sons —   O woe!
    [While Zion's children] who are comparable to fine gold,[9]
        are now like weasels in the bush   — woe, what has befallen us!

ב   [Zion's] precious children are run through by the sword — O woe!
    As are the Levite choristers and the priests who offer incense —
                                                        woe, what has befallen us!

ד   Youths and [priestly] blossoms [have fallen
        victim] to arrows and sabers —   O woe!
    Firstborn sons and pampered babies sigh in agony—
                                                        woe, what has befallen us!

ו   [The beleaguered priests] threw the keys [of the Temple heavenward]
        when they saw that they were beaten —   O woe!
    They melted in sin[10] and clapped [their] hands[11] [in anguish] —
                                                        woe, what has befallen us!

כַּפּוֹת וּבָזִיכִים, מֶנּוּ נִפְסָקִים,   אוֹיָה.

וּבָנַי נֶאֱנָקִים, בְּאֶרֶץ מֶרְחַקִּים,   אוֹי מֶה הָיָה לָנוּ.

חַי חוֹבוֹ גָּבָה, וְצִיץ טָהוֹר נִשְׁבָּה,   אוֹיָה.

נֵר מַעֲרָב כָּבָה, וְשִׂמְחַת בֵּית הַשּׁוֹאֵבָה,   אוֹי מֶה הָיָה לָנוּ.

זֵדִים בְּנֵי עֲדִינָה, עַל בְּנֵי מִי מָנָה,   אוֹיָה.

פְּאֵר בִּגְדֵי כְהֻנָּה, בְּיָדָם נִתָּנָה,   אוֹי מֶה הָיָה לָנוּ.

קְטֹרֶת נֶעֱדֶרֶת, וְאָרוֹן וְכַפֹּרֶת,   אוֹיָה.

תֻּכֵּן בַּזֶּרֶת,¹ תְּקֻבַּץ נִפְזֶרֶת,²   יְשׁוּעָה תִּהְיֶה לָנוּ.

לג.

אֵבֶל אֲעוֹרֵר, אֲנִינוּת אֲגָרֵר,   אוֹיָה לִי.

בְּבִכְי אֲמָרֵר, בַּחֲמַת צוֹרֵר, דְּרָכַי סוֹרֵר,³   אַלְלַי לִי.

גָּלוּת אָרַךְ, וְלִבִּי הֵרַךְ,⁴   אוֹיָה לִי.

דָּרַךְ וּפָרַךְ, נָחֲנִי נַחְשָׁרַךְ, וְצֵידוֹ חָרַךְ,   אַלְלַי לִי.

הַמְעַט מַבְאִישַׁי, חִלְּלוּ מִקְדָּשַׁי,   אוֹיָה לִי.

וְהֵם בָּזוּ קָדָשַׁי, הֶחֱלוּ מִמִּקְדָּשַׁי,⁵ וְזִלְזְלוּ קְדוֹשַׁי,   אַלְלַי לִי.

זְמַן שְׁנַת תַּתְנ"ו, בְּי"א לַמַּחֲזוֹר רנ"ו,*   אוֹיָה לִי.

חֲיָלוֹת זֵדִנוּ, מִקוֹמָם פִּנּוּ, כָּאַרְבֶּה נִמְנוּ,   אַלְלַי לִי.

טֶרֶף בִּקְיוֹ,⁶ וְעָלַי הִקְשׁוּ,⁷   אוֹיָה לִי.

יִרְאָתָם קִשְׁקְשׁוּ, וְאוֹתוֹת הִקִּישׁוּ, וְאוֹתִי עִקְּשׁוּ,   אַלְלַי לִי.

כִּפֵּר מָאָסוּ, וּנְפָשׁוֹת חָמָסוּ,   אוֹיָה לִי.

לְוִיַּי בּוֹסָסוּ, כֹּהֲנַי בּוֹשָׁסוּ, צְנוּעַי אָנָסוּ,   אַלְלַי לִי.

מְתֵי חֶרֶב מְהֻדָּמִים, בְּאֶפֶס דָּמִים,   אוֹיָה לִי.

נִבְלַת תְּמִימִים, בְּלִי מוּמִים, הָיוּ שׁוֹמֵמִים,   אַלְלַי לִי.

סָחוֹב וְהַשְׁלֵךְ,⁸ עֵרוֹם לְלַכְלֵךְ,   אוֹיָה לִי.

---

(1) Cf. *Isaiah* 40:12. (2) Cf. *Jeremiah* 50:17. (3) *Eichah* 3:11. (4) Cf. *Job* 23:16.
(5) Cf. *Ezekiel* 9:6. (6) Some editions read בִּקְשׁוּ טָעוּת, *they sought to misguide me.*
(7) Some editions read וְעָלַי הִקְשׁוּ, *they made my yoke heavy.* (8) *Jeremiah* 22:19.

אֵבֶל אֲעוֹרֵר — *I shall arouse mourning.* This *kinnah* bemoans the atrocities and calamities which befell the Jewish people during the First Crusade in the year 1096 C.E. (4856 from Creation). These events have already been described in much greater detail in *kinnah* 25. The author's signature appears in the acrostic after the *aleph-beis*; it reads אֲנֹכִי מְנַחֵם הָעָלוּב בְּרַבִּי מָכִיר, *I am Menachem, the unworthy one, the son of R' Machir.* The author's father, R' Machir, was a brother to Rabbeinu Gershom *Meor HaGolah.* His

Talmudic lexicon is quoted by Rashi. R' Menachem, together with his brother, compiled a halachic work called *Maaseh HaMachiri*, which is extensively cited in *Sefer HaPardes* and *Sefer HaOrah.* Although primarily a halachist, R' Menachem wrote other liturgical compositions, including: אָדָם בְּקוּם, recited in the *Selichos* for Taanis Esther; and כְּהוֹשַׁעְתָּ אָדָם, recited on the Sabbath of Succos.

שְׁנַת תַּתְנ"ו בְּי"א לְמַחֲזוֹר רנ"ו — *The year 4856 ... in the eleventh year of the 256th cycle.* There is

כ The incense spoons and ladles have been withdrawn from us — O woe!
   And my sons are screaming in a far-off land —
                                          woe, what has befallen us!

ח The Living One collected His debt, and the [Kohen Gadol's]
      forehead plate of pure [gold] was captured—   O woe!
   The Western Lamp was snuffed out, as is the joy of the Drawing
      of the Water —   woe, what has befallen us!

ו The wanton sons spoiled by luxury overpowered
      the sons [of Israel] too numerous to be counted—   O woe!
   The majestic priestly robes were given over into their hand
                                  — woe, what has befallen us!

ק The incense offering has vanished, as have the Ark and its Cover—
                                                              O woe!

   [O God] Who measures [the expanse of heaven] with a little finger,[1]
      gather the scattered[2]   and be a salvation unto us!

33.

א I shall arouse mourning, I shall drag out grief.   Woe unto me!

ב Through weeping, I am embittered, because of the fury of
   the tormentor, who has strewn my path with thorns.[3]   Alas for me!

ג He [God] lengthened the exile,
   and my heart grew timid.[4]   Woe unto me!

ד [The enemy] trampled and shattered, [Esau] the hunter led me
   [into captivity], and immobilized his prey.   Alas for me!

ה Is it then insignificant that those who sully me,
   also desecrated my Sanctuaries?   Woe unto me!

ו And they shamed my holy things, beginning with my holy people
   [the Kohanim],[5] they profaned my holy ones.   Alas for me!

ז The time was the year 4856 [from Creation]
   in the eleventh year of the 256th cycle* [of leap years]   Woe unto me!

ח Troops of soldiers armed themselves, they emptied out of their places
   as numerous as locusts   Alas for me!

ט While they sought provisions[6]
   they placed a severe burden on me[7]   Woe unto me!

י They gathered to their idols, wearing their [crucifix] symbols,
   and claimed that I was perverted.   Alas for me!

כ Ransom they rejected, but souls they snatched.   Woe unto me!

ל My Levites they stomped, my priests they trampled,
   and my modest women they ravished.   Alas for me!

מ The victims of the sword were cut to pieces,
   without a whit of guilt.   Woe unto me!

נ The corpses of the perfectly righteous, unblemished [by any sin],
   were abandoned [without burial].   Alas for me!

ס They were dragged around and thrown down[8]
   naked, to become filthy.   Woe unto me!

עוֹבְרֵי בְּכָל פֶּלֶךְ,' חֵיל יָרֵב מֶלֶךְ,² וְרָדוּ בְּפֶלֶךְ,　　　　אַלְלַי לִי.

פְּרִיעָה וּפְרִימָה, עַל תּוֹרָה תְּמִימָה,³　　　　אוֹיָה לִי.

צָר בְּיָד רָמָה, הַמִּשְׁכָּן תְּרוּמָה,⁴ נָם לְהַחֲרִימָה,　　　　אַלְלַי לִי.

קוֹל בָּתֵּי כְנֵסִיּוֹת, וּבָתֵּי תוּשִׁיּוֹת,　　　　אוֹיָה לִי.

רַחֲמָנִיּוֹת בִּידֵיהֶן נְקִיּוֹת, זִבְחֵי רְאִיּוֹת,　　　　אַלְלַי לִי.

שְׁלָמִים וְעוֹלוֹת, חֲתָנִים וְכַלּוֹת,　　　　אוֹיָה לִי.

תּוֹדוֹת וּבְלִילוֹת, בַּחוּרִים וּבְתוּלוֹת, וְטוֹבֵי קְהִלּוֹת,　　　　אַלְלַי לִי.

אַחִים גַּם יָחַד, נִשְׁפַּךְ דָּמָם כְּאֶחָד,　　　　אוֹיָה לִי.

כֵּן אֲחָיוֹת בְּפַחַד, בְּיִרְאַת שֵׁם הַמְּיֻחָד,

לַטֶּבַח לְהֶאָחָד,　　　　אַלְלַי לִי.

הוֹגֵי מִלְחֲמוֹת סֵפֶר, נֶשֶׁף וָצֶפֶר,　　　　אוֹיָה לִי.

חֵיךְ אִמְרֵי שֶׁפֶר,⁵ מָלֵא חָצָץ וָאֵפֶר,⁶

וְאַיֵּה שׁוֹקֵל וְסוֹקֵר,⁷　　　　אַלְלַי לִי.

הֲהָיְתָה זֹאת מֵאָז, עָלָה עַם עָז,　　　　אוֹיָה לִי.

לְהַשְׁמִיד הוּעַז, וְאָסַף עַם נוֹעָז,⁸ אֲרָם וְלוֹעֵז,⁹　　　　אַלְלַי לִי.

בִּקֵּשׁ עֵקֶר, רַק לַעֲקוֹר וּלְעַקֵּר,

(בְּקַר אַרְמָאִי מְשַׁקֵּר,)¹⁰ יָזַם הַזָּר¹¹ לְעַקֵּר,

וְלֹא לְגָרֵם לַבֹּקֶר,¹²　　　　אַלְלַי לִי.

מְקַיֵּם הַבְּרִית, לוּלֵי הוֹתִיר שְׁאֵרִית, בְּגֵיא נָכְרִית,　　　　(אוֹיָה לִי.)¹⁰

כְּשַׁר שַׁעֲרוּרִית, יְדִידַת עִבְרִית,

רַחֵם מֵהַכְרִית, וְיֵשׁ תִּקְוָה לְאַחֲרִית.¹³

לוֹבֵשׁ נְקָמָה, עוּרָה וְקוּמָה,

הָרִים שִׁפְלֵי קוֹמָה,

יָדִין גְּוִיּוֹת רְקָמָה.

וּשְׁכִינָה קָמָה עַל מְקוֹמָהּ.

---

(1) Some editions read עוֹבְרֵי, *those who passed;* others read עוֹבְדֵי לַמֶּלֶךְ, *those who worshiped the Molech.* (2) Cf. *Hosea* 5:13. (3) Cf. *Psalms* 19:8. (4) *Isaiah* 40:20. (5) Cf. *Genesis* 49:21. (6) Cf. *Eichah* 3:16. (7) Cf. *Isaiah* 33:18. (8) 33:19. (9) Some editions read בְּנֵי נָבָל וְלוֹעֵז, *the children of the irrelevant and speakers of foreign tongues,* a reading that completes the acrostic of the author's signature [see commentary]. (10) Some editions omit the words in parentheses. (11) Some editions read אֲרַמִי, *the Aramean,* instead of הַזָּר, *the alien.* (12) Cf. *Zephaniah* 3:3. (13) Cf. *Jeremiah* 31:16.

---

a period of about eleven days by which the solar year exceeds the lunar twelve months. The calendars can be brought into alignment by intercalating a thirteenth month (of thirty days) seven times every nineteen years. 255 of these nine nineteen-year cycles total 4845 years. Adding eleven years to this total brings us to 4856, the eleventh year in the 256th nineteen-year cycle.

ע Those who trod over me through every district;[1]
the army that fought with [God] the King[2]
and dominated all of the province   Alas for me!

פ Let your hair grow wild and rend your garments
over the perfect Torah[3] [desecrated by the enemy].   Woe unto me!

צ The tormentor with upraised hand,
accustomed to offering choice gifts [to his idols],[4]
now he announced [his intention] to demolish [the Torah]. Alas for me!

ק The sound of [mourning is heard in] the synagogues
and study halls.   Woe unto me!

ר Compassionate [mothers slaughtered their children] with their own
innocent hands, as if they were festival sacrifices.   Alas for me!

ש [Like] peace-offerings and burnt-offerings,
grooms and brides [were butchered]   Woe unto me!

ת Like thanksgiving-offerings and mixed flour-offerings, youths and
maidens and the elite community leaders [were sacrificed]. Alas for me!

א Brothers who lived in harmony,

ב their blood was shed as one.   Woe unto me!

כ Similarly, sisters who shared

י reverence for the awesome Name of the One and Only God, now shared
a common fate as they were slaughtered together   Alas for me!

מ Those who struggled to comprehend the lessons of the [Torah] volumes

נ from dusk to dawn.   Woe unto me!

ח The mouths which were filled with lovely [Torah] words[5]

ט were stuffed with dust and dirt;[6] and where are those who weighed
and measured [every Torah letter]?[7]   Alas for me!

ה Has similar [tragedy] occurred since days of yore,

ע that such a brazen nation should rise up [against God]?   Woe unto me!

ל With audacity to destroy [the Jews],

ו while they assembled fierce nations,[8]
Aram and others who spoken foreign languages.[9]   Alas for me!

כ These unworthy nations attempted

ר to uproot [us] and to leave us barren.   Woe unto me!

כ [With perverted justice the Aramean acted deceitfully][10]

י and the alien[11] plotted to uproot me
and to allow no bone to remain until the morning.[12]   Alas for me!

מ [O God] Who upholds the covenant,
if not for Your faithfulness which allowed a remnant
to survive in the deep valley of foreign exile;   [Woe unto me!][10]

כ When You observed the wretched misery

י of Your beloved Hebrews,

ר You mercifully saved [us] from annihilation
and there yet is hope for our future![13]
[O You] Who dons the robes of revenge, awaken and arise and elevate
the stature of the downtrodden, and do justice for the corpses
of elegant design [before being murdered],
and let the Divine Presence arise [and ascend] to its place.

לד.

יוֹם אַכְפִּי הִכְבַּדְתִּי,[1]* וַיִּכְפְּלוּ עֲוֹנִי,

בְּשָׁלְחִי יַד בְּדַם נָבִיא בַּחֲצַר אֵל מִקְדַּשׁ יהוה,

וְלֹא כִסָּתְהוּ אֲדָמָה עַד בֹּא חֶרֶב מוֹנִי,

וְלֹא שָׁקַט עֲדֵי הָקַם דַּם הַנָּבִיא זְכַרְיָה,

וַיֶּרֶב בְּבַת יְהוּדָה תַּאֲנִיָּה וַאֲנִיָּה.[2]

הָיָה הוֹלֵךְ וְסוֹעֵר, עַד בֹּא רַב טַבָּחִים,

וּבָא אֶל מִקְדַּשׁ יהוה, וּמָצָא דָמִים רוֹתְחִים,

וַיִּשְׁאַל בַּעֲבוּר זֶה, הַכֹּהֲנִים הַזּוֹבְחִים,

וַיַּעֲנוּהוּ כִּי זֶה הוּא, דַּם קָרְבַּן הַזְּבָחִים,

וַיְנַסֶּה בְּדַם פָּרִים וְדַם אֵילִים וְדַם מֵחִים,

וְגַם זֶבַח זֶבַח רַב, לַחֲקוֹר מֶה הָיָה,

וַיֶּרֶב בְּבַת יְהוּדָה תַּאֲנִיָּה וַאֲנִיָּה.

וּבְכָל זֹאת לֹא שָׁקַט, וְעוֹדוֹ כַיָּם נִגְרָשׁ,[3]

וַיְבַקֵּשׁ הַדָּבָר וַיִּמָּצֵא מְפֹרָשׁ,[4]

כִּי הוּא דַם אִישׁ הָאֱלֹהִים עַל לֹא חָמָס[5] שֹׁרָשׁ,

וַיֹּאמֶר נְבוּזַרְאֲדָן, גַּם דָּמוֹ הִנֵּה נִדְרָשׁ,[6]

אִסְפוּ לִי הַכֹּהֲנִים, וְהוֹצִיאוּם מִבֵּית יָהּ,

כִּי לֹא אֶשְׁקוֹט, עַד יִשְׁקוֹט, דַּם הַנָּבִיא זְכַרְיָה,

וַיֶּרֶב בְּבַת יְהוּדָה תַּאֲנִיָּה וַאֲנִיָּה..

דָּקַר יְשִׁישִׁים לְמֵאוֹת וּבַחוּרִים לִרְבֹּאוֹת,

וַיּוֹרֶד לַטֶּבַח כֹּהֲנֵי יהוה צְבָאוֹת,

וְאֵין שֶׁקֶט לְדַם נָבִיא, וַיְהִי לְמוֹפֵת וָאוֹת,　　וְהַבָּנִים נִשְׁחָטִים,

וְעֵינֵי אָבוֹת רוֹאוֹת,

וְאִמּוֹתָם לַטֶּבַח, גַּם אַחֲרֵיהֶם בָּאוֹת,

וָאֹמַר לְנַפְשִׁי זֶה חַטָּאתֵךְ וְזֶה פִּרְיָה,

וַיֶּרֶב בְּבַת יְהוּדָה תַּאֲנִיָּה וַאֲנִיָּה.

---

(1) Cf. *Job* 33:7. (2) *Eichah* 2:5. (3) Cf. *Isaiah* 57:20. (4) Cf. *Esther* 2:23.
(5) *Isaiah* 53:9. (6) Cf. *Genesis* 42:22.

יוֹם אַכְפִּי הִכְבַּדְתִּי — *On that day I increased my burden.* When Zechariah ben Jehoiada protested the introduction of a pagan idol into the Holy Temple, he was stoned to death in the Temple courtyard by the Jewish masses. This occurred during the time, and at the bidding, of the wicked King Joash. With this cold blooded murder the entire Jewish nation became guilty of a sevenfold crime: (1) The murder of an innocent person; (2) who was a *Kohen*; (3) a

34.

 י On that day I increased my burden,[1]*
     because I doubled my iniquity,
  When I stretched out my hand to spill the blood of the prophet
     in God's Courtyard, in HASHEM's Sanctuary.
  But the earth would not cover it until the sword of
     my tormentors entered;
  nor was the blood silent,
     until the blood of the prophet Zechariah was avenged.
                         And He increased within the daughter of Judah
                               moaning and mourning.[2]

ה [The blood] continued to churn and roil
     until the chief executioner arrived,
  He entered HASHEM's Sanctuary and found the blood boiling.
  He inquired about this from the priests
     who were slaughtering offerings.
  And they answered him,
     'Why, this is the blood of the sacrificial offerings.'
  And he tested [the seething blood by comparing it] with the blood
     of cows, the blood of rams, and the blood of fattened animals,
  and he slaughtered many animals, to determine what had occurred.
             And He increased within the daughter of Judah moaning and mourning.

ו Despite all this, the blood was not silent,
     but continued like the troubled sea.[3]
  The matter was investigated and clearly corroborated,[4]
     that this was the blood of the man of God
     who was ripped out by his roots for no reason.[5]
  Nebuzaradan then declared, 'Behold,
     his blood now demands [revenge]![6]
  Gather unto me the priests and remove them from God's House,
  for I shall not be silent, until the blood
     of the prophet Zechariah remains silent.'
             And He increased within the daughter of Judah moaning and mourning.

ז He stabbed elders by the hundreds
     and youths by the tens of thousands,
  and he dragged the priests of HASHEM, Master of Legions,
     to the slaughter.
  Yet the prophet's blood was not silent;
     and this was an amazing wonder and a clear sign.
  For the children were massacred
     while their fathers' eyes watched,
     and their mothers, too, followed them to the slaughter.
  And I said to myself,
     'This is your sin and this is its fruit!'
             And He increased within the daughter of Judah moaning and mourning.

הוֹסִיף לַהֲרוֹג נָשִׁים עִם יוֹנְקֵי שָׁדַיִם,

וְדָם עוֹלֶה בֵּינֵיהֶם, כְּדַם יְאוֹר מִצְרַיִם,

עֲדֵי נָשָׂא נְבוּזַרְאֲדָן לִבּוֹ לַשָּׁמַיִם,

וַיֹּאמֶר, הַאֵין דַּי בִּבְנוֹת יְרוּשָׁלַיִם,

הֲכָלָה אַתָּה עוֹשֶׂה לִשְׁאֵרִית הַשִּׁבְיָה,

וַיֶּרֶב בְּבַת יְהוּדָה תַּאֲנִיָּה וַאֲנִיָּה.

(לְךָ חָטָאנוּ אֱלֹהִים, הֶעֱוִינוּ וְהִרְשָׁעְנוּ,

וְהָרַגְנוּ נְבִיאֶךָ וְרֹשַׁעְנוּ יָדָעְנוּ,

יְהִי חַסְדְּךָ לְנַחֲמֵנוּ, כִּי מִשְּׁאוֹל שִׁוַּעְנוּ,

וּמִפְּרִי מַעֲלָלֵינוּ זֶה כַּמֶּה שָׂבָעְנוּ,

רַחֵם לֹא רֻחָמָה, הַסְּעָרָה עֲנִיָּה,

עֵינֶיהָ לְךָ תִשָּׂא, וְאֶת עֶזְרָתְךָ צוֹפִיָּה.)

לה.

שְׁכֻרַת וְלֹא מִיַּיִן[2] הַשְׁלִיכִי תְפֵּיךְ,

קָרְחִי נָא וָגְזִי[3] וְהַשְׁחִיתִי אַפֵּיךְ,

שְׂאִי עַל שְׁפָיִם קִינָה[4] וְסִבְבִי אֲגַפֵּיךְ.

וְצַעֲקִי לִפְנֵי יהוה עַל חֶרֶב סִפֵּיךְ,

עַל חֶרֶב סִפֵּיךְ, עַל נֶפֶשׁ עוֹלָלַיִךְ,[5] שְׂאִי אֵלָיו כַּפֵּיךְ.

אֵיכָה בָא צַר וְאוֹיֵב[6] בְּצִיּוֹן עִיר מַמְלֶכֶת,

אֵיכָה רֶגֶל זֵדִים אַדְמַת קֹדֶשׁ דּוֹרֶכֶת,

בְּבוֹאָם מָצְאוּ כֹהֲנִים שׁוֹמְרֵי הַמַּעֲרֶכֶת,

וְעַל מִשְׁמְרוֹתָם עָמְדוּ וְלֹא עָזְבוּ הַמְּלָאכֶת,

עַד אֲשֶׁר שָׁפַךְ דָּמָם כְּמֵימֵי הַמַּהְפֶּכֶת,

וּבָא עָרֵל וְטָמֵא[7] מִבֵּית לַפָּרֹכֶת,

---

prophet; (4) and a judge; (5) the desecration of the Temple Courtyard; (6) on Yom Kippur, (7) which was also a Sabbath day (see *II Chronicles* 24:20-21 and *Koheles Rabbah* 3:20).

The blood of Zechariah lay uncovered on the stone floor of the Temple Courtyard for one hundred and fifty years during which it continued to seethe and bubble as a sign of God's fury against the nation. The blood thus pointed an accusing finger, and demanded the retribution described in this *kinnah*, which is based on the following Talmudic account:

The Babylonian general Nebuzaradan was spurred on by the sight of the blood of the murdered prophet Zechariah seething on the floor of the Temple. At first, the Jews sought to conceal the true story connected with the blood. Eventually, however, they had to confess that it was the blood of a prophet who had prophesied the Destruction of the Temple, and had been slain by the people for his candor.

'I,' said Nebuzaradan, 'will appease him.' He ordered the scholars of the kingdom to be executed on that bloody spot, then the school

ה *He continued slaying women with [their] nurslings.*
And the blood surged up among them like
the [Nile] river of Egypt [at flood stage],
until Nebuzaradan lifted his heart towards heaven
and said, 'Are the daughters of Jerusalem not enough?
Is it Your intention to annihilate the remainder[1] of the captivity?'
    And He increased within the daughter of Judah moaning and mourning.

ל *(We have sinned to You, O God, we have been iniquitous and wicked;*
ו *we have murdered Your prophets and we recognize our evil.*
י *Let Your kindness comfort us, for we cry from the grave,*
and long have we been sated on the fruits of our misdeeds.
Be merciful with the unmercied, storm-tossed, afflicted one,
who lifts her eyes to You, and hopes for Your help.)

35.

[O Israel] drunk, but not from wine,[2]* throw down your tambourines!
Tear out your hair now and cut it off![3] Mutilate your face!
Raise a lament a lament upon the hills,[4] and circle around your borders.
And cry out before HASHEM about
  the destruction of your [Temple's] gateways
    about the destruction of your [Temple's] vessels,
    about the life of your young children,[5]
  lift your hands up to Him [in prayer].

O how was the enemy oppressor able to enter[6] Zion, the royal city;
how were the feet of the wanton able to tread on the holy ground?
When they entered they found the priests,
  the guardians of the sacrificial order
standing at their guard, not abandoning the service,
until their blood was spilled like the waters of [the Nile]
  that were changed [into blood].
Then the uncircumcised entered and contaminated[7]
  [the Holy of Holies] within the Paroches curtain,

---

(1) Cf. *Ezekiel* 11:13. (2) Cf. *Isaiah* 51:21. (3) Cf. *Micah* 1:16. (4) Cf. *Jeremiah* 7:29.
(5) Cf. *Eichah* 2:19. (6) 4:12. (7) Some editions read וּבָא כָּל עָרֵל וְטָמֵא, *Then all the uncircumsized and contaminated entered.*

---

children, and at last the young priests — more than ninety-four thousand in all.

But the blood of the prophet went on seething until Nebuzaradan exclaimed: 'Zechariah, Zechariah! I have destroyed the flower of them. Do you wish me to massacre them all?'

Only then did the blood rest.

Thoughts of repentance came to Nebuzaradan's mind: If the Jews, who killed one person only, have been so severely punished, what will be my fate?

He left, and ultimately converted to Judaism (*Sanhedrin* 96b).

This *kinnah* was composed by R' Yehudah

שֻׁכֻּרַת וְלֹא מִיַּיִן — *Drunk, but not from wine.* The prophet Isaiah foretells of the shock which will overcome Israel after the Destruction, a trauma that will delude their intellect:

Awaken! Awaken! Stand up, O Jerusalem! You have drunk from the hand of HASHEM the cup of His fury; you have drunk down to the very dregs the deep bowl which makes you stagger ... Therefore, now hear this, you who are afflicted, drunk, but not from wine! (Isaiah 51:17,21). The author here vividly describes the terrible cruelties that befell Israel and the destruction that numbed their hearts and their minds.

לַמָּקוֹם אֲשֶׁר כֹּהֵן גָּדוֹל יָרֵא שָׁם לָלֶכֶת,

וְהֶחֱרִיבוּ סִפֶּיךָ וְחַלּוֹנֵי שְׁקוּפֶיךָ.[1]

וְצַעֲקִי לִפְנֵי יהוה עַל חֻרְבַּן סִפֵּיךְ,

עַל חֻרְבַּן סִפֵּיךְ, עַל נֶפֶשׁ עוֹלָלַיִךְ, שְׂאִי אֵלָיו כַּפֵּיךְ.

קוֹל יְלָלַת בַּת צִיּוֹן מֵרָחוֹק נִשְׁמַעַת,

תִּזְעַק זַעֲקַת חֶשְׁבּוֹן[2] תִּבְכֶּה בְּכִי מֵיפַעַת,[3]

אֲהָהּ כִּי כוֹס שָׁתִיתִי וּמָצִיתִי קֻבַּעַת,[4]

אֲכָלוּנִי אֲרָיוֹת[5] חַדּוּדֵי מַלְתָּעַת,

בַּת בָּבֶל הַשְּׁדוּדָה וּבַת הַמִּרְשַׁעַת,

מַה תִּתְאוֹנְנִי צִיּוֹן וְחַטָּאתֵךְ נוֹדַעַת,

עַל רֹב עֲוֹנֵךְ[6] גָּלָה עַמֵּךְ מִבְּלִי דָעַת,[7]

עַל עָזְבֵךְ צוֹפַיִךְ וְשָׁמְעֵךְ קוֹל תִּרְפֶּיךְ.

וְצַעֲקִי לִפְנֵי יהוה עַל חֻרְבַּן סִפֵּיךְ,

עַל חֻרְבַּן סִפֵּיךְ, עַל נֶפֶשׁ עוֹלָלַיִךְ, שְׂאִי אֵלָיו כַּפֵּיךְ.

אַל תִּשְׂמְחִי אוֹיַבְתִּי, עַל שֶׁבֶר קַרְנִי,

כִּי נָפַלְתִּי קַמְתִּי[8] וַיהוה עֲזָרָנִי,[9]

הִנֵּה יַאַסְפֵנִי אֵלִי אֲשֶׁר פִּזְּרָנִי,

וְיִגְאָלֵנִי מִמֵּךְ צוּרִי אֲשֶׁר מְכָרָנִי,

וְגַם עָלַיִךְ תַּעֲבָר כּוֹס[10] אֲשֶׁר עֲבָרָנִי,

וְאָז בְּסַלְעֵי סְעִפַּיִךְ,

אֲנַפֵּץ אֶת טַפַּיִךְ.[11]

וְצַעֲקִי לִפְנֵי יהוה עַל חֻרְבַּן סִפֵּיךְ,

עַל חֻרְבַּן סִפֵּיךְ, עַל נֶפֶשׁ עוֹלָלַיִךְ, שְׂאִי אֵלָיו כַּפֵּיךְ.

---

(1) Cf. *I Kings* 6:4. (2) See *Jeremiah* 48:34. (3) See 48:21. (4) Cf. *Isaiah* 51:17.
(5) Some editions read . . . שִׁנֵּי אֲרָיוֹת, *the teeth of the sharp-fanged lions;* some read
שְׁנֵי אֲרָיוֹת, *the two . . . lions,* i.e., Babylon and Edom. (6) *Jeremiah* 30:14. (7) Cf. *Isaiah* 5:13.
(8) *Micah* 7:8. (9) *Psalms* 118:13. (10) Cf. *Eichah* 4:21. (11) Cf. *Psalms* 137:9.

The author's name שלמה, *Shlomo,* appears in   R' Shlomo ben Yitzchak of thirteenth-century
the first four words. He is usually identified as   Gerona, Spain.

the place where the High Priest feared to go,
and they destroyed your entranceways
    and your slotted windows.¹
            And cry out before HASHEM
            about the destruction of your [Temple's] gateways
                about the destruction of your [Temple's] vessels,
                about the life of your young children,
                lift your hands up to Him [in prayer].

The sound of Zion's daughter's wailing is heard from afar,
she cries out as Cheshbon once cried,²
    she weeps as Mephaath once wept.³
'Ah, woe! For I have drunk deeply of the cup [of retribution]
    and I have sucked out its bitter dregs!⁴
The sharp-fanged lions⁵ have consumed me,
the destructive daughter of Babylon,
    and the wicked daughter of Edom.
Why do you complain, O Zion, when your sins are well known!
Because of your many iniquities,⁶ your nation was exiled,
    for your ignorance [of God's ways];⁷
because you abandoned your seers,
    listened to the voice of your idolatrous oracles.
            And cry out before HASHEM
            about the destruction of your [Temple's] gateways
                about the destruction of your [Temple's] vessels,
                about the life of your young children,
                lift your hands up to Him [in prayer].

Do not rejoice, O my enemy,
    that my pride was broken,
for although I have fallen, I shall arise⁸
    and HASHEM shall assist me.⁹
Behold, it is the Almighty Who dispersed me,
    Who shall gather me in.
And my Creator Who sold me will redeem me from you.
Indeed, the cup [of retribution] that passed over me
    will also pass over you,¹⁰
and then upon the jagged edges of your rocks
    I will smash your infants [as you did mine]¹¹
            And cry out before HASHEM
            about the destruction of your [Temple's] gateways
                about the destruction of your [Temple's] vessels,
                about the life of your young children,
                lift your hands up to Him [in prayer].

לו.

צִיּוֹן הֲלֹא תִשְׁאֲלִי* לִשְׁלוֹם אֲסִירַיִךְ,

דּוֹרְשֵׁי שְׁלוֹמֵךְ[1] וְהֵם יֶתֶר עֲדָרָיִךְ.

מִיָּם וּמִזְרָח וּמִצָּפוֹן וְתֵימָן,[2]

שְׁלוֹם רָחוֹק וְקָרוֹב,[3] שְׂאִי מִכָּל עֲבָרָיִךְ.

וּשְׁלוֹם אֲסִיר תִּקְוָה,[4] נוֹתֵן דְּמָעָיו כְּטַל חֶרְמוֹן,[5]

וְנִכְסָף לְרִדְתָּם עַל הֲרָרָיִךְ.

לִבְכּוֹת עֱנוּתֵךְ אֲנִי תַנִּים,[6]

וְעֵת אֶחֱלוֹם שִׁיבַת שְׁבוּתֵךְ,[7] אֲנִי כִנּוֹר לְשִׁירָיִךְ.

לִבִּי לְבֵית אֵל, וְלִפְנֵי אֵל מְאֹד יֶהֱמֶה,

וּלְמַחֲנַיִם* וְכָל נִגְעֵי טְהוֹרָיִךְ.[8]

שָׁם הַשְּׁכִינָה שְׁכוּנָה לָךְ,

וְיוֹצְרֵךְ פָּתַח לְמוּל שַׁעֲרֵי שַׁחַק שְׁעָרָיִךְ.[9]

וּכְבוֹד יהוה לְבַד הָיָה מְאוֹרֵךְ,[10]

וְאֵין סַהַר וְשֶׁמֶשׁ וְכוֹכָבִים מְאוֹרָיִךְ.[11]

אֶבְחַר לְנַפְשִׁי לְהִשְׁתַּפֵּךְ,[12]

בְּמָקוֹם אֲשֶׁר רוּחַ אֱלֹהִים שְׁפוּכָה עַל בְּחִירָיִךְ.

אַתְּ בֵּית מְלוּכָה, וְאַתְּ כִּסֵּא כְבוֹד אֵל,[13]

וְאֵיךְ יָשְׁבוּ עֲבָדִים עֲלֵי כִסְאוֹת גְּבִירָיִךְ.

מִי יִתְּנֵנִי מְשׁוֹטֵט,

בִּמְקוֹמוֹת אֲשֶׁר נִגְלוּ אֱלֹהִים לְחוֹזַיִךְ וְצִירָיִךְ.

מִי יַעֲשֶׂה לִּי כְנָפַיִם[14] וְאַרְחִיק נְדוֹד,[15]

צִיּוֹן הֲלֹא תִשְׁאֲלִי — *O Zion, will you not inquire.* This very well-known *kinnah* was written by one of the greatest *paytanim* of all time, R' Yehudah (ben Shmuel) HaLevi. The beauty and passion of this *kinnah* reflects its author's life-long yearning to flee from the exile and to walk on the sacred soil of the Holy Land.

R' Yehudah HaLevi was born in Toledo, Spain (circa 1080) and received an intensive Torah education at the yeshivah of R' Yitzchak Alfasi (the *Rif*) in Lucena, Spain. In addition to studying Talmud, R' Yehudah became a master of literary style in Hebrew and Arabic. *Rashba* writes of him (Responsum 418): 'R' Yehudah HaLevi is foremost amongst all poetic singers in distinction and merit.' His greatest contribu-

tion to Torah knowledge was the *Kuzari*, a philosophical work telling of the king of the Khazar tribe who sought to determine the true religion by questioning a Christian, a Moslem and a Jewish scholar. The king was finally convinced of the authenticity of Judaism, which he, together with his entire kingdom, embraced as the true religion. In the course of the disputation, the Khazar king taunts the Jewish teacher that the Jews seem to pay insincere lip service to Zion, their homeland. They pray for the restoration of Zion three times daily, yet in practice they are not willing to leave behind the prosperity and comfort of the exile to live in *Eretz Yisrael.* Humiliated, the Jewish sage of the *Kuzari* resolves to tear himself away from the

36.

צִיּוֹן *O Zion, will you not inquire* about the welfare of your imprisoned,*
   who seek your welfare,[1] for they are the remnants of your flocks.
From west and east, from north and south,[2] carry [in your heart]
   the welfare of the distant and the near,[3] from your every side.
And the welfare of the prisoner who is yet full of hope,[4]
   who gives forth his tears like the dew of [Mount] Hermon,[5]
   and yearns to let them fall upon your hills.
Weeping over your suffering, I am like a sea monster,[6]
   but when I dream of the return of your captivity,[7]
   I am a harp for your songs.
My heart [longs] for God's Temple, and before God I long intensely,
   and for the [three] encampments* [of the Divine Presence,
   the Kohanim and Levites, the Israelites],
   and for all who approach your purity.[8]
For there [in Zion] the Divine Presence resides,
   and [there] your Creator has opened gates for you
   opposite the gates of heaven.[9]
And only the glory of God was your lamp,[10]
   but the moon, sun, and stars were not your luminaries.[11]
I would elect for my soul to be poured out[12] [in prayer],
   in the place where the prophetic spirit of God
   was poured out upon your chosen ones.
You are the royal palace and you are God's Throne of Glory.[13]
   How have slaves sat upon the thrones of your heroes?
If only I could be set adrift in the places where God
   was revealed to your seers and your emissaries.
Who shall make me wings[14] so that I might wander far away?[15]

---

(1) Cf. *Psalms* 122:6. (2) Cf. 107:3. (3) Cf. *Isaiah* 57:19. (4) Cf. *Zechariah* 9:12. (5) *Psalms* 133:5.
(6) Cf. *Micah* 1:8. (7) Cf. *Psalms* 126:1. (8) Some editions read פְּנֵי טְהוֹרָיִךְ, *the places where your pure ones prayed,* or *where your pure ones met.* (9) Cf. *Genesis* 28:17. (10) Cf. *Isaiah* 60:1. (11) Cf. 60:19.
(12) Cf. *Joel* 3:1. (13) Cf. *Jeremiah* 3:17. (14) Cf. *Proverbs* 23:5. (15) *Psalms* 55:8.

---

lands of the gentiles and to settle in *Eretz Yisrael.*

The author of the *Kuzari* took his own words to heart and prepared to make his way to the land for which he had always yearned. Had not Rabbi Yehudah HaLevi himself written, 'My heart is in the east while I am stranded in the farthest end of the west!' Despite many hardships he finally made his way to Damascus. An ancient manuscript states that R' Yehudah HaLevi composed this *kinnah* while journeying towards *Eretz Yisrael* and recited it when he reached Damascus, facing the direction of Zion. Tradition has it that when he finally reached Jerusalem (circa 1145), he fell to the ground, in a state of ecstasy to fulfill the verse כִּי רָצוּ עֲבָדֶיךָ

אֶת אֲבָנֶיהָ וְאֶת עֲפָרָהּ יְחֹנֵנוּ, *For Your servants had cherished her stones and been gracious to her dust* (*Psalms* 102:15).

As he was kissing and embracing the dust near the Temple Mount he was trampled and killed by an Arab horseman.

לְבֵית אֵל וְלִפְנֵי אֵל ... וּלְמַחֲנַיִם — *For God's Temple, and before God ... and for the [three] encampments.* Some editions read, לְבֵית־אֵל וְלִפְנִיאֵל, *For Bethel and for Peniel,* treating these words as place names. If so, מַחֲנַיִם is also a place name, *Mahanaim.* Each of these three places was named by the Patriarch Jacob: Bethel, after his dream of angels ascending and descending a ladder (*Genesis* 28:19); Mahanaim, after his

אָנִיד לְבִתְרֵי לְבָבִי בֵּין בְּתָרֶיךָ.

אֶפֹּל לְאַפִּי עֲלֵי אַרְצֶךָ,

וְאֶרְצֶה אֲבָנֶיךָ לִמְאֹד וַאֲחוֹנֵן אֶת עֲפָרֶיךָ.[1]

אַף כִּי בְּעָמְדִי עֲלֵי קִבְרוֹת אֲבוֹתַי,

וְאֶשְׁתּוֹמֵם עֲלֵי חֶבְרוֹן, מִבְחַר קְבָרֶיךָ.

הַר הָעֲבָרִים[2] וְהֹר הָהָר,[3]

אֲשֶׁר שָׁם שְׁנֵי אוֹרִים גְּדוֹלִים מְאוֹרֶיךָ וּמוֹרֶיךָ.

חַיֵּי נְשָׁמוֹת אֲוִיר אַרְצֶךָ,*

וּמִמָּר דְּרוֹר אַבְקַת עֲפָרֶךָ, וְנֹפֶת צוּף נְהָרֶיךָ.

יִנְעַם לְנַפְשִׁי הָלוֹךְ עָרוֹם וְיָחֵף,[4]

עֲלֵי חָרְבוֹת שְׁמָמָה, אֲשֶׁר הָיָה דְּבִירֶיךָ.

בִּמְקוֹם אֲרוֹנֶךָ אֲשֶׁר נִגְנַז וּבִמְקוֹם כְּרוּבֶיךָ,

אֲשֶׁר שָׁכְנוּ חַדְרֵי חֲדָרֶיךָ.

אָגוֹז וְאַשְׁלִיךְ פְּאֵר נֵזֶר[5] וְאֶקֹּב זְמָן,

חִלֵּל בְּאֶרֶץ בְּבֶל[6] אֶת נְזִירֶיךָ.

אֵיךְ יֶעֱרַב לִי אָכוֹל וְשָׁתוֹת בְּעֵת אֶחֱזֶה,

כִּי יִסְחֲבוּ הַכְּלָבִים אֶת כְּפִירֶיךָ.[7]

אוֹ אֵיךְ מְאוֹר יוֹם יְהִי מָתוֹק לְעֵינַי,[8]

בְּעוֹד אֶרְאֶה בְּפִי עוֹרְבִים פִּגְרֵי בְּשָׁרֶיךָ.[7]

כּוֹס הַיְּגוֹנִים לְאַט, הַרְפִּי מְעַט,

כִּי כְבָר מָלְאוּ כְסָלַי וְנַפְשִׁי[9] מִמְּרוֹרֶיךָ.

עֵת אֶזְכְּרָה אָהֳלָה[10] אֶשְׁתֶּה חֲמָרֶךָ,

וְאֶזְכּוֹר אָהֳלִיבָה, וְאִמְצֶה אֶת שְׁמָרֶיךָ.

צִיּוֹן כְּלִילַת יֹפִי,[11] אַהֲבָה וְחֵן עוֹרְרִי לִמְאֹד,[12]

וּבָךְ נִקְשְׁרוּ נַפְשׁוֹת חֲבֵרֶיךָ.

הֵם הַשְּׂמֵחִים לְשַׁלְוָתֵךְ,

וְהַכֹּאֲבִים עַל שׁוֹמְמוֹתֵךְ, וּבוֹכִים עַל שְׁבָרֶיךָ.

מִבּוֹר שְׁבִי שׁוֹאֲפִים נֶגְדֵּךְ,

וּמִשְׁתַּחֲוִים אִישׁ מִמְּקוֹמוֹ, עֲלֵי נֹכַח שְׁעָרֶיךָ.

---

encounter with an encampment of angels as he
returned to Canaan from Aram (ibid. 32:3); and
Peniel, after he wrestled with the angel and
prevailed (ibid. 32:31).

I would cause my shattered heart to wander
amidst your shattered ruins.
I would fall on my face upon your soil
and intensely cherish your stones and favor your dust.¹
Even as I stand by the graves of my Patriarchs,
I behold in sheer wonderment the choicest burial sites in Hebron.
Mount Abarim² and Mount Hor,³ the resting places
of your two great lights [Moses and Aaron],
your beacons and your guides.
A breath of life for [our] souls is the air of your land;*
the powder of your dust is finer than flowing myrrh
and your river is like the honeycomb's drippings.
My soul would be pleased walking naked and barefoot⁴
among the desolate ruins, where your Holy of Holies once stood.
In the place of your Ark, which was [later] hidden, and in the place
of your Cherubim, which resided in your innermost chamber.
I will clip and throw away my glorious crown⁵ [of hair in mourning]
and I will curse the time when your nazirim
were defiled in the land of Babylon.⁶
How can food and drink taste pleasant to me, when I witness
the dogs dragging away your leonine youth?⁷
Or how can the light of day be sweet to my eye⁸ when I must see
the flesh of your corpses in the mouth of ravens?⁷
O cup of misery, slow down, give me some respite! For my thoughts
and my soul have already had their fill⁹ of your bitterness.
When I remember Oholah [Shomron]¹⁰ I will drink your wine; and
when I recall Oholibah [Jerusalem] I shall sip it to the very lees.
O Zion, consummation of beauty,¹¹ with love and charm
have you aroused yourself¹² greatly, and the souls
of your dear friends are bound up with you.
It is they who rejoice over your serenity, and who are pained
by your destruction and weep over your devastation.
From the pit of captivity, they yearn for you, and everyone
at his place prostrates himself towards your gates.

---

(1) Cf. *Pslams* 102:15. (2) See *Deuteronomy* 32:49-50. (3) See *Numbers* 20:24-25. (4) *Isaiah* 20:2.
(5) Cf. *Jeremiah* 7:29. (6) This seems to be the censor's emandation; some editions read
בְּאֶרֶץ טְמֵאָה, *in an unclean land.* (7) Cf. *Jeremiah* 15:3. (8) Cf. *Ecclesiastes* 11:7.
(9) Cf. *Psalms* 38:8. (10) See commentary to *kinnah* 4. (11) *Eichah* 2:15. (12) Some editions
read עוֹרַרְתְּ, *you invigorated yourself;* some editions read תִּקְשְׁרִי מֵאָז, *you have bound from yore.*

חַיֵּי נִשְׁמוֹת אֲוִיר אַרְצֵךְ — *A breath of life for [our]*
souls is the air of your land. This stich can be
interpreted two ways. It may refer to the souls of
the living which receive an extra measure of
vitality from the very air of the Holy Land. This
is in accordance with the Talmudic dictum: The
air of Eretz Yisrael makes one wise (*Bava Basra*
158b). Or it may refer to the souls of the dead
who are buried in the Land of Israel. They will
rise immediately at the time of the Resuscitation
of the Dead. But those buried outside of the
Land will not arise until underground passages

עֶדְרֵי הֲמוֹנֶךָ, אֲשֶׁר גָּלוּ,

וְנִתְפַּזְּרוּ מֵהַר לְגִבְעָה וְלֹא שָׁכְחוּ גְדֵרֶיךָ.

הַמַּחֲזִיקִים בְּשׁוּלַיִךְ וּמִתְאַמְּצִים לַעֲלוֹת,

וְלֶאֱחוֹז בְּסַנְסִנֵּי תְמָרָיִךְ.²

שִׁנְעָר וּפַתְרוֹס, הַיַּעַרְכוּךְ בְּגָדְלָם,

וְאִם הֶבְלָם יְדַמּוּ לְתֻמַּיִךְ וְאוּרַיִךְ.*

אֵל מִי יְדַמּוּ מְשִׁיחַיִךְ, וְאֶל מִי נְבִיאַיִךְ,

וְאֶל מִי לְוִיַּיִךְ וְשִׁירָיִךְ.

יִשָּׁנֶה וְיַחֲלוֹף כְּלִיל כָּל מַמְלְכוֹת הָאֱלִילִים,³

חָסְנֵךְ לְעוֹלָם לְדוֹר וָדוֹר נְזִירַיִךְ.⁴

אָנָה לְמוֹשַׁב אֱלֹהָיִךְ,⁵

וְאַשְׁרֵי אֱנוֹשׁ יִבְחַר וִיקָרֵב וְיִשְׁכּוֹן בַּחֲצֵרָיִךְ.⁶

אַשְׁרֵי מְחַכֶּה וְיַגִּיעַ וְיִרְאֶה עֲלוֹת אוֹרֵךְ,

וְיִבָּקְעוּ עָלָיו שְׁחָרָיִךְ.⁷

לִרְאוֹת בְּטוֹבַת בְּחִירָיִךְ, לַעֲלוֹת בְּשִׂמְחָתֶךָ,

בְּשׁוּבֵךְ אֱלֵי קַדְמוּת נְעוּרָיִךְ.

---

are prepared for them to roll all the way to *Eretz Yisrael,* where they will be revived (see *Bereishis Rabbah* 96:5).

לְתֻמַּיִךְ וְאוּרַיִךְ — *To your Urim V'Tumim.* The חֹשֶׁן, *breastplate,* worn by the *Kohen Gadol* was made of linen; blue, purple and red wools; and gold threads. It was folded over and the *Urim V'Tumim* (see below) was inserted in the fold.

Twelve precious stones were attached to the front of the breastplate in four rows of three stones each, with each stone inscribed with the name of one of the tribes. When the *Urim V'Tumim* was consulted, the letters etched on the stones lit up and spelled out a message. Since the letters חטצק do not appear in the names of the tribes, the stones were also engraved with the names of the Patriarchs אַבְרָהָם יִצְחָק יַעֲקֹב,

The flocks of your masses who were exiled and scattered
    from mountain to hill,[1] they did not forget your sheepfolds.
Those who cling to your hems and exert themselves to climb
    and grasp the branches of your date palm.[2]
Can Shinar [Babylon] and Pathros [Egypt] compare with you
    despite their greatness, and can their worthless deities
    be likened to your Urim V'Tumim?*
To whom can your anointed ones be compared?
    To whom your prophets?
    And to whom your Levites and singers?
All idolatrous kingdoms shall pass on and disappear,[3]
    while your firm power is forever; your leaders [shall endure]
    for all generations.[4]
Your God desired you for His residence,[5]
    and fortunate is the man who chooses and draws near
    and dwells in your courtyards.[6]
Fortunate is he who waits and arrives and witnesses
    the rising of your light when your dawn bursts forth over him.[7]
To behold the goodness of your chosen ones,
    and exult in your joy when you return
    to the youthfulness of early times.

---

(1) Cf. Jeremiah 50:6. (2) Cf. Song of Songs 7:9. (3) Cf. Isaiah 2:18.
(4) Cf. Proverbs 27:24. (5) Cf. Psalms 132:13. (6) Cf. 65:5. (7) Cf. Isaiah 58:8.

Abraham, Isaac, Jacob, and the phrase שִׁבְטֵי
יְשֻׁרוּן, tribes of Yeshurun (another name for
Israel). This accounted for all twenty-two letters
of the aleph-beis.

According to Rashi the Urim V'Tumim was a
slip of parchment upon which the שֵׁם הַמְּפוֹרָשׁ,
Ineffable Four-Letter Name of HASHEM, was

written. This was the power that lit up the
letters on the breastplate. Ramban (Exodus
28:30) adds that this Name was written by
Moses in a manner entrusted by God to him
alone; it was considered a heavenly handicraft.
Ritva maintains that it was Divinely written
and given to Moses.

לז.

צִיּוֹן קְחִי* כָּל צֳרֵי גִלְעָד' לְצִירַיִךְ,

אֵין דַּי, לְמַעַן כַּיָּם גָּדְלוּ שְׁבָרָיִךְ.²

אֶרֶץ צְבִי אַתְּ³ בְּתוֹךְ גּוֹיִם נְתוּנָה,*⁴

וּמֵעֵדֶן מְקוֹם כָּל יָקָר יָצְאוּ נְהָרָיִךְ.⁵

וַיְהִי לְאוֹת, נַעֲמָן* רָחַץ בְּשָׂרוֹ בְּמֵי יַרְדֵּן,

אֲזַי נֶאֱסַף אַף כִּי טְהוֹרָיִךְ.

אַף לֹא יְסֻלֶּה עֲפַר אַרְצֵךְ בְּזָהָב וּפָז,⁶

יָקָר כְּמוֹ יָהֲלוֹם מַחְצַב הֲרָרָיִךְ.

כָּל תַּעֲנוּגִים* בְּבֹא בְּסָרֵךְ,

לֹא קָהֲתָה הַשֵּׁן' וְאוּלָם כִּצוּף מָתְקוּ מְרוֹרָיִךְ.

פִּרְיֵךְ לְמַרְפֵּא, וְכָל עָלֶה תַעֲלֶה,

הֲלֹא כְּיַעֲרַת הַדְּבַשׁ⁸ הָיוּ יְעָרָיִךְ.

עִם הַפְּתָנִים בְּרִית כָּרַתּוּ מְתַיִךְ וְאֵין שָׂטָן,

אֲבָל הֻשְׁלְמוּ לָהֶם כְּפִירָיִךְ.

בָּךְ כָּל בְּהֵמָה וְעוֹף חָכְמוּ, עֲדֵי כַּחֲמוֹר הָיָה לְפָנִים,

לְבֶן יָאִיר* הַמּוֹרָיִךְ.

בָּךְ אֵל לְבַדּוֹ וְאֵין בִּלְתּוֹ, וַיֵּצֵא שְׁמֵךְ'

עַד כִּי אֱלֹהִים אֱמֶת נוֹדַע בְּשִׁירָיִךְ.

צִיּוֹן קְחִי ❦ — O Zion, even if you took. This beautiful composition illustrates the unique natural gifts with which the Holy Land is so abundantly blessed. Indeed, it is this country which is closest in nature to the Garden of Eden itself. The waters of the land are endowed with curative powers; the earth is filled with precious gems and metals and every type of essential resource; the fruits and grain of Eretz Yisrael are as delicious and nutritious as can be. In this blessed environment the Torah nation developed the most perfect society ever known to mankind. Law and order reigned throughout the land, capably governed by a noble king and taught by holy priests and prophets. Alas, all this has fallen into the rapacious hands of our enemies, but we yearn for this splendor to return!

Scholars are in dispute regarding the authorship of this kinnah. It is variously attributed to R' Shlomo ibn Gabirol, R' Avraham HaChozeh, R' Avraham ibn Ezra, and R' Elyah ben Menachem HaZaken.

אַתְּ בְּתוֹךְ גּוֹיִם נְתוּנָה — You have been placed in the center of all nations. Eretz Yisrael is positioned in the center of the world; Jerusalem is at the center of Eretz Yisrael; the Temple is at the center of Jerusalem; the Heichal hall is at the center of the Temple; and the Holy Ark is at the center of the Heichal (Midrash Tanchuma, Kedoshim 10).

נַעֲמָן — Naaman. II Kings chapter 5 relates the story of Naaman, the great and victorious commander-in-chief of the Aramean army. Because of his excessive pride, God afflicted him with a painful leprous disease of the skin for which he could find no cure. Finally, out of sheer desperation he came to the prophet Elisha for help. At first Naaman adamantly refused to follow Elisha's instructions to bathe himself in the waters of the Jordan, exclaiming, 'Are not Amanah and Parpar, the rivers of (my homeland) Damascus, better than all the waters of Israel?' (ibid. v. 12). Finally, Naaman relented and humbly dipped himself seven times in the Jordan River and when he emerged, his flesh was

37.

צִיּוֹן O Zion, even if you took* all the balm of Gilead[1]
it would not be enough for your wounds,
because your ruination is as vast as the sea.[2]

O most desirable land,[3] you have been placed in the center
of all nations,[4]* and from Eden the source of
all splendor your rivers emanated.[5]

And this is the proof: Naaman* bathed his flesh in the waters
of the Jordan and his affliction disappeared; how much
more effective [are these waters] for your own pure people.

Indeed, even the value of the dust of your land cannot be measured
in comparison with plain gold or the purest gold,[6]
for even the coarse rocks hewn from your mountains
are as precious as yahalom gems.

All the delights* [of the world found their way to the Land of Israel]
and even your unripe fruits set no tooth on edge;[7] rather,
your most bitter fruits were as sweet as honey.

Your fruits had healing powers, and within every leaf was a cure;
indeed, your forests were thickets filled with sweet honey.[8]

Your citizens entered into a covenant with the vipers and none
were harmed; indeed, even your lions made peace with them.

Within you every animal and bird grew wise, to the point where
even the donkeys were as intelligent as the donkey of ben Yair.*

In your midst was God, Who is alone with none besides Him,
and your fame spread,[9] because the true God
was revealed through your songs.

---

(1) Cf. *Jeremiah* 8:22. (2) Cf. *Eichah* 2:13. (3) Cf. *Ezekiel* 20:6. (4) Cf. 5:5. (5) See *Genesis* 2:10.
(6) Cf. *Job* 28:16. (7) Cf. *Jeremiah* 31:28; *Ezekiel* 18:2. (8) I *Samuel* 14:27. (9) Cf. *Ezekiel* 16:14.

---

restored like the flesh of a small child (ibid. v.14).

כָּל תַּעֲנוּגִים — *All the delights.* The finest
agricultural area in the Land was adjacent to Lake
Kineret and was called גִינוֹסַר, *Gennosar,* which is
a contraction of גַּן שָׂרִים, *garden of Princes,* because its fruit and produce was desired by royalty
the world over (see *Pesachim* 8b and *Rashi* to
Genesis 49:21). The historian Josephus (*Wars of
the Jews,* Book III, 10:8) reports that the soil of
Gennosar is so fruitful that every type of tree can
grow on it: 'The temper of the air is so well mixed
that it agrees well with all sorts, particularly
walnuts, which require the coldest air, and
flourish there in vast plenty; there are also palm
trees which grow best in hot air. Fig trees and
olive trees which require more temperate air grow
near them. One may call this place the ambition
of nature, where it forces those plants which are
naturally enemies to abide together; it is a happy
contention of the seasons as if everyone of them
laid claim to the country at once.'

Even your lions made peace with them. The
Torah promised the Jews: *No man shall covet
your land when you go to appear before HASHEM
your God three times in the year* (*Exodus* 34:24).
The Talmud relates many wondrous examples of
how God protected the property that the pilgrims
left behind. A man once left his granary unprotected when he went to spend the festival in Jerusalem. When he returned he found everything
intact because a pride of lions was patroling his
premises, scaring away intruders. Another time, a
person left his chickens alone, unprotected from
hungry wolves. When he returned from
Jerusalem, he found dead wolves that had been
torn apart by his chickens. Another man came
home and found a deadly scorpion wrapped
around the doorknobs of his home, frightening
away all burglars (*Yerushalmi Peah* 3:7).

כַּחֲמוֹר... לְבֶן יָאִיר — *The donkey of ben Yair.* The
Talmud relates that one night robbers stole R'
Pinchas ben Yair's donkey. They hid the animal

מַה טּוֹב וְנָעִים,[1] בְּבֹא שִׁבְטֵי בְנֵי יַעֲקֹב

שָׁלֹשׁ פְּעָמִים[2] בְּכָל שָׁנָה בִּשְׁעָרֶיךְ.

בָּךְ סוֹד הַתְּעוּדָה וְסוֹד חַכְמוֹת,

וּבָאוּ בְנֵי קֶדֶם[3] וְחַכְמֵי שֵׁבָא לִכְתוֹב סְפָרֶיךְ.

שׁוֹטְרִים בְּכָל הַגְּבוּל, שׁוֹפְטִים בְּכָל עִיר וָעִיר,[4]

זִקְנֵי אֱמֶת הֵם וְאֵין מוֹרֶה כְּמוֹרֶיךְ.

מֶלֶךְ בְּקִרְבֵּךְ, וּבָךְ שָׂרֵי חֲיָלִים בְּכָל נֶשֶׁק,

וְעַל כָּל לְאֹם גָּבְרוּ גְבִירֶיךְ.

בִּימֵי בְחוּרוֹת, הֱיוֹת קֹדֶשׁ לָאֵל נִבְחָרוּ,

וּבְנֵי נְבִיאִים בְּנֵי אֵל חַי נְעָרֶיךְ.

בָּךְ הַתְּקוּפָה עֲלֵי קַו הָאֱמֶת נִשְׁקָלָה,

תְּכֶן שְׁנוֹת דּוֹר וָדוֹר[5] בִּשְׁנֵי אֲדָרֶיךְ.

מוֹלַד לְבָנָה כְּפִי אָרְכֵּךְ וְהַמַּחֲזֶה שׁוּמָה לְרָחְבֵּךְ,

וּבָהּ הֶרְאֵית סְתָרֶיךְ.

נִרְאֶה בְתַמּוּז כְּסִיל[65] בָּךְ יַעֲלֶה,

כִּי שָׁאַר כָּל הֶחֳדָשִׁים לְבַד זֶה בַּחֲדָרֶיךְ.

אַיֵּה דְבִירֵךְ מְקוֹם אָרוֹן,

וְאַיֵּה הֲדַר הֵיכָל וְהַמִּזְבְּחוֹת, וְאַיֵּה חֲצֵרֶיךְ.

אַיֵּה מְשִׁיחֵךְ, בְּעַד עַמֵּךְ יְכַפֵּר,

וּמֶה הָיָה לִילַדְרֵי קְהָת, וְאַיֵּה נְזִירֶיךְ.

אֵיפֹה נְבִיאִים בְּנֵי עֶלְיוֹן וְכָל יוֹעֲצַיִךְ אָבָדוּ,

וְהָלְכוּ שְׁבִי מַלְכֵּךְ וְשָׂרָיִךְ.

הָיִית יְפֵה נוֹף[7] וְרֹאשׁ עַפְרוֹת תֵּבֵל,[8]

בְּרֹושֵׁךְ לְנֵס, חֶטְאֵךְ סְחָפֵךְ, הֲלֹא קָצַר קְצִירָיִךְ.

אֶרֶץ מְאָסֵךְ וּמֵי נָכְרִים שְׁטָפוּךְ,

וְכָל רוּחַ הֱפִיצֵךְ, וְאֵשׁ בָּעֲרָה בְעָרֶיךְ.

---

(1) Cf. *Psalms* 133:1. (2) Cf. *Deuteronomy* 16:16. (3) *I Kings* 5:10. (4) Cf. *Deuteronomy* 16:18. (5) *Deuteronomy* 32:7. (65) See commentary to *kinnah* 5. (7) *Psalms* 48:3. (8) *Proverbs* 8:26.

for three days during which it refused to eat a thing, because it would never eat stolen goods. In desperation, the robbers released her and she made her way home to the rabbi's house. The family gave her barley to eat but again the donkey refused to partake. R' Pinchas asked, 'Are you certain that this barley was properly tithed?' The family responded, 'Father, you yourself ruled that we may follow the lenient opinion that exempts this type of produce from the tithe.' To

How good and pleasant[1] it was
  when the tribes the sons of Jacob entered your gates,
  three times each year.[2]
You are the repository of the secrets of [Torah] tradition
  and the secrets of wisdom, so the (wise) men of the Orient[3]
  and the scholars of Sheba came to transcribe your books.
Law enforcement officers were [posted] within all your borders
  and judges for each and every city;[4] these elders
  were men of truth and no teacher equaled your teachers.
A king was in your midst, and fully equipped military officers
  were in position; your warriors subdued every other nation.
In your youth, you were chosen to be consecrated unto God,
  and even your youngsters were disciples of the prophets,
  children of the Living God!
Through you the seasons of the year were balanced
  on a perfect time-line;
  the years were determined for generation upon generation[5]
  by intercalating the two months of Adar.
The birth of the new moon [fixes the new month]
  according to your longitude, and its visibility was measured
  according to your latitude, and through it was revealed
  your secret knowledge [of the heavens].
The constellation Orion[6] is visible everywhere [except in Israel]
  in the month of Tammuz, for it only ascends above
  you [Israel] during one of the other months [Sivan],
  while [in Tammuz] it remains concealed in your inner chambers.
O where is your Holy of Holies, the resting place of the Holy Ark?
  And where is the splendor of the Sanctuary and the Altars?
  And where are your courtyards?
And where is your anointed [High Priest,]
  who would effect atonement for your people?
  And what happened to [the Levite] children of Kehath?
  And where are your nazirites?
Where are the prophets, the sons of the Most High?
  All of your advisors have perished;
  your kings and nobles have gone into captivity.
You were the fairest of sites,[7] the first of the dusts of the earth,[8]
  your cypress tree is a banner;
  it is your sin that has drowned you,
  that has cut down your assassinated men.
The land abominated you and the alien waters swept you away,
  while every wind scattered you and fires raged in your cities.

מָרִית בְּצוּרֵךְ, אֲשֶׁר מִצָּר נִצְרֵךְ,

וְאָז זָרִים עֲכָרוּךְ, וְאַתְּ הָיִית בְּעוֹכְרַיִךְ.

אֵל הֶאֱמִירָךְ עֲדֵי נִקְרֵאת אֲרִיאֵל,*

וְאֵיךְ עָבַר בְּנֵוֶךְ אֲרִי טוֹרֵף עֲדָרַיִךְ.

שׁוּבִי לָאֵל בּוֹעֲלֵךְ, אַל תִּתְּנִי לוֹ דָמִי

עַד שׁוּב כְּבוֹדוֹ, עַד יִבְנֶה גְדֵרָיִךְ.

נַפְשִׁי מְאֹד נִכְסְפָה² לִרְאוֹת בְּזִיו זָהֳרֵךְ,

שָׁלוֹם יְהִי לָךְ וְרֹב שָׁלוֹם לְעוֹזְרָיִךְ.³

---

this R' Pinchas responded, 'Indeed, I personally
follow the lenient view, but what can I do if my
donkey wishes to accept the stricter opinion?'
(Yerushalmi Shekalim 5:1; see also Chullin 7a).

אֲרִיאֵל — Ariel [lit., the lion of God]. The Temple
is described thus because just as the lion is broad
in chest and small behind, so is the Temple wide
in front and narrow at the back.

The Midrash states: A lion came, in the month
of the lion and destroyed the lion of God.

'A lion came' refers to Nebuchadnezzar, the
wicked King of Babylon, of whom it is written:
A lion came forth from his thicket (Jeremiah
4:7).

'In the month of the lion,' means that the
Temple was destroyed in the month of Av
whose symbol in the Zodiac is the lion.

You rebelled against your Creator, He who had protected you
  from every foe. Therefore aliens distressed you,
  but it was you who brought this distress upon yourself.
*O how God elevated you! Until he bestowed upon you the title Ariel!**
  How then did He allow the lion to trespass your dwelling
  to tear apart your flocks?
Return to God, your devoted spouse, give Him no rest[1]
  [from entreaty], until His glory returns,
  until He rebuilds your walls.
My soul yearns intensely[2] to behold the splendor of your radiance;
  may peace be yours and abundant peace to those who help you![3]

---

(1) Cf. *Isaiah* 62:7. (2) *Psalms* 84:3. (3) *I Chronicles* 12:19.

'And destroyed the lion of God (Ariel)' refers to the Temple, as the prophet lamented: 'Woe *Ariel, Ariel, the city where David encamped'* (*Isaiah* 29:1).

The Midrash continues: In the end of time a lion shall come in the month of the lion, and rebuild the lion of God.

'A lion shall come' refers to Almighty God Himself.

'In the month of the lion' refers to the month of Av which will be transformed from sorrow to rejoicing.

'And rebuild the lion of God' refers to the Temple, as it says, *The Builder of Jerusalem is HASHEM, He will gather in the outcasts of Israel* (*Psalms* 147:2; *Pesikta* 13).

לח.

צִיּוֹן עֲטֶרֶת צְבִי[1] שִׂמְחַת הֲמוֹנָיִךְ,

שָׁלוֹם כְּנָהָר[2] קְחִי מֵאֵת אֲדוֹנָיִךְ.

אֵילֵי שְׁחָקִים אֲשֶׁר שׁוֹמְרִים לְחוֹמוֹת[3] נָחֵל[4]

לַיְלָה וָיוֹם יִדְרְשׁוּן[5] שָׁלוֹם לְמַחֲנָיִךְ.

גַּם הַנְּפוֹצִים בְּכָל אַרְבַּע קְצָוֹת,

וְהֵם דּוֹרְשֵׁי שְׁלוֹמֵךְ, בְּנוֹתָיִךְ וּבָנָיִךְ.

שׁוֹכְנֵי קְבָרִים מְחַכִּים וּמְצַפִּים לְיוֹם יִשְׁעֵךְ,

וְאָז יִצְמְחוּ יִחְיוּ יְשֵׁנָיִךְ.

וַאֲנִי בְּשָׁאֲלִי שְׁלוֹמֵךְ אֶקְרָא קוֹל בְּראשׁ הָרִים,

וְאֶדְמֶה לְעוֹף עַל רַעֲנָנָיִךְ.

שָׁלוֹם לְצִיּוֹן נְוֵה צֶדֶק[6] וְשָׁלוֹם עֲלֵי חֵילֵךְ

וְחוֹמוֹת יְקַר אַבְנֵי פְּנִינָיִךְ.

שָׁלוֹם לְאֶרֶץ צְבִי,[7]

שָׁלוֹם לְכָל הַגְּבוּל גִּלְעָד וְשׁוֹמְרוֹן, וְכָל יֶתֶר שְׁכֵנָיִךְ.

צִיּוֹן לְפָנִים הֲלֹא הָיִית יְפַת מַרְאֶה,

אֵיךְ נֶהְפְּכוּ לִשְׁחוֹר תָּאֳרֵךְ וּפָנָיִךְ.

כִּבְנוֹת מְלָכִים יְקָר עָטִית תְּהִלָּה,

וְאֵיךְ שַׂק תַּחְגְּרִי עַל חֲלָצַיִךְ וּמָתְנָיִךְ.

לַחְמֵי אֲנָחָה[8] בְּעֵת תַּעְדִּי אֵפֶר תַּחַת פְּאֵר,

(אֶפְעֶה)[9] וְאֶשְׁתֶּה יְגוֹנִי עֲלֵי יְגוֹנָיִךְ.

קוּמִי וְנַשְּׂא נְהִי, נִבְכֶּה דְמָעוֹת כַּיָּם,

יִזְּלוּ נְהָרוֹת, לְמִן עֵינַי לְעֵינָיִךְ.

עַל אַלְמְנוּתֵךְ אֲשֶׁר הָלַךְ יְדִידֵךְ,

וְהוּא הֶחֱרִיב דְּבִירוֹ וְכָל סִתְרֵי צְפוּנָיִךְ.

עֵת אֶרְאֶה יָפְיֵךְ אֶקְרָא מְשׁוֹרְרִים בְּשִׁיר,

עֵת אֶחֱזֶה עָנְיֵךְ אֶקְרָא מְקוֹנְנָיִךְ.

אֶבְחַר לָקַאת וְקִפּוֹד[10] יִשְׁכְּנוּ בָךְ,

צִיּוֹן עֲטֶרֶת צְבִי — *O Zion, most desirable crown.* The Destruction of the *Beis HaMikdash* has deprived the universe of God's favorite location, His garden of delights, the Holy Temple. The composer of this *kinnah* [R' Elazar, the son of R' Moshe HaDarshan, of

38.

צִיּוֹן   O Zion, most desirable crown,[1] joy for your multitudes;
   accept blessings of peace,
   [endless] as the river['s flow],[2] from your Lord.
The celestial angels who guard your walls[3] and cheil,[4]
   pray fervently by day and by night[5] for the welfare of your camp.
And those scattered to the four corners, they too beseech [God]
   on your behalf, for they are your sons and daughters.
Even those interred in graves wait and hope for the day
   of your salvation, and then those who slumber [in the earth]
   shall sprout forth and come [back] to life.
As for me, when I pray for your welfare, I shall cry out
   from the mountaintops, I shall be like a bird [singing aloud]
   from your verdant treetops.
Peace unto Zion, where righteousness resides,[6]
   and peace be upon your ramparts and walls
   whose stones are more precious than gems.
Peace unto [you] O desirable land,[7] and peace throughout
   all of your borders — reaching as far away as
   Gilead and Samaria, and the rest of your dwellings.
O Zion, did you not once enjoy fine appearance?
   How, then, has your form and your face
   become transfigured into blackness?
You were swathed in precious robes like the daughters of kings,
   O how you must gird yourself with sackcloth on your waist
   and on your loins!
My sighs [replace] my bread,[8] when you [Zion] cover yourself
   with ashes instead of splendor; (I shall cry out loud,)[9]
   and quaff my [cupful of] anguish for your anguish.
Arise, and let us arouse a lamentation; let us shed tears like the sea,
   let the tears flow like rivers, from my eyes to yours.
[I will cry over] your widowhood, for your Beloved has gone
   and He has destroyed His Temple residence
   and all the secret places of your concealment.
When I would behold your beauty, I would summon the singers
   to make song; [but] now when I witness your pain
   I summon those who chant your laments.
I would prefer that the pelican and porcupine[10]
   would dwell in your midst;

---

(1) *Isaiah* 28:5. (2) Cf. 48:18. (3) Cf. *Isaiah* 62:6. (4) Cf. *Eichah* 2:8. (5) Cf. *Isaiah* 58:2. (6) *Jeremiah* 50:7.
(7) Cf. *Ezekiel* 20:6. (8) Cf. *Job* 3:24. (9) Some editions omit the term in parentheses. (10) This
identification of these creatures of the wild may not be accurate.

Wurtzburg, Germany, early 13th century] de-   languishes to hear the herald of redemption and
scribes how he, a lover of Zion, yearns and   to witness the return of God to His Palace. He

וְאוֹי לִי אִם אֱדוֹם וַעֲרָב קֵנְנוּ בְקִנֶּיךָ.

עִיר הַמְּלוּכָה לְדָוִד וּשְׁלֹמֹה בְנוֹ* הָיִית בְּנוּיָה,
וְהֵם קֶדֶם מְכוֹנְנָיִךְ.

אַתְּ הִיא לְמִקְדָּשׁ לָאֵל, אַתְּ הִיא מְנוּחָה לְצוּר,
אַתְּ הִיא אֲשֶׁר יוֹם בְּיוֹם יָרַד לְגַנָּיִךְ.

שָׁם שֻׁלְחָן וּמְנוֹרָה, וַאֲרוֹן הַבְּרִית,*
אֵל בֵּין שָׁדֵי* אַהֲבָה, לָן בִּמְלוֹנָיִךְ.

עַל מִזְבְּחֵךְ עָמְדוּ כֹהֲנִים מְשָׁרְתִים,
בְּמוֹ זֶבַח וְעוֹלָה לְכַפֵּר עַל עֲוֹנָיִךְ.

רֹאשׁ הַכְּהֻנָּה אֲשֶׁר אֵפוֹד לְבוּשֵׁי יָקָר,
נִשְׁמַע בְּשׁוּלֵי מְעִיל קוֹל פַּעֲמוֹנָיִךְ.[1]

אַחַת בַּשָּׁנָה[2] פְּנִים הָלַךְ לְחַדְרֵי דְבִיר,
הֵבִיא קְטֹרֶת מָלֵא קֻמְצוֹ[3] וְחָפְנָיִךְ.[4]

קִדָּה וְקָנֶה, וְכָל רָאשֵׁי בְשָׂמִים,[5]
עֲדֵי עִיר הַתְּמָרִים, בְּבֹא רֵיחַ סַמָּנָיִךְ.*[6]

אַף הַלְוִיִּם אֲשֶׁר שׁוֹמְרִים שְׁעָרִים,
וְגַם הַמְשׁוֹרְרִים שִׁיר בְּפֶה עִם כָּל רְנָנָיִךְ.

---

calls upon all the angels in heaven above to join in the lament of the Jewish people who are scattered to the four corners of the earth.

לְדָוִד וּשְׁלֹמֹה בְנוֹ — *For David and Solomon his son.* David made all the preparations for Jerusalem and the Temple. At first the entire city was in the hands of Aravna the Jebusite. David collected fifty shekels from each of the twelve tribes of Israel, and paid a total of six hundred gold shekels for the city (*Zevachim* 116b). David also brought the place of the altar from Aravna for fifty silver shekels. David dug the foundations of the Temple especially for the place of the Altar (*Sukkah* 53a) and he laid down and consecrated the Temple's floor (*Zevachim* 24a). David assembled all the necessary money and materials in preparation for construction and he handed down to Solomon a comprehensive master plan describing how the Temple should be built, to the most scrupulous detail.

שֻׁלְחָן וּמְנוֹרָה וַאֲרוֹן הַבְּרִית — *The Table, the Menorah and the Ark of the Covenant.* God performs revealed miracles as a display of His love for the beneficiary of those miracles. Thus the supernatural events that occurred on a daily

basis in the *Beis HaMikdash* were clear demonstrations of God's extraordinary love for His Jewish people. The *Panim*-Bread was baked on Friday and arranged on the Table on Saturday, where it remained until the following Saturday. In good times the bread remained fresh and steaming hot until the last day, even though it was at least eight full days since it left the baking oven. This manifested God's intense and burning love for His people. The *Talmud* (*Chagigah* 26b) says that on the festivals the *Kohanim* would hold the Table aloft so that all the pilgrims could see the steaming hot bread and the *Kohanim* would say, 'Behold how beloved you are to God!'

The Menorah, too, had a perpetual miracle. One of its seven lamps, called the נֵר מַעֲרָבִי, *western lamp,* would be filled with the same quantity of oil and same size wick as the other six, yet it would continue to burn throughout the following day, long after the other lights had died out in the morning. This, says the *Talmud* (*Shabbos* 22b), was a public demonstration to the entire world that God's Holy Spirit settled over the people of Israel and caused miracles to occur.

Finally, the *Talmud* (*Yoma* 54a) teaches that

but woe unto me
   that Edom and Arabia make their home in your nest.
O Royal City! You were built expressly
      for David and Solomon his son,*
   and they were the first to lay down your foundations.
It is you who were a Sanctuary unto God; it is you
      who were a place of rest for the Creator; it is you,
      for to your gardens God descended every day.
There were the Table, the Menorah and the Ark of the Covenant;*
      there God dwelled lovingly in your Lodge between
      the staves of the Holy Ark.*
Upon your Altar stood the priests in [Divine] service,
   with animal sacrifices and burnt offerings
      to atone for your iniquities.
The High Priest was garbed in precious garments,
   from the edge of his tunic was heard the sound of your bells.[1]
Once a year [on Yom Kippur]² he entered into the Inner Chamber
   of the Sanctuary and offered [in addition to] his fistful³
   [of frankincense that accompanied the flour-offering
   of the tamid,] your double handful⁴ of incense.
The scent of the kaneh, kiddah and other primary spices⁵
   wafted to [Jericho] the City of Palms, where the
   fragrance of your spices reached.⁶*
Also [the sound of] the opening of the Temple gates
      by the Levite guards [was heard in Jericho],
      as well as the voices of the [Levite] singers
   who sang to the accompaniment of joyous instruments.

---

(1) See *Exodus* 28:33-35. (2) 30:10. (3) Cf. *Leviticus* 2:2. (4) Cf. 16:12.
(5) Cf. *Exodus* 30:23. (6) Some editions read שְׁמָנֶיךָ, *your oils*.

---

when God was pleased with the Jewish people that close love was symbolized by the golden *Cherubim* on top of the Holy Ark, for they would then embrace each other in a display of love and affection. However, when Israel's actions were contrary to the *mitzvos* of the Torah, the *Cherubim* would face away from one another.

בֵּין שָׁדַי — *Between the staves of the Holy Ark* [lit., *between the bosoms*]. The simile of שָׁדַיִם, *bosom*, and staves of the Ark is elaborated upon in the Talmud. Although the staves were very long they were *perceivable from without but could not be actually seen* (see *I Kings* 8:8), because the twin poles pressed against the Curtain from within, and only the twin bosom-like protrusions could be discerned from without (*Yoma* 54a; *Menachos* 98a).

The word לָן, *lodged*, infers a temporary situation as one who 'sleeps over' and then goes

his way. Similarly, God 'lodged' within the Sanctuary, but when Israel sinned, the *Shechinah* departed to its 'heavenly abode' and took up its lodging there.

עָרֵי עִיר הַתְּמָרִים בָּא רֵיחַ סַמָּנֵיךְ — *Wafted to [Jericho] the City of Palms, where the fragrance of your spices reached.* The Talmud lists many sounds and aromas from the Temple which were heard and smelled in Jericho, including the voice of the *Kohen Gadol* when he cried out God's name on Yom Kippur during the Temple service. *Raavad* (comm. ibid.) explains that the smell of the incense and the sounds of the Temple were only sensed in Jericho and not in any other areas around Jerusalem. This miracle was designed to demonstrate Jericho's special status and kinship to Jerusalem. Jericho was the first city to be conquered by Joshua so it achieved the sanctity of תְּרוּמָה, *the Kohen's due*, which is the first part of the crop that the Torah

נֶגְדָּם בְּנֵי מַעֲמָד* עוֹרְכִים תְּפִלָּה,

וְלוֹ יַעֲלֶה הַמּוֹנֵךְ בְּכָל פַּעֲמֵי זְמַנָּיִךְ.

בָּךְ הַנְּבִיאִים, הֲלֹא הָיוּ בְּסוֹד אֵל,[1]

וּבָךְ חַכְמֵי תְכוּנָה, וּבָךְ שִׁבְעִים זְקֵנָיִךְ.

אַרְצֵךְ מְלֵאָה בְּמוֹ עֶשֶׂר קְדֻשּׁוֹת,*

וְכָל מַעְשַׂר תְּרוּמָה וְגַם מִבְחַר דְּגָנָיִךְ.

עַתָּה שְׁמָמָה בְּלִי בָנִים וּבָנוֹת,

וְאָן מַלְכֵּךְ נְבִיאָיִךְ לְוִיָּיִךְ וְכֹהֲנָיִךְ.

מָתַי יְשׁוּבוּן וְיָבְוֹאוּ בְּתוֹךְ אָהֳלֵךְ,

הַמִּתְאַוִּים שְׁכוֹן תַּחַת עֲנָנָיִךְ.

(מִי יִתְּנֵנִי לְעֵת תֵּלְדִי יְלָדִים,

כְּמוֹ שִׁפְרָה וּפוּעָה מְיַלֶּדֶת בְּאַבְנָיִךְ.[2]

זֹאת אֶתְאַוֶּה לְיוֹם יָבָא חֲתָנֵךְ,

וְאַתְּ כַּלָּה וְהִתְפָּאֲרִי בַּעֲדִי עֲדָנָיִךְ.)[3]

לִבִּי יְאַוֶּה לְחַבֵּק בְּזְרוֹעוֹת עֲפַר אַרְצֵךְ,

וְאֶחְשׁוֹק בְּפִי נַשֵּׁק אֲבָנָיִךְ.

לוּ אֶרְאֵךְ בִּהְיוֹת נִבְנֵית בְּנֵין עָפֵךְ וָפוּךְ,

יֵרָאוּ לְצָפוֹן וְיָם גֹּבַהּ קְרָנָיִךְ.

אֶכְסוֹף וְאֶחְמוֹד לְנֶחָמָה,

וְתִשְׁמַעְנָה דִּבְרֵי מְבַשֵּׂר בְּקוֹל, אָזְנַי וְאָזְנָיִךְ.

הִתְעוֹרְרִי[4] לִקְרַאת דּוֹדֵךְ וְהִתְנַעֲרִי מִן הָאֲדָמָה[5]

בְּשׁוּבוֹ אֶל מְעוֹנָיִךְ.

<table>
<tr><td>

requires to be set aside. God wanted the inhabitants of Jericho to be aware of their city's status, so He gave them the ability to hear and smell things from Jerusalem which was many miles away.

בְּנֵי מַעֲמָד — *The maamad delegation.* The Mishnah explains that all the priests and the Levites were divided into twenty-four separate groups called *mishmaros* (watches; see commentary to *kinnah* 10) and each one served in the Temple for two weeks of the year and on the festivals. Corresponding to these *mishmaros*, all of the Israelites were divided into twenty-four groups. The Mishnah teaches: These are the *maamados.* Since the Torah states: *Command*

</td><td>

the Children of Israel and say to them, 'My sacrifice, My bread' (Numbers 28:2). Now, a person's sacrifice cannot be offered if he is not present. [So we require that all of Israel be represented in the sacrificial procedure.] Therefore, the early prophets (Samuel and David) instituted twenty-four *mishmaros* (of Priests and Levites). Corresponding to every single *mishmar* there was a *maamad* in Jerusalem of *Kohanim,* Levites and Israelites. When the time came for the *mishmar* to ascend, the *Kohanim* and Levites ascended to Jerusalem while the Israelites assigned to that *mishmar* would assemble in their own (specially designated) cities and read sections from the Story of Creation (in

</td></tr>
</table>

Facing them were the members of the maamad delegation*
  offering their prayers; and to [you,] your [pilgrim] masses
  ascended at every pilgrimage season.
Within you were the prophets, those who were privy
  to the secrets of God,[1]
  and within you were the experts of intercalation,
  together with your seventy elders.
Your land was permeated with holiness,
  with ten levels of sanctity;*
  tithes and priest's due were brought from your land,
  from the choicest of your grains.
But now you lie desolate, bereft of sons and daughters;
  and where are your kings, your prophets,
  your Levites and your priests?
O when will they return [from exile] and enter your tents,
  those who yearn to dwell under your [sheltering] clouds?
(Would that He allowed me to bear children,
  as [in the days of] Shifra and Puah,
  the midwives at the birthstone.[2]
For this I yearn, the day that your bridegroom will arrive,
  and you, the bride,
  will adorn yourself in jeweled ornaments.)[3]
My heart pines to embrace with my arms
  the very dust of your Land,
  and my passion is to kiss your stones with my mouth!
Would that I shall see you when you will be rebuilt
  with gemstones and jewels, when your lofty corner stones
  will be visible from north and west.
I yearn and languish for consolation.
  O that the loud proclamation of the herald [of redemption]
  be heard in my ears and yours!
Wake up[4] to greet your beloved!
  Shake yourself from the dust of the ground,[5]
  when He [God] returns to your palace!

---

(1) Cf. *Amos* 3:7. (2) Cf. *Exodus* 1:15-16. (3) Some editions omit
the two stanzas in parentheses. (4) *Isaiah* 51:17. (5) Cf. 52:2.

---

the Book of *Genesis*). Also, the men of the
maamad would fast four days a week, from
Monday through Thursday (*Taanis* 26a).

עֲשֶׂר קְדֻשּׁוֹת — *Ten levels of sanctity.* The
Mishnah teaches that in the dimension of space
there are ten levels of sanctity and enumerates
them in ascending order: (1) [The Land of Israel

and] its walled cities; (2) the area enclosed
within the walls of Jerusalem; (3) the Temple
Mount; (4) the enclosed area in front of the
Temple Courtyard; (5) the Women's Courtyard;
(6) the Israelites' courtyard; (7) the *Kohanim's*
Courtyard; (8) the area between the Altar and
the Sanctuary; (9) the great *Heichal* hall; and
(10) the Holy of Holies.

לט.

צִיּוֹן תְּקוֹנְנִי* עֲלֵי בֵיתֵךְ אֲשֶׁר נִשְׂרַף,

צָרְחִי בְּמֶרֶד עֲלֵי שִׁמְמוֹת גְּפָנֶיךָ.*

צִיּוֹן תְּעוֹרְרִי כְּאַלְמָנָה אֲשֶׁר הָיְתָה לָמַס[1]

לְכָל עוֹבְרִים מֵרֹב עֲוֹנֶיךָ.

עַל הַגְּבָעוֹת שְׂאִי קִינָה וְתַמְרוּר,

וְגַם נְהִי בְּקוֹל רָם אֲשֶׁר הִכּוּ הֲמוֹנֶיךָ.

אֵיכָה לְמוֹאָב בְּנֵי צִיּוֹן בְּאַף חָלְלוּ

עַל רֹב גְּאוֹנֶךְ, וְקִרְאִי אֶל מְקוֹנְנֶיךָ.

הֵילֵל וְקִינָה שְׂאִי צִיּוֹן בְּמַר וּנְהִי,

וּבְכִי שְׁמָמוֹת עֲלֵי שִׁמְמוֹת מְעוֹנֶיךָ.

קוֹנְנִי וְאַל תִּדְמִי קוֹלֵךְ בְּבִכְיֵי שְׂאִי,

דֶּבֶר וְחֶרֶב אֲשֶׁר שֻׁלַּח לְמַחֲנֶיךָ.

צָדוּ כְּצִפּוֹר[2] וְאֵין עוֹזֵר לְנֶגְדּוֹ,

אֲשֶׁר פָּרְשׂוּ רְשָׁתוֹת[3] לִגְלוֹת אֶת קְלוֹנֶיךָ.

וְאֵיךְ הִשְׁלִיךְ תִּפְאֶרֶת יִשְׂרָאֵל,[4]

וְלֹא זָכַר שְׁבוּעָה אֲשֶׁר כָּרַת לְאוֹמְנֶיךָ.

קוֹלֵךְ כְּקוֹל נַהֲמַת תַּנִּים,[5]

נְאוֹת יַעֲקֹב[6] בְּכִי וְקִינָה שְׂאִי, עַל רֹב תְּלוּנֶיךָ.

גַּזִּי נִזְרֵךְ וְהַשְׁלִיכִי[7] לְרֹאשֵׁךְ עֲלֵי אֶרֶץ,

וְשַׂק תִּקְשְׁרִי עָצְרֵי בְּמָתְנֶיךָ.

קוֹנְנִי בְּפֶשַׁע, וְאַל תִּתְּנִי מְנוּחָה וְקוֹנְנֵךְ אֶל שְׁפָיִם,[7]

שְׂאִי מֵרֹב מְעָנֶיךָ.

אֶרֶץ צְבִי צְבָאוֹת,[8] קִינָה וּנְהִי תְּעוֹרְרִי עַל שְׁפָיִם,

הֲלֹא תַּחַת שְׁשׁוֹנֶיךָ.

צִיּוֹן תְּקוֹנְנִי — *O Zion, lament.* In this *kinnah*, by R' Asher HaKohen, we cry out to Zion herself and implore her to weep and to wail over her own destruction, at the hand of the barbaric enemy which trampled over every one of Zion's precious treasures. The author concludes with a plea to Zion to approach the graves of the Patriarchs and Matriarchs to beg them to petition God on her behalf.

גְּפָנֶיךָ — *Your vines.* This refers to the Jewish people who are often compared to grapevines. The prophet *Isaiah* (5:1-7) devotes a number of passages to an allegory comparing Israel to a vineyard as does the prophet *Ezekiel* (ch. 15).

The Sages compare Israel to a vine in three respects: (1) The vine is alive, yet it is supported by posts of dead wood; similarly, Israel is bolstered by the merit of its forefathers, who are

39.

צִיּוֹן O Zion, lament* over your house which is burnt,
      cry out bitterly over the ruination of your vines.*
O Zion, intensify your wailing like a [helpless] widow
      who imposes a burden[1] [of charity] on all who pass her by;
      thus shall you weep over your many sins.
On the hills arouse a lamentation and bitterness;
      also moan very loud over your multitudes who were smitten.
Alas! For your sons of Zion are humiliated by Moab's fury
      which was aroused by your outstanding prominence;
      therefore summon those who will recite lamentations for you.
Arouse wailing and lamentation, O Zion,
      with bitterness and moaning, cry incessantly
      until you are devastated over the ruination of your palaces.
Lament and be not silent, raise your voice in weeping
      over the plague and the sword which were
      dispatched against your encampment.
The [enemy] ensnared you like a bird[2]
      and no one came to your assistance against them,
      when they spread out their nets[3] [to capture you]
      and to uncover your shame.
O how did God cast away the majesty of Israel,[4]
      while He failed to remember the oath of covenant
      which He made to [the Patriarchs] who nursed you.
Raise your voice like the howling of the serpents,[5]
      O congregation of Jacob;[6] arouse weeping and lamentation
      [over the tragedy you brought upon yourself]
      because of your many grievances.
Rip off your [crown of flowing] hair and throw[7] your head
      upon the ground; tie on a sackcloth and bind it to your loins.
Lament over the treachery [of your allies who betrayed you]
      and give yourself no rest [from mourning];
      carry your lamentations up to the barren hills[7]
      [and bemoan] the many who oppress you.
O land, desirable even to the host[8] [of gentile nations],
      arouse lamentations and moaning on your barren hills,
      indeed they now replace your former joys!

---

(1) Eichah 1:1. (2) Cf. 3:52. (3) Cf. 1:13. (4) Cf. 2:1. (5) Some editions read יְעֵנִים, ostriches.
(6) Eichah 2:2. (7) Jeremiah 7:29. (8) Cf. 3:19.

---

long dead (Shemos Rabbah 44); (2) If the vine fails to thrive on a given plot of soil, the farmer will uproot it and replant it elsewhere; similarly, if Israel sins in one land, God will uproot them and replant them on foreign soil (ibid.); (3) The grapes of the vine produce both sweet wine and sour vinegar; similarly, the fate of Israel may be sweet or it may be bitter. Under all circum-

קוֹנְנוּ מְלָכִים, וְהֵילִילוּ קְצִינִים

וְכָל יוֹשְׁבֵי מַעֲרָב וּמִזְרָח, עַל שִׁמְלוֹנָיִךְ.

פָּשְׁטוּ מְעִילֵךְ וְהַשְׁלִיכִי לָאָרֶץ,

וְחִגְרִי שַׂק וְגַם תֶּהֱמִי תַּחַת סְדִינָיִךְ.

בָּחוּר וְזָקֵן וְגַם עוֹלֵל וְיוֹנֵק,[1]

שְׂאוּ תַמְרוּר נֶפֶשׁ, לְעֵינֵי כָל זְקֵנָיִךְ.

צִיּוֹן שׁוֹשַׁנֵּךְ[2] הֲלֹא עָבַר כְּקוֹץ עֲלֵי מָיִם,

וְנֶהְפְּכוּ מֵרֹב זְדוֹנָיִךְ.

חָשְׁכוּ מְאוֹרוֹת וְגַם שְׁחָקִים,*

וְכָל דֶּרֶךְ מְלֵא נֶחְשַׁךְ, סָתוּם לְפָנָיִךְ.

כִּי הַשְּׁחָקִים מְאֹד זֹרוּ וְאָסְפוּ לְאוֹרָם,[3]

לִפְנֵי כָל שָׁאוֹן, עַל רֹב יְגוֹנָיִךְ.

צִיּוֹן בְּשׁוֹפָר תְּקַע,[4] עַל הַר וְגֶבַע בְּאִי,

צָרְחִי בְּמַר וּבְכִי, עַל מוֹת שָׂרָנָיִךְ.

שָׁלְחוּ שַׁלֶּךְ בָּאֵשׁ, צִיּוֹן לְמִרְמָס,

הֲלֹא טָבְעוּ שְׁעָרַיִךְ[5] בְּתוֹךְ אֶרֶץ אֲדָנָיִךְ.

הִנֵּה לְמִרְמָס נְתוּנָה בַּת יְהוּדָה,

וְאֵין מֵשִׁיב לְנַפְשָׁהּ,[6] עֲלֵי שִׁמְמוֹת שְׁמָנָיִךְ.

צִיּוֹן בְּמַר תִּבְכִּי מֵאֵין מְנַחֵם,[6]

אֲשֶׁר רָחַק מְאֹד מִקָּרוֹב נַחַם בְּחוּנָיִךְ.

קוֹלֵךְ כְּקוֹל יָם וְגַם תַּנִּין וְיַעֲנָה,[7]

וְקוֹל נְהִי וּבְכִי אֲשֶׁר תַּחַת סָלוֹנָיִךְ.

צִיּוֹן לַמָּרוֹם שְׂאִי עֵינָיִךְ,[8]

וְגַם תִּרְאִי סִפְדִי וְהֵילִילִי, עֲלֵי עָזְבֵךְ תּוֹאֲנָיִךְ.

---

stances, however, Israel blesses God for doing as He sees best (*Vayikra Rabbah* 36).

R' *S. R. Hirsch* (Commentary to *Psalms* 80:9) notes also that of all fruits, only the grape is so crushed and extensively altered from its natural state. But this very abuse serves to transform the grape into something far above what it had been — from an ordinary fruit into valuable, and treasured wine. Ultimately, the finished product, wine, intoxicates and overpowers the one who mangled the grape.

Similarly, Israel in the crucible of exile will eventually overcome their captors and tormentors.

חָשְׁכוּ מְאוֹרוֹת וְגַם שְׁחָקִים — *The celestial luminaries are plagued in darkness together with the dazzling skies.* The *Talmud* teaches in the name of Rav Chisda; since the day that the Holy Temple was destroyed the sky has never appeared in its pure (color) as it says, *I cloak the heavens with blackness, I make sackcloth their covering* (Isaiah 50:3; *Berachos* 59a).

Lament, O kings! Wail, O commanders!
   Together with all who dwell in east and west,
   over the [loss of] your protective cloak [the Temple].
Strip off your tunic and cast it to the ground;
   gird yourself with sackcloth instead of your
   fine linen wraps and continue your moaning.
Youth and elder, and also infant and suckling,[1]
   express the bitterness of your soul
   in the presence of all of your elders.
O Zion, your rose[2] has departed like a thorn in the water,
   so have you been transformed by
   the enormity of your wanton deeds.
The celestial luminaries are plunged in darkness together
   with the [once-dazzling] skies* and every path
   is shrouded in deep darkness and sealed off before you.
For the heavens are deeply alienated [from mankind],
   and therefore hold back their light[3]
   from the masses of nations
   as they [the skies] commiserate with your tremendous grief.
O Zion, sound the shofar's blast![4]
   Roll in the filth on mountain and hill!
   Scream bitterly and weep over the death of your leaders.
They cast your spoils into the fire and Zion to be trampled,
   indeed your gates sank[5] into the ground
   together with your foundations.
Behold, the beloved daughter of Judah [the city of Jerusalem]
   has been given over to be trampled.
   There is no one to restore her spirits[6]
   [from the shock] of the destruction of your finest inhabitants.
O Zion, weep bitterly!
   For there is none to offer you consolation;[6]
   He Who once was close is now much too distant
   to give comfort to [the Jews] who were so sorely tested.
Raise your [wailing] voice as loud as the raging sea,
   as loud as the cry of the serpent and the ostrich;[7]
   raise your voice in moaning and weeping
   like someone lying under your thorn[-like captors].
O Zion, raise your eyes on high and see [God's glory];[8]
   mourn and wail over your betrayal of your [God,]
   the First Cause [of the creation].

---

(1) Cf. *Deut.* 32:25. (2) Some editions read שְׂשׂוֹנֵךְ, *your joy.* (3) Cf. *Joel* 2:10.
(4) Cf. 2:15. (5) Cf. *Eichah* 2:9. (6) Cf. 1:16. (7) Cf. *Micah* 1:8. (8) Cf. *Isaiah* 40:26.

צִיּוֹן תְּקוֹנְנִי עֲלֵי אָבוֹת וְשַׁאֲלִי מְכוֹן בֵּיתֵךְ,

וְגַם עֶזְרֵךְ, חֹסֶן קְצִינָיִךְ.

אֶל הַמְּעָרָה לְכִי, צָרְחִי בְּמַר וּבְכִי,

עֲנוּ בָנַיִךְ וּבְנוֹתַיִךְ וְנִינָיִךְ.

שָׂרָה כְּשָׁמְעָה לְקוֹלֵךְ, גַּם מְבַכָּה עֲלֵי בָנִים,

אֲשֶׁר נִשְׁבּוּ אֶל כָּל שְׁכֵנָיִךְ.

רָחֵל וְלֵאָה* בָּכוּ, בִּלְהָה וְזִלְפָּה הֲלֹא קוֹנְנוּ,

וְקָרְאוּ בְּקוֹל, מְחִי בִּפְנָיִךְ.

כִּי הָאֱלֹהִים הֲלֹא לָנֶצַח וְלֹא יִזְנַח,[1]

כִּי תִקְוָה הִיא וְרֹב שָׁלוֹם לְבָנָיִךְ.[2]

רָחֵל וְלֵאָה — *Rachel and Leah.* When the Temple was destroyed, even the merit of the Patriarchs and the Matriarchs was not enough to prevent it. However, the arguments and pleas of the Matriarch Rachel did elicit from God a solemn pledge that the exiles of Israel would someday return. The Midrash (*Pesichta* to *Eichah Rabbasi* §24) records the logical argument which Rachel put before God: 'You know that your servant Jacob loved me intensely and worked for seven

hard years to earn my hand in marriage. But at the end of the seven long years of waiting, my father Laban wanted me to give up my rights to my beloved Jacob in favor of my older sister Leah. My heart ached, but I didn't want my sister to be humiliated. I suppressed all of my tender feelings and emotions and revealed to Leah all the secret identification signs that Jacob and I had agreed upon as guarantees that my father Laban would not trick him. Moreover, on

O Zion, lament to the Patriarchs [to seek]
*   for the reestablishment of your House,*
*   for He is your Helper, the One Who strengthens your leaders.*
א *Go to the Cave [of Machpelah], scream bitterly and cry*
*   [to the Patriarchs], because [the enemy] has tormented*
*   their sons and daughters and the descendants of their line.*
ש *Sarah [our Matriarch], when she hears your voice,*
*   she too will cry for [her] sons who were taken*
*   into captivity amongst all your [hostile] neighbors.*
ר *Rachel and Leah,* you cry too! Bilhah and Zilpah,*
*   surely you must lament! Cry out loud and beat on your faces.*
For indeed, God endures for eternity and He will never [totally]
*   abandon us.[1] Therefore, there surely is hope*
*   for abundant peace for your children.[2]*

---

(1) *Eichah* 3:31. (2) Cf. *Isaiah* 54:13.

the wedding night I hid under the bed and spoke instead of Leah who was together with Jacob, so that he wouldn't recognize her voice and reject her. Now, dear God, see how I acted even though I am a weak mortal of mere flesh and blood. Nevertheless, I overcame my inclination to be jealous of my rival, my sister. Certainly, You, O God, who are Infinite and Eternal and filled with compassion, can forgive my children, the Children of Israel, and not be jealous of the idols they worshiped instead of worshiping You!'

מ.

צִיּוֹן יְדִידוּת יְדִיד* צָעִיר לְשָׁרֶיךָ,¹

שָׁכַנְתְּ כְּתֵפָיו*² בְּרֹב עֲנוֹת הֲדָרֶיךָ.

צִיּוֹן הֲדַר כָּל חֲדַר מִטּוֹת,

וְכָל מִשְׁכַּב דּוֹדִים יְדִידֶךְ בְּבֹא חַדְרֵי חֲדָרֶיךָ.

צִיּוֹן בְּרוּכָה בְּרָכָה עֶלְיוֹנָה עֲלֵי רֹאשֶׁךְ,

לְמוֹלֵךְ מְחַטְּבִים שְׁעָרֶיךָ.

צִיּוֹן יְרֻשַּׁת זְאֵב עֶרֶב,³

שְׁבִי פְאֵרֵךְ בַּעֲדִי עֲדָיִים,⁴ עֲדִי עָלוּ כְתָרֶיךָ.

יָפִית בְּרֹב הוֹן וְהֵן רָבִית בְּדֵעוֹת,

וְהֵן מִזִּקְנֵי צוֹעֲנִים, חָכְמוּ נְעָרֶיךָ.

הָיִית יְפֵה מִכְלָל,⁵ נָאוָה בְּכָל מַהֲלָל,

עָלִית וְשָׁבִית שְׁלָל, מַלְכֵי מְגוּרָרֶיךָ.

בָּךְ בִּרְוָחָה אֱנוֹשׁ לָן* מִבְּלִי חֵטְא,

בָּךְ כֻּפַּר בְּקָרְבַּן תָּמִיד מְכַפָּרֶיךָ.

---

(1) Cf. *Psalms* 68:28. (2) Cf. *Deuteronomy* 33:12. (3) *Genesis* 49:27. (4) *Ezekiel* 16:7. (5) *Psalms* 50:2.

◆§ **צִיּוֹן יְדִידוּת יְדִיד** — *O Zion, . . . the Beloved's beloved.* Again we have a composition that sings the praises of Jerusalem and Zion, this time emphasizing the idea that the Temple was constructed on the territory of Benjamin, the youngest of Jacob's sons. The Second Temple was destroyed because of the senseless hatred which divided one Jew from another. This lack of brotherhood had its roots in the hatred displayed by Jacobs' sons for their brother Joseph, many centuries earlier. The only one of the twelve brothers who had nothing to do with this bitter feud was young Benjamin, and for this reason he was especially beloved to God. And for this reason the Temple, a symbol of national unity and brotherhood, was built in Benjamin's province.

Moreover, the Second Temple was destroyed by the Romans who were descendants of Esau. When Jacob encountered Esau with his entire family, Jacob, his wives, and his sons all bowed before Esau. Only Benjamin who was not born yet did not bow. Therefore, the Temple was built in Benjamin's portion so that it would not bend before Esau's onslaught.

Nevertheless, Israel's sins were so great that none of these merits could protect Zion and the Temple, when God's fury was aroused and the awesome day of reckoning arrived.

The composer of this *kinnah* is the otherwise unknown R' Yaakov.

יְדִידוּת יְדִיד — *The Beloved's beloved.* The Talmud (*Menachos* 53a) teaches that when the *Beis HaMikdash* was to be built, God said: 'Let the יְדִיד, *beloved*, son of the יְדִיד, come and build the יְדִיד for the יְדִיד in the portion of the יְדִיד, in order to bring atonement for the יְדִידִים.' This means: Let Solomon, who is called יְדִיד (*II Samuel* 12:24) the son, [i.e., descendant] of Abraham who is called יְדִיד (*Jeremiah* 11:15), come and build the *Beis HaMikdash* which is called יְדִיד (*Psalms* 84:2), for the Holy One, Blessed is He, Who is called יְדִיד (*Isaiah* 5:1), in the portion of Benjamin who is called יְדִיד (*Deuteronomy* 33:12), to bring atonement for Israel who are called יְדִידִים (*Jeremiah* 12:7).

From the first moment when God began His creation, His prime desire was to establish a place which would allow Him to dwell in the midst of His creatures on earth: The Temple is His *beloved*, therefore, because it is, so to speak, the culmination of God's aspirations (*Alshich*).

שָׁכַנְתְּ כְּתֵפָיו — *You [God] rest unobtrusively between his shoulders.* Moses gave his final blessing to the tribes of Israel. *Of Benjamin he said: 'May Hashem's beloved dwell securely by Him; He hovers above him all day long; and rests His Presence between his shoulders* (*Deuteronomy* 33:12). The Talmud (*Zevachim* 118b) explains that in this world God's presence was not permanently entrenched over the Temple, but in the future Third Temple of the Messianic Era,

40.

צִיּוֹן   O Zion, [Your Temple is] the Beloved's* beloved
          [because it is situated in the territory of Benjamin]
       the youngest of your [tribal] princes;[1] You [God]
       rest unobtrusively between his shoulders[2]*
       because your extreme humility is your greatest splendor.
O Zion, your splendor is that you are called 'the chamber of couches'
       [for God's Divine Presence rests within you],
       and when your beloved people [Israel]
       enter your inner chambers it is there
       that they rest in strong embrace [with God].
O Zion, you are blessed with the supreme celestial blessings
       which descend upon your head, for the heavenly gates
       are carved to be directly facing you.
O Zion, you are the heir [of Benjamin who is likened to]
       the wolf who hunts at dusk,[3]* your majestic tiara
       is encrusted with rows upon rows of gems,[4]
       but your [spiritual] crowns [of Torah, priesthood
       and monarchy] far surpass all jeweled adornment.
You are beautified by your abundant wealth,
       but even more so are you enriched by your vast wisdom,
       because even your youths are far wiser
       than the venerable elders of Tzoan [Egypt].
You were the consummation of beauty,[5]
       so lovely that you were worthy of every form of praise;
       you overwhelmed and captivated the kings
       who dwelled all around you.
Those who lodged within you found ample space*
       and were absolved from every sin, for the daily
       Tamid sacrifices atoned for the sins
       of all who required forgiveness.

God will dwell permanently and securely between the shoulders of Benjamin. Indeed, the
Holy Spirit of God dwelled among the Israelites
in three places and all three were in Benjamin's
territory. First the Tabernacle was in Shiloh, then
in Nob and Gibeon, and finally the Temple was
built in Jerusalem on the land belonging not to
Judah, but to the tribe of Benjamin. The Talmud
(Yoma 12a) explains that more than any other
tribe, Benjamin pined and yearned to host the
Divine Presence in his territory and therefore he
was granted his fervent wish. Elsewhere, the
Talmud (Sotah 38a) says that at the Sea of Reeds
the tribe of Benjamin displayed extraordinary
faith and devotion to God. Even before the
raging seawaters split, the Benjaminites eagerly
jumped into the sea in response to God's
command and in this merit the Divine Presence
dwelled in their midst. Finally, Sifri observes that
Benjamin's advantage was that he was the only

one of Jacob's sons born on the holy soil of Eretz
Yisrael and therefore merited to host God's holy
Shechinah.

וְאָב עֶרֶב — [Benjamin . . .] the wolf who hunts at
dusk. In Jacob's blessing to his son Benjamin, he
said: Benjamin is a predatory wolf; in the
morning he will devour prey and in the evening
he will distribute spoils (Genesis 49:2). According to Targum Onkelos this means that Benjamin
hungered for the Divine Presence as a wolf
hungers for its prey. Therefore the Temple, in
which the Kohanim offered sacrifices each morning and divided the remaining sacred portions in
the evening, stood in his territory.

בָּךְ בִּרְוָחָה אֱנוֹשׁ לָן — Those lodged within you
found ample space. The Mishnah (Avos 5:7) lists
ten miracles that were performed for our ancestors in the Holy Temple. One was that no man
ever said to his fellow, 'The space is insufficient

יְסַדְתָּ בְזִיו לְפָאֵר, חָרַבְתָּ בְּתוֹךְ אָב

בְּאַף אֶשַׁאף לְזֹאת אֶשְׁאַב, מִימֵי תַמְרוּרֶיךָ.

נִרְאוּ בְעִירֶךָ פְּנֵי קוֹנֶה,

בְּנֵי מַחֲנֶה רְצוֹן לְשׁוֹכְנִי סְנֶה,¹ בִּשְׁנֵי חֲצֵרֶיךָ.

עוֹשֵׂי מְלַאכְתֶּךָ בְּחוּט,

הִתְעַשְּׁרוּ בִּרְכוּשׁ כָּל הוֹן יָקָר נִמְצָא, לִקְהַל עֲשִׁירֶיךָ.

נִבְחַר מְקוֹמֶךָ לְצוּר בָּחַר בְּאֹם בְּחוּרָיו,

בָּחַר בְּמוֹצָאֶךָ, וּבַכֹּהֲנִים בְּחִירֶיךָ.²

בָּךְ דָּר בְּגִיל נֶהְדָּר, אַדְרֶךָ בְּכָל דּוֹר וָדוֹר,

עֶרְכֶּךָ בְּבֹא לַעֲדוֹר, עֶדְרֵי חֲבֵרֶיךָ.³

עָלָה גְבוּלֶךְ⁴ דְּבִיר צֶלַע יְבוּס,

לֹא לְעֵין עֵיטָם, לְבִלְתִּי שְׂאֵת כַּתְּפוֹת דְּבִירֶיךָ.

קָרָא יהוה שְׁמֶךָ עַל שֵׁם שְׁנֵי כֹהֲנִים,*

דָּוִד מְצָאֶךָ בְּחִיל בִּשְׂדֵי יְעָרֶיךָ.⁵

בָּנָה מְעוֹנֶךָ בְּנוֹ, וַיְחַנְּכֶךָ שֵׁם בְּשֵׁם אָבִיו אֲשֶׁר קִדְּמוֹ,

נֶחְתַּם בְּשִׁירֶיךָ.⁶

וּבְמַחְשְׁבוֹת בּוֹרְאָךְ עָלִית, בְּטֶרֶם בְּרֹא תֵבֵל,

וְשָׂחַק וְעוֹלָם* עַל עֲפָרֶיךָ.

וּבְמֵי מְרִיבָה בְּיוֹם זַעַם, אֲזַי טָהֲרָה אַרְצֶךָ,

וְלֹא גֻשְׁמָה⁷* בְּכָלוֹת יְצוּרֶיךָ.

יָרַד בְּעִתּוֹ מְטַר אַרְצֶךָ, זְמָן לַיְלָה בָּא לִבְרָכָה,

וְטַל לָן בִּקְצִירֶיךָ.

---

for me to stay overnight in Jerusalem,' i.e., despite the multitudes convening in Jerusalem for the festivals, there were sufficient accommodations for them all. Moreover, because of the sanctity of the city, God provided for all residents of Jerusalem, so that no one ever had to move to another city to seek a livelihood.

קָרָא ה' שְׁמֶךָ עַל שֵׁם שְׁנֵי כֹהֲנִים — HASHEM gave you the name [Jerusalem] based on the names [you were called] by the two priests [Shem and Abraham]. The Midrash (Bereishis Rabbah 5:1) notes that after the Akeidah, we read that Abraham named that site 'HASHEM Yireh [Hashem will see]' (Genesis 22:14), and earlier we read that Shem the son of Noah greeted Abraham in his role as Malchizedek, King of Shalem (Genesis 14:18). Both men were in the same

location and gave it different names reflecting different aspects of the unique sanctity of the holy mountain. Thus, God made a synthesis of Yireh and Shalem and called the city Yerushalem [יִרְאֶה שָׁלֵם = יְרוּשָׁלֵם = יְרוּשָׁלַיִם].

בְּטֶרֶם בְּרֹא תֵבֵל וְשַׂחַק וְעוֹלָם — Even before He created earth, heaven and the universe. The Talmud lists seven things that were created before the world itself: the Torah, the concept of teshuvah, Gan Eden, Gehinnom, the Throne of Glory, the Beis HaMikdash, and the name of the Messiah (Pesachim 54a)

אֲזַי טָהֲרָה אַרְצֶךָ וְלֹא גֻשְׁמָה — Only your land was deemed to be pure and was not rained upon. According to one view in the Talmud, the waters of Noah's Flood did not enter the area that was to become the Land of Israel (Zevachim 113a).

You were established in the bright [spring month of Iyar]
   to be a splendor, and you were destroyed with fury
   in the month of Av; therefore I gasp thirstily
   and drink deeply of your bitter waters.
The children of your camp [the Israelites] appeared
   in your city to be in the presence of your Maker;
   they entered the two courtyards [of the Temple]
   in order to find favor [in the eyes of] the One
   Who dwelt in the Burning Bush.[1]
Even those who worked for you [in the Temple]
   with the [weaver's] thread were enriched
   with many possessions, and every precious treasure
   was available for your community of prosperous people.
Your site was chosen for the One called 'the Rock',
   He selected the 'Chosen Ones' [Israel] for His Nation;
   He designated [David] whom He found [secluded with the sheep,
   to be His king], and for His priests He chose the finest
   [the seed of Aaron].[2]
Within you dwelt the One Who is majestic in joy,
   He remained your splendor for generation after generation;
   but your true value will be revealed when the flocks
   of your beloved [Israel] return to your fold.[3]
The borders of your Divine Residence ascended[4]
   only upward from the slopes of Yevus, but ultimately
   [the Temple was not built on the highest point called]
   the Fountain of Eitam so that the shoulders
   of your Divine Residence should not soar too high.
HASHEM gave you the name [Jerusalem],
   based on the names [you were called]
   by the two priests [Shem and Abraham].*
   David discovered you to be encircled [by mountains],
   in your forest fields.[5]
His son [King Solomon] built your palace [the Temple]
   and he dedicated it with the name of his father
   [David] who preceded him [and built the Temple's foundation]
   as is sealed in the inscription of your songs.[6]
You were conceived in the thoughts of your Creator even before
   He created earth, heaven and the universe* from your dust.
And on the day of wrath [at the time of the Flood] by the waters
   of strife, only your land was deemed to be pure and was not
   rained upon,[7]* while the [rest of God's creations] ceased to be.
The rain of your land descended in its proper time,
   it even fell at night [not to disturb wayfarers] as a blessing,
   and the dew came to rest [gently] on your harvests.

---

(1) Cf. *Deuteronomy* 33:16. (2) Cf. *I Samuel* 2:28. (3) Cf. *Song of Songs* 1:7.
(4) Cf. *Joshua* 15:8,9. (5) *Psalms* 132:6. (6) See *Psalms* 30:1. (7) Cf. *Ezekiel* 22:24.

הָיִיתָ לְשִׁית חוּג יְסוֹד, מִמֵּךְ תְּעוּדָה'

וְסוֹד קְדוּשׁ יַרְחֵךְ לְפִי עֵדִים מְעַבְּרָיִךְ.

בָּנִים וּבָנוֹת תְּשׁוּקָה, בַּשּׁוּק שׁוֹקְקוּ,

שָׂחֲקוּ וְהִשְׁתַּקְשְׁקוּ בַּסָךְ עוֹבְרָיִךְ.

בְּחַג פֶּסַח נִפְלָאוּ, פוּרִים בַּפָּז סֻלָּאוּ,²

טַל אוֹר וְחֵן נִמְלָאוּ, זַכּוּ נְזִירָיִךְ.³

אֵיךְ אֶשְׂמְחָה עוֹד בְּחַג, אֵיךְ אֶעֱלוֹז עוֹד בְּפוּר,

עַד כִּי יְבוֹאוּן, יְמֵי שָׂשׂוֹן לְפוּרָיִךְ.

אַרְצֵךְ חֲמוּדָה⁴ מְאֹד לֹא נֶחְמָדָה,⁵

בַּעֲלוֹת בָּנִים חֲמוּדִים, לְבֵית מַחְמַד מְגוּרָיִךְ.

נַעֲלָה עֲנַן הַקְּטְרֶת, מִמְּקוֹם מִקְדָּשׁ יָצָא מְקוֹמוֹ,

עָשַׁן אֵשׁ מִנְּדִחָיִךְ.

בִּקְרוֹב מְרֵעִים בָּעִיר,⁶ שִׁלְּחוּ בְכַרְמֵךְ בְּעִיר,⁷

עָרוּ וְעוֹרְרוּ,⁸ בְּעִיר וְקַדִּישׁ⁹ בְּעָרָיִךְ.

בַּרְזֶל בְּלִי נִשְׁמַע קוֹלוֹ¹⁰ בְּעֵת נִבְנֵית,*

אֵיךְ חַרְבוֹת צוּרִים, בָּךְ תָּקְעוּ מְצִירָיִךְ.

עַל זֹאת בַּשַּׂק עוֹבְרִים עֲבָרִים,

אֲבָל בּוֹטְחִים כִּי יִשְׂמְחוּ אַחֲרֵי חָתוּךְ בְּתָרָיִךְ.¹¹

לֵב מַדְוֶה יֶחֱלֶה, לְתַאֲוָה יִכְלֶה.

יִישַׁן עֲדֵי יַעֲלֶה, עַמּוּד שְׁחָרָיִךְ.

יְלֵל לְקוֹלִי, אֵלִי אֵיךְ תִּתְאַפָּקִי,

הֲלֹא קָרָא לְשַׂק וּבְכִי,¹² אַלּוּף נְעוּרָיִךְ.¹³

אָקוּם חֲצוֹת לַיְלָה,¹⁴ עַל מִשְׁמָרוֹת מַאֲפָל,

לִשְׁמוֹר לָאוֹר יֶאֱתֶה בְקֶר¹⁵ לְשַׁמְּרָיִךְ.

---

(1) Cf. *Micah* 4:2. (2) Cf. *Eichah* 4:2. (3) Cf. 4:7. (4) Cf. *Jeremiah* 3:19. (5) Cf. *Exodus* 34:24. (6) Cf. *Psalms* 27:2. (7) Cf. *Exodus* 22:4. (8) Cf. *Psalms* 137:7. (9) *Daniel* 4:10. (10) *I Kings* 6:7. (11) Some editions read הַתּוֹר בְּתוֹרָיִךְ, *the turtledove [which was not severed] is your portion,* a reference to the Covenant Between the Parts (*Genesis* 15:9-10 with *Rashi*); some read הַתּוֹר בְּשׁוֹרָיִךְ, *the guide [i.e., the herald] will inform you [of the Messiah's arrival].* (12) Cf. *Isaiah* 22:12. (13) Cf. *Jeremiah* 3:4. (14) Cf. *Psalms* 119:62. (15) Cf. *Isaiah* 21:12.

בַּרְזֶל בְּלִי נִשְׁמַע קוֹלוֹ בְּעֵת נִבְנֵית — *The sound of iron [tools] was not heard while you were under construction.* When Solomon constructed the First Temple, it is stated: *And the House, when it was being constructed, was built of stone finished at the quarry, and there was neither hammer, nor axe, nor any tool of iron heard in the House while*

it was under construction (I Kings 6:7). Rashi and *Radak* (based on *Sotah* 48b and *Gittin* 68a) explain that the stones for the Temple were hewn by a small, soft worm called שָׁמִיר, *shamir,* which has the amazing ability to cut through the hardest stones. The *shamir* was the size of a barleycorn and it was kept in a hollow lead pipe

You were the location of the Foundation Stone upon which
  the universe was established; from you went forth
  the [Torah] tradition.[1] The sanctification of the New Moon
  and the complexities of intercalation were determined
  [by the testimony] of your witnesses.
Darling sons and daughters merrily romped around the marketplace
  [bustling with pilgrims who journeyed there], they played
  amidst the clatter [of horses' hooves] and the [creaking of
  the] covered wagons of your [pilgrimage] travelers.
They displayed outstanding dedication [in braving the elements]
  to arrive for the Pesach celebration; from the Purim season
  they were already adorned with the finest of gold decoration;[2]
  thus dew and light and grace permeated them
  and purified your coronated people.[3]
O how can I rejoice any more on the festivals
  and how can I make merry on Purim day,
  until once again days of joy will return to your lot?
Although your land was most covetable,[4]
  [none dared] to usurp it [in the owner's absence
  during the festivals[5] when [your] coveted sons ascended
  to the coveted House where you took up residence.
The cloud of incense which once arose from your Holy Temple
  has now departed, in its place a furious flame
  smokes from your nostrils.
When evildoers approached the city,[6] they unleashed animals
  into your vineyards,[7] they aggravated and chased[8]
  the Alert Holy One[9] from your City.
The sound of iron [tools] was not heard[10]
  while you were under construction,*
  [for the wondrous shamir worm hewed your stones],
  how then were your tormentors allowed
  to pierce you with their sharpened swords?
For this, the Hebrews wander about in sackcloth;
  yet they maintain their firm faith that they are destined
  to rejoice when they see the one who decimated you cut down.[11]
The aching heart grows very sick,
  it pines away in [its] yearning,
  [therefore] it sinks into deep sleep
  until the breaking of your [Messianic] dawn.
[O all who hear] my voice, wail with me. How then [O Zion]
  can you restrain yourself? Has not the Mentor of your youth[12]
  ordained this day [Tishah B'Av] for sackcloth and crying?[13]
I will arise at midnight[14] during the gloomiest of the nightwatches,
  to keep vigil for the light which will arrive in the morning[15]
  for those who await you.

אָז תִּמְצָאִי צוּף דְּבַשׁ,[1] אָז לֹא תְקוֹנְנִי בְּרֹאשׁ,

כִּי תִתְכּוֹנְנִי בְּרֹאשׁ הָרִים הֲרָרָיִךְ.

יָבֹא כְּבוֹד הַלְּבָנוֹן לָךְ,[2]

וְתִתְלַבְּנִי כִּבְנֵי עֲדָרִים, בְּנֵי אָדָר גְּדָרָיִךְ.

עוּרִי וְהִתְנַעֲרִי[3] עֶרֶךְ יַעַר נוֹעָרִים,

נַעַר יָתָו אוֹת, לְעֵץ יַעַר[4] חֲזִירָיִךְ.[5]

(קוּמִי וְאוֹרִי לְכָל חוֹשְׁקֵי מְאוֹרֵךְ,

וְהֵם הוֹלְכֵי בְחוֹשֶׁךְ עֲדֵי אוֹרוֹ מְאוֹרָיִךְ.)[6]

צִיּוּן לְצִיּוּן נָאוֹת, עַז עוֹד תְּהִי וּלְנֵס עַמִּים,[7]

וְתִגְבְּהֶנָה רַגְלֵי מְבַשְּׂרָיִךְ.[8]

נַצְּלִי עֲדִי הֶעָנִי, וּתְנִי לְבוּשֵׁךְ שָׁנִי,

תּוֹלָעַ[9] כְּכַלָּה עֲדִי, לְקַשּׁוּר קִשּׁוּרָיִךְ.

אַל תֹּאמְרִי לִי, אֲשֶׁר זָקַנְתְּ הֱיוֹתֵךְ לְאִישׁ,[10]

עוֹד תִּתְעַדְּנִי חֲלוֹץ הַשַּׁד לְגוּרָיִךְ.[11]

תֵּלְדִי בְּנֵי שַׁעֲשׁוּעַיִךְ בְּעֵת עֶדְנָה,

תִּתְחַדְּשִׁי בִנְעוּרִים כַּנְּשָׁרָיִךְ.[12]

יַטֶּה לְטוֹב יִצְרֵךְ צוּר יוֹצְרֵךְ יְצָרֵךְ,

תְּהִי נְצוּרָה, כְּעִיר חֶבְרָה[13] לְמוֹרָיִךְ.

יִגְאַל בְּעֹז מִשְּׁבִי, לְהָשִׁיב לְאֶרֶץ הַצְּבִי,

וִיהִי עֲטֶרֶת צְבִי[14] לִשְׁאָר עֲדָרָיִךְ.

---

filled with rags and bran flour. This remarkable creature could split an entire mountain in half. Moses used it to cut the gemstones on the High Priest's breastplate and it was brought to Solomon from the Garden of Eden by an eagle (see also *Midrash Shocher Tov*).

Then you will discover [a contentment] as sweet as dripping honey,[1]
   no longer will you lament with [wormwood and] gall,
   for you will be firmly established on the summit
   of your foremost mountains.
י The glory of Lebanon shall return to you,[2]
   and you will be whitened as a flock.
   O children of [the Patriarchs who are] your [protective] walls.
ע Awaken [O Zion] and shake your dust,[3]
   you who are now like a forest stripped of its leaves;
   [in the future] a little child who can pen
   no more than one stroke [will be able to record
   the minuscule number of] your boarish enemies,[5]
   who will be] like a lone tree in the forest.[4]
(קב Arise and give light for all who seek your light,
   for they go in darkness, until your light will shine.)[6]
O Zion, you are destined to be an outstanding landmark
   and a signpost [of Divinity to the world];
   you will yet be a tower of strength and a banner unto the nations;[7]
   and the footsteps of your heralds will be lifted on high.[8]
Remove the rags of your poverty and don your robes of scarlet,
   swathe yourself in crimson[9] like a bride
   and bedeck yourself with ornaments.
Do not say to me that you are too old to have a husband,[10]
   for you will be rejuvenated and you will nurture your cubs.[11]
You will bear the children of your delight
   when you return to delicate smoothness,
   and you will renew your youth as do the eagles.[12]
The Creator, who fashioned all the inclinations
   of our impulsive nature, will incline your desires exclusively
   for the good, and you will be safeguarded [from evil]
   like a [fortified] city; [and you will be] bound[13] to your Master.
He [God] will powerfully redeem [you] from captivity,
   to return you to the desirable land,
   and He will be a desirable crown[14] for the remnants of your flock.

---

(1) *Proverbs* 16:24. (2) Cf. *Isaiah* 60:13. (3) Cf. 52:1,2. (4) Cf. 10:19.
(5) *Psalms* 80:14. (6) Some editions omit the stanza in parentheses.
(7) *Isaiah* 11:10. (8) Cf. 52:7. (9) Cf. *Exodus* 25:4. (10) Cf. *Ruth* 1:12.
(11) Cf. *Eichah* 4:3. (12) Cf. *Psalms* 103:5. (13) Cf. 122:3. (14) *Isaiah* 28:5.

מא.

שָׁאֲלִי שְׂרוּפָה בָאֵשׁ,* לִשְׁלוֹם אֲבֵלָיִךְ,
הַמִּתְאַוִּים שְׁכוֹן, בַּחֲצַר זְבוּלָיִךְ.

שָׁאֲלִי שְׂרוּפָה בָאֵשׁ — *O [Torah] by fire consumed, seek . . .* Twenty-four cartloads of the Talmud and its commentaries were publicly burned in the streets of Paris, France in the year 1242. The events leading to this tragedy give us a glimpse of the terrible persecution which hounded our ancestors in those dark times.

The French king, Louis IX (1226-1270), was a fanatical religious zealot, so much so, in fact, that he earned himself the title of Saint Louis. His piety, however, did not extend to his Jewish subjects, against whom he enacted many harsh and discriminatory laws. The king's pious zeal manifested itself most clearly in the favor he extended to apostates who abandoned Judaism. To encourage conversion, the king himself would often attend their baptisms.

Nicholas Donin of La Rochelle was an apostate who was especially vicious in his hatred for his former co-religionists, and who caused the forced baptism of the Jews of Anjou and Poitiers. Five hundred Jews from these cities surrendered before the threat of death and were baptized, while the majority of Jews, 3,000 martyrs in all, chose to meet their death while sanctifying God's Name.

Donin realized that the bulwark of firm Jewish faith was the holy Talmud, the repository of our traditions and teachings. He felt that if he could destroy the Talmud he could easily eradicate the Jews. To that end, he went to Pope Gregory IX in Rome, where he presented a formal accusation against the Talmud. He charged that it contained blasphemies against God and against Christianity, and that it alone was the cause of the Jews' steadfast refusal to accept the 'true' faith.

The Pope issued orders for a seizure of all copies of the Talmud and for a thorough examination and evaluation of its contents. The churchmen of France were only too eager to obey this decree, so on March 3, 1240, while the Jews were in their synagogues, all of their sacred tomes were seized and confiscated. On June 12th of that year a public debate was held in Paris between Donin and four of the most eminent rabbinical authorities in France.

The Jewish deputation was led by R' Yechiel ben Yosef (died 1268) who headed the Yeshiva in Paris. He was the father of Rabbeinu Asher (known as the *Rosh*) and many of the major sages of that period studied under him. These include R' Yitzchok of Corbeil (his son-in-law) and Maharam of Rothenburg.

The other representatives were R' Moshe of Coucy, R' Yehudah ben David of Melun and R' Shmuel ben Shlomo of Falaise.

Although R' Yechiel and his colleagues displayed great scholarship, courage, and dignity in their defense of the Talmud, the official verdict against them was a foregone conclusion. The Talmud would have been immediately consigned to the flames if not for the lone staunch ally the Jews had amongst the churchmen, the bishop of Sens (Shantz), whose arguments and pleas averted any evil decree for one year. At the year's end, while the good bishop was standing in the presence of King Louis, he suddenly convulsed and died in a most grotesque fashion. The anti-Semitic priests convinced the gullible king that this was actually an act of Divine retribution against the bishop for his heresy in defending the blasphemous Talmud. A tribunal of church elders condemned the Talmud to be burnt. Their agents eagerly searched and confiscated over 1200 manuscripts of the Talmud and commentaries. We must bear in mind that this occurred two centuries before the invention of the printing press. Each one of these volumes was a handwritten manuscript which took months, even years to write, at tremendous effort and expense. Moreover, many of the more recent works such as novellae by the *Tosafists* of France and their correspondence and halachic decisions were transcribed only in a limited number of copies and would be lost forever.

R' Yechiel recognized that this tragedy threatened the very survival of the French Jewish community. He therefore recorded the proceedings of his disputation in a work called simply וִיכּוּחַ, [*Vikuach*] *Debate*. In his introduction, paraphrasing the words of Jeremiah (*Eichah* 4:9), he states, כִּי הִנֵּה טוֹבִים חַלְלֵי חֶרֶב מֵהַיּוֹשְׁבִים שׁוֹמֵמִים בְּלִי תוֹרָה, *For those put to death by the sword were better off than those who sat in desolation without Torah.*

In 1242, on Friday, the day before the *Shabbos* when *Parashas Chukas* would be read, twenty-four wagonloads of holy *sefarim* were burnt.

R' Tzidkiyah ben Avrohom HaRofeh, who lived at that time, writes:

From Torah scholars who were involved, we heard that the Rabbis inquired of heaven by means of a dream (שְׁאֵלַת חֲלוֹם), to discover whether this terrible event had been so decreed by the Almighty. The heavenly reply was given in three words: ׳דָּא גְּזֵרַת אוֹרַיְיתָא, *This is the decree of the Torah,'* the Aramaic version of the opening words of that week's Torah reading — (וְאת חֻקַּת הַתּוֹרָה). R' Tzidkiyah further notes that, in commemoration of this tragic event, some pious people customarily fast on Erev Shabbos of *Parashas Chukas* every year (*Shibbolei HaLeket* 263).

The Ashes of the Rambam's Works

R' Hillel of Verona, Italy was an eyewitness to

41.

שַׁאֲלִי O [Torah] by fire consumed, seek* the welfare of your mourners,
of those who yearn to lodge in the courtyard of your dwelling;

these tragic events in Paris. He considered the burning of the Talmud as a clear sign of Divine anger and retribution for the destruction of the works of R' Moshe ben Maimon, known as the *Rambam* (Maimonides).

There were many great scholars, especially in southern France, who did not agree with many of *Rambam's* opinions in his *Moreh Nevuchim* (*Guide for the Perplexed*) and his philosophical observations in the first book of his *Yad HaChazakah* (*Sefer HaMada*). Some went so far as to place a ban on studying or even owning these works. A tremendous controversy erupted and the situation got out of control. The hysteria reached its terrible climax when members of the anti-*Rambam* camp submitted copies of his philosophical writings to the monks of the Dominican Order for the sake of determining whether these works contained heretical ideas.

The Dominicans, of course, swiftly concluded that the *Rambam's* writings were blasphemous and false. They publicly burned all copies of *Moreh Nevuchim* and *Sefer HaMada* that they could lay their hands on. This was done in Montpelier France in 1234. In the year 1242, fanatical churchmen once again burnt the *Rambam's* works in the streets of Paris.

In a letter recording these events, R' Hillel of Verona makes the following observations:

God looked down from heaven and avenged the honor of our holy master, *Rambam*, and his works. He poured His wrath upon the Jewish communities of France. You should not ask in wonderment, 'How did God disregard twelve hundred manuscripts of Talmud and Aggadah and allow them to be burnt as retribution for the *Moreh Nevuchim* and *Sefer HaMada*? Rather, you must bear in mind that R' Moshe ben Maimon was almost second in his generation to Moshe Rabbeinu, and the righteousness of the entire generation depended upon him . . . If you ask; 'Who can be sure that the Talmud was burned because of the burning of the *Rambam's* works?' I will answer you. This is the sign and proof. Take note of this: Not even forty days passed between the conflagration of the works of our master and the burning of the Talmud. On the very spot where the *Rambam's* works were destroyed, the Talmud was later burnt! The ashes of the burnt Talmud mingled with the ashes of the *Rambam's* volumes, for those ashes still remained in that very place. This served as a clear lesson to one and all, Jew and gentile alike.

The destruction of the Talmud was a crushing blow to the venerable and ancient Jewish community of France. It marked the beginning of its very rapid decline and eventual disintegration.

With the conditions of the Jews in France steadily worsening, R' Yechiel emigrated to *Eretz Yisrael* in 1260 together with a large group of French Talmudists. He settled in Acre, where he established the Talmudic academy *Midrash HaGadol d' Paris*. He is believed to have died in 1267.

One of the participants in the great Talmudic debate in Paris, R' Shmuel of Falaise summed up the enormity of the tragedy in the following elegy:

My spirit is gone, my strength is sapped, the light of my eyes has dimmed, because of the tyrant whose hand weighed very heavily upon us, when he seized the core of our soul and the delight of our eyes. Now we have no holy book in which to study and meditate. May the Almighty God avenge His people and may He say to our misery, 'It is enough!' (quoted in *Teshuvos Maharam MiRottenburg* 250).

In 1306, the glorious chapter of Jewish history in medieval France came an abrupt close, when King Philip IV (the Fair) expelled the Jews from all of France. French Jewry, which had enriched our eternal Torah legacy with the magnificent Talmudic commentaries of *Rashi* and *Tosafos*, was no longer.

The Maharam of Rothenburg

The author of this *kinnah* was R' Meir ben Baruch (1220-1293) better known as the Maharam of Rothenburg, who studied in the Yeshivah of Rabbeinu Yechiel of Paris and is said to have personally witnessed the tragic burning of the Talmud in 1242.

Born in Worms, Germany in the year 1220, Maharam first studied under the greatest *Tosafists* of that land including R' Yitzchak (author of *Or Zarua*) in Wurtzberg and R' Yehudah ben Moshe HaKohen of Mainz.

Maharam is considered to be one of the last important *Baalei Tosafos*, but his major contribution to Rabbinic literature was his prolific responsa in all areas of Halachah. Approximately one thousand of Maharam's responsa have been published and his rulings have been accepted by all subsequent generations as the opinion of a leading halachic authority.

From the seat of his rabbinate in Rothenburg, Maharam guided German Jewry throughout the second half of the thirteenth century. However, in his final years, he met with tragedy. The terrible burden of persecution was making life intolerable for the Jews of Germany. Taxation, pogroms, blood libels, harsh decrees — all of these spurred Jews to flee from this miserable exile and to make the arduous journey to *Eretz Yisrael*. Emperor Rudolph I did not wish to lose the Jews from whom he enjoyed extorting so much gold,

הַשּׁוֹאֲפִים בַּעֲפַר אֶרֶץ,[1]* וְהַכּוֹאֲבִים הַמְשׁתּוֹמְמִים,
עֲלֵי מוּקַד גְּלִילָיִךְ.[2]

הוֹלְכִים חֲשֵׁכִים וְאֵין נֹגַהּ,[3] וְקֹוִים לְאוֹר יוֹמָם,
אֲשֶׁר יִזְרַח עֲלֵיהֶם וְעָלָיִךְ.

וּשְׁלוֹם אֱנוֹשׁ נֶאֱנַח בּוֹכֶה בְּלֵב נִשְׁבָּר,
תָּמִיד מְקוֹנֵן עֲלֵי צִירֵי חֲבָלָיִךְ.

וְיִתְאוֹנֵן כַּתַּנִּים וּבְנוֹת יַעֲנָה,
וְיִקְרָא מִסְפֵּד מַר בִּגְלָלָיִךְ.

אֵיכָה נְתוּנָה בָּאֵשׁ אֻכְּלָה,[4]*
תֵּאָכֵל בָּאֵשׁ בָּשָׂר, וְלֹא נִכְווּ זָרִים בְּגַחֲלָיִךְ.

עַד אָן עֲדִינָה[5] תְּהִי שׁוֹכְנָה בְּרֹב הַשֶּׁקֶט,
וּפְנֵי פְרָחַי הֲלֹא כִסּוּ חֲרוּלָיִךְ.[6]

תֵּשֵׁב בְּרֹב גַּאֲוָה, לִשְׁפּוֹט בְּנֵי אֵל בְּכָל הַמִּשְׁפָּטִים,
וְתָבִיא בִּפְלִילָיִךְ.

עוֹד תִּגְזוֹר לִשְׂרוֹף דַּת אֵשׁ* וְחֻקִּים,
וְלָכֵן אַשְׁרֵי שֶׁיְּשַׁלֵּם לָךְ גְּמוּלָיִךְ.[7]

צוּרִי בְּלַפִּיד וָאֵשׁ,* הֲלְבַעֲבוּר זֶה נְתָנֵךְ כִּי בְּאַחֲרִיתֵךְ,
תְּלַהֵט אֵשׁ בְּשׁוּלָיִךְ.

סִינַי הַעַל כֵּן בָּךְ בָּחַר אֱלֹהִים,
וּמָאַס בִּגְדוֹלִים* וְזָרַח בִּגְבוּלָיִךְ.

לִהְיוֹת לְמוֹפֵת לְדָת, כִּי תִתְמַעֵט וְתֵרֵד מִכְּבוֹדָהּ,
וְהֵן אֶמְשׁוֹל מְשָׁלָיִךְ.

---

so, in the year 1286, he declared the Jews to be his personal property — *Servi Camerae*, serfs of the Emperor's Treasury. He prohibited Jews from leaving Germany and confiscated the property of those who did.

Maharam vigorously opposed this decree and together with his family attempted to flee Germany. Unfortunately, when he reached the border with Lombardy, he was recognized by a Jewish apostate who reported him to the royal agents. The Emperor imprisoned Maharam in the Castle of Ensishiem. He demanded an exorbitant ransom from the Jewish community if they were to obtain their leader's release.

German Jewry was prepared to pay the enormous sum of 23,000 talents of silver to redeem their Rav. However, Maharam refused to permit them to pay such an exorbitant sum, for the Mishnah (*Gittin* 45a) teaches; 'For the sake of public welfare it is prohibited to redeem Jewish captives for an exorbitant sum' (lest this encourage despots to kidnap other Jews for high ransom in the future). This noble act of self-sacrifice by Maharam achieved its purpose. Never again in Jewish history were great Rabbinic leaders held hostage in order to extort enormous ransom payments from the Jews.

Maharam died in prison in the year 1293, but his remains were not released for burial until they were ransomed fourteen years later by a wealthy Jew, Alexander Wimpton, whose sole request was that he be buried near this great leader.

הַשּׁוֹאֲפִים בַּעֲפַר אֶרֶץ — *Of those who long [to roll] in the dust of the [Holy] Land.* The Talmud (*Kesubos* 112a) relates that Rav Chiya bar Ganda would actually roll around in the dust of *Eretz Yisrael* to fulfill the dictate of the verse, *For Your*

of those who long [to roll] in the dust of the [Holy] Land;[1]*
of those distressed and bewildered by the incineration of your scrolls;[2]
of those who walk in the darkness [of exile], deprived of illumination;[3]
of those who wait hopefully for the light of day,
which will shine upon them and upon you.
[Seek] the welfare of the sighing mortal who cries with a broken heart,
who constantly laments over the excruciating pains of your suffering;
who howls like a serpent and ostriches
and cries out a bitter eulogy on your behalf.
O how did it come to pass [O Holy Torah] that you who were given
[by God] the All-Consuming Fire,[4]* should be consumed
by man-made fires — and yet, those alien intruders
[who burned you] escaped unscathed from your flaming coals?
Until when, O pampered [gentile nations],[5] will you lounge
in excessive serenity, while the faces of my
blossoming youths are covered with thistles?[6]
You sit with overbearing arrogance to judge the children
of God for every libelous accusation, and you drag us
before your judges.
In addition, you issued a decree to burn the fiery Law* and its statutes;
therefore praiseworthy is he who will repay you
with the punishment you deserve.[7]
O my Rock! [Who transmitted the Torah at Sinai] with flame and fire!*
Was it with this in mind that He [God] gave you [the Torah]
so that in the end the edges of your columns should be set ablaze?
O Sinai, was it for this reason that God chose you
while He spurned taller [mountains]* and made His light shine
within your boundaries?
[Did God choose you, Sinai, the lowest mountain]
to be an ominous sign for the Torah Law that it would be belittled
and forced to descend from its glory? Behold, I will illustrate
your condition with appropriate parables!

---

(1) Cf. *Amos* 2:7. (2) Some editions read גְוִילָיִךְ, *your parchments*. (3) Cf. *Isaiah* 50:10.
(4) *Deut.* 9:3. (5) *Isaiah* 47:8. (6) Cf. *Proverbs* 24:31. (7) *Psalms* 137:8.

---

servants had cherished her stones, and been gracious to her dust (Psalms 102:15).

אֵשׁ אוֹכְלָה — *The All-Consuming Fire*. Scripture refers to God as אֵשׁ אֹכְלָה, *an All-Consuming Flame* (Deuteronomy 9:3). The Talmud (*Yoma* 21b) identifies six types of fires which have different properties. The fire of the *Shechinah*, the Divine Presence, is so powerful that it can overwhelm any other flame — even that of the fiery ministering angels.

דָּת אֵשׁ — *The fiery Law*. The Torah was given, מִימִינוֹ אֵשׁ דָּת לָמוֹ, *From His right hand, the fiery Law* unto them (Deuteronomy 33:2). Rashi explains that when the Torah was given, the top of Mount Sinai was engulfed in flames; and the

Torah itself (as it appears before God in the highest celestial spheres) is black fire (in the shape of the letters) imposed upon white fire (which serves as the parchment).

בְּלַפִּיד וָאֵשׁ — *[Who transmitted the Torah at Sinai] with flame and fire!* The Torah states: *And Mount Sinai was engulfed in smoke, because* HASHEM *descended upon it in fire; and its smoke ascended like the smoke from a furnace and the entire mountain shook greatly* (Exodus 19:18). Elsewhere it is stated: *And the appearance of the glory of* HASHEM *was like an All-Consuming Fire at the top of the mountain in the eyes of the Children of Israel* (ibid. 24:17).

סִינַי ... בְּךָ בָּחַר אֱלֹהִים וּמָאַס בִּגְדוֹלִים — *Sinai ...*

מָשָׁל לְמֶלֶךְ, אֲשֶׁר בָּכָה לְמִשְׁתֵּה בְנוֹ,

צָפָה אֲשֶׁר יִגַּע כֵּן אֵת אֲתָ בִּמְלִיךְ.

תַּחַת מְעִיל, תִּתְכַּס סִינַי לְבוּשֵׁךְ בְּשַׂק,

תַּעֲטֶה לְבוּשׁ אַלְמָנוּת, תַּחֲלִיף שִׂמְלָיִךְ.

אוֹרִיד דְּמָעוֹת, עֲדֵי יִהְיוּ כְנַחַל,[1]

וְיַגִּיעוּ לְקִבְרוֹת שְׁנֵי שָׂרֵי אֲצִילָיִךְ.

מֹשֶׁה וְאַהֲרֹן בְּהֹר הָהָר,

וְאֶשְׁאַל הֲיֵשׁ תּוֹרָה חֲדָשָׁה, בְּכֵן נִשְׂרְפוּ גְלִילָיִךְ.

חֹדֶשׁ שְׁלִישִׁי וְהַקֶּשֶׁר הָרְבִיעִי,

לְהַשְׁחִית חֶמְדָּתֶךְ, וְכָל יְפִי כְּלִילָיִךְ.[2]

גֻּדַּע לֻלְחוֹת, וְעוֹד שָׁנָה בְּאוּלְתּוֹ,

לִשְׂרוֹף בָּאֵשׁ דָּת,[3] הֲזֶה תַשְׁלוּם כְּפָלָיִךְ.

אֶתְמַהּ לְנַפְשִׁי אֵיךְ יֶעֱרַב לְחִכִּי אָכוֹל,

אַחֲרֵי רְאוֹתִי, אֲשֶׁר אָסְפוּ שְׁלָלָיִךְ.

אֶל תּוֹךְ רְחוֹבָהּ כְּנִדַּחַת,* וְשָׂרְפוּ שְׁלַל עֶלְיוֹן,

אֲשֶׁר תִּמְאַס לָבֹא קְהָלָיִךְ.

לֹא אֵדְעָה לִמְצוֹא דֶּרֶךְ סְלוּלָה,[4]

הֲכִי הָיוּ אֲבֵלוֹת, נְתִיב יְשַׁר מְסִלָּיִךְ.

יֻמְתַּק בְּפִי מִדְּבַשׁ, לְמִסוֹךְ בְּמַשְׁקֶה דְּמָעוֹת,

וּלְרַגְלַי הֱיוֹת כָּבוּל כְּבָלָיִךְ.

יֶעֱרַב לְעֵינַי, שְׁאוֹב מֵימֵי דְמָעַי,

עֲדֵי כָלוּ לְכָל מַחֲזִיק בְּכַנַף מְעִילָיִךְ.[5]

אַךְ יֶחֱרְבוּ בְּרִדְתָּם עַל לְחָיַי,

עֲבוּר כִּי נִכְמְרוּ רַחֲמַי לִנְדוֹד בְּעָלָיִךְ.

לָקַח צְרוֹר כַּסְפּוֹ,*[6] הָלַךְ בְּדֶרֶךְ לְמֵרָחוֹק,[7]

וְעַמּוֹ הֲלֹא נָסוּ צְלָלָיִךְ.[8]

God chose you while He spurned taller (mountains). The *Talmud* (*Sotah* 5a) teaches that God rejected lofty mountains and summits and rested His Holy Presence upon Sinai because it is the lowest of all peaks. This emphasizes that no quality is more beloved to God than genuine humility. Moreover, even after God designated Sinai for greatness, the mountain remained low and humble (see *Megillah* 29a).

לִשְׂרוֹף בָּאֵשׁ דָּת — *By incinerating the Law in fire.* This refers to the Talmud's statement (*Taanis* 26b) that on the seventeenth of Tammuz, the gentile general Apostumus committed the terrible sacrilege of burning a *Sefer Torah.*

כְּנִדַּחַת — *Like the [condemned property of] an apostate city.* If an individual Jew is guilty of idolatry, he is condemned to death by stoning.

This may be compared to the king who wept
at his son's [wedding] feast because he foresaw his son's demise,
so too, [O Sinai,] did you foretell your fate in your own words.
Therefore, O Sinai, instead of a royal robe, garb yourself in sackcloth,
cloak yourself in widow's garb; change your attire!
And I will shed tears until they flow like a river[1]
that reaches to the gravesites of your two most noble princes.
They are Moses and Aaron [who were] on Mount Hor.
And I will ask them if there is perhaps a new Torah,
therefore your scrolls have been burnt!
[They accepted the Torah during Sivan,] the third month,
but [Tammuz] the fourth month revolted [against your Torah],
to destroy your delight and your most exquisite beauty.[2]
The Tablets of the Law were shattered [by Moses]
and [Tammuz'] folly was repeated by incinerating the Law in fire.[3]
Is this the payment of your double reward?
I wonder to myself, 'How can food ever again be pleasant to my taste
after I have seen what your plunderers gathered?'
Into the main public square [they heaped our Talmud scrolls]
like [the condemned property of] an apostate city;* there men,
rejected from entering your congregation, burned exalted spoils.
I know not how to find the straight road[4] [which will lead me
to fathom your ways]; has not your straight path
become shrouded in mourning?
It would be sweeter to my mouth than honey to mix tears
into [my] drink, and to have my feet chained in your shackles
[so that I might properly commiserate with your sorrow].
It would be pleasant to my eyes to absorb the waters of my tears,
until [the tears] would disappear for all those who cling
to edges of your robes.[5]
But they would evaporate as they rolled down my cheeks,
because my compassion is intense
over the wanderings of your Master.
[God] took His purseful of silver pieces[6]*
and embarked on a distant journey;[7] and behold,
when He departed, your sheltering shadows fled.[8]

---

(1) Cf. *Eichah* 2:18. (2) Cf. 2:15. (3) Cf. *Deuteronomy* 33:2. (4) Cf. *Jeremiah* 18:15.
(5) Cf. *I Samuel* 15:27. (6) Cf. *Proverbs* 7:20. (7) 7:19. (8) Cf. *Song of Songs* 2:17.

But if an entire city or a majority of its inhabitants are seduced by some of its citizens to worship idols, then this place is adjudged with the special laws of עִיר הַנִּדַּחַת, *an apostate city.* The idolaters are executed by the sword, whereas of the city the Torah says: *And you shall gather all of its contents into the middle of the main open place of the city and you shall burn with fire both the entire city and all of its contents, a total*

conflagration for HASHEM, *your God* (*Deuteronomy* 13:17). And that is just what happened to the Talmud volumes on that fateful Friday in Paris.

לָקַח צְרוֹר כַּסְפּוֹ — *[God] took His purseful of silver pieces.* The Talmud (*Sanhedrin* 96b) relates that Ammon and Moab are the most malicious enemies of the Jews. They heard that Nebuchadnezzar was apprehensive about de-

וַאֲנִי כְּשָׁכוּל וְגַלְמוּד, נִשְׁאַרְתִּי לְבַד מֵהֶם,

כְּתֹרֶן בְּרֹאשׁ הָהָר² מִגְּדוֹלָיִךְ.

לֹא אֶשְׁמַע עוֹד לְקוֹל שָׁרִים וְשָׁרוֹת,

עָלַי כִּי נִתְּקוּ, חֶבְלֵי תְּפֵי חֲלִילָיִךְ.

אֶלְבַּשׁ וְאֶתְכַּס בְּשַׂק, כִּי לִי מְאֹד יָקְרוּ,

עָצְמוּ כְּחוֹל יִרְבָּיוּן, נַפְשׁוֹת חֲלָלָיִךְ.

אֶתְמַהּ מְאֹד עַל מְאוֹר הַיּוֹם,

אֲשֶׁר יִזְרַח אֶל כֹּל, אֲבָל יַחֲשִׁיךְ אֵלַי וְאֵלָיִךְ.

זַעֲקִי בְּקוֹל מַר לְצוּר, עַל שִׁבְרוֹנֵךְ וְעַל חֳלָיֵךְ,

וְלוּ יִזְכֹּר אַהֲבַת כְּלוּלָיִךְ.³

חִגְרִי לִבוּשׁ שַׂק⁴ עֲלֵי הַהַבְעָרָה,

אֲשֶׁר יָצְתָה לְחַלֵּק וְסָפְתָה אֶת תְּלוּלָיִךְ.

כִּימֵי עֲנּוֹתֵךְ⁵ יְנַחֲמֵךְ צוּר,

וְיָשִׁיב שְׁבוּת שִׁבְטֵי יְשֻׁרוּן,⁶ וְיָרִים אֶת שְׁפָלָיִךְ.

עוֹד תַּעְדִּי⁷ בַּעֲדִי שָׁנִי וְתֹף תִּקְחִי,

תֵּלְכִי בְּמָחוֹל, וְצַהֲלִי בִּמְחוֹלָיִךְ.

יָרוּם לְבָבִי בְּעֵת צוּרֵךְ⁸ לְאוֹר לָךְ,

stroying the Temple. He was afraid that he would meet with the same ruinous disaster as others had before him when they had attempted to harm God's Holy Sanctuary. So Ammon and Moab assured him that he had nothing to fear for the God of the Jews had already abandoned

And I am left behind like someone bereft of all his children,
  utterly forlorn;[1] so have I been left all alone.
  I am like a [lone] flagstaff planted
  atop your towering mountain peak.[2]
No longer do I hear the sounds of [your] musicians, male and female,
  because the strings of your musical instruments have been torn.
I will clothe and cover myself with sackcloth, because [your martyrs]
  are very precious to me, and as powerful
  and numerous as the sand are the souls of your corpses.
I am deeply perplexed by the light of day which shines brightly
  towards everyone, yet towards you and me it casts only darkness.
O cry out to the Rock with bitter voice over your ruination
  and your debilitation; O if only He would remember
  the love of Your wedding day.[3]
Gird yourself with garments of sackcloth[4] over the conflagration
  which burst out and tore you to pieces,
  and wiped out your towering [Torah scholars].
May the Rock [of salvation] comfort you according to
  the days of your affliction,[5] and may He return the
  captivity of the Tribes of Jeshurun[6] and exalt your degraded ones.
Once again you will adorn yourself[7] with ornaments of scarlet,
  and you will take up the tambourine and go out in a circle
  dance and rejoice with your dancing.
At that time my heart will be uplifted, when your Rock will be a light
  unto you, to brighten your darkness[8] and to illuminate your gloom.

---

(1) Cf. *Isaiah* 49:21. (2) Cf. 30:17. (3) Cf. *Jeremiah* 2:2. (4) Cf. 6:26.
(5) Cf. *Psalms* 90:15. (6) Cf. *Jeremiah* 30:3. (7) 31:3. (8) Cf. *II Samuel* 22:29.

His Temple, as we read: *For the Man is not at home, He has gone on a faraway journey* (*Proverbs* 7:19). Still Nebuchadnezzar was reluctant. 'Perhaps there are still righteous men whose prayers will save the Jews and their Temple?' Again Ammon and Moab reassured him, for it is written, *He has taken a bag of silver with Him* (ibid. 7:20), i.e., in anticipation of the Destruction, God has removed the righteous who are as precious as silver coins!

מב.

צִיּוֹן צְפִירַת פְּאֵר[1]* חֶדְוַת אֲגוּדָיִךְ,
זַעֲקִי בְּרָמָה בְּקוֹלֵךְ[2] עַל אֲבוּדָיִךְ.
אֶל הַבְּנוּיָה לְבַקֵּשׁ וּלְחַנֵּן לָאֵל,
שָׁלוֹם יְשֻׁפּוֹת לָךְ[3] וְגַם לִבְנֵי בְחִירָיִךְ.
בְּעַל בְּחִירֵךְ אֲשֶׁר לָךְ אֲהֵבָתוֹ,
לְזָר נֶהְפַּךְ לְנֶגְדֵּךְ וְגַם נֶגֶד גְּדוּדָיִךְ.
גָּלַף וּפָתַח בְּלוּחַ לֵב, אֲזַי נִשְׁקַטְתְּ בֶּטַח
בְּשַׁלְוָה שְׁדוּכָה עַל רְדִידָיִךְ.
דַּבְּרִי נְכוֹחוֹת לְרֵעַיִךְ לְהָלִיץ עֲבוּרֵךְ,*
אַף תְּצַפְצְפִי לְהָרִים קוֹל הֲדָרָיִךְ.
הָשֵׁב יְדִידֵךְ לְמִטָּתֵךְ וְלָלוֹן בְּצִלֵּךְ,
וּלְטַיֵּל בְּסַגַּת גַּן וְרָדָיִךְ.
וְעַד בְּמְהַר וְקִדּוּשִׁין וְגַם בִּכְתֻבָּה,
לָךְ וּלְעֶזְרֵךְ וְהֵם בָּרוּר זְבָדָיִךְ.
זֶרַע וּבָנִים מְחֻטָּבִים לְאִישֵׁךְ הֲלֹא יָלַדְתְּ,
וְאֵיךְ נִשְׁכַּלְתְּ מִכָּל חֲסִידָיִךְ.
חָמַק וְעָבַר[4] וְגָז מִמֵּךְ וְלֹא נִשְׁלַחְתְּ,
לֹא בָא בְיָדֵךְ, שְׁטַר סֵפֶר טְרוּדָיִךְ.[5]
טוֹעֵן בְּטַעֲנַת מְמָאֶנֶת בְּמֶרֶד,
עָלַי כֵּן נִתְקַלַּסְתְּ וְהָשְׁפַּל עַם דּוֹדָיִךְ.
יוֹשֶׁבֶת בְּדוּדָה דְּמוּיָה כִּי חֲשׂוּפָה קְלוֹן שׁוּלָיִךְ,
וְנִגְלֵית וְנִדְלַל כְּבוֹדָיִךְ.
כָּל מַחֲזִיקִים בִּנְזָרֵךְ, הֵם יְצָאוּךְ,
דְּחוּפִים וּבְהוּלִים[6] וְהֵם הָיוּ לְבוּדָיִךְ.
לִבִּי הֲלֹא נֶחֱלַל[7] מֵאֵין הֲפוּגוֹת,[8]

---

(1) Cf. *Isaiah* 28:5. (2) Cf. *Jeremiah* 31:14. (3) Cf. *Isaiah* 26:12.
(5) Cf. *Isaiah* 50:1. (6) Cf. *Esther* 8:14. (7) Cf. *Psalms* 109:22. (8) *Eichah* 3:49.

ציון צְפִירַת פְּאֵר ◆§ — *O Zion, crown of splendor.*
The *paytan* urges terrestrial Zion to plead with
its celestial counterpart that it intervene with the
Heavenly Court to bring an end to Israel's exile
and dispersion.

The *kinnah* is arranged according to an

aleph-beis acrostic, each letter appearing twice:
as the initial of the first word of a line, and of
the last word of the preceding line. Then follows
the author's signature חָזָק מֵאִיר, *Meir, may he be
strong,* in a similar manner. The composer is
generally identified as R' Meir ben Elazar

42.

צִיּוֹן O Zion, crown of splendor,[1]* desire of your [diverse] groups,
      let your voice cry out to the highest [heavens][2]
   over your lost [populace].

א [Cry out] to the celestial Jerusalem built [on high],
      to beg and plead with God to settle you in peace,[3]
   as well as your chosen children.

ב [God,] the husband of your choice,
      whose love was [once exclusively] for you, has turned
   against you and against your soldiers like a total stranger.

ג As long as He was chiseled and engraved
      upon the tablet of your heart, you were quiet,
   confident and tranquil, relaxed on your mantle [the Holy Temple].

ד So speak to your friends [the angels Michael and Gabriel,
      and ask them] to intervene on your behalf,*
   and sing [like a bird] yourself, raising your
      splendid voice [in intensive prayer].

ה [And entreat] your Beloved to return to your [Temple] couch,
      to rest in your shade and to stroll in the garden
   hedged by your roses.

ו Bound together [with God, is Israel] through dowry [the Sabbath]
      and betrothal [the Ten Commandments] and also
   marriage contract [the Torah], [so that Israel is unto] you
      [the Holy Land] and your helpmate [the Temple],
   and they are your [choicest] portion.

ז [O Israel!] Have you not borne fine children for your spouse,
      sons hewn to perfection? How, then,
   are you now utterly bereft of your pious ones?

ח He [God] disappeared and went away[4]
      and severed Himself from you, although
   you were never formally released,
      for no official bill of your divorce was placed in your hand.

ט He [God] charges you with defiance and rebelliousness,
      therefore you, your Beloved's nation,
   are now disgraced and degraded.

י Now you sit solitary and silent, for the shame of your hems
      has been uncovered, and your honor has been diminished.

כ All who had supported your crown, fled from you speedily
      and confused,[6] — even though they had been connected to you.

ל Behold, my heart is hollow[7] within me without relief,[8]

Lombard HaDarshan who flourished early in
the thirteenth century.

דַּבְּרִי נְכוֹחוֹת לְרֵעַיִךְ לְהָלִיץ עֲבוּרֵךְ — *So speak to
your friends [the angels Michael and Gabriel
and ask them] to intervene on your behalf.* This
must not be misinterpreted as a prayer to the
angels to pray on our behalf. *Rambam* and
many others have clearly postulated that a Jew
must pray to God directly without any intermediaries. Rather, *in addition* to our own fervent

אֲשֶׁר הוּמַר וְנֶחֱלַף לְמַר מֶתֶק מִגְדָיִךְ.

מְלֹא דְמָעוֹת כַּמַּיִם נִשְׁטָפוּ,

נִמְלְאוּ דְמָעוֹת לֶחָיַי וְכָל עֵינֵי נְגִידָיִךְ.

נַפְשִׁי עֲטוּפָה בְּעֵת זָכְרִי לְאִשֵּׁךְ הֲלֹא נִכְבָּה,

וְלֹא יָכְלוּ לֶאֱפוֹת סְמִידָיִךְ.

סֶמֶךְ אֲשִׁישֵׁי עֵנָב מָהוּל בַּמַּיִם,*

וּפַס מִן הָרְפָתִים, בְּקַר זִבְחֵי עוֹבְדָיִךְ.

עֻדַּר וְנֶחֱרַשׁ יְסוֹדֵךְ* לִשְׂדֵה בוּר וְנִיר,

לְחֶכָה וְאָכְלָה סְבִיבֵךְ אֵשׁ פְּלָדָיִךְ.

פֶּלֶץ וְשָׁבָע לְבָשׂוּנִי, בְּעֵת אֶחֱזֶה מוֹנֵי שְׁקָטִים,

וְהֵם צָדוּ צְעָדָיִךְ.

צוֹעֵק אֲנִי לִמְקוֹנְנוֹת לִבְכּוֹת,

וּבְמַר לְזוֹעֵק נְהִי נִהְיָה, הוֹי עַל קְפָדָיִךְ.

קַלּוּ יְמֵי עָנְיִי, עֵת אֶחֱזֶה עֳנָיִךְ,

שׁוֹמְרִים מְצָאוּךְ, וְהֵם נָשְׂאוּ רְדִידָיִךְ.

רָחֲפוּ עֲצָמַי עֲלֵי בָנִים יְקָרִים

אֲשֶׁר כְּשִׂיד שְׂרוּפִים, בְּאוֹר אוּדֵי שְׂרִידָיִךְ.

שָׁקְדוּ וְיָקְדוּ גְּוִילֵי דַת מְשַׂנְאַי,

אוֹי אֵיךְ נִמְשַׁלְתְּ לְפַטִּישׁ תְּעוּדָיִךְ.

תּוֹהֶה לְבָבִי אֲשֶׁר נִרְצָה,

בְּאֶרֶץ טְמֵאָה לִנְדָבָה לִנְסוֹךְ יֵין תְּמִידָיִךְ.

צִיּוֹן עֲדִי אָן מְשִׂימָה אַתְּ לְפֶה אֶת יָדֵךְ,

אֵיכָה בְּיַד אוֹיְבַיִךְ נָפְלוּ נְגִידָיִךְ.

---

(1) Cf. *Psalms* 107:5. (2) Cf. *Song of Songs* 2:5. (3) Cf. *Isaiah* 1:22. (4) *Nahum* 2:4.
(5) Cf. *Eichah* 4:18. (6) Cf. *Song of Songs* 5:7. (7) Cf. *Jeremiah* 23:9. (8) Cf. *Job* 40:4.

prayers addressed directly and exclusively to God, we summon the defending angels to testify in our favor before the Heavenly Tribunal and to bring our good deeds and merits to God's attention in the most forceful fashion.

עֵנָב מָהוּל בַּמַּיִם — *Grape wine ... intermingled with the water.* This refers to the ritual of נִסּוּךְ הַמַּיִם, *the water libation,* which took place in the Temple on the Sukkos festival (see *Sukkah* 4:9). There were two bowls atop the Altar. A *Kohen* would pour wine into one bowl and water into the other. The liquids would flow out of the

bowls into two holes in the Altar's top. Eventually, they would mingle deep under the Altar. *Vilna Gaon* explains that strong wine symbolizes God's Attribute of Strict Justice whereas sweet, pure water represents God's Attribute of Mercy. When the strong wine is diluted by the water it symbolizes God's desire to temper His Strict Justice with tender and compassionate Mercy.

יְסוֹדֵךְ ... עֻדַּר — *Your foundations were hacked away.* Five terrible tragedies befell the Jewish people on Tishah B'Av. They culminated with because spoiled and turned into bitterness are your sweet fruit.

מ Full of tears flowing like flooding waters, my cheeks, as well as
the eyes of all your princes, have become filled with tears.

נ My spirit is weakened[1] when I remember
your [Altar] fire that is now extinguished!
And no longer can they bake your fine-flour offerings.

ס [Gone are] the pitches[2] of grape wine [for the libations]
that intermingled with the water* [libation[3]
during the Festival of Sukkos];
and absent from the pens are the cattle
for the sacrifices of those who serve You.

ע Your foundations were hacked away*
and plowed under [by the Roman Turnus Rufus]
into a plowed yet fallow field; your tongues of flame
licked at you from every side.[4]

פ I am clad with trembling and revulsion,
when I observe my tormentors [lounging] in tranquility;
those [murderers] who hunted down
those who followed in Your footsteps.[5]

צ I scream to the wailing-women to weep and to cry bitterly,
'O woe! Alas! Ho!' for your [citizens who were] cut off.

ק My days of suffering feel light, when I see your suffering;
the [hostile] watchmen caught you
and they carried off your mantle.[6]

ר A shudder passes through my bones[7] for the precious children
who were burnt like limestone ash; those very survivors
who [originally were saved] like a fire-brand from the fire.

ש My avowed enemies made all haste
to burn the parchments of the Law.
Woe! How did this befall you [O Torah]
who are likened to a hammer
[which destroys every obstacle in its path]?

ת My heart is thrown into turmoil when I consider that You
prefer to send beneficial rains down on the defiled lands
of the gentiles more than You desire the pouring
of the wine libations of the daily [Temple] sacrifice.
O Zion! How long will you clasp your hand to your mouth[8]
[to ensure your silence]? O how did you allow your princes
to fall into the hands of your foes?

---

the obliteration of every last vestige of the
Temple by the wicked Roman governor Turnus
Rufus some sixty years after the Temple was
destroyed. He plowed over the Temple mount
and its surroundings in fulfillment of the
prophet; threat: צִיּוֹן שָׂדֶה תֵחָרֵשׁ, Zion will be
plowed over like a field (Micah 3:12; Taanis 29a;
Rambam, Hilchos Taanis 5:3).

מִמֵּךְ אֲבוּדִים יְלָדִים חֲמוּדִים כְּפָז,

עַל זֹאת בְּמֶרֶר בְּכִי יִלְלַת מְרוּדָיִךְ.

אֵיכָה מְעֻכָּב זְמַן לְדָתֵךְ,

וְעַד אָן תְּהִי אַתְּ נִקְשֶׁרֶת בְּחִיל צִירֵי אֲחוּדָיִךְ.

יוֹלְדוֹת לְתִשְׁעָה יְרָחִים עֵת נְשֵׁי כָל,

וְאֵיךְ רַבּוּ שְׁנוֹתֵךְ אֲשֶׁר הָרִית יְלָדָיִךְ.

רָנִּי לְשׁוֹמֵר לְאַיָּלָה חֲבָלִים,

וְהוּא יַתִּיר לְצִירֵךְ עֲלֵי רֶבֶד רְפִידָיִךְ.

חוֹשֵׁב זְמַן יַעֲלֵי סֶלַע לְהַתִּיר,

וְלֹא חָשַׁב זְמַנֵּךְ לְהָסִיר כָּל חֲרָדָיִךְ.

זְמַן בְּיָדוֹ פִּתַּח אַרְבַּע נְעוּלִים,*

וְגַם כֵּן יִפְתַּח גִּנְזֵי אוֹצַר זְבוּלָיִךְ.

קוֹל יַשְׁמִיעַ לְקַבֵּץ הָאֱמוּנִים,

וְאָז דְּלָתָיו פָּתוֹחַ יַפְקִידֵם עַל קְלִידָיִךְ.

צִיּוֹן מִעֲשִׂים בְּצַעֲרֵךְ וּבְיָפְיֵךְ מְעֻשָּׁתִים,

אֲשֶׁר יִזְרַח חֶרֶס חֲדוּדָיִךְ.[2]

צִיּוֹן בְּמִנְחָה יְכַפְּרוּן אֶת פְּנֵי זַעֲמֶךְ,

אָז יִשְׁתַּחֲווּ לְכַף רַגְלֵךְ חֲרָדָיִךְ.

צִיּוֹן עֲדִי עֶדְיֵךְ[3] רִקְמַת בִּגְדֵךְ,[4]

וְגַם עֹז וְזְרוֹעַ[5] פְּאֵר בִּגְדֵי חֲמוּדָיִךְ.

פִּתַּח אַרְבַּע נְעוּלִים — *In his hands are the keys to unlock the four sealed vaults.* The Talmud (*Taanis* 2a; *Sanhedrin* 113a) teaches that although God has entrusted all of the blessings of nature to angels intermediaries, three "keys" remain in His hand because there natural phenomenon require intimate Divine Providence. The three are rainfall, resurrection and childbirth. *Tur Shulchan Aruch* (*Orach Chaim* #114, based on the *Jerusalem Talmud*) adds a fourth key — that of livelihood. *Tur* notes that the word מַפְתֵּחַ, *key,* is an acronym for these four blessings: מָטָר, *rainfall;* פַּרְנָסָה, *livelihood;* תְּחִיָּה, *resurrection;* and חַיָּה, *child-bearing mother* (see ArtScroll, *Shemoneh Esrei,* p. 70).

מ Your children, as precious as the finest gold have vanished,
  therefore your anguished wailing is mixed with bitter weeping.

א O how long will your rebirth be delayed? And until when will you
  be gripped by the excruciating travails of birth which grip you?

י A birth process terminating in nine months is the norm for all women,
  why then have the years since you conceived
  your children extended for so much longer?

ר Cry out prayerfully to He Who even watches over the hind[1]
  in her birth travail, certainly He will release you from the pain
  you suffer over [the loss of] your couch like Temple.

ח Although He even calculates with precision the moment
  the mountain goat delivers its offspring,[1]
  He nevertheless refrained from determining the final time
  [of your redemption] to spare you from [prolonged] terror.

ז prepared in His hands are the keys to the four sealed
  [celestial] vaults;* and also He [alone holds the key]
  to open the hidden treasures of the Temple Dwelling.

ק He will issue a call to gather in the faithful,
  and then He will command the gatekeepers
  to leave the doors [of Jerusalem] wide open.

  O Zion! Those who are heartbroken over your pains
  will be thrilled by your [future] beauty,
  when the dazzling rays of your sun will shine.[2]

  O Zion! [The gentile nations] shall attempt
  to appease your wrath with a gift-offering,
  then those who made you shudder with fear
  will bow down to the bottoms of your feet.

  O Zion! Adorn yourself with ornaments,[3]
  with your embroidered robes,[4]
  and gird yourself, too, with power and might[5]
  and the splendor of your precious garments.

---

(1) Cf. 39:1. (2) Cf. 41:22. (3) Cf. *Jeremiah* 4:30. (4) Cf. *Ezekiel* 16:18. (5) *Isaiah* 51:9.

מג.

צִיּוֹן בְּמִשְׁפָּט לְכִי לָךְ עִם מְעוֹנְנָיִךְ,
הִתְעוֹךְ בְּכָזָב וְלֹא גִלּוּ עֲוֹנָיִךְ.[1]

אָכֵן בְּנֵי עַוְלָה עִנּוּךְ וִירָשׁוּךְ,
נְוֵה צֶדֶק הָיִית אֵל כָּל שְׁכֵנָיִךְ.

בָּזִית מַמְלִיכֵךְ, וְלֹא הִקְשַׁבְתְּ לְמוֹרֵךְ לְטוֹב,
בִּשְׁכֹּן בְּאַרְצֵךְ קְדוֹשֵׁךְ בְּמִלּוֹנָיִךְ.

גָּלִית קְלוֹנֵךְ וְטֻמְאָתֵךְ בְּשׁוּלָיִךְ[3]
וְגַם טִמֵּאת דַּרְכֵּךְ, מְאֹד הִרְבֵּית זְנוּנָיִךְ.

דֶּרֶךְ אֲחוֹתֵךְ הֲלֹא הָלַכְתְּ,
וְזָנִית בְּתַזְנוּתָהּ, וְהִזְנֵית בְּנוֹתַיִךְ וּבָנָיִךְ.

הֻכֵּית וְנִגַּפְתְּ לְאֵין מַרְפֵּא,
וְהָשְׁלַכְתְּ כְּטִיט חוּצוֹת,[4] וְהִנֵּךְ שְׂחוֹק לִבְנֵי מְעַנָּיִךְ.

וַתְּהִי נְגִינָה בְּפִי זֵדִים אֲרוּרִים,
אֲשֶׁר אָמְרוּ לְנַפְשֵׁךְ שְׁחִי[5] הֲרוֹס לְשִׁנָּיִךְ.

זִכְרִי עָנְיֵךְ בְּלֵב נִשְׁבָּר,
וְזַעֲקִי עֲלֵי מַכֵּךְ וְנוֹגְשֵׁךְ אֲשֶׁר גָּדַע קַרְנָיִךְ.[6]

חַכִּי בֶּאֱמֶת לְאֵל צוּרֵךְ וּבוֹרְאֵךְ,
וְהוֹחִילִי לְמַלְכֵּךְ לְבַד כִּי הוּא אֲדוֹנָיִךְ.

טַהֲרִי לְבָבֵךְ וְכַפַּיִךְ,
וְשׁוּבִי עֲדֵי אִישֵׁךְ קְדוֹשֵׁךְ, וְלוֹ הַרְבִּי רְנָנָיִךְ.

יוֹמָם וָלַיְלָה תְּנִי קוֹל בִּבְכִי מַר,
עֲלֵי קִרְיַת מְלוּכָה[7] וְעַל תֵּל אַרְמוֹנָיִךְ.

כָּבוֹד וְהָדָר וְרֹב יְפִי בְּתוֹכֵךְ,
הֲלֹא נִמְצָא פְּנֵי קְדוֹשֵׁךְ וְהֵן נָתַן לְעוֹנָיִךְ.

---

(1) Cf. *Eichah* 2:14. (2) *Jeremiah* 31:22. (3) Cf. *Eichah* 1:9. (4) *Psalms* 18:43.
(5) *Isaiah* 51:23. (6) Cf. *Eichah* 2:3. (7) Cf. *Psalms* 48:3.

•⊷ צִיּוֹן בְּמִשְׁפָּט ⊷• — *O Zion, enter into litigation.*
This *kinnah* was written by R' Yosef bar Chaim
HaKohen who highlights the tragic fact that the
Jewish people were misguided and led to sin by
false prophets and corrupt leaders. Indeed, corruption and perversion of justice was one of the
primary causes of our nation's decline and

ultimate banishment. As the Talmud (*Shabbos*
118b) graphically describes, the leaders and
judges of the Temple era were afraid to offend
the rich and the powerful so they twisted the
law in their favor.

Isaiah the prophet lamented this saying: *How
has the faithful city become a harlot? It had*

43.

צִיּוֹן O Zion, enter into litigation against your false prophets
who deliberately misled you with deceit and who failed
to expose your iniquities[1] [and deprived you of
an opportunity for repentance and salvation].

א Indeed, men of iniquity tortured and exploited you,
even though you were once a haven of righteousness[2]
for all of your neighbors.

ב [Because] you disgraced [God] who invested you
with sovereignty, and you did not listen to those
who attempted to guide you towards goodness,
while you were settled in your land and your sacred [God]
dwelt in your abode [the Temple].

ג You uncovered your own shame and your impurity is spread out
over your garments;[3] you even sullied your pathway,
because you increased your acts of harlotry.

ד Have you not followed in the path of your sister
[the Northern Kingdom], and strayed after her harlotry?
Moreover, you even perverted the ways of your daughters
and sons and caused them to take up harlotry.

ה Therefore, you were beaten and plagued beyond any cure,
and were thrown out like mud in the streets,[4]
and you have become a laughing stock for the sons
of those who torment you.

ו And you were the butt of the taunting songs in the mouths
of the accused wanton ones who said to you,
'Bend over so that we may smash your teeth!'

ז Remember the impoverished one [Israel] with her broken heart,
and cry out over your abusers and taskmasters
who tore away your dignity.

ח Look forward sincerely for [salvation at the hand of] God
who is your Rock and your Creator, and yearn exclusively
for your King for only He is your Lord.

ט Purify your heart and your hands and return [in penitence]
to your [Divine] Helpmate, your Holy One;
and intensify towards Him your joyous songs.

י Day and night, raise your voice with bitter weeping
over [Jerusalem] the city of royalty[7]
and the heaped ruins of your Temple palace.

כ Glory and splendor and bountiful beauty were in your midst,
all these were displayed before your holy one [Israel],
but now they have been given over to your malicious enemies.

---

been filled with justice, righteousness lodged in
it; but now — murderers! (Isaiah 1:21). The

prophet goes on to predict that in the future God
will purge Jerusalem of its crooked leaders and

לָמָה לְגַלִּים, מְעוֹן תַּנִּים,[1]

וּמוֹרַשׁ קָאַת וְקִפּוֹד,[2] וְגַם אַגְמֵי מַיִם מַעְיָנָיִךְ.

מֵאַנְתְּ שְׁמֽוֹעַ לְקוֹל מוּסָר מְיַסְּרָךְ,

בְּכֶן שָׁתִית וּמָצִית,[3] שְׁמָנַיִךְ שְׁמָרָיִךְ.

נֹכַח פְּנֵי עֶלְיוֹן שִׁפְכִי לִבֵּךְ[4] כְּמֵי נָהָר,

וְאַל תִּתְּנִי פוּגַת[5] לְעֵינָיִךְ.

סֽׄבִּי וְהֽוֹמִי בְעִיר,[6] קִרְאִי מְקוֹנֽנוֹת[7]

וְכָל נָשִׁים מְבַכּוֹת, בְּכִי גָדוֹל מְקוֹנְנָיִךְ.

עָלֵי צְנִיף מַלְכֵּךְ[8] עַד אָן לְמִרְמָס יְהִי,

עַד מֶה בְּיַד צָר בְּנֵי שָׂרִים סְגָנָיִךְ.

פְּתַח לְבָנוֹן שְׁעָרָיִךְ,[9]* אֲשֶׁר טָבְעוּ בָאָרֶץ[10]

נְשִׂיָּה[11] וְאֵין מָלוֹן לְכֹהֲנָיִךְ.

צִיּוֹן עֲלֵיהֶם נְהִי נִהְיָה,[12] וְלֹא תֶחֱשִׁי,

אַסְפִי וְקַבְּצִי זְקֵנוֹת וּזְקֵנָיִךְ.

קָרְחִי וָגֽוֹזִי כַּנֶּֽשֶׁר עַל בְּנֵי תַעֲנוּגָיִךְ,[13]

וְעַל כָּל נְשִׂיאַיִךְ וְרוֹזְנָיִךְ.

רָמוּ וְגָדְלוּ כְּמוֹ גַלִּים בְּלֵב יָם מְזוֹרָרָיִךְ,

בְּלֵיל שָׁדְדוּ[14] טוּרֵי אֲבָנָיִךְ.

שָׁדַד מְלוֹנֵךְ וְכָל מַחֲמַד יְקָרֵךְ,

בְּאֵין אוּרִים וְתֻמִּים[15] אֲשֶׁר גֻּלּוּ צְפוּנָיִךְ.

תָּבוֹר וְכַרְמֶל כְּהָרֵי גִלְבּֽעַ*

בְּלִי טַלֵּךְ וּמְטָרֵךְ,[16] וְלֹא אוֹר עֲנָנָיִךְ.[17]

צִיּוֹן יְגוֹנֵךְ נְשִׁי, טַהֲרִי וְהִתְקַדְּשִׁי,

עֲדִי יְקָר לִבְשִׁי, תַּמְרוּק שְׁמָנָיִךְ.

---

that will lead to the redemption. *And I shall restore your judges as in earliest times and your counselors at first. Afterwards you shall be called the city of righteousness, the faithful city* (Isaiah 1:26).

This kinnah ends off on a note of hope that after Zion is purified it will once again be regarded as 'the most precious treasure of monarchs and kingdoms.'

פְּתַח לְבָנוֹן שְׁעָרָיִךְ — *Open your gates, O [Levanon] Whitened One!* This is based on the words of the prophet who said: פְּתַח לְבָנוֹן דְּלָתֶיךָ, *Open your doors, O [Levanon] Whitened One!* (Zechariah 11:1). The Talmud (Yoma 39b) teaches that forty years before the destruction of the Second Temple, the Temple itself exhibited many signs and omens of its impending doom. One of the portents was that the Temple gates would swing open all by themselves as if to invite the enemy to enter and destroy it. Rabban Yochanan ben Zakkai saw this and addressed the Temple: Sanctuary, O Sanctuary! Why do

ל Why has it [Jerusalem] been turned into a mound of rubble,
   a den of serpents,[1] the domain of the wild birds of the night?[2]
   Even your springs have turned into swamps.

מ You stubbornly refused to heed the warning voice
   of those who admonished you, therefore you have drunk deep
   and drained[3] the very grease and the lees.

נ In the presence of the Exalted God, pour out your heart[4]
   like waters of the river and give no rest to your eyes.[5]

ס Go around and moan all over the city.[6]
   Summon forth the wailing-women[7] and all the women
   who know how to weep. Let your lamenters weep copiously!

ע [To bemoan] your royal tiara,[8] O how long will it be trampled over?
   Until when will the children of your nobles, your ministers,
   remain in the hands of your tormentors?

פ Open your gates, O [Levanon,] Whitened One![9]*
   The ones that sank into the forgotten[11] land[10]
   for [now] there is no [longer] a lodging house for your priests.

צ O Zion engage in pitiful cries of doleful lamentation[12]
   over their plight and be not silent. Gather together
   and assemble your old women and old men [to join in mourning].

ק Make yourself bald as an eagle as you tear out your hair
   over the children of your pleasure[13]
   and for all your princes and advisers.

ר Your ugly wounds became swollen and bloated like billowing waves
   in the heart of the sea, on the night when the rows of your precious
   gems were plundered[14] [from the High Priest's breastplate].

ש Your lodging place [the Temple] was plundered together
   with your most precious treasures, you are bereft of
   your Urim V'Tumim[15] which revealed all things hidden.

ת Tabor and Carmel have become like the mountains of Gilboa*
   which are devoid of your dew and your rain[16]
   and deprived of the light of your [protective] clouds.[17]

י O Zion! You will ultimately forget your agony.
   Purify and prepare yourself in sanctity!
   Adorn yourself with precious Jewels and with your perfumed oils.

---

(1) Jeremiah 9:10. (2) Cf. Isaiah 34:11. (3) 51:17. (4) Cf. Eichah 2:19. (5) 2:18.
(6) Cf. Isaiah 23:16. (7) Jeremiah 9:16. (8) Cf. Isaiah 62:3. (9) Cf. Zechariah 11:1.
(10) Eichah 2:9. (11) Psalms 88:13. (12) Micah 2:4. (13) Cf. 1:16.
(14) Cf. Isaiah 15:1. (15) Exodus 28:30. (16) Cf. II Samuel 1:21. (17) Cf. Job 37:11.

---

you take such pains to terrify yourself? I know full well that you are destined to be destroyed as indeed the prophet Zechariah foretold when he said, *Open your doors, O [Levanon] Whitened One, so that the fire many consume your cedars!* [But why must you fulfill this prophecy so early and prematurely?]. The *Talmud* concludes: And

why is the Temple referred to as לְבָנוֹן, *Levanon* [Whitened One]? Because it is there that the Jewish nation finds atonement and the stain of their sins is whitened and cleansed!

תָבוֹר וְכַרְמֶל כְּהָרֵי גִלְבּוֹעַ — *Tabor and Carmel have become like the mountains of Gilboa.* Tabor and Carmel were fertile mountains cov-

צִיּוֹן וְשָׁלְמוּ יְמֵי אֶבְלֵךְ בְּשָׂשׂוֹן וָגִיל,
כִּי תַם עֲוֹנֵךְ וּמִשְׁנֶה שברוֹנָיִךְ.
צִיּוֹן סְגֻלַּת מְלָכִים וּמְדִינוֹת[2] תְּהִי עוֹד,
יִזְּלוּ מֵי מְנוּחוֹת[3] מַעְיָנָיִךְ.
צִיּוֹן פְּדוּתֵךְ צָפִי. עוֹד יִקְרָאוּךְ צְפִירַת תִּפְאָרָה,[4]
בְּפִי יְשָׁרִים וְנוֹגְנָיִךְ.[5]
צִיּוֹן בְּרָכָה וְחַיִּים,[6] בָּךְ אֲבִיר יַעֲקֹב,[7]
צִוָּה לְעוֹלָם[6] וְעוֹד יֹאמְרוּ בְּאָזְנָיִךְ.
צִיּוֹן הֲמוֹן כֹּהֲנִים הֵמָּה יְשָׁרְתוּנֵךְ,
וְגַם יוֹסִיף יהוה קָנוֹת שֵׁנִית קְצִינָיִךְ.[8]

---

(1) *Isaiah* 60:20. (2) *Ecclesiates* 2:8. (3) *Psalms* 23:2. (4) *Isaiah* 28:5.
(5) Cf. *Psalms* 68:26. (6) Cf. 133:3. (7) *Genesis* 49:24. (8) Cf. *Isaiah* 11:11.

ered with grass and trees. Gilboa, however, was cursed and barren for it was on Gilboa that King Saul died in his final battle with the Philistines.

In his passionate eulogy for Saul, David cursed Mount Gilboa forever: *O mountains of Gilboa let there be no dew nor rain upon you, nor shall*

ו   O Zion! Your era of mourning will come to an end[1]
      with joy and jubilation, for your sins will be entirely absolved
      and your double Destruction will be concluded.

ט   O Zion! Once again you will be considered
      the most precious treasure
      by all the monarchs[2] and kingdoms,
      and tranquil waters will flow[3] from your fountain springs.

נ   O Zion! Look forward to your redemption!
      You will again be called a crown of splendor[4]
      by the mouth of the upright and by your musicians [the Levites].[5]

     O Zion! [God] the Mighty One of Jacob[7] has decreed blessing
      and life for you forever[6] and [mankind]
      is destined to say that in your ears.

   — O Zion! A multitude of priests shall serve you!
      And HASHEM will once again take charge of your leaders.[8]

---

your fields produce heave offerings for there the   Saul was as though not anointed with oil [II
shield of the mighty was rejected, the shield of   Samuel 1:21].

מד.

צִיּוֹן גְּבֶרֶת לְמַמְלְכוֹת מְצִירַיִךְ,

רַבֵּי שְׁלוֹמִים שְׂאִי, מֵאֵת אֲסִירַיִךְ.

יֶחֱמַץ לְבָבִי לְקוֹל נָתְנוּ רְאֵמִים,

בְּנֵי שֵׂעִיר וּמוֹאָב, בְּתוֹךְ הֵיכַל דְּבִירַיִךְ.

לָבְּסוּ מְשִׁיחַי בְּדַם קָדְקֹד סְגָנִים

טָרוֹף שׁוֹעַ וְקוֹעַ, רְמוֹס עַמִּי בְּחִירַיִךְ.

עָרִים בְּצוּרוֹת תִּפוֹשׂ דָּיֵק וְסוֹלָל שָׁפוּךְ,

אַרְזֵי לְבָנוֹן כְּרוּת, מַעֲצֵי יְעָרַיִךְ.

חָזוּ נְבִיאִים בְּשָׁוְא דִּבְּרוּ בְּשֵׁם עִיר קָדוֹשׁ יַעֲקֹב לְשָׁלוֹם,

וְלֹא חָבְּשׁוּ מְזוֹרַיִךְ.

יִתַּר לְבָבִי עֲלֵי אָרוֹן וּמִשְׁכָּן וְצִיץ זָהָב וְאֵפוֹד,

וְשֵׁם קֹדֶשׁ סְתָרַיִךְ.

אִיִּם יַחֲווּ לְרָז אוֹתוֹת וּמוֹפֵת,

עֲלֵי שִׁבְרֵךְ יֵרָפְאוּ, אֱלֵי מִשְׁנֶה שְׁבָרַיִךְ.

שֶׁמֶשׁ וְכָל כּוֹכְבֵי שַׁחַק בְּעֵמֶק דָּמוּ,

קוֹלֵךְ בְּרָמָה שְׂאִי, קוֹל תַּמְרוּרַיִךְ.

סַהַר וְכִימָה וְעָשׁ וּכְסִיל לָזאת יִבְכּוּ,

נַגְהָם אֲשֶׁר אָסְפוּ, כּוֹכְבֵי שְׁחָרַיִךְ.

מַטֵּה רְשָׁעִים כְּקָם, שָׂרִים בְּיָדָם תְּלוּת,

שָׁבַת מְשׂוֹשֵׂךְ וְגִיל וּכְלֵי זְמָרַיִךְ.

אָבַל לְבָנוֹן וְגִיל כַּרְמֶל בְּלִי נִשְׁמַע חָפְרוּ סְגָנִים,

בְּבֹא צַר בִּשְׁעָרַיִךְ.

חָכְמַת נְבוֹנִים בְּיוֹם אָבְדָה וְאָסְרוּ קְצִינַיִךְ,

וְשָׁחוּ בְּנֵי צִיּוֹן יְקָרַיִךְ.

צִיּוֹן גְּבֶרֶת — O Zion, you were once the mistress. In this kinnah we bemoan Zion's terrible fall from prominence to pitiful wretchedness. Once Zion was the center of the entire world, mistress to all the nations but now she lies downtrodden beneath the heel of her former vassals.

Indeed it seems as if God has lost all interest in Jerusalem (Zion) and has abandoned it to heathen marauders, but in truth, God still cares deeply for Israel and Jerusalem, only He is hidden from our view. For this reason we sing kinnos such as this one, to arouse God to reveal His Presence once more.

The Talmud (Menachos 87a) states that even after the destruction of Zion, God protected this sacred site by posting guardian angels around it. As the prophet says, Upon your walls, O

44.

צִיּוֹן O Zion! You who were once the mistress over the nations[1]
    who are now your tormentors, accept abundant wishes
  for peace from your captive [people].
My heart is in ferment[2] when I hear the roar of the royal monarchs,
    the sons of Seir and Moab, inside the hall of your Sanctuary.
My anointed ones [the High Priest and the king] were besmirched
    by the blood which splattered from the [smashed]
    skulls of the slain [Jewish] princes.
    Shoa and Koa [fierce gentile princes] tore them to pieces[3]
    and trampled over my nation, your chosen ones.
They seized the fortified cities by building siege towers and by
    paving assault roads;[4] they chopped down the cedars of
    Lebanon from the woods of your forests [for construction materials].
The [corrupt] prophets prophesied falsely,[5]
    saying in the Name of God that [Jerusalem]
    the city of the Holy One of Jacob[6] would be left in peace.
    Thus, your festering [spiritual] wounds were not bandaged
    [and you did not repent].
My heart pounded [in terror] over the loss of the Ark, the Tabernacle,
    the golden Headplate [of the High Priest], the sacred Ephod robe
    and Your concealed Holy Name.
Even the inhabitants of the most remote islands
    acknowledge your power to reveal secrets through the signs
    [of the Urim V'Tumim breastplate] and the wonders
    [of your prophets]. These [wondrous faces] could have cured
    your wounds, now instead we wail over your two-fold devastation![7]
The Sun and the all the heavenly stars were plunged
    into deepest silence, so raise up your voice in Ramah,
    the voice of your bitter wailing.[8]
The moon and the constellations of Pleaides, Ursa and Orion,[9]
    let them all weep over this, that your morning stars
    have withheld their radiance.[10]
When the powerful staff of the wicked[11] arose,
    they commanded the [Jewish] princes to be hung
    by their own hands; at that moment Your gladness
    and joy ceased,[12] together with the instruments of your music.
Lebanon [the Temple] mourns, and the joy of Carmel [the Temple]
    is no longer heard, the deputies were disgraced
    when the enemy entered your gates.
The wisdom of the sages[13] vanished on that day
    [of the Temple's destruction] and your leaders were imprisoned,
    and your precious ones, the sons of Zion were bent low.[14]

---

(1) Isaiah 47::5. (2) Cf. Psalms 73:21. (3) Cf. Deuteronomy 33:20. (4) Cf. Ezekiel 4:2.
(5) Cf. Eichah 2:14. (6) Isaiah 29:23. (7) Cf. Jeremiah 17:18. (8) Cf. Jeremiah 31:14. (9) Cf. Job 9:9.
(10) Cf. Joel 2:10. (11) Isaiah 14:5. (12) Cf. Eichah 5:15. (13) Cf. Isaiah 29:14. (14) Cf. Eichah 4:2.

מִכְּלַל מְלָכִים לְבוּשׁ בָּנוֹת רְעוּלוֹת,

פְּאֵר רָאמוֹת וְגָבִישׁ,[1] וְאַף סַפִּיר גְּזָרַיִךְ.[2]

בָּזְאוּ נְהָרִים[3] בְּתוֹךְ קִרְיָה עַלִּיזָה,[4]

לְאֵין קֵץ לִתְכוּנָה[5] וְסוֹף, פָּרְצוּ גְדֵרַיִךְ.[6]

גִּבְעָה וְעֵץ רַעֲנָן,[7]

אֵלֶּה מְקוֹם פִּגּוּל מְלֵאִים מֵחֲלַל פְּגָרַיִךְ.

יֶהֱמוּ קְרָבַי כַּיָּם, יִזְּלוּ דְמָעַי

כְּמֵי נְמָרִים[8] לַבָּאִים בְּיוֹם טָרְפוּ כְּפִירַיִךְ.[9]

יִסְעַר לְבָבִי כְּמוֹ סוּפָה וָסַעַר,

כְּמוֹץ גֹּרֶן יְסוֹעַר,[10] עֲלֵי אַשְׁמוֹת כְּמָרַיִךְ.

הוּמַר בְּשָׂרִי לְיוֹם נֵאַר קְדוֹשׁ יַעֲקֹב

מִקְדָּשׁ וּמִזְבְּחוֹ,[11] בְּלִי בוֹא בַּחֲצֵרַיִךְ.

שׂוֹרֵק וּנְטַע נַעֲמָן[12] הָיִית,

וּבְקֶר כְּצָץ פֶּרַח וְנִצָּה, תְּשַׁגְשְׁגִי זְמוֹרַיִךְ.

שׁוּבִי צְבִיָּה לְאֵל יוֹצְרֵךְ, יְכוֹנְנֵךְ לְדוֹר וָדוֹר,

בְּתוֹכֵךְ שְׁכוֹן בָּעַל נְעוּרַיִךְ.

אַרְיֵה בְּנֶךְ לְכַל יַעֲלֶה[13] מְסִלּוֹת,

וְצִי אַדִּיר וְשַׁיִט לְבַל יַעֲבוֹר[14] יְאוֹרַיִךְ.

נַפְשִׁי שְׁלוֹמֵךְ דְּרוֹשׁ אוֹתָהּ כְּחוֹם צַח עֲלֵי אוֹר,

כְּעָב טַל בְּחוֹם[15] יוֹם, נֵד קְצִירַיִךְ.[16]

אֶשְׂמַח וְאָשִׂישׂ בְּיוֹם אֶשְׁמַע מְבַשֵּׂר בְּקוֹל,[17]

שָׁלוֹם מְנוּחָה דְּרוֹשׁ, וּשְׁלוֹם אֲסִירַיִךְ.

Jerusalem, I posted sentries all day and all
night; they will ever be silent; all those who
remember HASHEM be not still! (Isaiah 62:6).
What do these angels say as they stand guard?
Either they recite the verse, 'You will arise and
show Zion mercy' (Psalms 102:14), or they recite
the verse, 'The builder of Jerusalem is HASHEM'

(ibid. 147:2).
     What did the angels say before the destruc-
tion? They recited the verse, 'For HASHEM has
chosen Zion, it He desired for His dwelling
place' (ibid. 132:13). And when the Temple is
rebuilt, Rashi comments, they will recite that
verse once again.

The crown of [Jewish] kings is now worn by gentile daughters;
   [the crown] resplendent with precious stones,[1]
   even [inlaid] with skillfully cut sapphires.[2]

Streams [of gentile hordes] utterly pillaged[3] the [once] joyous city,[4]
   [multitudes] without end[5] or limit to their numbers,
   and they breached your walls.

On every hill and beneath every flourishing tree,[7]
   all places where idolatrous abominations [once] stood,
   are now filled with the corpses of your slaughtered.

My innards churn like the sea, my tears flow like water courses,
   because of the [barbaric gentiles who attacked Jews like]
   leopards[8] and lions on the day they tore apart
   the [young Jewish] cubs.[9]

My heart is in turmoil as if struck by a tempest and a storm,
   swirling like the chaff flying wildly from the threshing floor,[10]
   because of the guilt of your idolatrous priests [who led Israel astray].

The appearance of my flesh has changed [by suffering] since the day
   on which the Holy One of Jacob rejected the Temple and its Altar,[11]
   and prevented our entry into Your courtyards

[O Israel] at one time you were a sturdy vine,[12] a choice planting,
   at the dawn [of your history] when your buds blossomed
   and flowered, your vine's tendrils got entangled
   [in the destructive thorns of sin].

Return, O lovely hind, to God, Your Creator, and He will establish
   You firmly for generation upon generation, when He,
   the husband of your youth will dwell in your midst.

The lion [Nebuchadnezzar] will no longer march up the highways[13]
   [to attack] your Temple dwelling, nor will any mighty naval fleet
   or any sailing vessel trespass[14] your waterways

My soul yearns to seek your welfare [as people] long for a day
   radiant with brilliant sunshine[15] or as [they pine] for a cloud of dew
   on the day of intense heat[16] at the time of your harvest.

I will rejoice and exalt on the day that I hear the herald who proclaims[17]
   [the Redemption] out loud, and strives to bring tranquility and peace
   and [above all] seeks the peace and welfare of your captives.

---

(1) Job 28:18. (2) Cf. Eichah 4:7. (3) Isaiah 18:7. (4) 22:2. (5) Nahum 2:10. (6) Cf. Psalms 80:13.
(7) Cf. Jeremiah 2:20. (8) Isaiah 15:6. (9) Cf. Nahum 2:14. (10) Cf. Hosea 13:3. (11) Cf. Eichah 2:7.
(12) Cf. Jeremiah 2:21. (13) Cf. Isaiah 34:9. (14) Cf. 33:21. (15) 18:4. (16) Cf. 17:11. (17) Cf. 52:7.

קינות לזכרון הקדושים של חורבן איירופא

זִכְרוּ נָא וְקוֹנֲנוּ כָּל יִשְׂרָאֵל, קוֹלְכֶם יִשָּׁמַע בָּרָמָה,

כִּי הִשְׁמִידָה גֶּרְמַנְיָא אֶת עַמֵּנוּ בִּימֵי זַעַם הַמִּלְחָמָה,

בְּמִיתוֹת מְשֻׁנּוֹת אַכְזָרִיּוֹת, בָּרָעָב וּבַצָּמָא,

אַל תִּשְׁכְּחוּ בְּכָל הַדּוֹרוֹת, עֲדֵי תִזְכּוּ לִרְאוֹת בַּנֶּחָמָה.

צַעֲקָתָם וּבְכִיּוֹתֵיהֶם, צְפוּפִים וּסְגוּרִים בַּקְּרוֹנִים,

כַּצֹּאן לַטֶּבַח יוּבָלוּ, לִשְׂרֵפָה בַּכִּשְׁרוֹנִים,

קוֹל שַׁוְעָם יִזָּכֵר תָּמִיד לִפְנֵי שׁוֹכֵן מְעוֹנִים.

בְּקָרְאָם שְׁמַע יִשְׂרָאֵל, מָסְרוּ נַפְשָׁם לַאֲדוֹנֵי הָאֲדוֹנִים.

רָאשֵׁי יְשִׁיבוֹת וְתַלְמִידֵיהֶם, וְהַמוֹנֵי עַמְּךָ שָׁמָּה,

הֶעֱבִידוּם בְּעִנּוּיִים קָשִׁים, וַהֲרָגוּם בְּיָד רָמָה,

דְּמֵי יְלָדִים רַכִּים צוֹעֲקִים אֵלֶךְ מִן הָאֲדָמָה,

נְקוֹם נִקְמַת טַף וְנָשִׁים, לֹא תְחַיֶּה כָּל נְשָׁמָה.

עַל שְׂרֵפַת אַלְפֵי מִדְרָשׁוֹת וּבָתֵּי כְנֵסִיּוֹת,

רִבְבוֹת סִפְרֵי תוֹרָה וְלוֹמְדֶהָ, נְקוֹנֵן בִּשְׁאִיּוֹת,

שָׁלְחוּ בָאֵשׁ מִקְדְּשֵׁי אֵל, הִצִּיתוּ וְעֵינֵנוּ צוֹפִיּוֹת,

יְשַׁלֵּם הַמַּבְעִיר אֶת הַבְּעֵרָה, יָדִין בַּגּוֹיִם מָלֵא גְוִיּוֹת.

זַעֲקוּ שָׁמַיִם וַאֲדָמָה, עַל אַלְפֵי עֲיָרוֹת מִבְצְרֵי תוֹרָה,

אַרְצוֹת אֵירוֹפָּא וּקְהִלּוֹתֶהָ, נוֹחֲלֵי וּמְקַיְּמֵי מְסוֹרָה,

צַדִּיקִים זְקֵנִים וַחֲסִידִים, דְּבֵקֵי אֱמוּנָה טְהוֹרָה,

מִיּוֹם גָּלִינוּ מֵאַרְצֵנוּ לֹא הָיָה כָזֶה כִּלָּיוֹן נוֹרָא.

◆§ The destruction of European Jewry by the Nazis during World War II was the most massive calamity to befall our people since the Destruction of the Second Temple. As explained in the prefatory notes to *kinnah* 25, which laments the devastation of the Crusades, Torah Jews recognize that all Jewish misfortunes have their roots in the tragic events of Tishah B'Av. Therefore we designate no new days of mourning to commemorate later events, but include them in our Tishah B'Av *kinnos* service.

The Bobover Rav, Admor HaRav Shlomo Halberstam, שליט״א, is a scion of Sanz, one of the most illustrious Rabbinic and Chassidic dynasties. The Rav lost everything in the Holocaust — family, friends, followers, disciples and students in the thousands. A lone survivor,

the Rebbe arrived in America after the war with nothing but the clothes on his back and a burning determination to rebuild what the Nazis destroyed. With the help of Hashem the glory of the House of Bobov has been restored and one will find dozens of Bobov institutions and thousands of Bobover Chassidim in every corner of the globe.

In 1984, the Bobover Rav composed a special *kinnah* to bemoan the tragedy of *Churban Europa*, and it is recited in many congregations. When the Rav was asked for permission to include his *kinnah* and its translation in this edition of *kinnos*, he graciously conceded. Then he explained why he had written it: 'For years I had wanted to express my grief over my personal loss and *Klal Yisrael's* loss, in a special

KINNOS IN MEMORY OF THE MARTYRS OF CHURBAN EUROPE

זִכְרוּ נָא *Remember, please, and lament, O all of Israel,*
let your voices be heard on high.
For Germany has destroyed our people,
during stormy days of the World War;
with killings, horrible and cruel,
with starvation and thirst.
For all generations, do not forget,
until you will merit witnessing the [ultimate] consolation.
[Remember] their screams and their weeping as they were
    tightly packed and locked into the train's [cattle] cars.
Like sheep to the slaughter they were led to be
    incinerated in the crematorium ovens.
May the sound of their pleading cries be eternally remembered,
    by the One Who dwells in the Heavens.
When they proclaimed, 'Shema Yisrael'
    they offered up their lives to the Lord of lords.

Roshei Yeshiva and their students, and the
    multitudes of Your people were there.
They enslaved them with brutal tortures,
    and they slaughtered them with high-handed arrogance.
The blood of tender babes cries out to You from the earth, [saying;]
    'Exact vengeance for the children and the women;
    let no living soul escape alive!'

For the burning of thousands of study halls and synagogues,
    and for myriad of Torah scrolls and their students,
    we shall lament with raised and screaming voices.
They set God's sanctuaries aflame, they ignited them,
    and our eyes witnessed this.
Let those who lit the fire suffer retribution;
    may God judge the corpse-filled nations.

Cry out loud, O heaven and earth, for the thousands of cities,
    citadels of Torah,
for the countries of Europe and their Jewish communities,
    the heirs and trustees of our traditions,
for righteous tzaddikim, elders, pious chassidim,
    all those who cleaved unto a faith so pure.
From the day we were exiled from our homeland,
    there was never an annihilation as awesome as this.

---

kinnah, but I hesitated. I felt that in order to
compose a kinnah one must be on the exalted
level of R' Elazar HaKalir, who wrote with
Ruach HaKodesh, Divine inspiration. Moreover,

he was a master of Kabbalistic secrets and knew
the mystical incantations of the ministering
angels. Still, many chassidim requested a vehicle
to convey their personal sorrow on this bitter

רַחֵם עַל שְׁאֵרִיתֵנוּ, הַבֶּט נָא מִשָּׁמַיִם,
לְמַחֲנוֹת הַקְּדוֹשִׁים, פִּי עֶשֶׂר כְּיוֹצְאֵי מִצְרָיִם,
קוֹמֵס בֵּית קָדְשֵׁנוּ, וְנַחֲמֵנוּ בְּכִפְלַיִם,
רוֹמְמֵנוּ, וַהֲבִיאֵנוּ לְצִיּוֹן וִירוּשָׁלָיִם.

🦋 🦋 🦋

הַזּוֹכֵר מַזְכִּירָיו,   דּוֹר דּוֹר וְקָדוֹשָׁיו,
מֵעֵת אֲשֶׁר אָז בְּחַרְתָּנוּ,
יִזְכּוֹר דְּרָאוֹן,   שֶׁל דּוֹר אַחֲרוֹן,
אוֹיָה מֶה הָיָה לָנוּ.

שְׁטוּפֵי מַבּוּל דָם,   שֶׁמָּסְרוּ נַפְשׁוֹתָם,
כָּל שְׁקוּעֵי עִמְקֵי הַבָּכָא,
יִפְקְדֵם אֱלֹהִים,   בְּאַרְצוֹת הַחַיִּים,
וַעֲדֵי עַד זִכְרָם לִבְרָכָה.

שְׂאוּ אֵלָיו כַּפַּיִם,   אֲהָהּ, אִי שָׁמַיִם,
הוֹי עַל מֵיטַב שִׁבְטֵי יִשְׂרָאֵל,
עֵדוֹת וּקְהִלּוֹת,   עָרִים וּגְלִילוֹת,
חֲבוּרוֹת, מוֹסָדוֹת, כָּל מוֹעֲדֵי אֵל.

מִי יִתֵּן פַּלְגֵי מַיִם,   תֵּרַדְנָה עֵינַיִם,
אֶל אַשְׁדוֹת נַחֲלֵי הַדְּמָעוֹת,
עֲלֵי אַלְפֵי אֲלָפִים,   גּוּפִים נִשְׂרָפִים,
בְּמוֹ אֵשׁ הַחֻרְבָּן וּזְוָעוֹת.

---

day, but I held back, because I felt genuinely unworthy.

Then, one day, I was studying the laws of Tishah B'Av in the book *Seder HaYom* [by R' Moshe ben Yehudah Makir, Rosh Yeshivah in Safed, and a colleague of the *Arizal* and R' Yosef Karo]. He writes as follows:

iiiWhoever can wail on this day should wail, and whoever can recite *kinnos* should recite *kinnos* — either those already recorded in the holy books, one the *kinnos* he himself composed with the intellect God has granted him. It is a mitzvah for each and every individual to compose kinnos for weeping and moaning and to recite them on this bitter day. One who does this is considered most righteous and is worthy of being described as one of Jerusalem's mourners and one of her holy men. But one who is *not* capable of composing his personal *kinnos*, should recite the *kinnos* written by others.iii

'When I read these words,' the Rav concluded, 'I saw a clear sign from heaven that the time had come to compose a *kinnah* over the last *churban*. For doesn't the *Seder HaYom* say clearly that any

compassionate with our remnant; look down upon us,
   please, from heaven,
at the [death] camps of the martyrs,
   ten times as many as those who left Egypt.
Rebuild our holy Temple, and provide us with double consolation,
Exalt us, and bring us back to Zion and Jerusalem.

🦋 🦋 🦋

הַזּוֹכֵר   He, Who remembers those who remember Him,
         Each generation and its holy ones —
since the time You have chosen us —
May He remember the gruesome fate
of the last generation.
Woe! what has happened to us!

Those who were swept away by the flood of blood —
who sacrificed their lives —
All who were submerged in valleys of tears,
May God think of them in the lands of eternal life.
May their memory be a blessing for all eternity.

Lift up your hands to Him, woe O you Heavens!
Woe over the best of Israel's tribes,
Communities and congregations, cities and districts,
fraternities, foundations, all rendezvous with God.

If only streams of water could pour down from eyes
towards waterfalls of the rivers of tears,
for the thousands times thousands of corpses
consumed in the fire of destructions and horrors.

---

person, even the smallest, should express his own feelings in his original *kinnah*.'

◆§ הַזּוֹכֵר — *He, Who remembers.* Rav Shimon Schwab, שליט"א, widely recognized as an eloquent spokesman for Torah Jewry, joined the Rabbinate of Congregation K'hal Adas Jeshurun in the Washington Heights neighborhood of New York, in 1958, in association with the late revered Rav Dr. Joseph Breuer, זצ"ל.

Rav Schwab was born in Frankfurt-am-Main, Germany, in 1908, and studied at several well-known Eastern European *yeshivos*, including Telshe and Mir. In those years, Rav Schwab had the opportunity to meet with and learn from the foremost *Gedolim* of the time, including the holy Chafetz Chaim of Radin.

In the early 1930's, Rav Schwab was an eyewitness to the rise of Hitler Nazism in Germany and the systematic oppression of the Jews. In 1936, the persecution of the Nazis forced him to leave his pulpit in Germany. He came to the United States where he assumed a position in the Baltimore Rabbinate.

Rav Schwab relates that in 1959, as Tishah B'Av approached, the late Rav Breuer made a request of him, 'Please compose a special Tishah B'Av *kinnah* for our *kehillah*. Each and every one of us is either a refugee or a Holocaust survivor. We have all lost family and friends in this *churban*, and we German Jews bore the brunt of Hitler's fury. We must not forget, nor can we allow our children to forget. Eight centuries ago German Jewry was slaughtered by the Crusaders.

וְעַל שָׂרֵי הַתּוֹרָה,　וּמַחֲזִיקֵי מָסוֹרָה,
וְעַל פִּרְחֵי הַכְּהוּנָה הַצְּעִירִים,
וְעַל חוֹבְשֵׁי מִדְרָשׁוֹת,　וּמוֹרִים וּמוֹרוֹת,
תִּינוֹקוֹת בֵּית רַבָּן יַקִּירִים.

עַל בָּנוֹת בּוֹטְחוֹת,　וְסָבִים וְסָבוֹת,
וְעַל זַרְעָם וְטַפָּם שֶׁיָּלָדוּ,
וְגַם לָרַבּוֹת,　רִבְבוֹת נֶאֱהָבִים בַּחַיִּים,
בְּמוֹתָם לֹא נִפְרָדוּ.

אֶת דָּמָם דְּרוֹשׁ,　כִּי תִשָּׂא אֶת רֹאשׁ,
שֶׁל כָּל נִדָּף לְעָלִים הַטְּרוּפִים.
כָּל נַפְשׁוֹת מֵת,　בִּימֵי שֶׁבֶר וָשֵׁאת,
שִׁשָּׁה אַלְפֵי פְעָמִים אֲלָפִים.

שְׁלִישִׁיָּה לְבָעֵר,　בִּבְרַק זַעַם סוֹעֵר,
מִכַּרְמֵי הַחֶמֶד אָהָבְתָּ,
גּוֹאֵל הַדָּם,　נָא זְכֹר צַעֲרָם,
אַל תִּמְחֶה מִסֵּפֶר כְּתַבְתָּ.

זְכֹר הַנְּאָקוֹת,　וְרַעַשׁ צְעָקוֹת,
אָז יוּבְלוּ לָרֶצַח,
יְאוֹרֵי דְמֵיהֶם,　וְדִמְעוֹת פְּנֵיהֶם,
לֹא תִשָּׁכַחְנָה לָנֶצַח.

כָּל חֵיל וּגְנִיחָה,　וּנְהִי צְרִיחָה,
מִשְּׁדוּדֵי לַהֲקוֹת הַכְּלָבִים,
זְכֹר וּסְפֹר,　בְּנֹאדְךָ צְרוֹר,
עַד עֵת נְקֹם עֶלְבּוֹן עֲלוּבִים.

בְּמַחֲנוֹת הַפְּרָאִים,　כְּאֵב וּנְגָעִים,
וּפַחֵי נְפָשׁוֹת עֲגוּמוֹת,
חֲרָפוֹת וּצְחוֹק,　כְּלִימוֹת וָרוֹק,
פִּצְעֵי הַכָּאוֹת אֵימוֹת.

According to historians, how many Jews were killed? Perhaps 5,000. In World War II more than one thousand times that number were killed! In just one day at Aushchwitz more than 5,000 Jews

For the princes of Torah, the pillars of tradition,
for the young flowers of the priesthood,
for the diligent scholars, the men teachers and women,
and the precious children in school.

The trusting daughters, the elderly grandparents,
and their offspring,
and the infants whom they bore, everyone —
including the myriads beloved in life,
not parted by death.

Seek out their blood when You take the count
of all the scattered, rent leaves, of every life perished
in the days of destruction and calamity —
six thousand times a thousand.
An entire third to be destroyed,
by the Blitzkrieg's fury,
of the cherished vineyards You dearly loved.
O Avenger of blood!
The memory of their misery, please
do not erase from the book You have written.

Remember the moans and tumultuous screams,
when they were herded for slaughter —
May the rivers of their blood
and the tears on their faces:
not be forgotten forever.

Every tremble, every groan, every piercing cry
of those torn asunder by hoards of dogs,
remember and count them,
collect them into Your flask,
Till the time the degraded ones' shame is avenged.

In the barbarian's camps
were pain and sickness,
the anguish of mortified souls;
insults and mockery, shame and spit,
searing wounds from horrible blows.

---

were brutally gassed and murdered. If German Jewry composed *kinnos* to commemorate the evil that befell us during the Crusades, how much more so must we compose one over the Holocaust!'

In deference to this request, Rav Schwab composed the following *kinnah* which, in Khal Adas Jeshurun, is recited by the Rav on Tishah

B'Av night at the conclusion of the *kinnos* service after the passage which begins with תְּרַחֵם צִיּוֹן, *Have mercy on Zion.* Although Rav Schwab only composed this *kinnah* to be said in his *kehillah,* many other congregations have adopted the custom of reciting it on Tishah B'Av, either at night or by day, as a memorial of our most recent *Churban.*

וּרְעָבוֹן, צִמָּאוֹן, שִׁגָּעוֹן, עִצָּבוֹן,
וְכִשָּׁלוֹן נֶחֱשָׁלִים בְּלִי כֹחַ,
וְכָל נַאֲקוֹת חָלָל, מִכָּל יָחִיד אֻמְלָל,
חָלִילָה לְךָ מִלִּשְׁכֹּחַ.

וְתִימְרוֹת עָשָׁן, וְקִיטוֹר מִכִּבְשָׁן,
תִּלֵּי תִלִּים עֲצָמוֹת וְגִידִים,
וְחַדְרֵי הָרַעַל, קוֹל שַׁאֲגוֹת מִקָּהֵל
הַנֶּחְנָקִים תּוֹךְ תָּאֵי הָאֵדִים.

וְסִרְחוֹן גּוּפוֹת, וּגְוִיּוֹת סְגוּפוֹת,
גְּלַל דִּמֶן אַדְמַת נוֹאָצִים,
אֵיךְ הָפְכוּ טוֹרְפֵיהֶם, לִבְרִית חֶלְבֵּיהֶם,
וְעוֹר אִישׁ לְקִשּׁוּטֵי הַנָּשִׁים.

וּקְרִיצַת אֶצְבָּעוֹת, שֶׁל רָאשֵׁי הַפְּרָעוֹת,
לִימִין שֶׁעֲבוּד פֶּרֶךְ, צַלְמָוֶת לִשְׂמֹאול.
וְאֵיךְ יָרוּ יְרִיּוֹת עַל חוֹפְרֵי הַבּוֹרוֹת,
בְּיִסּוּרֵי חִבּוּט קֶבֶר הוֹרְדוּם שְׁאֹול.

אֵיךְ עֻנּוּ אַחְיוֹתֵינוּ, וְסֹרְסוּ בְּנוֹתֵינוּ,
כּוֹסוֹת תַּרְעֵלָה מִידֵי רוֹפְאִים אַכְזָרִים.
וּפְלִיטֵי הַשְּׂרִידִים בְּמַחֲלוֹת וּסְתָרִים,
וְטֻמְיוֹן יְלָדִים בְּבָתֵּי שְׁמַד כְּמָרִים.

שֶׂה תָמִים לָעוֹלָה, דַּם בְּנֵי הַגּוֹלָה,
הוֹי אֲרִיאֵל מִנִּבְלַת חֲסִידֶיךָ,
צֹאן קֳדָשִׁים מִי יִמְנֶה, אֲשֶׁר אָשָׁם לֹא תִכְבֶּה,
בְּחוּנֶיךָ הָיוּ מְקַדְּשֵׁי שְׁמֶךָ.

בְּקוֹל שְׁמַע יִשְׂרָאֵל, מָסְרוּ נֶפֶשׁ לָאֵל,
שֶׁהוּא יַאַסְפֵם, וְעַד יוֹם אַחֲרוֹן,
הִצְדִּיקוּ דִין, וְאַף אֲנִי מַאֲמִין
עָנוּ, וְשָׁרוּ שִׁירַת בִּטָּחוֹן.

Hunger, thirst, frenzy, sorrow,
the faint stumbling without any strength;
every death-rattle of every forlorn one,
far be it from You to forget.

The pillars of smoke, the fumes from furnace,
Piles and piles of bones and sinews,
poison-filled halls,
the roaring sound of the multitude,
choking in gas chamber.

The stench of the bodies, the tortured corpses,
fertilizers for the soil of the blasphemers.
How the tormentors turned
their fat into soap,
and human skin into feminine adornments.

[Remember] the finger motions
of the savage officers.
To the right — slave labor!
To the left — the shadow of death.
[Remember] how the sharpshooters shot
at those digging [their own] graves,
lowering them to the depths in the agony of the grave.

And how they afflicted our sisters
and mutilated our daughters,
doses of poison from sadistic doctors,
And fugitive survivors
in burrows and bunkers,
and the disappearance of children
in houses of apostasy, in monasteries.

Unblemished sheep, completely consumed,
the blood of the Diaspora's children,
Woe! O Ariel, for the corpses of your devout ones.
Who could count the sacred flock,
whose flame will never be extinguished,
Your tested ones were Sanctifiers of Your name.

With the cry of 'Shema Yisrael,'
they gave up their lives for God,
so that He might gather them in.
And until the very last day,
they justified His judgment,
and called out, 'I believe...'
and sang a song of trust.

וּבְכֵן נִשְׁאַר עָם,   כְּיָתוֹם נִדְהָם,
בְּלִי קְבָרִים לְהִשְׁתַּטֵּחַ,
וְלֹא מַצֵּבוֹת,   אֵיפֹה לִבְכּוֹת,
יְכַבּוֹת לֵבָב רוֹתֵחַ.

רַק נִסְכֵּי הַדָּם,   אַזְכָּרוֹתָם,
תּוֹסְסִים בְּלִי שׁוֹכֵחַ,
וְהָרֵי אֶפְרֵי עֲקֵדָתָם,
תְּרוּמוֹת דִּשְׁנֵי מִזְבֵּחַ.

מִי יְמַלֵּל   צַעַר יִשְׂרָאֵל,
אֲשֶׁר דַּעְתּוֹ מִכְּאֵב נִטְרֶפֶת,
וּשְׁאֵרִית הַפְּאֵר,   כִּמְעַט מִזְּעֵיר,
וְאֵיךְ קוֹמָתָה הַיּוֹם נִכְפֶּפֶת.

אֵל חַי מְרַחֵם,   עֲדָתְךָ נַחֵם,
אֲשֶׁר לְךָ מְאֹד נִכְסֶפֶת,
אוֹר חָדָשׁ תַּזְרִיחַ,   קַרְנֵי הוֹד תַּצְמִיחַ,
וְרוּחַ אֱלֹהִים מְרַחֶפֶת.

And now, a people is left,
bewildered as an orphan —
without graves at which to pray,
without tombstones
where to weep
the laments of emotion-filled hearts.

Only blood libations
are their memorials
boiling, unforgettable —
and the mounds of ashes from their Akeidah,
are tributes from the Altar's ashes.

Who can express
Israel's torment,
whose mind is frenzied by misery?
The remnants of its splendor
is a fraction of a bit,
how its pride is humbled today!

O Living God! Merciful One!
Comfort Your congregation
that yearns for You so mightily,
Let new light shine,
let rays of glory grow,
And may God's spirit hover.

מה.

The congregation rises and recites the following *kinnah* responsively with the *chazzan*.

אֱלִי צִיּוֹן* וְעָרֶיהָ, כְּמוֹ אִשָּׁה בְּצִירֶיהָ,
וְכִבְתוּלָה חֲגֻרַת שַׂק עַל בַּעַל נְעוּרֶיהָ.[1]

עֲלֵי אַרְמוֹן אֲשֶׁר נֻטַּשׁ בְּאַשְׁמַת צֹאן עֲדָרֶיהָ,
וְעַל בִּיאַת מְחָרְפֵי אֵל בְּתוֹךְ מִקְדַּשׁ חֲדָרֶיהָ,

אֱלִי צִיּוֹן וְעָרֶיהָ, כְּמוֹ אִשָּׁה בְּצִירֶיהָ,
וְכִבְתוּלָה חֲגֻרַת שַׂק עַל בַּעַל נְעוּרֶיהָ.

עֲלֵי גָלוּת מְשָׁרְתֵי אֵל, מַנְעִימֵי שִׁיר זְמָרֶיהָ,[2]
וְעַל דָּמָם אֲשֶׁר שֻׁפַּךְ, כְּמוֹ מֵימֵי יְאוֹרֶיהָ,

אֱלִי צִיּוֹן וְעָרֶיהָ, כְּמוֹ אִשָּׁה בְּצִירֶיהָ,
וְכִבְתוּלָה חֲגֻרַת שַׂק עַל בַּעַל נְעוּרֶיהָ.

עֲלֵי הֶגְיוֹן מְחוֹלֶיהָ, אֲשֶׁר דָּמַם בְּעָרֶיהָ,
וְעַל וַעַד אֲשֶׁר שָׁמֵם וּבִטּוּל סַנְהֶדְרֶיהָ,

אֱלִי צִיּוֹן וְעָרֶיהָ, כְּמוֹ אִשָּׁה בְּצִירֶיהָ,
וְכִבְתוּלָה חֲגֻרַת שַׂק עַל בַּעַל נְעוּרֶיהָ.

עֲלֵי זִבְחֵי תְמִידֶיהָ, וּפִדְיוֹנֵי בְּכוֹרֶיהָ,*
וְעַל חִלּוּל כְּלֵי הֵיכָל וּמִזְבַּח קְטוֹרֶיהָ,

אֱלִי צִיּוֹן וְעָרֶיהָ, כְּמוֹ אִשָּׁה בְּצִירֶיהָ,
וְכִבְתוּלָה חֲגֻרַת שַׂק עַל בַּעַל נְעוּרֶיהָ.

עֲלֵי טַפֵּי מְלָכֶיהָ, בְּנֵי דָוִד גְּבִירֶיהָ,
וְעַל יָפְיָם אֲשֶׁר חָשַׁךְ בְּעֵת סָרוּ כְתָרֶיהָ,

אֱלִי צִיּוֹן וְעָרֶיהָ, כְּמוֹ אִשָּׁה בְּצִירֶיהָ,
וְכִבְתוּלָה חֲגֻרַת שַׂק עַל בַּעַל נְעוּרֶיהָ.

אֱלִי צִיּוֹן ‫≈‬ — *Wail, O Zion.* This final *kinnah* is chanted to a traditional heart-rending melody that expresses the full measure of our sorrow. Once again, in this last lament, we list all that we lost at the time of the Destruction, both materially and spiritually. However, the opening line of the *kinnah* (which is repeated either as a refrain after every second line, or once at the end of the *kinnah*) provides a ray of hope: 'Wail, O Zion and her cities, like a woman suffering from birth travail.' Israel's suffering is not in vain, rather the Destruction and Exile should be viewed as a period of embryonic development and gestation leading to the rebirth of our nation. No pain is more excruciating than birth travail, yet the mother accepts it because it heralds the exhilarating joy of birth. Similarly, Israel's suffering has been indescribable but we must accept it as the travail which precedes the glorious rebirth of our people.

עֲלֵי זִבְחֵי תְמִידֶיהָ וּפִדְיוֹנֵי בְּכוֹרֶיהָ — *. . . for her daily [Tamid] offerings, and for the redemption of her*

45.

The congregation rises and recites the following *kinnah* responsively with the *chazzan*.

אֱלִי צִיּוֹן *Wail, O Zion* and her cities,*
like a woman suffering from birth travail,
and like a maiden girded in sackcloth,
[lamenting] for the husband of her youth. . .[1]

א ... *for the palace that is abandoned because of*
the sin of the sheep of her flocks,

ב *and for the entrance of the blasphemers of God*
into the chambers of her Sanctuary.

> *Wail, O Zion and her cities, like a woman suffering from birth travail,*
> *and like a maiden girded in sackcloth, [lamenting] for the husband of her youth...*

ג ... *for the exile of [the Kohanim,] the servants of God*
[and the Levites] who sweetly sang the song of her praise,[2]

ד *and for their blood that was spilt like the waters of her canals.*

> *Wail, O Zion and her cities, like a woman suffering from birth travail,*
> *and like a maiden girded in sackcloth, [lamenting] for the husband of her youth...*

ה ... *for the lyrics of her dances, that have been stilled in her cities,*

ו *and for the assembly chamber that is abandoned,*
with the disbandment of her Sanhedrin.

> *Wail, O Zion and her cities, like a woman suffering from birth travail,*
> *and like a maiden girded in sackcloth, [lamenting] for the husband of her youth...*

ז ... *for her daily [Tamid] offerings,*
and for the redemption of her firstborn sons,*

ח *and for the desecration of the Temple's vessels and her incense Altar.*

> *Wail, O Zion and her cities, like a woman suffering from birth travail,*
> *and like a maiden girded in sackcloth, [lamenting] for the husband of her youth...*

ט ... *for young children of her kings,*
the sons of David, her royal sovereigns,

י *and for their beauty which was darkened*
when her crowns were taken from her.

> *Wail, O Zion and her cities, like a woman suffering from birth travail,*
> *and like a maiden girded in sackcloth, [lamenting] for the husband of her youth...*

(1) *Joel* 1:8. (2) Cf. *II Samuel* 23:1.

firstborn sons. This statement is very puzzling. True, the daily *Tamid* offerings are dependent on the existence of the Temple, but the *mitzvah* of redeeming the firstborn son is not a function of the Temple. Indeed, it is in full force today and is practiced wherever Jews may live! This question has prodded some commentaries to suggest that the text be emended from פִּדְיוֹנֵי to בְּכוּרֶיהָ, בִּיכּוּרֵי בִּיכּוּרֵי בִּיכּוּרֵי, *her bikkurim fruits,* i.e., the *mitzvah* of bringing the first fruits to the *Kohen* in the Temple is no longer possible. Others explain that the redemption of the

firstborn here alludes to the Levites who served as the original objects by which the firstborn Israelites were redeemed in the Wilderness (see *Numbers* 3:11-13, 44-51). Thus, the first stich of this line, זִבְחֵי תְמִידֶיהָ, refers to the *Kohanim* who offered the *Tamid,* while the second stich speaks of the *Leviim.*

However, the passage may also be explained in its simplest and most literal reading. Regarding the *mitzvah* of redeeming the firstborn, the Torah states: כֹּל בְּכוֹר בָּנֶיךָ תִּפְדֶּה וְלֹא יֵרָאוּ פָנַי רֵיקָם, *Every firstborn of your sons you shall*

עֲלֵי **כָבוֹד**, אֲשֶׁר גָּלָה בְּעֵת חֻרְבַּן דְּבִירֶיהָ,
וְעַל **לוֹחֵץ** אֲשֶׁר לָחַץ, וְשָׁם שַׂקִּים חֲגוֹרֶיהָ,

אֱלִי צִיּוֹן וְעָרֶיהָ, כְּמוֹ אִשָּׁה בְּצִירֶיהָ,
וְכִבְתוּלָה חֲגֻרַת שַׂק עַל בַּעַל נְעוּרֶיהָ.

עֲלֵי **מַחַץ** וְרֹב מַכּוֹת' אֲשֶׁר הֻכּוּ נְזִירֶיהָ,
וְעַל **נִפּוּץ** עֲלֵי סֶלַע עוֹלָלֶיהָ' וּנְעָרֶיהָ,

אֱלִי צִיּוֹן וְעָרֶיהָ, כְּמוֹ אִשָּׁה בְּצִירֶיהָ,
וְכִבְתוּלָה חֲגֻרַת שַׂק עַל בַּעַל נְעוּרֶיהָ.

עֲלֵי **שִׂמְחַת** אוֹיְבֶיהָ, שָׂחֲקוּ עַל שְׁבָרֶיהָ,
וְעַל **עֱנוּי** בְּנֵי חוֹרִין נְדִיבֶיהָ טְהוֹרֶיהָ,

אֱלִי צִיּוֹן וְעָרֶיהָ, כְּמוֹ אִשָּׁה בְּצִירֶיהָ,
וְכִבְתוּלָה חֲגֻרַת שַׂק עַל בַּעַל נְעוּרֶיהָ.

עֲלֵי **פֶשַׁע** אֲשֶׁר עֻוְּתָה עוֹתָה סְלוּל דֶּרֶךְ אֲשׁוּרֶיהָ,
וְעַל **צִבְאוֹת** קְהָלֶיהָ שְׁזוּפֶיהָ שְׁחוֹרֶיהָ,

אֱלִי צִיּוֹן וְעָרֶיהָ, כְּמוֹ אִשָּׁה בְּצִירֶיהָ,
וְכִבְתוּלָה חֲגֻרַת שַׂק עַל בַּעַל נְעוּרֶיהָ.

עֲלֵי **קוֹלוֹת** מְחָרְפֶיהָ, בְּעֵת רַבּוּ פְגָרֶיהָ,
וְעַל **רִגְשַׁת** מְגַדְּפֶיהָ, בְּתוֹךְ מִשְׁכַּן חֲצֵרֶיהָ,

אֱלִי צִיּוֹן וְעָרֶיהָ, כְּמוֹ אִשָּׁה בְּצִירֶיהָ,
וְכִבְתוּלָה חֲגֻרַת שַׂק עַל בַּעַל נְעוּרֶיהָ.

עֲלֵי **שִׁמְךָ** אֲשֶׁר חֻלַּל בְּפִי קָמֵי מְצִירֶיהָ,
וְעַל **תַּחַן** יְצַוְּחוּ לָךְ קְשׁוֹב וּשְׁמַע אֲמָרֶיהָ,

אֱלִי צִיּוֹן וְעָרֶיהָ, כְּמוֹ אִשָּׁה בְּצִירֶיהָ,
וְכִבְתוּלָה חֲגֻרַת שַׂק עַל בַּעַל נְעוּרֶיהָ.

---

redeem, and none shall appear before Me empty (Exodus 34:20). *Rabbeinu Bachya* (ibid.) comments: Why did the Torah juxtapose the *mitzvah* of redeeming the firstborn son with the *mitzvah* of appearing before God in the Temple on the festivals? To teach that the firstborn who

is redeemed is assured that he will merit the privilege of seeing the construction of the Temple and he will witness God's presence therein.

Thus, the purpose of the firstborn's redemption is to prepare him for an encounter with God

כ   ... for the [Divine] glory which was exiled
     at the time of the Destruction of her Temples,
ל   and for the tyrant who persecuted her
     and caused her to gird herself in sackcloth.
> Wail, O Zion and her cities, like a woman suffering from birth travail,
> and like a maiden girded in sackcloth, [lamenting] for the husband of her youth. . .

מ   ... for the pounding and the numerous blows[1]
     with which her aristocrats were beaten,
נ   and for the smashing on the rock of her infants[2] and her youths.
> Wail, O Zion and her cities, like a woman suffering from birth travail,
> and like a maiden girded in sackcloth, [lamenting] for the husband of her youth. . .

ס   ... for the joy of her enemies when they made sport of her calamities,
ע   and for the tormenting of her free-spirited men,
     her noble-minded and pure-hearted people.
> Wail, O Zion and her cities, like a woman suffering from birth travail,
> and like a maiden girded in sackcloth, [lamenting] for the husband of her youth. . .

פ   ... for the sin which corrupted her,
     and diverted her footsteps from the straight path,
צ   and for the legions of her congregations
     whose [faces] now are wrinkled and blackened
     [by the flames of the Temple's destruction].
> Wail, O Zion and her cities, like a woman suffering from birth travail,
> and like a maiden girded in sackcloth, [lamenting] for the husband of her youth. . .

ק   ... for the cries of those who vilified her
     when the number of her corpses increased,
ר   and for the clamor of those who cursed her,
     inside the Courtyards of her Tabernacle.
> Wail, O Zion and her cities, like a woman suffering from birth travail,
> and like a maiden girded in sackcloth, [lamenting] for the husband of her youth. . .

ש   ... for Your Name which was profaned by the mouth
     of those who arose to torment her,
ת   and to the pleaful prayer which they cry out to You,
     listen carefully and heed her words.

Wail, O Zion and her cities,
   like a woman suffering from birth travail,
and like a maiden girded in sackcloth,
   [lamenting] for the husband of her youth. . .

---

(1) Cf. *Isaiah* 30:26. (2) Cf. *Psalms* 137:9.

---

in the Temple so that he will 'belong' to the
Temple and be one of *her* firstborn sons. In this
kinnah, we lament the fact that today, in the 0.1
absence of the Temple, the firstborn sons cannot
achieve this encounter, the ultimate purpose of
their redemption.

מו.

שׁוֹמְרוֹן קוֹל תִּתֵּן מְצָאוּנִי עֲוֹנַי,[1]
לְאֶרֶץ אַחֶרֶת יְצָאוּנִי בָנַי,[2]
וְאָהֳלִיבָה תִּזְעַק נִשְׂרְפוּ אַרְמוֹנַי,[3]
וַתֹּאמֶר צִיּוֹן עֲזָבַנִי יהוה.[4]

לֹא לָךְ אָהֳלִיבָה חֲשׁוֹב עֲנָיֵךְ כְּעָנְיִי,
הֲתַמְשִׁילִי חָלְיֵךְ לְשִׁבְרִי וּלְחָלְיִי,
אֲנִי אָהֳלָה סוּרָה בָּגַדְתִּי בִקְשָׁיִי,
וְקָם עָלַי כַּחֲשִׁי וְעָנָה בִי מֶרְיִי,[5]
וּלְמִקְצַת הַיָּמִים שְׁלַחְתִּי נְשָׁיִי,
וְתִגְלַת פִּלְאֶסֶר[6] אָכַל אֶת פִּרְיִי,
חֶמְדָּתִי פָּשַׁט וְהִצִּיל אֶת עֶדְיִי,[7]*
וְלַחֲלַח וְחָבוֹר[8] נָשָׂא אֶת שִׁבְיִי,
דְּמִי אָהֳלִיבָה וְאַל תִּבְכִּי כְּבִכְיִי,
שְׁנוֹתַיִךְ אָרְכוּ וְלֹא אָרְכוּ שָׁנַי.*

וְאָהֳלִיבָה תִּזְעַק נִשְׂרְפוּ אַרְמוֹנַי,
וַתֹּאמֶר צִיּוֹן עֲזָבַנִי יהוה.

מְשִׁיבָה אָהֳלִיבָה אֲנִי כֵן נֶעְקַשְׁתִּי,
וּבְאַלּוּף נְעוּרַי[9] כְּאָהֳלָה בָּגַדְתִּי,
דְּמִי אָהֳלָה כִּי יְגוֹנִי זָכַרְתִּי,
נָדַדְתְּ אַתְּ אַחַת וְרַבּוֹת נָדַדְתִּי,
הִנֵּה בְּיַד הַכַּשְׂדִּים פַּעֲמַיִם נִלְכַּדְתִּי,
וּשְׁבִיָּה עֲנִיָּה לְבָבֶל יָרַדְתִּי,

שׁוֹמְרוֹן ◆§ — *Shomron*. This *kinnah* is based on chapter 23 of *Ezekiel*, where God bids the prophet to expose the sins of the Jewish people. Then unfolds the shocking parable of two faithless wives who seek fulfillment of their unnatural lusts through numerous lovers. Ezekiel tells of two sisters, אָהֳלָה, *Oholah*, and אָהֳלִיבָה, *Oholivah*, who are both married to the same man. Oholah is identified as Shomron [Samaria, capital of the Northern Kingdom, also called the Kingdom of Israel, which comprised ten of the tribes] and Oholivah as Jerusalem [capital of the Southern Kingdom, also called the Kingdom of Judah, which comprised Judah and Benjamin]. Both are 'wed' to one 'husband', God, but both brazenly betray Him.

The names, אָהֳלָה, *Oholah*, and אָהֳלִיבָה, *Oholivah*, are both derived from אֹהֶל, a *tent* or *dwelling place*. However, אָהֳלָה, is a contraction of הָאֹהֶל שֶׁלָּה, *her tent*, because God had no part in the tabernacles of Shomron. They were 'her own tents' which she had dedicated to the golden calves Jeroboam ben Nevat had erected (see *I Kings* 12:28). On the other hand, אָהֳלִיבָה is

46.

שׁוֹמְרוֹן *Shomron gives forth [her] voice,*
   'The deserts of my sins have found me![1]
My children have gone forth from me[2] *to another land!'*
Then Oholivah screams, 'My palaces were burnt down!'[3]
And Zion says, 'HASHEM has abandoned me!'[4]

ל *[Oholah:] 'It is not right for you, Oholivah,*
 to consider your suffering as mine!
Can you compare your sickness to my fracture and sickness?
I, Oholah, [am now] displaced, I have rebelled in my stubbornness,
but now my deceitfulness has risen against me,[5]
and my defiance has testified against me,
and after a short time I paid my debts [for my sins].
[The Assyrian king] Tiglath-pileser[6] *devoured my [womb's] fruits,*
he stripped away my precious possessions
 and confiscated my jewelry,[7]***
then [his successor Shalmaneser] carried away my captives
 to Halah and Habor.[8]
[Therefore,] Oholivah be silent and weep not as I weep!
Your years [in the Land] were prolonged,
but my years were not prolonged!*
      Then Oholivah screams, 'My palaces were burnt down!'
      And Zion says, 'HASHEM has abandoned me!'

מ *Oholivah responds: 'I too deviated,*
 and like Oholah, I betrayed [God,] the Mentor of my youth![9]
Be still, Oholah, for I remember my agony.
You were exiled but once, while I was exiled repeatedly.
Behold, by the hands of the Chaldeans I was taken twice;
as a miserable captive I descended to Babylon;

---

(1) Cf. *II Kings* 7:9. (2) Cf. *Jeremiah* 10:20. (3) Cf. *II Chronicles* 36:19. (4) *Isaiah* 49:14.
(5) Cf. *Job* 16:8. (6) *II Kings* 15:29. (7) Cf. *Exodus* 33:6. (8) See *II Kings* 17:3-6. (9) Cf. *Jeremiah* 3:4.

a contraction of הָאֹהֶל שֶׁלִּי בָהּ, *My Tent is within her*, i.e., the Tent of God, the *Beis HaMikdash*. These names place Judah, in which God's Temple stood, in sharp contrast to Shomron.

The wicked city of Shomron, with the abominations of its citizens, epitomizes all of the evil of the Ten Tribes. That segment of Israel became so corrupted that to this day those tribes are lost in exile and the possibility of their ultimate return remains the subject of considerable Talmudic debate (see *Sanhedrin* 110b and *Ramban, Sefer HaGeulah*, shaar I).

In this *kinnah*, the author compares the tragedies which befell both Judah and Samaria by means of a debate raging between the two. Each capital claims — and vehemently defends

its claim — that it suffered more at the hand of the marauding enemy.

The composer of the *kinnah*, R' Shlomo ibn Gabirol (11th-century Spain), used the letters of his name שלמה to begin the respective stanzas.

חֲמַדְתִּי . . . עֶדְיִי — *My precious possessions . . . my jewelry.* Some commentators understand these expressions as allusions to the two Temples. We have rejected that interpretation because Oholah is the speaker, but the Temples had stood in Oholivah's estate.

שְׁנוֹתַיִךְ אָרְכוּ וְלֹא אָרְכוּ שָׁנָי — *Your years [in the Land] were prolonged, but my years were not prolonged!* Oholah, the Northern Kingdom of Samaria, was exiled more than one hundred

וְנִשְׂרַף הַהֵיכָל אֲשֶׁר בּוֹ נִכְבַּדְתִּי,

וְלְשִׁבְעִים שָׁנָה בְּבָבֶל נִפְקַדְתִּי,

וְשַׁבְתִּי לְצִיּוֹן עוֹד וְהֵיכָל יָסַדְתִּי,

גַּם זֹאת הַפַּעַם מְעַט לֹא עָמַדְתִּי,

עַד לְקָחַנִי אֱדוֹם וְכִמְעַט אָבַדְתִּי,

וְעַל כָּל הָאֲרָצוֹת נָפְצוּ הֲמוֹנַי,

וְאָהֳלִיבָה תִּזְעַק נִשְׂרְפוּ אַרְמוֹנַי,

וַתֹּאמֶר צִיּוֹן עֲזָבַנִי יהוה.

הַחוֹמֵל עַל דַּל חֲמוֹל עַל דַּלּוּתָם,*

וּרְאֵה שְׁמְמוֹתָם' וְאָרֵךְ גָּלוּתָם,

אַל תִּקְצוֹף עַד מְאֹד² וּרְאֵה שִׁפְלוּתָם,

וְאַל לָעַד תִּזְכּוֹר עֲוֹנָם² וְסִכְלוּתָם,

רְפָא נָא אֶת שִׁבְרָם³ וְנַחֵם אֲבֵלוּתָם,

כִּי אַתָּה סִבְרָם וְאַתָּה אֱיָלוּתָם,

חַדֵּשׁ יָמֵינוּ כִּימֵי קַדְמוֹנִי,⁴

כְּנֶאֱמַךְ בּוֹנֵה יְרוּשָׁלַיִם יהוה.⁵

תְּרַחֵם צִיּוֹן כַּאֲשֶׁר אָמַרְתָּ, וּתְכוֹנְנֶהָ כַּאֲשֶׁר דִּבַּרְתָּ, תְּמַהֵר יְשׁוּעָה וְתָחִישׁ גְּאֻלָּה, וְתָשׁוּב לִירוּשָׁלַיִם בְּרַחֲמִים רַבִּים.

כַּכָּתוּב עַל יַד נְבִיאֶךָ, לָכֵן כֹּה אָמַר יהוה, שַׁבְתִּי לִירוּשָׁלַיִם בְּרַחֲמִים, בֵּיתִי יִבָּנֶה בָּהּ, נְאֻם יהוה צְבָאוֹת, וְקָו יִנָּטֶה עַל יְרוּשָׁלָיִם.⁶

וְנֶאֱמַר, עוֹד קְרָא לֵאמֹר, כֹּה אָמַר יהוה צְבָאוֹת, עוֹד תְּפוּצֶנָה עָרַי מִטּוֹב, וְנִחַם יהוה עוֹד אֶת צִיּוֹן, וּבָחַר עוֹד בִּירוּשָׁלָיִם.⁷

וְנֶאֱמַר, כִּי נִחַם יהוה צִיּוֹן, נִחַם כָּל חָרְבֹתֶיהָ, וַיָּשֶׂם מִדְבָּרָהּ כְּעֵדֶן, וְעַרְבָתָהּ כְּגַן יהוה, שָׂשׂוֹן וְשִׂמְחָה יִמָּצֵא בָהּ, תּוֹדָה וְקוֹל זִמְרָה.⁸

(1) Cf. *Daniel* 9:18. (2) Cf. *Isaiah* 64:8. (3) Cf. *Psalms* 60:4. (4) Cf. *Eichah* 5:21. (5) *Psalms* 147:2. (6) *Zechariah* 1:16. (7) 1:17. (8) *Isaiah* 51:3.

and the Sanctuary by which I was honored
   was burnt down.
After seventy years in Babylon I was recalled [by God];
I returned once again to Zion
   and established the [Second] Temple.
This time, too, I did not last long
before Edom seized me and I was all but annihilated.
Through all the lands were my multitudes dispersed.'

> Then Oholivah screams, 'My palaces were burnt down!'
> And Zion says, 'HASHEM has abandoned me!'

ה O You Who takes pity on the pauper,
   take pity on their poverty.*
See their desolation[1] and the length of their exile.
Do not be overly angered,[2] rather take note of their degradation.
Do not eternally remember their sins[2] and their foolishness.
Please heal their wounds[3] and assuage their mourning;
for You are their Hope and You are their Strength.

> Renew our days as the days of my youth;[4]
> as You have said: 'The Builder of Jerusalem is HASHEM.'[5]

Show Zion mercy as You have said, and establish her as You have spoken. Hasten salvation and speed redemption and return to Jerusalem with abundant compassion.

As it is written by the hand of Your prophet: Therefore, thus says HASHEM, 'I shall return to Jerusalem with compassion, My House shall be rebuilt within it,' says HASHEM, Master of Legions, 'and a [measuring] string shall be stretched over Jerusalem.'[6]

And it is said: Call out again, saying, Thus says HASHEM, Master of Legions, 'My cities shall again overflow with beneficence, and again HASHEM will assuage Zion and again He will choose Jerusalem.'[7]

And it is said: For HASHEM comforts Zion, He comforts her ruins, and He will make her wilderness like Eden, and her wastes like a garden of HASHEM; gladness and joy shall be found there, thanksgiving and the sound of music.[8]

---

thirty years before Oholivah, the Southern Kingdom of Judah.

דַּלּוּתָם — *Their poverty.* Until this point, the *kinnah* has been a one-on-one debate between Oholah and Oholivah. Thus, the statements are all in first or second person singular. The last stanza, however, is the *paytan*'s supplication for the restitution of both, and consequently is couched in third person plural. Finally, the last line prays for the reunification of the two Kingdoms with Jerusalem as the focal point as it was in 'the days of my youth.'

❧ אשרי – ובא לציון ❧

אַ֫שְׁרֵי יוֹשְׁבֵי בֵיתֶ֑ךָ, עוֹד יְהַלְל֥וּךָ סֶּֽלָה.¹ אַשְׁרֵי הָעָם שֶׁכָּֽכָה לּוֹ, אַשְׁרֵי הָעָם שֶׁיהוה אֱלֹהָיו.²

תהלים קמה

תְּהִלָּה לְדָוִד,

אֲרוֹמִמְךָ אֱלוֹהַי הַמֶּֽלֶךְ, וַאֲבָרְכָה שִׁמְךָ לְעוֹלָם וָעֶד.

בְּכָל יוֹם אֲבָרְכֶֽךָּ, וַאֲהַלְלָה שִׁמְךָ לְעוֹלָם וָעֶד.

גָּדוֹל יהוה וּמְהֻלָּל מְאֹד, וְלִגְדֻלָּתוֹ אֵין חֵֽקֶר.

דּוֹר לְדוֹר יְשַׁבַּח מַעֲשֶֽׂיךָ, וּגְבוּרֹתֶֽיךָ יַגִּֽידוּ.

הֲדַר כְּבוֹד הוֹדֶֽךָ, וְדִבְרֵי נִפְלְאֹתֶֽיךָ אָשִֽׂיחָה.

וֶעֱזוּז נוֹרְאוֹתֶֽיךָ יֹאמֵֽרוּ, וּגְדוּלָּתְךָ אֲסַפְּרֶֽנָּה.

זֵֽכֶר רַב טוּבְךָ יַבִּֽיעוּ, וְצִדְקָתְךָ יְרַנֵּֽנוּ.

חַנּוּן וְרַחוּם יהוה, אֶֽרֶךְ אַפַּֽיִם וּגְדָל חָֽסֶד.

טוֹב יהוה לַכֹּל, וְרַחֲמָיו עַל כָּל מַעֲשָׂיו.

יוֹדֽוּךָ יהוה כָּל מַעֲשֶֽׂיךָ, וַחֲסִידֶֽיךָ יְבָרְכֽוּכָה.

כְּבוֹד מַלְכוּתְךָ יֹאמֵֽרוּ, וּגְבוּרָתְךָ יְדַבֵּֽרוּ.

לְהוֹדִֽיעַ לִבְנֵי הָאָדָם גְּבוּרֹתָיו, וּכְבוֹד הֲדַר מַלְכוּתוֹ.

מַלְכוּתְךָ מַלְכוּת כָּל עֹלָמִים, וּמֶמְשַׁלְתְּךָ בְּכָל דּוֹר וָדֹר.

סוֹמֵךְ יהוה לְכָל הַנֹּפְלִים, וְזוֹקֵף לְכָל הַכְּפוּפִים.

עֵינֵי כֹל אֵלֶֽיךָ יְשַׂבֵּֽרוּ, וְאַתָּה נוֹתֵן לָהֶם אֶת אָכְלָם בְּעִתּוֹ.

While reciting the verse פּוֹתֵחַ, concentrate intently on its meaning.

פּוֹתֵֽחַ אֶת יָדֶֽךָ,

וּמַשְׂבִּֽיעַ לְכָל חַי רָצוֹן.

צַדִּיק יהוה בְּכָל דְּרָכָיו, וְחָסִיד בְּכָל מַעֲשָׂיו.

קָרוֹב יהוה לְכָל קֹרְאָיו, לְכֹל אֲשֶׁר יִקְרָאֻֽהוּ בֶאֱמֶת.

רְצוֹן יְרֵאָיו יַעֲשֶׂה, וְאֶת שַׁוְעָתָם יִשְׁמַע וְיוֹשִׁיעֵם.

שׁוֹמֵר יהוה אֶת כָּל אֹהֲבָיו, וְאֵת כָּל הָרְשָׁעִים יַשְׁמִיד.

❖ תְּהִלַּת יהוה יְדַבֶּר פִּי, וִיבָרֵךְ כָּל בָּשָׂר שֵׁם קָדְשׁוֹ לְעוֹלָם וָעֶד.

וַאֲנַֽחְנוּ נְבָרֵךְ יָהּ, מֵעַתָּה וְעַד עוֹלָם, הַלְלוּיָהּ.³

PSALM 20, לַמְנַצֵּחַ, IS OMITTED.

---

(1) *Psalms* 84:5. (2) 144:15. (3) 115:8.

⊰{ ASHREI — UVA L'TZION }⊱

אַשְׁרֵי *Praiseworthy are those who dwell in Your house; may they always praise You, Selah![1] Praiseworthy is the people for whom this is so, praiseworthy is the people whose God is HASHEM.[2]*

Psalm 145   *A psalm of praise by David:*

א *I will exalt You, my God the King,*
      and I will bless Your Name forever and ever.

ב *Every day I will bless You, and I will laud Your Name forever and ever.*

ג *HASHEM is great and exceedingly lauded,*
      and His greatness is beyond investigation.

ד *Each generation will praise Your deeds to the next*
      and of Your mighty deeds they will tell.

ה *The splendrous glory of Your power*
      and Your wondrous deeds I shall discuss.

ו *And of Your awesome power they will speak,*
      and Your greatness I shall relate.

ז *A recollection of Your abundant goodness they will utter*
      and of Your righteousness they will sing exultantly.

ח *Gracious and merciful is HASHEM,*
      slow to anger, and great in [bestowing] kindness.

ט *HASHEM is good to all; His mercies are on all His works.*

י *All Your works shall thank You, HASHEM,*
      and Your devout ones will bless You.

כ *Of the glory of Your kingdom they will speak,*
      and of Your power they will tell;

ל *To inform human beings of His mighty deeds,*
      and the glorious splendor of His kingdom.

מ *Your kingdom is a kingdom spanning all eternities,*
      and Your dominion is throughout every generation.

ס *HASHEM supports all the fallen ones and straightens all the bent.*

ע *The eyes of all look to You with hope*
      and You give them their food in its proper time;

פ *You open Your hand, and satisfy*   While reciting the verse, 'You open . . .'
      the desire of every living thing.   concentrate intently on its meaning.

צ *Righteous is HASHEM in all His ways*
      and magnanimous in all His deeds.

ק *HASHEM is close to all who call upon Him —*
      to all who call upon Him sincerely.

ר *The will of those who fear Him He will do;*
      and their cry He will hear, and save them.

ש *HASHEM protects all who love Him; but all the wicked He will destroy.*

ת Chazzan— *May my mouth declare the praise of HASHEM*
      and may all flesh bless His Holy Name forever and ever.

We will bless God from this time and forever, Halleluyah![3]

PSALM 20, לַמְנַצֵּחַ, IS OMITTED.

The primary part of וּבָא לְצִיּוֹן is the *Kedushah* recited by the angels. These verses are presented in bold type and it is preferable that the congregation recite them aloud and in unison. However, the interpretive translation in Aramaic (which follows the verses in bold type) should be recited softly.

THE VERSE וַאֲנִי זֹאת, IS OMITTED.

וּבָא לְצִיּוֹן גּוֹאֵל, וּלְשָׁבֵי פֶשַׁע בְּיַעֲקֹב, נְאֻם יהוה. [...]

❖ וְאַתָּה קָדוֹשׁ יוֹשֵׁב תְּהִלּוֹת יִשְׂרָאֵל.[1] וְקָרָא זֶה אֶל זֶה וְאָמַר:

קָדוֹשׁ, קָדוֹשׁ, קָדוֹשׁ יהוה צְבָאוֹת, מְלֹא כָל הָאָרֶץ כְּבוֹדוֹ.[2]

וּמְקַבְּלִין דֵּין מִן דֵּין וְאָמְרִין:

קַדִּישׁ בִּשְׁמֵי מְרוֹמָא עִלָּאָה בֵּית שְׁכִינְתֵּהּ,

קַדִּישׁ עַל אַרְעָא עוֹבַד גְּבוּרְתֵּהּ,

קַדִּישׁ לְעָלַם וּלְעָלְמֵי עָלְמַיָּא, יהוה צְבָאוֹת,

מַלְיָא כָל אַרְעָא זִיו יְקָרֵהּ.[3]

❖ וַתִּשָּׂאֵנִי רוּחַ, וָאֶשְׁמַע אַחֲרַי קוֹל רַעַשׁ גָּדוֹל:

בָּרוּךְ כְּבוֹד יהוה מִמְּקוֹמוֹ.[4]

וּנְטָלַתְנִי רוּחָא, וְשִׁמְעֵת בַּתְרַי קָל זִיעַ סַגִּיא דִּמְשַׁבְּחִין וְאָמְרִין:

בְּרִיךְ יְקָרָא דַיהוה מֵאֲתַר בֵּית שְׁכִינְתֵּהּ.[5]

יהוה יִמְלֹךְ לְעֹלָם וָעֶד.[6]

יהוה מַלְכוּתֵהּ קָאֵם לְעָלַם וּלְעָלְמֵי עָלְמַיָּא.[7]

יהוה אֱלֹהֵי אַבְרָהָם יִצְחָק וְיִשְׂרָאֵל אֲבֹתֵינוּ, שָׁמְרָה זֹּאת לְעוֹלָם, לְיֵצֶר מַחְשְׁבוֹת לְבַב עַמֶּךָ, וְהָכֵן לְבָבָם אֵלֶיךָ.[8] וְהוּא רַחוּם, יְכַפֵּר עָוֹן וְלֹא יַשְׁחִית, וְהִרְבָּה לְהָשִׁיב אַפּוֹ, וְלֹא יָעִיר כָּל חֲמָתוֹ.[9] כִּי אַתָּה אֲדֹנָי טוֹב וְסַלָּח, וְרַב חֶסֶד לְכָל קֹרְאֶיךָ.[10] צִדְקָתְךָ צֶדֶק לְעוֹלָם, וְתוֹרָתְךָ אֱמֶת.[11] תִּתֵּן אֱמֶת לְיַעֲקֹב, חֶסֶד לְאַבְרָהָם, אֲשֶׁר נִשְׁבַּעְתָּ לַאֲבֹתֵינוּ מִימֵי קֶדֶם.[12] בָּרוּךְ אֲדֹנָי יוֹם יוֹם יַעֲמָס לָנוּ, הָאֵל יְשׁוּעָתֵנוּ סֶלָה.[13] יהוה צְבָאוֹת עִמָּנוּ, מִשְׂגָּב לָנוּ אֱלֹהֵי יַעֲקֹב סֶלָה.[14] יהוה צְבָאוֹת, אַשְׁרֵי אָדָם בֹּטֵחַ בָּךְ.[15] יהוה הוֹשִׁיעָה, הַמֶּלֶךְ יַעֲנֵנוּ בְיוֹם קָרְאֵנוּ.[16]

בָּרוּךְ הוּא אֱלֹהֵינוּ שֶׁבְּרָאָנוּ לִכְבוֹדוֹ, וְהִבְדִּילָנוּ מִן הַתּוֹעִים, וְנָתַן לָנוּ תּוֹרַת אֱמֶת, וְחַיֵּי עוֹלָם נָטַע בְּתוֹכֵנוּ. הוּא יִפְתַּח לִבֵּנוּ בְּתוֹרָתוֹ, וְיָשֵׂם בְּלִבֵּנוּ אַהֲבָתוֹ וְיִרְאָתוֹ וְלַעֲשׂוֹת רְצוֹנוֹ וּלְעָבְדוֹ בְּלֵבָב שָׁלֵם, לְמַעַן לֹא נִיגַע לָרִיק, וְלֹא נֵלֵד לַבֶּהָלָה.[17]

The primary part of וּבָא לְצִיּוֹן, 'A redeemer shall come . . .', is the Kedushah recited by the angels. These verses are presented in bold type and it is preferable that the congregation recite them aloud and in unison. However, the interpretive translation in Aramaic (which follows the verses in bold type) should be recited softly.

THE VERSE וַאֲנִי זֹאת, IS OMITTED.

וּבָא לְצִיּוֹן   'A redeemer shall come to Zion and to those of Jacob who repent from willful sin,' the words of HASHEM. [...]
Chazzan— You are the Holy One, enthroned upon the praises of Israel.[1] And one [angel] will call another and say:

**'Holy, holy, holy is HASHEM, Master of Legions,
the whole world is filled with His glory.'[2]**
And they receive permission from one another and say:
'Holy in the most exalted heaven, the abode of His Presence;
holy on earth, product of His strength;
holy forever and ever is HASHEM, Master of Legions —
the entire world is filled with the radiance of His glory.'[3]
∴ And a wind lifted me; and I heard behind me the sound of a great noise:
'Blessed is the glory of HASHEM from His place.'[4]
And a wind lifted me and I heard behind me the sound
of the powerful movement of those who praised saying:
'Blessed is the honor of HASHEM
from the place of the abode of His Presence.'[5]
HASHEM shall reign for all eternity.[6]
HASHEM — His kingdom is established forever and ever.[7]

HASHEM, God of Abraham, Isaac, and Israel, our forefathers, may You preserve this forever as the realization of the thoughts in Your people's heart, and may You direct their heart to You.[8] He, the Merciful One, is forgiving of iniquity and does not destroy; frequently He withdraws His anger, not arousing His entire rage.[9] For You, my Lord, are good and forgiving, and abundantly kind to all who call upon You.[10] Your righteousness remains righteous forever, and Your Torah is truth.[11] Grant truth to Jacob, kindness to Abraham, as You swore to our forefathers from ancient times.[12] Blessed is my Lord for every single day, He burdens us with blessings, the God of our salvation, Selah.[13] HASHEM, Master of Legions, is with us, a stronghold for us is the God of Jacob, Selah.[14] HASHEM, Master of Legions, praiseworthy is the man who trusts in You.[15] HASHEM, save! May the King answer us on the day we call.[16]

Blessed is He, our God, Who created us for His glory, separated us from those who stray, gave us the Torah of truth and implanted eternal life within us. May He open our heart through His Torah and imbue our heart with love and awe of Him and that we may do His will and serve Him wholeheartedly, so that we do not struggle in vain nor produce for futility.[17]

---

(1) Psalms 22:4. (2) Isaiah 6:3. (3) Targum Yonasan to Isaiah 6:3. (4) Ezekiel 3:12.
(5) Targum Yonasan to Ezekiel 3:12. (6) Exodus 15:18. (7) Targum Onkelos to Exodus 15:18.
(8) I Chronicles 29:18. (9) Psalms 78:38. (10) 86:5. (11) 119:142. (12) Micah 7:20.
(13) Psalms 68:20. (14) 46:8. (15) 84:13. (16) 20:10. (17) Cf. Isaiah 65:23.

יְהִי רָצוֹן מִלְּפָנֶיךָ יהוה אֱלֹהֵינוּ וֵאלֹהֵי אֲבוֹתֵינוּ, שֶׁנִּשְׁמֹר
חֻקֶּיךָ בָּעוֹלָם הַזֶּה, וְנִזְכֶּה וְנִחְיֶה וְנִרְאֶה וְנִירַשׁ טוֹבָה וּבְרָכָה
לִשְׁנֵי יְמוֹת הַמָּשִׁיחַ וּלְחַיֵּי הָעוֹלָם הַבָּא. לְמַעַן יְזַמֶּרְךָ כָבוֹד וְלֹא
יִדֹּם, יהוה אֱלֹהַי לְעוֹלָם אוֹדֶךָּ.¹ בָּרוּךְ הַגֶּבֶר אֲשֶׁר יִבְטַח בַּיהוה,
וְהָיָה יהוה מִבְטַחוֹ.² בִּטְחוּ בַיהוה עֲדֵי עַד, כִּי בְּיָהּ יהוה צוּר
עוֹלָמִים.³ ❖ וְיִבְטְחוּ בְךָ יוֹדְעֵי שְׁמֶךָ, כִּי לֹא עָזַבְתָּ דֹרְשֶׁיךָ, יהוה.⁴
יהוה חָפֵץ לְמַעַן צִדְקוֹ, יַגְדִּיל תּוֹרָה וְיַאְדִּיר.⁵

קַדִּישׁ שָׁלֵם בְּלֹא תִּתְקַבַּל. The chazzan recites

יִתְגַּדַּל וְיִתְקַדַּשׁ שְׁמֵהּ רַבָּא. (.Cong – אָמֵן.) בְּעָלְמָא דִּי בְרָא כִרְעוּתֵהּ.
וְיַמְלִיךְ מַלְכוּתֵהּ, בְּחַיֵּיכוֹן וּבְיוֹמֵיכוֹן וּבְחַיֵּי דְכָל בֵּית יִשְׂרָאֵל,
בַּעֲגָלָא וּבִזְמַן קָרִיב. וְאִמְרוּ: אָמֵן.

(.Cong – אָמֵן. יְהֵא שְׁמֵהּ רַבָּא מְבָרַךְ לְעָלַם וּלְעָלְמֵי עָלְמַיָּא.)
יְהֵא שְׁמֵהּ רַבָּא מְבָרַךְ לְעָלַם וּלְעָלְמֵי עָלְמַיָּא.

יִתְבָּרַךְ וְיִשְׁתַּבַּח וְיִתְפָּאַר וְיִתְרוֹמַם וְיִתְנַשֵּׂא וְיִתְהַדָּר וְיִתְעַלֶּה
וְיִתְהַלָּל שְׁמֵהּ דְּקֻדְשָׁא בְּרִיךְ הוּא (.Cong – בְּרִיךְ הוּא) – לְעֵלָּא מִן כָּל
בִּרְכָתָא וְשִׁירָתָא תֻּשְׁבְּחָתָא וְנֶחֱמָתָא, דַּאֲמִירָן בְּעָלְמָא. וְאִמְרוּ: אָמֵן.
(.Cong – אָמֵן.)

יְהֵא שְׁלָמָא רַבָּא מִן שְׁמַיָּא, וְחַיִּים עָלֵינוּ וְעַל כָּל יִשְׂרָאֵל. וְאִמְרוּ:
אָמֵן. (.Cong – אָמֵן.)

Take three steps back. Bow left and say . . . עֹשֶׂה; bow right and say . . . הוּא; bow forward and say
וְעַל כָּל . . . אָמֵן. Remain standing in place for a few moments, then take three steps forward.

עֹשֶׂה שָׁלוֹם בִּמְרוֹמָיו, הוּא יַעֲשֶׂה שָׁלוֹם עָלֵינוּ, וְעַל כָּל יִשְׂרָאֵל.
וְאִמְרוּ: אָמֵן. (.Cong – אָמֵן.)

עלינו

Stand while reciting עָלֵינוּ.

עָלֵינוּ לְשַׁבֵּחַ לַאֲדוֹן הַכֹּל, לָתֵת גְּדֻלָּה לְיוֹצֵר בְּרֵאשִׁית,
שֶׁלֹּא עָשָׂנוּ כְּגוֹיֵי הָאֲרָצוֹת, וְלֹא שָׂמָנוּ כְּמִשְׁפְּחוֹת
הָאֲדָמָה. שֶׁלֹּא שָׂם חֶלְקֵנוּ כָּהֶם, וְגוֹרָלֵנוּ כְּכָל הֲמוֹנָם. (שֶׁהֵם
מִשְׁתַּחֲוִים לְהֶבֶל וָרִיק, וּמִתְפַּלְּלִים אֶל אֵל לֹא יוֹשִׁיעַ.⁶) וַאֲנַחְנוּ

Bow while reciting
וַאֲנַחְנוּ כּוֹרְעִים וּמִשְׁתַּחֲוִים.

כּוֹרְעִים וּמִשְׁתַּחֲוִים וּמוֹדִים, לִפְנֵי מֶלֶךְ מַלְכֵי
הַמְּלָכִים הַקָּדוֹשׁ בָּרוּךְ הוּא. שֶׁהוּא נוֹטֶה שָׁמַיִם וְיֹסֵד אָרֶץ,⁷
וּמוֹשַׁב יְקָרוֹ בַּשָּׁמַיִם מִמַּעַל, וּשְׁכִינַת עֻזּוֹ בְּגָבְהֵי מְרוֹמִים. הוּא

May it be Your will, HASHEM, our God and the God of our fore-fathers, that we observe Your decrees in This World, and merit that we live and see and inherit goodness and blessing in the years of Messianic times and for the life of the World to Come. So that my soul might sing to You and not be stilled, HASHEM, my God, forever will I thank You.[1] Blessed is the man who trusts in HASHEM, then HASHEM will be his security.[2] Trust in HASHEM forever, for in God, HASHEM, is the strength of the worlds.[3] Chazzan— *Those knowing Your Name will trust in You, and You forsake not those Who seek You, HASHEM.[4] HASHEM desired, for the sake of its [Israel's] righteousness, that the Torah be made great and glorious.[5]*

The chazzan recites the following Kaddish.

יִתְגַּדַּל *May His great Name grow exalted and sanctified* (Cong.— *Amen.*) *in the world that He created as He willed. May He give reign to His kingship in your lifetimes and in your days, and in the lifetimes of the entire Family of Israel, swiftly and soon. Now respond: Amen.*

(Cong.— *Amen. May His great Name be blessed forever and ever.*)
May His great Name be blessed forever and ever.

Blessed, praised, glorified, exalted, extolled, mighty, upraised, and lauded be the Name of the Holy One, Blessed is He (Cong.— *Blessed is He*) — *beyond any blessing and song, praise and consolation that are uttered in the world. Now respond: Amen.* (Cong.— *Amen.*)

May there be abundant peace from Heaven, and life, upon us and upon all Israel. Now respond: Amen. (Cong.— *Amen.*)

Take three steps back. Bow left and say, 'He Who makes peace . . .';
bow right and say, 'may He . . .'; bow forward and say, 'and upon all Israel . . .'
Remain standing in place for a few moments, then take three steps forward.

He Who makes peace in His heights, may He make peace upon us, and upon all Israel. Now respond: Amen. (Cong.— *Amen.*)

ALEINU

Stand while reciting עָלֵינוּ, 'It is our duty . . .'

עָלֵינוּ *It is our duty to praise the Master of all, to ascribe greatness to the Molder of primeval creation, for He has not made us like the nations of the lands, and has not emplaced us like the families of the earth; for He has not assigned our portion like theirs nor our lot like all their multitudes. (For they bow to vanity and emptiness and pray to a*

Bow while reciting
'But we bend our knees.'

god which helps not.[6]) But we bend our knees, bow, and acknowledge our thanks before the King Who reigns over kings, the Holy One, Blessed is He. He stretches out heaven and establishes earth's foundation,[7] the seat of His homage is in the heavens above and His powerful Presence is in the loftiest heights. He

---

(1) *Psalms* 30:13. (2) *Jeremiah* 17:7. (3) *Isaiah* 26:4.
(4) *Psalms* 9:11. (5) *Isaiah* 42:21. (6) *Isaiah* 45:20. (7) 51:13.

אֱלֹהֵינוּ, אֵין עוֹד. אֱמֶת מַלְכֵּנוּ, אֶפֶס זוּלָתוֹ, כַּכָּתוּב בְּתוֹרָתוֹ: וְיָדַעְתָּ הַיּוֹם וַהֲשֵׁבֹתָ אֶל לְבָבֶךָ, כִּי יהוה הוּא הָאֱלֹהִים בַּשָּׁמַיִם מִמַּעַל וְעַל הָאָרֶץ מִתָּחַת, אֵין עוֹד.[1]

עַל כֵּן נְקַוֶּה לְּךָ יהוה אֱלֹהֵינוּ לִרְאוֹת מְהֵרָה בְּתִפְאֶרֶת עֻזֶּךָ, לְהַעֲבִיר גִּלּוּלִים מִן הָאָרֶץ, וְהָאֱלִילִים כָּרוֹת יִכָּרֵתוּן, לְתַקֵּן עוֹלָם בְּמַלְכוּת שַׁדַּי. וְכָל בְּנֵי בָשָׂר יִקְרְאוּ בִשְׁמֶךָ, לְהַפְנוֹת אֵלֶיךָ כָּל רִשְׁעֵי אָרֶץ. יַכִּירוּ וְיֵדְעוּ כָּל יוֹשְׁבֵי תֵבֵל, כִּי לְךָ תִּכְרַע כָּל בֶּרֶךְ, תִּשָּׁבַע כָּל לָשׁוֹן.[2] לְפָנֶיךָ יהוה אֱלֹהֵינוּ יִכְרְעוּ וְיִפֹּלוּ, וְלִכְבוֹד שִׁמְךָ יְקָר יִתֵּנוּ. וִיקַבְּלוּ כֻלָּם אֶת עוֹל מַלְכוּתֶךָ, וְתִמְלֹךְ עֲלֵיהֶם מְהֵרָה לְעוֹלָם וָעֶד. כִּי הַמַּלְכוּת שֶׁלְּךָ הִיא וּלְעוֹלְמֵי עַד תִּמְלוֹךְ בְּכָבוֹד, כַּכָּתוּב בְּתוֹרָתֶךָ: יהוה יִמְלֹךְ לְעֹלָם וָעֶד.[3] ❖ וְנֶאֱמַר: וְהָיָה יהוה לְמֶלֶךְ עַל כָּל הָאָרֶץ, בַּיּוֹם הַהוּא יִהְיֶה יהוה אֶחָד וּשְׁמוֹ אֶחָד.[4]

Some congregations recite the following after עלינו.

אַל תִּירָא מִפַּחַד פִּתְאֹם, וּמִשֹּׁאַת רְשָׁעִים כִּי תָבֹא.[5] עֻצוּ עֵצָה וְתֻפָר, דַּבְּרוּ דָבָר וְלֹא יָקוּם, כִּי עִמָּנוּ אֵל.[6] וְעַד זִקְנָה אֲנִי הוּא, וְעַד שֵׂיבָה אֲנִי אֶסְבֹּל, אֲנִי עָשִׂיתִי וַאֲנִי אֶשָּׂא, וַאֲנִי אֶסְבֹּל וַאֲמַלֵּט.[7]

קדיש יתום

In the presence of a *minyan*, mourners recite קַדִּישׁ יָתוֹם, the Mourner's *Kaddish* (see Laws §132-134).

יִתְגַּדַּל וְיִתְקַדַּשׁ שְׁמֵהּ רַבָּא. (.Cong – אָמֵן.) בְּעָלְמָא דִּי בְרָא כִרְעוּתֵהּ. וְיַמְלִיךְ מַלְכוּתֵהּ, בְּחַיֵּיכוֹן וּבְיוֹמֵיכוֹן וּבְחַיֵּי דְכָל בֵּית יִשְׂרָאֵל, בַּעֲגָלָא וּבִזְמַן קָרִיב. וְאִמְרוּ: אָמֵן.

(.Cong – אָמֵן. יְהֵא שְׁמֵהּ רַבָּא מְבָרַךְ לְעָלַם וּלְעָלְמֵי עָלְמַיָּא.)

יְהֵא שְׁמֵהּ רַבָּא מְבָרַךְ לְעָלַם וּלְעָלְמֵי עָלְמַיָּא.

יִתְבָּרַךְ וְיִשְׁתַּבַּח וְיִתְפָּאַר וְיִתְרוֹמַם וְיִתְנַשֵּׂא וְיִתְהַדָּר וְיִתְעַלֶּה וְיִתְהַלָּל שְׁמֵהּ דְּקֻדְשָׁא בְּרִיךְ הוּא (.Cong – בְּרִיךְ הוּא) – לְעֵלָּא מִן כָּל בִּרְכָתָא וְשִׁירָתָא תֻּשְׁבְּחָתָא וְנֶחֱמָתָא, דַּאֲמִירָן בְּעָלְמָא. וְאִמְרוּ: אָמֵן. (.Cong – אָמֵן.)

יְהֵא שְׁלָמָא רַבָּא מִן שְׁמַיָּא, וְחַיִּים עָלֵינוּ וְעַל כָּל יִשְׂרָאֵל. וְאִמְרוּ: אָמֵן. (.Cong – אָמֵן.)

Take three steps back. Bow left and say . . . עֹשֶׂה; bow right and say . . . הוּא; bow forward and say וְעַל כָּל . . . אָמֵן. Remain standing in place for a few moments, then take three steps forward.

עֹשֶׂה שָׁלוֹם בִּמְרוֹמָיו, הוּא יַעֲשֶׂה שָׁלוֹם עָלֵינוּ, וְעַל כָּל יִשְׂרָאֵל. וְאִמְרוּ: אָמֵן. (.Cong – אָמֵן.)

The recitation of שִׁיר שֶׁל יוֹם, the Song of the Day, is postponed until Minchah.
After midday it is permissible to sit on a regular seat.

is our God and there is none other. True is our King, there is nothing beside Him, as it is written in His Torah: 'You are to know this day and take to your heart that HASHEM is the only God — in heaven above and on the earth below — there is none other.'[1]

עַל כֵּן Therefore we put our hope in You, HASHEM, our God, that we may soon see Your mighty splendor, to remove detestable idolatry from the earth, and false gods will be utterly cut off, to perfect the universe through the Almighty's sovereignty. Then all humanity will call upon Your Name, to turn all the earth's wicked toward You. All the world's inhabitants will recognize and know that to You every knee should bend, every tongue should swear.[2] Before You, HASHEM, our God, they will bend every knee and cast themselves down and to the glory of Your Name they will render homage, and they will all accept upon themselves the yoke of Your kingship that You may reign over them soon and eternally. For the kingdom is Yours and You will reign for all eternity in glory as it is written in Your Torah: HASHEM shall reign for all eternity.[3] Chazzan— And it is said: HASHEM will be King over all the world — on that day HASHEM will be One and His Name will be One.[4]

Some congregations recite the following after Aleinu.

אַל תִּירָא Do not fear sudden terror, or the holocaust of the wicked when it comes.[5] Plan a conspiracy and it will be annulled; speak your piece and it shall not stand, for God is with us.[6] Even till your seniority, I remain unchanged; and even till your ripe old age, I shall endure. I created you and I shall bear you; I shall endure and rescue.[7]

MOURNER'S KADDISH

In the presence of a *minyan,* mourners recite קַדִּישׁ יָתוֹם, the Mourner's *Kaddish* (see *Laws* 132-134).
[A transliteration of this *Kaddish* appears on page 486.]

יִתְגַּדַּל May His great Name grow exalted and sanctified (Cong.— Amen.) in the world that He created as He willed. May He give reign to His kingship in your lifetimes and in your days, and in the lifetimes of the entire Family of Israel, swiftly and soon. Now respond: Amen.

(Cong.— Amen. May His great Name be blessed forever and ever.)
May His great Name be blessed forever and ever.

Blessed, praised, glorified, exalted, extolled, mighty, upraised, and lauded be the Name of the Holy One, Blessed is He (Cong.— Blessed is He) — beyond any blessing and song, praise and consolation that are uttered in the world. Now respond: Amen. (Cong.— Amen).

May there be abundant peace from Heaven, and life, upon us and upon all Israel. Now respond: Amen. (Cong.— Amen.)

Take three steps back. Bow left and say, 'He Who makes peace . . .';
bow right and say, 'may He . . .'; bow forward and say, 'and upon all Israel . . .'
Remain standing in place for a few moments, then take three steps forward.

He Who makes peace in His heights, may He make peace upon us, and upon all Israel. Now respond: Amen. (Cong.— Amen.)

The recitation of שִׁיר שֶׁל יוֹם, the Song of the Day, is postponed until Minchah.
After midday it is permissible to sit on a regular seat.

---

(1) *Deuteronomy* 4:39. (2) Cf. *Isaiah* 45:23. (3) *Exodus* 15:18.
(4) *Zechariah* 14:9. (5) *Proverbs* 3:25. (6) *Isaiah* 8:10. (7) 46:4.

﴾ **מנחה** ﴿

The *Paroches* is returned to the Ark.

﴾ **עטיפת טלית** ﴿

Before donning the *tallis*, inspect the *tzitzis*, while reciting these verses:

בָּרְכִי נַפְשִׁי אֶת יהוה, יהוה אֱלֹהַי גָּדַלְתָּ מְּאֹד, הוֹד וְהָדָר לָבָשְׁתָּ. עֹטֶה אוֹר כַּשַּׂלְמָה, נוֹטֶה שָׁמַיִם כַּיְרִיעָה.[1]

Many recite the following declaration of intent before donning the *tallis*:

לְשֵׁם יִחוּד קֻדְשָׁא בְּרִיךְ הוּא וּשְׁכִינְתֵּהּ, בִּדְחִילוּ וּרְחִימוּ לְיַחֵד שֵׁם י"ה בּו"ה בְּיִחוּדָא שְׁלִים, בְּשֵׁם כָּל יִשְׂרָאֵל.

הֲרֵינִי מִתְעַטֵּף גּוּפִי בַּצִּיצַת, כֵּן תִּתְעַטֵּף נִשְׁמָתִי וּרְמַ"ח אֵבָרַי וּשְׁסָ"ה גִידַי בְּאוֹר הַצִּיצַת הָעוֹלֶה תַרְיַ"ג. וּכְשֵׁם שֶׁאֲנִי מִתְכַּסֶּה בְּטַלִּית בָּעוֹלָם הַזֶּה, כַּךְ אֶזְכֶּה לַחֲלוּקָא דְרַבָּנָן וּלְטַלִּית נָאֶה לָעוֹלָם הַבָּא בְּגַן עֵדֶן. וְעַל יְדֵי מִצְוַת צִיצַת תִּנָּצֵל נַפְשִׁי וְרוּחִי וְנִשְׁמָתִי וּתְפִלָּתִי מִן הַחִיצוֹנִים. וְהַטַּלִּית יִפְרוֹשׂ כְּנָפָיו עֲלֵיהֶם וְיַצִּילֵם כְּנֶשֶׁר יָעִיר קִנּוֹ, עַל גּוֹזָלָיו יְרַחֵף.[2] וּתְהֵא חֲשׁוּבָה מִצְוַת צִיצַת לִפְנֵי הַקָּדוֹשׁ בָּרוּךְ הוּא כְּאִלּוּ קִיַּמְתֵּיהָ בְּכָל פְּרָטֶיהָ וְדִקְדּוּקֶיהָ וְכַוָּנוֹתֶיהָ וְתַרְיַ"ג מִצְוֹת הַתְּלוּיִם בָּהּ. אָמֵן סֶלָה.

Unfold the *tallis*, hold it in readiness to wrap around yourself, and recite the following blessing:

בָּרוּךְ אַתָּה יהוה אֱלֹהֵינוּ מֶלֶךְ הָעוֹלָם, אֲשֶׁר קִדְּשָׁנוּ בְּמִצְוֹתָיו, וְצִוָּנוּ לְהִתְעַטֵּף בַּצִּיצַת.

Wrap the *tallis* around your head and body, then recite:

מַה יָּקָר חַסְדְּךָ אֱלֹהִים, וּבְנֵי אָדָם בְּצֵל כְּנָפֶיךָ יֶחֱסָיוּן. יִרְוְיֻן מִדֶּשֶׁן בֵּיתֶךָ, וְנַחַל עֲדָנֶיךָ תַשְׁקֵם. כִּי עִמְּךָ מְקוֹר חַיִּים, בְּאוֹרְךָ נִרְאֶה אוֹר. מְשֹׁךְ חַסְדְּךָ לְיֹדְעֶיךָ, וְצִדְקָתְךָ לְיִשְׁרֵי לֵב.[3]

﴾ **סדר הנחת תפילין** ﴿

Many recite the following declaration of intent before putting on *tefillin*:

לְשֵׁם יִחוּד קֻדְשָׁא בְּרִיךְ הוּא וּשְׁכִינְתֵּהּ, בִּדְחִילוּ וּרְחִימוּ לְיַחֵד שֵׁם י"ה בּו"ה בְּיִחוּדָא שְׁלִים, בְּשֵׁם כָּל יִשְׂרָאֵל.

הִנְנִי מְכַוֵּן בַּהֲנָחַת תְּפִלִּין לְקַיֵּם מִצְוַת בּוֹרְאִי, שֶׁצִּוָּנוּ לְהָנִיחַ תְּפִלִּין, כַּכָּתוּב בְּתוֹרָתוֹ: וּקְשַׁרְתָּם לְאוֹת עַל יָדֶךָ, וְהָיוּ לְטֹטָפֹת בֵּין עֵינֶיךָ[4] וְהֵם אַרְבַּע פָּרָשִׁיּוֹת אֵלּוּ – שְׁמַע, וְהָיָה אִם שָׁמֹעַ, קַדֶּשׁ,

⊰ MINCHAH ⊱

The *Paroches* is returned to the Ark.

⊰ DONNING THE TALLIS ⊱

Before donning the *tallis*, inspect the *tzitzis*, while reciting these verses:

בָּרְכִי נַפְשִׁי *Bless HASHEM, O my soul; HASHEM, my God, You are very great; You have donned majesty and splendor; cloaked in light as with a garment, stretching out the heavens like a curtain.*[1]

Many recite the following declaration of intent before donning the *tallis:*

לְשֵׁם יִחוּד *For the sake of the unification of the Holy One, Blessed is He, and His Presence, in fear and love to unify the Name — yud-kei with vav-kei — in perfect unity, in the name of all Israel.*

הֲרֵינִי *I am ready to wrap my body in tzitzis, so may my soul, my two hundred forty-eight organs and my three hundred sixty-five sinews be wrapped in the illumination of tzitzis which has the numerical value of six hundred thirteen. Just as I cover myself with a tallis in This World, so may I merit the rabbinical garb and a beautiful cloak in the World to Come in the Garden of Eden. Through the commandment of tzitzis may my life-force, spirit, soul, and prayer be rescued from the external forces. May the tallis spread its wings over them and rescue them like an eagle rousing his nest, fluttering over his eaglets.*[2] *May the commandment of tzitzis be worthy before the Holy One, Blessed is He, as if I had fulfilled it in all its details, implications, and intentions, as well as the six hundred thirteen commandments that are dependent upon it. Amen, Selah!*

Unfold the *tallis*, hold it in readiness to wrap around yourself, and recite the following blessing:

בָּרוּךְ *Blessed are You, HASHEM, our God, King of the universe, Who has sanctified us with His commandments and has commanded us to wrap ourselves in tzitzis.*

Wrap the *tallis* around your head and body, then recite:

מַה יָּקָר *How precious is Your kindness, O God! The sons of man take refuge in the shadows of Your wings. May they be sated from the abundance of Your house; and may You give them to drink from the stream of Your delights. For with You is the source of life — by Your light we shall see light. Extend Your kindness to those who know You, and Your charity to the upright of heart.*[3]

⊰ ORDER OF PUTTIN ON TEFILLIN ⊱

Many recite the following declaration of intent before putting on *tefillin:*

לְשֵׁם יִחוּד *For the sake of the unification of the Holy One, Blessed is He, and His Presence, in fear and love, to unify the Name — yud-kei with vav-kei — in perfect unity, in the name of all Israel.*

הִנְנִי מְכַוֵּן *Behold, in putting on tefillin I intend to fulfill the commandment of my Creator, Who has commanded us to put on tefillin, as is written in His Torah: 'Bind them as a sign upon your arm and let them be tefillin between your eyes.'*[4] *These four portions [contained in the tefillin] — [1] 'Shema (Deuteronomy 6:4-9); [2] 'And it will come to pass, if you will hearken' (Deuteronomy 11:13-21); [3] 'Sanctify (Exodus 13:1-10)*

---

(1) *Psalms* 104:1-2. (2) *Deuteronomy* 32:11. (3) *Psalms* 36:8-11. (4) *Deuteronomy* 6:8.

וְהָיָה כִּי יְבִאֲךָ – שֶׁיֵּשׁ בָּהֶם יִחוּדוֹ וְאַחְדוּתוֹ יִתְבָּרַךְ שְׁמוֹ בָּעוֹלָם; וְשֶׁנִּזְכּוֹר נִסִּים וְנִפְלָאוֹת שֶׁעָשָׂה עִמָּנוּ בְּהוֹצִיאֵנוּ מִמִּצְרָיִם; וַאֲשֶׁר לוֹ הַכֹּחַ וְהַמֶּמְשָׁלָה בָּעֶלְיוֹנִים וּבַתַּחְתּוֹנִים לַעֲשׂוֹת בָּהֶם כִּרְצוֹנוֹ. וְצִוָּנוּ לְהָנִיחַ עַל הַיָּד, לְזִכָּרוֹן זְרוֹעַ הַנְּטוּיָה, וְשֶׁהִיא נֶגֶד הַלֵּב, לְשַׁעְבֵּד בָּזֶה תַּאֲוַת וּמַחְשְׁבוֹת לִבֵּנוּ לַעֲבוֹדָתוֹ, יִתְבָּרַךְ שְׁמוֹ. וְעַל הָרֹאשׁ נֶגֶד הַמּוֹחַ, שֶׁהַנְּשָׁמָה שֶׁבְּמוֹחִי, עִם שְׁאָר חוּשַׁי וְכֹחוֹתַי, כֻּלָּם יִהְיוּ מְשֻׁעְבָּדִים לַעֲבוֹדָתוֹ, יִתְבָּרַךְ שְׁמוֹ. וּמִשֶּׁפַע מִצְוַת תְּפִלִּין יִתְמַשֵּׁךְ עָלַי לִהְיוֹת לִי חַיִּים אֲרוּכִים, וְשֶׁפַע קֹדֶשׁ, וּמַחְשָׁבוֹת קְדוֹשׁוֹת בְּלִי הִרְהוּר חֵטְא וְעָוֹן כְּלָל; וְשֶׁלֹּא יְפַתֵּנוּ וְלֹא יִתְגָּרֶה בָּנוּ יֵצֶר הָרָע, וְיַנִּיחֵנוּ לַעֲבֹד אֶת יהוה כַּאֲשֶׁר עִם לְבָבֵנוּ. וִיהִי רָצוֹן מִלְּפָנֶיךָ, יהוה אֱלֹהֵינוּ וֵאלֹהֵי אֲבוֹתֵינוּ, שֶׁתְּהֵא חֲשׁוּבָה מִצְוַת הֲנָחַת תְּפִלִּין לִפְנֵי הַקָּדוֹשׁ בָּרוּךְ הוּא כְּאִלּוּ קִיַּמְתִּיהָ בְּכָל פְּרָטֶיהָ וְדִקְדּוּקֶיהָ וְכַוָּנוֹתֶיהָ, וְתַרְיַ״ג מִצְוֹת הַתְּלוּיִים בָּהּ. אָמֵן סֶלָה.

Stand while putting on tefillin. Place the arm-tefillin upon the left biceps (or the right biceps of one who writes left-handed), hold it in place ready for tightening, then recite the following blessing:

בָּרוּךְ אַתָּה יהוה אֱלֹהֵינוּ מֶלֶךְ הָעוֹלָם, אֲשֶׁר קִדְּשָׁנוּ בְּמִצְוֹתָיו, וְצִוָּנוּ לְהָנִיחַ תְּפִלִּין.

Tighten the arm-tefillin and wrap the strap seven times around the arm. Without any interruption whatsoever, put the head-tefillin in place, above the hairline and opposite the space between the eyes. Before tightening the head-tefillin recite the following blessing:

בָּרוּךְ אַתָּה יהוה אֱלֹהֵינוּ מֶלֶךְ הָעוֹלָם, אֲשֶׁר קִדְּשָׁנוּ בְּמִצְוֹתָיו, וְצִוָּנוּ עַל מִצְוַת תְּפִלִּין.

Tighten the head-tefillin and recite:

בָּרוּךְ שֵׁם כְּבוֹד מַלְכוּתוֹ לְעוֹלָם וָעֶד.

After the head-tefillin is securely in place, recite:

וּמֵחָכְמָתְךָ אֵל עֶלְיוֹן, תַּאֲצִיל עָלַי; וּמִבִּינָתְךָ תְּבִינֵנִי; וּבְחַסְדְּךָ תַּגְדִּיל עָלַי; וּבִגְבוּרָתְךָ תַּצְמִית אֹיְבַי וְקָמַי. וְשֶׁמֶן הַטּוֹב תָּרִיק עַל שִׁבְעָה קְנֵי הַמְּנוֹרָה, לְהַשְׁפִּיעַ טוּבְךָ לִבְרִיּוֹתֶיךָ. פּוֹתֵחַ אֶת יָדֶךָ, וּמַשְׂבִּיעַ לְכָל חַי רָצוֹן.[1]

Wrap the strap around the middle finger and hand according to your custom. While doing this, recite:

וְאֵרַשְׂתִּיךְ לִי לְעוֹלָם, וְאֵרַשְׂתִּיךְ לִי בְּצֶדֶק וּבְמִשְׁפָּט וּבְחֶסֶד וּבְרַחֲמִים. וְאֵרַשְׂתִּיךְ לִי בֶּאֱמוּנָה, וְיָדַעַתְּ אֶת יהוה.[2]

and [4] *'And it will come to pass when He shall bring you' (Exodus 13:11-16)* — *contain His Oneness and Unity, may His Name be blessed, in the universe; so that we will recall the miracles and wonders that He did with us when He removed us from Egypt; and that He has the strength and dominion over those above and those below to do with them as He wishes. He has commanded us to put [tefillin] upon the arm to recall the 'outstretched arm' [of the Exodus] and that it be opposite the heart thereby to subjugate the desires and thoughts of our heart to His service, may His Name be blessed; and upon the head opposite the brain, so that the soul that is in my brain, together with my other senses and potentials, may all be subjugated to His service, may His Name be blessed. May some of the spiritual influence of the commandment of tefillin be extended upon me so that I have a long life, a flow of holiness, and holy thoughts, without even an inkling of sin or iniquity; and that the Evil Inclination will not seduce us nor incite against us, and that it permit us to serve HASHEM as is our hearts' desire. May it be Your will, HASHEM, our God and the God of our forefathers, that the commandment of putting on tefillin be considered as worthy before the Holy One, Blessed is He, as if I had fulfilled it in all its details, implications, and intentions, as well as the six hundred thirteen commandments that are dependent upon it. Amen, Selah.*

Stand while putting on *tefillin*. Place the arm-*tefillin* upon the left biceps (or the right biceps of one who writes left-handed), hold it in place ready for tightening, then recite the following blessing:

בָּרוּךְ *Blessed are You, HASHEM, our God, King of the universe, Who has sanctified us with His commandments and has commanded us to put on tefillin.*

Tighten the arm-*tefillin* and wrap the strap seven times around the arm. Without any interruption whatsoever, put the head-*tefillin* in place, above the hairline and opposite the space between the eyes. Before tightening the head-*tefillin* recite the following blessing:

בָּרוּךְ *Blessed are You, HASHEM, our God, King of the universe, Who has sanctified us with His commandments and has commanded us regarding the commandment of tefillin.*

Tighten the head-*tefillin* and recite:

Blessed is the Name of His glorious kingdom for all eternity.

After the head-*tefillin* is securely in place, recite:

וּמֵחָכְמָתְךָ *From Your wisdom, O supreme God, may You imbue me; from Your understanding give me understanding; with Your kindness do greatly with me; with Your power cut down my foes and rebels. [May] You pour goodly oil upon the seven arms of the menorah, to cause Your good to flow to Your creatures. [May] You open Your hand and satisfy the desire of every living thing.[1]*

Wrap the strap around the middle finger and hand according to your custom.
While doing this, recite:

וְאֵרַשְׂתִּיךְ *I will betroth you to Me forever, and I will betroth you to Me with righteousness, justice, kindness, and mercy. I will betroth you to Me with fidelity, and you shall know HASHEM.[2]*

(1) *Psalms* 145:16. (2) *Hoshea* 2:21-22.

PORTIONS OMITTED FROM SHACHARIS (EXCEPT לַמְנַצֵּחַ AND תַּחֲנוּן) ARE RECITED HERE.

‎א‎ שִׁיר שֶׁל יוֹם ‎א‎

A different apsalm is assigned as the Song of the Day for each day of the week.

SUNDAY

הַיּוֹם יוֹם רִאשׁוֹן בַּשַּׁבָּת, שֶׁבּוֹ הָיוּ הַלְוִיִּם אוֹמְרִים בְּבֵית הַמִּקְדָּשׁ:

תהלים כד

לְדָוִד מִזְמוֹר, לַיהוה הָאָרֶץ וּמְלוֹאָהּ, תֵּבֵל וְיֹשְׁבֵי בָהּ. כִּי הוּא עַל יַמִּים
יְסָדָהּ, וְעַל נְהָרוֹת יְכוֹנְנֶהָ. מִי יַעֲלֶה בְהַר יהוה, וּמִי יָקוּם בִּמְקוֹם
קָדְשׁוֹ. נְקִי כַפַּיִם וּבַר לֵבָב, אֲשֶׁר לֹא נָשָׂא לַשָּׁוְא נַפְשִׁי, וְלֹא נִשְׁבַּע
לְמִרְמָה. יִשָּׂא בְרָכָה מֵאֵת יהוה, וּצְדָקָה מֵאֱלֹהֵי יִשְׁעוֹ. זֶה דּוֹר דֹּרְשָׁיו,
מְבַקְשֵׁי פָנֶיךָ יַעֲקֹב סֶלָה. שְׂאוּ שְׁעָרִים רָאשֵׁיכֶם, וְהִנָּשְׂאוּ פִּתְחֵי עוֹלָם,
וְיָבוֹא מֶלֶךְ הַכָּבוֹד. מִי זֶה מֶלֶךְ הַכָּבוֹד, יהוה עִזּוּז וְגִבּוֹר, יהוה גִּבּוֹר
מִלְחָמָה. ‎❖‎ שְׂאוּ שְׁעָרִים רָאשֵׁיכֶם, וּשְׂאוּ פִּתְחֵי עוֹלָם, וְיָבֹא מֶלֶךְ הַכָּבוֹד.
מִי הוּא זֶה מֶלֶךְ הַכָּבוֹד, יהוה צְבָאוֹת, הוּא מֶלֶךְ הַכָּבוֹד סֶלָה.

The service continues with קַדִּישׁ יָתוֹם, the Mourner's Kaddish (page 414).

TUESDAY

הַיּוֹם יוֹם שְׁלִישִׁי בַּשַּׁבָּת, שֶׁבּוֹ הָיוּ הַלְוִיִּם אוֹמְרִים בְּבֵית הַמִּקְדָּשׁ:

תהלים פב

מִזְמוֹר לְאָסָף, אֱלֹהִים נִצָּב בַּעֲדַת אֵל, בְּקֶרֶב אֱלֹהִים יִשְׁפֹּט. עַד
מָתַי תִּשְׁפְּטוּ עָוֶל, וּפְנֵי רְשָׁעִים תִּשְׂאוּ סֶלָה. שִׁפְטוּ דָל וְיָתוֹם,
עָנִי וָרָשׁ הַצְדִּיקוּ. פַּלְּטוּ דַל וְאֶבְיוֹן, מִיַּד רְשָׁעִים הַצִּילוּ. לֹא יָדְעוּ וְלֹא
יָבִינוּ, בַּחֲשֵׁכָה יִתְהַלָּכוּ, יִמּוֹטוּ כָּל מוֹסְדֵי אָרֶץ. אֲנִי אָמַרְתִּי אֱלֹהִים אַתֶּם,
וּבְנֵי עֶלְיוֹן כֻּלְּכֶם. אָכֵן כְּאָדָם תְּמוּתוּן, וּכְאַחַד הַשָּׂרִים תִּפֹּלוּ. ‎❖‎ קוּמָה
אֱלֹהִים שָׁפְטָה הָאָרֶץ, כִּי אַתָּה תִנְחַל בְּכָל הַגּוֹיִם.

The service continues with קַדִּישׁ יָתוֹם, the Mourner's Kaddish (page 414).

THURSDAY

הַיּוֹם יוֹם חֲמִישִׁי בַּשַּׁבָּת, שֶׁבּוֹ הָיוּ הַלְוִיִּם אוֹמְרִים בְּבֵית הַמִּקְדָּשׁ:

תהלים פא

לַמְנַצֵּחַ עַל הַגִּתִּית לְאָסָף. הַרְנִינוּ לֵאלֹהִים עוּזֵּנוּ, הָרִיעוּ לֵאלֹהֵי
יַעֲקֹב. שְׂאוּ זִמְרָה וּתְנוּ תֹף, כִּנּוֹר נָעִים עִם נָבֶל. תִּקְעוּ בַחֹדֶשׁ
שׁוֹפָר, בַּכֶּסֶה לְיוֹם חַגֵּנוּ. כִּי חֹק לְיִשְׂרָאֵל הוּא, מִשְׁפָּט לֵאלֹהֵי יַעֲקֹב.
עֵדוּת בִּיהוֹסֵף שָׂמוֹ, בְּצֵאתוֹ עַל אֶרֶץ מִצְרָיִם, שְׂפַת לֹא יָדַעְתִּי אֶשְׁמָע.
הֲסִירוֹתִי מִסֵּבֶל שִׁכְמוֹ, כַּפָּיו מִדּוּד תַּעֲבֹרְנָה. בַּצָּרָה קָרָאתָ, וָאֲחַלְּצֶךָּ,
אֶעֶנְךָ בְּסֵתֶר רַעַם, אֶבְחָנְךָ עַל מֵי מְרִיבָה, סֶלָה. שְׁמַע עַמִּי וְאָעִידָה בָּךְ,
יִשְׂרָאֵל אִם תִּשְׁמַע לִי. לֹא יִהְיֶה בְךָ אֵל זָר, וְלֹא תִשְׁתַּחֲוֶה לְאֵל נֵכָר. אָנֹכִי

PORTIONS OMITTED FROM SHACHARIS (EXCEPT תַּחֲנוּן AND לַמְנַצֵּחַ) ARE RECITED HERE.

⁂{ SONG OF THE DAY }⁂

A different psalm is assigned as the Song of the Day for each day of the week.

SUNDAY

*Today is the first day of the Sabbath,
on which the Levites would recite in the Holy Temple:*

Psalm 24

לְדָוִד *Of David a psalm. HASHEM's is the earth and its fullness, the inhabited land and those who dwell in it. For He founded it upon seas, and established it upon rivers. Who may ascend the mountain of HASHEM, and who may stand in the place of His sanctity? One with clean hands and pure heart, who has not sworn in vain by My soul and has not sworn deceitfully. He will receive a blessing from HASHEM and just kindness from the God of his salvation. This is the generation of those who seek Him, those who strive for Your Presence — Jacob, Selah. Raise up your heads, O gates, and be uplifted, you everlasting entrances, so that the King of Glory may enter. Who is this King of Glory? — HASHEM, the mighty and strong, HASHEM, the strong in battle.* Chazzan— *Raise up your heads, O gates, and raise up, you everlasting entrances, so that the King of Glory may enter. Who then is the King of Glory? HASHEM, Master of Legions, He is the King of Glory. Selah!*

The service continues with קַדִּישׁ יָתוֹם, *the Mourner's Kaddish (p. 414).*

TUESDAY

*Today is the third day of the Sabbath,
on which the Levites would recite in the Holy Temple:*

Psalm 82

מִזְמוֹר *A psalm of Assaf: God stands in the Divine assembly, in the midst of judges shall He judge. Until when will you judge lawlessly and favor the presence of the wicked, Selah? Judge the needy and the orphan, vindicate the poor and impoverished. Rescue the needy and destitute, from the hand of the wicked deliver them. They do not know nor do they understand, in darkness they walk; all foundations of the earth collapse. I said, 'You are angelic, sons of the Most High are you all.' But like men you shall die, and like one of the princes you shall fall.* Chazzan— *Arise, O God, judge the earth, for You allot the heritage among all the nations.*

The service continues with קַדִּישׁ יָתוֹם, *the Mourner's Kaddish (p. 414).*

THURSDAY

*Today is the fifth day of the Sabbath,
on which the Levites would recite in the Holy Temple:*

Psalm 81

לַמְנַצֵּחַ *For the Conductor, upon the gittis, by Assaf. Sing joyously to the God of our might, call out to the God of Jacob. Raise a song and sound the drum, the sweet harp with the lyre. Blow the shofar at the moon's renewal, at the time appointed for our festive day. Because it is a decree for Israel, a judgment day for the God of Jacob. He imposed it as a testimony for Joseph when he went forth over the land of Egypt — 'I understood a language I never knew!' I removed his shoulder from the burden, his hands let go of the kettle. In distress you called out, and I released you, I answered you with thunder when you hid, I tested you at the Waters of Strife, Selah. Listen, My nation, and I will attest to you; O Israel, if you would but listen to Me. There shall be no strange god within you, nor shall you bow before an alien god. I am*

יהוה אֱלֹהֶיךָ, הַמַּעַלְךָ מֵאֶרֶץ מִצְרָיִם, הַרְחֶב פִּיךָ וַאֲמַלְאֵהוּ. וְלֹא שָׁמַע
עַמִּי לְקוֹלִי, וְיִשְׂרָאֵל לֹא אָבָה לִי. וָאֲשַׁלְּחֵהוּ בִּשְׁרִירוּת לִבָּם, יֵלְכוּ
בְּמוֹעֲצוֹתֵיהֶם. לוּ עַמִּי שֹׁמֵעַ לִי, יִשְׂרָאֵל בִּדְרָכַי יְהַלֵּכוּ. כִּמְעַט אוֹיְבֵיהֶם
אַכְנִיעַ, וְעַל צָרֵיהֶם אָשִׁיב יָדִי. מְשַׂנְאֵי יהוה יְכַחֲשׁוּ לוֹ, וִיהִי עִתָּם לְעוֹלָם.
❖ וַיַּאֲכִילֵהוּ מֵחֵלֶב חִטָּה, וּמִצּוּר דְּבַשׁ אַשְׂבִּיעֶךָ.

The service continues with קַדִּישׁ יָתוֹם, *the Mourner's Kaddish* (below).

קדיש יתום

In the presence of a *minyan*, mourners recite קַדִּישׁ יָתוֹם, the Mourner's *Kaddish* (see *Laws §132-134*):

יִתְגַּדַּל וְיִתְקַדַּשׁ שְׁמֵהּ רַבָּא. (.Cong – אָמֵן.) בְּעָלְמָא דִּי בְרָא כִרְעוּתֵהּ.
וְיַמְלִיךְ מַלְכוּתֵהּ, בְּחַיֵּיכוֹן וּבְיוֹמֵיכוֹן וּבְחַיֵּי דְכָל בֵּית יִשְׂרָאֵל,
בַּעֲגָלָא וּבִזְמַן קָרִיב. וְאִמְרוּ: אָמֵן.

(.Cong – אָמֵן. יְהֵא שְׁמֵהּ רַבָּא מְבָרַךְ לְעָלַם וּלְעָלְמֵי עָלְמַיָּא.)
יְהֵא שְׁמֵהּ רַבָּא מְבָרַךְ לְעָלַם וּלְעָלְמֵי עָלְמַיָּא.

יִתְבָּרַךְ וְיִשְׁתַּבַּח וְיִתְפָּאַר וְיִתְרוֹמַם וְיִתְנַשֵּׂא וְיִתְהַדָּר וְיִתְעַלֶּה וְיִתְהַלָּל
שְׁמֵהּ דְּקֻדְשָׁא בְּרִיךְ הוּא (.Cong – בְּרִיךְ הוּא) – לְעֵלָּא מִן כָּל בִּרְכָתָא
וְשִׁירָתָא תֻּשְׁבְּחָתָא וְנֶחֱמָתָא, דַּאֲמִירָן בְּעָלְמָא. וְאִמְרוּ: אָמֵן. (.Cong – אָמֵן.)
יְהֵא שְׁלָמָא רַבָּא מִן שְׁמַיָּא, וְחַיִּים עָלֵינוּ וְעַל כָּל יִשְׂרָאֵל.
וְאִמְרוּ: אָמֵן. (.Cong – אָמֵן.)

Take three steps back. Bow left and say . . . עֹשֶׂה; bow right and say . . . הוּא; bow forward and say
וְעַל כָּל . . . אָמֵן. Remain standing in place for a few moments, then take three steps forward.

עֹשֶׂה שָׁלוֹם בִּמְרוֹמָיו, הוּא יַעֲשֶׂה שָׁלוֹם עָלֵינוּ, וְעַל כָּל יִשְׂרָאֵל.
וְאִמְרוּ: אָמֵן. (.Cong – אָמֵן.)

אַשְׁרֵי יוֹשְׁבֵי בֵיתֶךָ, עוֹד יְהַלְלוּךָ סֶּלָה.[1] אַשְׁרֵי הָעָם שֶׁכָּכָה לּוֹ,
אַשְׁרֵי הָעָם שֶׁיהוה אֱלֹהָיו.[2]
תְּהִלָּה לְדָוִד,

תהלים קמה

אֲרוֹמִמְךָ אֱלוֹהַי הַמֶּלֶךְ, וַאֲבָרְכָה שִׁמְךָ לְעוֹלָם וָעֶד.
בְּכָל יוֹם אֲבָרְכֶךָּ, וַאֲהַלְלָה שִׁמְךָ לְעוֹלָם וָעֶד.
גָּדוֹל יהוה וּמְהֻלָּל מְאֹד, וְלִגְדֻלָּתוֹ אֵין חֵקֶר.
דּוֹר לְדוֹר יְשַׁבַּח מַעֲשֶׂיךָ, וּגְבוּרֹתֶיךָ יַגִּידוּ.
הֲדַר כְּבוֹד הוֹדֶךָ, וְדִבְרֵי נִפְלְאֹתֶיךָ אָשִׂיחָה.
וֶעֱזוּז נוֹרְאֹתֶיךָ יֹאמֵרוּ, וּגְדוּלָּתְךָ אֲסַפְּרֶנָּה.
זֵכֶר רַב טוּבְךָ יַבִּיעוּ, וְצִדְקָתְךָ יְרַנֵּנוּ.
חַנּוּן וְרַחוּם יהוה, אֶרֶךְ אַפַּיִם וּגְדָל חָסֶד.

(1) *Psalms* 84:5. (2) 144:15.

HASHEM, your God, who elevated you from the land of Egypt, open wide your mouth and I will fill it. But My people did not heed My voice and Israel did not desire Me. So I let them follow their heart's fantasies, they follow their own counsels. If only My people would heed Me, if Israel would walk in My ways. In an instant I would subdue their foes, and against their tormentors turn My hand. Those who hate HASHEM lie to Him — so their destiny is eternal. Chazzan— *But He would feed him with the cream of the wheat, and with honey from a rock sate you.*

The service continues with קַדִּישׁ יָתוֹם, *the Mourner's Kaddish* (below).

MOURNER'S KADDISH

In the presence of a *minyan*, mourners recite קַדִּישׁ יָתוֹם, *the Mourner's Kaddish* (see *Laws* §132-134):

[A transliteration of this *Kaddish* appears on p. 486.]

יִתְגַּדַּל *May His great Name grow exalted and sanctified* (Cong.— *Amen.*) *in the world that He created as He willed. May He give reign to His kingship in your lifetimes and in your days, and in the lifetimes of the entire Family of Israel, swiftly and soon. Now respond: Amen.*

(Cong.— *Amen. May His great Name be blessed forever and ever.*)

May His great Name be blessed forever and ever.

Blessed, praised, glorified, exalted, extolled, mighty, upraised, and lauded be the Name of the Holy One, Blessed is He (Cong.— *Blessed is He*) — *beyond any blessing and song, praise and consolation that are uttered in the world. Now respond: Amen.* (Cong.— *Amen*).

May there be abundant peace from Heaven, and life, upon us and upon all Israel. Now respond: Amen. (Cong.— *Amen.*)

Take three steps back. Bow left and say, 'He Who makes peace . . .';
bow right and say, 'may He . . .'; bow forward and say, 'and upon all Israel . . .'
Remain standing in place for a few moments, then take three steps forward.

He Who makes peace in His heights, may He make peace upon us, and upon all Israel. Now respond: Amen. (Cong.— *Amen.*)

אַשְׁרֵי *Praiseworthy are those who dwell in Your house; may they always praise You, Selah!*[1] *Praiseworthy is the people for whom this is so, praiseworthy is the people whose God is* HASHEM.[2]

Psalm 145   *A psalm of praise by David:*

א *I will exalt You, my God the King,*
      and I will bless Your Name forever and ever.

ב *Every day I will bless You,*
      and I will laud Your Name forever and ever.

ג HASHEM *is great and exceedingly lauded,*
      and His greatness is beyond investigation.

ד *Each generation will praise Your deeds to the next*
        and of Your mighty deeds they will tell.

ה *The splendrous glory of Your power*
        and Your wondrous deeds I shall discuss.

ו *And of Your awesome power they will speak,*
      and Your greatness I shall relate.

ז *A recollection of Your abundant goodness they will utter*
      and of Your righteousness they will sing exultantly.

ח *Gracious and merciful is* HASHEM,
      slow to anger, and great in [bestowing] kindness.

טוֹב יהוה לַכֹּל, וְרַחֲמָיו עַל כָּל מַעֲשָׂיו.

יוֹדוּךָ יהוה כָּל מַעֲשֶׂיךָ, וַחֲסִידֶיךָ יְבָרְכִוּכָה.

כְּבוֹד מַלְכוּתְךָ יֹאמֵרוּ, וּגְבוּרָתְךָ יְדַבֵּרוּ.

לְהוֹדִיעַ לִבְנֵי הָאָדָם גְּבוּרֹתָיו, וּכְבוֹד הֲדַר מַלְכוּתוֹ.

מַלְכוּתְךָ מַלְכוּת כָּל עֹלָמִים, וּמֶמְשַׁלְתְּךָ בְּכָל דּוֹר וָדֹר.

סוֹמֵךְ יהוה לְכָל הַנֹּפְלִים, וְזוֹקֵף לְכָל הַכְּפוּפִים.

עֵינֵי כֹל אֵלֶיךָ יְשַׂבֵּרוּ, וְאַתָּה נוֹתֵן לָהֶם אֶת אָכְלָם בְּעִתּוֹ.

פּוֹתֵחַ אֶת יָדֶךָ,

While reciting the verse פּוֹתֵחַ, *concentrate intently on its meaning.*

וּמַשְׂבִּיעַ לְכָל חַי רָצוֹן.

צַדִּיק יהוה בְּכָל דְּרָכָיו, וְחָסִיד בְּכָל מַעֲשָׂיו.

קָרוֹב יהוה לְכָל קֹרְאָיו, לְכֹל אֲשֶׁר יִקְרָאֻהוּ בֶאֱמֶת.

רְצוֹן יְרֵאָיו יַעֲשֶׂה, וְאֶת שַׁוְעָתָם יִשְׁמַע וְיוֹשִׁיעֵם.

שׁוֹמֵר יהוה אֶת כָּל אֹהֲבָיו, וְאֵת כָּל הָרְשָׁעִים יַשְׁמִיד.

תְּהִלַּת יהוה יְדַבֶּר פִּי, וִיבָרֵךְ כָּל בָּשָׂר שֵׁם קָדְשׁוֹ לְעוֹלָם וָעֶד.

וַאֲנַחְנוּ נְבָרֵךְ יָהּ, מֵעַתָּה וְעַד עוֹלָם, הַלְלוּיָהּ.

The chazzan recites Half-Kaddish:

יִתְגַּדַּל וְיִתְקַדַּשׁ שְׁמֵהּ רַבָּא. (.Cong – אָמֵן.) בְּעָלְמָא דִּי בְרָא כִרְעוּתֵהּ. וְיַמְלִיךְ מַלְכוּתֵהּ, בְּחַיֵּיכוֹן וּבְיוֹמֵיכוֹן וּבְחַיֵּי דְכָל בֵּית יִשְׂרָאֵל, בַּעֲגָלָא וּבִזְמַן קָרִיב. וְאִמְרוּ: אָמֵן.

(.Cong – אָמֵן. יְהֵא שְׁמֵהּ רַבָּא מְבָרַךְ לְעָלַם וּלְעָלְמֵי עָלְמַיָּא.)

יְהֵא שְׁמֵהּ רַבָּא מְבָרַךְ לְעָלַם וּלְעָלְמֵי עָלְמַיָּא.

יִתְבָּרַךְ וְיִשְׁתַּבַּח וְיִתְפָּאַר וְיִתְרוֹמַם וְיִתְנַשֵּׂא וְיִתְהַדָּר וְיִתְעַלֶּה וְיִתְהַלָּל שְׁמֵהּ דְּקֻדְשָׁא בְּרִיךְ הוּא (.Cong – בְּרִיךְ הוּא) – לְעֵלָּא מִן כָּל בִּרְכָתָא וְשִׁירָתָא תֻּשְׁבְּחָתָא וְנֶחֱמָתָא, דַּאֲמִירָן בְּעָלְמָא. וְאִמְרוּ: אָמֵן.
(.Cong – אָמֵן.)

∗{ הוֹצָאַת סֵפֶר תּוֹרָה }∗

From the moment the Ark is opened until the Torah is returned to it, one must conduct himself with the utmost respect, and avoid unnecessary conversation. It is commendable to kiss the Torah as it is carried to the bimah [reading table] and back to the Ark. All rise and remain standing until the Torah is placed on the bimah. The Ark is opened. Before the Torah is removed the congregation recites:

וַיְהִי בִּנְסֹעַ הָאָרֹן וַיֹּאמֶר מֹשֶׁה, קוּמָה יהוה וְיָפֻצוּ אֹיְבֶיךָ וְיָנֻסוּ מְשַׂנְאֶיךָ מִפָּנֶיךָ.׳ כִּי מִצִּיּוֹן תֵּצֵא תוֹרָה, וּדְבַר יהוה מִירוּשָׁלָיִם.׳ בָּרוּךְ שֶׁנָּתַן תּוֹרָה לְעַמּוֹ יִשְׂרָאֵל בִּקְדֻשָּׁתוֹ.

ט *HASHEM is good to all; His mercies are on all His works.*

י *All Your works shall thank You, HASHEM,*
  and Your devout ones will bless You.

כ *Of the glory of Your kingdom they will speak,*
  and of Your power they will tell;

ל *To inform human beings of His mighty deeds,*
  and the glorious splendor of His kingdom.

מ *Your kingdom is a kingdom spanning all eternities,*
  and Your dominion is throughout every generation.

ס *HASHEM supports all the fallen ones and straightens all the bent.*

ע *The eyes of all look to You with hope*
  and You give them their food in its proper time;

פ *You open Your hand,*   While reciting the verse, 'You open . . .' concentrate
  and satisfy the desire of every living thing.   intently on its meaning.

צ *Righteous is HASHEM in all His ways*
  and magnanimous in all His deeds.

ק *HASHEM is close to all who call upon Him —*
  to all who call upon Him sincerely.

ר *The will of those who fear Him He will do;*
  and their cry He will hear, and save them.

ש *HASHEM protects all who love Him; but all the wicked He will destroy.*

ת Chazzan— *May my mouth declare the praise of HASHEM*
  and may all flesh bless His Holy Name forever and ever.

We will bless God from this time and forever, Halleluyah![1]

The chazzan recites Half-*Kaddish:*

יִתְגַּדַּל *May His great Name grow exalted and sanctified* (Cong.— *Amen.*) *in*
      the world that He created as He willed. May He give reign to His
kingship in your lifetimes and in your days, and in the lifetimes of the entire
Family of Israel, swiftly and soon. Now respond: Amen.

   (Cong.— *Amen. May His great Name be blessed forever and ever.)*
      May His great Name be blessed forever and ever.

   Blessed, praised, glorified, exalted, extolled, mighty, upraised, and lauded
be the Name of the Holy One, Blessed is He (Cong.— *Blessed is He*) *— beyond any*
blessing and song, praise and consolation that are uttered in the world. Now
respond: Amen. (Cong.— *Amen.*)

⧏ **REMOVAL OF THE TORAH FROM THE ARK** ⧐

From the moment the Ark is opened until the Torah is returned to it, one must conduct himself with
the utmost respect, and avoid unnecessary conversation. It is commendable to kiss the Torah as it
is carried to the *bimah* [reading table] and back to the Ark. All rise and remain standing until the Torah
is placed on the *bimah*. The Ark is opened. Before the Torah is removed the congregation recites:

וַיְהִי בִּנְסֹעַ *When the Ark would travel, Moses would say, 'Arise,*
      HASHEM, and let Your foes be scattered, let those who hate
You flee from You.'[2] *For from Zion the Torah will come forth and the word*
of HASHEM from Jerusalem.[3] *Blessed is He Who gave the Torah to His*
people Israel in His holiness.

---
(1) *Psalms* 115:18. (2) *Numbers* 10:35. (3) *Isaiah* 2:3.

זוהר ויקהל שס:א

בְּרִיךְ שְׁמֵהּ דְּמָרֵא עָלְמָא, בְּרִיךְ כִּתְרָךְ וְאַתְרָךְ. יְהֵא רְעוּתָךְ עִם עַמָּךְ יִשְׂרָאֵל לְעָלַם, וּפֻרְקַן יְמִינָךְ אַחֲזֵי לְעַמָּךְ בְּבֵית מַקְדְּשָׁךְ, וּלְאַמְטוּיֵי לָנָא מִטּוּב נְהוֹרָךְ, וּלְקַבֵּל צְלוֹתָנָא בְּרַחֲמִין. יְהֵא רַעֲוָא קֳדָמָךְ, דְּתוֹרִיךְ לָן חַיִּין בְּטִיבוּתָא, וְלֶהֱוֵי אֲנָא פְקִידָא בְּגוֹ צַדִּיקַיָּא, לְמִרְחַם עֲלַי וּלְמִנְטַר יָתִי וְיָת כָּל דִּי לִי, וְדִי לְעַמָּךְ יִשְׂרָאֵל. אַנְתְּ הוּא זָן לְכֹלָּא, וּמְפַרְנֵס לְכֹלָּא, אַנְתְּ הוּא שַׁלִּיט עַל כֹּלָּא. אַנְתְּ הוּא דְּשַׁלִּיט עַל מַלְכַיָּא, וּמַלְכוּתָא דִּילָךְ הִיא. אֲנָא עַבְדָּא דְּקֻדְשָׁא בְּרִיךְ הוּא, דְּסָגִידְנָא קַמֵּהּ וּמִקַּמָּא דִּיקַר אוֹרַיְתֵהּ בְּכָל עִדָּן וְעִדָּן. לָא עַל אֱנָשׁ רָחִיצְנָא, וְלָא עַל בַּר אֱלָהִין סָמִיכְנָא, אֶלָּא בֶּאֱלָהָא דִשְׁמַיָּא, דְּהוּא אֱלָהָא קְשׁוֹט, וְאוֹרַיְתֵהּ קְשׁוֹט, וּנְבִיאוֹהִי קְשׁוֹט, וּמַסְגֵּא לְמֶעְבַּד טַבְוָן וּקְשׁוֹט. בֵּהּ אֲנָא רָחִיץ, וְלִשְׁמֵהּ קַדִּישָׁא יַקִּירָא אֲנָא אֵמַר תֻּשְׁבְּחָן. יְהֵא רַעֲוָא קֳדָמָךְ, דְּתִפְתַּח לִבָּאי בְּאוֹרַיְתָא, וְתַשְׁלִים מִשְׁאֲלִין דְּלִבָּאי, וְלִבָּא דְכָל עַמָּךְ יִשְׂרָאֵל, לְטַב וּלְחַיִּין וְלִשְׁלָם. (אָמֵן.)

The Torah is removed from the Ark and presented to the *chazzan*, who accepts it in his right arm. He then turns to the Ark, bows while raising the Torah, and recites:

גַּדְּלוּ לַיהוה אִתִּי וּנְרוֹמְמָה שְׁמוֹ יַחְדָּו.[1]

The *chazzan* turns to his right and carries the Torah to the *bimah*, as the congregation responds:

לְךָ יהוה הַגְּדֻלָּה וְהַגְּבוּרָה וְהַתִּפְאֶרֶת וְהַנֵּצַח וְהַהוֹד כִּי כֹל בַּשָּׁמַיִם וּבָאָרֶץ, לְךָ יהוה הַמַּמְלָכָה וְהַמִּתְנַשֵּׂא לְכֹל לְרֹאשׁ.[2] רוֹמְמוּ יהוה אֱלֹהֵינוּ, וְהִשְׁתַּחֲווּ לַהֲדֹם רַגְלָיו, קָדוֹשׁ הוּא. רוֹמְמוּ יהוה אֱלֹהֵינוּ, וְהִשְׁתַּחֲווּ לְהַר קָדְשׁוֹ, כִּי קָדוֹשׁ יהוה אֱלֹהֵינוּ.[3]

אַב הָרַחֲמִים הוּא יְרַחֵם עַם עֲמוּסִים, וְיִזְכֹּר בְּרִית אֵיתָנִים, וְיַצִּיל נַפְשׁוֹתֵינוּ מִן הַשָּׁעוֹת הָרָעוֹת, וְיִגְעַר בְּיֵצֶר הָרָע מִן הַנְּשׂוּאִים, וְיָחֹן אוֹתָנוּ לִפְלֵיטַת עוֹלָמִים, וִימַלֵּא מִשְׁאֲלוֹתֵינוּ בְּמִדָּה טוֹבָה יְשׁוּעָה וְרַחֲמִים.

The Torah is placed on the *bimah* and prepared for reading. The *gabbai* uses the following formula to call a *Kohen* to the Torah:

וְתִגָּלֶה וְתֵרָאֶה מַלְכוּתוֹ עָלֵינוּ בִּזְמַן קָרוֹב, וְיָחֹן פְּלֵיטָתֵנוּ וּפְלֵיטַת עַמּוֹ בֵּית יִשְׂרָאֵל לְחֵן וּלְחֶסֶד וּלְרַחֲמִים וּלְרָצוֹן. וְנֹאמַר אָמֵן. הַכֹּל הָבוּ גֹדֶל לֵאלֹהֵינוּ וּתְנוּ כָבוֹד לַתּוֹרָה. כֹּהֵן° קְרָב, יַעֲמֹד (insert name) הַכֹּהֵן.

°If no *Kohen* is present, the *gabbai* says: "אִין כָּאן כֹּהֵן, יַעֲמֹד (name) יִשְׂרָאֵל (לֵוִי) בִּמְקוֹם כֹּהֵן."

Zohar, Vayakhel 369a

בְּרִיךְ שְׁמֵהּ Blessed is the Name of the Master of the universe,
blessed is Your crown and Your place. May Your favor
remain with Your people Israel forever; may You display the salvation
of Your right hand to Your people in Your Holy Temple, to benefit
us with the goodness of Your luminescence and to accept our prayers with mercy. May it be Your will that You extend our lives with
goodness and that I be numbered among the righteous; that You have
mercy on me and protect me, all that is mine and that is Your people
Israel's. It is You Who nourishes all and sustains all; You control
everything. It is You Who controls kings, and kingship is Yours. I am
a servant of the Holy One, Blessed is He, and I prostrate myself before
Him and before the glory of His Torah at all times. Not in any man
do I put trust, nor on any angel do I rely — only on the God of heaven Who
is the God of truth, Whose Torah is truth and Whose prophets are true
and Who acts liberally with kindness and truth. In Him do I trust, and
to His glorious and holy Name do I declare praises. May it be Your will
that You open my heart to the Torah and that You fulfill the wishes of
my heart and the heart of Your entire people Israel for good, for life, and
for peace. (Amen.)

The Torah is removed from the Ark and presented to the chazzan, who accepts it in his right arm.
He turns to the Ark, bows while raising the Torah, and recites:

Declare the greatness of HASHEM with me,
and let us exalt His Name together.[1]

The chazzan turns to his right and carries the Torah to the bimah, as the congregation responds:

לְךָ Yours, HASHEM, is the greatness, the strength, the splendor, the
triumph, and the glory; even everything in heaven and earth; Yours,
HASHEM, is the kingdom, and the sovereignty over every leader.[2] Exalt
HASHEM, our God, and bow at His footstool; He is Holy! Exalt HASHEM,
our God, and bow to His holy mountain; for holy is HASHEM, our God.[3]

אַב הָרַחֲמִים May the Father of compassion have mercy on the
nation that is borne by Him, and may He remember the
covenant of the spiritually mighty. May He rescue our souls from the bad
times, and upbraid the evil inclination to leave those borne by Him,
graciously make us an eternal remnant, and fulfill our requests in good
measure, for salvation and mercy.

The Torah is placed on the bimah and prepared for reading.
The gabbai uses the following formula to call a Kohen to the Torah:

וְתִגָּלֶה And may His kingship over us be revealed and become visible soon,
and may He be gracious to our remnant and the remnant of His people
the Family of Israel, for graciousness, kindness, mercy, and favor. And let us
respond, Amen. All of you ascribe greatness to our God and give honor to the
Torah. Kohen,° approach. Stand (name) son of (father's name) the Kohen.

°If no Kohen is present, the gabbai says: 'There is no Kohen present,
stand (name) son of (father's name) an Israelite (Levite) in place of the Kohen.'

(1) Psalms 34:4. (2) I Chronicles 29:11. (3) Psalms 99:5,9.

בָּרוּךְ שֶׁנָּתַן תּוֹרָה לְעַמּוֹ יִשְׂרָאֵל בִּקְדֻשָּׁתוֹ. (תּוֹרַת יהוה תְּמִימָה מְשִׁיבַת נָפֶשׁ, עֵדוּת יהוה נֶאֱמָנָה מַחְכִּימַת פֶּתִי. פִּקּוּדֵי יהוה יְשָׁרִים מְשַׂמְּחֵי לֵב, מִצְוַת יהוה בָּרָה מְאִירַת עֵינָיִם.[1] יהוה עֹז לְעַמּוֹ יִתֵּן, יהוה יְבָרֵךְ אֶת עַמּוֹ בַשָּׁלוֹם.[2] הָאֵל תָּמִים דַּרְכּוֹ, אִמְרַת יהוה צְרוּפָה, מָגֵן הוּא לְכֹל הַחוֹסִים בּוֹ.[3])

Congregation, then *gabbai:*

וְאַתֶּם הַדְּבֵקִים בַּיהוה אֱלֹהֵיכֶם, חַיִּים כֻּלְּכֶם הַיּוֹם.[4]

The reader shows the *oleh* (person called to the Torah) the place in the Torah. The *oleh* touches the Torah with a corner of his *tallis,* or the belt or mantle of the Torah, and kisses it. He then begins the blessing, bowing at בָּרְכוּ, and straightening up at 'ה.

בָּרְכוּ אֶת יהוה הַמְּבֹרָךְ.

Congregation, followed by *oleh,* responds, bowing at בָּרוּךְ, and straightening up at 'ה.

בָּרוּךְ יהוה הַמְּבֹרָךְ לְעוֹלָם וָעֶד.

Oleh continues:

בָּרוּךְ אַתָּה יהוה אֱלֹהֵינוּ מֶלֶךְ הָעוֹלָם, אֲשֶׁר בָּחַר בָּנוּ מִכָּל הָעַמִּים, וְנָתַן לָנוּ אֶת תּוֹרָתוֹ. בָּרוּךְ אַתָּה יהוה, נוֹתֵן הַתּוֹרָה. (Cong.– אָמֵן.)

After his Torah portion has been read, the *oleh* recites:

בָּרוּךְ אַתָּה יהוה אֱלֹהֵינוּ מֶלֶךְ הָעוֹלָם, אֲשֶׁר נָתַן לָנוּ תּוֹרַת אֱמֶת, וְחַיֵּי עוֹלָם נָטַע בְּתוֹכֵנוּ. בָּרוּךְ אַתָּה יהוה, נוֹתֵן הַתּוֹרָה. (Cong.– אָמֵן.)

PRAYER FOR A SICK PERSON / מי שברך לחולה

מִי שֶׁבֵּרַךְ אֲבוֹתֵינוּ אַבְרָהָם יִצְחָק וְיַעֲקֹב, מֹשֶׁה אַהֲרֹן דָּוִד וּשְׁלֹמֹה,

for a man	for a woman
הוּא יְבָרֵךְ וִירַפֵּא אֶת הַחוֹלֶה	הוּא יְבָרֵךְ וִירַפֵּא אֶת הַחוֹלָה
(patient's name) בֶּן (mother's name)	(patient's name) בַּת (mother's name)
בַּעֲבוּר שֶׁ(supplicant's name) יִתֵּן	בַּעֲבוּר שֶׁ(supplicant's name) יִתֵּן
לִצְדָקָה בַּעֲבוּרוֹ.°° בִּשְׂכַר זֶה,	לִצְדָקָה בַּעֲבוּרָהּ.°° בִּשְׂכַר זֶה,
הַקָּדוֹשׁ בָּרוּךְ הוּא יִמָּלֵא רַחֲמִים	הַקָּדוֹשׁ בָּרוּךְ הוּא יִמָּלֵא רַחֲמִים
עָלָיו, לְהַחֲלִימוֹ וּלְרַפְּאתוֹ	עָלֶיהָ, לְהַחֲלִימָהּ וּלְרַפְּאתָהּ
לְהַחֲזִיקוֹ וּלְהַחֲיוֹתוֹ, וְיִשְׁלַח לוֹ	וּלְהַחֲזִיקָהּ וּלְהַחֲיוֹתָהּ, וְיִשְׁלַח לָהּ
מְהֵרָה רְפוּאָה שְׁלֵמָה מִן הַשָּׁמַיִם,	מְהֵרָה רְפוּאָה שְׁלֵמָה מִן הַשָּׁמַיִם,
לִרְמַ״ח אֵבָרָיו, וּשְׁסָ״ה גִּידָיו, בְּתוֹךְ	לְכָל אֵבָרֶיהָ, וּלְכָל גִּידֶיהָ, בְּתוֹךְ

שְׁאָר חוֹלֵי יִשְׂרָאֵל, רְפוּאַת הַנֶּפֶשׁ, וּרְפוּאַת הַגּוּף, הַשְׁתָּא, בַּעֲגָלָא וּבִזְמַן קָרִיב. וְנֹאמַר: אָמֵן. (Cong.– אָמֵן.)

°°Many congregations substitute:

בַּעֲבוּר שֶׁכָּל הַקָּהָל מִתְפַּלְּלִים בַּעֲבוּרוֹ (בַּעֲבוּרָהּ)

Blessed is He Who gave the Torah to His people Israel in His holiness. (The Torah of HASHEM is perfect, restoring the soul; the testimony of HASHEM is trustworthy, making the simple one wise. The orders of HASHEM are upright, gladdening the heart; the command of HASHEM is clear, enlightening the eyes.[1] HASHEM will give might to His nation; HASHEM will bless His nation with peace.[2] The God Whose way is perfect, the promise of HASHEM is flawless, He is a shield for all who take refuge in Him.[3])

Congregation, then *gabbai:*

You who cling to HASHEM, your God, you are all alive today.[4]

The reader shows the *oleh* (person called to the Torah) the place in the Torah. The *oleh* touches the Torah with a corner of his *tallis,* or the belt or mantle of the Torah, and kisses it. He then begins the blessing, bowing at *'Bless,'* and straightening up at *'HASHEM.'*

Bless HASHEM, the blessed One.

Congregation, followed by *oleh,* responds, bowing at 'Blessed,' and straightening up at 'HASHEM.'

Blessed is HASHEM, the blessed One, for all eternity.

Oleh continues:

בָּרוּךְ   *Blessed are You, HASHEM, our God, King of the universe, Who selected us from all the peoples and gave us His Torah. Blessed are You, HASHEM, Giver of the Torah.*   (Cong.— Amen.)

After his Torah portion has been read, the *oleh* recites:

בָּרוּךְ   *Blessed are You, HASHEM, our God, King of the universe, Who gave us the Torah of truth and implanted eternal life within us. Blessed are You, HASHEM, Giver of the Torah.*   (Cong.— Amen.)

PRAYER FOR A SICK PERSON

מִי שֶׁבֵּרַךְ   *He Who blessed our forefathers Abraham, Isaac and Jacob, Moses and Aaron, David and Solomon — may He bless and heal the sick person (* patient's Hebrew name *) son/daughter of (* patient's mother's Hebrew name *) because (* name of supplicant *) will contribute to charity on his/her behalf.°° In reward for this, may the Holy One, Blessed is He, be filled with*

for a man	for a woman
compassion for him to restore his health, to heal him, to strengthen him, and to revivify him. And may He send him speedily a complete recovery from heaven for his two hundred forty-eight organs and three hundred sixty-five blood vessels, among the other	*compassion for her to restore her health, to heal her, to strengthen her, and to revivify her. And may He send her speedily a complete recovery from heaven for all her organs and all her blood vessels, among the other*

sick people of Israel, a recovery of the body and a recovery of the spirit, may a recovery come speedily, swiftly and soon. Now let us respond: Amen.

          (Cong.—Amen.)

°°Many congregations substitute:
because the entire congregation prays for him (her)

(1) *Psalms* 19:8-9. (2) 29:11. (3) 18:31. (4) *Deuteronomy* 4:4.

❖ קריאת התורה ❖

שמות לב:יא-יד; לד:א-י

Upon reaching the phrases in bold type, the reader pauses.
The congregation recites the phrases, after which they are recited by the reader.

כהן – וַיְחַ֣ל מֹשֶׁ֔ה אֶת־פְּנֵ֖י יהוה אֱלֹהָ֑יו וַיֹּ֗אמֶר לָמָ֤ה יהוה֙ יֶחֱרֶ֤ה אַפְּךָ֙ בְּעַמֶּ֔ךָ אֲשֶׁ֤ר הוֹצֵ֨אתָ֙ מֵאֶ֣רֶץ מִצְרַ֔יִם בְּכֹ֥חַ גָּד֖וֹל וּבְיָ֥ד חֲזָקָֽה: לָ֣מָּה יֹאמְר֣וּ מִצְרַ֡יִם לֵאמֹר֩ בְּרָעָ֨ה הוֹצִיאָ֜ם לַהֲרֹ֣ג אֹתָ֗ם בֶּֽהָרִים֙ **וּֽלְכַלֹּתָ֔ם מֵעַ֖ל פְּנֵ֣י הָֽאֲדָמָ֑ה שׁ֚וּב מֵחֲר֣וֹן אַפֶּ֔ךָ וְהִנָּחֵ֥ם עַל־הָֽרָעָ֖ה לְעַמֶּֽךָ:** זְכֹ֡ר לְאַבְרָהָם֩ לְיִצְחָ֨ק וּלְיִשְׂרָאֵ֜ל עֲבָדֶ֗יךָ אֲשֶׁ֨ר נִשְׁבַּ֣עְתָּ לָהֶם֮ בָּךְ֒ וַתְּדַבֵּ֣ר אֲלֵהֶ֔ם אַרְבֶּה֙ אֶֽת־זַרְעֲכֶ֔ם כְּכוֹכְבֵ֖י הַשָּׁמָ֑יִם וְכָל־הָאָ֨רֶץ הַזֹּ֜את אֲשֶׁ֣ר אָמַ֗רְתִּי אֶתֵּן֙ לְזַרְעֲכֶ֔ם וְנָחֲל֖וּ לְעֹלָֽם: וַיִּנָּ֖חֶם יהוה עַל־הָ֣רָעָ֑ה אֲשֶׁ֥ר דִּבֶּ֖ר לַעֲשׂ֥וֹת לְעַמּֽוֹ:

לוי – וַיֹּ֤אמֶר יהוה֙ אֶל־מֹשֶׁ֔ה פְּסָל־לְךָ֛ שְׁנֵֽי־לֻחֹ֥ת אֲבָנִ֖ים כָּרִֽאשֹׁנִ֑ים וְכָתַבְתִּי֙ עַל־הַלֻּחֹ֔ת אֶת־הַדְּבָרִ֔ים אֲשֶׁ֥ר הָי֛וּ עַל־הַלֻּחֹ֥ת הָרִֽאשֹׁנִ֖ים אֲשֶׁ֥ר שִׁבַּֽרְתָּ: וֶהְיֵ֥ה נָכ֖וֹן לַבֹּ֑קֶר וְעָלִ֤יתָ בַבֹּ֨קֶר֙ אֶל־הַ֣ר סִינַ֔י וְנִצַּבְתָּ֥ לִ֛י שָׁ֖ם עַל־רֹ֥אשׁ הָהָֽר: וְאִישׁ֙ לֹֽא־יַעֲלֶ֣ה עִמָּ֔ךְ וְגַם־אִ֥ישׁ אַל־יֵרָ֖א בְּכָל־הָהָ֑ר גַּם־הַצֹּ֤אן וְהַבָּקָר֙ אַל־יִרְע֔וּ אֶל־מ֖וּל הָהָ֥ר הַהֽוּא:

מפטיר – וַיִּפְסֹ֡ל שְׁנֵֽי־לֻחֹ֨ת אֲבָנִ֜ים כָּרִֽאשֹׁנִ֗ים וַיַּשְׁכֵּ֨ם מֹשֶׁ֤ה בַבֹּ֨קֶר֙ וַיַּ֨עַל֙ אֶל־הַ֣ר סִינַ֔י כַּאֲשֶׁ֛ר צִוָּ֥ה יהוה אֹת֑וֹ וַיִּקַּ֣ח בְּיָד֔וֹ שְׁנֵ֖י לֻחֹ֥ת אֲבָנִֽים: וַיֵּ֤רֶד יהוה֙ בֶּֽעָנָ֔ן וַיִּתְיַצֵּ֥ב עִמּ֖וֹ שָׁ֑ם וַיִּקְרָ֥א בְשֵׁ֖ם יהוה: וַיַּעֲבֹ֨ר יהוה ׀ עַל־פָּנָיו֮ וַיִּקְרָא֒ **יהוה ׀ יהוה אֵ֥ל רַח֖וּם וְחַנּ֑וּן אֶ֥רֶךְ אַפַּ֖יִם וְרַב־חֶ֥סֶד וֶאֱמֶֽת: נֹצֵ֥ר חֶ֨סֶד֙ לָאֲלָפִ֔ים נֹשֵׂ֥א עָוֹ֛ן וָפֶ֖שַׁע וְחַטָּאָ֑ה וְנַקֵּה֙ לֹ֣א יְנַקֶּ֔ה** פֹּקֵ֣ד ׀ עֲוֹ֣ן אָב֗וֹת עַל־בָּנִים֙ וְעַל־בְּנֵ֣י בָנִ֔ים עַל־שִׁלֵּשִׁ֖ים וְעַל־רִבֵּעִֽים: וַיְמַהֵ֖ר מֹשֶׁ֑ה וַיִּקֹּ֥ד אַ֖רְצָה וַיִּשְׁתָּֽחוּ: וַיֹּ֡אמֶר אִם־נָא֩ מָצָ֨אתִי חֵ֤ן בְּעֵינֶ֨יךָ֙ אֲדֹנָ֔י יֵֽלֶךְ־נָ֥א אֲדֹנָ֖י בְּקִרְבֵּ֑נוּ כִּ֤י עַם־קְשֵׁה־עֹ֨רֶף֙ ה֔וּא **וְסָלַחְתָּ֛ לַעֲוֹנֵ֥נוּ וּלְחַטָּאתֵ֖נוּ וּנְחַלְתָּֽנוּ:** וַיֹּ֗אמֶר הִנֵּ֣ה אָנֹכִי֮ כֹּרֵ֣ת בְּרִית֒ נֶ֤גֶד כָּֽל־עַמְּךָ֙ אֶעֱשֶׂ֣ה נִפְלָאֹ֔ת אֲשֶׁ֛ר לֹֽא־נִבְרְא֥וּ בְכָל־הָאָ֖רֶץ וּבְכָל־הַגּוֹיִ֑ם וְרָאָ֣ה כָל־הָ֠עָם אֲשֶׁר־אַתָּ֨ה בְקִרְבּ֜וֹ אֶת־מַעֲשֵׂ֤ה יהוה כִּֽי־נוֹרָ֣א ה֔וּא אֲשֶׁ֥ר אֲנִ֖י עֹשֶׂ֥ה עִמָּֽךְ:

❧ Torah Reading

The afternoon Torah reading for Tishah B'Av is the same as that read on the other fast days. Rather than an admonition that outlines the national weaknesses that cause the sorts of tragedy commemorated by the fast day, this reading might be described as an "antidote" to the calamity.

❧ TORAH READING ❧

Exodus 32:11-14; 34:1-10

Kohen – Moses prayed before HASHEM, his God, and he said, "Why, HASHEM, shall Your wrath burn against Your people, whom You have taken out of Egypt with great might and with a strong hand? Why should Egypt say as follows, 'Under an evil fate did He take them out to kill them in the mountains and to exterminate them from upon the face of the earth?' Turn back from Your burning wrath and relent from this evil to Your people. Remember for the sake of Abraham, Isaac, and Jacob, Your servants, what You swore to them by Your Person, and You spoke to them, 'I shall multiply your offspring like the stars of heaven, and this entire land of which I spoke I shall give to your offspring, and they shall have it as a heritage forever.'"

HASHEM relented over the evil that He had said He would do to His people.

Levi – HASHEM said to Moses, 'Carve for yourself two stone tablets like the first ones, and I shall write upon the tablets the words that were on the first tablets, which you smashed. And be ready in the morning; you shall ascend in the morning to Mount Sinai and stand before Me there on the mountaintop. No man shall ascend with you, nor shall any man be seen on the entire mountain, even the sheep and cattle shall not graze opposite that mountain.'

Maftir – He carved two stone tablets like the first ones; and Moses arose early in the morning and ascended Mount Sinai, as HASHEM had commanded him; and in his hand he took two stone tablets. HASHEM descended in a cloud and stood there with him, and He called out with the Name HASHEM. And HASHEM passed before him and proclaimed, "HASHEM, HASHEM, God, Compassionate and Gracious, Slow to anger, and Abundant in Kindness and Truth. Preserver of kindness for thousands of generations, Forgiver of iniquity, willful sin, and error; and Cleanses but does not cleanse [entirely], remembering the iniquity of parents upon children and grandchildren to the third and fourth generations.'

Moses hastened and bowed his head and prostrated himself. He said, 'If I have now found favor in Your eyes, my Lord, may my Lord go among us, for it is a stiff-necked people. May you forgive our iniquities and our errors and make us Your heritage.'

He said, 'Behold! I seal a covenant: Before all your people I shall perform such wonders as have never been created in all the world or in any nation; and the entire people in whose midst you are will recognize the handiwork of HASHEM that it is awesome, that I perform with you.

While Moses was on Mount Sinai receiving the Torah and the Tablets of the Law, his people in the Wilderness were making the Golden Calf and giving it their allegiance. God told Moses that the purpose of his mission no longer existed; he was the representative of Israel, but his nation had betrayed God. He told Moses that He would destroy the nation, and begin anew with Moses and his offspring. But in making this chilling declaration to Moses, God Asked Moses to "permit Him" to do so — this implied that Moses could prevent the destruction of Israel (see *Rashi*

הגבהה וגלילה

The Torah Scroll is raised and each person looks at the Torah and recites aloud:

וְזֹאת הַתּוֹרָה אֲשֶׁר שָׂם מֹשֶׁה לִפְנֵי בְּנֵי יִשְׂרָאֵל,¹ עַל פִּי יהוה בְּיַד מֹשֶׁה.²

Some add:

עֵץ חַיִּים הִיא לַמַּחֲזִיקִים בָּהּ, וְתֹמְכֶיהָ מְאֻשָּׁר.³ דְּרָכֶיהָ דַרְכֵי נֹעַם, וְכָל נְתִיבוֹתֶיהָ שָׁלוֹם.⁴ אֹרֶךְ יָמִים בִּימִינָהּ, בִּשְׂמֹאלָהּ עֹשֶׁר וְכָבוֹד.⁵ יהוה חָפֵץ לְמַעַן צִדְקוֹ, יַגְדִּיל תּוֹרָה וְיַאְדִּיר.⁶

After the Torah Scroll has been wound, tied and covered, he *maftir* recites the *Haftarah* blessings.

ברכה קודם ההפטרה

בָּרוּךְ אַתָּה יהוה אֱלֹהֵינוּ מֶלֶךְ הָעוֹלָם, אֲשֶׁר בָּחַר בִּנְבִיאִים טוֹבִים, וְרָצָה בְדִבְרֵיהֶם הַנֶּאֱמָרִים בֶּאֱמֶת, בָּרוּךְ אַתָּה יהוה, הַבּוֹחֵר בַּתּוֹרָה וּבְמֹשֶׁה עַבְדּוֹ, וּבְיִשְׂרָאֵל עַמּוֹ, וּבִנְבִיאֵי הָאֱמֶת וָצֶדֶק: (Cong.— אָמֵן.)

◈ הפטרה ◈

ישעיה נה:ו-נו:ח

[Although the Divine Name יהוה is pronounced as if it were spelled אֲדֹנָי, when it is vowelized יֱהֹוִה, it is pronounced as if it were spelled אֱלֹהִים.]

דִּרְשׁוּ יהוה בְּהִמָּצְאוֹ קְרָאֻהוּ בִּהְיוֹתוֹ קָרוֹב: יַעֲזֹב רָשָׁע דַּרְכּוֹ וְאִישׁ אָוֶן מַחְשְׁבֹתָיו וְיָשֹׁב אֶל־יהוה וִירַחֲמֵהוּ וְאֶל־אֱלֹהֵינוּ כִּי־יַרְבֶּה לִסְלוֹחַ: כִּי לֹא מַחְשְׁבוֹתַי מַחְשְׁבוֹתֵיכֶם וְלֹא דַרְכֵיכֶם דְּרָכָי נְאֻם יהוה: כִּי־גָבְהוּ שָׁמַיִם מֵאָרֶץ כֵּן גָּבְהוּ דְרָכַי מִדַּרְכֵיכֶם וּמַחְשְׁבֹתַי מִמַּחְשְׁבֹתֵיכֶם: כִּי כַּאֲשֶׁר יֵרֵד הַגֶּשֶׁם וְהַשֶּׁלֶג מִן־הַשָּׁמַיִם וְשָׁמָּה לֹא יָשׁוּב כִּי אִם־הִרְוָה אֶת־הָאָרֶץ וְהוֹלִידָהּ וְהִצְמִיחָהּ וְנָתַן זֶרַע לַזֹּרֵעַ וְלֶחֶם לָאֹכֵל: כֵּן יִהְיֶה דְבָרִי אֲשֶׁר יֵצֵא מִפִּי לֹא־יָשׁוּב אֵלַי רֵיקָם כִּי אִם־עָשָׂה אֶת־אֲשֶׁר חָפַצְתִּי וְהִצְלִיחַ אֲשֶׁר שְׁלַחְתִּיו: כִּי־בְשִׂמְחָה תֵצֵאוּ וּבְשָׁלוֹם תּוּבָלוּן הֶהָרִים וְהַגְּבָעוֹת יִפְצְחוּ לִפְנֵיכֶם רִנָּה וְכָל־עֲצֵי הַשָּׂדֶה יִמְחֲאוּ־כָף:

to *Exodus* 32:10). From this, Moses understood that his prayers could save Israel, and he immediately begged God to spare them.

The first portion of this reading is his prayer on the mountain; after returning to the camp, he smashed the Tablets and took charge of a mass repentance, which made Israel worthy to receive the Second Tablets. The rest of the reading skips to God's command that Moses fashion a pair of tablets, upon which God would inscribe the Ten Commandments a second time. In the context of the fast days, the significance of the passage is

that in it God taught Moses the Thirteen Attributes of Mercy, which are now the central theme of the fast day Selichos (except for Tishah B'Av) and of the evening and Neilah services of Yom Kippur. According to R' Yochanan (*Rosh Hashana* 17b), Moses thought that Israel's sin was so grievous that there was no possibility for him to intercede on their behalf. Thereupon God appeared to him in the form of a chazzan wrapped in a tallis and taught him the Thirteen Attributes. God said, "Whenever Israel sins, let them recite this in its proper order and I shall

HAGBAHAH AND GELILAH

The Torah Scroll is raised and each person looks at the Torah and recites aloud:

This is the Torah that Moses placed before the Children of Israel,[1] upon the command of HASHEM, through Moses' hand.[2]

Some add:

עֵץ *It is a tree of life for those who grasp it, and its supporters are praise-worthy.[3] Its ways are ways of pleasantness and all its paths are peace.[4] Lengthy days are at its right; at its left are wealth and honor.[5] HASHEM desired, for the sake of its [Israel's] righteousness, that the Torah be made great and glorious.[6]*

After the Torah Scroll has been wound, tied and covered, the *maftir* recites the *Haftarah* blessings.

BLESSING BEFORE THE HAFTARAH

בָּרוּךְ *Blessed are You, HASHEM, our God, King of the universe, Who has chosen good prophets and was pleased with their words that were uttered with truth. Blessed are You, HASHEM, Who chooses the Torah; Moses, His servant; Israel, His nation; and the prophets of truth and righteousness.* (Cong.— Amen.)

⊰ HAFTARAH ⊱

Isaiah 55:6-56:8

Seek HASHEM when He can be found; call Him when He is near. Let the wicked one forsake his way and the iniquitous man his thoughts; and let him return to HASHEM and He will show him mercy, to our God for He will be abundantly forgiving. For My thoughts are not your thoughts, and your ways are not My ways, the words of HASHEM. As high as the heavens over the earth, so are My ways higher than your ways, and thoughts than your thoughts. For just as the rain and snow descend from heaven and will not return there, but it waters the earth and causes it to produce and sprout, and gives seed to the sower and food to the eater; so shall be My word that emanates from My mouth, it shall not return to Me unfulfilled unless it will have accomplished what I desired and brought success where I sent it. For in gladness shall you go out and in peace shall you arrive, the mountains and hills will break out in glad song before you, and all the trees of the field will clap hands.

---

(1) *Deuteronomy* 4:44. (2) *Numbers* 9:23. (3) *Proverbs* 3:18. (4) 3:17. (5) 3:16. (6) *Isaiah* 42:21.

forgive them." Thus the appeal found in this Torah reading reassures us that repentance is always possible and that God is always awaits our return.

Since it is axiomatic that punishment and exile are always the result of Jewish shortcomings, and as Rambam teaches, we fast to remind ourselves that no Jewish suffering is coincidental, this Torah reading teaches us the way to curtail the suffering and end the exile.

⊰§ The Haftarah

As noted above, fast days represent a call to repentance and a the Torah reading is the encouraging message that God is always ready — indeed, anxious — to accept our prayers. The Haftarah is an eloquent expression of that theme. It begins by urging us to seek God where He can be found and when He is near. The commentators explain that these times are before He brings punishment upon us, for then He longs for us to repent and thereby remove the root of His anger; and they are also times when we are ready to seek Him with all our hearts.

God declares that we should not project our own base, human frailties onto our perceptions of Him. God is merciful. He guarantees us that everyone who is sincere and ready to serve Him wholeheartedly has a place at His table. Even those who are barren — literally or figuratively — will blossom if they join themselves to Him. The aliens who leave their origins to become Jews

תַּחַת הַנַּעֲצוּץ יַעֲלֶה בְרוֹשׁ וְתַחַת הַסִּרְפַּד יַעֲלֶה הֲדַס וְהָיָה לַיהוה
לְשֵׁם לְאוֹת עוֹלָם לֹא יִכָּרֵת: כֹּה אָמַר יהוה שִׁמְרוּ מִשְׁפָּט וַעֲשׂוּ
צְדָקָה כִּי־קְרוֹבָה יְשׁוּעָתִי לָבוֹא וְצִדְקָתִי לְהִגָּלוֹת: אַשְׁרֵי אֱנוֹשׁ
יַעֲשֶׂה־זֹּאת וּבֶן־אָדָם יַחֲזִיק בָּהּ שֹׁמֵר שַׁבָּת מֵחַלְּלוֹ וְשֹׁמֵר יָדוֹ
מֵעֲשׂוֹת כָּל־רָע: וְאַל־יֹאמַר בֶּן־הַנֵּכָר הַנִּלְוָה אֶל־יהוה לֵאמֹר
הַבְדֵּל יַבְדִּילַנִי יהוה מֵעַל עַמּוֹ וְאַל־יֹאמַר הַסָּרִיס הֵן אֲנִי עֵץ יָבֵשׁ:
כִּי־כֹה ׀ אָמַר יהוה לַסָּרִיסִים אֲשֶׁר יִשְׁמְרוּ אֶת־שַׁבְּתוֹתַי וּבָחֲרוּ
בַּאֲשֶׁר חָפָצְתִּי וּמַחֲזִיקִים בִּבְרִיתִי: וְנָתַתִּי לָהֶם בְּבֵיתִי וּבְחוֹמֹתַי
יָד וָשֵׁם טוֹב מִבָּנִים וּמִבָּנוֹת שֵׁם עוֹלָם אֶתֶּן־לוֹ אֲשֶׁר לֹא יִכָּרֵת:
וּבְנֵי הַנֵּכָר הַנִּלְוִים עַל־יהוה לְשָׁרְתוֹ וּלְאַהֲבָה אֶת־שֵׁם יהוה
לִהְיוֹת לוֹ לַעֲבָדִים כָּל־שֹׁמֵר שַׁבָּת מֵחַלְּלוֹ וּמַחֲזִיקִים בִּבְרִיתִי:
וַהֲבִיאוֹתִים אֶל־הַר קָדְשִׁי וְשִׂמַּחְתִּים בְּבֵית תְּפִלָּתִי עוֹלֹתֵיהֶם
וְזִבְחֵיהֶם לְרָצוֹן עַל־מִזְבְּחִי כִּי בֵיתִי בֵּית־תְּפִלָּה יִקָּרֵא לְכָל־
הָעַמִּים: נְאֻם אֲדֹנָי יֱהֹוִה מְקַבֵּץ נִדְחֵי יִשְׂרָאֵל עוֹד אֲקַבֵּץ עָלָיו
לְנִקְבָּצָיו:

ברכות לאחר ההפטרה

After the *Haftarah* is read, the *oleh* recites the following blessings.

בָּרוּךְ אַתָּה יהוה אֱלֹהֵינוּ מֶלֶךְ הָעוֹלָם, צוּר כָּל הָעוֹלָמִים,
צַדִּיק בְּכָל הַדּוֹרוֹת, הָאֵל הַנֶּאֱמָן הָאוֹמֵר וְעֹשֶׂה, הַמְדַבֵּר
וּמְקַיֵּם, שֶׁכָּל דְּבָרָיו אֱמֶת וָצֶדֶק. נֶאֱמָן אַתָּה הוּא יהוה אֱלֹהֵינוּ,
וְנֶאֱמָנִים דְּבָרֶיךָ, וְדָבָר אֶחָד מִדְּבָרֶיךָ אָחוֹר לֹא יָשׁוּב רֵיקָם, כִּי
אֵל מֶלֶךְ נֶאֱמָן (וְרַחֲמָן) אָתָּה. בָּרוּךְ אַתָּה יהוה, הָאֵל הַנֶּאֱמָן בְּכָל
דְּבָרָיו. (Cong.– אָמֵן.)

רַחֵם עַל צִיּוֹן כִּי הִיא בֵּית חַיֵּינוּ, וְלַעֲלוּבַת נֶפֶשׁ תּוֹשִׁיעַ
בִּמְהֵרָה בְיָמֵינוּ. בָּרוּךְ אַתָּה יהוה, מְשַׂמֵּחַ צִיּוֹן בְּבָנֶיהָ. (Cong.– אָמֵן.)

שַׂמְּחֵנוּ יהוה אֱלֹהֵינוּ בְּאֵלִיָּהוּ הַנָּבִיא עַבְדֶּךָ, וּבְמַלְכוּת בֵּית
דָּוִד מְשִׁיחֶךָ, בִּמְהֵרָה יָבֹא וְיָגֵל לִבֵּנוּ, עַל כִּסְאוֹ לֹא
יֵשֶׁב זָר וְלֹא יִנְחֲלוּ עוֹד אֲחֵרִים אֶת כְּבוֹדוֹ, כִּי בְשֵׁם קָדְשְׁךָ
נִשְׁבַּעְתָּ לּוֹ, שֶׁלֹּא יִכְבֶּה נֵרוֹ לְעוֹלָם וָעֶד. בָּרוּךְ אַתָּה יהוה, מָגֵן
דָּוִד. (Cong.– אָמֵן.)

In place of the thorn-bush, a cypress will rise; and in place of the nettle, a myrtle will rise. This will be a monument to HASHEM, an eternal sign never to be cut down.

So said HASHEM: Observe justice and perform righteousness, for My salvation is at hand to come and My righteousness to be revealed. Praiseworthy is the man who does this and the son of man who grasps it tightly: Whoever guards the Sabbath against desecration and guards his hand against doing any evil.

Let not the alien, who has joined himself to HASHEM, say: "HASHEM shall utterly separate me from His people;" and let not the barren one say: "Behold I am a shriveled tree." For so says HASHEM to the barren ones who observe My Sabbaths and choose what I desire, and grasp My covenant tightly. In My House and within My walls I shall give them a place and renown, better than sons and daughters; eternal renown shall I give them, never to be cut down; and the aliens who join HASHEM to serve Him and to love the Name of HASHEM to become His servants, whoever guards the Sabbath against desecration and grasps My covenant tightly — I shall bring them to My holy mountain, and I shall gladden them in My house of prayer, their elevation-offerings and their feast-offerings will find favor on My Altar, for My House shall be a house of prayer for all the peoples.

The words of my Lord, HASHEM/ELOHIM, Who gathers in the dispersed of Israel, "I shall gather to him even more than those already gathered."

BLESSINGS AFTER THE HAFTARAH

After the *Haftarah* is read, the *oleh* recites the following blessings.

בָּרוּךְ Blessed are You, HASHEM, King of the universe, Rock of all eternities, Righteous in all generations, the trustworthy God, Who says and does, Who speaks and fulfills, all of Whose words are true and righteous. Trustworthy are You, HASHEM, our God, and trustworthy are Your words, not one of Your words is turned back to its origin unfulfilled, for You are God, trustworthy (and compassionate) King. Blessed are You, HASHEM, the God Who is trustworthy in all His words.   (Cong.— Amen.)

רַחֵם Have mercy on Zion for it is the source of our life; to the one who is deeply humiliated bring salvation speedily, in our days. Blessed are You, HASHEM, Who gladdens Zion through her children.

(Cong.— Amen.)

שַׂמְּחֵנוּ Gladden us, HASHEM, our God, with Elijah the prophet, Your servant, and with the kingdom of the House of David, Your anointed, may he come speedily and cause our heart to exult. On his throne let no stranger sit nor let others continue to inherit his honor, for by Your holy Name You swore to him that his heir will not be extinguished forever and ever. Blessed are You, HASHEM, Shield of David.

(Cong.— Amen.)

---

are no longer aliens. To the contrary they will be the forerunners of the masses who will flock to the truth when the time of redemption finally arrives.

הכנסת ספר תורה

Chazzan takes the Torah in his right arm and recites:

יְהַלְלוּ אֶת שֵׁם יהוה, כִּי נִשְׂגָּב שְׁמוֹ לְבַדּוֹ –

Congregation responds:

– הוֹדוֹ עַל אֶרֶץ וְשָׁמָיִם. וַיָּרֶם קֶרֶן לְעַמּוֹ, תְּהִלָּה לְכָל חֲסִידָיו, לִבְנֵי יִשְׂרָאֵל עַם קְרֹבוֹ, הַלְלוּיָהּ.[1]

As the Torah is carried to the Ark, congregation recites Psalm 24, לְדָוִד מִזְמוֹר.

לְדָוִד מִזְמוֹר, לַיהוה הָאָרֶץ וּמְלוֹאָהּ, תֵּבֵל וְיֹשְׁבֵי בָהּ. כִּי הוּא עַל יַמִּים יְסָדָהּ, וְעַל נְהָרוֹת יְכוֹנְנֶהָ. מִי יַעֲלֶה בְהַר יהוה, וּמִי יָקוּם בִּמְקוֹם קָדְשׁוֹ. נְקִי כַפַּיִם וּבַר לֵבָב, אֲשֶׁר לֹא נָשָׂא לַשָּׁוְא נַפְשִׁי וְלֹא נִשְׁבַּע לְמִרְמָה. יִשָּׂא בְרָכָה מֵאֵת יהוה, וּצְדָקָה מֵאֱלֹהֵי יִשְׁעוֹ. זֶה דּוֹר דֹּרְשָׁיו, מְבַקְשֵׁי פָנֶיךָ, יַעֲקֹב, סֶלָה. שְׂאוּ שְׁעָרִים רָאשֵׁיכֶם, וְהִנָּשְׂאוּ פִּתְחֵי עוֹלָם, וְיָבוֹא מֶלֶךְ הַכָּבוֹד. מִי זֶה מֶלֶךְ הַכָּבוֹד, יהוה עִזּוּז וְגִבּוֹר, יהוה גִּבּוֹר מִלְחָמָה. שְׂאוּ שְׁעָרִים רָאשֵׁיכֶם, וּשְׂאוּ פִּתְחֵי עוֹלָם, וְיָבֹא מֶלֶךְ הַכָּבוֹד. מִי הוּא זֶה מֶלֶךְ הַכָּבוֹד, יהוה צְבָאוֹת הוּא מֶלֶךְ הַכָּבוֹד, סֶלָה.

As the Torah is placed into the Ark, congregation recites the following verses:

וּבְנֻחֹה יֹאמַר, שׁוּבָה יהוה רִבְבוֹת אַלְפֵי יִשְׂרָאֵל.[2] קוּמָה יהוה לִמְנוּחָתֶךָ, אַתָּה וַאֲרוֹן עֻזֶּךָ. כֹּהֲנֶיךָ יִלְבְּשׁוּ צֶדֶק, וַחֲסִידֶיךָ יְרַנֵּנוּ. בַּעֲבוּר דָּוִד עַבְדֶּךָ אַל תָּשֵׁב פְּנֵי מְשִׁיחֶךָ.[3] כִּי לֶקַח טוֹב נָתַתִּי לָכֶם, תּוֹרָתִי אַל תַּעֲזֹבוּ.[4] ❖ עֵץ חַיִּים הִיא לַמַּחֲזִיקִים בָּהּ, וְתֹמְכֶיהָ מְאֻשָּׁר.[5] דְּרָכֶיהָ דַרְכֵי נֹעַם, וְכָל נְתִיבוֹתֶיהָ שָׁלוֹם.[6] הֲשִׁיבֵנוּ יהוה אֵלֶיךָ וְנָשׁוּבָה, חַדֵּשׁ יָמֵינוּ כְּקֶדֶם.[7]

חצי קדיש

The Ark is closed and the chazzan recites חֲצִי קַדִּישׁ.

יִתְגַּדַּל וְיִתְקַדַּשׁ שְׁמֵהּ רַבָּא. (.Cong– אָמֵן) בְּעָלְמָא דִּי בְרָא כִרְעוּתֵהּ. וְיַמְלִיךְ מַלְכוּתֵהּ, בְּחַיֵּיכוֹן וּבְיוֹמֵיכוֹן וּבְחַיֵּי דְכָל בֵּית יִשְׂרָאֵל, בַּעֲגָלָא וּבִזְמַן קָרִיב. וְאִמְרוּ: אָמֵן.

(.Cong– אָמֵן. יְהֵא שְׁמֵהּ רַבָּא מְבָרַךְ לְעָלַם וּלְעָלְמֵי עָלְמַיָּא.)

יְהֵא שְׁמֵהּ רַבָּא מְבָרַךְ לְעָלַם וּלְעָלְמֵי עָלְמַיָּא.

יִתְבָּרַךְ וְיִשְׁתַּבַּח וְיִתְפָּאַר וְיִתְרוֹמַם וְיִתְנַשֵּׂא וְיִתְהַדָּר וְיִתְעַלֶּה וְיִתְהַלָּל שְׁמֵהּ דְּקֻדְשָׁא בְּרִיךְ הוּא (.Cong– בְּרִיךְ הוּא) – לְעֵלָּא מִן כָּל בִּרְכָתָא וְשִׁירָתָא תֻּשְׁבְּחָתָא וְנֶחֱמָתָא, דַּאֲמִירָן בְּעָלְמָא, וְאִמְרוּ: אָמֵן. (.Cong– אָמֵן)

---

(1) *Psalms* 148:13-14. (2) *Numbers* 10:36. (3) *Psalms* 132:8-10.
(4) *Proverbs* 4:2. (5) 3:18. (6) 3:17. (7) *Lamentations* 5:21.

RETURNING THE TORAH

Chazzan takes the Torah in his right arm and recites:

Let them praise the Name of HASHEM,
for His Name alone will have been exalted —

Congregation responds:

— His glory is above earth and heaven. And He will have exalted the pride of His people, causing praise for all His devout ones, for the Children of Israel, His intimate nation. Halleluyah![1]

As the Torah is carried to the Ark, congregation recites Psalm 24, 'Of David a psalm.'

לְדָוִד Of David a psalm. HASHEM's is the earth and its fullness, the inhabited land and those who dwell in it. For He founded it upon seas, and established it upon rivers. Who may ascend the mountain of HASHEM, and who may stand in the place of His sanctity? One with clean hands and pure heart, who has not sworn in vain by My soul and has not sworn deceitfully. He will receive a blessing from HASHEM and just kindness from the God of his salvation. This is the generation of those who seek Him, those who strive for Your Presence — Jacob, Selah. Raise up your heads, O gates, and be uplifted, you everlasting entrances, so that the King of Glory may enter. Who is this King of Glory? — HASHEM, the mighty and strong, HASHEM, the strong in battle. Raise up your heads, O gates, and raise up, you everlasting entrances, so that the King of Glory may enter. Who then is the King of Glory? HASHEM, Master of Legions, He is the King of Glory. Selah!

As the Torah is placed into the Ark, congregation recites the following verses:

וּבְנֻחֹה And when it rested he would say, 'Return, HASHEM, to the myriad thousands of Israel.'[2] Arise, HASHEM, to Your resting place, You and the Ark of Your strength. Let Your priests be clothed in righteousness, and Your devout ones will sing joyously. For the sake of David, Your servant, turn not away the face of Your anointed.[3] For I have given you a good teaching, do not forsake My Torah.[4] Chazzan— It is a tree of life for those who grasp it, and its supporters are praiseworthy.[5] Its ways are ways of pleasantness and all its paths are peace.[6] Bring us back to You, HASHEM, and we shall return, renew our days as of old.[7]

HALF KADDISH

The Ark is closed and the chazzan recites Half-Kaddish.

יִתְגַּדַּל May His great Name grow exalted and sanctified (Cong.— Amen.) in the world that He created as He willed. May He give reign to His kingship in your lifetimes and in your days, and in the lifetimes of the entire Family of Israel, swiftly and soon. Now respond: Amen.

(Cong.— Amen. May His great Name be blessed forever and ever.)

May His great Name be blessed forever and ever.

Blessed, praised, glorified, exalted, extolled, mighty, upraised, and lauded be the Name of the Holy One, Blessed is He (Cong.— Blessed is He) — beyond any blessing and song, praise and consolation that are uttered in the world. Now respond: Amen. (Cong.— Amen.)

שמונה עשרה – עמידה

Take three steps backward, then three steps forward. Remain standing with feet together while reciting *Shemoneh Esrei*. Recite it with quiet devotion and without interruption, verbal or otherwise. Although it should not be audible to others, one must pray loudly enough to hear himself.

כִּי שֵׁם יהוה אֶקְרָא, הָבוּ גֹדֶל לֵאלֹהֵינוּ.[1]
אֲדֹנָי שְׂפָתַי תִּפְתָּח, וּפִי יַגִּיד תְּהִלָּתֶךָ.[2]

אבות

Bend the knees at בָּרוּךְ; bow at אַתָּה; straighten up at ה'.

בָּרוּךְ אַתָּה יהוה אֱלֹהֵינוּ וֵאלֹהֵי אֲבוֹתֵינוּ, אֱלֹהֵי אַבְרָהָם, אֱלֹהֵי יִצְחָק, וֵאלֹהֵי יַעֲקֹב, הָאֵל הַגָּדוֹל הַגִּבּוֹר וְהַנּוֹרָא, אֵל עֶלְיוֹן, גּוֹמֵל חֲסָדִים טוֹבִים וְקוֹנֵה הַכֹּל, וְזוֹכֵר חַסְדֵי אָבוֹת, וּמֵבִיא גוֹאֵל לִבְנֵי בְנֵיהֶם, לְמַעַן שְׁמוֹ בְּאַהֲבָה. מֶלֶךְ עוֹזֵר וּמוֹשִׁיעַ וּמָגֵן.

Bend the knees at בָּרוּךְ; bow at אַתָּה; straighten up at ה'.

בָּרוּךְ אַתָּה יהוה, מָגֵן אַבְרָהָם.

גבורות

אַתָּה גִּבּוֹר לְעוֹלָם אֲדֹנָי, מְחַיֶּה מֵתִים אַתָּה, רַב לְהוֹשִׁיעַ. מְכַלְכֵּל חַיִּים בְּחֶסֶד, מְחַיֶּה מֵתִים בְּרַחֲמִים רַבִּים, סוֹמֵךְ נוֹפְלִים, וְרוֹפֵא חוֹלִים, וּמַתִּיר אֲסוּרִים, וּמְקַיֵּם אֱמוּנָתוֹ לִישֵׁנֵי עָפָר. מִי כָמוֹךָ בַּעַל גְּבוּרוֹת, וּמִי דְוֹמֶה לָּךְ, מֶלֶךְ מֵמִית וּמְחַיֶּה וּמַצְמִיחַ יְשׁוּעָה. וְנֶאֱמָן אַתָּה לְהַחֲיוֹת מֵתִים. בָּרוּךְ אַתָּה יהוה, מְחַיֶּה הַמֵּתִים.

During the *chazzan's* repetition, *Kedushah* (below) is recited at this point.

קדושה

When reciting *Kedushah*, one must stand with his feet together and avoid any interruptions. One should rise on his toes when saying the words קָדוֹשׁ, קָדוֹשׁ, קָדוֹשׁ; בָּרוּךְ (of בָּרוּךְ כְּבוֹד); and יִמְלֹךְ.

נְקַדֵּשׁ – Cong. then Chazzan אֶת שִׁמְךָ בָּעוֹלָם, כְּשֵׁם שֶׁמַּקְדִּישִׁים אוֹתוֹ בִּשְׁמֵי מָרוֹם, כַּכָּתוּב עַל יַד נְבִיאֶךָ, וְקָרָא זֶה אֶל זֶה וְאָמַר:

קָדוֹשׁ קָדוֹשׁ קָדוֹשׁ יהוה צְבָאוֹת, מְלֹא כָל הָאָרֶץ כְּבוֹדוֹ.[3] – All

לְעֻמָּתָם בָּרוּךְ יֹאמֵרוּ: – Chazzan

בָּרוּךְ כְּבוֹד יהוה, מִמְּקוֹמוֹ.[4] – All

וּבְדִבְרֵי קָדְשְׁךָ כָּתוּב לֵאמֹר: – Chazzan

יִמְלֹךְ יהוה לְעוֹלָם, אֱלֹהַיִךְ צִיּוֹן לְדֹר וָדֹר, הַלְלוּיָהּ.[5] – All

לְדוֹר וָדוֹר נַגִּיד גָּדְלֶךָ וּלְנֵצַח נְצָחִים קְדֻשָּׁתְךָ – Chazzan only concludes נַקְדִּישׁ, וְשִׁבְחֲךָ אֱלֹהֵינוּ מִפִּינוּ לֹא יָמוּשׁ לְעוֹלָם וָעֶד, כִּי אֵל מֶלֶךְ גָּדוֹל וְקָדוֹשׁ אָתָּה. בָּרוּךְ אַתָּה יהוה, הָאֵל הַקָּדוֹשׁ.

Chazzan continues . . . אַתָּה חוֹנֵן (page 432).

ᴥᴥ SHEMONEH ESREI — AMIDAH ᴥᴥ

Take three steps backward, then three steps forward. Remain standing with feet together while reciting *Shemoneh Esrei*. Recite it with quiet devotion and without interruption, verbal or otherwise. Although it should not be audible to others, one must pray loudly enough to hear himself.

When I call out the Name of Hashem, ascribe greatness to our God.[1]
My Lord, open my lips, that my mouth may declare Your praise.[2]

PATRIARCHS

Bend the knees at *'Blessed'*; bow at *'You'*; straighten up at *'Hashem.'*

בָּרוּךְ **Blessed** are You, Hashem, our God and the God of our fore-fathers, God of Abraham, God of Isaac, and God of Jacob; the great, mighty, and awesome God, the supreme God, Who bestows beneficial kindnesses and creates everything, Who recalls the kindnesses of the Patriarchs and brings a Redeemer to their children's children, for His Name's sake, with love. O King, Helper, Savior, and Shield.

Bend the knees at *'Blessed'*; bow at *'You'*; straighten up at *'Hashem.'*

Blessed are You, Hashem, Shield of Abraham.

GOD'S MIGHT

אַתָּה **You** are eternally mighty, my Lord, the Resuscitator of the dead are You; abundantly able to save. He sustains the living with kindness, resuscitates the dead with abundant mercy, supports the fallen, heals the sick, releases the confined, and maintains His faith to those asleep in the dust. Who is like You, O Master of mighty deeds, and who is comparable to You, O King Who causes death and restores life and makes salvation sprout! And You are faithful to resuscitate the dead. Blessed are You, Hashem, Who resuscitates the dead.

During the *chazzan's* repetition, *Kedushah* (below) is recited at this point.

KEDUSHAH

When reciting *Kedushah*, one must stand with his feet together and avoid any interruptions. One should rise on his toes when saying *Holy, holy, holy; Blessed is;* and *Hashem shall reign.*

Cong. — נְקַדֵּשׁ **We** shall sanctify Your Name in this world, just as they
then   sanctify it in heaven above, as it is written by Your prophet,
Chazzan   *"And one [angel] will call another and say:*

All —*'Holy, holy, holy is Hashem, Master of Legions, the whole world is filled with His glory.'* "[3]

Chazzan —*Those facing them say 'Blessed':*

All —*'Blessed is the glory of Hashem from His place.'*[4]

Chazzan —*And in Your holy Writings the following is written:*

All —*'Hashem shall reign forever — your God, O Zion — from generation to generation, Halleluyah!'*[5]

Chazzan only concludes— *From generation to generation we shall relate Your greatness and for infinite eternities we shall proclaim Your holiness. Your praise, our God, shall not leave our mouth forever and ever, for You, O God, are a great and holy King. Blessed are You, Hashem, the holy God.*

Chazzan continues אַתָּה חוֹנֵן, *You graciously endow . . .* (page 432).

---

(1) *Deuteronomy* 32:3. (2) *Psalms* 51:17. (3) *Isaiah* 6:3. (4) *Ezekiel* 3:12. (5) *Psalms* 146:10.

קדושת השם

אַתָּה קָדוֹשׁ וְשִׁמְךָ קָדוֹשׁ, וּקְדוֹשִׁים בְּכָל יוֹם יְהַלְלוּךָ סֶּלָה. בָּרוּךְ אַתָּה יהוה, הָאֵל הַקָּדוֹשׁ.

בינה

אַתָּה חוֹנֵן לְאָדָם דַּעַת, וּמְלַמֵּד לֶאֱנוֹשׁ בִּינָה. חָנֵּנוּ מֵאִתְּךָ דֵּעָה בִּינָה וְהַשְׂכֵּל. בָּרוּךְ אַתָּה יהוה, חוֹנֵן הַדָּעַת.

תשובה

הֲשִׁיבֵנוּ אָבִינוּ לְתוֹרָתֶךָ, וְקָרְבֵנוּ מַלְכֵּנוּ לַעֲבוֹדָתֶךָ, וְהַחֲזִירֵנוּ בִּתְשׁוּבָה שְׁלֵמָה לְפָנֶיךָ. בָּרוּךְ אַתָּה יהוה, הָרוֹצֶה בִּתְשׁוּבָה.

סליחה

Strike the left side of the chest with the right fist while reciting the words חָטָאנוּ and פָּשָׁעְנוּ.

סְלַח לָנוּ אָבִינוּ כִּי חָטָאנוּ, מְחַל לָנוּ מַלְכֵּנוּ כִּי פָשָׁעְנוּ, כִּי מוֹחֵל וְסוֹלֵחַ אָתָּה. בָּרוּךְ אַתָּה יהוה, חַנּוּן הַמַּרְבֶּה לִסְלוֹחַ.

גאולה

רְאֵה בְעָנְיֵנוּ, וְרִיבָה רִיבֵנוּ, וּגְאָלֵנוּ[1] מְהֵרָה לְמַעַן שְׁמֶךָ, כִּי גּוֹאֵל חָזָק אָתָּה. בָּרוּךְ אַתָּה יהוה, גּוֹאֵל יִשְׂרָאֵל.

During his repetition the chazzan recites עֲנֵנוּ at this point. See Laws §61-63.
[If he forgot to recite it at this point, he may insert it in שְׁמַע קוֹלֵנוּ, p. 436].

עֲנֵנוּ יהוה עֲנֵנוּ, בְּיוֹם צוֹם תַּעֲנִיתֵנוּ, כִּי בְצָרָה גְדוֹלָה אֲנָחְנוּ. אַל תֵּפֶן אֶל רִשְׁעֵנוּ, וְאַל תַּסְתֵּר פָּנֶיךָ מִמֶּנּוּ, וְאַל תִּתְעַלַּם מִתְּחִנָּתֵנוּ. הֱיֵה נָא קָרוֹב לְשַׁוְעָתֵנוּ, יְהִי נָא חַסְדְּךָ לְנַחֲמֵנוּ, טֶרֶם נִקְרָא אֵלֶיךָ עֲנֵנוּ, כַּדָּבָר שֶׁנֶּאֱמַר: וְהָיָה טֶרֶם יִקְרָאוּ וַאֲנִי אֶעֱנֶה, עוֹד הֵם מְדַבְּרִים וַאֲנִי אֶשְׁמָע.[2] כִּי אַתָּה יהוה הָעוֹנֶה בְּעֵת צָרָה, פּוֹדֶה וּמַצִּיל בְּכָל עֵת צָרָה וְצוּקָה. בָּרוּךְ אַתָּה יהוה, הָעוֹנֶה בְּעֵת צָרָה.

רפואה

רְפָאֵנוּ יהוה וְנֵרָפֵא, הוֹשִׁיעֵנוּ וְנִוָּשֵׁעָה, כִּי תְהִלָּתֵנוּ אָתָּה,[3] וְהַעֲלֵה רְפוּאָה שְׁלֵמָה לְכָל מַכּוֹתֵינוּ, °°כִּי אֵל מֶלֶךְ רוֹפֵא נֶאֱמָן וְרַחֲמָן אָתָּה. בָּרוּךְ אַתָּה יהוה, רוֹפֵא חוֹלֵי עַמּוֹ יִשְׂרָאֵל.

°°At this point one may interject a prayer for one who is ill:

יְהִי רָצוֹן מִלְּפָנֶיךָ יהוה אֱלֹהַי וֵאלֹהֵי אֲבוֹתַי, שֶׁתִּשְׁלַח מְהֵרָה רְפוּאָה שְׁלֵמָה מִן הַשָּׁמַיִם, רְפוּאַת הַנֶּפֶשׁ וּרְפוּאַת הַגּוּף

for a male—לַחוֹלֶה (patient's name) בֶּן (mother's name) בְּתוֹךְ שְׁאָר חוֹלֵי יִשְׂרָאֵל.
for a female—לַחוֹלָה (patient's name) בַּת (mother's name) בְּתוֹךְ שְׁאָר חוֹלֵי יִשְׂרָאֵל.
Continue—כִּי אֵל ...

HOLINESS OF GOD'S NAME

אַתָּה **You** are holy and Your Name is holy, and holy ones praise
You every day, forever. Blessed are You, HASHEM, the holy God.

INSIGHT

אַתָּה **You** graciously endow man with wisdom and teach insight to a
frail mortal. Endow us graciously from Yourself with wisdom,
insight, and discernment. Blessed are You, HASHEM, gracious Giver of
wisdom.

REPENTANCE

הֲשִׁיבֵנוּ **Bring** us back, our Father, to Your Torah, and bring us near,
our King, to Your service, and influence us to return in perfect
repentance before You. Blessed are You, HASHEM, Who desires
repentance.

FORGIVENESS

Strike the left side of the chest with the right fist while reciting the words 'erred' and 'sinned.'

סְלַח **Forgive** us, our Father, for we have erred; pardon us, our King,
for we have willfully sinned; for You pardon and forgive. Blessed
are You, HASHEM, the gracious One Who pardons abundantly.

REDEMPTION

רְאֵה **Behold** our affliction, take up our grievance, and redeem us[1]
speedily for Your Name's sake, for You are a powerful
Redeemer. Blessed are You, HASHEM, Redeemer of Israel.

During his repetition the chazzan recites עֲנֵנוּ, 'Answer us,' at this point. See Laws §61-63.
[If he forgot to recite it at this point, he may insert it in שְׁמַע קוֹלֵנוּ, 'Hear our voice' (p. 436).]

עֲנֵנוּ **Answer** us, HASHEM, answer us, on this day of our fast, for we are in
great distress. Do not pay attention to our wickedness; do not hide
Your Face from us; and do not ignore our supplication. Please be near to our
outcry; please let Your kindness comfort us — before we call to You answer
us, as it is said: 'And it will be that before they call, I will answer; while they
yet speak, I will hear.'[2] For You, HASHEM, are the One Who responds in time
of distress, Who redeems and rescues in every time of distress and woe.
Blessed are You, HASHEM, Who responds in time of distress.

HEALTH AND HEALING

רְפָאֵנוּ **Heal** us, HASHEM — then we will be healed; save us — then
we will be saved, for You are our praise.[3] Bring complete
recovery for all our ailments, °°for You are God, King, the faithful and
compassionate Healer. Blessed are You, HASHEM, Who heals the sick of
His people Israel.

°°At this point one may interject a prayer for one who is ill:

May it be Your will, HASHEM, my God, and the God of my forefathers, that You
quickly send a complete recovery from heaven, spiritual healing and physical healing
to the patient (name) son/daughter of (mother's name) among the other patients of
Israel.   Continue: For You are God ...

(1) Cf. Psalms 119:153-154. (2) Isaiah 65:24. (3) Cf. Jeremiah 17:14.

ברכת השנים

בָּרֵךְ עָלֵינוּ יהוה אֱלֹהֵינוּ אֶת הַשָּׁנָה הַזֹּאת וְאֶת כָּל מִינֵי תְבוּאָתָהּ לְטוֹבָה, וְתֵן בְּרָכָה עַל פְּנֵי הָאֲדָמָה, וְשַׂבְּעֵנוּ מִטּוּבֶךְ, וּבָרֵךְ שְׁנָתֵנוּ כַּשָּׁנִים הַטּוֹבוֹת. בָּרוּךְ אַתָּה יהוה, מְבָרֵךְ הַשָּׁנִים.

קיבוץ גליות

תְּקַע בְּשׁוֹפָר גָּדוֹל לְחֵרוּתֵנוּ, וְשָׂא נֵס לְקַבֵּץ גָּלֻיּוֹתֵינוּ, וְקַבְּצֵנוּ יַחַד מֵאַרְבַּע כַּנְפוֹת הָאָרֶץ.[1] בָּרוּךְ אַתָּה יהוה, מְקַבֵּץ נִדְחֵי עַמּוֹ יִשְׂרָאֵל.

דין

הָשִׁיבָה שׁוֹפְטֵינוּ כְּבָרִאשׁוֹנָה, וְיוֹעֲצֵינוּ כְּבַתְּחִלָּה,[2] וְהָסֵר מִמֶּנּוּ יָגוֹן וַאֲנָחָה, וּמְלוֹךְ עָלֵינוּ אַתָּה יהוה לְבַדְּךָ בְּחֶסֶד וּבְרַחֲמִים, וְצַדְּקֵנוּ בַּמִּשְׁפָּט. בָּרוּךְ אַתָּה יהוה, מֶלֶךְ אוֹהֵב צְדָקָה וּמִשְׁפָּט.

ברכת המינים

וְלַמַּלְשִׁינִים אַל תְּהִי תִקְוָה, וְכָל הָרִשְׁעָה כְּרֶגַע תֹּאבֵד, וְכָל אֹיְבֶיךָ מְהֵרָה יִכָּרֵתוּ, וְהַזֵּדִים מְהֵרָה תְעַקֵּר וּתְשַׁבֵּר וּתְמַגֵּר וְתַכְנִיעַ בִּמְהֵרָה בְיָמֵינוּ. בָּרוּךְ אַתָּה יהוה, שׁוֹבֵר אֹיְבִים וּמַכְנִיעַ זֵדִים.

צדיקים

עַל הַצַּדִּיקִים וְעַל הַחֲסִידִים, וְעַל זִקְנֵי עַמְּךָ בֵּית יִשְׂרָאֵל, וְעַל פְּלֵיטַת סוֹפְרֵיהֶם, וְעַל גֵּרֵי הַצֶּדֶק וְעָלֵינוּ, יֶהֱמוּ רַחֲמֶיךָ יהוה אֱלֹהֵינוּ, וְתֵן שָׂכָר טוֹב לְכָל הַבּוֹטְחִים בְּשִׁמְךָ בֶּאֱמֶת, וְשִׂים חֶלְקֵנוּ עִמָּהֶם לְעוֹלָם, וְלֹא נֵבוֹשׁ כִּי בְךָ בָּטָחְנוּ. בָּרוּךְ אַתָּה יהוה, מִשְׁעָן וּמִבְטָח לַצַּדִּיקִים.

בנין ירושלים

וְלִירוּשָׁלַיִם עִירְךָ בְּרַחֲמִים תָּשׁוּב, וְתִשְׁכּוֹן בְּתוֹכָהּ כַּאֲשֶׁר דִּבַּרְתָּ, וּבְנֵה אוֹתָהּ בְּקָרוֹב בְּיָמֵינוּ בִּנְיַן עוֹלָם, וְכִסֵּא דָוִד מְהֵרָה לְתוֹכָהּ תָּכִין. נַחֵם יהוה אֱלֹהֵינוּ אֶת אֲבֵלֵי צִיּוֹן, וְאֶת אֲבֵלֵי יְרוּשָׁלַיִם, וְאֶת הָעִיר הָאֲבֵלָה וְהַחֲרֵבָה וְהַבְּזוּיָה וְהַשּׁוֹמֵמָה. הָאֲבֵלָה מִבְּלִי בָנֶיהָ, וְהַחֲרֵבָה מִמְּעוֹנוֹתֶיהָ, וְהַבְּזוּיָה מִכְּבוֹדָהּ, וְהַשּׁוֹמֵמָה מֵאֵין יוֹשֵׁב. וְהִיא יוֹשֶׁבֶת וְרֹאשָׁהּ חָפוּי

YEAR OF PROSPERITY

בָּרֵךְ *Bless on our behalf — O* HASHEM, *our God — this year and all its kinds of crops for the best, and give a blessing on the face of the earth, and satisfy us from Your bounty, and bless our year like the best years. Blessed are You,* HASHEM, *Who blesses the years.*

INGATHERING OF EXILES

תְּקַע *Sound the great shofar for our freedom, raise the banner to gather our exiles and gather us together from the four corners of the earth.[1] Blessed are You,* HASHEM, *Who gathers in the dispersed of His people Israel.*

RESTORATION OF JUSTICE

הָשִׁיבָה *Restore our judges as in earliest times and our counselors as at first;[2] remove from us sorrow and groan; and reign over us — You,* HASHEM, *alone — with kindness and compassion, and justify us through judgment. Blessed are You,* HASHEM, *the King Who loves righteousness and judgment.*

AGAINST HERETICS

וְלַמַּלְשִׁינִים *And for slanderers let there be no hope; and may all wickedness perish in an instant; and may all Your enemies be cut down speedily. May You speedily uproot, smash, cast down, and humble the wanton sinners — speedily in our days. Blessed are You,* HASHEM, *Who breaks enemies and humbles wanton sinners.*

THE RIGHTEOUS

עַל הַצַּדִּיקִים *On the righteous, on the devout, on the elders of Your people the Family of Israel, on the remnant of their scholars, on the righteous converts and on ourselves — may Your compassion be aroused,* HASHEM, *our God, and give goodly reward to all who sincerely believe in Your Name. Put our lot with them forever, and we will not feel ashamed, for we trust in You. Blessed are You,* HASHEM, *Mainstay and Assurance of the righteous.*

REBUILDING JERUSALEM

וְלִירוּשָׁלַיִם *And to Jerusalem, Your city, may You return in compassion, and may You rest within it, as You have spoken. May You rebuild it soon in our days as an eternal structure, and may You speedily establish the throne of David within it. O* HASHEM, *our God, console the mourners of Zion and the mourners of Jerusalem, and the city that is mournful, ruined, scorned, and desolate: mournful without her children, ruined without her abodes, scorned without her glory, and desolate without inhabitant. She sits with covered head*

---

(1) Cf. *Isaiah* 11:12. (2) Cf. 1:26.

כְּאִשָּׁה עֲקָרָה שֶׁלֹּא יָלָדָה. וַיְבַלְּעוּהָ לִגְיוֹנוֹת, וַיִּרָשׁוּהָ עוֹבְדֵי זָרִים, וַיַּטִּילוּ אֶת עַמְּךָ יִשְׂרָאֵל לֶחָרֶב, וַיַּהַרְגוּ בְזָדוֹן חֲסִידֵי עֶלְיוֹן. עַל כֵּן צִיּוֹן בְּמַר תִּבְכֶּה, וִירוּשָׁלַיִם תִּתֵּן קוֹלָהּ. לִבִּי לִבִּי עַל חַלְלֵיהֶם, מֵעַי מֵעַי עַל חַלְלֵיהֶם, כִּי אַתָּה יהוה בָּאֵשׁ הִצַּתָּהּ, וּבָאֵשׁ אַתָּה עָתִיד לִבְנוֹתָהּ, כָּאָמוּר: וַאֲנִי אֶהְיֶה לָּהּ, נְאֻם יהוה, חוֹמַת אֵשׁ סָבִיב וּלְכָבוֹד אֶהְיֶה בְתוֹכָהּ.[1] בָּרוּךְ אַתָּה יהוה, מְנַחֵם צִיּוֹן וּבוֹנֵה יְרוּשָׁלָיִם.

מלכות בית דוד

אֶת צֶמַח דָּוִד עַבְדְּךָ מְהֵרָה תַצְמִיחַ, וְקַרְנוֹ תָּרוּם בִּישׁוּעָתֶךָ, כִּי לִישׁוּעָתְךָ קִוִּינוּ כָּל הַיּוֹם. בָּרוּךְ אַתָּה יהוה, מַצְמִיחַ קֶרֶן יְשׁוּעָה.

קבלת תפלה

שְׁמַע קוֹלֵנוּ יהוה אֱלֹהֵינוּ, חוּס וְרַחֵם עָלֵינוּ, וְקַבֵּל בְּרַחֲמִים וּבְרָצוֹן אֶת תְּפִלָּתֵנוּ, כִּי אֵל שׁוֹמֵעַ תְּפִלּוֹת וְתַחֲנוּנִים אָתָּה. וּמִלְּפָנֶיךָ מַלְכֵּנוּ רֵיקָם אַל תְּשִׁיבֵנוּ,

---

During the silent *Shemoneh Esrei* individuals recite עֲנֵנוּ, *'Answer us,'* at this point.
[If he forgotten, *Shemoneh Esrei* is not repeated. See Laws §61-63.]

עֲנֵנוּ יהוה עֲנֵנוּ, בְּיוֹם צוֹם תַּעֲנִיתֵנוּ, כִּי בְצָרָה גְדוֹלָה אֲנָחְנוּ. אַל תֵּפֶן אֶל רִשְׁעֵנוּ, וְאַל תַּסְתֵּר פָּנֶיךָ מִמֶּנּוּ, וְאַל תִּתְעַלַּם מִתְּחִנָּתֵנוּ. הֱיֵה נָא קָרוֹב לְשַׁוְעָתֵנוּ, יְהִי נָא חַסְדְּךָ לְנַחֲמֵנוּ, טֶרֶם נִקְרָא אֵלֶיךָ עֲנֵנוּ, כַּדָּבָר שֶׁנֶּאֱמַר: וְהָיָה טֶרֶם יִקְרָאוּ וַאֲנִי אֶעֱנֶה, עוֹד הֵם מְדַבְּרִים וַאֲנִי אֶשְׁמָע.[2] כִּי אַתָּה יהוה הָעוֹנֶה בְּעֵת צָרָה, פּוֹדֶה וּמַצִּיל בְּכָל עֵת צָרָה וְצוּקָה.
כִּי אַתָּה ... — Continue

∞During the silent *Shemoneh Esrei* one may insert either or both of these personal prayers.

For livelihood:

אַתָּה הוּא יהוה הָאֱלֹהִים, הַזָּן וּמְפַרְנֵס וּמְכַלְכֵּל מִקַּרְנֵי רְאֵמִים עַד בֵּיצֵי כִנִּים. הַטְרִיפֵנִי לֶחֶם חֻקִּי, וְהַמְצֵא לִי וּלְכָל בְּנֵי בֵיתִי מְזוֹנוֹתַי קוֹדֶם שֶׁאֶצְטָרֵךְ לָהֶם, בְּנַחַת וְלֹא בְצַעַר, בְּהֶתֵּר וְלֹא בְאִסּוּר, בְּכָבוֹד וְלֹא בְבִזָּיוֹן, לְחַיִּים וּלְשָׁלוֹם, מִשֶּׁפַע בְּרָכָה וְהַצְלָחָה, וּמִשֶּׁפַע בְּרָכָה עֶלְיוֹנָה, כְּדֵי שֶׁאוּכַל לַעֲשׂוֹת רְצוֹנֶךָ וְלַעֲסוֹק בְּתוֹרָתֶךָ וּלְקַיֵּם מִצְוֹתֶיךָ. וְאַל תַּצְרִיכֵנִי לִידֵי מַתְּנַת בָּשָׂר וָדָם. וִיקֻיַּם בִּי מִקְרָא שֶׁכָּתוּב: פּוֹתֵחַ אֶת יָדֶךָ, וּמַשְׂבִּיעַ לְכָל חַי רָצוֹן.[3] וְכָתוּב: הַשְׁלֵךְ עַל יהוה יְהָבְךָ וְהוּא יְכַלְכְּלֶךָ.[4]
כִּי אַתָּה ... — Continue

For forgiveness:

אָנָּא יהוה, חָטָאתִי עָוִיתִי וּפָשַׁעְתִּי לְפָנֶיךָ, מִיּוֹם הֱיוֹתִי עַל הָאֲדָמָה עַד הַיּוֹם הַזֶּה (וּבִפְרָט בַּחֵטְא ....). אָנָּא יהוה, עֲשֵׂה לְמַעַן שִׁמְךָ הַגָּדוֹל, וּתְכַפֶּר לִי עַל עֲוֹנִי וַחֲטָאַי וּפְשָׁעַי שֶׁחָטָאתִי וְשֶׁעָוִיתִי וְשֶׁפָּשַׁעְתִּי לְפָנֶיךָ, מִנְּעוּרַי עַד הַיּוֹם הַזֶּה. וּתְמַלֵּא כָּל הַשֵּׁמוֹת שֶׁפָּגַמְתִּי בְּשִׁמְךָ הַגָּדוֹל.

*like a barren woman who never gave birth. Legions have devoured her,
and idolaters have conquered her; they have cast Your people Israel to
the sword and wantonly murdered the devout servants of the Supreme
One. Therefore, Zion weeps bitterly and Jerusalem raises her voice. My
heart, my heart — [it aches] for their slain! My innards, my innards —
[they ache] for their slain! For You* HASHEM, *with fire You consumed her
and with fire You will rebuild her, as it is said: 'I will be for her, the
words of* HASHEM, *a wall of fire around and I will be glorious in her
midst.'¹ Blessed are You,* HASHEM, *Who consoles Zion and rebuilds
Jerusalem.*

DAVIDIC REIGN

אֶת צֶמַח *The offspring of Your servant David may You speedily
cause to flourish, and enhance his pride through Your
salvation, for we hope for Your salvation all day long. Blessed are You,*
HASHEM, *Who causes the pride of salvation to flourish.*

ACCEPTANCE OF PRAYER

שְׁמַע *Hear our voice,* HASHEM *our God, pity and be compassionate to us, and accept — with compassion and favor — our
prayer, for God Who hears prayers and supplications are You.
From before Yourself, our King, turn us not away empty-handed,*

During the silent *Shemoneh Esrei* individuals recite עֲנֵנוּ, '*Answer us,*' at this point.
[If he forgotten, *Shemoneh Esrei* is not repeated. See *Laws* §61-63.]

עֲנֵנוּ *Answer us,* HASHEM, *answer us, on this day of our fast, for we are in
great distress. Do not pay attention to our wickedness; do not hide
Your Face from us; and do not ignore our supplication. Please be near to our
outcry; please let Your kindness comfort us — before we call to You answer
us, as it is said: 'And it will be that before they call, I will answer; while they
yet speak, I will hear.'² For You,* HASHEM, *are the One Who responds in time
of distress, Who redeems and rescues in every time of distress and woe.*

Continue: *For You hear the prayer . . .*

°°During the silent *Shemoneh Esrei* one may insert either or both of these personal prayers.

For forgiveness:	For livelihood:

אָנָּא *Please, O* HASHEM, *I have
erred, been iniquitous, and
willfully sinned before You, from
the day I have existed on earth until
this very day (and especially with
the sin of . . .). Please,* HASHEM, *act
for the sake of Your Great Name
and grant me atonement for my
iniquities, my errors, and my willful
sins through which I have erred,
been iniquitous, and willfully sinned
before You, from my youth until
this day. And make whole all the
Names that I have blemished in
Your Great Name.*

אַתָּה *It is You,* HASHEM *the God, Who nourishes, sustains, and supports, from the horns of re'eimim
to the eggs of lice. Provide me with my allotment of
bread; and bring forth for me and all members of my
household, my food, before I have need for it; in
contentment but not in pain, in a permissible but not
a forbidden manner, in honor but not in disgrace, for
life and for peace; from the flow of blessing and success
and from the flow of the Heavenly spring, so that I
be enabled to do Your will and engage in Your Torah
and fulfill Your commandments. Make me not needful
of people's largesse; and may there be fulfilled in me
the verse that states, 'You open Your hand and satisfy
the desire of every living thing'³ and that states, 'Cast
Your burden upon* HASHEM *and He will support you.'⁴*

Continue: *For You hear the prayer . . .*

---

(1) *Zechariah* 2:9. (2) *Isaiah* 65:24. (3) *Psalms* 145:16. (4) 55:23.

°° כִּי אַתָּה שׁוֹמֵעַ תְּפִלַּת עַמְּךָ יִשְׂרָאֵל בְּרַחֲמִים. בָּרוּךְ אַתָּה יהוה, שׁוֹמֵעַ תְּפִלָּה.

עבודה

רְצֵה יהוה אֱלֹהֵינוּ בְּעַמְּךָ יִשְׂרָאֵל וּבִתְפִלָּתָם, וְהָשֵׁב אֶת הָעֲבוֹדָה לִדְבִיר בֵּיתֶךָ. וְאִשֵּׁי יִשְׂרָאֵל וּתְפִלָּתָם בְּאַהֲבָה תְקַבֵּל בְּרָצוֹן, וּתְהִי לְרָצוֹן תָּמִיד עֲבוֹדַת יִשְׂרָאֵל עַמֶּךָ.

וְתֶחֱזֶינָה עֵינֵינוּ בְּשׁוּבְךָ לְצִיּוֹן בְּרַחֲמִים. בָּרוּךְ אַתָּה יהוה, הַמַּחֲזִיר שְׁכִינָתוֹ לְצִיּוֹן.

הודאה

Bow at מוֹדִים; straighten up at ה'. In his repetition the *chazzan* should recite the entire מוֹדִים aloud, while the congregation recites מוֹדִים דְּרַבָּנָן softly.

מוֹדִים אֲנַחְנוּ לָךְ, שָׁאַתָּה הוּא יהוה אֱלֹהֵינוּ וֵאלֹהֵי אֲבוֹתֵינוּ לְעוֹלָם וָעֶד. צוּר חַיֵּינוּ, מָגֵן יִשְׁעֵנוּ אַתָּה הוּא לְדוֹר וָדוֹר. נוֹדֶה לְּךָ וּנְסַפֵּר תְּהִלָּתֶךָ עַל חַיֵּינוּ הַמְּסוּרִים בְּיָדֶךָ, וְעַל נִשְׁמוֹתֵינוּ הַפְּקוּדוֹת לָךְ, וְעַל נִסֶּיךָ שֶׁבְּכָל יוֹם עִמָּנוּ, וְעַל נִפְלְאוֹתֶיךָ וְטוֹבוֹתֶיךָ שֶׁבְּכָל עֵת, עֶרֶב וָבֹקֶר וְצָהֳרָיִם. הַטּוֹב כִּי לֹא כָלוּ רַחֲמֶיךָ, וְהַמְרַחֵם כִּי לֹא תַמּוּ חֲסָדֶיךָ, מֵעוֹלָם קִוִּינוּ לָךְ.

מודים דרבנן

מוֹדִים אֲנַחְנוּ לָךְ, שָׁאַתָּה הוּא יהוה אֱלֹהֵינוּ וֵאלֹהֵי אֲבוֹתֵינוּ, אֱלֹהֵי כָל בָּשָׂר, יוֹצְרֵנוּ, יוֹצֵר בְּרֵאשִׁית. בְּרָכוֹת וְהוֹדָאוֹת לְשִׁמְךָ הַגָּדוֹל וְהַקָּדוֹשׁ, עַל שֶׁהֶחֱיִיתָנוּ וְקִיַּמְתָּנוּ. כֵּן תְּחַיֵּינוּ וּתְקַיְּמֵנוּ, וְתֶאֱסוֹף גָּלֻיּוֹתֵינוּ לְחַצְרוֹת קָדְשֶׁךָ, לִשְׁמוֹר חֻקֶּיךָ וְלַעֲשׂוֹת רְצוֹנֶךָ, וּלְעָבְדְּךָ בְּלֵבָב שָׁלֵם, עַל שֶׁאֲנַחְנוּ מוֹדִים לָךְ. בָּרוּךְ אֵל הַהוֹדָאוֹת.

וְעַל כֻּלָּם יִתְבָּרַךְ וְיִתְרוֹמַם שִׁמְךָ מַלְכֵּנוּ תָּמִיד לְעוֹלָם וָעֶד.

Bend the knees at בָּרוּךְ; bow at אַתָּה; straighten up at ה'.

וְכֹל הַחַיִּים יוֹדוּךָ סֶּלָה, וִיהַלְלוּ אֶת שִׁמְךָ בֶּאֱמֶת, הָאֵל יְשׁוּעָתֵנוּ וְעֶזְרָתֵנוּ סֶלָה. בָּרוּךְ אַתָּה יהוה, הַטּוֹב שִׁמְךָ וּלְךָ נָאֶה לְהוֹדוֹת.

°° *for You hear the prayer of Your people Israel with compassion. Blessed are You, HASHEM, Who hears prayer.*

TEMPLE SERVICE

רְצֵה *Be favorable, HASHEM, our God, toward Your people Israel and their prayer and restore the service to the Holy of Holies of Your Temple. The fire-offerings of Israel and their prayer accept with love and favor, and may the service of Your people Israel always be favorable to You.*

וְתֶחֱזֶינָה *May our eyes behold Your return to Zion in compassion. Blessed are You, HASHEM, Who restores His Presence to Zion.*

THANKSGIVING [MODIM]

Bow at 'We gratefully thank You'; straighten up at 'HASHEM.' In his repetition the chazzan should recite the entire Modim aloud, while the congregation recites Modim of the Rabbis softly.

מוֹדִים *We gratefully thank You, for it is You Who are HASHEM, our God and the God of our forefathers for all eternity; Rock of our lives, Shield of our salvation are You from generation to generation. We shall thank You and relate Your praise[1] — for our lives, which are committed to Your power and for our souls that are entrusted to You; for Your miracles that are with us every day; and for Your wonders and favors in every season — evening, morning, and afternoon. The Beneficent One, for Your compassions were never exhausted, and the Compassionate One, for Your kindnesses never ended[2] — always have we put our hope in You.*

> **MODIM OF THE RABBIS**
>
> **מוֹדִים** *We gratefully thank You, for it is You Who are HASHEM, our God and the God of our forefathers, the God of all flesh, our Molder, the Molder of the universe. Blessings and thanks are due Your great and holy Name for You have given us life and sustained us. So may You continue to give us life and sustain us and gather our exiles to the Courtyards of Your Sanctuary, to observe Your decrees, to do Your will and to serve You wholeheartedly. [We thank You] for inspiring us to thank You. Blessed is the God of thanksgivings.*

For all these, may Your Name be blessed and exalted, our King, continually forever and ever.

Bend the knees at 'Blessed'; bow at 'You'; straighten up at 'HASHEM.'

Everything alive will gratefully acknowledge You, Selah! and praise Your Name sincerely, O God of our salvation and help, Selah! Blessed are You, HASHEM, Your Name is 'The Beneficent One' and to You it is fitting to give thanks.

---

(1) Cf. *Psalms* 79:13. (2) Cf. *Lamentations* 3:22.

ברכת כהנים

The *chazzan* recites the following during his repetition.
He faces right at וְיִשְׁמְרֶךָ; faces left at אֵלֶיךָ וִיחֻנֶּךָּ; faces the Ark for the rest of the blessings.

אֱלֹהֵינוּ, וֵאלֹהֵי אֲבוֹתֵינוּ, בָּרְכֵנוּ בַבְּרָכָה הַמְשֻׁלֶּשֶׁת בַּתּוֹרָה
הַכְּתוּבָה עַל יְדֵי מֹשֶׁה עַבְדֶּךָ, הָאֲמוּרָה מִפִּי אַהֲרֹן וּבָנָיו,
כֹּהֲנִים עַם קְדוֹשֶׁךָ, כָּאָמוּר:

יְבָרֶכְךָ יהוה, וְיִשְׁמְרֶךָ.   (.כֵּן יְהִי רָצוֹן —Cong.)

יָאֵר יהוה פָּנָיו אֵלֶיךָ וִיחֻנֶּךָּ.   (.כֵּן יְהִי רָצוֹן —Cong.)

יִשָּׂא יהוה פָּנָיו אֵלֶיךָ וְיָשֵׂם לְךָ שָׁלוֹם.[1]   (.כֵּן יְהִי רָצוֹן —Cong.)

שלום

שִׂים שָׁלוֹם, טוֹבָה, וּבְרָכָה, חֵן, וָחֶסֶד וְרַחֲמִים עָלֵינוּ וְעַל
כָּל יִשְׂרָאֵל עַמֶּךָ. בָּרְכֵנוּ אָבִינוּ, כֻּלָּנוּ כְּאֶחָד
בְּאוֹר פָּנֶיךָ, כִּי בְאוֹר פָּנֶיךָ נָתַתָּ לָּנוּ, יהוה אֱלֹהֵינוּ, תּוֹרַת חַיִּים
וְאַהֲבַת חֶסֶד, וּצְדָקָה, וּבְרָכָה, וְרַחֲמִים, וְחַיִּים, וְשָׁלוֹם. וְטוֹב
בְּעֵינֶיךָ לְבָרֵךְ אֶת עַמְּךָ יִשְׂרָאֵל, בְּכָל עֵת וּבְכָל שָׁעָה בִּשְׁלוֹמֶךָ.
בָּרוּךְ אַתָּה יהוה, הַמְבָרֵךְ אֶת עַמּוֹ יִשְׂרָאֵל בַּשָּׁלוֹם.

יִהְיוּ לְרָצוֹן אִמְרֵי פִי וְהֶגְיוֹן לִבִּי לְפָנֶיךָ, יהוה צוּרִי וְגֹאֲלִי.[2]

Chazzan's repetition of Shemoneh Esrei ends here. Individuals continue below:

אֱלֹהַי, נְצוֹר לְשׁוֹנִי מֵרָע, וּשְׂפָתַי מִדַּבֵּר מִרְמָה,[3] וְלִמְקַלְלַי
נַפְשִׁי תִדּוֹם, וְנַפְשִׁי כֶּעָפָר לַכֹּל תִּהְיֶה. פְּתַח לִבִּי
בְּתוֹרָתֶךָ, וּבְמִצְוֹתֶיךָ תִּרְדּוֹף נַפְשִׁי. וְכָל הַחוֹשְׁבִים עָלַי רָעָה,
מְהֵרָה הָפֵר עֲצָתָם וְקַלְקֵל מַחֲשַׁבְתָּם. עֲשֵׂה לְמַעַן שְׁמֶךָ, עֲשֵׂה
לְמַעַן יְמִינֶךָ, עֲשֵׂה לְמַעַן קְדֻשָּׁתֶךָ, עֲשֵׂה לְמַעַן תּוֹרָתֶךָ. לְמַעַן
יֵחָלְצוּן יְדִידֶיךָ, הוֹשִׁיעָה יְמִינְךָ וַעֲנֵנִי.[4]

Some recite verses pertaining to their names here. See page 492.

יִהְיוּ לְרָצוֹן אִמְרֵי פִי וְהֶגְיוֹן לִבִּי לְפָנֶיךָ, יהוה צוּרִי וְגֹאֲלִי.[2]

עֹשֶׂה שָׁלוֹם בִּמְרוֹמָיו, הוּא יַעֲשֶׂה שָׁלוֹם
עָלֵינוּ, וְעַל כָּל יִשְׂרָאֵל. וְאִמְרוּ: אָמֵן.

Bow and take three steps back.
Bow left and say . . . עֹשֶׂה; bow
right and say . . . הוּא יַעֲשֶׂה; bow
forward and say אָמֵן . . . וְעַל כָּל.

יְהִי רָצוֹן מִלְּפָנֶיךָ יהוה אֱלֹהֵינוּ וֵאלֹהֵי אֲבוֹתֵינוּ, שֶׁיִּבָּנֶה בֵּית
הַמִּקְדָּשׁ בִּמְהֵרָה בְיָמֵינוּ, וְתֵן חֶלְקֵנוּ בְּתוֹרָתֶךָ. וְשָׁם נַעֲבָדְךָ
בְּיִרְאָה, כִּימֵי עוֹלָם וּכְשָׁנִים קַדְמוֹנִיּוֹת. וְעָרְבָה לַיהוה מִנְחַת יְהוּדָה
וִירוּשָׁלָיִם, כִּימֵי עוֹלָם וּכְשָׁנִים קַדְמוֹנִיּוֹת.[5]

THE INDIVIDUAL'S RECITATION OF *SHEMONEH ESREI* ENDS HERE.

The individual remains standing in place until the *chazzan* reaches *Kedushah* — or at least until the
chazzan begins his repetition — then he takes three steps forward. The *chazzan* himself, or one who
is praying alone, should remain in place for a few moments before taking three steps forward.

THE PRIESTLY BLESSING

The chazzan recites the following during his repetition.

אֱלֹהֵינוּ Our God and the God of our forefathers, bless us with the three-verse blessing in the Torah that was written by the hand of Moses, Your servant, that was said by Aaron and his sons, the Kohanim, Your holy people, as it is said:

May HASHEM bless you and safeguard you.   (Cong.— So may it be.)

May HASHEM illuminate His countenance for you and be gracious to you.   (Cong.— So may it be.)

May HASHEM turn His countenance to you and establish peace for you.[1]

(Cong.— So may it be.)

PEACE

שִׂים שָׁלוֹם Establish peace, goodness, blessing, graciousness, kindness, and compassion upon us and upon all of Your people Israel. Bless us, our Father, all of us as one, with the light of Your countenance, for with the light of Your countenance You gave us, HASHEM, our God, the Torah of life and a love of kindness, righteousness, blessing, compassion, life, and peace. And may it be good in Your eyes to bless Your people Israel at every time and every hour with Your peace. Blessed are You, HASHEM, Who blesses His people Israel with peace.

May the expressions of my mouth and the thoughts of my heart find favor before You, HASHEM, my Rock and my Redeemer.[2]

Chazzan's repetition of Shemoneh Esrei ends here. Individuals continue below:

אֱלֹהַי My God, guard my tongue from evil and my lips from speaking deceitfully.[3] To those who curse me, let my soul be silent; and let my soul be like dust to everyone. Open my heart to Your Torah, then my soul will pursue Your commandments. As for all those who design evil against me, speedily nullify their counsel and disrupt their design. Act for Your Name's sake; act for Your right hand's sake; act for Your sanctity's sake; act for Your Torah's sake. That Your beloved ones may be given rest; let Your right hand save, and respond to me.[4]

Some recite verses pertaining to their names at this point. See page 492. May the expressions of my mouth and the thoughts of my heart find favor before You, HASHEM, my Rock and my Redeemer.[2] °°He Who makes peace in His heights, may He make peace upon us, and upon all Israel. Now respond: Amen.

Bow and take three steps back. Bow left and say, 'He Who makes peace ...'; bow right and say, 'may He make peace ...'; bow forward and say, 'and upon ... Amen.'

יְהִי רָצוֹן May it be Your will, HASHEM, our God and the God of our forefathers, that the Holy Temple be rebuilt, speedily in our days. Grant us our share in Your Torah, and may we serve You there with reverence, as in days of old and in former years. Then the offering of Judah and Jerusalem will be pleasing to HASHEM, as in days of old and in former years.[5]

THE INDIVIDUAL'S RECITATION OF SHEMONEH ESREI ENDS HERE.

The individual remains standing in place until the chazzan reaches Kedushah — or at least until the chazzan begins his repetition — then he takes three steps forward. The chazzan himself, or one who is praying alone, should remain in place for a few moments before taking three steps forward.

(1) Numbers 6:24-26. (2) Psalms 19:15. (3) Cf. 34:14. (4) 60:7; 108:7. (5) Malachi 3:4.

קדיש שלם

The *chazzan* recites קַדִּישׁ שָׁלֵם.

יִתְגַּדַּל וְיִתְקַדַּשׁ שְׁמֵהּ רַבָּא. (Cong.– אָמֵן.) בְּעָלְמָא דִּי בְרָא כִרְעוּתֵהּ.
וְיַמְלִיךְ מַלְכוּתֵהּ, בְּחַיֵּיכוֹן וּבְיוֹמֵיכוֹן וּבְחַיֵּי דְכָל בֵּית יִשְׂרָאֵל,
בַּעֲגָלָא וּבִזְמַן קָרִיב. וְאִמְרוּ: אָמֵן.

(Cong.– אָמֵן. יְהֵא שְׁמֵהּ רַבָּא מְבָרַךְ לְעָלַם וּלְעָלְמֵי עָלְמַיָּא.)

יְהֵא שְׁמֵהּ רַבָּא מְבָרַךְ לְעָלַם וּלְעָלְמֵי עָלְמַיָּא.
יִתְבָּרַךְ וְיִשְׁתַּבַּח וְיִתְפָּאַר וְיִתְרוֹמַם וְיִתְנַשֵּׂא וְיִתְהַדָּר וְיִתְעַלֶּה
וְיִתְהַלָּל שְׁמֵהּ דְּקֻדְשָׁא בְּרִיךְ הוּא (Cong.– בְּרִיךְ הוּא) – לְעֵלָּא מִן כָּל
בִּרְכָתָא וְשִׁירָתָא תֻּשְׁבְּחָתָא וְנֶחֱמָתָא, דַּאֲמִירָן בְּעָלְמָא. וְאִמְרוּ: אָמֵן.
(Cong.– אָמֵן.)

(Cong.– קַבֵּל בְּרַחֲמִים וּבְרָצוֹן אֶת תְּפִלָּתֵנוּ.)

תִּתְקַבֵּל צְלוֹתְהוֹן וּבָעוּתְהוֹן דְּכָל בֵּית יִשְׂרָאֵל קֳדָם אֲבוּהוֹן דִּי
בִשְׁמַיָּא. וְאִמְרוּ: אָמֵן. (Cong.– אָמֵן.)

(Cong.– יְהִי שֵׁם יהוה מְבֹרָךְ, מֵעַתָּה וְעַד עוֹלָם.)

יְהֵא שְׁלָמָא רַבָּא מִן שְׁמַיָּא, וְחַיִּים עָלֵינוּ וְעַל כָּל יִשְׂרָאֵל. וְאִמְרוּ:
אָמֵן. (Cong.– אָמֵן.)

(Cong.– עֶזְרִי מֵעִם יהוה, עֹשֵׂה שָׁמַיִם וָאָרֶץ.)

Take three steps back. Bow left and say . . . עֹשֶׂה; bow right and say . . . הוּא; bow forward and say
וְעַל כָּל . . . אָמֵן. Remain standing in place for a few moments, then take three steps forward.

עֹשֶׂה שָׁלוֹם בִּמְרוֹמָיו, הוּא יַעֲשֶׂה שָׁלוֹם עָלֵינוּ, וְעַל כָּל יִשְׂרָאֵל.
וְאִמְרוּ: אָמֵן. (Cong.– אָמֵן.)

עלינו

Stand while reciting עָלֵינוּ.

עָלֵינוּ לְשַׁבֵּחַ לַאֲדוֹן הַכֹּל, לָתֵת גְּדֻלָּה לְיוֹצֵר בְּרֵאשִׁית,
שֶׁלֹּא עָשָׂנוּ כְּגוֹיֵי הָאֲרָצוֹת, וְלֹא שָׂמָנוּ כְּמִשְׁפְּחוֹת
הָאֲדָמָה. שֶׁלֹּא שָׂם חֶלְקֵנוּ כָּהֶם, וְגוֹרָלֵנוּ כְּכָל הֲמוֹנָם. (שֶׁהֵם
מִשְׁתַּחֲוִים לְהֶבֶל וָרִיק, וּמִתְפַּלְלִים אֶל אֵל לֹא יוֹשִׁיעַ.) וַאֲנַחְנוּ
כּוֹרְעִים וּמִשְׁתַּחֲוִים וּמוֹדִים, לִפְנֵי מֶלֶךְ מַלְכֵי
Bow while reciting
וַאֲנַחְנוּ כּוֹרְעִים וּמִשְׁתַּחֲוִים.
הַמְּלָכִים הַקָּדוֹשׁ בָּרוּךְ הוּא. שֶׁהוּא נוֹטֶה שָׁמַיִם וְיֹסֵד אָרֶץ,
וּמוֹשַׁב יְקָרוֹ בַּשָּׁמַיִם מִמַּעַל, וּשְׁכִינַת עֻזּוֹ בְּגָבְהֵי מְרוֹמִים. הוּא
אֱלֹהֵינוּ, אֵין עוֹד. אֱמֶת מַלְכֵּנוּ, אֶפֶס זוּלָתוֹ, כַּכָּתוּב בְּתוֹרָתוֹ:
וְיָדַעְתָּ הַיּוֹם וַהֲשֵׁבֹתָ אֶל לְבָבֶךָ, כִּי יהוה הוּא הָאֱלֹהִים בַּשָּׁמַיִם
מִמַּעַל וְעַל הָאָרֶץ מִתָּחַת, אֵין עוֹד.

FULL KADDISH

The *chazzan* recites the Full *Kaddish*.

יִתְגַּדַּל May His great Name grow exalted and sanctified (Cong.— Amen.)
in the world that He created as He willed. May He give reign to His
kingship in your lifetimes and in your days, and in the lifetimes of the entire
Family of Israel, swiftly and soon. Now respond: Amen.

(Cong.— Amen. May His great Name be blessed forever and ever.)
May His great Name be blessed forever and ever.

Blessed, praised, glorified, exalted, extolled, mighty, upraised, and lauded be
the Name of the Holy One, Blessed is He (Cong.— Blessed is He) — beyond any
blessing and song, praise and consolation that are uttered in the world. Now
respond: Amen. (Cong.— Amen.)

(Cong.— Accept our prayers with mercy and favor.)

May the prayers and supplications of the entire Family of Israel be accepted
before their Father Who is in Heaven. Now respond: Amen. (Cong.— Amen.)

(Cong.— Blessed be the Name of HASHEM, from this time and forever.[1])

May there be abundant peace from Heaven, and life, upon us and upon all
Israel. Now respond: Amen. (Cong.— Amen.)

(Cong.— My help is from HASHEM, Maker of heaven and earth.[2])

Take three steps back. Bow left and say, 'He Who makes peace . . .';
bow right and say, 'may He . . .'; bow forward and say, 'and upon all Israel . . .'
Remain standing in place for a few moments, then take three steps forward.

He Who makes peace in His heights, may He make peace upon us, and
upon all Israel. Now respond: Amen. (Cong.— Amen.)

ALEINU

Stand while reciting עָלֵינוּ, 'It is our duty . . .'

עָלֵינוּ It is our duty to praise the Master of all, to ascribe greatness to
the Molder of primeval creation, for He has not made us like the
nations of the lands, and has not emplaced us like the families of the
earth; for He has not assigned our portion like theirs nor our lot like
all their multitudes. (For they bow to vanity and emptiness and pray to

Bow while reciting   a god which helps not.[3]) But we bend our knees,
'But we bend our knees.'   bow, and acknowledge our thanks before the King
Who reigns over kings, the Holy One, Blessed is He. He stretches out
heaven and establishes earth's foundation,[4] the seat of His homage is in
the heavens above and His powerful Presence is in the loftiest heights.
He is our God and there is none other. True is our King, there is nothing
beside Him, as it is written in His Torah: 'You are to know this day and
take to your heart that HASHEM is the only God — in heaven above and
on the earth below — there is none other.'[5]

(1) *Psalms* 113:2. (2) 121:2. (3) *Isaiah* 45:20. (4) 51:13. (5) *Deuteronomy* 4:39.

עַל כֵּן נְקַוֶּה לְּךָ יהוה אֱלֹהֵינוּ לִרְאוֹת מְהֵרָה בְּתִפְאֶרֶת עֻזֶּךָ, לְהַעֲבִיר גִּלּוּלִים מִן הָאָרֶץ, וְהָאֱלִילִים כָּרוֹת יִכָּרֵתוּן, לְתַקֵּן עוֹלָם בְּמַלְכוּת שַׁדַּי. וְכָל בְּנֵי בָשָׂר יִקְרְאוּ בִשְׁמֶךָ, לְהַפְנוֹת אֵלֶיךָ כָּל רִשְׁעֵי אָרֶץ. יַכִּירוּ וְיֵדְעוּ כָּל יוֹשְׁבֵי תֵבֵל, כִּי לְךָ תִּכְרַע כָּל בֶּרֶךְ, תִּשָּׁבַע כָּל לָשׁוֹן.[1] לְפָנֶיךָ יהוה אֱלֹהֵינוּ יִכְרְעוּ וְיִפֹּלוּ, וְלִכְבוֹד שִׁמְךָ יְקָר יִתֵּנוּ. וִיקַבְּלוּ כֻלָּם אֶת עוֹל מַלְכוּתֶךָ, וְתִמְלֹךְ עֲלֵיהֶם מְהֵרָה לְעוֹלָם וָעֶד. כִּי הַמַּלְכוּת שֶׁלְּךָ הִיא וּלְעוֹלְמֵי עַד תִּמְלוֹךְ בְּכָבוֹד, כַּכָּתוּב בְּתוֹרָתֶךָ: יהוה יִמְלֹךְ לְעֹלָם וָעֶד.[2] ❖ וְנֶאֱמַר: וְהָיָה יהוה לְמֶלֶךְ עַל כָּל הָאָרֶץ, בַּיּוֹם הַהוּא יִהְיֶה יהוה אֶחָד וּשְׁמוֹ אֶחָד.[3]

Some congregations recite the following after עלינו:

אַל תִּירָא מִפַּחַד פִּתְאֹם, וּמִשֹּׁאַת רְשָׁעִים כִּי תָבֹא.[4] עֻצוּ עֵצָה וְתֻפָר, דַּבְּרוּ דָבָר וְלֹא יָקוּם, כִּי עִמָּנוּ אֵל.[5] וְעַד זִקְנָה אֲנִי הוּא, וְעַד שֵׂיבָה אֲנִי אֶסְבֹּל, אֲנִי עָשִׂיתִי וַאֲנִי אֶשָּׂא, וַאֲנִי אֶסְבֹּל וַאֲמַלֵּט.[6]

קדיש יתום

In the presence of a *minyan*, mourners recite קַדִּישׁ יָתוֹם, the Mourner's *Kaddish* (see *Laws* §132-134).

יִתְגַּדַּל וְיִתְקַדַּשׁ שְׁמֵהּ רַבָּא. (Cong.– אָמֵן.) בְּעָלְמָא דִּי בְרָא כִרְעוּתֵהּ. וְיַמְלִיךְ מַלְכוּתֵהּ, בְּחַיֵּיכוֹן וּבְיוֹמֵיכוֹן וּבְחַיֵּי דְכָל בֵּית יִשְׂרָאֵל, בַּעֲגָלָא וּבִזְמַן קָרִיב. וְאִמְרוּ: אָמֵן.

(Cong.– אָמֵן. יְהֵא שְׁמֵהּ רַבָּא מְבָרַךְ לְעָלַם וּלְעָלְמֵי עָלְמַיָּא.)

יְהֵא שְׁמֵהּ רַבָּא מְבָרַךְ לְעָלַם וּלְעָלְמֵי עָלְמַיָּא.

יִתְבָּרַךְ וְיִשְׁתַּבַּח וְיִתְפָּאַר וְיִתְרוֹמַם וְיִתְנַשֵּׂא וְיִתְהַדָּר וְיִתְעַלֶּה וְיִתְהַלָּל שְׁמֵהּ דְּקֻדְשָׁא בְּרִיךְ הוּא (Cong.– בְּרִיךְ הוּא) – לְעֵלָּא מִן כָּל בִּרְכָתָא וְשִׁירָתָא תֻּשְׁבְּחָתָא וְנֶחֱמָתָא, דַּאֲמִירָן בְּעָלְמָא, וְאִמְרוּ: אָמֵן. (Cong.– אָמֵן.)

יְהֵא שְׁלָמָא רַבָּא מִן שְׁמַיָּא, וְחַיִּים עָלֵינוּ וְעַל כָּל יִשְׂרָאֵל. וְאִמְרוּ: אָמֵן. (Cong.– אָמֵן.)

Take three steps back. Bow left and say . . . עֹשֶׂה; bow right and say . . . הוּא; bow forward and say וְעַל כָּל . . . אָמֵן. Remain standing in place for a few moments, then take three steps forward.

עֹשֶׂה שָׁלוֹם בִּמְרוֹמָיו, הוּא יַעֲשֶׂה שָׁלוֹם עָלֵינוּ, וְעַל כָּל יִשְׂרָאֵל. וְאִמְרוּ: אָמֵן. (Cong.– אָמֵן.)

עַל כֵּן *Therefore we put our hope in You, HASHEM, our God, that we may soon see Your mighty splendor, to remove detestable idolatry from the earth, and false gods will be utterly cut off, to perfect the universe through the Almighty's sovereignty. Then all humanity will call upon Your Name, to turn all the earth's wicked toward You. All the world's inhabitants will recognize and know that to You every knee should bend, every tongue should swear.[1] Before You, HASHEM, our God, they will bend every knee and cast themselves down and to the glory of Your Name they will render homage, and they will all accept upon themselves the yoke of Your kingship that You may reign over them soon and eternally. For the kingdom is Yours and You will reign for all eternity in glory as it is written in Your Torah: HASHEM shall reign for all eternity.[2]* Chazzan— *And it is said: HASHEM will be King over all the world — on that day HASHEM will be One and His Name will be One.[3]*

Some congregations recite the following after *Aleinu.*

אַל תִּירָא *Do not fear sudden terror, or the holocaust of the wicked when it comes.[4] Plan a conspiracy and it will be annulled; speak your piece and it shall not stand, for God is with us.[5] Even till your seniority, I remain unchanged; and even till your ripe old age, I shall endure. I created you and I shall bear you; I shall endure and rescue.[6]*

MOURNER'S KADDISH

In the presence of a *minyan,* mourners recite קַדִּישׁ יָתוֹם, the Mourner's *Kaddish* (see *Laws* 132-133).

[A transliteration of this *Kaddish* appears on page 496.]

יִתְגַּדַּל *May His great Name grow exalted and sanctified* (Cong.— *Amen.*) *in the world that He created as He willed. May He give reign to His kingship in your lifetimes and in your days, and in the lifetimes of the entire Family of Israel, swiftly and soon. Now respond: Amen.*

(Cong.— *Amen. May His great Name be blessed forever and ever.*)

May His great Name be blessed forever and ever.

Blessed, praised, glorified, exalted, extolled, mighty, upraised, and lauded be the Name of the Holy One, Blessed is He (Cong.— *Blessed is He*) — *beyond any blessing and song, praise and consolation that are uttered in the world. Now respond: Amen.* (Cong.— *Amen*).

May there be abundant peace from Heaven, and life, upon us and upon all Israel. Now respond: Amen. (Cong.— *Amen.*)

Take three steps back. Bow left and say, 'He Who makes peace . . .';
bow right and say, 'may He . . .'; bow forward and say, 'and upon all Israel . . .'
Remain standing in place for a few moments, then take three steps forward.

He Who makes peace in His heights, may He make peace upon us, and upon all Israel. Now respond: Amen. (Cong.— *Amen.*

---

(1) Cf. *Isaiah* 45:23. (2) *Exodus* 15:18. (3) *Zechariah* 14:9. (4) *Proverbs* 3:25. (5) *Isaiah* 8:10. (6) 46:4.

❊ מעריב למוצאי תשעה באב ❊

Congregation, then *chazzan:*

וְהוּא רַחוּם יְכַפֵּר עָוֹן וְלֹא יַשְׁחִית, וְהִרְבָּה לְהָשִׁיב אַפּוֹ, וְלֹא יָעִיר כָּל חֲמָתוֹ.[1] יהוה הוֹשִׁיעָה, הַמֶּלֶךְ יַעֲנֵנוּ בְיוֹם קָרְאֵנוּ.[2]

In some congregations the *chazzan* chants a melody during his recitation of בָּרְכוּ, so that the congregation can then recite יִתְבָּרַךְ.

Chazzan bows at בָּרְכוּ and straightens up at 'ה.

יִתְבָּרַךְ וְיִשְׁתַּבַּח וְיִתְפָּאַר וְיִתְרוֹמַם וְיִתְנַשֵּׂא שְׁמוֹ שֶׁל מֶלֶךְ מַלְכֵי הַמְּלָכִים, הַקָּדוֹשׁ בָּרוּךְ הוּא. שֶׁהוּא רִאשׁוֹן וְהוּא אַחֲרוֹן, וּמִבַּלְעָדָיו אֵין אֱלֹהִים.[3] סֶלוּ, לָרֹכֵב

בָּרְכוּ אֶת יהוה הַמְבֹרָךְ ּ

Congregation, followed by *chazzan,* responds, bowing at בָּרוּךְ and straightening up at 'ה.

בָּרוּךְ יהוה הַמְבֹרָךְ לְעוֹלָם וָעֶד.

בָּעֲרָבוֹת, בְּיָהּ שְׁמוֹ, וְעִלְזוּ לְפָנָיו.[4] וְשִׁמוֹ מְרוֹמַם עַל כָּל בְּרָכָה וּתְהִלָּה.[5] בָּרוּךְ שֵׁם כְּבוֹד מַלְכוּתוֹ לְעוֹלָם וָעֶד. יְהִי שֵׁם יהוה מְבֹרָךְ, מֵעַתָּה וְעַד עוֹלָם.[6]

ברכות קריאת שמע

בָּרוּךְ אַתָּה יהוה אֱלֹהֵינוּ מֶלֶךְ הָעוֹלָם, אֲשֶׁר בִּדְבָרוֹ מַעֲרִיב עֲרָבִים, בְּחָכְמָה פּוֹתֵחַ שְׁעָרִים, וּבִתְבוּנָה מְשַׁנֶּה עִתִּים, וּמַחֲלִיף אֶת הַזְּמַנִּים, וּמְסַדֵּר אֶת הַכּוֹכָבִים בְּמִשְׁמְרוֹתֵיהֶם בָּרָקִיעַ כִּרְצוֹנוֹ. בּוֹרֵא יוֹם וָלָיְלָה, גּוֹלֵל אוֹר מִפְּנֵי חֹשֶׁךְ וְחֹשֶׁךְ מִפְּנֵי אוֹר. וּמַעֲבִיר יוֹם וּמֵבִיא לָיְלָה, וּמַבְדִּיל בֵּין יוֹם וּבֵין לָיְלָה, יהוה צְבָאוֹת שְׁמוֹ. ❖ אֵל חַי וְקַיָּם, תָּמִיד יִמְלוֹךְ עָלֵינוּ, לְעוֹלָם וָעֶד. בָּרוּךְ אַתָּה יהוה, הַמַּעֲרִיב עֲרָבִים. (אָמֵן. –Cong.)

אַהֲבַת עוֹלָם בֵּית יִשְׂרָאֵל עַמְּךָ אָהָבְתָּ. תּוֹרָה וּמִצְוֹת, חֻקִּים וּמִשְׁפָּטִים, אוֹתָנוּ לִמַּדְתָּ. עַל כֵּן יהוה אֱלֹהֵינוּ, בְּשָׁכְבֵנוּ וּבְקוּמֵנוּ נָשִׂיחַ בְּחֻקֶּיךָ, וְנִשְׂמַח בְּדִבְרֵי תוֹרָתֶךָ, וּבְמִצְוֹתֶיךָ לְעוֹלָם וָעֶד. ❖ כִּי הֵם חַיֵּינוּ, וְאֹרֶךְ יָמֵינוּ, וּבָהֶם נֶהְגֶּה יוֹמָם וָלָיְלָה. וְאַהֲבָתְךָ, אַל תָּסִיר מִמֶּנּוּ לְעוֹלָמִים. בָּרוּךְ אַתָּה יהוה, אוֹהֵב עַמּוֹ יִשְׂרָאֵל. (אָמֵן. –Cong.)

שמע

Immediately before its recitation, concentrate on fulfilling the positive commandment of reciting the *Shema* twice daily. It is important to enunciate each word clearly and not to run words together. For this reason, vertical lines have been placed between two words that are prone to be slurred into one and are not separated by a comma or a hyphen. See Laws §95-109.

⊰{ MAARIV FOR THE CONCLUSION OF TISHAH B'AV }⊱

Congregation, then *chazzan:*

וְהוּא רַחוּם *He, the Merciful One, is forgiving of iniquity and does not destroy. Frequently He withdraws His anger, not arousing His entire rage.[1] HASHEM, save! May the King answer us on the day we call.[2]*

In some congregations the *chazzan* chants a melody during his recitation of *Borchu*, so that the congregation can then recite 'Blessed, praised . . .'

Chazzan bows at 'Bless,' and straightens up at 'HASHEM.'

Bless HASHEM, the blessed One.

Congregation, followed by *chazzan*, responds, bowing at 'Blessed' and straightening up at 'HASHEM.'

Blessed is HASHEM, the blessed One,
for all eternity.

Blessed, praised, glorified, exalted and upraised is the Name of the King Who rules over kings — the Holy One, Blessed is He. For He is the First and He is the Last and aside from Him there is no god.[3] Extol Him — Who rides the highest heavens — with His Name, YAH, and exult before Him.[4] His Name is exalted beyond every blessing and praise.[5] Blessed is the Name of His glorious kingdom for all eternity. Blessed be the Name of HASHEM from this time and forever.[6]

BLESSINGS OF THE SHEMA

בָּרוּךְ *Blessed are You, HASHEM, our God, King of the universe, Who by His word brings on evenings, with wisdom opens gates, with understanding alters periods, changes the seasons, and orders the stars in their heavenly constellations as He wills. He creates day and night, removing light before darkness and darkness before light. He causes day to pass and brings night, and separates between day and night — HASHEM, Master of Legions, is His Name.* Chazzan— *May the living and enduring God continuously reign over us, for all eternity. Blessed are You, HASHEM, Who brings on evenings.*   (Cong.— Amen.)

אַהֲבַת *With an eternal love have You loved the House of Israel, Your nation. Torah and commandments, decrees and ordinances have You taught us. Therefore HASHEM, our God, upon our retiring and arising, we will discuss Your decrees and we will rejoice with the words of Your Torah and with Your commandments for all eternity.* Chazzan— *For they are our life and the length of our days and about them we will meditate day and night. May You not remove Your love from us forever. Blessed are You, HASHEM, Who loves His nation Israel.* (Cong.— Amen.)

THE SHEMA

Immediately before its recitation, concentrate on fulfilling the positive commandment of reciting the *Shema* twice daily. It is important to enunciate each word clearly and not to run words together.
See *Laws* §95-109.

---

(1) *Psalms* 78:38. (2) 20:10. (3) Cf. *Isaiah* 44:6. (4) *Psalms* 68:5.
(5) Cf. *Nehemiah* 9:5. (6) *Psalms* 113:2.

When praying without a *minyan*, begin with the following three-word formula:

אֵל מֶלֶךְ נֶאֱמָן.

Recite the first verse aloud, with the right hand covering the eyes,
and concentrate intently upon accepting God's absolute sovereignty.

שְׁמַע ׀ יִשְׂרָאֵל, יְהוָה ׀ אֱלֹהֵינוּ, יְהוָה ׀ אֶחָד:

In an undertone — בָּרוּךְ שֵׁם כְּבוֹד מַלְכוּתוֹ לְעוֹלָם וָעֶד.

While reciting the first paragraph (דברים ו:ה-ט), concentrate on
accepting the commandment to love God.

וְאָהַבְתָּ אֵת ׀ יְהוָה ׀ אֱלֹהֶיךָ, בְּכָל-לְבָבְךָ, וּבְכָל-
נַפְשְׁךָ, וּבְכָל-מְאֹדֶךָ: וְהָיוּ הַדְּבָרִים הָאֵלֶּה, אֲשֶׁר ׀ אָנֹכִי מְצַוְּךָ הַיּוֹם,
עַל-לְבָבֶךָ: וְשִׁנַּנְתָּם לְבָנֶיךָ, וְדִבַּרְתָּ בָּם, בְּשִׁבְתְּךָ בְּבֵיתֶךָ, וּבְלֶכְתְּךָ
בַדֶּרֶךְ, וּבְשָׁכְבְּךָ וּבְקוּמֶךָ: וּקְשַׁרְתָּם לְאוֹת ׀ עַל-יָדֶךָ, וְהָיוּ לְטֹטָפֹת
בֵּין ׀ עֵינֶיךָ: וּכְתַבְתָּם ׀ עַל-מְזֻזוֹת בֵּיתֶךָ, וּבִשְׁעָרֶיךָ:

While reciting the second paragraph (דברים יא:יג-כא), concentrate on
accepting all the commandments and the concept of reward and punishment.

וְהָיָה, אִם-שָׁמֹעַ תִּשְׁמְעוּ אֶל-מִצְוֹתַי, אֲשֶׁר ׀ אָנֹכִי מְצַוֶּה ׀ אֶתְכֶם
הַיּוֹם, לְאַהֲבָה אֶת-יְהוָה ׀ אֱלֹהֵיכֶם וּלְעָבְדוֹ, בְּכָל-
לְבַבְכֶם, וּבְכָל-נַפְשְׁכֶם: וְנָתַתִּי מְטַר-אַרְצְכֶם בְּעִתּוֹ, יוֹרֶה וּמַלְקוֹשׁ,
וְאָסַפְתָּ דְגָנֶךָ וְתִירֹשְׁךָ וְיִצְהָרֶךָ: וְנָתַתִּי ׀ עֵשֶׂב ׀ בְּשָׂדְךָ לִבְהֶמְתֶּךָ,
וְאָכַלְתָּ וְשָׂבָעְתָּ: הִשָּׁמְרוּ לָכֶם, פֶּן-יִפְתֶּה לְבַבְכֶם, וְסַרְתֶּם וַעֲבַדְתֶּם
׀ אֱלֹהִים ׀ אֲחֵרִים, וְהִשְׁתַּחֲוִיתֶם לָהֶם: וְחָרָה ׀ אַף-יְהוָה בָּכֶם, וְעָצַר
׀ אֶת-הַשָּׁמַיִם, וְלֹא-יִהְיֶה מָטָר, וְהָאֲדָמָה לֹא תִתֵּן אֶת-יְבוּלָהּ,
וַאֲבַדְתֶּם ׀ מְהֵרָה מֵעַל הָאָרֶץ הַטֹּבָה ׀ אֲשֶׁר ׀ יְהוָה נֹתֵן לָכֶם:
וְשַׂמְתֶּם ׀ אֶת-דְּבָרַי ׀ אֵלֶּה, עַל-לְבַבְכֶם וְעַל-נַפְשְׁכֶם, וּקְשַׁרְתֶּם ׀
אֹתָם לְאוֹת ׀ עַל-יֶדְכֶם, וְהָיוּ לְטוֹטָפֹת בֵּין ׀ עֵינֵיכֶם: וְלִמַּדְתֶּם ׀ אֹתָם
׀ אֶת-בְּנֵיכֶם, לְדַבֵּר בָּם, בְּשִׁבְתְּךָ בְּבֵיתֶךָ, וּבְלֶכְתְּךָ בַדֶּרֶךְ, וּבְשָׁכְבְּךָ
וּבְקוּמֶךָ: וּכְתַבְתָּם ׀ עַל-מְזוּזוֹת בֵּיתֶךָ, וּבִשְׁעָרֶיךָ: לְמַעַן ׀ יִרְבּוּ ׀
יְמֵיכֶם וִימֵי בְנֵיכֶם, עַל הָאֲדָמָה, אֲשֶׁר נִשְׁבַּע ׀ יְהוָה לַאֲבֹתֵיכֶם
לָתֵת לָהֶם, כִּימֵי הַשָּׁמַיִם ׀ עַל-הָאָרֶץ:

במדבר טו:לז-מא

וַיֹּאמֶר ׀ יְהוָה ׀ אֶל-מֹשֶׁה לֵּאמֹר: דַּבֵּר ׀ אֶל-בְּנֵי ׀ יִשְׂרָאֵל,
וְאָמַרְתָּ אֲלֵהֶם, וְעָשׂוּ לָהֶם צִיצִת, עַל-כַּנְפֵי בִגְדֵיהֶם
לְדֹרֹתָם, וְנָתְנוּ ׀ עַל-צִיצִת הַכָּנָף, פְּתִיל תְּכֵלֶת: וְהָיָה לָכֶם לְצִיצִת,
וּרְאִיתֶם ׀ אֹתוֹ, וּזְכַרְתֶּם ׀ אֶת-כָּל-מִצְוֹת יְהוָה, וַעֲשִׂיתֶם ׀ אֹתָם,

When praying without a *minyan*, begin with the following three-word formula:
God, trustworthy King.
Recite the first verse aloud, with the right hand covering the eyes,
and concentrate intently upon accepting God's absolute sovereignty.

Hear, O Israel: HASHEM is our God, HASHEM, the One and Only.[1]

In an undertone— *Blessed is the Name of His glorious kingdom for all eternity.*

While reciting the first paragraph (*Deuteronomy* 6:5-9), concentrate on
accepting the commandment to love God.

וְאָהַבְתָּ *You shall love HASHEM, your God, with all your heart, with all your soul and with all your resources. Let these matters that I command you today be upon your heart. Teach them thoroughly to your children and speak of them while you sit in your home, while you walk on the way, when you retire and when you arise. Bind them as a sign upon your arm and let them be tefillin between your eyes. And write them on the doorposts of your house and upon your gates.*

While reciting the second paragraph (*Deuteronomy* 11:13-21), concentrate on
accepting all the commandments and the concept of reward and punishment.

וְהָיָה *And it will come to pass that if you continually hearken to My commandments that I command you today, to love HASHEM, your God, and to serve Him, with all your heart and with all your soul — then I will provide rain for your land in its proper time, the early and late rains, that you may gather in your grain, your wine, and your oil. I will provide grass in your field for your cattle and you will eat and be satisfied. Beware lest your heart be seduced and you turn astray and serve gods of others and bow to them. Then the wrath of HASHEM will blaze against you. He will restrain the heaven so there will be no rain and the ground will not yield its produce. And you will swiftly be banished from the goodly land which HASHEM gives you. Place these words of Mine upon your heart and upon your soul; bind them for a sign upon your arm and let them be tefillin between your eyes. Teach them to your children, to discuss them, while you sit in your home, while you walk on the way, when you retire and when you arise. And write them on the doorposts of your house and upon your gates. In order to prolong your days and the days of your children upon the ground that HASHEM has sworn to your ancestors to give them, like the days of the heaven on the earth.*

Numbers 15:37-41

וַיֹּאמֶר *And HASHEM said to Moses saying: Speak to the Children of Israel and say to them that they are to make themselves tzitzis on the corners of their garments, throughout their generations. And they are to place upon the tzitzis of each corner a thread of techeiles. And it shall constitute tzitzis for you, that you may see it and remember all the commandments of HASHEM and perform them;*

---

(1) *Deuteronomy* 6:4.

וְלֹא תָתוּרוּ ן אַחֲרֵי לְבַבְכֶם וְאַחֲרֵי ן עֵינֵיכֶם, אֲשֶׁר־אַתֶּם זֹנִים ן
אַחֲרֵיהֶם: לְמַעַן תִּזְכְּרוּ, וַעֲשִׂיתֶם ן אֶת־כָּל־מִצְוֹתָי, וִהְיִיתֶם
קְדֹשִׁים לֵאלֹהֵיכֶם: אֲנִי יהוה ן אֱלֹהֵיכֶם, Concentrate on fulfilling the
commandment of remember-
אֲשֶׁר הוֹצֵאתִי ן אֶתְכֶם ן מֵאֶרֶץ מִצְרַיִם, ing the Exodus from Egypt.
לִהְיוֹת לָכֶם לֵאלֹהִים, אֲנִי ן יהוה ן אֱלֹהֵיכֶם: אֱמֶת —

Although the word אֱמֶת belongs to the next paragraph,
it is appended to the conclusion of the previous one.

יהוה אֱלֹהֵיכֶם אֱמֶת. — *Chazzan repeats*

וֶאֱמוּנָה כָּל זֹאת, וְקַיָּם עָלֵינוּ, כִּי הוּא יהוה אֱלֹהֵינוּ וְאֵין
זוּלָתוֹ, וַאֲנַחְנוּ יִשְׂרָאֵל עַמּוֹ. הַפּוֹדֵנוּ מִיַּד מְלָכִים,
מַלְכֵּנוּ הַגּוֹאֲלֵנוּ מִכַּף כָּל הֶעָרִיצִים. הָאֵל הַנִּפְרָע לָנוּ מִצָּרֵינוּ,
וְהַמְשַׁלֵּם גְּמוּל לְכָל אֹיְבֵי נַפְשֵׁנוּ. הָעֹשֶׂה גְדֹלוֹת עַד אֵין חֵקֶר,
וְנִפְלָאוֹת עַד אֵין מִסְפָּר. הַשָּׂם נַפְשֵׁנוּ בַּחַיִּים, וְלֹא נָתַן לַמּוֹט
רַגְלֵנוּ. הַמַּדְרִיכֵנוּ עַל בָּמוֹת אוֹיְבֵינוּ, וַיָּרֶם קַרְנֵנוּ עַל כָּל שֹׂנְאֵינוּ.
הָעֹשֶׂה לָּנוּ נִסִּים וּנְקָמָה בְּפַרְעֹה, אוֹתוֹת וּמוֹפְתִים בְּאַדְמַת בְּנֵי
חָם. הַמַּכֶּה בְעֶבְרָתוֹ כָּל בְּכוֹרֵי מִצְרָיִם, וַיּוֹצֵא אֶת עַמּוֹ יִשְׂרָאֵל
מִתּוֹכָם לְחֵרוּת עוֹלָם. הַמַּעֲבִיר בָּנָיו בֵּין גִּזְרֵי יַם סוּף, אֶת
רוֹדְפֵיהֶם וְאֶת שׂוֹנְאֵיהֶם בִּתְהוֹמוֹת טִבַּע. וְרָאוּ בָנָיו גְּבוּרָתוֹ,
שִׁבְּחוּ וְהוֹדוּ לִשְׁמוֹ. ❖ וּמַלְכוּתוֹ בְּרָצוֹן קִבְּלוּ עֲלֵיהֶם. מֹשֶׁה וּבְנֵי
יִשְׂרָאֵל לְךָ עָנוּ שִׁירָה, בְּשִׂמְחָה רַבָּה, וְאָמְרוּ כֻלָּם:

מִי כָמֹכָה בָּאֵלִים יהוה, מִי כָּמֹכָה נֶאְדָּר בַּקֹּדֶשׁ, נוֹרָא
תְהִלֹּת, עֹשֵׂה פֶלֶא.[3] ❖ מַלְכוּתְךָ רָאוּ בָנֶיךָ בּוֹקֵעַ יָם
לִפְנֵי מֹשֶׁה, זֶה אֵלִי עָנוּ וְאָמְרוּ:

יהוה יִמְלֹךְ לְעֹלָם וָעֶד.[5] ❖ וְנֶאֱמַר: כִּי פָדָה יהוה אֶת יַעֲקֹב,
וּגְאָלוֹ מִיַּד חָזָק מִמֶּנּוּ.[6] בָּרוּךְ אַתָּה יהוה, גָּאַל יִשְׂרָאֵל.
(אָמֵן.) — *Cong.*

הַשְׁכִּיבֵנוּ יהוה אֱלֹהֵינוּ לְשָׁלוֹם, וְהַעֲמִידֵנוּ מַלְכֵּנוּ לְחַיִּים,
וּפְרוֹשׂ עָלֵינוּ סֻכַּת שְׁלוֹמֶךָ, וְתַקְּנֵנוּ בְּעֵצָה טוֹבָה
מִלְּפָנֶיךָ, וְהוֹשִׁיעֵנוּ לְמַעַן שְׁמֶךָ. וְהָגֵן בַּעֲדֵנוּ, וְהָסֵר מֵעָלֵינוּ
אוֹיֵב, דֶּבֶר, וְחֶרֶב, וְרָעָב, וְיָגוֹן, וְהָסֵר שָׂטָן מִלְּפָנֵינוּ וּמֵאַחֲרֵינוּ,
וּבְצֵל כְּנָפֶיךָ תַּסְתִּירֵנוּ,[7] כִּי אֵל שׁוֹמְרֵנוּ וּמַצִּילֵנוּ אָתָּה, כִּי אֵל

and not explore after your heart and after your eyes after which you
stray. So that you may remember and perform all My commandments;

Concentrate on fulfill-
ing the commandment
of remembering the
Exodus from Egypt.

and be holy to your God. I am HASHEM, your God,
Who has removed you from the land of Egypt to be
a God to you; I am HASHEM your God — it is true —

Although the word אֱמֶת, 'it is true,' belongs to the next paragraph,
it is appended to the conclusion of the previous one.

Chazzan repeats: **HASHEM, your God, is true.**

וֶאֱמוּנָה And faithful is all this, and it is firmly established for us
that He is HASHEM our God, and there is none but Him, and we
are Israel, His nation. He redeems us from the power of kings, our King
Who delivers us from the hand of all the cruel tyrants. He is the God Who
exacts vengeance for us from our foes and Who brings just retribution
upon all enemies of our soul; Who performs great deeds that are beyond
comprehension, and wonders beyond number.[1] Who set our soul in life
and did not allow our foot to falter.[2] Who led us upon the heights of our
enemies and raised our pride above all who hate us; Who wrought for us
miracles and vengeance upon Pharaoh; signs and wonders on the land of
the offspring of Ham; Who struck with His anger all the firstborn of
Egypt and removed His nation Israel from their midst to eternal
freedom; Who brought His children through the split parts of the Sea of
Reeds while those who pursued them and hated them He caused to sink
into the depths. When His children perceived His power, they lauded
and gave grateful praise to His Name. Chazzan— And His Kingship they
accepted upon themselves willingly. Moses and the Children of Israel
raised their voices to You in song with abundant gladness — and said
unanimously:

מִי כָמֹכָה Who is like You among the heavenly powers, HASHEM! Who
is like You, mighty in holiness, too awesome for praise, doing
wonders![3] Chazzan— Your children beheld Your majesty, as You split the
sea before Moses: 'This is my God!'[4] they exclaimed, then they said:

יהוה 'HASHEM shall reign for all eternity!'[5] Chazzan— And it is further
said: 'For HASHEM has redeemed Jacob and delivered him from a
power mightier than he.'[6] Blessed are You, HASHEM, Who redeemed
Israel.   (Cong.— Amen.)

הַשְׁכִּיבֵנוּ Lay us down to sleep, HASHEM our God, in peace, raise us
erect, our King, to life; and spread over us the shelter of
Your peace. Set us aright with good counsel from before Your Presence,
and save us for Your Name's sake. Shield us, remove from us foe,
plague, sword, famine, and woe; and remove spiritual impediment
from before us and behind us, and in the shadow of Your wings
shelter us[7] — for God Who protects and rescues us are You; for God,

(1) Job 9:10. (2) Psalms 66:9. (3) Exodus 15:11. (4) 15:2. (5) 15:18. (6) Jeremiah 31:10. (7) Cf. Psalms 17:8.

מֶלֶךְ חַנּוּן וְרַחוּם אָתָּה.¹ ❖ וּשְׁמוֹר צֵאתֵנוּ וּבוֹאֵנוּ, לְחַיִּים וּלְשָׁלוֹם מֵעַתָּה וְעַד עוֹלָם.² בָּרוּךְ אַתָּה יהוה, שׁוֹמֵר עַמּוֹ יִשְׂרָאֵל לָעַד.

(.אָמֵן —Cong.)

Some congregations omit the following prayers and continue with Half-*Kaddish* (below).

בָּרוּךְ יהוה לְעוֹלָם, אָמֵן וְאָמֵן.³ בָּרוּךְ יהוה מִצִּיּוֹן, שֹׁכֵן יְרוּשָׁלָיִם, הַלְלוּיָהּ.⁴ בָּרוּךְ יהוה אֱלֹהִים אֱלֹהֵי יִשְׂרָאֵל, עֹשֵׂה נִפְלָאוֹת לְבַדּוֹ. וּבָרוּךְ שֵׁם כְּבוֹדוֹ לְעוֹלָם, וְיִמָּלֵא כְבוֹדוֹ אֶת כָּל הָאָרֶץ, אָמֵן וְאָמֵן.⁵ יְהִי כְבוֹד יהוה לְעוֹלָם, יִשְׂמַח יהוה בְּמַעֲשָׂיו.⁶ יְהִי שֵׁם יהוה מְבֹרָךְ, מֵעַתָּה וְעַד עוֹלָם.⁷ כִּי לֹא יִטֹּשׁ יהוה אֶת עַמּוֹ בַּעֲבוּר שְׁמוֹ הַגָּדוֹל, כִּי הוֹאִיל יהוה לַעֲשׂוֹת אֶתְכֶם לוֹ לְעָם.⁸ וַיַּרְא כָּל הָעָם וַיִּפְּלוּ עַל פְּנֵיהֶם, וַיֹּאמְרוּ, יהוה הוּא הָאֱלֹהִים, יהוה הוּא הָאֱלֹהִים.⁹ וְהָיָה יהוה לְמֶלֶךְ עַל כָּל הָאָרֶץ, בַּיּוֹם הַהוּא יִהְיֶה יהוה אֶחָד וּשְׁמוֹ אֶחָד.¹⁰ יְהִי חַסְדְּךָ יהוה עָלֵינוּ, כַּאֲשֶׁר יִחַלְנוּ לָךְ.¹¹ הוֹשִׁיעֵנוּ יהוה אֱלֹהֵינוּ, וְקַבְּצֵנוּ מִן הַגּוֹיִם, לְהֹדוֹת לְשֵׁם קָדְשֶׁךָ, לְהִשְׁתַּבֵּחַ בִּתְהִלָּתֶךָ.¹² כָּל גּוֹיִם אֲשֶׁר עָשִׂיתָ יָבוֹאוּ וְיִשְׁתַּחֲווּ לְפָנֶיךָ אֲדֹנָי, וִיכַבְּדוּ לִשְׁמֶךָ. כִּי גָדוֹל אַתָּה וְעֹשֵׂה נִפְלָאוֹת, אַתָּה אֱלֹהִים לְבַדֶּךָ.¹³ וַאֲנַחְנוּ עַמְּךָ וְצֹאן מַרְעִיתֶךָ, נוֹדֶה לְּךָ לְעוֹלָם, לְדוֹר וָדֹר נְסַפֵּר תְּהִלָּתֶךָ.¹⁴ בָּרוּךְ יהוה בַּיּוֹם. בָּרוּךְ יהוה בַּלָּיְלָה. בָּרוּךְ יהוה בְּשָׁכְבֵנוּ. בָּרוּךְ יהוה בְּקוּמֵנוּ. כִּי בְיָדְךָ נַפְשׁוֹת הַחַיִּים וְהַמֵּתִים. אֲשֶׁר בְּיָדוֹ נֶפֶשׁ כָּל חָי, וְרוּחַ כָּל בְּשַׂר אִישׁ.¹⁵ בְּיָדְךָ אַפְקִיד רוּחִי, פָּדִיתָה אוֹתִי, יהוה אֵל אֱמֶת.¹⁶ אֱלֹהֵינוּ שֶׁבַּשָּׁמַיִם יַחֵד שְׁמֶךָ, וְקַיֵּם מַלְכוּתְךָ תָּמִיד, וּמְלוֹךְ עָלֵינוּ לְעוֹלָם וָעֶד.

יִרְאוּ עֵינֵינוּ וְיִשְׂמַח לִבֵּנוּ וְתָגֵל נַפְשֵׁנוּ בִּישׁוּעָתְךָ בֶּאֱמֶת, בֶּאֱמֹר לְצִיּוֹן מָלַךְ אֱלֹהָיִךְ.¹⁷ יהוה מֶלֶךְ,¹⁸ יהוה מָלָךְ,¹⁹ יהוה יִמְלֹךְ לְעֹלָם וָעֶד.²⁰ כִּי הַמַּלְכוּת שֶׁלְּךָ הִיא, וּלְעוֹלְמֵי עַד תִּמְלוֹךְ בְּכָבוֹד, כִּי אֵין לָנוּ מֶלֶךְ אֶלָּא אָתָּה. בָּרוּךְ אַתָּה יהוה, הַמֶּלֶךְ בִּכְבוֹדוֹ תָּמִיד יִמְלוֹךְ עָלֵינוּ לְעוֹלָם וָעֶד, וְעַל כָּל מַעֲשָׂיו.

(.אָמֵן —Cong.)

the Gracious and Compassionate King, are You.[1] Chazzan— *Safeguard our*
going and coming, for life and for peace from now to eternity.[2] *Blessed*
are You, HASHEM, Who protects His people Israel forever.

(Cong.— *Amen.*)

Some congregations omit the following prayers and continue with Half-*Kaddish* (below).

בָּרוּךְ *Blessed is HASHEM forever, Amen and Amen.*[3] *Blessed is*
HASHEM from Zion, Who dwells in Jerusalem, Halleluyah![4]
Blessed is HASHEM, God, the God of Israel, Who alone does wondrous
things. Blessed is His glorious Name forever, and may all the earth be
filled with His glory, Amen and Amen.[5] *May the glory of HASHEM*
endure forever, let HASHEM rejoice in His works.[6] *Blessed be the Name of*
HASHEM from this time and forever.[7] *For HASHEM will not cast off His*
nation for the sake of His Great Name, for HASHEM has vowed to make
you His own people.[8] *Then the entire nation saw and fell on their faces*
and said, 'HASHEM — only He is God! HASHEM — only He is God!'[9]
Then HASHEM will be King over all the world, on that day HASHEM will
be One and His Name will be One.[10] *May Your kindness, HASHEM, be*
upon us, just as we awaited You.[11] *Save us, HASHEM, our God, gather us*
from the nations, to thank Your Holy Name and to glory in Your
praise![12] *All the nations that You made will come and bow before You,*
My Lord, and shall glorify Your Name. For You are great and work
wonders; You alone, O God.[13] *Then we, Your nation and the sheep of*
Your pasture, shall thank You forever; for generation after generation
we will relate Your praise.[14] *Blessed is HASHEM by day; Blessed is*
HASHEM by night; Blessed is HASHEM when we retire; Blessed is HASHEM
when we arise. For in Your hand are the souls of the living and the
dead. He in Whose hand is the soul of all the living and the spirit of
every human being.[15] *In Your hand I shall entrust my spirit, You*
redeemed me, HASHEM, God of truth.[16] *Our God, Who is in heaven, bring*
unity to Your Name; establish Your kingdom forever and reign over us
for all eternity.

יִרְאוּ *May our eyes see, our heart rejoice and our soul exult in Your*
salvation in truth, when Zion is told, 'Your God has reigned!'[17]
HASHEM reigns,[18] *HASHEM has reigned,*[19] *HASHEM will reign for*
all eternity.[20] Chazzan— *For the kingdom is Yours and for all eternity*
You will reign in glory, for we have no King but You. Blessed are You,
HASHEM, the King in His glory — He shall constantly reign over us
forever and ever, and over all His creatures.   (Cong.— *Amen.*)

---

(1) Cf. *Nehemiah* 9:31. (2) Cf. *Psalms* 121:8. (3) *Psalms* 89:53. (4) 135:21.
(5) 72:18-19. (6) 104:31. (7) 113:2. (8) *I Samuel* 12:22. (9) *I Kings* 18:39. (10) *Zechariah* 14:9.
(11) *Psalms* 33:22. (12) 106:47. (13) 86:9-10. (14) 79:13. (15) *Job* 12:10. (16) *Psalms* 31:6.
(17) Cf. *Isaiah* 52:7. (18) *Psalms* 10:16. (19) 93:1 et al. (20) *Exodus* 15:18.

יִתְגַּדַּל וְיִתְקַדַּשׁ שְׁמֵהּ רַבָּא. (.Cong – אָמֵן) בְּעָלְמָא דִּי בְרָא כִרְעוּתֵהּ,
וְיַמְלִיךְ מַלְכוּתֵהּ, בְּחַיֵּיכוֹן וּבְיוֹמֵיכוֹן וּבְחַיֵּי דְכָל בֵּית יִשְׂרָאֵל,
בַּעֲגָלָא וּבִזְמַן קָרִיב. וְאִמְרוּ: אָמֵן.

(.Cong – אָמֵן. יְהֵא שְׁמֵהּ רַבָּא מְבָרַךְ לְעָלַם וּלְעָלְמֵי עָלְמַיָּא.)

יְהֵא שְׁמֵהּ רַבָּא מְבָרַךְ לְעָלַם וּלְעָלְמֵי עָלְמַיָּא.

יִתְבָּרַךְ וְיִשְׁתַּבַּח וְיִתְפָּאַר וְיִתְרוֹמַם וְיִתְנַשֵּׂא וְיִתְהַדָּר וְיִתְעַלֶּה וְיִתְהַלָּל שְׁמֵהּ
דְּקֻדְשָׁא בְּרִיךְ הוּא (.Cong – בְּרִיךְ הוּא) – לְעֵלָּא מִן כָּל בִּרְכָתָא וְשִׁירָתָא
תֻּשְׁבְּחָתָא וְנֶחֱמָתָא, דַּאֲמִירָן בְּעָלְמָא, וְאִמְרוּ: אָמֵן. (.Cong – אָמֵן.)

שְׁמוֹנֶה עֶשְׂרֵה – עֲמִידָה

Take three steps backward, then three steps forward. Remain standing with the feet together while reciting *Shemoneh Esrei*. Recite it with quiet devotion and without interruption, verbal or otherwise. Although its recitation should not be audible to others, one must pray loudly enough to hear himself.

אֲדֹנָי שְׂפָתַי תִּפְתָּח, וּפִי יַגִּיד תְּהִלָּתֶךָ.

אבות

Bend the knees at בָּרוּךְ; bow at אַתָּה; straighten up at ה'.

בָּרוּךְ אַתָּה יהוה אֱלֹהֵינוּ וֵאלֹהֵי אֲבוֹתֵינוּ, אֱלֹהֵי אַבְרָהָם, אֱלֹהֵי
יִצְחָק, וֵאלֹהֵי יַעֲקֹב, הָאֵל הַגָּדוֹל הַגִּבּוֹר וְהַנּוֹרָא, אֵל
עֶלְיוֹן, גּוֹמֵל חֲסָדִים טוֹבִים וְקוֹנֵה הַכֹּל, וְזוֹכֵר חַסְדֵי אָבוֹת, וּמֵבִיא
גוֹאֵל לִבְנֵי בְנֵיהֶם, לְמַעַן שְׁמוֹ בְּאַהֲבָה. מֶלֶךְ עוֹזֵר וּמוֹשִׁיעַ וּמָגֵן.

Bend the knees at בָּרוּךְ; bow at אַתָּה; straighten up at ה'.

בָּרוּךְ אַתָּה יהוה, מָגֵן אַבְרָהָם.

גבורות

אַתָּה גִּבּוֹר לְעוֹלָם אֲדֹנָי, מְחַיֵּה מֵתִים אַתָּה, רַב לְהוֹשִׁיעַ.
מְכַלְכֵּל חַיִּים בְּחֶסֶד, מְחַיֵּה מֵתִים בְּרַחֲמִים רַבִּים, סוֹמֵךְ
נוֹפְלִים, וְרוֹפֵא חוֹלִים, וּמַתִּיר אֲסוּרִים, וּמְקַיֵּם אֱמוּנָתוֹ לִישֵׁנֵי
עָפָר. מִי כָמוֹךָ בַּעַל גְּבוּרוֹת, וּמִי דוֹמֶה לָּךְ, מֶלֶךְ מֵמִית וּמְחַיֶּה
וּמַצְמִיחַ יְשׁוּעָה. וְנֶאֱמָן אַתָּה לְהַחֲיוֹת מֵתִים. בָּרוּךְ אַתָּה יהוה,
מְחַיֵּה הַמֵּתִים.

קדושת השם

אַתָּה קָדוֹשׁ וְשִׁמְךָ קָדוֹשׁ, וּקְדוֹשִׁים בְּכָל יוֹם יְהַלְלוּךָ סֶּלָה.
בָּרוּךְ אַתָּה יהוה, הָאֵל הַקָּדוֹשׁ.

בינה

אַתָּה חוֹנֵן לְאָדָם דַּעַת, וּמְלַמֵּד לֶאֱנוֹשׁ בִּינָה. חָנֵּנוּ מֵאִתְּךָ דֵּעָה
בִּינָה וְהַשְׂכֵּל. בָּרוּךְ אַתָּה יהוה, חוֹנֵן הַדָּעַת.

The chazzan recites Half-Kaddish.

יִתְגַּדַּל *May His great Name grow exalted and sanctified* (Cong.— Amen.) *in the world that He created as He willed. May He give reign to His kingship in your lifetimes and in your days, and in the lifetimes of the entire Family of Israel, swiftly and soon. Now respond: Amen.*

(Cong.— Amen. May His great Name be blessed forever and ever.)

May His great Name be blessed forever and ever.

Blessed, praised, glorified, exalted, extolled, mighty, upraised, and lauded be the Name of the Holy One, Blessed is He (Cong.— Blessed is He) — *beyond any blessing and song, praise and consolation that are uttered in the world. Now respond: Amen.* (Cong.— Amen.)

⁘ SHEMONEH ESREI – AMIDAH ⁘

Take three steps backward, then three steps forward. Remain standing with the feet together while reciting Shemoneh Esrei. Recite it with quiet devotion and without interruption, verbal or otherwise. Although its recitation should not be audible to others, one must pray loudly enough to hear himself.

My Lord, open my lips, that my mouth may declare Your praise.[1]

PATRIARCHS

Bend the knees at 'Blessed'; bow at 'You'; straighten up at 'HASHEM.'

בָּרוּךְ *Blessed are You, HASHEM, our God and the God of our fore-fathers, God of Abraham, God of Isaac, and God of Jacob; the great, mighty, and awesome God, the supreme God, Who bestows beneficial kindnesses and creates everything, Who recalls the kindnesses of the Patriarchs and brings a Redeemer to their children's children, for His Name's sake, with love. O King, Helper, Savior, and Shield.*

Bend the knees at 'Blessed'; bow at 'You'; straighten up at 'HASHEM.'

Blessed are You, HASHEM, Shield of Abraham.

GOD'S MIGHT

אַתָּה *You are eternally mighty, my Lord, the Resuscitator of the dead are You; abundantly able to save. He sustains the living with kindness, resuscitates the dead with abundant mercy, supports the fallen, heals the sick, releases the confined, and maintains His faith to those asleep in the dust. Who is like You, O Master of mighty deeds, and who is comparable to You, O King Who causes death and restores life and makes salvation sprout! And You are faithful to resuscitate the dead. Blessed are You, HASHEM, Who resuscitates the dead.*

HOLINESS OF GOD'S NAME

אַתָּה *You are holy and Your Name is holy, and holy ones praise You every day, forever. Blessed are You, HASHEM, the holy God.*

INSIGHT

אַתָּה *You graciously endow man with wisdom and teach insight to a frail mortal. Endow us graciously from Yourself with wisdom, insight, and discernment. Blessed are You, HASHEM, gracious Giver of wisdom.*

---

(1) *Psalms* 51:17.

תשובה

הֲשִׁיבֵנוּ אָבִינוּ לְתוֹרָתֶךָ, וְקָרְבֵנוּ מַלְכֵּנוּ לַעֲבוֹדָתֶךָ, וְהַחֲזִירֵנוּ בִּתְשׁוּבָה שְׁלֵמָה לְפָנֶיךָ. בָּרוּךְ אַתָּה יהוה, הָרוֹצֶה בִּתְשׁוּבָה.

סליחה

Strike the left side of the chest with the right fist while reciting the words פְּשָׁעְנוּ and חָטָאנוּ.

סְלַח לָנוּ אָבִינוּ כִּי חָטָאנוּ, מְחַל לָנוּ מַלְכֵּנוּ כִּי פָשָׁעְנוּ, כִּי מוֹחֵל וְסוֹלֵחַ אָתָּה. בָּרוּךְ אַתָּה יהוה, חַנּוּן הַמַּרְבֶּה לִסְלוֹחַ.

גאולה

רְאֵה בְעָנְיֵנוּ, וְרִיבָה רִיבֵנוּ, וּגְאָלֵנוּ[1] מְהֵרָה לְמַעַן שְׁמֶךָ, כִּי גוֹאֵל חָזָק אָתָּה. בָּרוּךְ אַתָּה יהוה, גּוֹאֵל יִשְׂרָאֵל.

רפואה

רְפָאֵנוּ יהוה וְנֵרָפֵא, הוֹשִׁיעֵנוּ וְנִוָּשֵׁעָה, כִּי תְהִלָּתֵנוּ אָתָּה,[2] וְהַעֲלֵה רְפוּאָה שְׁלֵמָה לְכָל מַכּוֹתֵינוּ, °°כִּי אֵל מֶלֶךְ רוֹפֵא נֶאֱמָן וְרַחֲמָן אָתָּה. בָּרוּךְ אַתָּה יהוה, רוֹפֵא חוֹלֵי עַמּוֹ יִשְׂרָאֵל.

ברכת השנים

בָּרֵךְ עָלֵינוּ יהוה אֱלֹהֵינוּ אֶת הַשָּׁנָה הַזֹּאת וְאֶת כָּל מִינֵי תְבוּאָתָהּ לְטוֹבָה, וְתֵן בְּרָכָה עַל פְּנֵי הָאֲדָמָה, וְשַׂבְּעֵנוּ מִטּוּבֶךָ, וּבָרֵךְ שְׁנָתֵנוּ כַּשָּׁנִים הַטּוֹבוֹת. בָּרוּךְ אַתָּה יהוה, מְבָרֵךְ הַשָּׁנִים.

קיבוץ גליות

תְּקַע בְּשׁוֹפָר גָּדוֹל לְחֵרוּתֵנוּ, וְשָׂא נֵס לְקַבֵּץ גָּלֻיּוֹתֵינוּ, וְקַבְּצֵנוּ יַחַד מֵאַרְבַּע כַּנְפוֹת הָאָרֶץ.[3] בָּרוּךְ אַתָּה יהוה, מְקַבֵּץ נִדְחֵי עַמּוֹ יִשְׂרָאֵל.

דין

הָשִׁיבָה שׁוֹפְטֵינוּ כְּבָרִאשׁוֹנָה, וְיוֹעֲצֵינוּ כְּבַתְּחִלָּה,[4] וְהָסֵר מִמֶּנּוּ יָגוֹן וַאֲנָחָה, וּמְלוֹךְ עָלֵינוּ אַתָּה יהוה לְבַדְּךָ בְּחֶסֶד וּבְרַחֲמִים, וְצַדְּקֵנוּ בַּמִּשְׁפָּט. בָּרוּךְ אַתָּה יהוה, מֶלֶךְ אוֹהֵב צְדָקָה וּמִשְׁפָּט.

°°At this point one may interject a prayer for one who is ill:

יְהִי רָצוֹן מִלְּפָנֶיךָ יהוה אֱלֹהַי וֵאלֹהֵי אֲבוֹתַי, שֶׁתִּשְׁלַח מְהֵרָה רְפוּאָה שְׁלֵמָה מִן הַשָּׁמַיִם, רְפוּאַת הַנֶּפֶשׁ וּרְפוּאַת הַגּוּף

for a male—לַחוֹלֶה (patient's name) בֶּן (mother's name) בְּתוֹךְ שְׁאָר חוֹלֵי יִשְׂרָאֵל.
for a female—לַחוֹלָה (patient's name) בַּת (mother's name) בְּתוֹךְ שְׁאָר חוֹלֵי יִשְׂרָאֵל.
continue—כִּי אֵל . . .

REPENTANCE

הֲשִׁיבֵנוּ *Bring us back, our Father, to Your Torah, and bring us near,
our King, to Your service, and influence us to return in perfect
repentance before You. Blessed are You, HASHEM, Who desires
repentance.*

FORGIVENESS

Strike the left side of the chest with the right fist while reciting the words 'erred' and 'sinned.'

סְלַח *Forgive us, our Father, for we have erred; pardon us, our King,
for we have willfully sinned; for You pardon and forgive. Blessed
are You, HASHEM, the gracious One Who pardons abundantly.*

REDEMPTION

רְאֵה *Behold our affliction, take up our grievance, and redeem us[1]
speedily for Your Name's sake, for You are a powerful Redeemer.
Blessed are You, HASHEM, Redeemer of Israel.*

HEALTH AND HEALING

רְפָאֵנוּ *Heal us, HASHEM — then we will be healed; save us — then
we will be saved, for You are our praise.[2] Bring complete
recovery for all our ailments, °°for You are God, King, the faithful and
compassionate Healer. Blessed are You, HASHEM, Who heals the sick of
His people Israel.*

YEAR OF PROSPERITY

בָּרֵךְ *Bless on our behalf — O HASHEM, our God — this year and
all its kinds of crops for the best, and give a blessing on the face
of the earth, and satisfy us from Your bounty, and bless our year like the
best years. Blessed are You, HASHEM, Who blesses the years.*

INGATHERING OF EXILES

תְּקַע *Sound the great shofar for our freedom, raise the banner to
gather our exiles and gather us together from the four corners of
the earth.[3] Blessed are You, HASHEM, Who gathers in the dispersed of His
people Israel.*

RESTORATION OF JUSTICE

הָשִׁיבָה *Restore our judges as in earliest times and our counselors
as at first;[4] remove from us sorrow and groan; and reign over
us — You, HASHEM, alone — with kindness and compassion, and justify
us through judgment. Blessed are You, HASHEM, the King Who loves
righteousness and judgment.*

°°At this point one may interject a prayer for one who is ill:

*May it be Your will, HASHEM, my God, and the God of my forefathers, that You
quickly send a complete recovery from heaven, spiritual healing and physical
healing to the patient* (name) *son/daughter of* (mother's name) *among the other
patients of Israel.* Continue: For You are God . . .

---

(1) Cf. *Psalms* 119:153-154. (2) Cf. *Jeremiah* 17:14. (3) Cf. *Isaiah* 11:12. (4) Cf. 1:26.

ברכת המינים

וְלַמַּלְשִׁינִים אַל תְּהִי תִקְוָה, וְכָל הָרִשְׁעָה כְּרֶגַע תֹּאבֵד, וְכָל אֹיְבֶיךָ מְהֵרָה יִכָּרֵתוּ, וְהַזֵּדִים מְהֵרָה תְעַקֵּר וּתְשַׁבֵּר וּתְמַגֵּר וְתַכְנִיעַ בִּמְהֵרָה בְיָמֵינוּ. בָּרוּךְ אַתָּה יהוה, שׁוֹבֵר אֹיְבִים וּמַכְנִיעַ זֵדִים.

צדיקים

עַל הַצַּדִּיקִים וְעַל הַחֲסִידִים, וְעַל זִקְנֵי עַמְּךָ בֵּית יִשְׂרָאֵל, וְעַל פְּלֵיטַת סוֹפְרֵיהֶם, וְעַל גֵּרֵי הַצֶּדֶק וְעָלֵינוּ, יֶהֱמוּ רַחֲמֶיךָ יהוה אֱלֹהֵינוּ, וְתֵן שָׂכָר טוֹב לְכָל הַבּוֹטְחִים בְּשִׁמְךָ בֶּאֱמֶת, וְשִׂים חֶלְקֵנוּ עִמָּהֶם לְעוֹלָם, וְלֹא נֵבוֹשׁ כִּי בְךָ בָּטָחְנוּ. בָּרוּךְ אַתָּה יהוה, מִשְׁעָן וּמִבְטָח לַצַּדִּיקִים.

בנין ירושלים

וְלִירוּשָׁלַיִם עִירְךָ בְּרַחֲמִים תָּשׁוּב, וְתִשְׁכּוֹן בְּתוֹכָהּ כַּאֲשֶׁר דִּבַּרְתָּ, וּבְנֵה אוֹתָהּ בְּקָרוֹב בְּיָמֵינוּ בִּנְיַן עוֹלָם, וְכִסֵּא דָוִד מְהֵרָה לְתוֹכָהּ תָּכִין. בָּרוּךְ אַתָּה יהוה, בּוֹנֵה יְרוּשָׁלָיִם.

מלכות בית דוד

אֶת צֶמַח דָּוִד עַבְדְּךָ מְהֵרָה תַצְמִיחַ, וְקַרְנוֹ תָּרוּם בִּישׁוּעָתֶךָ, כִּי לִישׁוּעָתְךָ קִוִּינוּ כָּל הַיּוֹם. בָּרוּךְ אַתָּה יהוה, מַצְמִיחַ קֶרֶן יְשׁוּעָה.

קבלת תפלה

שְׁמַע קוֹלֵנוּ יהוה אֱלֹהֵינוּ, חוּס וְרַחֵם עָלֵינוּ, וְקַבֵּל בְּרַחֲמִים וּבְרָצוֹן אֶת תְּפִלָּתֵנוּ, כִּי אֵל שׁוֹמֵעַ תְּפִלּוֹת וְתַחֲנוּנִים אָתָּה. וּמִלְּפָנֶיךָ מַלְכֵּנוּ רֵיקָם אַל תְּשִׁיבֵנוּ,°°

°°During the silent *Shemoneh Esrei* one may insert either or both of these personal prayers.

For livelihood:	For forgiveness:

אַתָּה הוּא יהוה הָאֱלֹהִים, הַזָּן וּמְפַרְנֵס וּמְכַלְכֵּל מִקַּרְנֵי רְאֵמִים עַד בֵּיצֵי כִנִּים. הַטְרִיפֵנִי לֶחֶם חֻקִּי, וְהַמְצֵא לִי וּלְכָל בְּנֵי בֵיתִי מְזוֹנוֹתַי קוֹדֶם שֶׁאֶצְטָרֵךְ לָהֶם, בְּנַחַת וְלֹא בְצַעַר, בְּהֶתֵּר וְלֹא בְאִסּוּר, בְּכָבוֹד וְלֹא בְבִזָּיוֹן, לְחַיִּים וּלְשָׁלוֹם, מִשֶּׁפַע בְּרָכָה וְהַצְלָחָה, וּמִשֶּׁפַע בְּרָכָה עֶלְיוֹנָה, כְּדֵי שֶׁאוּכַל לַעֲשׂוֹת רְצוֹנֶךָ וְלַעֲסוֹק בְּתוֹרָתֶךָ וּלְקַיֵּם מִצְוֹתֶיךָ. וְאַל תַּצְרִיכֵנִי לִידֵי מַתְּנַת בָּשָׂר וָדָם. וִיקֻיַּם בִּי מִקְרָא שֶׁכָּתוּב: פּוֹתֵחַ אֶת יָדֶךָ, וּמַשְׂבִּיעַ לְכָל חַי רָצוֹן.[1] וְכָתוּב: הַשְׁלֵךְ עַל יהוה יְהָבְךָ וְהוּא יְכַלְכְּלֶךָ.[2]

אָנָּא יהוה, חָטָאתִי עָוִיתִי וּפָשַׁעְתִּי לְפָנֶיךָ, מִיּוֹם הֱיוֹתִי עַל הָאֲדָמָה עַד הַיּוֹם הַזֶּה (וּבִפְרָט בְּחֵטְא..........). אָנָּא יהוה, עֲשֵׂה לְמַעַן שִׁמְךָ הַגָּדוֹל, וּתְכַפֶּר לִי עַל עֲוֹנַי וַחֲטָאַי וּפְשָׁעַי שֶׁחָטָאתִי וְשֶׁעָוִיתִי וְשֶׁפָּשַׁעְתִּי לְפָנֶיךָ, מִנְּעוּרַי עַד הַיּוֹם הַזֶּה. וּתְמַלֵּא כָּל הַשֵּׁמוֹת שֶׁפָּגַמְתִּי בְּשִׁמְךָ הַגָּדוֹל.

Continue — כִּי אַתָּה ...

AGAINST HERETICS

וְלַמַּלְשִׁינִים *And for slanderers let there be no hope; and may all wickedness perish in an instant; and may all Your enemies be cut down speedily. May You speedily uproot, smash, cast down, and humble the wanton sinners — speedily in our days. Blessed are You, HASHEM, Who breaks enemies and humbles wanton sinners.*

THE RIGHTEOUS

עַל הַצַּדִּיקִים *On the righteous, on the devout, on the elders of Your people the Family of Israel, on the remnant of their scholars, on the righteous converts and on ourselves — may Your compassion be aroused, HASHEM, our God, and give goodly reward to all who sincerely believe in Your Name. Put our lot with them forever, and we will not feel ashamed, for we trust in You. Blessed are You, HASHEM, Mainstay and Assurance of the righteous.*

REBUILDING JERUSALEM

וְלִירוּשָׁלַיִם *And to Jerusalem, Your city, may You return in compassion, and may You rest within it, as You have spoken. May You rebuild it soon in our days as an eternal structure, and may You speedily establish the throne of David within it. Blessed are You, HASHEM, the Builder of Jerusalem.*

DAVIDIC REIGN

אֶת צֶמַח *The offspring of Your servant David may You speedily cause to flourish, and enhance his pride through Your salvation, for we hope for Your salvation all day long. Blessed are You, HASHEM, Who causes the pride of salvation to flourish.*

ACCEPTANCE OF PRAYER

שְׁמַע *Hear our voice, HASHEM our God, pity and be compassionate to us, and accept — with compassion and favor — our prayer, for God Who hears prayers and supplications are You. From before Yourself, our King, turn us not away empty-handed,°°*

°°*During the silent Shemoneh Esrei one may insert either or both of these personal prayers.*

For forgiveness:

אָנָּא *Please, O HASHEM, I have erred, been iniquitous, and willfully sinned before You, from the day I have existed on earth until this very day (and especially with the sin of . . .). Please, HASHEM, act for the sake of Your Great Name and grant me atonement for my iniquities, my errors, and my willful sins through which I have erred, been iniquitous, and willfully sinned before You, from my youth until this day. And make whole all the Names that I have blemished in Your Great Name.*

For livelihood:

אַתָּה *It is You, HASHEM the God, Who nourishes, sustains, and supports, from the horns of re'eimim to the eggs of lice. Provide me with my allotment of bread; and bring forth for me and all members of my household, my food, before I have need for it; in contentment but not in pain, in a permissible but not a forbidden manner, in honor but not in disgrace, for life and for peace; from the flow of blessing and success and from the flow of the Heavenly spring, so that I be enabled to do Your will and engage in Your Torah and fulfill Your commandments. Make me not needful of people's largesse; and may there be fulfilled in me the verse that states, 'You open Your hand and satisfy the desire of every living thing'[1] and that states, 'Cast Your burden upon HASHEM and He will support you.'[2]*

Continue: For You hear the prayer . . .

---

(1) *Psalms* 145:16. (2) 55:23.

כִּי אַתָּה שׁוֹמֵעַ תְּפִלַּת עַמְּךָ יִשְׂרָאֵל בְּרַחֲמִים. בָּרוּךְ אַתָּה יהוה, שׁוֹמֵעַ תְּפִלָּה.

עבודה

רְצֵה יהוה אֱלֹהֵינוּ בְּעַמְּךָ יִשְׂרָאֵל וּבִתְפִלָּתָם, וְהָשֵׁב אֶת הָעֲבוֹדָה לִדְבִיר בֵּיתֶךָ. וְאִשֵּׁי יִשְׂרָאֵל וּתְפִלָּתָם בְּאַהֲבָה תְקַבֵּל בְּרָצוֹן, וּתְהִי לְרָצוֹן תָּמִיד עֲבוֹדַת יִשְׂרָאֵל עַמֶּךָ.

וְתֶחֱזֶינָה עֵינֵינוּ בְּשׁוּבְךָ לְצִיּוֹן בְּרַחֲמִים. בָּרוּךְ אַתָּה יהוה, הַמַּחֲזִיר שְׁכִינָתוֹ לְצִיּוֹן.

הודאה

Bow at מוֹדִים; straighten up at ה'.

מוֹדִים אֲנַחְנוּ לָךְ שָׁאַתָּה הוּא יהוה אֱלֹהֵינוּ וֵאלֹהֵי אֲבוֹתֵינוּ לְעוֹלָם וָעֶד. צוּר חַיֵּינוּ, מָגֵן יִשְׁעֵנוּ אַתָּה הוּא לְדוֹר וָדוֹר. נוֹדֶה לְּךָ וּנְסַפֵּר תְּהִלָּתֶךָ[1] עַל חַיֵּינוּ הַמְּסוּרִים בְּיָדֶךָ, וְעַל נִשְׁמוֹתֵינוּ הַפְּקוּדוֹת לָךְ, וְעַל נִסֶּיךָ שֶׁבְּכָל יוֹם עִמָּנוּ, וְעַל נִפְלְאוֹתֶיךָ וְטוֹבוֹתֶיךָ שֶׁבְּכָל עֵת, עֶרֶב וָבֹקֶר וְצָהֳרָיִם. הַטּוֹב כִּי לֹא כָלוּ רַחֲמֶיךָ, וְהַמְרַחֵם כִּי לֹא תַמּוּ חֲסָדֶיךָ[2] מֵעוֹלָם קִוִּינוּ לָךְ. וְעַל כֻּלָּם יִתְבָּרַךְ וְיִתְרוֹמַם שִׁמְךָ מַלְכֵּנוּ תָּמִיד לְעוֹלָם וָעֶד.

Bend the knees at בָּרוּךְ; bow at אַתָּה; straighten up at ה'.

וְכֹל הַחַיִּים יוֹדוּךָ סֶּלָה, וִיהַלְלוּ אֶת שִׁמְךָ בֶּאֱמֶת, הָאֵל יְשׁוּעָתֵנוּ וְעֶזְרָתֵנוּ סֶלָה. בָּרוּךְ אַתָּה יהוה, הַטּוֹב שִׁמְךָ וּלְךָ נָאֶה לְהוֹדוֹת.

שלום

שָׁלוֹם רָב עַל יִשְׂרָאֵל עַמְּךָ תָּשִׂים לְעוֹלָם, כִּי אַתָּה הוּא מֶלֶךְ אָדוֹן לְכָל הַשָּׁלוֹם. וְטוֹב בְּעֵינֶיךָ לְבָרֵךְ אֶת עַמְּךָ יִשְׂרָאֵל, בְּכָל עֵת וּבְכָל שָׁעָה בִּשְׁלוֹמֶךָ. בָּרוּךְ אַתָּה יהוה, הַמְבָרֵךְ אֶת עַמּוֹ יִשְׂרָאֵל בַּשָּׁלוֹם.

יִהְיוּ לְרָצוֹן אִמְרֵי פִי וְהֶגְיוֹן לִבִּי לְפָנֶיךָ, יהוה צוּרִי וְגוֹאֲלִי[3].

אֱלֹהַי, נְצוֹר לְשׁוֹנִי מֵרָע, וּשְׂפָתַי מִדַּבֵּר מִרְמָה[4], וְלִמְקַלְלַי נַפְשִׁי תִדּוֹם, וְנַפְשִׁי כֶּעָפָר לַכֹּל תִּהְיֶה. פְּתַח לִבִּי בְּתוֹרָתֶךָ, וּבְמִצְוֹתֶיךָ תִּרְדּוֹף נַפְשִׁי. וְכָל הַחוֹשְׁבִים עָלַי רָעָה, מְהֵרָה הָפֵר עֲצָתָם וְקַלְקֵל מַחֲשַׁבְתָּם. עֲשֵׂה לְמַעַן שְׁמֶךָ, עֲשֵׂה לְמַעַן יְמִינֶךָ, עֲשֵׂה לְמַעַן קְדֻשָּׁתֶךָ, עֲשֵׂה לְמַעַן תּוֹרָתֶךָ. לְמַעַן יֵחָלְצוּן יְדִידֶיךָ, הוֹשִׁיעָה יְמִינְךָ וַעֲנֵנִי[5].

for You hear the prayer of Your people Israel with compassion. Blessed
are You, HASHEM, Who hears prayer.

TEMPLE SERVICE

רְצֵה Be favorable, HASHEM, our God, toward Your people Israel and
their prayer and restore the service to the Holy of Holies of Your
Temple. The fire-offerings of Israel and their prayer accept with love
and favor, and may the service of Your people Israel always be favorable
to You.

וְתֶחֱזֶינָה May our eyes behold Your return to Zion in compassion.
Blessed are You, HASHEM, Who restores His Presence to Zion.

THANKSGIVING [MODIM]
Bow at 'We gratefully thank You'; straighten up at 'HASHEM.'

מוֹדִים We gratefully thank You, for it is You Who are HASHEM, our
God and the God of our forefathers for all eternity; Rock of our
lives, Shield of our salvation are You from generation to generation. We
shall thank You and relate Your praise[1] — for our lives, which are
committed to Your power and for our souls that are entrusted to You; for
Your miracles that are with us every day; and for Your wonders and
favors in every season — evening, morning, and afternoon. The
Beneficent One, for Your compassions were never exhausted, and the
Compassionate One, for Your kindnesses never ended[2] — always have
we put our hope in You.

For all these, may Your Name be blessed and exalted, our King,
continually forever and ever.

Bend the knees at 'Blessed'; bow at 'You'; straighten up at 'HASHEM.'

Everything alive will gratefully acknowledge You, Selah! and praise
Your Name sincerely, O God of our salvation and help, Selah! Blessed are
You, HASHEM, Your Name is 'The Beneficent One' and to You it is fitting
to give thanks.

PEACE

שָׁלוֹם Establish abundant peace upon Your people Israel forever, for
You are King, Master of all peace. May it be good in Your eyes
to bless Your people Israel at every time and every hour with Your peace.
Blessed are You, HASHEM, Who blesses His people Israel with peace.

*May the expressions of my mouth and the thoughts of my heart
find favor before You, HASHEM, my Rock and my Redeemer.[3]*

אֱלֹהַי My God, guard my tongue from evil and my lips from speaking
deceitfully.[4] To those who curse me, let my soul be silent; and
let my soul be like dust to everyone. Open my heart to Your Torah,
then my soul will pursue Your commandments. As for all those who
design evil against me, speedily nullify their counsel and disrupt their
design. Act for Your Name's sake; act for Your right hand's sake; act
for Your sanctity's sake; act for Your Torah's sake. That Your beloved
ones may be given rest; let Your right hand save, and respond to me.[5]

(1) Cf. *Psalms* 79:13. (2) Cf. *Lamentations* 3:22. (2) *Psalms* 19:15. (4) Cf. 34:14. (5) 60:7; 108:7.

Some recite verses pertaining to their names here. See page 482.

יִהְיוּ לְרָצוֹן אִמְרֵי פִי וְהֶגְיוֹן לִבִּי לְפָנֶיךָ, יהוה צוּרִי וְגֹאֲלִי.¹

Bow and take three steps back.
Bow left and say . . . עֹשֶׂה; bow
right and say . . . הוּא יַעֲשֶׂה; bow
forward and say וְעַל כָּל . . . אָמֵן.

עֹשֶׂה שָׁלוֹם בִּמְרוֹמָיו, הוּא יַעֲשֶׂה שָׁלוֹם עָלֵינוּ, וְעַל כָּל יִשְׂרָאֵל. וְאִמְרוּ: אָמֵן.

יְהִי רָצוֹן מִלְּפָנֶיךָ יהוה אֱלֹהֵינוּ וֵאלֹהֵי אֲבוֹתֵינוּ, שֶׁיִּבָּנֶה בֵּית הַמִּקְדָּשׁ בִּמְהֵרָה בְיָמֵינוּ, וְתֵן חֶלְקֵנוּ בְּתוֹרָתֶךָ. וְשָׁם נַעֲבָדְךָ בְּיִרְאָה, כִּימֵי עוֹלָם וּכְשָׁנִים קַדְמוֹנִיּוֹת. וְעָרְבָה לַיהוה מִנְחַת יְהוּדָה וִירוּשָׁלָיִם, כִּימֵי עוֹלָם וּכְשָׁנִים קַדְמוֹנִיּוֹת.²

SHEMONEH ESREI ENDS HERE.

Remain standing in place for at least a few moments before taking three steps forward.

Chazzan recites קַדִּישׁ שָׁלֵם.

יִתְגַּדַּל וְיִתְקַדַּשׁ שְׁמֵהּ רַבָּא. (Cong. – אָמֵן.) בְּעָלְמָא דִּי בְרָא כִרְעוּתֵהּ. וְיַמְלִיךְ מַלְכוּתֵהּ, בְּחַיֵּיכוֹן וּבְיוֹמֵיכוֹן וּבְחַיֵּי דְכָל בֵּית יִשְׂרָאֵל, בַּעֲגָלָא וּבִזְמַן קָרִיב. וְאִמְרוּ: אָמֵן.

(Cong. – אָמֵן. יְהֵא שְׁמֵהּ רַבָּא מְבָרַךְ לְעָלַם וּלְעָלְמֵי עָלְמַיָּא.)

יְהֵא שְׁמֵהּ רַבָּא מְבָרַךְ לְעָלַם וּלְעָלְמֵי עָלְמַיָּא.

יִתְבָּרַךְ וְיִשְׁתַּבַּח וְיִתְפָּאַר וְיִתְרוֹמַם וְיִתְנַשֵּׂא וְיִתְהַדָּר וְיִתְעַלֶּה וְיִתְהַלָּל שְׁמֵהּ דְּקֻדְשָׁא בְּרִיךְ הוּא (Cong. – בְּרִיךְ הוּא) – לְעֵלָּא מִן כָּל בִּרְכָתָא וְשִׁירָתָא תֻּשְׁבְּחָתָא וְנֶחֱמָתָא, דַּאֲמִירָן בְּעָלְמָא. וְאִמְרוּ: אָמֵן. (Cong.– אָמֵן.)

(Cong. – קַבֵּל בְּרַחֲמִים וּבְרָצוֹן אֶת תְּפִלָּתֵנוּ.)

תִּתְקַבֵּל צְלוֹתְהוֹן וּבָעוּתְהוֹן דְּכָל בֵּית יִשְׂרָאֵל קֳדָם אֲבוּהוֹן דִּי בִשְׁמַיָּא. וְאִמְרוּ: אָמֵן. (Cong. – אָמֵן.)

(Cong. – יְהֵא שְׁמָא יהוה מְבֹרָךְ, מֵעַתָּה וְעַד עוֹלָם.³)

יְהֵא שְׁלָמָא רַבָּא מִן שְׁמַיָּא, וְחַיִּים עָלֵינוּ וְעַל כָּל יִשְׂרָאֵל. וְאִמְרוּ: אָמֵן. (Cong. – אָמֵן.)

(Cong. – עֶזְרִי מֵעִם יהוה, עֹשֵׂה שָׁמַיִם וָאָרֶץ.⁴)

Take three steps back. Bow left and say . . . עֹשֶׂה; bow right and say . . . הוּא; bow forward and say וְעַל כָּל . . . אָמֵן. Remain standing in place for a few moments, then take three steps forward.

עֹשֶׂה שָׁלוֹם בִּמְרוֹמָיו, הוּא יַעֲשֶׂה שָׁלוֹם עָלֵינוּ, וְעַל כָּל יִשְׂרָאֵל. וְאִמְרוּ: אָמֵן. (Cong. – אָמֵן.)

The congregation stands while reciting עָלֵינוּ.

עָלֵינוּ לְשַׁבֵּחַ לַאֲדוֹן הַכֹּל, לָתֵת גְּדֻלָּה לְיוֹצֵר בְּרֵאשִׁית, שֶׁלֹּא עָשָׂנוּ כְּגוֹיֵי הָאֲרָצוֹת, וְלֹא שָׂמָנוּ כְּמִשְׁפְּחוֹת הָאֲדָמָה. שֶׁלֹּא שָׂם חֶלְקֵנוּ כָּהֶם, וְגוֹרָלֵנוּ כְּכָל הֲמוֹנָם. (שֶׁהֵם מִשְׁתַּחֲוִים לְהֶבֶל וָרִיק, וּמִתְפַּלְּלִים אֶל אֵל לֹא יוֹשִׁיעַ.⁵) וַאֲנַחְנוּ כּוֹרְעִים וּמִשְׁתַּחֲוִים

Bow while reciting וַאֲנַחְנוּ כּוֹרְעִים וּמִשְׁתַּחֲוִים.

וּמוֹדִים, לִפְנֵי מֶלֶךְ מַלְכֵי הַמְּלָכִים הַקָּדוֹשׁ בָּרוּךְ הוּא. שֶׁהוּא נוֹטֶה שָׁמַיִם וְיֹסֵד אָרֶץ,⁶ וּמוֹשַׁב יְקָרוֹ בַּשָּׁמַיִם

Some recite verses pertaining to their names at this point. See page 482.

May the expressions of my mouth and the thoughts of my heart find favor before You, HASHEM, my Rock and my Redeemer.[1] He Who makes peace in His heights, may He make peace upon us, and upon all Israel. Now respond: Amen.

Bow and take three steps back. Bow left and say, 'He Who makes peace . . .'; bow right and say, 'may He make peace . . .'; bow forward and say, 'and upon . . . Amen.'

יְהִי רָצוֹן **May** it be Your will, HASHEM, our God and the God of our forefathers, that the Holy Temple be rebuilt, speedily in our days. Grant us our share in Your Torah, and may we serve You there with reverence, as in days of old and in former years. Then the offering of Judah and Jerusalem will be pleasing to HASHEM, as in days of old and in former years.[2]

SHEMONEH ESREI ENDS HERE.

Remain standing in place for at least a few moments before taking three steps forward.

Chazzan recites the Full Kaddish.

יִתְגַּדַּל **May** His great Name grow exalted and sanctified (Cong.— Amen.) in the world that He created as He willed. May He give reign to His kingship in your lifetimes and in your days, and in the lifetimes of the entire Family of Israel, swiftly and soon. Now respond: Amen.

(Cong.— Amen. May His great Name be blessed forever and ever.)

May His great Name be blessed forever and ever.

Blessed, praised, glorified, exalted, extolled, mighty, upraised, and lauded be the Name of the Holy One, Blessed is He (Cong.— Blessed is He) — beyond any blessing and song, praise and consolation that are uttered in the world. Now respond: Amen. (Cong.— Amen.)

(Cong.— Accept our prayers with mercy and favor.)

May the prayers and supplications of the entire Family of Israel be accepted before their Father Who is in Heaven. Now respond: Amen. (Cong.— Amen.)

(Cong.— Blessed be the Name of HASHEM, from this time and forever.[3])

May there be abundant peace from Heaven, and life, upon us and upon all Israel. Now respond: Amen. (Cong.— Amen.)

(Cong.— My help is from HASHEM, Maker of heaven and earth.[4])

Take three steps back. Bow left and say, 'He Who makes peace . . .';
bow right and say, 'may He . . .'; bow forward and say, 'and upon all Israel . . .'
Remain standing in place for a few moments, then take three steps forward.

He Who makes peace in His heights, may He make peace upon us, and upon all Israel. Now respond: Amen. (Cong.— Amen.)

The congregation stands while reciting עָלֵינוּ, 'It is our duty . . .'

עָלֵינוּ **It** is our duty to praise the Master of all, to ascribe greatness to the Molder of primeval creation, for He has not made us like the nations of the lands, and has not emplaced us like the families of the earth; for He has not assigned our portion like theirs nor our lot like all their multitudes. (For they bow to vanity and emptiness and pray to a god which helps not.[5]) But we bend our knees, bow, and acknowledge our thanks before the King Who reigns over kings, the Holy One, Blessed is He. He stretches out heaven and establishes earth's foundation,[6] the seat of His homage is in the heav-

Bow while reciting 'But we bend our knees.'

---

(1) Psalms 19:15. (2) Malachi 3:4. (3) Psalms 113:2.
(4) 121:2. (5) Isaiah 45:20. (6) 51:13.

מִמַּעַל, וּשְׁכִינַת עֻזּוֹ בְּגָבְהֵי מְרוֹמִים. הוּא אֱלֹהֵינוּ, אֵין עוֹד. אֱמֶת
מַלְכֵּנוּ, אֶפֶס זוּלָתוֹ, כַּכָּתוּב בְּתוֹרָתוֹ: וְיָדַעְתָּ הַיּוֹם וַהֲשֵׁבֹתָ אֶל
לְבָבֶךָ, כִּי יהוה הוּא הָאֱלֹהִים בַּשָּׁמַיִם מִמַּעַל וְעַל הָאָרֶץ מִתָּחַת,
אֵין עוֹד.[1]

עַל כֵּן נְקַוֶּה לְּךָ יהוה אֱלֹהֵינוּ לִרְאוֹת מְהֵרָה בְּתִפְאֶרֶת עֻזֶּךָ,
לְהַעֲבִיר גִּלּוּלִים מִן הָאָרֶץ, וְהָאֱלִילִים כָּרוֹת יִכָּרֵתוּן,
לְתַקֵּן עוֹלָם בְּמַלְכוּת שַׁדַּי. וְכָל בְּנֵי בָשָׂר יִקְרְאוּ בִשְׁמֶךָ, לְהַפְנוֹת
אֵלֶיךָ כָּל רִשְׁעֵי אָרֶץ. יַכִּירוּ וְיֵדְעוּ כָּל יוֹשְׁבֵי תֵבֵל, כִּי לְךָ תִּכְרַע
כָּל בֶּרֶךְ, תִּשָּׁבַע כָּל לָשׁוֹן.[2] לְפָנֶיךָ יהוה אֱלֹהֵינוּ יִכְרְעוּ וְיִפֹּלוּ,
וְלִכְבוֹד שִׁמְךָ יְקָר יִתֵּנוּ. וִיקַבְּלוּ כֻלָּם אֶת עוֹל מַלְכוּתֶךָ, וְתִמְלֹךְ
עֲלֵיהֶם מְהֵרָה לְעוֹלָם וָעֶד. כִּי הַמַּלְכוּת שֶׁלְּךָ הִיא וּלְעוֹלְמֵי עַד
תִּמְלוֹךְ בְּכָבוֹד, כַּכָּתוּב בְּתוֹרָתֶךָ: יהוה יִמְלֹךְ לְעֹלָם וָעֶד.[3]
✧ וְנֶאֱמַר: וְהָיָה יהוה לְמֶלֶךְ עַל כָּל הָאָרֶץ, בַּיּוֹם הַהוּא יִהְיֶה יהוה
אֶחָד וּשְׁמוֹ אֶחָד.[4]

אַל תִּירָא מִפַּחַד פִּתְאֹם, וּמִשֹּׁאַת רְשָׁעִים כִּי תָבֹא.[5] עֻצוּ עֵצָה
וְתֻפָר, דַּבְּרוּ דָבָר וְלֹא יָקוּם, כִּי עִמָּנוּ אֵל.[6] וְעַד זִקְנָה אֲנִי
הוּא, וְעַד שֵׂיבָה אֲנִי אֶסְבֹּל, אֲנִי עָשִׂיתִי וַאֲנִי אֶשָּׂא, וַאֲנִי אֶסְבֹּל וַאֲמַלֵּט.[7]

קדיש יתום

.קַדִּישׁ יָתוֹם Mourners recite

יִתְגַּדַּל וְיִתְקַדַּשׁ שְׁמֵהּ רַבָּא. (.Cong – אָמֵן.) בְּעָלְמָא דִּי בְרָא כִרְעוּתֵהּ.
וְיַמְלִיךְ מַלְכוּתֵהּ, בְּחַיֵּיכוֹן וּבְיוֹמֵיכוֹן וּבְחַיֵּי דְכָל בֵּית יִשְׂרָאֵל,
בַּעֲגָלָא וּבִזְמַן קָרִיב. וְאִמְרוּ: אָמֵן.

(.Cong – אָמֵן. יְהֵא שְׁמֵהּ רַבָּא מְבָרַךְ לְעָלַם וּלְעָלְמֵי עָלְמַיָּא.)

יְהֵא שְׁמֵהּ רַבָּא מְבָרַךְ לְעָלַם וּלְעָלְמֵי עָלְמַיָּא.

יִתְבָּרַךְ וְיִשְׁתַּבַּח וְיִתְפָּאַר וְיִתְרוֹמַם וְיִתְנַשֵּׂא וְיִתְהַדָּר וְיִתְעַלֶּה וְיִתְהַלָּל
שְׁמֵהּ דְּקֻדְשָׁא בְּרִיךְ הוּא (.Cong – בְּרִיךְ הוּא) – לְעֵלָּא מִן כָּל בִּרְכָתָא
וְשִׁירָתָא תֻּשְׁבְּחָתָא וְנֶחֱמָתָא, דַּאֲמִירָן בְּעָלְמָא. וְאִמְרוּ: אָמֵן. (.Cong – אָמֵן.)
יְהֵא שְׁלָמָא רַבָּא מִן שְׁמַיָּא, וְחַיִּים עָלֵינוּ וְעַל כָּל יִשְׂרָאֵל. וְאִמְרוּ:
אָמֵן. (.Cong – אָמֵן.)

Take three steps back. Bow left and say . . . עֹשֶׂה; bow right and say . . . הוּא; bow forward and say
וְעַל כָּל . . . אָמֵן. Remain standing in place for a few moments, then take three steps forward.

עֹשֶׂה שָׁלוֹם בִּמְרוֹמָיו, הוּא יַעֲשֶׂה שָׁלוֹם עָלֵינוּ, וְעַל כָּל יִשְׂרָאֵל.
וְאִמְרוּ: אָמֵן. (.Cong – אָמֵן.)

---

(1) *Deuteronomy* 4:39. (2) Cf. *Isaiah* 45:23. (3) *Exodus* 15:18.
(4) *Zechariah* 14:9. (5) *Proverbs* 3:25. (6) *Isaiah* 8:10. (7) 46:4.

ens above and His powerful Presence is in the loftiest heights. He is our God and there is none other. True is our King, there is nothing beside Him, as it is written in His Torah: 'You are to know this day and take to your heart that HASHEM is the only God — in heaven above and on the earth below — there is none other.'[1]

עַל כֵּן Therefore we put our hope in You, HASHEM, our God, that we may soon see Your mighty splendor, to remove detestable idolatry from the earth, and false gods will be utterly cut off, to perfect the universe through the Almighty's sovereignty. Then all humanity will call upon Your Name, to turn all the earth's wicked toward You. All the world's inhabitants will recognize and know that to You every knee should bend, every tongue should swear.[2] Before You, HASHEM, our God, they will bend every knee and cast themselves down and to the glory of Your Name they will render homage, and they will all accept upon themselves the yoke of Your kingship that You may reign over them soon and eternally. For the kingdom is Yours and You will reign for all eternity in glory as it is written in Your Torah: HASHEM shall reign for all eternity.[3] Chazzan— And it is said: HASHEM will be King over all the world — on that day HASHEM will be One and His Name will be One.[4]

אַל תִּירָא Do not fear sudden terror, or the holocaust of the wicked when it comes.[5] Plan a conspiracy and it will be annulled; speak your piece and it shall not stand, for God is with us.[6] Even till your seniority, I remain unchanged; and even till your ripe old age, I shall endure. I created you and I shall bear you; I shall endure and rescue.[7]

MOURNER'S KADDISH

In the presence of a *minyan*, mourners recite קַדִּישׁ יָתוֹם, the Mourner's *Kaddish* (see *Laws* 132-134).
[A transliteration of this *Kaddish* appears on page 486.]

יִתְגַּדַּל May His great Name grow exalted and sanctified (Cong.— Amen.) in the world that He created as He willed. May He give reign to His kingship in your lifetimes and in your days, and in the lifetimes of the entire Family of Israel, swiftly and soon. Now respond: Amen.

(Cong.— Amen. May His great Name be blessed forever and ever.)
May His great Name be blessed forever and ever.

Blessed, praised, glorified, exalted, extolled, mighty, upraised, and lauded be the Name of the Holy One, Blessed is He (Cong.— Blessed is He) — beyond any blessing and song, praise and consolation that are uttered in the world. Now respond: Amen. (Cong.— Amen.)

May there be abundant peace from Heaven, and life, upon us and upon all Israel. Now respond: Amen. (Cong.— Amen.)

Take three steps back. Bow left and say, 'He Who makes peace . . .';
bow right and say, 'may He . . .'; bow forward and say, 'and upon all Israel . . .'
Remain standing in place for a few moments, then take three steps forward.

He Who makes peace in His heights, may He make peace upon us, and upon all Israel. Now respond: Amen. (Cong.— Amen.)

❖ הבדלה ❖

When Tishah B'Av falls on Sunday Havdalah is recited. Spices and a flame are not used.

סַבְרִי מָרָנָן וְרַבָּנָן וְרַבּוֹתַי:

בָּרוּךְ אַתָּה יהוה אֱלֹהֵינוּ מֶלֶךְ הָעוֹלָם, בּוֹרֵא פְּרִי הַגָּפֶן.

(אָמֵן. –all present respond)

בָּרוּךְ אַתָּה יהוה אֱלֹהֵינוּ מֶלֶךְ הָעוֹלָם, הַמַּבְדִּיל בֵּין קֹדֶשׁ לְחוֹל,

בֵּין אוֹר לְחֹשֶׁךְ, בֵּין יִשְׂרָאֵל לָעַמִּים, בֵּין יוֹם הַשְּׁבִיעִי

לְשֵׁשֶׁת יְמֵי הַמַּעֲשֶׂה. בָּרוּךְ אַתָּה יהוה, הַמַּבְדִּיל בֵּין קֹדֶשׁ לְחוֹל.

(אָמֵן. –all present respond)

The one who recited Havdalah, or someone else present for Havdalah,
should drink most of the wine from the cup.

❖ קידוש לבנה ❖

תהלים קמח:א-ו

הַלְלוּיָהּ, הַלְלוּ אֶת יהוה מִן הַשָּׁמַיִם, הַלְלוּהוּ בַּמְּרוֹמִים. הַלְלוּהוּ

כָל מַלְאָכָיו, הַלְלוּהוּ כָּל צְבָאָיו. הַלְלוּהוּ שֶׁמֶשׁ וְיָרֵחַ,

הַלְלוּהוּ כָּל כּוֹכְבֵי אוֹר. הַלְלוּהוּ שְׁמֵי הַשָּׁמָיִם, וְהַמַּיִם אֲשֶׁר מֵעַל

הַשָּׁמָיִם. יְהַלְלוּ אֶת שֵׁם יהוה, כִּי הוּא צִוָּה וְנִבְרָאוּ. וַיַּעֲמִידֵם לָעַד

לְעוֹלָם, חָק נָתַן וְלֹא יַעֲבוֹר. הֲרֵינִי מוּכָן וּמְזוּמָּן לְקַיֵּם הַמִּצְוָה לְקַדֵּשׁ

הַלְּבָנָה. לְשֵׁם יִחוּד קֻדְשָׁא בְּרִיךְ הוּא וּשְׁכִינְתֵּיהּ עַל יְדֵי הַהוּא טָמִיר

וְנֶעְלָם, בְּשֵׁם כָּל יִשְׂרָאֵל.

One should look at the moon before reciting this blessing:

בָּרוּךְ אַתָּה יהוה, אֱלֹהֵינוּ מֶלֶךְ הָעוֹלָם, אֲשֶׁר בְּמַאֲמָרוֹ בָּרָא

שְׁחָקִים, וּבְרוּחַ פִּיו כָּל צְבָאָם. חֹק וּזְמַן נָתַן לָהֶם שֶׁלֹּא יְשַׁנּוּ

אֶת תַּפְקִידָם. שָׂשִׂים וּשְׂמֵחִים לַעֲשׂוֹת רְצוֹן קוֹנָם, פּוֹעֵל אֱמֶת שֶׁפְּעֻלָּתוֹ

אֱמֶת. וְלַלְּבָנָה אָמַר שֶׁתִּתְחַדֵּשׁ עֲטֶרֶת תִּפְאֶרֶת לַעֲמוּסֵי בָטֶן, שֶׁהֵם

עֲתִידִים לְהִתְחַדֵּשׁ כְּמוֹתָהּ, וּלְפָאֵר לְיוֹצְרָם עַל שֵׁם כְּבוֹד מַלְכוּתוֹ. בָּרוּךְ

אַתָּה יהוה, מְחַדֵּשׁ חֳדָשִׁים.

Recite three times – בָּרוּךְ יוֹצְרֵךְ, בָּרוּךְ עוֹשֵׂךְ, בָּרוּךְ קוֹנֵךְ, בָּרוּךְ בּוֹרְאֵךְ.

Upon reciting the next verse, rise on the toes as if in dance:

Recite three times – כְּשֵׁם שֶׁאֲנִי רוֹקֵד כְּנֶגְדֵּךְ וְאֵינִי יָכוֹל לִנְגּוֹעַ בָּךְ כָּךְ

לֹא יוּכְלוּ כָּל אוֹיְבַי לִנְגּוֹעַ בִּי לְרָעָה.

Recite three times – תִּפֹּל עֲלֵיהֶם אֵימָתָה וָפַחַד, בִּגְדֹל זְרוֹעֲךָ יִדְּמוּ כָּאָבֶן.¹

Recite three times – כָּאָבֶן יִדְּמוּ זְרוֹעֲךָ בִּגְדֹל וָפַחַד אֵימָתָה עֲלֵיהֶם תִּפֹּל.

◆§ Laws of Kiddush Levanah

It is preferable that *Kiddush Levanah* be recited: (a) under the open sky; (b) with a *minyan*;

(c) at the departure of the Sabbath. When these optimal conditions are not feasible, they may be waived (e.g., a shut-in may recite it indoors if he

⁓❴ HAVDALAH ❵⁓

When Tishah B'Av falls on Sunday *Havdalah* is recited. Spices and a flame are not used.

By your leave, my masters and teachers:

בָּרוּךְ *Blessed are You, HASHEM, our God, King of the universe, Who creates the fruit of the vine.* (All present respond— Amen.)

בָּרוּךְ *Blessed are You, HASHEM our God, King of the universe, Who separates between holy and secular, between light and darkness, between Israel and the nations, between the seventh day and the six days of labor. Blessed are You, HASHEM, Who separates between holy and secular.* (All present respond— Amen.)

The one who recited *Havdalah*, or someone else present for *Havdalah*, should drink most of the wine from the cup.

⁓❴ SANCTIFICATION OF THE MOON/KIDDUSH LEVANAH ❵⁓

Psalms 148:1-6

הַלְלוּיָהּ *Halleluyah! Praise HASHEM from the heavens; praise Him in the heights. Praise Him, all His angels; praise Him, all His legions. Praise Him, sun and moon; praise Him, all bright stars. Praise Him, the most exalted of the heavens and the waters that are above the heavens. Let them praise the Name of HASHEM, for He commanded and they were created. And He established them forever and ever, He issued a decree that will not change. Behold I am prepared and ready to perform the commandment to sanctify the moon. For the sake of the unification of the Holy One, Blessed is He, and His Presence, through Him Who is hidden and inscrutable — [I pray] in the name of all Israel.*

One should look at the moon before reciting this blessing:

בָּרוּךְ *Blessed are You, HASHEM, our God, King of the Universe, Who with His utterance created the heavens, and with the breath of His mouth all their legion. A decree and a schedule did He give them that they not alter their assigned task. They are joyous and glad to perform the will of their Owner — the Worker of truth Whose work is truth. To the moon He said that it should renew itself, which will be a crown of splendor for those borne [by Him] from the womb, those who are destined to renew themselves like it, and to glorify their Molder for the name of His glorious kingdom. Blessed are You, HASHEM, Who renews the months.*

Recite three times — *Blessed is your Molder; blessed is your Maker; blessed is your Owner; blessed is your Creator.*

Upon reciting the next verse, rise on the toes as if in dance:

Recite three times — *Just as I dance toward you but cannot touch you, so may none of my enemies be able to touch me for evil.*

Recite three times — *Let fall upon them fear and terror; at the greatness of Your arm, let them be still as stone.*[1]

Recite three times — *As stone let them be still, at Your arm's greatness; terror and fear, upon them let fall.*

---

(1) *Exodus* 15:16.

---

can see the moon through a window or door; one who cannot form a *minyan*; the sky is cloudy at the departure of the Sabbath).

The earliest time for reciting *Kiddush Levanah* is seventy-two hours after the *molad* (new moon), although some authorities delay its recitation until seven full days after the *molad*. The latest

time is mid-month, i.e., fourteen days, eighteen hours and twenty-two minutes (some authorities extend this limit to fifteen full days) after the *molad*. Those who follow the latter opinion do not recite *Kiddush Levanah* during the month of Sivan until after Shavuos.

Kiddush Levanah should not be recited on a

דָּוִד מֶלֶךְ יִשְׂרָאֵל חַי וְקַיָּם. — Recite three times

שָׁלוֹם עֲלֵיכֶם — Extend greetings to three different people

עֲלֵיכֶם שָׁלוֹם. — who, in turn, respond

סִמָּן טוֹב וּמַזָּל טוֹב יְהֵא לָנוּ וּלְכָל יִשְׂרָאֵל. אָמֵן. — Recite three times

קוֹל דּוֹדִי הִנֵּה זֶה בָּא מְדַלֵּג עַל הֶהָרִים מְקַפֵּץ עַל הַגְּבָעוֹת. דּוֹמֶה דוֹדִי לִצְבִי אוֹ לְעֹפֶר הָאַיָּלִים הִנֵּה זֶה עוֹמֵד אַחַר כָּתְלֵנוּ, מַשְׁגִּיחַ מִן הַחַלֹּנוֹת, מֵצִיץ מִן הַחֲרַכִּים.[1]

תהלים קכא

שִׁיר לַמַּעֲלוֹת, אֶשָּׂא עֵינַי אֶל הֶהָרִים, מֵאַיִן יָבֹא עֶזְרִי. עֶזְרִי מֵעִם יהוה, עֹשֵׂה שָׁמַיִם וָאָרֶץ. אַל יִתֵּן לַמּוֹט רַגְלֶךָ, אַל יָנוּם שֹׁמְרֶךָ. הִנֵּה לֹא יָנוּם וְלֹא יִישָׁן, שׁוֹמֵר יִשְׂרָאֵל. יהוה שֹׁמְרֶךָ, יהוה צִלְּךָ עַל יַד יְמִינֶךָ. יוֹמָם הַשֶּׁמֶשׁ לֹא יַכֶּכָּה וְיָרֵחַ בַּלָּיְלָה. יהוה יִשְׁמָרְךָ מִכָּל רָע, יִשְׁמֹר אֶת נַפְשֶׁךָ. יהוה יִשְׁמָר צֵאתְךָ וּבוֹאֶךָ, מֵעַתָּה וְעַד עוֹלָם.

תהלים קנ

הַלְלוּיָהּ, הַלְלוּ אֵל בְּקָדְשׁוֹ, הַלְלוּהוּ בִּרְקִיעַ עֻזּוֹ. הַלְלוּהוּ בִגְבוּרֹתָיו, הַלְלוּהוּ כְּרֹב גֻּדְלוֹ. הַלְלוּהוּ בְּתֵקַע שׁוֹפָר, הַלְלוּהוּ בְּנֵבֶל וְכִנּוֹר. הַלְלוּהוּ בְּתֹף וּמָחוֹל, הַלְלוּהוּ בְּמִנִּים וְעֻגָב. הַלְלוּהוּ בְצִלְצְלֵי שָׁמַע, הַלְלוּהוּ בְּצִלְצְלֵי תְרוּעָה. כֹּל הַנְּשָׁמָה תְּהַלֵּל יָהּ, הַלְלוּיָהּ.

תָּנָא דְּבֵי רַבִּי יִשְׁמָעֵאל: אִלְמָלֵי לֹא זָכוּ יִשְׂרָאֵל אֶלָּא לְהַקְבִּיל פְּנֵי אֲבִיהֶם שֶׁבַּשָּׁמַיִם פַּעַם אַחַת בַּחֹדֶשׁ, דַּיָּם. אָמַר אַבַּיֵּי: הִלְכָּךְ צָרִיךְ לְמֵימְרָא מְעֻמָּד. מִי זֹאת עֹלָה מִן הַמִּדְבָּר מִתְרַפֶּקֶת עַל דּוֹדָהּ.[2]

וִיהִי רָצוֹן מִלְּפָנֶיךָ יהוה אֱלֹהַי וֵאלֹהֵי אֲבוֹתַי, לְמַלֹּאות פְּגִימַת הַלְּבָנָה, וְלֹא יִהְיֶה בָּהּ שׁוּם מִעוּט, וִיהִי אוֹר הַלְּבָנָה כְּאוֹר הַחַמָּה, וּכְאוֹר שִׁבְעַת יְמֵי בְרֵאשִׁית[4] כְּמוֹ שֶׁהָיְתָה קֹדֶם מִעוּטָהּ, שֶׁנֶּאֱמַר: אֶת שְׁנֵי הַמְּאֹרֹת הַגְּדֹלִים.[4] וְיִתְקַיֵּם בָּנוּ מִקְרָא שֶׁכָּתוּב: וּבִקְשׁוּ אֶת יהוה אֱלֹהֵיהֶם, וְאֵת דָּוִיד מַלְכָּם.[5] אָמֵן.

תהלים סז

לַמְנַצֵּחַ בִּנְגִינֹת מִזְמוֹר שִׁיר. אֱלֹהִים יְחָנֵּנוּ וִיבָרְכֵנוּ, יָאֵר פָּנָיו אִתָּנוּ סֶלָה. לָדַעַת בָּאָרֶץ דַּרְכֶּךָ, בְּכָל גּוֹיִם יְשׁוּעָתֶךָ. יוֹדוּךָ עַמִּים אֱלֹהִים, יוֹדוּךָ עַמִּים כֻּלָּם. יִשְׂמְחוּ וִירַנְּנוּ לְאֻמִּים, כִּי תִשְׁפֹּט עַמִּים מִישׁוֹר, וּלְאֻמִּים בָּאָרֶץ תַּנְחֵם סֶלָה. יוֹדוּךָ עַמִּים אֱלֹהִים, יוֹדוּךָ עַמִּים כֻּלָּם. אֶרֶץ נָתְנָה יְבוּלָהּ, יְבָרְכֵנוּ אֱלֹהִים אֱלֹהֵינוּ. יְבָרְכֵנוּ אֱלֹהִים, וְיִירְאוּ אוֹתוֹ כָּל אַפְסֵי אָרֶץ.

In most congregations, עָלֵינוּ (page 462), followed by the Mourner's *Kaddish,* is recited at this point.

Recite three times — *David, King of Israel, is alive and enduring.*
Extend greetings to three different people — *Peace upon you—*
who, in turn, respond — *Upon you, peace.*
Recite three times — *May there be a good sign and a good fortune for us and for all Israel. Amen.*

קוֹל *The voice of my beloved — Behold! It came suddenly, leaping over mountains, skipping over hills. My beloved is like a gazelle or a young hart. Behold! He was standing behind our wall, observing through the windows, peering through the lattices.*[1]

Psalm 121

שִׁיר לַמַּעֲלוֹת *A song to the ascents. I raise my eyes to the mountains; whence will come my help? My help is from HASHEM, Maker of heaven and earth. He will not allow your foot to falter; your Guardian will not slumber. Behold, He neither slumbers nor sleeps — the Guardian of Israel. HASHEM is your Guardian; HASHEM is your Shade at your right hand. By day the sun will not harm you, nor the moon by night. HASHEM will protect you from every evil; He will guard your soul. HASHEM will guard your departure and your arrival, from this time and forever.*

Psalm 150

הַלְלוּיָהּ *Halleluyah! Praise God in His Sanctuary; praise Him in the firmament of His power. Praise Him for His mighty acts; praise Him as befits His abundant greatness. Praise Him with the blast of the shofar; praise Him with lyre and harp. Praise Him with drum and dance; praise Him with organ and flute. Praise Him with clanging cymbals; praise him with resonant trumpets. Let all souls praise God, Halleluyah!*

תָּנָא *The Academy of Rabbi Yishmael taught: Had Israel not been privileged to greet the countenance of their Father in Heaven except for once a month — it would have sufficed them. Abaye said: Therefore one must recite it while standing. Who is this who rises from the desert clinging to her Beloved?*[2] *May it be Your will, HASHEM, my God and the God of my forefathers, to fill the flaw of the moon that there be no diminution in it. May the light of the moon be like the light of the sun and like the light of the seven days of creation,*[3] *as it was before it was diminished, as it is said: 'The two great luminaries.'*[4] *And may there be fulfilled upon us the verse that is written: They shall seek HASHEM, their God, and David, their king.*[5] *Amen.*

Psalm 67

לַמְנַצֵּחַ *For the Conductor, upon Neginos, a psalm, a song. May God favor us and bless us, may He illuminate His countenance with us, Selah. To make known Your way on earth, among all the nations Your salvation. The peoples will acknowledge You, O God, the peoples will acknowledge You, all of them. Nations will be glad and sing for joy, because You will judge the peoples fairly and guide the nations on earth, Selah. Then peoples will acknowledge You, O God, the peoples will acknowledge You, all of them. The earth has yielded its produce, may God, our own God, bless us. May God bless us and may all the ends of the earth fear Him.*

In most congregations, *Aleinu* (page 462), followed by the Mourner's *Kaddish*, is recited at this point.

---

(1) *Song of Songs* 2:8-9. (2) 8:5. (3) Cf. *Isaiah* 30:26. (4) *Genesis* 1:16. (5) *Hosea* 3:5.

Sabbath or a Festival unless it is the last remaining night before the mid-month deadline.
    If one cannot recite *Kiddush Levanah* with a minyan, he should try to do so in the presence of at least three others. If this, too, is not possible, he may recite it by himself.

✑§ Selected Tishah B'Av Laws and Customs

compiled by Rabbi Hersh Goldwurm

Although most of the applicable laws are cited in the main text of the prayers, in some cases they are too involved or too lengthy to be given fully where they apply. A selection of such laws is compiled here. This digest cannot cover all eventualities and should be regarded merely as a guide; in case of doubt, one should consult a competent halachic authority. When a particular *halachah* is in dispute, we generally follow the ruling of the *Mishnah Berurah*. On occasion, however (usually when *Mishnah Berurah* does not give a definitive ruling or when a significant number of congregations do not follow *Mishnah Berurah's* ruling), we cite more than one opinion. As a general rule, each congregation is bound by its tradition and the ruling of its authorities.

These laws and customs have been culled, in the main, from the most widely accepted authorities: the *Shulchan Aruch Orach Chaim* [here abbreviated *O.C.*] and *Mishnah Berurah* [*M.B.*]. We have also included many of the general laws of prayer that also apply to Tishah B'Av. They are meant only as a learning and familiarizing tool. For halachic questions, one should consult the *Shulchan Aruch* and its commentaries and/or a halachic authority.

EREV TISHAH B'AV — TISHAH B'AV EVE

✑§ The Afternoon

1. The afternoon before the Tishah B'Av fast takes on some of the mourning aspects of the fast day itself. One should not go on a pleasure trip or even on a pleasurable stroll. [Rather, one should devote his time to reflect on the theme of the upcoming day.] (*Rama O.C.* 553:2).

2. Similarly, from the hour of noon before the fast it is customary to learn only the Torah subjects that one may learn on Tishah B'Av itself (see §38), i.e. matters that pertain to the fast or to mourning. Therefore, even when Tishah B'Av falls on the Sabbath (so that the fast is observed on Sunday) or Sunday, it is customary to refrain from learning matters other than those permitted on Tishah B'Av on the Sabbath afternoon before the fast; the recitation of *Pirkei Avos* is deferred to the following week (*Rama O.C.* 553:2). However, many *poskim* point out that the custom has no Talmudic basis and argue that it is better to study whatever Torah subjects one wishes, rather than to desist from learning altogether. Therefore if one wishes to be lenient in this matter we do not deter him (*M.B.* 553:8).

✑§ Minchah

3. The *Minchah* prayer should be recited early enough to allow time to eat a small meal — the *se'udah hamafsekes* (see §5) — between the prayer and the beginning of the fast.

4. *Minchah* is recited in the usual manner, *Tachanun* is omitted. Since Tishah B'Av itself has the status of a quasi-festival on which *Tachanun* is omitted, it is also omitted at *Minchah* of the preceding afternoon (*O.C.* 552:2).

✑§ The Se'udah Hamafsekes

5. The meal that immediately precedes the fast — the *se'udah hamafsekes*, literally the *meal that interposes* — should reflect the mourning theme of the impending fast day. The *Gemara* (*Taanis* 30a) relates that on the eve of

Tishah B'Av, the Tanna R' Yehudah bar Ilai's meal consisted only of stale bread with salt and a jug of water, which he would consume while seated between the oven and the stove. *Rambam* writes (*Taanis* 5:9): 'The following was the practice of the devout people of ancient times: On the eve of Tishah B'Av one would be served dry bread ... and after it, drink a jug of water, in sadness, desolation, and with tears, like one who has the body of a dear one in his presence. This, or [a practice] resembling this, should be the practice of Torah scholars. In all my life I have not eaten a cooked dish on the eve of Tishah B'Av — even one of lentils — except when [Tishah B'Av or its eve] falls on the Sabbath.'

6. The above practices, however, were the stringent practices of the extremely devout; they are not binding upon every Jew. The *halachah* follows the Mishnah (*Taanis* 26b), which states that at the final meal before the fast, one may not eat more than one cooked dish. Meat and wine are entirely forbidden. (The ban upon meat and wine need not concern us, since it is customary to refrain from these foods from Rosh Chodesh Av.) It should be noted that in this context fish is also categorized as meat.Thus, even fish may not be eaten at the *se'udah hamafsekes* (*O.C.* 352:2).

7. The *Gemara* (30a) applies two qualifications to the food restrictions in the meals of Tishah B'Av eve: (a) They apply only to meals eaten after the hour of noon; and (b) only to the meal that immediately precedes the fast — hence, the restrictions apply only to the *se'udah hamafsekes*, provided it is eaten in the afternoon. Hence, if one eats more than one meal in the afternoon, the restrictions apply to the final full meal of the day, and if one's last meal was eaten before noon, it is not subject to these restrictions (*O.C.* 552:9).

8. One may eat even many different types of raw fruit and vegetables (*O.C.* 552:4), but not two cooked fruit or vegetable dishes; even if they are also fit to be eaten raw (e.g. apple sauce), they qualify as cooked dishes (O.C. 552:3). Therefore, some poskim prohibit hot coffee or tea at the se'udah hamafsekes (in addition to one cooked dish). Some permit this, arguing that the prohibition applies only to solid foods, not to drinks (Shaarei Teshuvah 552:1).

9. Roasted (and fried) foods are considered cooked dishes in this regard (O.C. 552:3), as are also pickled foods (Shaarei Teshuvah 552:1).

10. Even two batches of the same food could be considered two dishes in this regard: if they were cooked in two different pots and thereby differ in some way, even if the difference is only in consistency, e.g. one has a thick texture while the other is more watery. But if both batches are identical they are considered one food (O.C. 552:3 with M.B. §8).

11. Two foods that were cooked together are considered two dishes, unless it is customary to cook these foods together year round, e.g. peas with onions (O.C. 552:3).

12. One should also curtail one's pleasure at this meal, by cutting down on the amount and type of drinks consumed. Beer and other intoxicating drinks should be avoided completely. One should not eat salads after the meal, as is the custom year round (O.C. 552:1).

13. The prevalent custom, which is also the ancient Ashkenazic custom, is to eat a regular meal in the afternoon before Minchah. There are no restrictions on this meal, and it is customary to eat well at this meal so that fasting will not be difficult the next day. However, if one feels that the fast will not harm him and he wishes to be stringent in this matter, he is to be commended. After Minchah, the seudah hamafsekes is eaten, subject to the restrictions noted above (Rama O.C. 552:9). Moreover, one should take care not to overeat at the first meal, because if one has no appetite to eat afterwards, the meal may be considered as inconsequential, so that the first meal will be the actual se'udah hamafsekes.

◆§ Customs of the Se'udah Hamafsekes

14. At the se'udah hamafsekes it is customary to eat [bread and] a hard-boiled egg, because eggs are a mourner's food. At the conclusion of the meal one dips a piece of bread in ashes and says, 'This is the Tishah B'Av meal' (O.C. 552:5, 6, with M.B.).

15. The meal is eaten sitting on the ground or a low seat, but one need not remove one's shoes. After the meal, however, one may sit on a chair (O.C. 552:7).

16. Three males should not sit together during the meal, so that they will not have to recite Birkas Hamazon together with zimun. Even if

they did eat together, they should nevertheless not say zimun (O.C. 552:8 with M.B.).

◆§ After the Se'udah Hamafsekes

17. After the meal has been concluded and Birkas Hamazon been recited, until sundown one may still eat and do other things that are prohibited on the fast itself (O.C. 553:1).

18. If, however, one explicitly (i.e. orally) expressed the resolve not to eat anymore, he is considered to have taken the fast upon himself, and is obligated to observe all the strictures of the fast (eating, drinking, washing, etc.) — except for the wearing of shoes, which is permitted until sundown (O.C. 553:1 with M.B. §4). The same is true if one did not mention 'eating,' but said that he accepts the fast upon himself (M.B. §1).

19. The above-mentioned acceptance of the fast is valid only if it is done before plag haminchah, i.e. within approximately one and one half hours before sundown (or more precisely, 5/48 of the time between sunrise and sunset). Consequently, if the resolve not to eat was expressed prior to that time, one need not observe all the strictures of the fast, but, in accordance with his explicit vow, one is forbidden to eat (M.B. §4).

20. According to the Shulchan Aruch (O.C. 553:1) only an oral declaration has validity, so that if one resolved only mentally not to eat or to accept the fast, one may still eat thereafter. Some poskim dispute this ruling, however, and obligate one to fast even if he made merely a mental resolution to fast; but if he resolved mentally not to eat, the resolution is not binding. In view of the above, it is advisable to declare (either orally or mentally) at the conclusion of the meal that one does not wish to accept the fast prematurely (M.B. §2).

21. Immediately upon sundown, the fast takes effect, and all of its strictures apply. Therefore one must take care to stop eating and drinking before sundown, but there is no obligation to 'add' from the daytime to the fast, as there is on the eve of the Sabbaths and festivals (O.C. 553:2 with M.B. §3).

22. Since wearing shoes is prohibited on Tishah B'Av, one must take off his shoes before sundown. Moreover if Maariv is recited before sundown, the shoes should be taken off before borchu (i.e. the beginning of the service) is recited. Some advise that the shoes be taken off before one goes to the synagogue. However, once the sun sets one must remove them even if one has not yet gone to the synagogue (O.C. 553:2 with M.B. §5).

◆§ Tishah B'Av Eve on the Sabbath

23. When Tishah B'Av occurs on Sunday or on the Sabbath itself (so that the fast is observed on Sunday), none of the strictures regarding the *se'udah hamafsekes* apply. One may eat meat and drink wine and set the table 'as King Solomon did in his time.' Moreover, it is a sin to deprive oneself of these foods if one does so in observance of the mourning of Tishah B'Av (*O.C.* 552:10 with *M.B.* §23). [It goes without saying that customs such as sitting on the ground, eating a hard-boiled egg and dipping the bread in ashes are not observed.]

24. Some say that one should not eat the third meal of Sabbath — the *se'udah shlishis* — together with a group, but others argue that if one always eats this meal together with his associates (e.g. the group meets in the synagogue for a public *se'udah shlishis*), one must also do so now, for to refrain would be a public observance of mourning on the Sabbath. All agree that at home the meal should be eaten with the family sitting together, and that *Birkas Hamazon* be recited with *zimun* (*O.C.* 552:10 with *M.B.* §23).

25. As on a weekday, the fast begins at sundown (*O.C.* 552:10 with *M.B.* §24). At this time all eating, drinking, etc. must stop, and the five restrictions are observed. However, wearing of shoes is permitted until *borchu* is recited. The members of the congregation remove their shoes after the recitation and the *chazzan* does so before it; they should first recite the formula: בָּרוּךְ הַמַּבְדִּיל בֵּין קוֹדֶשׁ לְחוֹל, *Blessed*

is He Who separates between holy and secular (*O.C.* 553:2). [Nowadays it is customary in many congregations to recite *Maariv* some time after the Sabbath has ended, so that people will have time to remove their shoes and change into their weekday clothing at home, before they go to the synagogue. They should of course recite the above-mentioned formula first.]

26. Regarding Torah study on Tishah B'Av eve when it occurs on the Sabbath, see above §2.

27. The verses of צִדְקָתֶךָ, *Tzidkas'cha*, which are said at the conclusion of the *chazzan's* repetition of the Sabbath *Minchah*, are omitted (*O.C.* 552:12).

⋖§ Tishah B'Av on the Sabbath

28. Even when Tishah B'Av falls on the Sabbath itself, none of the restrictions of the fast day apply, because to observe them would be a public manifestation of mourning on the Sabbath. Regarding marital relations see *O.C.* 554:19. *M.B.* §39-40.

29. Torah study is permitted until noon (*M.B.* 553:9). Thereafter, the restrictions are the same as those of a Tishah B'Av eve that falls on the Sabbath; see above §2.

30. The prayer *Av Harachamim* is recited after the Torah reading (*M.B.* 552:30).

THINGS PROHIBITED ON THE FAST DAY

⋖§ The Five Restrictions

31. Fasting on Tishah B'Av is a broader concept than mere abstention from food and drink. It includes abstention from five activities: (1) eating and drinking; (2) washing one's body; (3) anointing oneself; (4) wearing leather shoes; and (5) marital relations. It is not within the scope of this summary to discuss in detail the ramifications of the restrictions that do not pertain to the prayer service. However, a few words about the restriction on washing, especially about washing the hands before a prayer service, are appropriate here.

32. It is absolutely forbidden to wash even a minute part of the body, whether in hot or cold water, or even to dip one's finger in water (*O.C.* 554:7). However, one may wash his hands three times upon arising in the morning [נְטִילַת יָדַיִם] except that one may wash only the minimum-required area — the fingers, but not the palm of the hand (*O.C.* 554:10).

33. If one has performed his bodily functions and is returning to his prayers (i.e. to recite the *Shemoneh Esrei*), he may also wash his fingers (as above; *O.C.* 554:9, 613:2, *M.B.* 4). If it is his custom all year round to wash three times, he

may wash his fingers three times (*Matteh Ephraim* 613:5). One may also wash his hands in preparation for *Minchah* (*M.B.* 554:21).

34. However, if one has merely urinated and will not recite the *Shemoneh Esrei*, it is questionable whether he may wash his hands. In order to avoid this problem, one should touch a covered part of the body, thus incurring an unquestionable obligation to wash his hands before reciting the blessing of אֲשֶׁר יָצַר (see *O.C.* 613:3, *M.B.* 4,6).

35. One who merely entered a bathroom may not wash his hands, even if this is one's practice throughout the year. Rather one should wipe his hands, on a clean cloth or board, in lieu of washing (*M.E.* 613:7). However, if one is upset at praying with unwashed hands, one may wash them (*Eleph LaMatteh* 613:7). [Presumably the device of touching oneself on a covered part of the body is applicable here too.]

36. If one has touched a covered part of the body and wishes to pray or recite a blessing, one should wash all the fingers of that hand. But if one has touched dirt or mud, he may wash only the soiled area (*O. C.* 554:9, *M.B.* 613:6).

37. Although it is customary to wash one's face and rinse one's mouth every morning before praying, it is forbidden to do so on Tishah B'Av. However, if one has mucous on his eyes, he may moisten his fingers and rub them over his eyes (O.C. 554:11).

✦§ Other Prohibitions

38. Though we cannot detail all the laws of Tishah B'Av here, the following is a brief listing: One may not study Torah, except for things pertaining to mourning of Tishah B'Av, because the study of Torah brings joy. One may study, with commentary, the Biblical books of Job, the 'unpleasant' passages in Jeremiah (omitting the verses of consolation), and Eichah. One may also study the Midrash to Eichah, the third chapter of Moed Kattan (which discusses the laws of mourning), the passages in the Talmud (Gittin 55b-58a) that discuss the destruction of the Temple, and the story of the destruction of the Temple in the book of Yossipon (O.C. 554:1-2, M.B. §3).

39. One does not greet his fellows on Tishah B'Av; not even to say good morning. If one is greeted by someone who is unaware of this law, one should answer quietly and with a serious mien. It is better to tell him that on Tishah B'Av one does not extend greetings. One should also not give a present on Tishah B'Av (O.C. 554:20; M.B. 41-2).

40. Work should be avoided until noon. See O.C. 554:22-4. If possible, one should refrain from smoking on Tishah B'Av. If this is very difficult, one may smoke in private after the hour of noon (M.B. 555:8).

41. On the night of Tishah B'Av and on the morning, until noon, one sits on the ground or on a low stool (O.C. 559:3; M.B. §3).

MAARIV

42. Maariv begins in the usual manner. After בָּרְכוּ the congregation sits on the floor or on low stools and the lights are dimmed. The paroches is removed from the front of the Holy Ark. On Tishah B'Av the prayers are said slowly and tearfully, in the manner of mourners (O.C. 559:1).

43. The regular Maariv service is recited [on Saturday night with the addition of אַתָּה חוֹנַנְתָּנוּ]. After Shemoneh Esrei the Full Kaddish is recited [including the verse תִּתְקַבַּל] (M.B. 559:4).

44. On Saturday night, although Havdalah is not recited [see below], a multi-wicked candle is lit and the blessing בּוֹרֵא מְאוֹרֵי הָאֵשׁ is recited (O.C. 556:1).

45. Eichah (the Book of Lamentations) is chanted aloud by the reader. The prevalent custom is that the entire congregation reads along in an undertone (see M.B. 559:15. See also Taz, Magen Avraham, and Pri Megadim to 559:4). After Eichah has been concluded, the evening Kinnos are recited.

46. After the Kinnos, the congregation recites וְאַתָּה קָדוֹשׁ, omitting the verse וַאֲנִי זֹאת בְּרִיתִי; the reader recites the Full Kaddish, but omits the verse תִּתְקַבַּל; and the congregation recites עָלֵינוּ, followed by the Mourner's Kaddish. [At the end of the Sabbath, וִיהִי נֹעַם and וְיִתֶּן לְךָ are omitted, and Havdalah is postponed until Sunday night.]

SHACHARIS

47. Candles are not lit at the chazzan's lectern for Shacharis, but they are lit for Minchah (M.B. 559:15).

48. Donning of the tallis and tefillin is postponed until Minchah. The tallis kattan (tzitzis) is worn, however, but the accompanying blessing is omitted. (O.C. 555:1)

49. The morning blessings (p. 72) are recited as usual. Although the blessing שֶׁעָשָׂה לִי כָּל צָרְכִּי was instituted to thank God for providing us with shoes, it is the general custom among Ashkenazim to recite it even though shoes are not worn on Tishah B'Av (M.B. 554:31, see Shaarei Teshuvah and Pri Megadim to O.C. 46:8). However, Sephardim omit the blessing (see Kaf HaChaim 46:17), and the Vilna Gaon (Maaseh Rav) is reported to have recited the blessing only at night, after the fast.

50. The entire prayer service which precedes פְּסוּקֵי דְזִמְרָה (the Verses of Praise), including אֵיזֶהוּ מְקוֹמָן, may be said [Although Eizehu Mekoman is a chapter of Mishnah — which may not be studied on Tishah B'Av — it is part of the regular prayer order, and is therefore not omitted.] (O.C. 554:4, M.B. 7). However, Rama states (O.C. 559:4) that פִּטוּם הַקְּטוֹרֶת is omitted (because, M.B. explains, its recitation is not considered to be sufficiently widespread for it to be considered part of the 'order of the day').

Mishnah Berurah (554:7) maintains that according to Rama's view, the passage of Tamid is the only Scriptural passage referring to offerings that may be recited. Nevertheless, in many communities the entire service is recited, without omission, as already indicated.

51. Individuals recite Shemoneh Esrei at Shacharis as usual, without any additions.

The *chazzan*, however, inserts the blessing עֲנֵנוּ in his repetition. See §61 for laws pertaining to this blessing. *Birkas Kohanim* is omitted (see *Dagul Merevavah* to O.C. 559) as is *tachanun*.

52. The prayer service continues with reading from the Torah, followed by the Half *Kaddish* and *Haftarah*. The Torah is returned to the Ark and *Kinnos* are recited. It is preferable that their recitation extend until close to noon (O.C. 559:2).

53. After the recitation of *Kinnos*, the prayer service continues with אַשְׁרֵי and וּבָא לְצִיּוֹן (with the omission of the verse . . . וַאֲנִי זֹאת), the

Full *Kaddish*, with the omission of תִּתְקַבֵּל; followed by עָלֵינוּ and the Mourner's *Kaddish*. The Song of the Day is deferred until *Minchah*.

54. During the recitation of *Kinnos*, one should not talk about extraneous matters nor leave the synagogue, in order to fully concentrate on mourning for the destruction of the Temple (O.C. 559:5).

55. It is commendable that every individual read *Eichah* again during the daytime (*Shelah* cited by *Magen Avraham*, beginning of 559).

MINCHAH

56. Candles are lit at the *chazzan's* lectern for *Minchah* (*Pri Megadim* in *Eishel Avraham* 559:3). The *paroches* [Ark curtain] is put back in place (*Kaf HaChaim* 559:19).

57. The *talis* and *tefillin* are donned (O.C. 555:1), and the remainder of the *Shacharis* prayer is said.

58. *Minchah* on Tishah B'Av is the same as that of a regular fast day (except that נַחֵם, *Nacheim*, is inserted in the Shemoneh Esrei (see §64). The Torah reading and the *Haftarah* are identical to that of a regular fast day, with the exception of *Avinu Malkeinu* and *tachanun*, which are omitted.

59. In *Shemoneh Esrei*, עֲנֵנוּ, *Aneinu*, [*Answer us*] is inserted, as on other fast days. In addition, נַחֵם, *Nacheim*, [*comfort*] is inserted. See below §64.

60. The *chazzan* repeats the *Shemoneh Esrei* as usual and inserts the above two prayers (see below). He also recites the Priestly Blessing, as on other fast days (*Kitzur Shulchan Aruch* 124:19). The *Shemoneh Esrei* is followed by the Full *Kaddish* (with תִּתְקַבֵּל), then עָלֵינוּ, and the Mourner's *Kaddish*.

עֲנֵנוּ / Aneinu

61. A special fast-day prayer — עֲנֵנוּ — is interjected both in the silent *Shemoneh Esrei* and in the *chazzan's* repetition. This prayer may be recited only by one who is fasting; for someone not fasting to recite this prayer which refers specifically to 'our public fast' would be fraudulent (see O.C. 565:3 in *Rama*). This insertion is made by the *chazzan* in his repetition of both *Shacharis* and *Minchah*, but in the silent *Shemoneh Esrei* it is recited only during *Minchah* (O.C. 565:3). In the *chazzan's* prayer, *Aneinu* takes the form of a complete benediction, concluding with הָעוֹנֶה בְּעֵת צָרָה, *Blessed . . . Who responds in time of distress* (O.C. 566:1), . . . בָּרוּךְ רְפָאֵנוּ and גוֹאֵל יִשְׂרָאֵל. The individual's recitation is included in the benediction שְׁמַע קוֹלֵנוּ (O.C. 565:1).

blessing in his repetition of the *Shemoneh Esrei*, there must be ten congregants who are fasting. Some authorities rule that it is sufficient that there be seven fasting individuals (O.C. 566:3, M.B. §14). Individuals recite *Aneinu* in their own *Shemoneh Esrei* even if no one else is fasting.

62. If an individual forgot to insert עֲנֵנוּ in its proper place and has already said the word *Hashem* in the concluding blessing of שְׁמַע קוֹלֵנוּ, he must conclude with שׁוֹמֵעַ תְּפִלָּה and continue with רְצֵה. He may insert עֲנֵנוּ at the end of the *Shemoneh Esrei* before אֱלֹהַי נְצוֹר. If he finished *Shemoneh Esrei* before realizing his error, he should not repeat the *Shemoneh Esrei* (M.B. 119:16,19).

63. If the *chazzan* forgot to insert עֲנֵנוּ in its proper place, but has not yet said the word *HASHEM* of the concluding blessing of רְפָאֵנוּ, he should interrupt his recitation, and recite עֲנֵנוּ. Thereafter he should begin רְפָאֵנוּ again and continue. If he has already uttered the word *HASHEM*, he must conclude the blessing רוֹפֵא חוֹלֵי and continue his prayer as usual. In this case, the *chazzan* inserts עֲנֵנוּ in the benediction שְׁמַע קוֹלֵנוּ, as do individuals in the silent prayer, but omits the concluding formula בָּרוּךְ הָעוֹנֶה בְּעֵת צָרָה. If he realized his error after he uttered the word *HASHEM* in the concluding formula of שְׁמַע קוֹלֵנוּ, he must continue with שׁוֹמֵעַ תְּפִלָּה. In that case, he may recite עֲנֵנוּ (omitting the concluding blessing) after הַמְבָרֵךְ אֶת עַמּוֹ יִשְׂרָאֵל בַּשָּׁלוֹם (O.C. 119:4 M.B. §16,19).

נַחֵם / Nacheim

64. In addition to עֲנֵנוּ, a special prayer (נַחֵם, *Comfort*), mourning the destruction of the Holy Temple and supplicating that it be rebuilt, is inserted in the benediction וְלִירוּשָׁלַיִם, *and to Jerusalem* (both in the silent and *Chazzan's Shemoneh Esrei*) of *Minchah*. The concluding blessing of וְלִירוּשָׁלַיִם is changed (both for individuals and for the *chazzan*) to בָּרוּךְ . . . מְנַחֵם, *Blessed . . . Who consoles Zion and rebuilds Jerusalem*. If one forgot to recite this prayer in its appropriate place, he inserts it in the benediction רְצֵה, before the word וְתֶחֱזֶינָה, but in that case one omits the concluding formula ... מְנַחֵם צִיּוֹן (O.C. 557:1, M.B. §2). However, if one recited נַחֵם erroneously in the benediction שְׁמַע קוֹלֵנוּ, it need not be repeated in

רְצֵה (Be'ur Halachah). If one has already concluded the רְצֵה benediction with הַמַּחֲזִיר שְׁכִינָתוֹ לְצִיּוֹן (or even said the word Hashem), he continues his prayer, and need not repeat Shemoneh Esrei (O.C. 557).

AFTERNOON

65. Although some restrictions are relaxed in the afternoon, e.g. one may sit on a chair etc., this applies only to practices that are based on custom. However, all halachic strictures

that apply to the fast, i.e. eating, drinking, wearing shoes, studying Torah, et al., are in force until nightfall, when stars become visible (M.B. 553:3).

MAARIV

66. The regular Maariv is recited. On Sunday night, Havdalah is recited, with the following exceptions: a) Havdalah commences with the blessing over wine; the preliminary verses that are reciting at the end of the Sabbath are omitted; b) The blessings over spices and the candles are omitted. Even those who do not drink the Havdalah wine during the nine days may do so now; they need not give the wine to a child to drink. [One should not eat before reciting Havdalah.] (O.C. 556:1, M.B. §3).

with a minyan, some permit its recitation even if one has not yet broken his fast (Shaar HaTziyun §9).

⋅◦§ The Night After the Fast

68. The strictures that were observed during the Nine Days apply also to the night following Tishah B'Av and the next day until noon. Thus, one does not eat meat, take a haircut, wash clothing, etc. until noon of the next day (O.C. 558:1, M.B. §3).

However if Tishah B'Av was on Thursday, one may wash clothing and take a haircut or shave on Friday morning in preparation for the Sabbath (M.B. 558:3), Shaarei Teshuvah §2).

⋅◦§ Kiddush Levanah

67. According to Rama (O.C. 426:2), Kiddush Levanah should not be recited on the night following Tishah B'Av, because it should be recited joyously, but we are still in mourning. However, many poskim dispute this ruling and permit the recitation of Kiddush Levanah. Nevertheless, one should first eat something and don his shoes (M.B. §11). However, if this is the only time he will be able to recite Kiddush Levanah

69. If Tishah B'Av fell on the Sabbath so that the fast was observed on the tenth of Av, one need not observe the strictures of the Nine Days on the night after the fast. However, one should abstain from meat and wine on the night itself (O.C. 558:1, M.B. §4).

GENERAL LAWS OF PRAYER

⋅◦§ The Obligation

70. Prayer is a major ingredient of every Jew's daily religious life. The Sages teach us that in the post-Temple era, prayer was substituted for the Temple service, and according to some authorities it is a Scriptural obligation to pray every single day (see Rambam, Hil. Tefillah 1:1).

71. Before praying, one should set aside a few minutes to collect his thoughts and to prepare himself mentally to stand before his Maker. Also, one should not rush away immediately after ending his prayer so as not to give the impression that he regards prayer as a burdensome task (O.C. 93:1).

72. Before beginning to pray, one should meditate upon God's infinite greatness and man's insignificance, and thereby remove from his heart any thoughts of physical pleasure (O.C. 98:1). By pondering God's works, man recognizes His infinite wisdom and comes to love and laud Him. This makes man cognizant of his

own puny intelligence and flawed nature and puts him in a proper frame of mind to plead for God's mercy (Rambam, Yesodei HaTorah 2:2).

73. The prayers should be said with a feeling of awe and humility, and surely not in an atmosphere of levity, frivolity, or mundane concerns, nor should one pray while angry. Rather, one should pray with the feeling of happiness brought on by the knowledge of God's historic kindness to Israel and His mercy to all creatures (O.C. 93:2).

⋅◦§ Concentration on the Prayers

74. During Shemoneh Esrei one should imagine that he is in the Holy Temple and concentrate his feelings and thoughts toward Heaven, clearing his mind of all extraneous matters (O.C. 95:2). His eyes should be directed downward, either closed or reading from the machzor (O.C. 95:2, M.B. 5). One should not look up during Shemoneh Esrei, but when he feels his concentration failing, he should raise his eyes heavenward to renew his inspiration (*M.B.* 90:8).

75. One should know the meaning of his prayers. If one had an audience with a human ruler he would take the utmost care in his choice of words and be aware of their meaning. Surely, therefore, when one stands before the King of kings Who knows his innermost thoughts, he must be careful how he speaks (*O.C.* 98:1). Especially in regard to the benedictions of *Shemoneh Esrei*, one should at least meditate on the meaning of the concluding sentence of each benediction, which summarizes its theme (e.g., בָּרוּךְ . . . הָאֵל הַקָּדוֹשׁ, *Blessed . . . the holy God; M.B.* 101:1). The first benediction of the *Shemoneh Esrei* is treated with special stringency in this regard. According to the *halachah* as stated in the Talmud, this benediction must be repeated if it was said without concentration on its meaning (*O.C.* 101:1). However, *Rama* (loc. cit.) rules that it is best *not* to repeat the benediction because it is likely that one will not concentrate properly even during the repetition. *Chayei Adam* (cited in *M.B.* 101:4) advises that if one realized his inattentiveness before saying the word HASHEM in the concluding formula of the first blessing (בָּרוּךְ . . . מָגֵן אַבְרָהָם), he should start over from אֱלֹהֵי אַבְרָהָם. Thus, it is of utmost importance that one learn the meaning of the prayers in order to develop his power of concentration (*M.B.* 101:2).

76. On Tishah B'Av a lengthy selection of lamentation liturgy — *Kinnos* — is a central part of the *Shacharis* service. It is important that one familiarize himself with these prayers prior to the fast day, some of which use unfamiliar language and contain numerous allusions to Midrashic sources.

⇥§ Women's Obligation to Pray

77. Women are obligated to pray, and according to *Rambam* and *Shulchan Aruch* (*O.C.*

106:1) this obligation has Scriptural status. However, there are various opinions regarding the extent of their obligation.

According to the views preferred by *M.B.* (106:4), women are required to recite the *Shemoneh Esrei* of *Shacharis* and *Minchah*; they must recall the Exodus by reciting אֱמֶת וְיַצִּיב, *true and certain* (the prayer after the *Shacharis* recitation of *Shema*), and אֱמֶת וֶאֱמוּנָה, *true and faithful* (the parallel prayer after the *Maariv* recitation of *Shema*), because it recalls the Exodus (*M.B.* 70:2); and it is urged that they recite at least the first verse of *Shema* because it constitutes קַבָּלַת עוֹל מַלְכוּת שָׁמַיִם, *acceptance of God's sovereignty* (*O.C.* 70:1).

Some authorities rule that women should also recite all the morning benedictions. According to one view, *Pesukei D'zimrah* is introductory to *Shemoneh Esrei* and, consequently, is obligatory upon women too (*M.B.* 70:2).

Women should recite בִּרְכַּת הַתּוֹרָה, *blessings of the Torah* (*O.C.* 47:14, see *Be'ur Halachah*).

According to *Magen Avraham* (*O.C.* 106:2), women are required by the Torah to pray once a day and they may formulate the prayer as they wish. In many countries, this ruling became the basis for the custom that women recite a brief prayer early in the morning and do not recite any of the formal prayers from the *Siddur*.

⇥§ Miscellaneous Laws

78. One may not pray in the presence of immodestly clad women, or facing a window through which they can be observed (see *O.C.* 75 for details).

79. It is forbidden to pray while one feels the need to discharge his bodily functions (*O.C.* 92:1-3).

80. One must wash his hands before praying, but no benediction is required (*O.C.* 92:4).

On Tishah B'Av, certain strictures must be observed when washing one's hands before prayer; see §32-36.

PRAYER WITH THE CONGREGATION

⇥§ Prayer with a Minyan of Ten

81. One should do his utmost to pray in the synagogue together with the congregation (*O.C.* 90:9), for the Almighty does not reject the prayer of the many. Contrary to the popular misconception that it is sufficient to respond to בָּרְכוּ and קְדוּשָׁה, the main objective of prayer with a *minyan* is to recite *Shemoneh Esrei* with the *minyan*. Therefore one must arrive at the synagogue early enough to keep up with the congregation (*M.B.* §28).

⇥§ Instructions for Latecomers

82. If one arrived at the synagogue too late to recite the entire order of the prayer and still recite the *Shemoneh Esrei* together with the congregation, he may omit certain parts of the

service and recite them after the end of *Shacharis*. If time is extremely short, it suffices to recite the benedictions אֱלֹהַי נְשָׁמָה; אֲשֶׁר יָצַר; עַל נְטִילַת יָדַיִם; the benedictions over the Torah; בָּרוּךְ שֶׁאָמַר; אַשְׁרֵי; and from יִשְׁתַּבַּח through *Shemoneh Esrei*. If time permits, the following sections (listed in descending order of importance) should be recited:

(1) הַלְלוּיָהּ הַלְלוּ אֵל בְּקָדְשׁוֹ;
(2) הַלְלוּיָהּ הַלְלוּ אֶת ה' מִן הַשָּׁמַיִם;
(3) the other three הַלְלוּיָהּ psalms;
(4) from וַיְבָרֶךְ דָּוִיד until לְשֵׁם תִּפְאַרְתֶּךָ;
(5) וְהוּא רַחוּם until הוֹדוּ;
(6) the rest of *Pesukei D'zimrah* (*O.C.* 52:1, *M.B.* 4, *Ba'er Heitev* §3).

83. The above is only an emergency solution. One should not rely on this to arrive late for the *Pesukei D'zimrah*, because the proper order of the prayers is of utmost importance. Indeed, some authorities contend that recitation of the prayers in their proper order takes priority over the obligation to recite *Shemoneh Esrei* together with the congregation (M.B. 52:1).

RESPONSES DURING THE PRAYER

◄§ During Pesukei D'zimrah

84. Other than the exceptions noted below, it is prohibited to interrupt from the beginning of בָּרוּךְ שֶׁאָמַר until the conclusion of the *Shemoneh Esrei* (O.C. 51:4). Wherever one may not talk, it is forbidden to do so even in Hebrew (M.B. 51:7).

85. With the exception of *Shemoneh Esrei*, parts of *Shacharis* may be interrupted for certain responses to the *chazzan* or for certain blessings, but the rules vary widely, depending on the section of *Shacharis* and the response. In this regard, the most lenient part of *Shacharis* is *Pesukei D'zimrah*, i.e., the unit that includes the verses between בָּרוּךְ שֶׁאָמַר and יִשְׁתַּבַּח. There, one may respond with *Amen* to any benediction, but may not say בָּרוּךְ הוּא וּבָרוּךְ שְׁמוֹ. It is permitted to respond to *Kedushah* and מוֹדִים (in the repetition of *Shemoneh Esrei*), בָּרְכוּ, and *Kaddish*. If the congregation is reciting the *Shema*, one should recite the first verse (*Shema Yisrael . . .*) together with them. If one discharged his bodily functions, he may recite the benediction אֲשֶׁר יָצַר (M.B. 51:8).

86. If one did not yet recite the *Shema* and calculates that the congregation will reach it after the deadline (see §109 below) or if he had forgotten to say the daily *berachos* on the Torah, he should say them in the *Pesukei D'zimrah* (M.B. 51:10).

◄§ During the Pesukei D'zimrah Blessings

87. The second level of stringency regarding interruptions includes the two benedictions of *Pesukei D'zimrah* — בָּרוּךְ שֶׁאָמַר and יִשְׁתַּבַּח.

בָּרוּךְ שֶׁאָמַר is composed of three parts:
(a) From בָּרוּךְ שֶׁאָמַר until the first 'ה אַתָּה בָּרוּךְ is but a preamble; all responses are permitted.
(b) From the first 'ה אַתָּה בָּרוּךְ until the final one, all the interruptions permitted in §85 for the rest of *Pesukei D'zimrah* are also permitted here. However, the following interruptions are *not* permitted at this point: אֲשֶׁר יָצַר and the *Amen* after the benedictions בָּרוּךְ שֶׁאָמַר and יִשְׁתַּבַּח.
(c) The last, brief blessing, בָּרוּךְ . . . בְּתִשְׁבָּחוֹת, during which no interruption at all is permitted (M.B. 51:2).

יִשְׁתַּבַּח is composed of two parts:
(a) From the beginning of יִשְׁתַּבַּח to 'ה אַתָּה בָּרוּךְ which has the same rules as (b) above.
(b) From 'ה אַתָּה בָּרוּךְ to the end, which has the same rules as (c) above (M.B. 51:2, 65:11, 54:11).

◄§ Between the Shema Blessings of Shacharis and Maariv

88. The third level of stringency concerns the 'intervals' between the various sections of the *Shema* and the benedictions bracketing it. The intervals are as follows: After בָּרוּךְ . . . יוֹצֵר בָּרוּךְ; after הַמְּאוֹרוֹת . . . בָּאַהֲבָה; and after the first and second sections of the *Shema*. [The end of the *Shema* is immediately followed by the first word of the following paragraph (אֱמֶת) so that there is no 'interval' there. Similarly, it is forbidden to interrupt between the benediction גָּאַל יִשְׂרָאֵל and *Shemoneh Esrei* (O.C. 66:5,9).]

Corresponding 'intervals' exist in *Maariv* following each blessing and after the first and second sections of the *Shema* (M.B. 66:27; *Be'ur Halachah* there).

89. During the 'intervals' one may respond with *Amen* to all benedictions (M.B. 66:23). Regarding קָדִישׁ, קְדוּשָׁה, בָּרְכוּ, and other interruptions, the 'intervals' are treated in the same way as are interruptions in the fourth level (see below §90). During the interval between בָּאַהֲבָה and שְׁמַע, however, only the *Amen* after בָּאַהֲבָה is permitted (*Derech HaChaim*; see M.B. 59:25).

◄§ During the Shema and Its Blessings in Shacharis and Maariv

90. The fourth level concerns the *Shema* itself and the benedictions bracketing it. The benedictions may be separated into two parts for this purpose: (1) During the concluding, brief blessing, and during the verses of שְׁמַע . . . אֶחָד and בָּרוּךְ שֵׁם, no interruption whatever is permitted (O.C. 66:1; M.B. §11, 12). (2) During the rest of the fourth level, one may respond with *Amen* only to the two blessings הָאֵל הַקָּדוֹשׁ and שׁוֹמֵעַ תְּפִלָּה in *Shemoneh Esrei*. It is permitted to respond to בָּרְכוּ of both the *chazzan* and one who is called up to the Torah. In *Kaddish* one may respond with . . . אָמֵן יְהֵא שְׁמֵהּ רַבָּא and with the *Amen* to דַאֲמִירָן בְּעָלְמָא. In *Kedushah* one may say only the verses beginning קָדוֹשׁ and בָּרוּךְ. To *Modim*, one may respond only with the three words מוֹדִים אֲנַחְנוּ לָךְ (O.C 66:3; M.B. §17,18).

A person who is reciting the *Shema* or its benedictions should not be called up to the Torah, even if he is the only *Kohen* or Levite present; in such a case it is preferable that he leave the room. However, if he *was* called up to the Torah, he may recite the benedictions, but should not read along with the reader. If possible he should attempt to get to an 'interval' in his prayers before doing so (M.B. 66:26).

If one had to discharge his bodily functions he should merely wash his hands and defer the recitation of אֲשֶׁר יָצַר until after *Shemoneh Esrei* (M.B. 66:23).

91. If one has not yet responded to בָּרְכוּ, קְדוּשָׁה or מוֹדִים and is nearly up to *Shemoneh Esrei*, he should stop before שִׁירָה

חֲדָשָׁה in order to make the responses. If he has already said שִׁירָה חֲדָשָׁה, but has not yet concluded the benediction, he may respond, but after the response he should start again from שִׁירָה חֲדָשָׁה (*M.B.* 66:52).

92. Regarding גָּאַל יִשְׂרָאֵל of *Shacharis*, *Rama*, followed by most Ashkenazic congregations, rules that it is permitted to answer *Amen*, while others, particularly Chassidic congregations, follow R' Yosef Caro's ruling against *Amen* at this point. To avoid the controversy, many individuals recite the blessing in unison with the *chazzan* (*O.C.* 66:7, *M.B.* §35).

93. The fifth level concerns the *Shemoneh Esrei* prayer. Here, any interruption is forbidden. Even motioning to someone is prohibited (*O.C.* 104:1; *M.B.* §1). If the *chazzan* is up to

בָּרְכוּ, or קְדוּשָׁה, קָדִישׁ, one should stop and listen silently to the *chazzan's* recitation; his own silent concentration is considered as if he had responded (*O.C.* 104:7; *M.B.* §26-28).

94. From the time one has concluded the last benediction of *Shemoneh Esrei* with בְּשָׁלוֹם until the end of the standard prayers (i.e., אֱלֹהַי נְצוֹר at the end of יִהְיוּ לְרָצוֹן), one is restricted to the responses listed in level four. However, whenever possible, one should hurry to say the verse וְגוֹאֲלִי . . . יִהְיוּ לְרָצוֹן before making any kind of response. It is preferable to take the usual three steps backward before making the responses (*O.C.* 122:1; *M.B.* §2-4). [Once one has concluded the *Shemoneh Esrei* by taking three steps backward, he may make any response, even if he has not yet recited אֱלֹהַי נְצוֹר.]

LAWS OF RECITING THE SHEMA

95. It is a Scriptural precept to recite the *Shema* twice daily, once in the morning and again in the evening. When one recites the *Shema* he must have in mind that he is fulfilling a Scriptural precept; otherwise it must be repeated (*O.C.* 60:4). However, if the circumstances make it obvious that the intention was present — e.g., he recited it during the prayer with the benedictions preceding and following it — he need not repeat the *Shema* even if he did not make a mental declaration of purpose (*M.B.* 60:10).

96. The third section of *Shema*, whose recitation is Rabbinical in origin according to almost all authorities, contains a verse whose recitation fulfills the Scriptural obligation to commemorate the Exodus from Egypt twice daily (see *Berachos* 12b; *Rambam, Hil. Kerias Shema* 1:3). The above rule concerning a mental declaration of intent applies here, too.

97. One should concentrate on the meaning of all the words, and read them with awe and trepidation (*O.C.* 61:1). He should read the *Shema* as if it were a new proclamation containing teachings never yet revealed (*O.C.* 61:2). The first verse of *Shema* is the essential profession of our faith. Therefore, the utmost concentration on its meaning is necessary. If one said it without such concentration, he has not fulfilled his obligation and must repeat it (*O.C.* 60:5, 63:4), but he should repeat the verse quietly, for one may not (publicly) say the first verse of *Shema* repeatedly (ibid.).

98. While reciting the first verse, it is customary to cover the eyes with the right hand to avoid distraction and to enhance concentration (*O.C.* 61:5).

99. Although *Shema* may be recited quietly, one should recite it loudly enough to hear himself. However, one has discharged his obligation even if he does not hear himself, as long as he has enunciated the words (*O.C.* 62:3).

100. The last word of the first verse, אֶחָד,

must be pronounced with special emphasis, while one meditates on God's exclusive sovereignty over the seven heavens and earth, and the four directions — east, south, west, and north (*O.C.* 61:6).

101. Some consider it preferable to recite the entire *Shema* aloud (except for the passage בָּרוּךְ שֵׁם) while others say it quietly; our custom follows the latter usage. However, the first verse should be said aloud in order to arouse one's full concentration (*O.C.* 61:4,26). It is customary for the *chazzan* to lead the congregation in the recitation of the first verse so that they all proclaim the Kingdom of Heaven together (*Kol Bo* cited in *Darkei Moshe* to *O.C.* 61; *Levush*).

102. Every word must be enunciated clearly and uttered with the correct grammatical pronunciation (*O.C.* 62:1, 61:23, 16-19). It is especially important to enunciate each word clearly and to avoid run-on words by pausing briefly between words ending and beginning with the same consonant, such as וַאֲבַדְתֶּם מְהֵרָה, בְּכָל לְבָבְכֶם, and to pause between a word that ends with a consonant and the next one that begins with a silent letter [i.e., א or ע], such as אֲשֶׁר אָנֹכִי, הַיּוֹם עַל, וּרְאִיתֶם אֹתוֹ (*O.C.* 61:20, 21).

103. Although it is not the universal custom to chant the *Shema* with the cantillation melody used during the synagogue Torah reading, it is laudable to do so, unless one finds that such chanting interferes with his concentration. In any event, the proper punctuation must be followed so that words are grouped into the proper phrases in accordance with the syntax of each word-group and verse (*O.C.* 61:24, *M.B.* §37,38).

104. While reciting the first two portions of the *Shema*, one may not communicate with someone else by winking or motioning with his lips or fingers (*O.C.* 63:6, *M.B.* §18).

105. It is incumbent that each paragraph of the *Shema* be read word for word as it appears in the Torah. If one erred and skipped a word, he must return to the place of his error and continue the section from there (O.C. 64:1-2).

106. The *Shema* should be said in one uninterrupted recitation, but, if one interrupted, whether by talking or waiting silently, he does not have to repeat the *Shema*. However, if the interruption was involuntary in nature [e.g., one had to relieve himself], and the interruption was long enough for him to have recited all three paragraphs of the *Shema* at his own normal speed, he must repeat the entire *Shema* (*Rama O.C.* 65:1). Multiple interruptions interspersed in the recitation of *Shema* are not added together to constitute one long, invalidating interruption (*M.B.* 65:4).

107. If one is present in the synagogue when the congregation recites the *Shema*, he must recite at least the first verse and the verse בָּרוּךְ שֵׁם together with them. If he is in the midst of a prayer that he may not interrupt (see above §87-92), he should at least give the appearance of saying *Shema* by praying loudly in the tune the congregation uses for the *Shema* (*O.C.* 65:2,3; *M.B.* §10).

108. During morning services, one ordinarily gathers together the four *tzitzis* when he says the words וַהֲבִיאֵנוּ לְשָׁלוֹם מֵאַרְבַּע כַּנְפוֹת הָאָרֶץ, *Bring us in peacefulness from the four corners of the earth,* in the paragraph preceding the *Shema.* [The *tzitzis* are then held in the hand and kissed at specific points of the *Shema* recitation and the blessing which follows it. On Tishah B'Av, however, this is not done.]

109. It is absolutely required that the *Shema* be recited within the requisite time — the first quarter of the day. There are various opinions among the *poskim* as to how to calculate the first quarter of a day, and these are noted in many Jewish calendars. If the congregation begins *Shacharis* late, one should be careful to check the deadline for *K'rias Shema* and, if necessary, recite all three passages of the *Shema* before the communal prayers.

◈§ The Chazzan's Repetition of the Shemoneh Esrei

110. The *chazzan's* repetition of *Shemoneh Esrei* is a congregational, rather than an individual, worship. By definition, a 'congregation' consists of a *minyan* (quorum of at least ten males over *bar mitzvah,* including the *chazzan*), present and listening to the recitation. If the congregants do not pay attention, it is almost as if the *chazzan* were taking God's Name in vain. Every person should imagine that there are only ten congregants present and that he is one of the nine attentive whose listening is vital to the recitation (*O.C.* 124:4).

If one of the ten is in the middle of the silent *Amidah,* he may still be counted as part of the *minyan.* However, it is preferable that not more than one such person be included (*M.B.* 55:32-34).

111. One should respond with *Amen* to every benediction he hears, and should teach his young children to do so (*O.C.* 124:6,7).

112. When one says *Amen,* it is important to enunciate all of the vowels and consonants distinctly. One should not respond until the *chazzan* has concluded the benediction, and then the response should be immediate (*O.C.* 124:8). *Mishnah Berurah* (§17) cautions even against Torah study or recitation of psalms and other prayers during the *chazzan's* recitation of the *Shemoneh Esrei.*

113. It is absolutely forbidden to talk during the repetition of *Shemoneh Esrei* even if one makes sure to respond with *Amen* at the conclusion of each benediction (*O.C.* 124:7).

THE READING OF THE TORAH

114. On Tishah B'Av, as on every fast day, three people are called to the Torah at the *Shacharis* prayer, and three at the *Minchah* prayer. One may not add to the prescribed amount of *aliyos* (*O.C.* 282:1, *M.B.* §6).

115. The first *aliyah* belongs to a *Kohen* and the second to a *Levi* (if any are present). If no *Kohen* is present, there is no obligation to call a *Levi* in his place, but if no *Levi* is present the same *Kohen* who has been called for his own *aliyah* is called again to replace the *Levi.* He recites both blessings again (*O.C.* 135:10; *M.B.* §35).

◈§ Procedure of the Aliyah

116. Before the person called to the Torah for an *aliyah* recites the benediction, he must open the Torah and find the passage that will be read for him (*O.C.* 139:4). In order to dispel any notion that he is reading the benedictions from the Torah, one should avert his face while reciting them; it is preferable to turn to the left side (*Rama* there). Some authorities maintain that it is better to face the Torah while saying the benedictions but to close his eyes (*M.B.* §19). Others say that it is better to close the Torah during the recitation of the benedictions (*Be'ur Halachah* there). All three modes are practiced today in various congregations.

117. In many congregations it is customary to touch the Torah with a *tallis* (or the Torah's mantle or girdle) at the beginning of the passage to be read, and to kiss the edge which touched the Torah (*Sha'arei Ephraim* 4:3). One should be careful not to rub on the Torah script forcefully for this can cause words to become erased and thus invalidate the Torah scroll.

118. It is extremely important that the benedictions be said loud enough for the congregation to hear (O.C. 139:6). If the congregation did not hear the recitation of בָּרְכוּ, they may not respond with בָּרוּךְ... וָעֶד (Be'ur Halachah to O.C. 57:1). However, if the congregation (or at least a *minyan*) heard בָּרְכוּ, then even someone who has not heard בָּרְכוּ may respond along with the congregation (M.B. 57:2).

119. While reciting the benedictions, one should hold the poles (atzei chaim) upon which the Torah is rolled. During the reading, the reader holds one pole and the person called to the Torah holds the other one (O.C. 139:11; M.B. §35). *Arizal* says one should hold the *atzei chaim* with both hands during the benedictions and with the right hand only during the reading (cited in *Magen Avraham* 139:13).

120. Upon completion of the reading it is customary for the person who has been called up to touch the Torah with a *tallis* (or the Torah's mantle or girdle) and to kiss the edge that has touched the Torah (see M.B. 139:35).

121. After the Torah passage has been read, he closes the Torah scroll and then recites the benediction (Rama O.C. 139:5). If the Torah reading will not be resumed immediately (e.g., a מִי שֶׁבֵּרַךְ is said), then a covering should be spread out over the Torah (M.B. 139:21).

122. In Talmudic times the person called for an *aliyah* would also read aloud from the Torah. This practice was still followed in Greek and Turkish communities up to the sixteenth century (see Beis Yosef to Tur O.C. 141), and the tradition persists to this day in Yemenite communities. However, since ancient times the Ashke-nazic custom has been for a designated reader (baal korei) to read the Torah aloud to the congregation (see Rosh cited in Tur loc. cit). Nevertheless, the person who recites the benedictions should read quietly along with the reader (O.C. 141:2).

123. The reader and the one called up to the Torah must stand while reading the Torah in public. It is forbidden even to lean upon something (O.C. 141:1).

124. When going up to the *bimah* to recite the benedictions one should pick the shortest route possible, and when returning to his seat, he should take a longer route. If two routes are equidistant, one should go to the *bimah* via the route which is to his right and descend via the opposite route (O.C. 141:7).

125. After one has finished reciting the concluding benediction he should not return to his place at least until the next person called up to the Torah has come to the *bimah* (O.C. 141:7). However, it is customary to wait until the next person has finished his passage of the Torah (M.B. §26).

126. It is forbidden to talk or even to discuss Torah topics while the Torah is being read (O.C. 146:2).

127. It is forbidden to leave the synagogue while the Torah is being read (O.C. 146:1), even if one has already heard the reading of the passage elsewhere (M.B. §1). However, if necessary, one may leave during the pause between one portion and the next (O.C. 146:1), provided that a *minyan* remains in the synagogue (M.B. §2).

KADDISH

128. The conclusion of a section of prayer is usually signified by the recitation of the Kaddish. Many of these Kaddish recitations are the privilege of mourners (within the eleven months following the death or burial of a parent, or in some instances, of other close relatives), or of those observing yahrzeit, i.e., the anniversary of the death of a parent (and in some congregations, of a grandparent who has no living sons; see Matteh Ephraim, Dinei Kaddish 3:14). However, many recitations of Kaddish are exclusively the prerogative of the chazzan.

129. Basically there are four types of Kaddish:
(a) חֲצִי קַדִּישׁ, Half-Kaddish, which ends with דַּאֲמִירָן בְּעָלְמָא וְאִמְרוּ אָמֵן;
(b) קַדִּישׁ יָתוֹם, the Mourner's Kaddish, which consists of the Half-Kaddish, with the addition of עֹשֶׂה שָׁלוֹם and יְהֵא שְׁלָמָא;
(c) קַדִּישׁ שָׁלֵם, the Full Kaddish, the same as the Mourner's Kaddish with the addition of תִּתְקַבֵּל before יְהֵא שְׁלָמָא; and
(d) קַדִּישׁ דְּרַבָּנָן, the Rabbis' Kaddish, the same as the Mourner's Kaddish with the addition of עַל יִשְׂרָאֵל.

130. The function of the Half-Kaddish is to link different segments of the prayer, e.g., it is recited between Pesukei D'zimrah and the Shema benedictions, between Shemoneh Esrei (or Tachanun) and the prayers that conclude the service (Pri Megadim in Mishbetzos Zahav, Orach Chaim 55:1). Thus, it is recited by the chazzan.

Nevertheless, in some congregations it is customary for a mourner to recite the Kaddish following the reading of the Torah if he has been called to the Torah for the concluding segment (Sha'arei Ephraim 10:9). The rationale for this custom is that the person called to the Torah is also a chazzan of sorts, since he too must read from the Torah, albeit quietly. In some congregations, a mourner recites this Kaddish even if he was not called to the Torah.

131. The Full Kaddish is recited only after the communal recitation of Shemoneh Esrei (or Selichos). It includes the chazzan's prayer that the just-concluded service be accepted by God. Consequently it must be recited by the chazzan.

132. The Mourner's *Kaddish* is recited after the recital of Scriptural verses that supplement the main body of prayer. The recital of *Kaddish* after this portion of the service is not obligatory, and is not recited if no mourners are present. Since *Kaddish* in these parts of the service is recited exclusively by mourners, it has become customary that one whose parents are living should not recite it, since this would be a mark of disrespect to his parents (see *Rama O.C.* 132:2; *Pis'chei Teshuvah, Yoreh Deah* 376:4).

If no mourners are present, the Mourner's *Kaddish* is not recited. After *Aleinu*, which also contains Scriptural verses, *Kaddish* should be recited even if no mourner is present. In such a case, it should be recited by the *chazzan* or one of the congregants, preferably one whose parents are no longer alive, or one whose parents have not explicitly expressed their opposition to his recitation of *Kaddish* (*O.C.* 132:2 with *M.B.* §11).

133. Ideally, each Mourner's *Kaddish* should be recited by only one person. Where more than one mourner is present, the *poskim* developed a system of rules establishing an order of priorities for those who must recite *Kaddish* (see *M.B.* in *Be'ur Halachah* to *O.C.* 132, et al.). However, since adherence to these rules can often cause discord in the congregation, it has become widely accepted for all the mourners to recite the *Kaddish* simultaneously (see *Aruch HaShulchan*

O.C. 132:8; *Siddur R' Yaakov Emden; Teshuvos Chasam Sofer, O. C.* 159).

134. In many congregations it is customary that someone observing a *yahrzeit* is given the exclusive privilege of reciting a *Kaddish*, usually the one after *Aleinu*. In that case, an additional psalm (usually *Psalm* 24) is recited at the conclusion of the services so that all the mourners can recite *Kaddish* after it.

135. The Rabbis' *Kaddish* (*Kaddish D'Rabbanan*) is recited after segments of the Oral Torah (e.g., Talmud) have been studied or recited by a quorum of ten adult males (*Rambam, Seder Tefilos Kol HaShanah*). The Talmud (*Sotah* 49a) refers to the great significance of יְהֵא שְׁמֵיהּ רַבָּא (a reference to *Kaddish*) that is said after *Aggadah*, indicating that this *Kaddish* has a special relevance to the Midrashic portion of the Torah. Therefore, it is customary to append a brief Aggadic selection to Torah study and then to recite the Rabbis' *Kaddish* (*M.B.* 54:9).

136. Although *Kaddish D'Rabbanan* is not reserved for mourners and may be recited even by one whose parents are alive (*Pischei Teshuvah, Yoreh Deah* 376:4), it is generally recited by mourners. However, when one celebrates the completion of a tractate of the Talmud, or when the rabbi delivers a *derashah* (homiletical discourse), it is customary for the celebrant or the rabbi to recite the *Kaddish* himself.

﴾ VERSES FOR PEOPLE'S NAMES / פסוקים לשמות אנשים ﴿

Kitzur Sh'lah teaches that it is a source of merit to recite a Scriptural verse symbolizing one's name before יִהְיוּ לְרָצוֹן at the end of *Shemoneh Esrei*. The verse should either contain the person's name, or else begin and end with the first and last letters of the name.

Following is a selection of first and last letters of names, with appropriate verses:

א...א   אָנָּא יהוה הוֹשִׁיעָה נָּא, אָנָּא יהוה הַצְלִיחָה נָּא.[1]

א...ה   אַשְׁרֵי מַשְׂכִּיל אֶל דָּל, בְּיוֹם רָעָה יְמַלְּטֵהוּ יהוה.[2]

א...ו   אַשְׁרֵי שֶׁאֵל יַעֲקֹב בְּעֶזְרוֹ, שִׂבְרוֹ עַל יהוה אֱלֹהָיו.[3]

א...י   אִמְרֵי הַאֲזִינָה יהוה בִּינָה הֲגִיגִי.[4]

א...ך   אָמַרְתְּ לַיהוה אֲדֹנָי אָתָּה, טוֹבָתִי בַּל עָלֶיךָ.[5]

א...ל   אֶרֶץ רָעֲשָׁה אַף שָׁמַיִם נָטְפוּ מִפְּנֵי אֱלֹהִים זֶה סִינַי, מִפְּנֵי אֱלֹהִים אֱלֹהֵי יִשְׂרָאֵל.[6]

א...ם   אַתָּה הוּא יהוה הָאֱלֹהִים, אֲשֶׁר בָּחַרְתָּ בְּאַבְרָם, וְהוֹצֵאתוֹ מֵאוּר כַּשְׂדִּים, וְשַׂמְתָּ שְּׁמוֹ אַבְרָהָם.[7]

א...ן   אֵלֶיךָ יהוה אֶקְרָא, וְאֶל אֲדֹנָי אֶתְחַנָּן.[8]

א...ע   אָמַר בְּלִבּוֹ בַּל אֶמּוֹט, לְדֹר וָדֹר אֲשֶׁר לֹא בְרָע.[9]

א...ר   אֵלֶּה בָרֶכֶב וְאֵלֶּה בַסּוּסִים, וַאֲנַחְנוּ בְּשֵׁם יהוה אֱלֹהֵינוּ נַזְכִּיר.[10]

ב...א   בְּרִיתִי הָיְתָה אִתּוֹ הַחַיִּים וְהַשָּׁלוֹם, וָאֶתְּנֵם לוֹ מוֹרָא וַיִּירָאֵנִי, וּמִפְּנֵי שְׁמִי נִחַת הוּא.[11]

ב...ה   בַּעֲבוּר יִשְׁמְרוּ חֻקָּיו, וְתוֹרֹתָיו יִנְצֹרוּ, הַלְלוּיָהּ.[12]

ב...ז   בְּיוֹם קָרָאתִי וַתַּעֲנֵנִי, תַּרְהִבֵנִי בְנַפְשִׁי עֹז.[13]

ב...ך   בָּרוּךְ אַתָּה יהוה, לַמְּדֵנִי חֻקֶּיךָ.[14]

ב...ל   בְּמַקְהֵלוֹת בָּרְכוּ אֱלֹהִים, אֲדֹנָי מִמְּקוֹר יִשְׂרָאֵל.[15]

ב...ן   בָּרוּךְ יהוה אֱלֹהֵי יִשְׂרָאֵל מֵהָעוֹלָם וְעַד הָעוֹלָם, אָמֵן וְאָמֵן.[16]

ב...ע   בְּחֶסֶד וֶאֱמֶת יְכֻפַּר עָוֹן, וּבְיִרְאַת יהוה סוּר מֵרָע.[17]

ג...ה   גּוֹל עַל יהוה דַּרְכֶּךָ, וּבְטַח עָלָיו וְהוּא יַעֲשֶׂה.[18]

ג...ל   גַּם אֲנִי אוֹדְךָ בִכְלִי נֶבֶל, אֲמִתְּךָ אֱלֹהָי אֲזַמְּרָה לְּךָ בְכִנּוֹר, קְדוֹשׁ יִשְׂרָאֵל.[19]

ג...ן   גַּם בְּנֵי אָדָם גַּם בְּנֵי אִישׁ, יַחַד עָשִׁיר וְאֶבְיוֹן.[20]

ד...ב   דִּרְשׁוּ יהוה בְּהִמָּצְאוֹ, קְרָאֻהוּ בִּהְיוֹתוֹ קָרוֹב.[21]

ד...ד   דִּרְשׁוּ יהוה וְעֻזּוֹ, בַּקְּשׁוּ פָנָיו תָּמִיד.[22]

ד...ה   דְּאָגָה בְלֶב אִישׁ יַשְׁחֶנָּה, וְדָבָר טוֹב יְשַׂמְּחֶנָּה.[23]

ד...ל   דָּן יָדִין עַמּוֹ, כְּאַחַד שִׁבְטֵי יִשְׂרָאֵל.[24]

ה...א   הַצּוּר תָּמִים פָּעֳלוֹ, כִּי כָל דְּרָכָיו מִשְׁפָּט, אֵל אֱמוּנָה וְאֵין עָוֶל, צַדִּיק וְיָשָׁר הוּא.[25]

ה...ה   הַסְתֵּר פָּנֶיךָ מֵחֲטָאָי, וְכָל עֲוֹנֹתַי מְחֵה.[26]

ה...ל   הַקְשִׁיבָה לְקוֹל שַׁוְעִי מַלְכִּי וֵאלֹהָי, כִּי אֵלֶיךָ אֶתְפַּלָּל.[27]

ז...ב   זֵכֶר צַדִּיק לִבְרָכָה, וְשֵׁם רְשָׁעִים יִרְקָב.[28]

ז...ה   זֹאת מְנוּחָתִי עֲדֵי עַד, פֹּה אֵשֵׁב כִּי אִוִּתִיהָ.[29]

ז...ח   זָכַרְתִּי יָמִים מִקֶּדֶם, הָגִיתִי בְכָל פָּעֳלֶךָ, בְּמַעֲשֵׂה יָדֶיךָ אֲשׂוֹחֵחַ.[30]

ז...ן   זְבוּלֻן לְחוֹף יַמִּים יִשְׁכֹּן, וְהוּא לְחוֹף אֳנִיּוֹת וְיַרְכָתוֹ עַל צִידֹן.[31]

---

(1) *Psalms* 118:25. (2) 41:2. (3) 146:5. (4) 5:2. (5) 16:2. (6) 68:9. (7) *Nehemiah* 9:7. (8) *Psalms* 30:9. (9) 10:6. (10) 20:8. (11) *Malachi* 2:5. (12) *Psalms* 105:45. (13) 138:3. (14) 119:12. (15) 68:27. (16) 41:14. (17) *Proverbs* 16:6. (18) *Psalms* 37:5. (19) 71:22. (20) 49:3. (21) *Isaiah* 55:6. (22) *Psalms* 105:4. (23) *Proverbs* 12:25. (24) *Genesis* 49:16. (25) *Deuteronomy* 32:4. (26) *Psalms* 51:11. (27) 5:3. (28) *Proverbs* 10:7. (29) *Psalms* 132:14. (30) 143:5. (31) *Genesis* 49:13.

ח...ה חָגְרָה בְעוֹז מָתְנֶיהָ, וַתְּאַמֵּץ זְרוֹעֹתֶיהָ.¹

ח...ך חֲצוֹת לַיְלָה אָקוּם לְהוֹדוֹת לָךְ, עַל מִשְׁפְּטֵי צִדְקֶךָ.²

ח...ם חֹנֶה מַלְאַךְ יהוה סָבִיב לִירֵאָיו, וַיְחַלְּצֵם.³

ט...א טוֹב יַנְחִיל בְּנֵי בָנִים, וְצָפוּן לַצַּדִּיק חֵיל חוֹטֵא.⁴

ט...ה טָמְנוּ גֵאִים פַּח לִי, וַחֲבָלִים פָּרְשׂוּ רֶשֶׁת לְיַד מַעְגָּל, מֹקְשִׁים שָׁתוּ לִי סֶלָה.⁵

י...א יִשְׂרָאֵל בְּטַח בַּיהוה, עֶזְרָם וּמָגִנָּם הוּא.⁶

י...ב יַעַנְךָ יהוה בְּיוֹם צָרָה, יְשַׂגֶּבְךָ שֵׁם אֱלֹהֵי יַעֲקֹב.⁷

י...ד יָסַד אֶרֶץ עַל מְכוֹנֶיהָ, בַּל תִּמּוֹט עוֹלָם וָעֶד.⁸

י...ה יהוה הַצִּילָה נַפְשִׁי מִשְּׂפַת שֶׁקֶר, מִלָּשׁוֹן רְמִיָּה.⁹

י...י יהוה לִי בְּעֹזְרָי, וַאֲנִי אֶרְאֶה בְשֹׂנְאָי.¹⁰

י...ל יְמִין יהוה רוֹמֵמָה, יְמִין יהוה עֹשָׂה חָיִל.¹¹

י...ם יַעְלְזוּ חֲסִידִים בְּכָבוֹד, יְרַנְּנוּ עַל מִשְׁכְּבוֹתָם.¹²

י...ן יָשֵׂם נְהָרוֹת לְמִדְבָּר, וּמֹצָאֵי מַיִם לְצִמָּאוֹן.¹³

י...ע יָחֹס עַל דַּל וְאֶבְיוֹן, וְנַפְשׁוֹת אֶבְיוֹנִים יוֹשִׁיעַ.¹⁴

י...ף יהוה יִגְמֹר בַּעֲדִי, יהוה חַסְדְּךָ לְעוֹלָם, מַעֲשֵׂי יָדֶיךָ אַל תֶּרֶף.¹⁵

י...ץ יְבָרְכֵנוּ אֱלֹהִים וְיִירְאוּ אוֹתוֹ כָּל אַפְסֵי אָרֶץ.¹⁶

י...ק יוֹצִיאֵם מֵחֹשֶׁךְ וְצַלְמָוֶת, וּמוֹסְרוֹתֵיהֶם יְנַתֵּק.¹⁷

י...ר יהוה שִׁמְךָ לְעוֹלָם, יהוה זִכְרְךָ לְדֹר וָדֹר.¹⁸

י...ת יהוה שֹׁמֵר אֶת גֵּרִים, יָתוֹם וְאַלְמָנָה יְעוֹדֵד, וְדֶרֶךְ רְשָׁעִים יְעַוֵּת.¹⁹

כ...ב כִּי לֹא יִטֹּשׁ יהוה עַמּוֹ, וְנַחֲלָתוֹ לֹא יַעֲזֹב.²⁰

כ...ל כִּי מֶלֶךְ כָּל הָאָרֶץ אֱלֹהִים, זַמְּרוּ מַשְׂכִּיל.²¹

ל...א לֹא תִהְיֶה מְשַׁכֵּלָה וַעֲקָרָה בְּאַרְצֶךָ, אֶת מִסְפַּר יָמֶיךָ אֲמַלֵּא.²²

ל...ה לְדָוִד בָּרוּךְ יהוה צוּרִי הַמְלַמֵּד יָדַי לַקְרָב, אֶצְבְּעוֹתַי לַמִּלְחָמָה.²³

ל...י לוּלֵי תוֹרָתְךָ שַׁעֲשֻׁעָי, אָז אָבַדְתִּי בְעָנְיִי.²⁴

ל...ת לַמְנַצֵּחַ עַל שֹׁשַׁנִּים לִבְנֵי קֹרַח, מַשְׂכִּיל שִׁיר יְדִידֹת.²⁵

מ...א מִי כָמֹכָה בָּאֵלִם יהוה מִי כָּמֹכָה נֶאְדָּר בַּקֹּדֶשׁ, נוֹרָא תְהִלֹּת עֹשֵׂה פֶלֶא.²⁶

מ...ה מַחֲשָׁבוֹת בְּעֵצָה תִכּוֹן, וּבְתַחְבֻּלוֹת עֲשֵׂה מִלְחָמָה.²⁷

מ...ו מַה דּוֹדֵךְ מִדּוֹד הַיָּפָה בַּנָּשִׁים, מַה דּוֹדֵךְ מִדּוֹד שֶׁכָּכָה הִשְׁבַּעְתָּנוּ.²⁸

מ...י מָה אָהַבְתִּי תוֹרָתֶךָ, כָּל הַיּוֹם הִיא שִׂיחָתִי.²⁹

מ...ל מַה טֹּבוּ אֹהָלֶיךָ יַעֲקֹב, מִשְׁכְּנֹתֶיךָ יִשְׂרָאֵל.³⁰

מ...ם מְאוֹר עֵינַיִם יְשַׂמַּח לֵב, שְׁמוּעָה טוֹבָה תְּדַשֶּׁן עָצֶם.³¹

מ...ר מִי זֶה הָאִישׁ יְרֵא יהוה, יוֹרֶנּוּ בְּדֶרֶךְ יִבְחָר.³²

נ...א נַפְשֵׁנוּ חִכְּתָה לַיהוה עֶזְרֵנוּ וּמָגִנֵּנוּ הוּא.³³

נ...ה נָחַלְתִּי עֵדְוֹתֶיךָ לְעוֹלָם, כִּי שְׂשׂוֹן לִבִּי הֵמָּה.³⁴

נ...י נִדְבוֹת פִּי רְצֵה נָא יהוה, וּמִשְׁפָּטֶיךָ לַמְּדֵנִי.³⁵

נ...ל נֶחְשַׁבְתִּי עִם יוֹרְדֵי בוֹר, הָיִיתִי כְּגֶבֶר אֵין אֱיָל.³⁶

נ...ם נַחֲמוּ נַחֲמוּ עַמִּי, יֹאמַר אֱלֹהֵיכֶם.³⁷

---

(1) Proverbs 31:17. (2) Psalms 119:62. (3) 34:8. (4) Proverbs 13:22. (5) Psalms 140:6. (6) 115:9. (7) 20:2. (8) 104:5. (9) 120:2. (10) 118:7. (11) 118:16. (12) 149:5. (13) 107:33. (14) 72:13. (15) 138:8. (16) 67:8. (17) 107:14. (18) 135:13. (19) 146:9. (20) 94:14. (21) 47:8. (22) Exodus 23:26. (23) Psalms 144:1. (24) 119:92. (25) 45:1. (26) Exodus 15:11. (27) Proverbs 20:18. (28) Song of Songs 5:9. (29) Psalms 119:97. (30) Numbers 24:5. (31) Proverbs 15:30. (32) Psalms 25:12. (33) 33:20. (34) 119:111. (35) 119:108. (36) 88:5. (37) Isaiah 40:1.

נ...ן   נֵר יהוה נִשְׁמַת אָדָם, חֹפֵשׂ כָּל חַדְרֵי בֶטֶן.[1]

ס...ה   סֹבּוּ צִיּוֹן וְהַקִּיפוּהָ סִפְרוּ מִגְדָּלֶיהָ.[2]

ס...י   סַעֲפִים שָׂנֵאתִי, וְתוֹרָתְךָ אָהָבְתִּי.[3]

ע...א   עַתָּה אָקוּם, יֹאמַר יהוה, עַתָּה אֵרוֹמָם, עַתָּה אֶנָּשֵׂא.[4]

ע...ב   עַד אֶמְצָא מָקוֹם לַיהוה, מִשְׁכָּנוֹת לַאֲבִיר יַעֲקֹב.[5]

ע...ה   עָזִּי וְזִמְרָת יָהּ, וַיְהִי לִי לִישׁוּעָה.[6]

ע...ל   עַל דַּעְתְּךָ כִּי לֹא אֶרְשָׁע, וְאֵין מִיָּדְךָ מַצִּיל.[7]

ע...ס   עֲרֹב עַבְדְּךָ לְטוֹב, אַל יַעַשְׁקֻנִי זֵדִים.[8]

ע...ר   עֹשֶׂה גְדֹלוֹת וְאֵין חֵקֶר, נִפְלָאוֹת עַד אֵין מִסְפָּר.[9]

פ...ה   פִּתְחוּ לִי שַׁעֲרֵי צֶדֶק, אָבֹא בָם אוֹדֶה יָהּ.[10]

פ...ל   פֶּן יִטְרֹף כְּאַרְיֵה נַפְשִׁי, פֹּרֵק וְאֵין מַצִּיל.[11]

פ...ס   פֶּלֶס וּמֹאזְנֵי מִשְׁפָּט לַיהוה, מַעֲשֵׂהוּ כָּל אַבְנֵי כִיס.[12]

פ...ץ   פִּנִּיתָ לְפָנֶיהָ וַתַּשְׁרֵשׁ שָׁרָשֶׁיהָ וַתְּמַלֵּא אָרֶץ.[13]

צ...ה   צִיּוֹן בְּמִשְׁפָּט תִּפָּדֶה, וְשָׁבֶיהָ בִּצְדָקָה.[14]

צ...ח   צִיּוֹן יִשְׁאָלוּ דֶּרֶךְ הֵנָּה פְנֵיהֶם, בֹּאוּ וְנִלְווּ אֶל יהוה, בְּרִית עוֹלָם לֹא תִשָּׁכֵחַ.[15]

צ...י   צַר וּמָצוֹק מְצָאוּנִי, מִצְוֹתֶיךָ שַׁעֲשֻׁעָי.[16]

ק...ל   קַמְתִּי אֲנִי לִפְתֹּחַ לְדוֹדִי, וְיָדַי נָטְפוּ מוֹר וְאֶצְבְּעֹתַי מוֹר עֹבֵר עַל כַּפּוֹת הַמַּנְעוּל.[17]

ק...ן   קוֹלִי אֶל יהוה אֶזְעָק, קוֹלִי אֶל יהוה אֶתְחַנָּן.[18]

ק...ת   קָרוֹב אַתָּה יהוה, וְכָל מִצְוֹתֶיךָ אֱמֶת.[19]

ר...ה   רִגְזוּ וְאַל תֶּחֱטָאוּ, אִמְרוּ בִלְבַבְכֶם עַל מִשְׁכַּבְכֶם, וְדֹמּוּ סֶלָה.[20]

ר...ל   רְאוּ עַתָּה כִּי אֲנִי אֲנִי הוּא, וְאֵין אֱלֹהִים עִמָּדִי, אֲנִי אָמִית וַאֲחַיֶּה, מָחַצְתִּי וַאֲנִי אֶרְפָּא, וְאֵין מִיָּדִי מַצִּיל.[21]

ר...ן   רְאֵה זֶה מָצָאתִי, אָמְרָה קֹהֶלֶת, אַחַת לְאַחַת לִמְצֹא חֶשְׁבּוֹן.[22]

ש...א   שַׂמֵּחַ נֶפֶשׁ עַבְדֶּךָ, כִּי אֵלֶיךָ אֲדֹנָי נַפְשִׁי אֶשָּׂא.[23]

ש...ה   שְׂאוּ יְדֵכֶם קֹדֶשׁ, וּבָרְכוּ אֶת יהוה.[24]

ש...ח   שָׁמַע יהוה תְּחִנָּתִי, יהוה תְּפִלָּתִי יִקָּח.[25]

ש...י   שָׂנֵאתִי הַשֹּׁמְרִים הַבְלֵי שָׁוְא, וַאֲנִי אֶל יהוה בָּטָחְתִּי.[26]

ש...ל   שָׁלוֹם רָב לְאֹהֲבֵי תוֹרָתֶךָ וְאֵין לָמוֹ מִכְשׁוֹל.[27]

ש...ם   שְׁמָר תָּם וּרְאֵה יָשָׁר, כִּי אַחֲרִית לְאִישׁ שָׁלוֹם.[28]

ש...ן   שִׁיתוּ לִבְּכֶם לְחֵילָה פַּסְּגוּ אַרְמְנוֹתֶיהָ, לְמַעַן תְּסַפְּרוּ לְדוֹר אַחֲרוֹן.[29]

ש...ר   שְׂפַת אֱמֶת תִּכּוֹן לָעַד, וְעַד אַרְגִּיעָה לְשׁוֹן שָׁקֶר.[30]

ש...ת   שִׁיר הַמַּעֲלוֹת, הִנֵּה בָּרְכוּ אֶת יהוה כָּל עַבְדֵי יהוה, הָעֹמְדִים בְּבֵית יהוה בַּלֵּילוֹת.[31]

ת...ה   תַּעֲרֹךְ לְפָנַי שֻׁלְחָן נֶגֶד צֹרְרָי, דִּשַּׁנְתָּ בַשֶּׁמֶן רֹאשִׁי, כּוֹסִי רְוָיָה.[32]

ת...י   תּוֹצִיאֵנִי מֵרֶשֶׁת זוּ, טָמְנוּ לִי, כִּי אַתָּה מָעוּזִּי.[33]

ת...ם   תְּנוּ עֹז לֵאלֹהִים עַל יִשְׂרָאֵל גַּאֲוָתוֹ, וְעֻזּוֹ בַּשְּׁחָקִים.[34]

---

(1) Proverbs 20:27. (2) Psalms 48:13. (3) 119:113. (4) Isaiah 33:10. (5) Psalms 132:5. (6) 118:14. (7) Job 10:7. (8) Psalms 119:122. (9) Job 5:9. (10) Psalms 118:19. (11) 7:3. (12) Proverbs 16:11. (13) Psalms 80:10. (14) Isaiah 1:27. (15) Jeremiah 50:5. (16) Psalms 119:143. (17) Song of Songs 5:5. (18) Psalms 142:2. (19) 119:151. (20) 5:4. (21) Deuteronomy 32:39. (22) Ecclesiastes 7:27. (23) Psalms 86:4. (24) 134:2. (25) 6:10. (26) 31:7. (27) 119:165. (28) 37:37. (29) 48:14. (30) Proverbs 12:19. (31) Psalms 134:1. (32) 23:5. (33) 31:5. (34) 68:35.

◆§ THE RABBIS' KADDISH / KADDISH D'RABBANAN §◆

TRANSLITERATED WITH ASHKENAZIC PRONUNCIATION

Yisgadal v'yiskadash sh'mei rabbaw (Cong.— Amein).
   B'allmaw dee v'raw chir'usei v'yamlich malchusei,
b'chayeichon, uv'yomeichon, uv'chayei d'chol beis yisroel,
ba'agawlaw u'vizman kawriv, v'imru: Amein.
   (Cong.—Amein. Y'hei sh'mei rabbaw m'vawrach l'allam u'l'allmei allmayaw.)
Y'hei sh'mei rabbaw m'vawrach, l'allam u'l'allmei allmayaw.

Yis'bawrach, v'yishtabach, v'yispaw'ar, v'yisromam, v'yis'nasei,
v'yis'hadar, v'yis'aleh, v'yis'halawl
sh'mei d'kudshaw b'rich hu (Cong.— b'rich hu).
L'aylaw l'aylaw mikol bir'chawsaw v'shirawsaw,
tush'b'chawsaw v'nechemawsaw,
da'ami'rawn b'allmaw, v'imru: Amein (Cong.— Amein).
Al yisroel v'al rabaw'nawn v'al talmidei'hon,
v'al kol talmidei salmidei'hon,
v'al kol mawn d'awskin b'oray'saw,
dee v'as'raw haw'dain, v'dee b'chol asar va'asar.
Y'hei l'hon u'l'chon shlaw'maw rabbaw,
chee'naw v'chisdaw v'rachamin,
v'chayin arichin, u'm'zonei r'vichei,
u'furkawnaw min kaw'dawm a'vu'hone dee vi'sh'ma'yaw
v'imru: Amein (Cong.— Amein).
Y'hei shlawmaw rabbaw min sh'mayaw,
v'chayim awleinu v'al kol yisroel, v'imru: Amein (Cong.— Amein).

Take three steps back, bow left and say, 'Oseh . . .'; bow right and say,
'hu b'rachamawv ya'aseh . . .'; bow forward and say, 'v'al kol yisroel v'imru: Amein.

Oseh shawlom bim'ro'mawv,
hu b'rachamawv ya'aseh shawlom awleinu,
v'al kol yisroel v'imru: Amein (Cong.— Amein).

Remain standing in place for a few moments, then take three steps forward.